The Next Level of Preparation

NEET PG 2016–22

The Next Level of Preparation

NEET PG 2016–22

Fourth Edition

Thameem Saif
Leading Faculty of Medicine

Apurv Mehra
Leading Faculty of Orthopedics

Akhil Monga
MD (Radiodiagnosis), AIIMS, New Delhi

Kavan Parikh
MBBS MD (Radiodiagnosis), BJMC, Ahmedabad, Gujarat

Chief Editors

Saurabh Taneja MD FNB (Critical Care Medicine)
Consultant, Sir Ganga Ram Hospital, New Delhi

Dipin Sudhakaran MD (Radiodiagnosis), AIIMS, New Delhi

Vishnu Prasad MD (Radiodiagnosis), AIIMS, New Delhi

Deepankar Srigyan MD (Microbiology), AIIMS, New Delhi

Mandakini Gupta MBBS BRD Medical College, Gorakhpur, Uttar Pradesh

JAYPEE

JAYPEE BROTHERS MEDICAL PUBLISHERS

The Health Sciences Publisher

New Delhi | London

JAYPEE Jaypee Brothers Medical Publishers (P) Ltd

Headquarters

Jaypee Brothers Medical Publishers (P) Ltd
EMCA House, 23/23-B
Ansari Road, Daryaganj
New Delhi 110 002, India
Landline: +91-11-23272143, +91-11-23272703
+91-11-23282021, +91-11-23245672
Email: jaypee@jaypeebrothers.com

Corporate Office

Jaypee Brothers Medical Publishers (P) Ltd
4838/24, Ansari Road, Daryaganj
New Delhi 110 002, India
Phone: +91-11-43574357
Fax: +91-11-43574314
Email: jaypee@jaypeebrothers.com

Overseas Office

JP Medical Ltd
83 Victoria Street, London
SW1H 0HW (UK)
Phone: +44 20 3170 8910
Fax: +44 (0)20 3008 6180
Email: info@jpmedpub.com

Website: www.jaypeebrothers.com
Website: www.jaypeedigital.com

Inquiries for bulk sales may be solicited at: jaypee@jaypeebrothers.com

The Next Level of Preparation: NEET PG 2016–22

First Edition: 2019, Second Edition: 2020, Third Edition: 2021

Fourth Edition: **2022**

ISBN: 978-93-5465-999-7

Printed at Rajkamal Electric Press, Kundli, Haryana.

Dedication

I dedicate this book to all my students who have enabled me to become a better student of this awesome subject of medicine.

Thameem Saif

I dedicate this book to my students, my teachers and my patients who helped me evolve into a better teacher and Orthopedic Surgeon.

Apurv Mehra

I dedicate this book to my parents.

Akhil Monga

I dedicate this book to my parents and teachers (with special thanks to Dr Apurv Sir) who shaped my life and contributed to my growth.

Kavan Parikh

PREFACE

After the great response that our AIIMS Review Book: INI CET The Precise Version received from our friends preparing for the PG Entrance Exams, the demand for release of The NEET PG Exam book since then, has upscaled.

As promised by Dr Apurv Mehra's Team, *NEET PG: The Next Level of Preparation* is just like the AIIMS Book. Our authors have worked assiduously to overcome the herculean task of fitting all that you need to revise for the NEET PG Exam in a single book covering important topics of all subjects along with inclusion of previous year questions, important images, flowcharts and in just 781 pages…!!!

Remember, how we sometimes yearn for a nice cup of coffee in the morning and yet we find ourselves too lazy to make one and end up going to the vending machine even though it tastes pathetic. It seems to be too much work to collect all ingredients, get up early, go through the steps and be able to figure out the right combination. What if, you woke up to a new machine that dispensed just the perfect cup!

Despite all the content being available to students, in the form of detailed review books, hours and hours of offline and online classes, subjectwise ready-made notes and thousands of MCQ questions, they usually find themselves at a loss few months before the exam. Everything that they had read seems to have suddenly evaporated and revising all the subjects again feels like an impossible task. Except for a few, students are unable to develop a concise revision material for themselves as it is difficult to have a good insight about the important topics after just one reading. What if, it was delivered to your doorstep? Miracle…?…Yes it is indeed a miracle!!!

The *NEET PG: The Next Level of Preparation* book is a compilation of all the topics, spanning all 19 subjects, that you need to revise before you enter the examination hall. It will help you attempt most of the questions and make sure you do not make silly mistakes in easy questions (90% of the questions are like that!!). It makes sure that you have the time to revise all subjects equally. A balanced revision is the key before any examination and there are no extra marks for solving the most difficult questions. Every attempt has been made to include all important concepts and facts without overburdening the student.

Medical science is ever evolving and it is important for every student to stay updated with the knowledge they have. In the face of changing exam patterns and emphasis on horizontal and vertical integration, in the 4th edition, we have tried to provide more of conceptual explanations to help you integrate the subjects better. This book will hereafter serve to develop a better approach towards learning alongwith knowledge and information.

This book in our view will be of great utility to anybody aspiring to crack the NEET PG entrance exam and we hope to fulfil the expectations of our students who have been eagerly waiting for it.

HAPPY LEARNING!!

Thameem Saif
Apurv Mehra
Akhil Monga
Kavan Parikh

ACKNOWLEDGMENTS

We express sincere gratitude and are thankful to all Faculties, Subject Specialists, NEET PG and INI-CET Toppers who have also been Our Students for coming together on a single platform and sharing our mission to help and guide PG aspirants to fulfill their dream of securing a PG seat.

We as a team will be always grateful for the support provided in helping us throughout and suggesting appropriate changes to enhance output through this book.

We would like to thank Dr Amit Gupta for his hard work and contribution to the book in first and second edition.

Dr. Apurv Mehra

For Any Academic / Nonacademic Doubt write to **drapurv@gmail.com**

Dr. Apurv Mehra – The Orthopedic Surgeon

Dr. Apurv Mehra is an Internationally Trained & Experienced Computer Navigation Joint Replacement & Arthroscopy Surgeon
He is an Orthopedic Consultant at Max Institute of Bone & Joint Care at Patparganj, Delhi
Dr.Apurv Mehra is the Founder & Director of Vidya Jeevan Ortho Pedics Centre, Delhi – India's most Trusted Orthopedic Centre as per Leading Clinicians.
He has exceptional academic skills, his clear logical thoughts & approach to complex surgical issues makes him a standout in Knee Arthoplasty & Ligament Reconstructions. His surgical skills & compassionate behavior helps his patients to return back to routine activities & lead a normal life. His clinical skills are exemplary, he achieves good outcomes, and his patients love him.

Dr. Apurv Mehra – Renowned Author, Leading Faculty, Inspirational & Motivational Speaker

Dr. Apurv Mehra is The Leading Faculty of Orthopedics & is recognized Nationally & Internationally as an outstanding teacher, world class scholar & dedicated mentor. Dr. Apurv Mehra is also Co-Founder of Cerebellum Academy To Guide Students Preparing for Medical Entrance Exams. He is best known for his stupendous efforts in teaching, motivating & inspiring budding doctors.
The quality that sets him apart is his unique style of teaching with fun & passion. He is the Author of many International Bestsellers across South East Asia. Apart from Orthopedics Quick Review, he has also written AIIMS The Precise Version; NEET PG The Next Level of Preparation & Review of Pediatrics All of his books are being highly appreciated across the globe.
Dr. Apurv Mehra is a youth icon, guide, mentor & role model for aspiring doctors. He is known for his highly inspirational & motivational Speeches.
He has a vision & aims to provide high content resources needed to take students to the next level of education.
Thousands of students have been benefitted by his Orthopedic live lectures named Ortho Dhoom Dhadaka. His lectures are highly recommended by PG Toppers Dr. Apurv inspires students to work hard, he builds trust in them & helps them to achieve their goals. His Orthopedics App has been the Best Seller in Online Education since its inception in September 2018.
Inspired from his lectures, students not only learn but also follow his advice & guidance in their day to day lives.

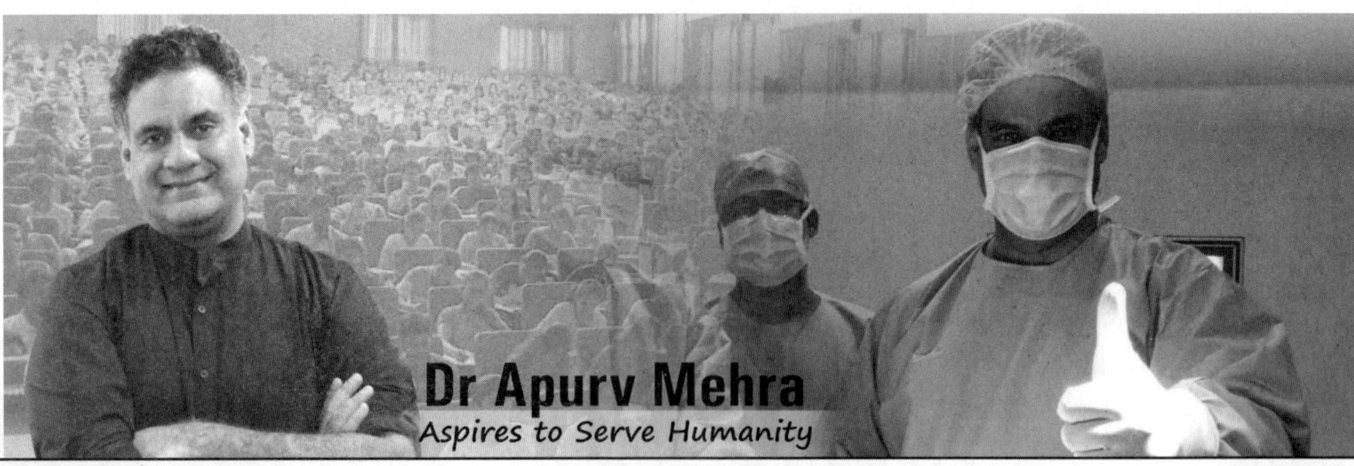

Why This Book... NEET PG
The Precise Content

The Idea behind the book stems from the age-old principle of competition exams – "***What has been asked will be asked again!***"

This idea has been commonly misinterpreted by various teachers and students alike. It does not mean that the same questions shall be repeated in future exams. Though, old questions are sometimes repeated as it is, they are not sufficient to get you across the line.

With a team of toppers behind this book, we do understand that **it is not the questions but the topics that are repeated**. They were similar when **Dr Thameem Saif** and **Dr Apurv Mehra** appeared for the exam, also when NEET PG Topper Dr Swasti Pathak wrote NEET PG in 2016 and so did Dr Ashraf and Dr Kavan Parikh. The list has remained almost the same over the last 5 years with a few additions. This conclusion has never been challenged by people who have aced the exam.

We realized the lacunae in the **exam-oriented revision material available to the students**. An effort has been made to remove redundancy and repetitiveness to make things as crisp as possible, which gives **extra time to the students to revise more and catch up on sleep**. The book flows like a river and allows you to read for long hours without getting bored or tired.

This book aims at providing an insight to the pattern of NEET PG exam and at the same time equipping students with a **topic-based quick review** of the most important concepts and facts that have been labelled **high-yield** by our team of toppers. FREQUENT REVISIONS have been emphasized as a key determinant to success in NEET-PG by all faculties and toppers. The most important aspect while revising is the ART OF PRIORITIZING the content. Many students find it difficult to determine which topics to stress upon in revision and which ones to leave. At that juncture, this book will be the saviour for you. Alongwith highlighting the MUST KNOW TOPICS for exams, it will also help you quickly brush up the most vital information that you cannot afford to miss. It will help you build up confidence because you will be sure that you have read what was supposed to be read!

We aim to reduce the burden on students for preparing their own revision material. This book can act as the base, with students adding their own updates, mnemonics, sticky notes and cheat sheets to it. We firmly believe that it is important to **strengthen your knowledge at the end, rather than looking for more**.

The immense hard work of the authors, co-authors and the contributing faculties and students has made this a **must-read book** for all medical students preparing for the NEET PG exam.

This book has been made with an intent to help our juniors as **we understand the turmoil** that hits their lives during this phase. We hope you have a great time reading the book and find it useful in your preparation.

Best Wishes
Dr Apurv Mehra

All Students reading this book are invited to join
Dr Apurv Mehra Platforms

To know latest updates/Important Topics/High Yield Questions/Pearls to stimulus your preparation

Mail All Your Doubts & Queries to
drapurv@gmail.com
To be directly answered By Dr Apurv Mehra

CONTENTS

Latest NEET 2022

NEET PG 2022

ANATOMY

1. Identify the tissue: *(NEET 2022)*

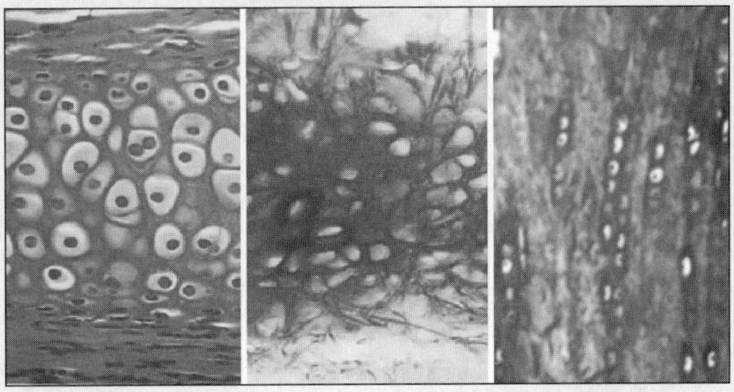

a. Hyaline
b. Fibrous
c. Articular
d. Elastic

Ans. is 'B'. Fibrous

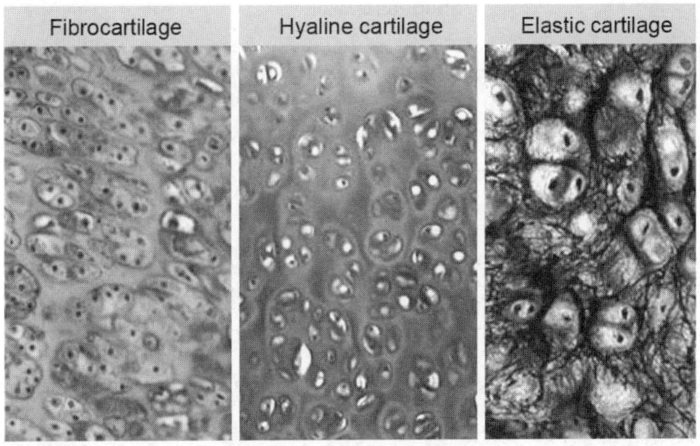

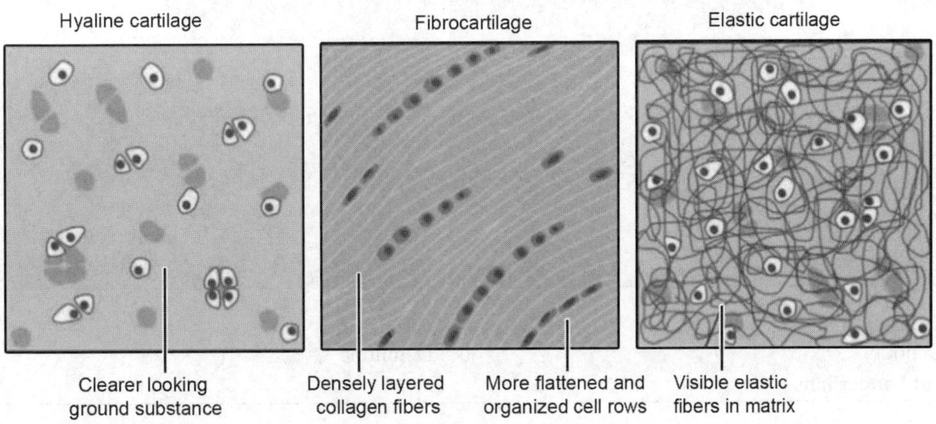

2. Which of the following is derived from the arrowed structure? *(NEET 2022)*

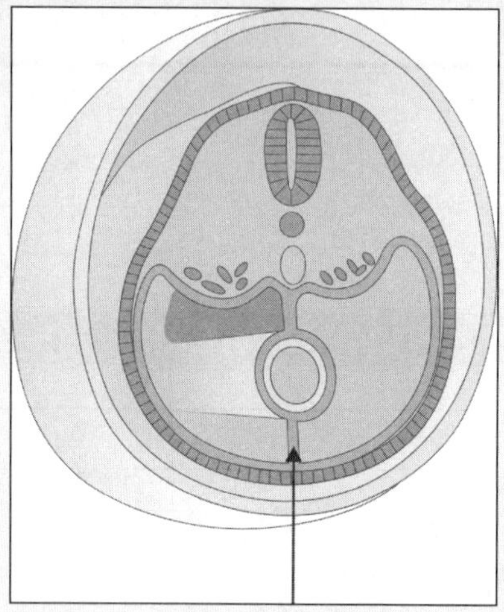

a. Falciform ligament
b. Lienorenal ligament
c. Gastrosplenic ligament
d. Phrenicocolic ligament

Ans. is 'a' Falciform ligament

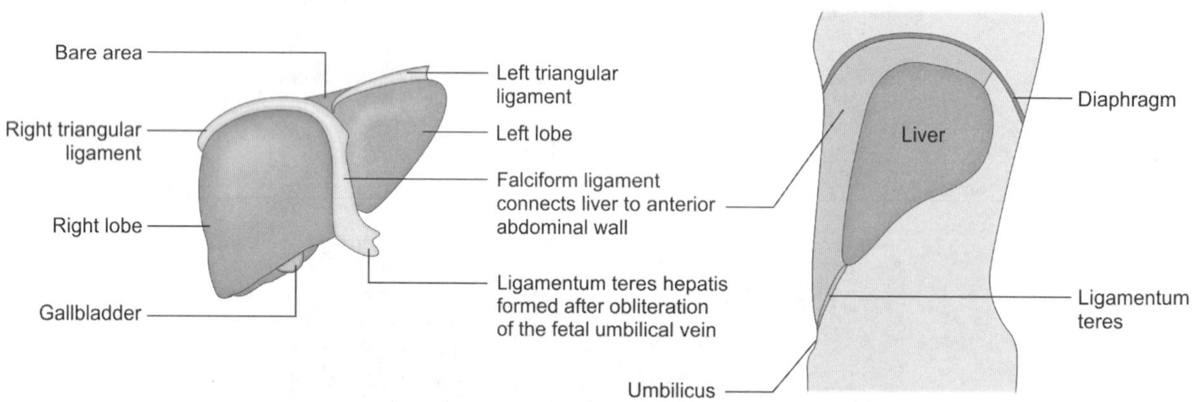

Falciform ligament

Falciform ligament is derived from the ventral mesentry. It connects the anterior abdominal wall to liver.

3. Identify the tissue: *(NEET 2022)*

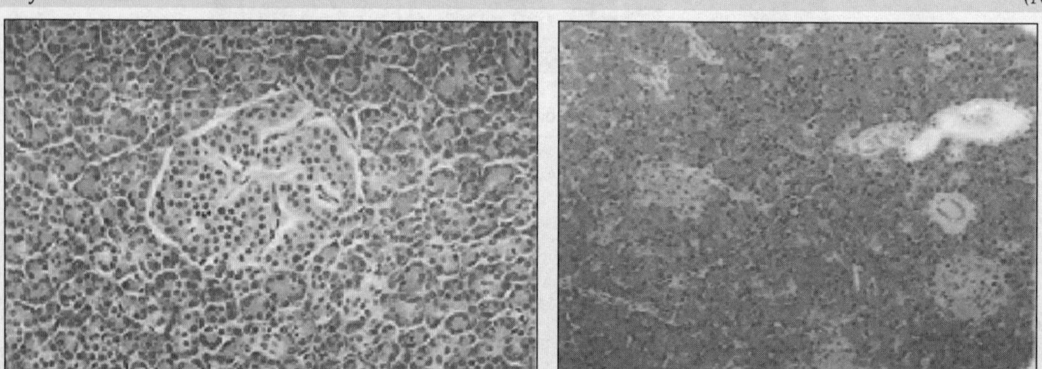

a. Islets of Langerhans
b. Glomerulus
c. Lymph node
d. Demilune

Ans. is 'a' Islets of Langerhans

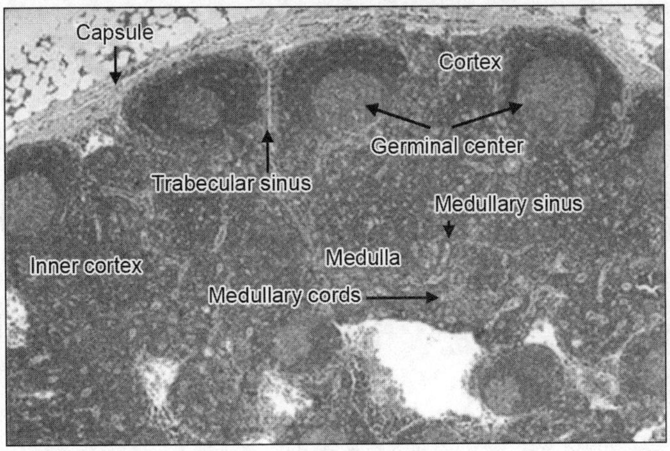

Histology of lymph node

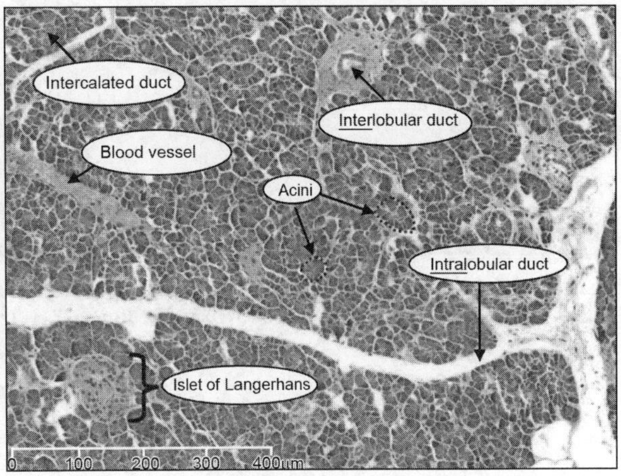

Histology of pancreas

4. Most common site for intraperitoneal abscess: *(NEET 2022)*

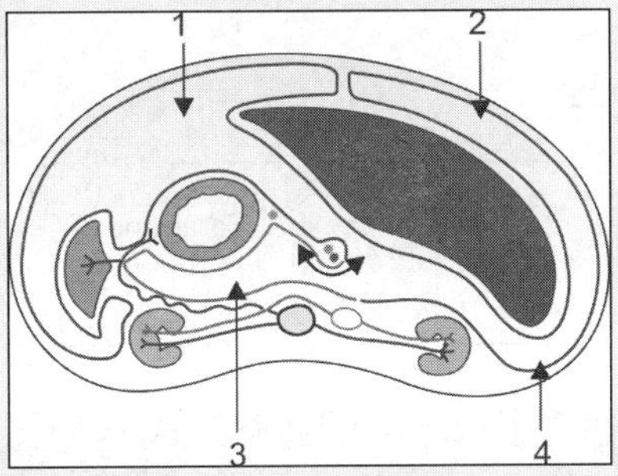

a. 1 b. 2 c. 3 d. 4

Ans. is 'd' 4

1 & 2 = left and right subphrenic spaces

3 = lesser sac/mental bursa

4 = Morrison's pouch/heaptorenal pouch

Morrison's pouch is the most common site of intrapersonal abscess.

Sitting/standing/ambulatory patients = pelvic cavity

5. A patient presents with a unilateral throbbing headache, photophobia, and excessive lacrimation. He also complains of hemifacial pain on clenching of teeth. On examination, pupillary reaction, light reflex, and accommodation reflex are normal. Which of the following marked nerves is involved in the above scenario? *(NEET 2022)*

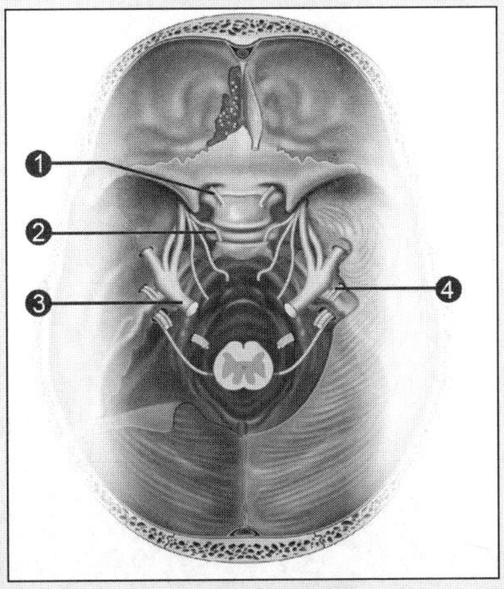

a. 1 b. 2 c. 3 d. 4

Ans. is 'c' 3

1 = Optic nerve
2 = Oculomotor nerve
3 = Trigeminal nerve
4 = Facial nerve

PHYSIOLOGY

6. Which type of signaling is shown in the figure? *(NEET 2022)*

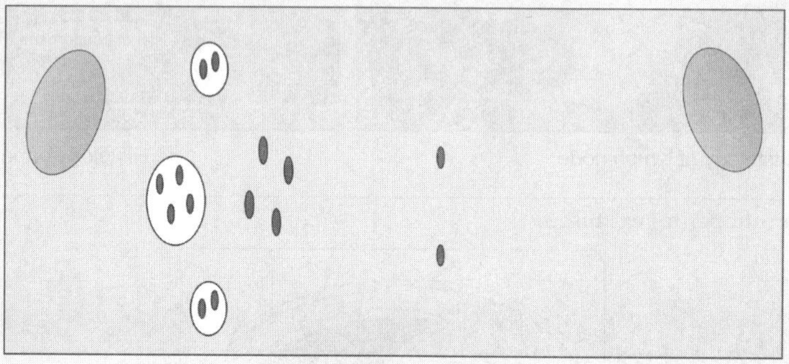

a. Autocrine
b. Paracrine
c. Merocrine
d. Endocrine

Ans. is 'b' Paracrine

Forms of chemical signaling	
Autocrine	A cell targets itself
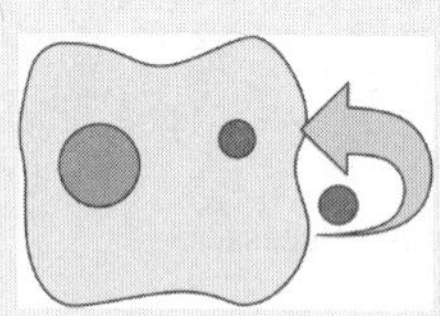	
Signaling across gap junctions	A cell targets a cell connected by gap junctions
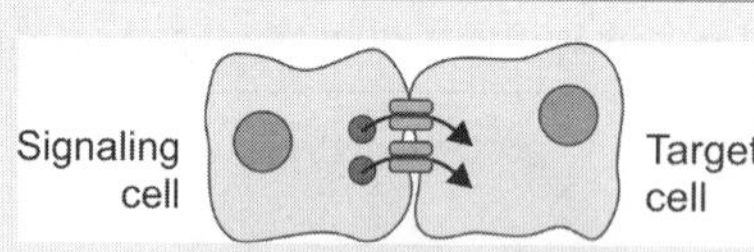	
Paracrine	A cell targets a nearby cell
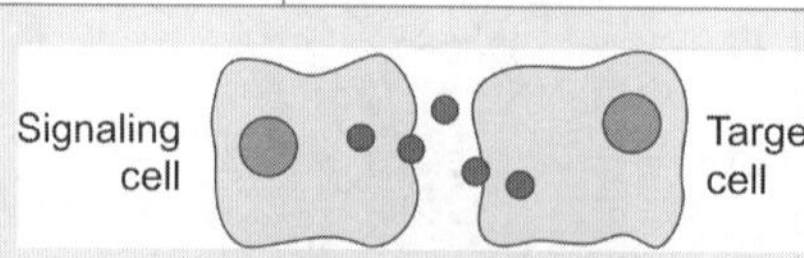	
Endocrine	A cell targets a distant cell through the bloodstream
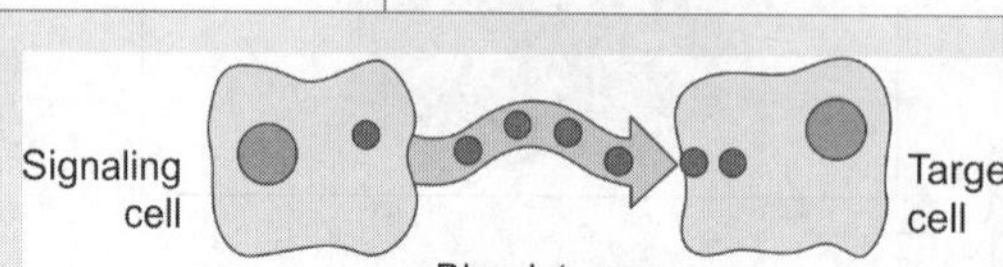	

7. Which of the following will cause a decrease in extracellular K^+? *(NEET 2022)*

a. Lactic acid
b. Epinephrine
c. Glucagon
d. Atropine

Ans. is 'b' Epinephrine

Hypokalemia	*Hyperkalemia*
• Insulin	• Glucagon
• Alkalosis	• Acidosis
• Sympathomimetic stimulation	• Atropine
• Aldosterone	• CKD/AKI
• RTA type 1&2	• Addison's disease
• Vomiting	• Gordon syndrome
• Diarrhoea	
• Barter's, Gitelman	

8. Which of the following will involved in baroreceptor reflex? *(NEET 2022)*

a. Negative feedback
b. Positive feedback
c. Adaptive control
d. Feed forward

Ans. is 'a' Negative feedback

The baroreceptor reflex is a classic example of negative feedback in which stimulation of baroreceptors leads to a decrease in blood pressure and inhibition of baroreceptors leads to increase in blood pressure.

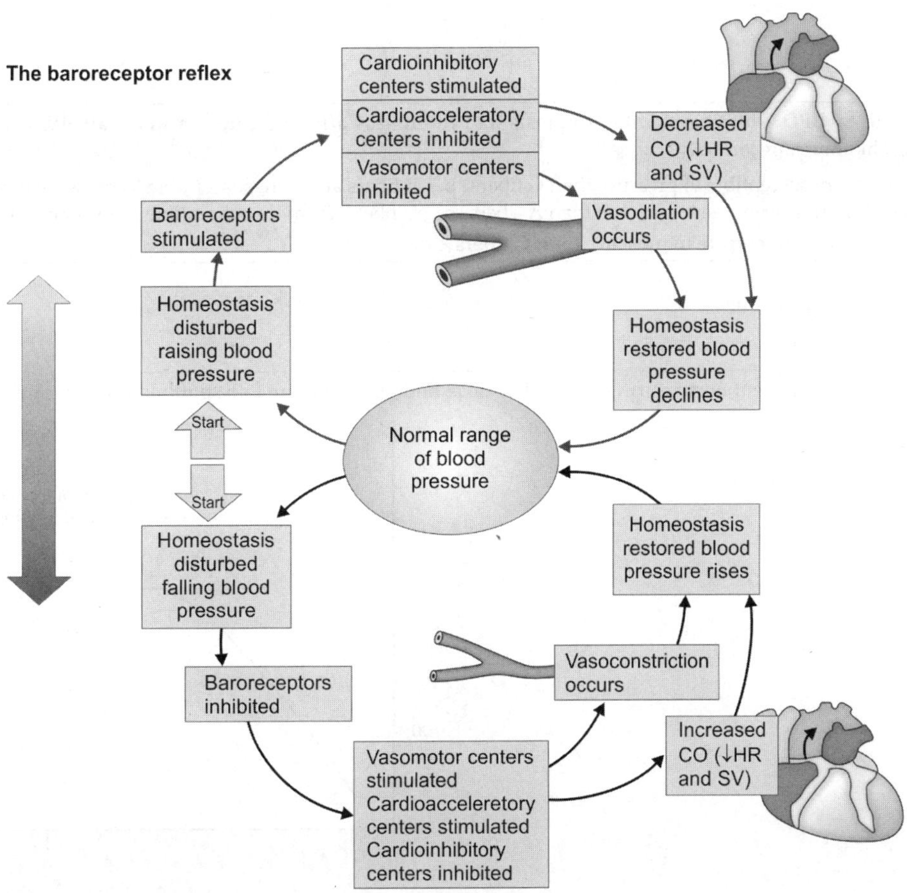

9. True about following figure: *(NEET 2022)*

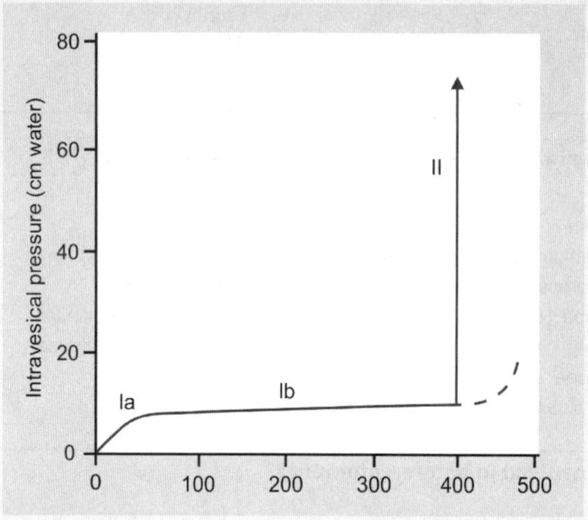

a. Dotted line represents pressure with no micturition
b. Segment 1a denotes pressure due to residual urine
c. Segment 1b represents Laplace Law
d. Micturition reflex is inhibited at phase II

Ans. is 'c' Segment 1b represents Laplace Law

Cystometrogram

- 1a = residual volume in bladder and slight raise in pressure
- 1b = obeys Laplace law
- 2 = steep rise in pressure with increase in volume

Laplace Law

P = 2T/R

10. A patient came to OPD with complaints of paresis and numbness after sleeping on his chair. Which of the following explains the phenomenon correctly? *(NEET 2022)*

a. A fibers are more susceptible to pressure than C fibers
b. B fibers are more susceptible to pressure than A fibers
c. C fibers and more susceptible to hypoxia than A fibers
d. C fibers are more susceptible to pressure than A fibers

Ans. is 'a' A fibers are more susceptible to pressure than C fibers

- Most pressure sensitive: A Fibers
- Most hypoxia sensitive: B Fibers
- Most LA sensitive: C Fibers

11. Which of the following event occur during phase B to raise body temperature to hypothalamus set point? *(NEET 2022)*

a. Shivering
b. Sweating
c. Decrease in thermogenesis
d. Cutaneous vasodilation

Ans. is 'a' Shivering

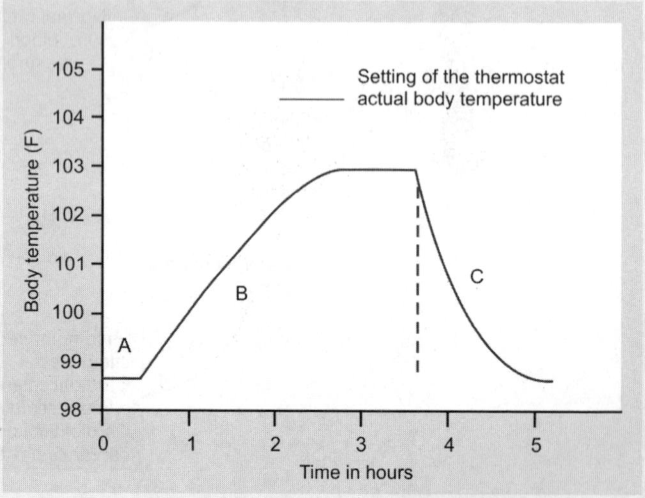

The question asks 'to raise body temperature' by hypothalamus is done by shivering which leads to increase in body temperature. In the graph.

A = normal physiological body temperature

B = rise of the body temperature to a new set point (this phenomenon leads to chills and rigours) and hypothalamus uses shivering thermogenesis for the new set body temperature.

BIOCHEMISTRY

12. The following histological image is seen in the patient who is complaining of growth failures and abdominal distension. Signs found were anemia, thrombocytopenia & bony pain. Which enzyme is deficient in is this patient? *(NEET 2022)*

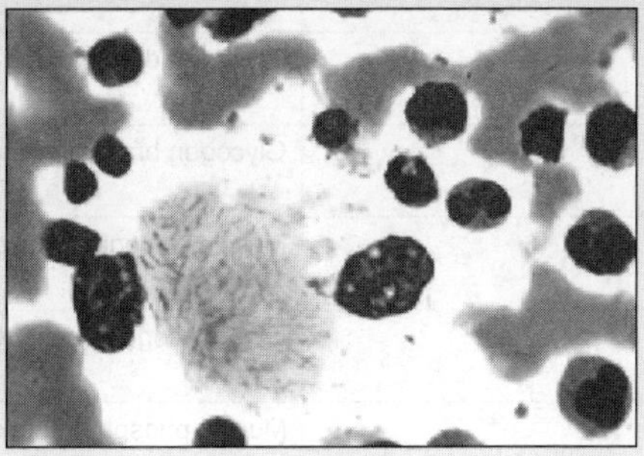

a. Beta Glucocerebrosidase
b. Sphingomyelinase
c. Hexosaminidase
d. Glu-6-phosphatase alpha glucocerebrosidase

Ans. is 'a' Beta Glucocerebrosidase

Diagnosis: Gaucher's disease

Clinical features: Avascular necrosis, bone pain, multiple fractures, anemia, thrombocytopenia

HPE: Crumpled/crinkled tissue paper appearance

Radiological investigation: Femur = Erlenmeyer flask deformity

*most common type = Type 1 Gaucher's disease

13. DNA packing is done by: *(NEET 2022)*

a. Histone
b. Glycoprotein
c. Nucleic acid
d. Helicases
e. Cytochromes

Ans. is 'a' Histone

Glycoprotein = complex of carbohydrates and protein

Helicases = enzymes that unwind/separate the two strands of DNA helix

Histone = packing of DNA

Cytochrome = hemoproteins undergoing reduction and oxidation

14. A patient factory worker working since 20 years c/o joint pain, insomnia, fatigue, constipation, headache. He is found to have anemia. Enzyme affected is: *(NEET 2022)*

a. Uroporphyrinogen III synthase
b. Uroporphyrinogen I synthase
c. ALA synthase
d. Ferrochelatase

Ans. is 'd' Ferrochelatase

For detail see explanation on pages 133–134

15. Complex 4 inhibitor: *(NEET 2022)*

a. Cyanide
b. Carbon dioxide
c. Oligomycin
d. Antimycin

Ans. is 'a' Cyanide

For detail see explanation on pages 112–113

16. Enzyme defect in McArdle's disease: *(NEET 2022)*

a. Myophosphorylase
b. Glucose-6-phosphatase
c. Glycogen phosphorylase
d. Hexokinase

Ans. is 'a' Myophosphorylase

Glycogen storage disease	*Enzyme defects*
GSD TYPE 0	Glycogen synthase
VON GIERKE'S DISEASE GSD TYPE 1A	Glucose-6-phosphatase
GSD TYPE 1B	ER glucose-6-phosphatase
POMPE'S DISEASE GSD TYPE 2	Lysosomal alpha1,4; alpha 1,6 glucosidase
CORI/FORBE'S GSD TYPE 3	Glycogen debranching enzyme
ANDERSON DISEASE GSD TYPE 4	Glycogen branching enzyme
MCARDLE DISEASE GSD TYPE 5	Muscle glycogen phosphorylase
HER'S DISEASE GSD TYPE 6	Liver glycogen phosphorylase
TARUI'S DISEASE GSD TYPE 7	Muscle phosphofructokinase

17. An Alcoholic patient on anti-tubercular drugs for the past 3 months complains of numbness, tingling and burning sensation in all the extremities. What could be vitamin deficiency? *(NEET 2022)*

a. Vitamin A
b. Vitamin B_{12}
c. Vitamin B_1
d. Vitamin D

Ans. is 'c' Vitamin B_1

Alcoholics on ATT have deficiency: B1 earlier than B6

Non-alcoholics on ATT have deficiency: B6 > B1

18. Cherry red spots on retina and mental retardation is seen in: *(NEET 2022)*

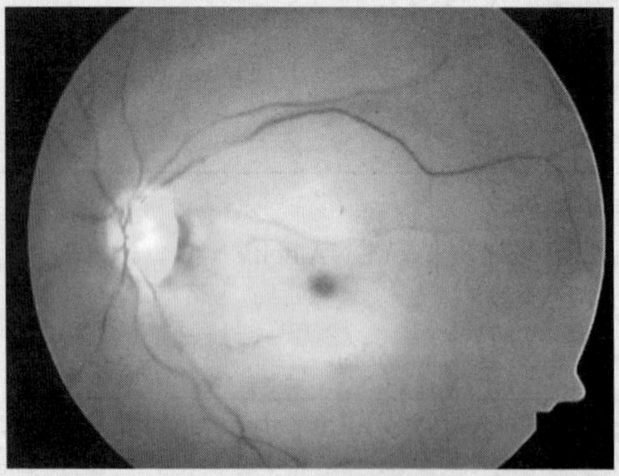

For colour version see Plate 1

a. Gaucher's disease
b. Tay Sachs disease
c. Hunter syndrome
d. Krabbe's disease

Ans. is 'b' Tay Sachs disease

Tay Sachs Disease

- Deficiency: Beta hexosaminidase A deficiency
- Accumulation: GM2
- Clinical features: Mental retardation, exaggerated startle response/hyperacusis, cherry red spot
- *Cherry red spot with no hepatomegaly = Tay Sachs disease
- Cherry red spot with organomegaly = Niemann-Pick disease

19. FAD status in body is determined by: *(NEET 2022)*

a. Thiamine
b. Glutathione reductase
c. Hexokinase
d. Transketolase

Ans. is 'b' Glutathione reductase

Vitamin	Assay and test
B1Z (THIAMINE)	RBC Transketolase
B2 (RIBOFLAVIN/FAD)	RBC glutathione reductase
B6 (PYRIDOXINE)	RBC transaminase
B9 (FOLIC ACID)	FIGLU excretion/Histidine load test
B12 (COBALAMINE)	Serum methyl malonate level

20. A mediterrangean person didn't receive primaquine. Which pathway is affected by G6PD enzyme deficiency? *(NEET 2022)*

a. HMP pathway
b. Glycolysis
c. Gluconeogenesis
d. Krebs cycle

Ans. is 'a' HMP pathway

For detail see explanation on page 109

21. Condition shown below is due to which vitamin deficiency? *(NEET 2022)*

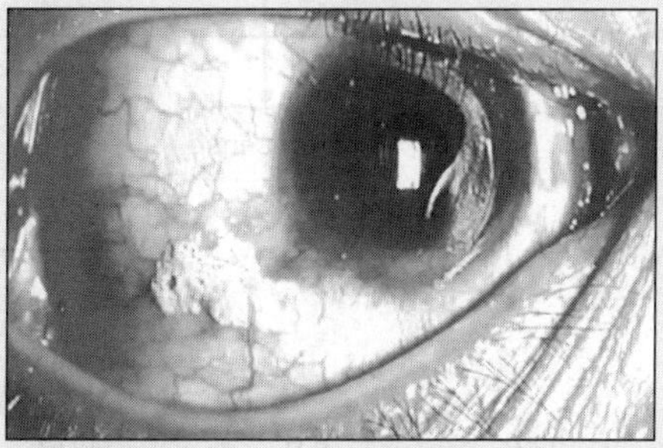

a. Vitamin A
b. Vitamin B
c. Vitamin C
d. Vitamin K

Ans. is 'a' Vitamin A

The Who Classification of vitamin A deficiency is as follows:

XN	Night blindness
X1A	Conjunctival xerosis
X1B	Bitot's spot
X2	Corneal xerosis
X3A	Corneal ulceration/keratomalacia involving one-third or less of the cornea
X3B	Corneal ulceration/keratomalacia involving one-half or more of the cornea
XS	Corneal scar
XF	Xerophthalmic fundus

22. Fatty acid transport through mitochondrial membrane is via: *(NEET 2022)*

a. Carnitine
b. Acyl carrier protein
c. Cholesterol transporter
d. LCAT

Ans. is 'a' Carnitine

For detail see explanation on page 116

23. A woman on anti-depressants presents with bleeding. She gives a history of bulky stools which stick to the pan. Which of the following vitamin deficiency can cause bleeding in this condition? *(NEET 2022)*

a. Vitamin A
b. Vitamin D
c. Vitamin E
d. Vitamin K

Ans. is 'd' Vitamin K

- The patient presents with steatorrhea and bleeding.
- Steatorrhea is presence of fat in stools due to malabsorption. Hence, fat soluble vitamins (vitamin A,D,E,K) are deficient in the body.
- Vitamin K is required for clotting factors-2,7,9,10, protein C and protein S. Hence, deficiency of vitamin K will present as bleeding.

PATHOLOGY

24. Single nucleotide change resulting in stop codon called: *(NEET 2022)*

a. Missense
b. Nonsense
c. Point mutation
d. Silent

Ans. is 'b' Nonsense

Single Nucleotide Changes

Results	*Mutation*
Same product at protein level	Silent mutation
Different product at protein level	Missense Mutation
No product due to STOP CODON	Nonsense Mutation

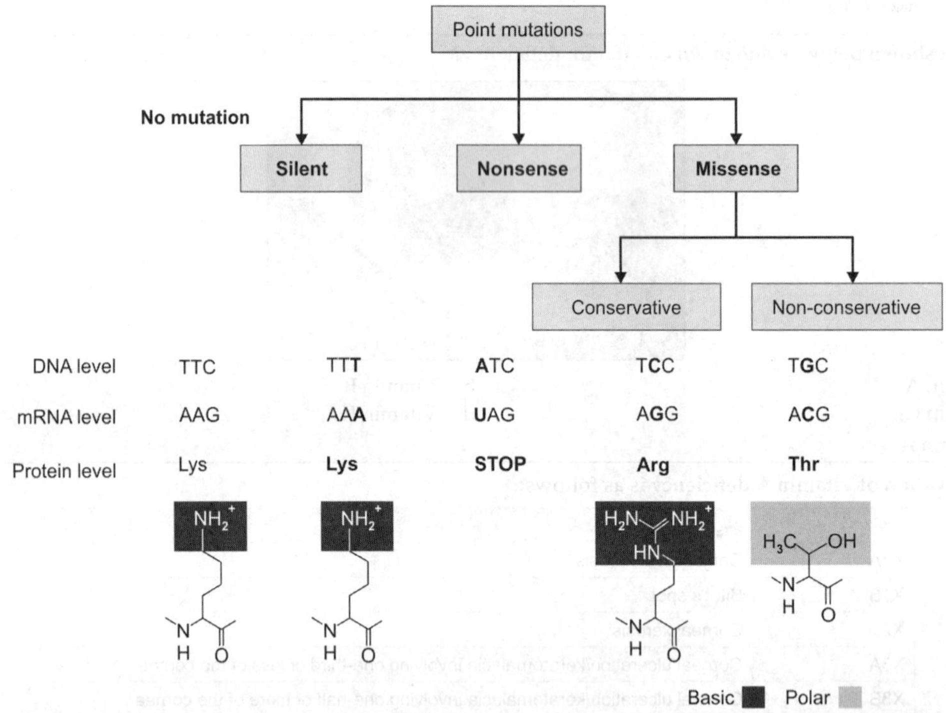

25. A trauma patient was to undergo Emergency laparotomy, they wanted to monitor the coagulation studies, which is the investigation of choice? *(NEET 2022)*

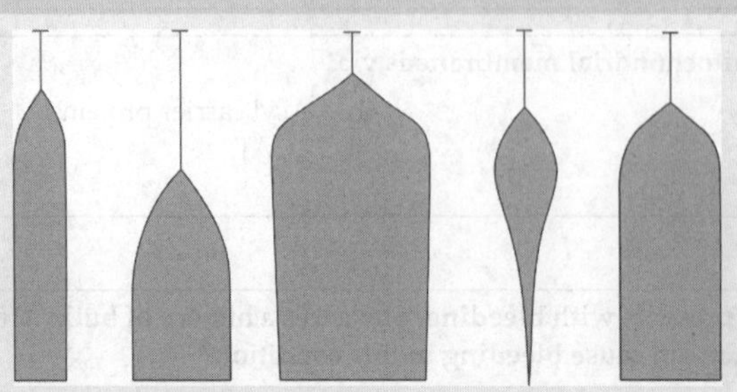

a. Elastography
b. Thromboelastography
c. None of the above
d. All of the above

Ans. is 'b' Thromboelastography

Coagulation status	TEG tracing	R value	K and a value	Maximum amplitude	Treatment algorithm
Normal hemostasis	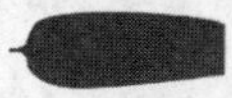	Normal	Normal	Normal	Attain surgical hemostasis using sutures
Hemodilution or clotting factor deficiency	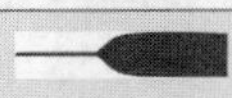	High	Low or normal	Low or normal	Administer fresh frozen plasma If indicated
Fibrinogen deficiency	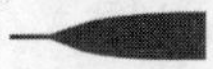	Normal or high	Low	Low or normal	Administer cryoprecipitate
Low or dysfunctional platelets	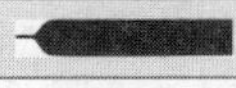	Normal	Normal	Low	Administer platelets
Primary fibrinolysis	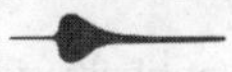	Normal	Normal	Low	Administer antifibrinolytics or tranexamic acid as indicated
Secondary fibrinolysis hypercoagulopathy with fibrinolysis	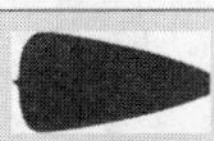	Low	High	High	Treat disseminated intravascular coagulopathy
Thrombosis		Low	High	High	Administer anticoagulant indicated

Common clotting disorders. Thromboelastography (TEG) Tracina Example. Characteristic Values.

26. What will increase life span? *(NEET 2022)*

a. Regular exercise (walking for 30 mins)
b. Decreasing stress
c. Decrease calorie by 30%
d. All of the above

Ans. is 'c' Decrease calorie by 30%

Proven method to Decrease the process of ageing by decrease calorie intake.

Calorie restriction leads to stimulation of sirtuin.

SIRTUIN is also induced by red wine.

Mechanism of action of SIRTUIN:

- Decreases free radical injury
- Increase proper protein folding
- Decrease apoptosis
- Increase insulin sensitivity that increases glucose metabolism
- Decreases overall metabolism

27. Which is AR inheritance? *(NEET 2022)*

a. Cystic fibrosis
b. Huntington ds
c. Achondroplasia
d. Teacher Colin

Ans. is 'a' Cystic fibrosis

Autosomal Recessive Conditions

- Cystic fibrosis
- Phenylketonuria
- Galactosemia
- Homocystinuria
- Lysosomal storage disorder
- Alpha 1 antitrypsin deficiency
- Wilson disease
- Hemochromatosis
- Glycogen storage disorders
- Sickle cell anemia
- Thalassemias
- Alkaptonuria
- Friedrich ataxia

Autosomal Recessive Disorders

- m-ABCDEFGH
- **A**lbinism, **A**taxia telangiectasia, **A**lkaptonuria
- **B**eta Thalassemia

- Cystic Fibrosis, Congenital Adrenal Hyperplasia
- Distal spinal muscular atrophy 1, Dubin Johnson syndrome
- Emphysema (Alpha-1 antitrypsin deficiency)
- Friedreich ataxia
- Galactosemia, Glycogen storage disorders
- Hemochromatosis, Homocystinuria

28. True about NET are all, *except*? *(NEET 2022)*

a. Seen in sepsis
b. Seen with bacteria
c. Mitochondrial DNA is seen
d. It is chromatin with antibacterial enzymes

Ans. is 'c' Mitochondrial DNA is seen

Neutrophil Extracellular Trap

Functions:

- Anti-microbial
- Nuclear chromatin exposed that leads to formation of anti-nuclear antibodies. Therefore associated with autoimmunity.
- DVT

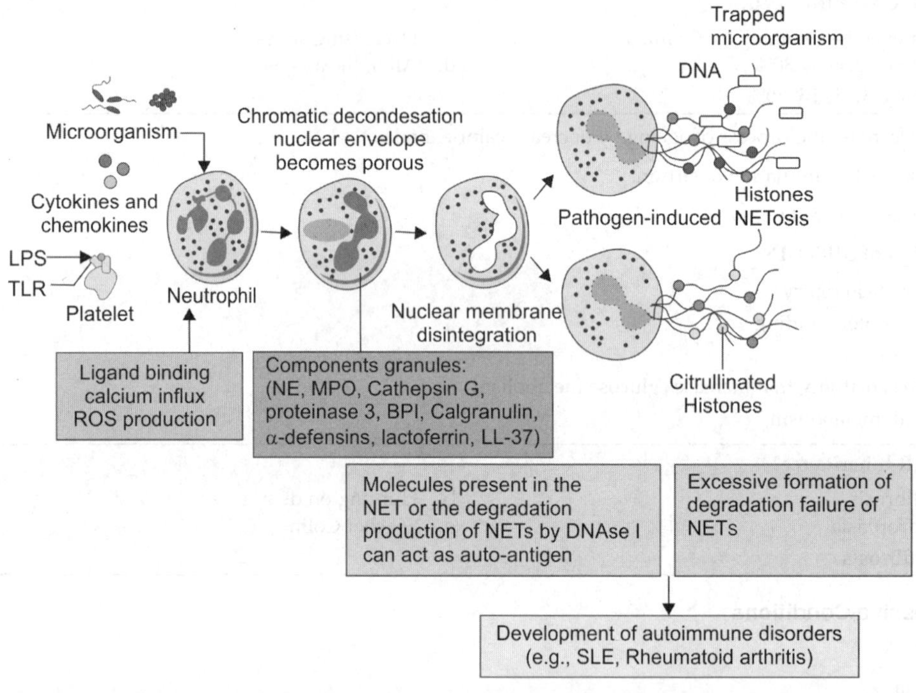

29. Case of hypochromic microcytic anemia with reduced RBC indices and target cells present. RBC count of 5.2 × 109/uL. What is the next best investigation? *(NEET 2022)*

a. HbA_2
b. Serum ferritin
c. Serum Folate
d. RDW

Ans. is 'a' HbA_2

- To differentiate between IDA and Thalassemia minor is by calculating Mentzer index.
- Mentzer index = MCV/RBC COUNT
- <13 = Thalassemia minor
- >13 = IDA
- As in the above question, RBC indices are low with normal RBC count so Mentzer index would be less than 13.
- Diagnosis: Thalassemia minor
- Investigation: To detect the levels of HbA_2, HbA and HbF
- HbF = Normal
- HbA_2 = Increases

❖ HbA = decreases

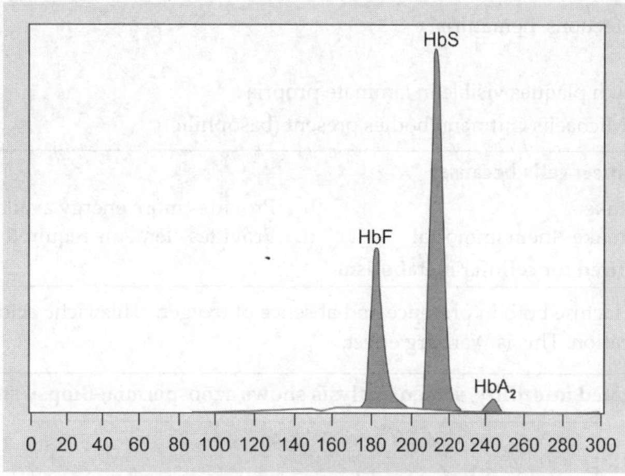

30. A 56-year-old male patient presented with dragging sensation in abdomen. O/e there is massive splenomegaly. Laboratory reports show increased hemoglobin, total WBC count and platelet counts. PS show metamyelocytes and myelocytes. Which chromosomal translocation is associated with this condition? *(NEET 2022)*

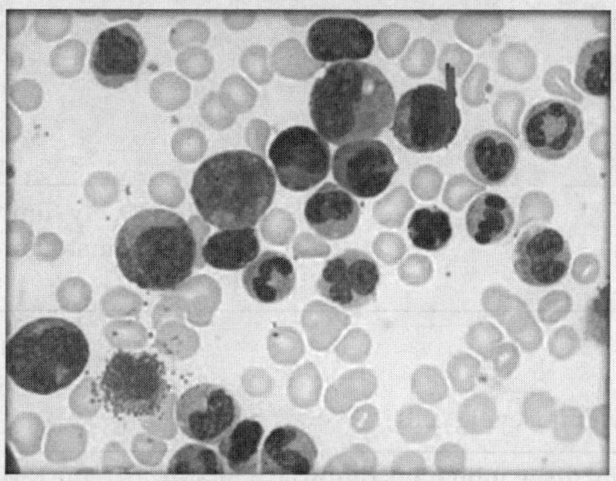

a. t9,22
b. 8,14
c. 8,11
d. 8,22

Ans. is 'a' t9,22

❖ This is a case of CML
❖ Philadelphia chromosome is associated with CML t9;22
❖ HPE: Garden party appearance/college girl appearance

31. A patient was underwent cystoscopy which showed multiple yellow white plaque in bladder, the HPE shows infiltrated in the lamina propria layer as shown below. What is your diagnosis? *(NEET 2022)*

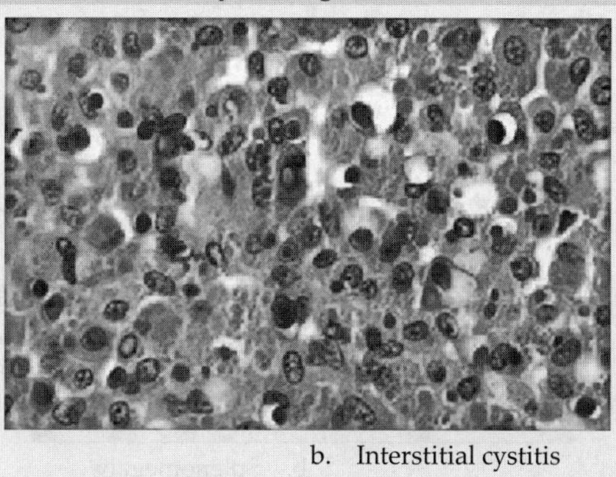

For colour version see Plate 1

a. Malakoplakia
b. Interstitial cystitis
c. Acute cystitis
d. Chronic cystitis

Ans. is 'a' Malakoplakia

Malakoplakia

- *Clinical features:* Urinary tract infections, hematuria
- *Etiology:* Proteus, E. coli
- *Cystoscopy:* Multiple yellow brown plaques visible in laminate propria
- *HPE:* Dark blue-black bodies = Michaelis Gutmann bodies present (basophilic)

32. Warburg effect is used by cancer cells because: *(NEET 2022)*

a. Reduced the glucose uptake
b. Provides more energy available to cancer cells (ATP)
c. Prevents apoptosis and makes them immortal
d. Provides elements required for cellular metabolism

Ans. is 'd' Provides elements required for cellular metabolism

Tumour cells metabolise glucose to lactose both in presence and absence of oxygen. This lactic acid provides to be a source of cellular metabolites for the cancer cell replication. This is Warburg effect.

33. A 30-year-old male investigated infertility, semen analysis shows azoospermia, Biopsy shows: *(NEET 2022)*

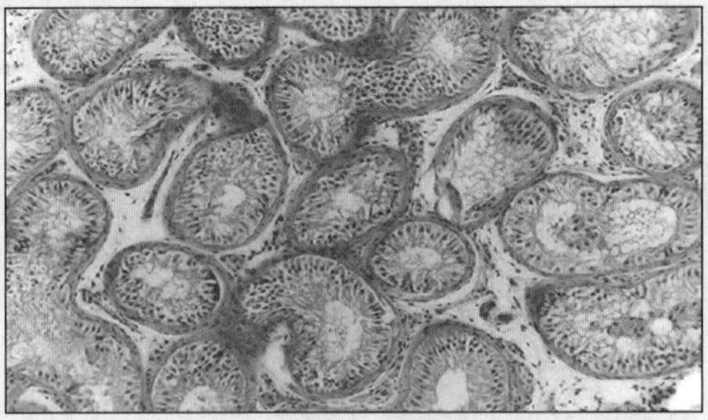

a. Orchitis
b. Sertoli cell only tumor
c. Testicular atrophy
d. Nonseminomatous germ cell tumor

Ans. is 'b' Sertoli cell only tumor

- This is a case of serotli cell tumour
- *Clinical features:* Infertility
- *HPE:* Seminiferous tubules are seen with no leydig cells

34. A 40-year-old female arthralgia, oral ulcer, joint pain, oliguria, hematuria. Urine RM shows RBC casts. What is the diagnosis? *(NEET 2022)*

a. PSGN
b. MGN
c. Lupus nephritis
d. IgA nephropathy

Ans. is 'c' Lupus nephritis

- Arthralgia, oral ulcer, joint pain, hematuria, oliguria with RBC casts in urine = SLE.
- Lupus nephritis is seen in SLE.

35. A patient presented with anemia and hemoglobinuria. Lab investigations revealed raised LDH and Elevated bilirubin levels. Peripheral smear is as shown below. Which of the following findings is likely to be present in this patient? *(NEET 2022)*

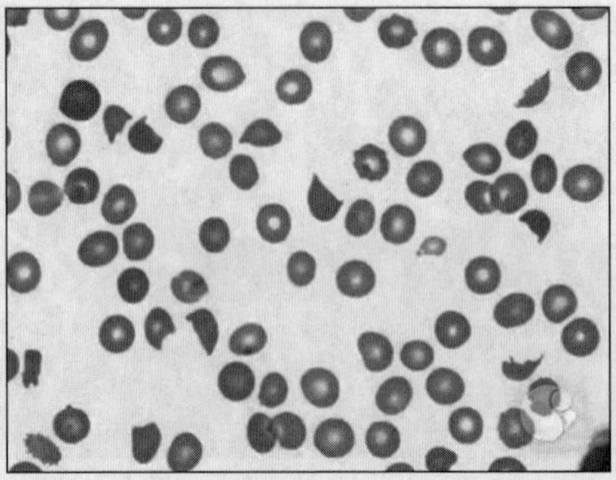

a. Goiters
b. Splenomegaly
c. Raised HbA_2
d. Mechanical 2nd Heart sounds

Ans. is 'd' Mechanical 2nd Heart sounds

- Raised LDH + elevated bilirubin + hemoglobinuria = MAHA
- MAHA = Micro Angiopathic Hemolytic Anemia
- MAHA can occur in patient having prosthetic heart valves.

36. A middle aged female died of COVID-19 while she was on ventilator. Which of the following microscopic findings is attributable to her cause of death? *(NEET 2022)*

a. Thick fibrin lining alveoli
b. Intracytoplasmic and intranuclear inclusion bodies
c. Acute and chronic hemorrhages
d. PAS+ bodies in bronchoalveolar lavage

Ans. is 'a' Thick fibrin lining alveoli

COVID

Mechanism of lung injury: ADRS - Alveolar membrane damage via deposition of fibrin.

37. A patient with long standing hemorrhoids came to the hospital for the routine check-up. On blood investigations, Hb was 7 g/dL. On peripheral blood smear following findings are seen. What is the most likely diagnosis? *(NEET 2022)*

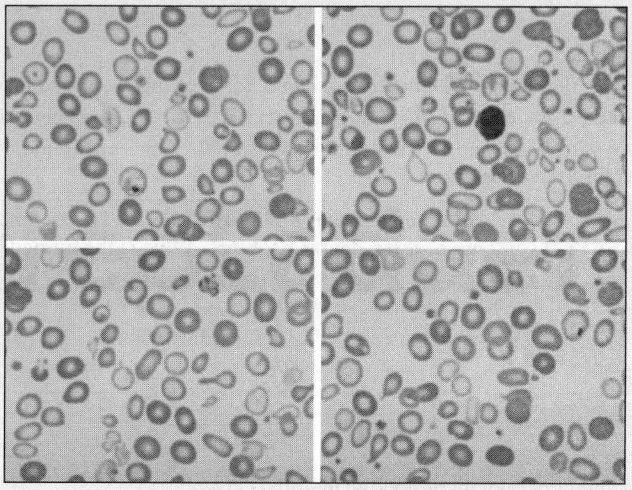

a. Iron deficiency anemia
b. Sideroblastic anemia
c. Megaloblastic anemia
d. Hemolytic anemia

Ans. is 'a' Iron deficiency anemia

Iron Deficiency Anemia

PBS:

- Microcytic hypochromic RBCs
- Pencil cells (occasionally)
- Target cells

PHARMACOLOGY

38. A patient was given intravenous botulinum toxin and the patient died. Mechanism of botulinum toxin overdose is: *(NEET 2022)*

a. Inhibits release of acetylcholine
b. Inhibit reuptake of nor-epinephrine
c. Blockade of post synaptic nicotinic cholinergic receptors
d. Inhibit entry of acetylcholine in vesicle

Ans. is 'a' Inhibits release of acetylcholine

- Botulinum toxin inhibits release of acetylcholine
- Hemicholinium inhibits choline uptake (rate limiting step)
- Vesamicol inhibits vesicular uptake of acetylcholine
- Physostigmine is acetylcholinesterase inhibitor

39. Drug of choice in paracetamol overdose is: *(NEET 2022)*

a. N-acetylcysteine
b. Dopamine
c. Hydralazine
d. Furosemide

Ans. is 'a' N-acetylcysteine

- Drug of choice in Paracetamol overdose is N-acetylcysteine.
- NAC provides a Cysteine group for glutathione synthesis.
- NAPQ1 produced after paracetamol metabolism, binds to glutathione and hence cannot bind to any SH group (toxic).

40. A young female presented with left sided severe throbbing headache associated with nausea, vomiting, photophobia and phonophobia. Which of the following drug can provide immediate relief to this patient? *(NEET 2022)*

a. Propranolol
b. Sumatriptan
c. Topiramate
d. Flunarizine

Ans. is 'b' Sumatriptan

Triptans

- These are 5-HT ID/IB receptor agonists.
- Sumatriptan is the 1st triptan to be developed. It is the drug of choice for aborting an acute attack of migraine.
- Other triptans include almotriptan, eletriptan, frovatriptan, rizatriptan, naratriptan, and zolmitriptan.
- All triptans can cause coronary vasospasm and are contraindicated in IHD. Other contraindications are hypertension, epilepsy, hepatic or renal impairment and during pregnancy.

41. A patient on digoxin therapy accidently consumed 8 tablets of digoxin 0.25 mg. Two hours later, he presented to emergency with heart rate of 54 bpm and ECG evidence of third-degree AV block. What is the immediate management of this patient? *(NEET 2022)*

a. Digoxin immune Fab
b. Lignocaine
c. Phenytoin
d. DC cardioversion

Ans. is 'a' Digoxin immune Fab

Treatment of digoxin toxicity:

- *Mild toxicity:* KCL infusion given
- *Severe toxicity:* Purified Fab fragments of digitalis antibody/DIGIBIND given

42. An 82-year-old patient presented with acute episode of breathlessness. Chest X-ray shows pulmonary edema. History reveals that the patient has uncontrolled hypertension and is not taking the medication regularly. Which should be the management of this patient? *(NEET 2022)*

a. Intravenous nitroglycerine
b. Salbutamol nebulization
c. Intravenous salbutamol
d. Intravenous antibiotics plus oxygen

Ans. is 'a' Intravenous nitroglycerine

43. Which of the following hypolipidemic drug acts by inhibition of PCSK-9? *(NEET 2022)*

a. Atorvastatin
b. Evolocumab
c. Ezetimibe
d. Lomitapide

Ans. is 'b' Evolocumab

New drugs for treating hyperlipidaemia:

- MTP inhibitor—Lomitapide
- CETP inhibitor—Anacetrapib
- PCSK9 inhibitor—Alirocumab, Evolocumab

44. A patient presents with pituitary tumor that overproduces growth hormone. Surgical removal of the tumor was incomplete. What is the first line treatment of this patient? *(NEET 2022)*

a. Leuprolide
b. Octreotide
c. Nafarelin
d. Goserelin

Ans. is 'b' Octreotide

Uses of subcutaneous octreotide:

- Used in acromegaly
- Used in islet cell tumour

- Secretory diarrhoea
- Esophageal varices

45. A 40-year-old male presents with protrusion of chin, excessive sweating, impaired glucose tolerance and enlargement of hands and feet. Which of the following drugs is a growth hormone receptor antagonist used to treat this condition? *(NEET 2022)*

a. Pegvisomant
b. Octreotide
c. Cabergoline
d. Olcegepant

Ans. is 'a' Pegvisomant

Treatment of acromegaly:

- Subcutaneous octreotide (GH inhibiting hormone)
- Oral cabergoline (D2 analogue) = DOC
- *Pegvisomant:* Long acting growth hormone receptor blocking drug (somatotropin antagonist). It affects vision.

46. A female presented with galactorrhea. Her urine pregnancy test was negative. MRI of head revealed a large pituitary tumor. Patient refused to undergo surgery for the tumor. Which of the following is the best drug for the treatment of this patient? *(NEET 2022)*

a. Octreotide
b. Bromocriptine
c. Promethazine
d. Clozapine

Ans. is 'b' Bromocriptine

This is a case of Prolactinoma. It presents as galactorrhea or infertility.

Treatment of prolactinoma:

- Drugs-bromocriptine (when the female wants to conceive/already pregnant) or oral cabergoline.
- Surgical resection (if medical methods fail or no improvement in symptoms/decrease in tumour size/onset of visual symptoms).

47. A patient with opioid poisoning presents with severe respiratory depression. What is the most effective drug for treatment of this patient? *(NEET 2022)*

a. Fomepizole
b. Naltrexone
c. Flumazenil
d. Naloxone

Ans. is d. Naloxone

Treatment of opioid poisoning:

- *Acute poisoning:* IV naloxone
- *To prevent relapse:* Oral naltrexone
- *To prevent withdrawal symptoms:* Methadone
- *To treat withdrawal symptoms:* Beta blockers
- *To treat seizures (withdrawal symptoms):* Benzodiazepines

48. A patient presents with tremors, rigidity and bradykinesia. Which of the following drugs can be used for the treatment of this patient? *(NEET 2022)*

a. Selegiline
b. Donepezil
c. Fluoxetine
d. Haloperidol

Ans. is 'a' Selegiline

- This is a case of parkinsonism
- Selegiline is MAO-B inhibitor (Predominantly in brain) used for treatment of Parkinsonism
- Also Transdermal patch of Selegiline is approved for depression but not Parkinsonism
- Haloperidol: Antipsychotic
- Fluoxetine: SSRIs
- Donepezil: Acetylcholine Estrase—DOC—Senile dementia

49. An 11-year-old boy presented to emergency with vomiting. Parents gave history of consuming 10–15 tablets of ferrous sulphate a day before. What is the antidote of iron for treatment of this patient? *(NEET 2022)*

a. Dimercaprol
b. Deferiprone
c. d-Penicillamine
d. Activated charcoal

Ans. is 'b' Deferiprone

Treatment of iron poisoning:

- Acute poisoning ivy Desferrioxamine
- Chronic poisoning oral Desferipirone
- Penicillamine: Copper poisoning/Wilson disease

50. A deep vein thrombosis patient was started on an anticoagulant therapy. Next day, the patient presented with the features shown in the diagram below. Likely drug implicated for this adverse effect is: *(NEET 2022)*

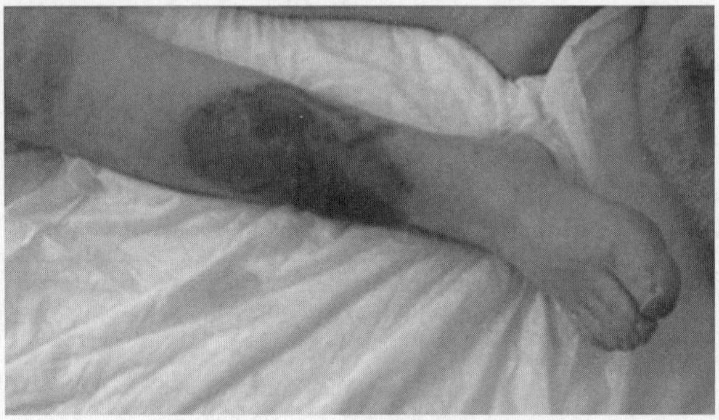

a. Heparin
b. Rivaroxaban
c. Warfarin
d. Dabigatran

Ans. is 'c' Warfarin

- Warfarin inactivates factor 2,7,9,10 and protein C and S.
- On giving warfarin, new factor does not get activated and already activated factor finishes according to their half-lives. Therefore, action of warfarin comes late in about 4 to 5 days.
- Protein C finishes earlier therefore, there is increased risk of clotting and hence dermal vascular necrosis occurs.

51. A patient with COPD was given intravenous aminophylline therapy following which the patient developed diuresis. This is due to action on which effector: *(NEET 2022)*

a. Adenosine receptors
b. Beta 2 adrenergic receptors
c. IL-10
d. Histone deacetylase

Ans. is 'a' Adenosine receptors

Aminophylline has three modes of actions:

1. PDE inhibition
   PDE3 inhibition: Causes relaxation of bronchial smooth muscles
   PDE4 inhibition: Causes inhibition of cytokines and chemokines which decreases immune cell migration and activation
2. Adenosine receptor blocking inhibits bronco constriction and acts at afferent arteriole and PCT which leads to dieresis.
3. Activate histone Deacetylase 2 anti-inflammatory action.

52. A female with ovarian cancer was on cisplatin therapy. She presented to hospital with several episodes of vomiting. After giving an antiemetic drug, the patient developed dystonia. The anti-emetic drug most likely to be responsible for these features is: *(NEET 2022)*

a. Metoclopramide
b. Meclizine
c. Ondansetron
d. Scopolamine

Ans. is 'a' Metoclopramide

Metoclopramide crosses blood brain barrier and blocks

- D2 in the brain, causing extrapyramidal symptoms
- Dystonia is the most common side-effect
- It can also cause hyperprolactinemia

Metoclopramide has additional effects as 5HT3 blocker and 5HT4 stimulator

53. A pregnant female with urinary tract infection took antimicrobials for the same. The baby of this female developed tendon rupture and arthropathy. What is the likely mechanism of action of the antimicrobial consumed by the pregnant female? *(NEET 2022)*

a. Folic acid synthesis inhibitor
b. Mycolic acid synthesis inhibitor
c. DNA gyrase inhibitor
d. DNA inhibitor

Ans. is 'c' DNA gyrase inhibitor

The drug given in the question is a Quinolone.
Quinolone acts by inhibiting DNA Gyrase which helps in replication in bacteria.

54. A 48-year-old patient presented to OPD with tingling and numbness of fingers. The patient is chronic alcoholic and was recently started on antitubercular treatment. What should be the treatment of this patient? *(NEET 2022)*

a. Vitamin B_3
b. Vitamin B_6
c. Vitamin B_1
d. Vitamin B_{12}

Ans. is 'b' Vitamin B_6

- Antitubercular drug causing pyridoxine deficiency is ISONIAZID(H). It is metabolised by acetylation.
- Pyridoxine (B6) is given along with isoniazid to treat and prevent peripheral neuropathy which causes tingling and peripheral neuropathy.

55. In MDR tuberculosis, which of following drug combinations show resistance? *(NEET 2022)*

a. Rifampicin and Fluoroquinolones
b. Isoniazid and rifampicin
c. Isoniazid and Pyrazinamide
d. Rifampicin and kanamycin

Ans. is 'b' Isoniazid and rifampicin

Drug-resistant TB

- *Mono drug resistance:* Bacteria is resistant to only firstline drug except rifampicin
- *Poly drug resistance:* >1 first line drug resistance except rifampicin
- MDR-bacteria resistant to both ISONIAZID and RIFAMPICIN
- XDR-resistance to ISONIAZID & RIFAMPICIN +1 fluoroquinolones +1 of the injectables.

56. Which of the following drugs have least adverse effect on pleura? *(NEET 2022)*

a. Bromocriptine
b. Metformin
c. Nitrofurantoin
d. Methysergide

Ans. is 'b' Metformin

MICROBIOLOGY

57. A female presented with curdy white discharge. Sample microscopy showed budding yeast cell with pseudohyphae. Which medium is used to differentiate the species of the causative organism? *(NEET 2022)*

a. Bird seed agar
b. Chrome agar
c. SDA
d. PDA

Ans. is 'b' Chrome agar

- Chrome agar is used to differentiate the species of the causative Organism-Candida.
- Bird seed agar is used for blastomycosis.
- SDA agar is used for isolation of Fungi.

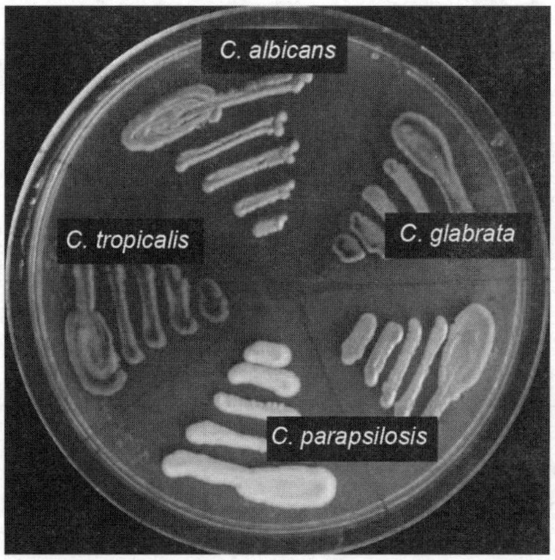

58. A farmer is presented with sinuses with a discharging granule on the leg. The granules were crushed and examined, which of the following statement is correct regarding this scenario? *(NEET 2022)*

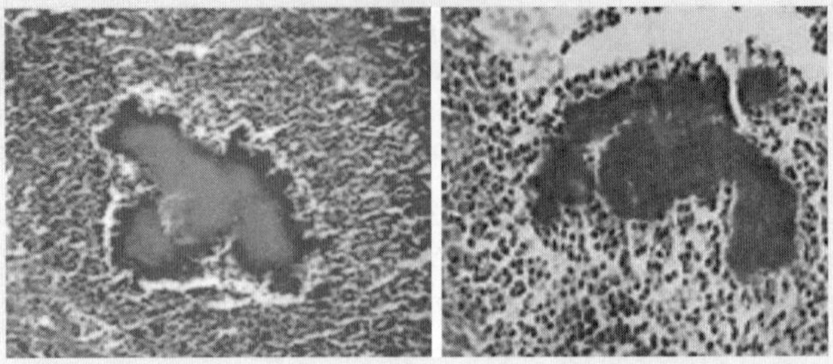

a. Can be caused by Bacteria and Fungi
b. Involves skin only. No deeper tissue involvement
c. Lymphocyte accumulation is present
d. Spread by hematogenous route

Ans. is 'a' Can be caused by Bacteria and Fungi

The given case is of Madura foot. It can be caused both by bacteria and Fungi.

Feature	***Eumycetoma***	***Actinomycetoma***
Ethological agent	Fungus	Bacteria
Site	• Extremities, most commonly foot • Trunk and head involvement almost nil	• Most commonly on foot • Trunk and head involvement may be seen
Progression lesions	• Slow • Well-encapsulated • Clear margin • Less inflammatory • Less destructive	• Rapid • Diffuse • Margins not very clear • More inflammatory • More destructive
Sinuses	**Few**	**Many**
Grains	• **Usually black** • **Pale grains may be seen** • **Never red**	• **Usually pale yellow to white** • **Red gains may be seen** • **Never black**
Underlying structures	• Bone invasion is late • Multiple punched out lytic lesions on a radiograph	• Earlier invasion of bones • Both osteolytic and osteosclerotic lesions on radiograph

59. A woodworker presented with Chronic localized infection of the skin on lower legs and feet which were irregular, rough, cauliflower-like lesions, Microscopy of biopsy shows Copper penny/muriform cells/medial bodies, etiological agent is: *(NEET 2022)*

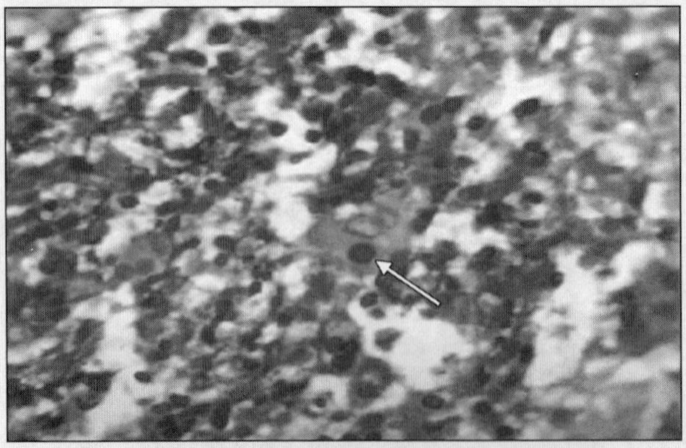

a. Chromoblastomycosis
b. Phaeohyphomycosis
c. Chromomycosis
d. Rhinosporidiosis

Ans. is 'a' Chromoblastomycosis

- *Chromoblastomycosis:* Verrucous Dermatitis
- *Clinical features:* Warty, resemble florets of a cauliflower
- *Risk factors:* Agricultural workers, woodcutters, barefoot (traumatic implantation)
- *Microscopy:* Copper/medlar/muriform/sclerotic body

60. In a patient with rice water diarrhea, which will be involved? *(NEET 2022)*

a. GM1 ganglioside
b. GM2 ganglioside
c. Both A and B
d. None of the above

Ans. is 'a' GM1 ganglioside

- *Cholera toxin has two fragments:* A and B
- *Fragment A:* Increases cAMP that causes watery diarrhoea
- *Fragment B:* Binds to GM1 ganglioside

61. A young boy presented with fever, sore throat, malaise and abdominal pain, conjunctival suffusion and calf tenderness. No history of cough, vomiting, hemorrhage and travel. What is the diagnosis? *(NEET 2022)*

a. Chikungunya
b. Leptospira
c. Dengue hemorrhagic fever
d. Hepatic encephalopathy with hepatitis A

Ans. is 'b' Leptospira

- Leptospira interrogans belongs to spirochetes, causes leptospirosis a zoonotic infection.
- The 3 important epidemiological determinants for leptospirosis include exposure to rodents, rainfall and rice field.
- Weil's disease (Hepato-renal-hemorrhagic syndrome), a severe form of icteric illness occurs in 10% patients.
- *Specimens for diagnosis:* CSF, blood and urine.
- Dark-field microscopy or by immunofluorescence or light microscopy after silver impregnation staining used for diagnosis of leptospirosis.
- EMJH (Ellinghausen, McCullough, Johnson, Harris) medium, Korthof's and Fletcher's media used for culture.
- Microscopic agglutination test (MAT) (Gold Standard and reference test) detects antibodies against specific serovars of L. interrogans and also Macroscopic agglutination test used for diagnosis.
- Treatment with Doxycycline and Penicillin.

62. Which of the following is the best way to diagnose a Clostridium associated Diarrhea? *(NEET 2022)*

a. Stool culture
b. Toxin demonstration
c. Blood culture
d. None of the above

Ans. is 'b' Toxin demonstration

Detection of toxin A and B in stools by PCR or culture is the best way to diagnose a clostridium associated diarrhoea.

63. A 24-year-old male who recently returned from Africa reported with Jaundice and Hemorrhagic fever & having torres body, Symptomatic treatment was given but the patient died. Which vaccine must have prevented this occurrence? *(NEET 2022)*

a. Edmonston-Zagreb vaccine
b. RA27/3 vaccine
c. Jeryl Lynn vaccine
d. 17 D vaccine

Ans. is 'd' 17 D vaccine

Inclusion Bodies

Intracytoplasmic	Acidophilic	Negri bodies	Rabies
		• Guarnieri bodies • Bollinger bodies • Henderson-Peterson bodies • Paschen • Halberstaedter Prowazek (HD body)	• Variola, vaccinia • Fowlpox • Molluscum contagiosum • Smallpox • Chlamydia trachomatis
	Basophilic	Levinthal Cole Lillie (LCL Body)	Chlamydia psittaci
Intranuclear	Acidophilic	• Cowdry type A (granular)	• Herpes, Chickenpox, CMV, Yellow fever
		• Torres bodies	• Yellow fever
		• Cowdry type B	• Polio virus
	Basophilic	• Cowdry type B	• Adenovirus
Both intracytoplasmic and intranuclear		• Warthin-Finkeldey	• Measles

Note: CMV produces intranuclear 'owl's eye' inclusion body.

64. A police officer admitted to hospital with Fever and myalgia. Physical examination revealed rash which is exclusively absent on palm and soles. Which of the following lice infestation best explains this feature? *(NEET 2022)*

a. R. Prowazekii
b. R. Akari
c. R. Typhi
d. R. Conorii

Ans. is 'a' R. Prowazekii

Rickettsial Diseases

Disease	Agent	Insect vector	Mammalian reservoir
Typhus group epidemic typhus • Murine typhus (Endemic typhus) • Scrub typhus	R. prowazekii R. typhi R. tsutsugamushi	Louse Flea Mite	Humans, Rodents
Spotted fever group Indian tick typhus • Rocky mountain spotted fever • Rickettsial pox	R. conori R. rickettsiae R. akari	Tick Tick Mite	Rodents, dogs Mice
Others Q fever • Trench fever	Coxiella burnetii Bartonella quintana	Nil Louse	Cattle, sheep, goats, humans

65. A HIV patient presented with fever, cough and breathlessness, red pigment with TLC-2500, the isolated organism was a fungi showing yeast from at 37C and mold form at 25C as shown in the image. What is the causative agent? *(NEET 2022)*

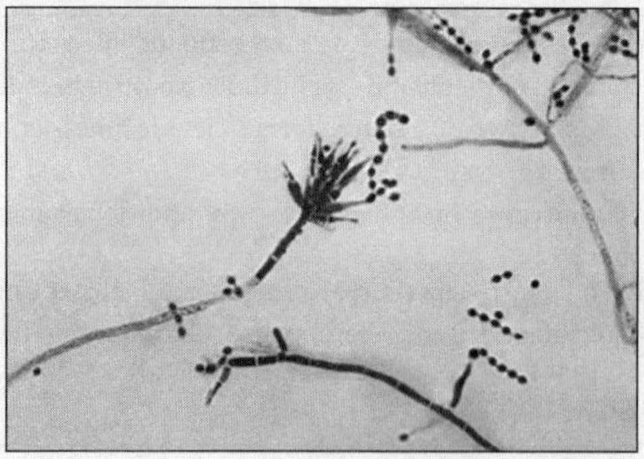

a. Pneumocystis
b. Talaromyces marneffei
c. Blastomyces
d. Aspergillus versicolor

Ans. is 'b' Talaromyces marneffei

Talaromyces Marneffei/Penicillium

- ❖ Yeast like form
- ❖ Pseudomycelia absent
- ❖ Brush like conidia
- ❖ Chain of spores

66. A new born of a HIV infected mother has diarrhea. Which test is to be done to identify causative organism? *(NEET 2022)*

a. HIV Antibody in neonate
b. GDH
c. Stool microscopy
d. HIV RNA PCR to determine viral load

Ans. is 'd' HIV RNA PCR to determine viral load

HIV RNA PCR is done to determine the viral load in an infant who is at high risk of acquiring HIV infection from mother.

67. A red pigment producing pencil shaped macroconidia? *(NEET 2022)*

a. Trichophyton rubrum
b. Trichophyton violaceum
c. Trichophyton tonsurans
d. Trichophyton schoenleinii

Ans. is 'a' Trichophyton rubrum

Trichophyton are Pencil-shaped macroconidia:

- ❖ *Rubrum:* Red
- ❖ *Violaceum:* Port wine
- ❖ *Schoenleinii:* White
- ❖ *Tonsurans:* Pale yellow

68. Microfilaria with a sheath surrounding it and two big nuclei at its tail tip. Identify: *(NEET 2022)*

a. Wuchereria bancrofti
b. Brugia malayi
c. Loa Loa
d. Onchocerca volvulus

Ans. is 'b' Brugia malayi

In Brugia malayi, headspace is twice as long as it is broad, nuclei in body appears crowded and tail tapers around to 2 nuclei that appears to be connected by a fine thread.

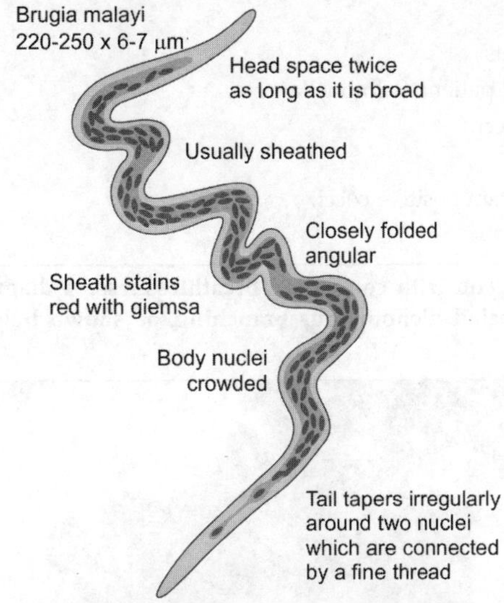

69. A 28-year-old lady with HBsAg positive, IgM HBc positive, IgG HBS and IgG HBe negative, anti-HCV negative. What is the diagnosis? *(NEET 2022)*

a. Acute HBV infection
b. Chronic HBV infection
c. Acute HCV infection
d. Chronic HCV infection

Ans. is 'a' Acute HBV infection

HBsAg	HBeAg	Anti-HBe	Anti-HBc	Anti-HBs	Interpretation	Infectivity of blood
+	+	–	–	–	Incubation period or early acute period during hepatitis B	High
+	+	–	+	–	Acute hepatitis B or chronic carrier	High
+	–	+	+	–	Late during hepatitis B or chronic state	Low
–	–	+	+	+	Convalescent from acute hepatitis B infection	None
–	–	–	+	+	Recovered from past hepatitis B infection	None
–	–	–	–	+	Immunized without infection, repeatedly exposed to HBsAg without infection, or recovered from past hepatitis B infection	None

70. Broken vaccine vials to be segregated in which colour bag? *(NEET 2022)*

a. Yellow
b. Puncture proof blue
c. White
d. Red

Ans. is 'b' Puncture proof blue

- ❖ Call glassware and metallic body implants are segregated of in puncture proof blue bags/containers.
- ❖ They are treated with sodium hypochlorite/autoclaving/microwaving/hydro cleaving followed by recycling and then disposed.

71. A child with sickle cell disease presented with pain and swelling of the knee joint. X-ray showed lytic lesions and sclerotic borders. Joint aspirate was collected which showed the following picture. What is the causative agent? *(NEET 2022)*

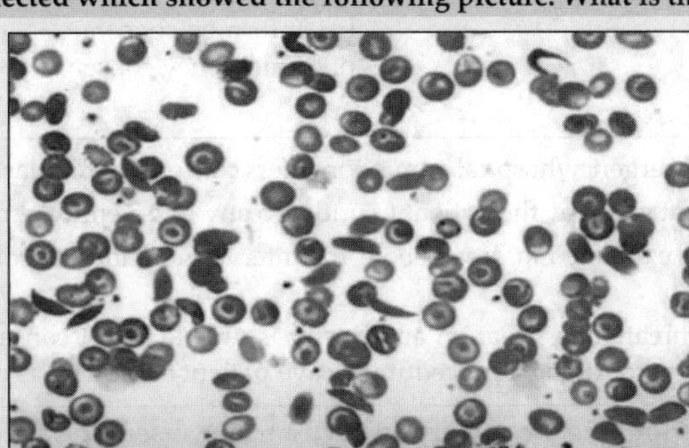

a. Staphylococcus
b. Streptococcus
c. Salmonella
d. E. coli

Ans. is 'c' Salmonella

- This is a case of OsteoMyelitis
- Most common cause of OM: Staph aureus
- Most common cause of OM in sickle cell patient: Salmonella
- The given slide shows gram negative cocci.
- Salmonella is gram negative cocci.
- Staphylococcus and streptococcus are gram positive cocci.
- E. coli is gram negative rod.

72. A diabetic truck driver presents to you with cough and breathlessness. A diagnosis of pneumonia was confirmed, and histopathological examination revealed dichotomous branching, as shown below. What is the likely causative agent? *(NEET 2022)*

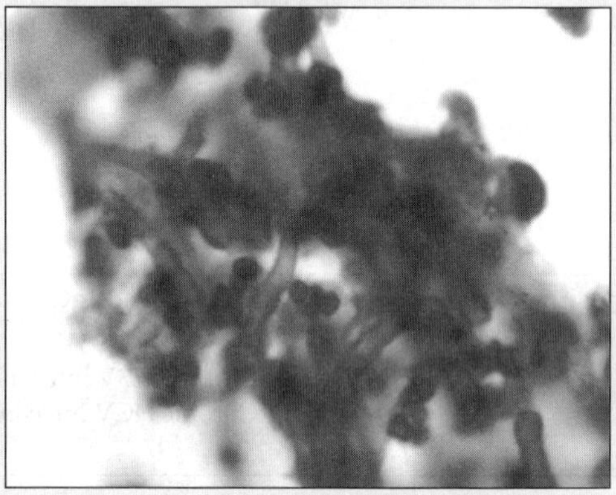

a. Rhizopus
b. Mucor
c. Candida
d. Aspergillus

Ans. is 'd' Aspergillus

Solution: Already mentioned in the book

73. A diabetic patient with COVID-19, on treatment with steroids, presented with complaints of facial pain, blurry vision, and loosening of teeth. Which of the following is most likely implicated? *(NEET 2022)*

a. Rhinosporidiosis
b. Coccidioidomycosis
c. Blastomycosis
d. Mucormycosis

Ans. is 'd' Mucormycosis

Solution: Already mentioned in book

FORENSIC MEDICINE

74. A female has come to gynecologist for hysterectomy. The doctor explains the benefits & risks of the procedure & obtained consent. This type of consent is: *(NEET 2022)*

a. Implied consent
b. Informed consent
c. Blanket consent
d. Emergency consent

Ans. is 'b' Informed consent

- *Implied consent:* Presentation at pod/emergency/hospital admission infers consent for regular diagnostic and treatment interventions.
- *Expressed consent:* Oral/written consent given by the patient to undergo any interventional medical procedure.
- *Informed consent:* When the patient is explained in detail about the intervention and it's complications by the doctor and then the consent is obtained.
- *Emergency consent:* When it's a life threatening situation and doctor is unable to get consent both from the patient and relatives, doctor is not compelled to take consent for doing a procedure to save patient's life. This is defined as 92 IPC.

75. A doctor who is drunk, while performing the surgery, injured a major vessel & Death of patient. This is: *(NEET 2022)*

a. Civil negligence
b. Criminal negligence
c. Therapeutic misadventure
d. Dichotomy

Ans. is 'b' Criminal negligence

- *Civil negligence:* Simple lack of care and skill from the doctor
- *Criminal negligence:* When the doctor performs surgery or any intervention in drunk/intoxicated state then it is said to be Gross negligent act resulting in damage to the patient
- *Therapeutic misadventure:* Any accidental damage to the patient during the treatment
- *Dichotomy:* Fee splitting/commission when a patient is sent to any hospital or lab.

76. A 45-year-old male came with acute loss of hair in head & madarosis. The wife had given history of behavioral changes. The doctor examined the nails & made the diagnosis. The condition is: *(NEET 2022)*

a. Arsenic poisoning
b. Thallium poisoning
c. Mercury poisoning
d. Lead poisoning

Ans. is 'b' Thallium poisoning

- Thallium poisoning > ideal homicidal poison
- Clinical features:
- *Early:* GIT symptoms, joint pain
- *Late:* Hair loss, neuropathies, Aldrich mees lines, cranial nerve impairment, psychosis/behavioural changes

Treatment

- Antidote = Prussian blue
- Severe/refractory poisoning = hemodialysis

77. The injury is suggestive of: *(NEET 2022)*

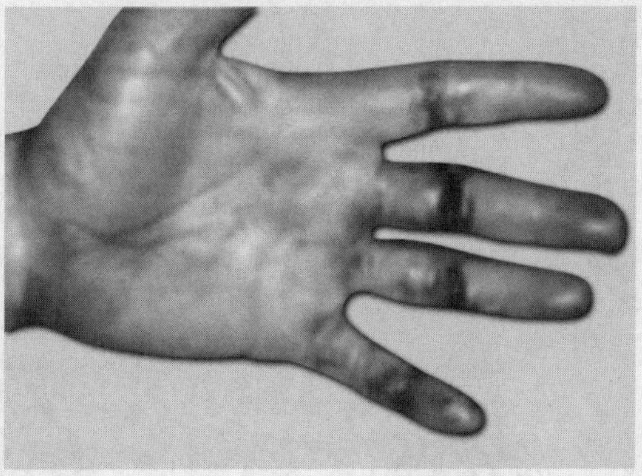

a. Postmortem wound
b. Self-inflicted cut
c. Defence cuts
d. Hesitational cut

Ans. is 'c' Defence cuts

Defence Wounds

- Deep cuts to the palm and fingers of the hand
- Irregular and ragged cuts result from the hand held in a gripping position causing the palm skin to become loose and folded
- They may be duplicated by the thrust and withdrawal of the weapon

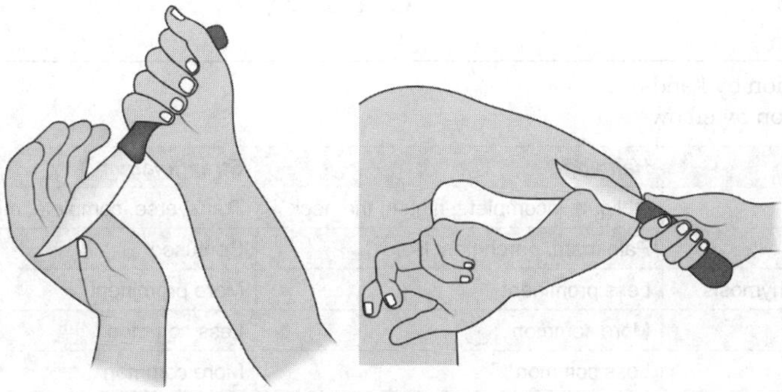

78. This type of hymen is: *(NEET 2022)*

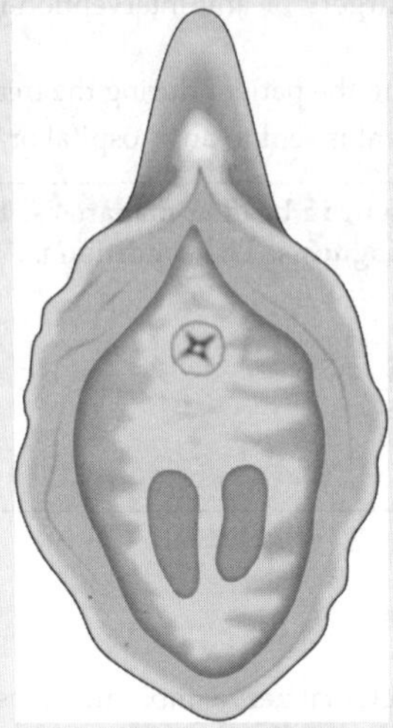

a. Septate
b. Fimbriate
c. Annular
d. Semilunar

Ans. is 'a' Septate

Hymen types

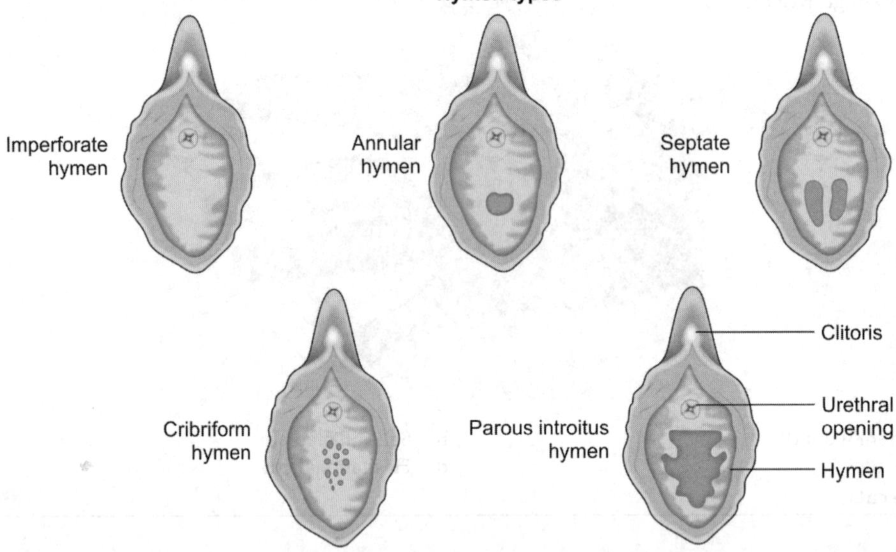

79. A dead body is brought with ligature mark over neck, which is encircling the neck, transverse, below the thyroid cartilage. No salivary dribbling noted. This condition is: *(NEET 2022)*

a. Throttling
b. Mugging
c. Ligature strangulation
d. Hanging

Ans. is 'c' Ligature strangulation

- *Throttling:* Manual strangulation by hands
- *Mugging:* Manual strangulation by elbows

Sr. No	*Trait*	*Hanging*	*Strangulation*
1	Ligature mark	Oblique, incomplete, high in the neck	Transverse, complete, mid-level or below thyroid cartilage
2	Base	Pale, hard, parchment like	Contused
3	Abrasion, contusion & Ecchymosis	Less prominent	More prominent
4	Hyoid fracture	More common	Less common
5	Thyroid cartilage	Less common	More common

80. Identify the range: *(NEET 2022)*

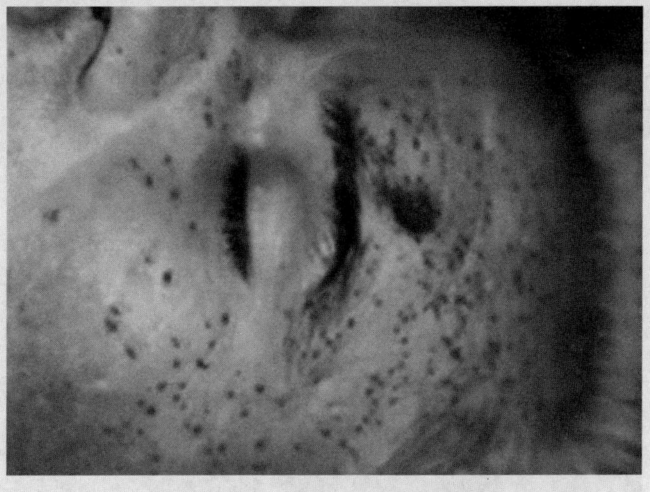

a. Pistol near range
b. Rifle closer range
c. Pistol close range
d. Shot gun intermediate

Ans. is 'a' Pistol near range

For detail see explanation on pages 365-366

81. In a court trial, leading questions are not permitted in all the following, *except*: *(NEET 2022)*

a. Re-examination
b. Cross examination
c. Dying declaration
d. Direct examination

Ans. is 'b' Cross examination

- *Direct examination/Examination in chief:* The process of questioning of a witness by the lawyer that called such witness in a trial.
- *Cross examination:* Questioning the opposing party's witness who has already testified (direct examination)
- *Re Examination:* The process of questioning one's own witness again, after cross examination by the opposing counsel.

OPHTHALMOLOGY

82. A patient comes with history of rheumatoid arthritis and ocular finding as shown in this image. What is the diagnosis? *(NEET 2022)*

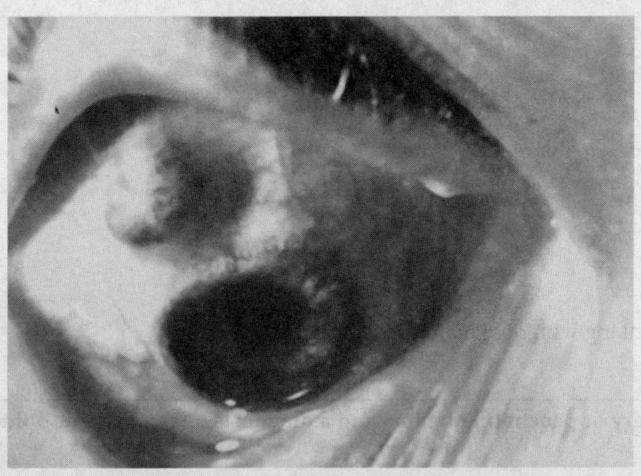

a. Ciliary staphyloma
b. Scleromalacia perforans
c. Coloboma
d. Staphyloma

Ans. is 'b' Scleromalacia perforans

Scleromalacia Perforans

- Anterior scleritis which is necrotising but without inflammation.
- Common in patients of seropositive RA
- *Clinical features:* Development of necrotic patch leads to thinning of sclera by which the uveal tissue gets exposed.

83. For what condition is this surgery as shown in picture, done for? *(NEET 2022)*

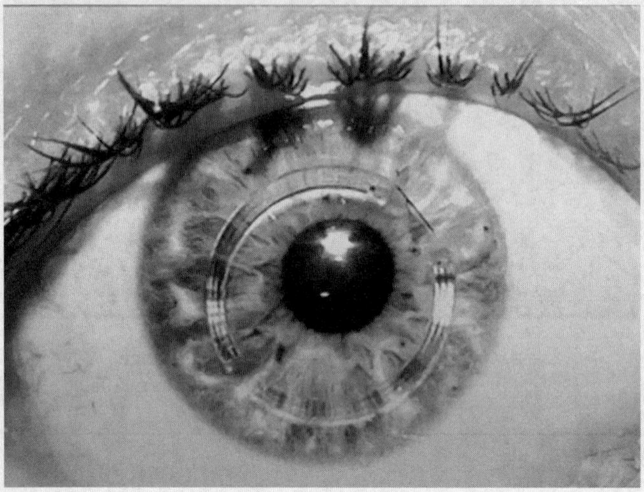

a. Keratoconus
b. Keratoglobus
c. Vogt's limbal girdle
d. Corneal dystrophy

Ans. is 'a' Keratoconus

The given image shows INTACS: (intracorneal ring segments) = 2 clear plastic ring segments placed in cornea to flatten it, used in keratoconus.

Keratoconus

- Autosomal dominant
- Ectatic dystrophy of cornea: Corneal protrusion
- Slow progression
- *Clinical features:* Diminished vision
- *On examination:*
  - Fleischer's ring
  - Munson's sign
  - Corneal topography
  - Retinoscopy: Scissor's reflex
  - Prominent corneal nerves due to thinning of cornea
  - Break in descemet's membrane = VOGT's stria

Treatment:

- Specks
- Contact lens/INTACS
- C3R = corneal collagen cross linking with riboflavin (it arrests progression)
- Penetrating keratoplasty

84. A patient comes with history of penetrating trauma and a diagnosis of sympathetic ophthalmitis was made. Which of the following will be seen? *(NEET 2022)*

a. Acute anterior uveitis
b. Chronic anterior uveitis
c. Pars planitis
d. Pan uveitis

Ans. is 'd' Pan uveitis

Sympathetic ophthalmitis perforating injury in one eye causing uveitis in other eye.

Etiology:

- Due to autoimmune reaction towards uveal tissue
- Granulomatous panuveitis
- Not before 2 weeks

Symptoms: Difficulty in near vision, decreased accommodation, photophobia.

- Ciliary body (dangerous area of eye) = any trauma in this area has a very high risk of sympathetic ophthalmitis.

85. A diabetic patient comes to you with preretinal haemorrhages and neovascularization of disc. What is the treatment? *(NEET 2022)*

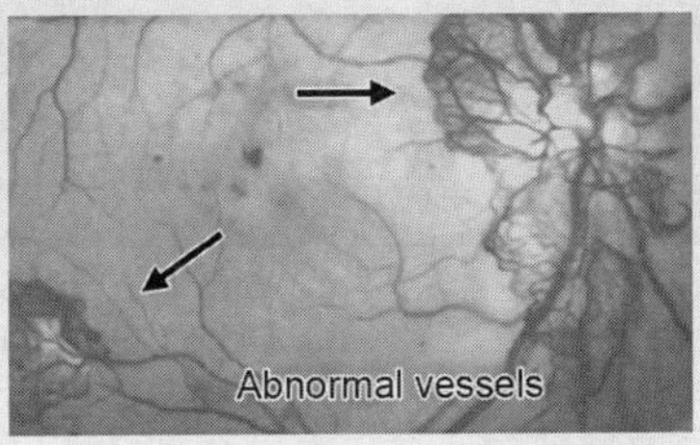

a. Pan retinal photocoagulation
b. Grid laser photocoagulation
c. Focal laser photocoagulation
d. Anti VEGF drugs

Ans. is 'a' Pan retinal photocoagulation

- This is a case of proliferation diabetic retinopathy
- *Treatment of choice*: Panretinal
- Photocoagulation
  - 2000–2500 burns
  - Start from the inferior quadrant
  - With sparing of macula

86. What is the diagnosis? *(NEET 2022)*

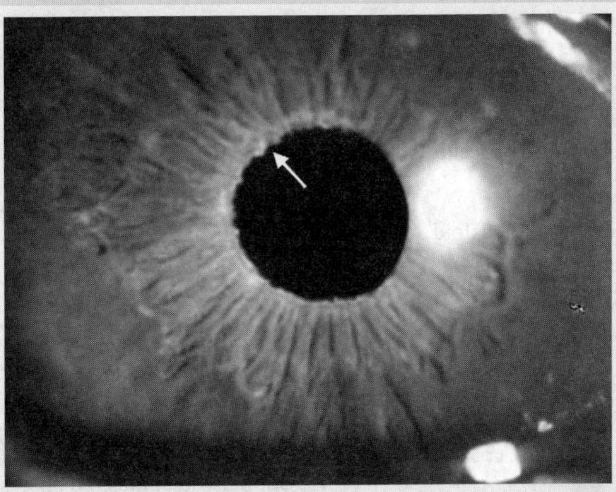

a. Intraocular foreign body
b. Pseudoexfoliation syndrome
c. Ocular trauma
d. Vossius ring

Ans. is 'b' Pseudoexfoliation syndrome

- The diagnosis based on the image given is pseudoexfoliation syndrome.
- Pseudoexfoliation syndrome is an age-related degenerative disorder, more commonly seen in women. It is marked by the deposition of exfoliative material on the iris, ciliary region, and lens capsule. They appear as flakes on the anterior lens capsule and edge of the iris.
- The material can get collected in the anterior chamber angle and impede the aqueous humor drainage. Patients affected by this condition are at an increased risk of developing open-angle glaucoma. Rarely, angle-closure glaucoma can also be seen. Other ocular symptoms include iris sphincter atrophy, anisocoria, and heterochromia. Systemic manifestations due to abnormal fibrillary deposition may also be seen.

ENT

87. A Patient came with Swelling under the ear lobe as shown below in the image. The Swelling was nontender & Firm. What is the most likely Diagnosis? *(NEET 2022)*

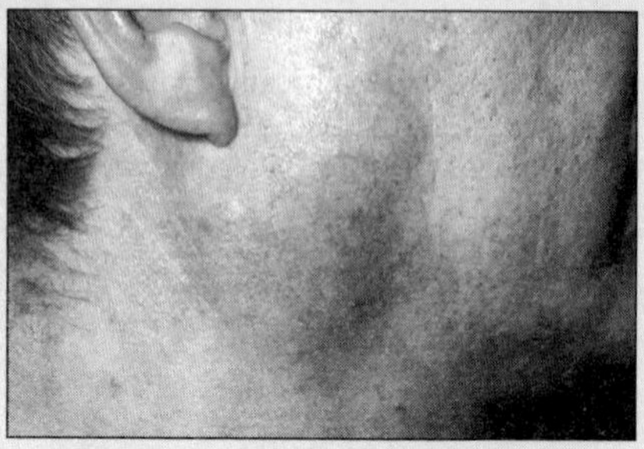

a. Bezold Abscess
b. Parotid gland Swelling
c. Osteoid Osteoma
d. Deep Cervical Lymph Node Enlargement

Ans. is 'b' Parotid gland Swelling

Osteoid Osteoma

- Diaphyseal bone tumour
- Typical history: Night pain relieved on salicylates

Deep Cervical LN Enlargement

- Most commonly due to TB
- Most common level: Level 2 (upper deep cervical LN)
- Location: In the neck behind the ear
- Palpating: Nontender and firm

Parotid Gland Swelling

- Swelling: Lifts the ear lobe, non-tender, firm
- On examination: Deep lobe enlargement leads to tonsillitis fossa being pushed medially

Bezold Abscess

- Extracranial complication of unsafe ear/CSOM
- Clinical features: Tender swelling, fever, Torricelli swelling, purulent otorrhea

Extracranial complications of unsafe ear/CSOM:

- *Bezold's abscess:* Abscess along sternocleidomastoid
- *Citteli's abscess:* Abscess along digastric muscle
- *Luc's abscess:* Abscess in external auditory canal
- Subperiosteal abscess
- Zygomatic abscess
- Occipital abscess

Abscesses in relation to mastoid	
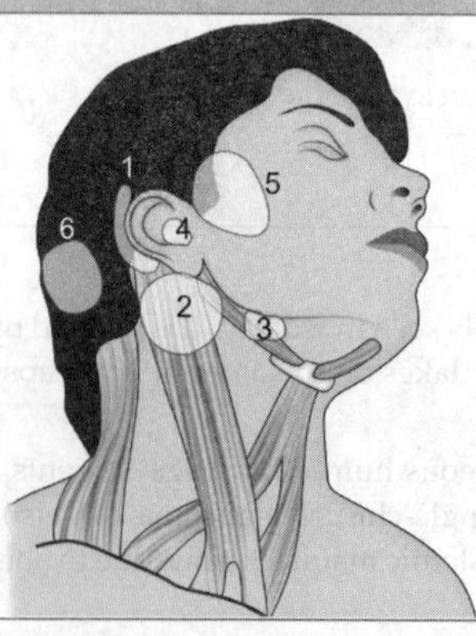 	❖ Subperiosteal mastoid abscess ❖ Bezold abscess ❖ Cittell's abscess ❖ Luc abscess ❖ Zygomatic abscess ❖ Occipital abscess

88. A Mother brought her 6 years old child to ENT OPD with complaints of recurrent crying & hearing loss. On Otoscopic examination, following findings are seen. Identify the diagnosis: *(NEET 2022)*

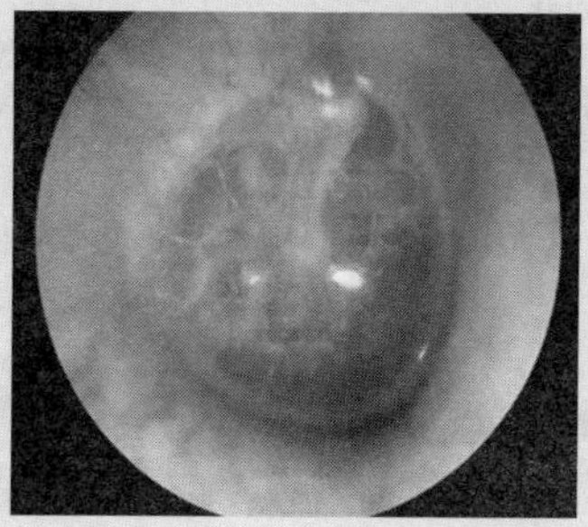

a. Bullous myringitis
b. Chronic Suppurative Otitis Media (CSOM)
c. Otitis Media with Effusion (OME)
d. Pneumotympanum

Ans. is 'c' Otitis Media with Effusion (OME)

- *OM with effusion:* Page 442
- *Bullous myringitis:* Blistering lesions
- CSOM: Blood stained purulent discharge, presence of perforation

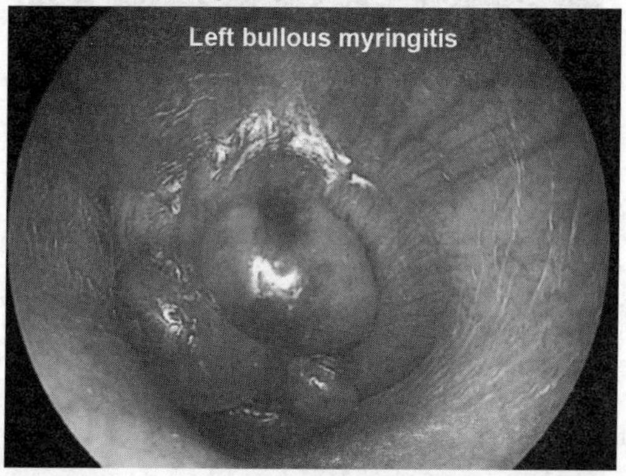

89. An 18 years old male presented with chief complaint of Recurrent Epistaxis with nasal blockage. On examination, a Polypoidal mass is seen going from nose to nasopharynx, completely occupying the posterior choana as seen in following image. On CT Scan enhanced uptake of Contrast is seen. Most Likely Diagnosis is: *(NEET 2022)*

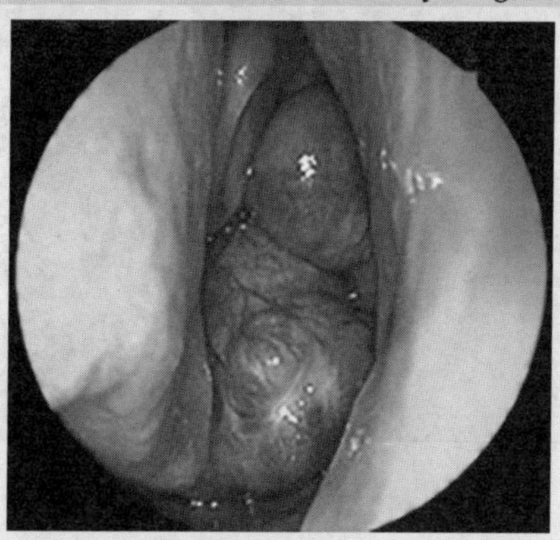

a. Nasopharyngeal Angiofibroma
b. Rhinoscleroma
c. Rhinosporidiosis
d. Antrochoanal polyp

Ans. is 'a' Nasopharyngeal Angiofibroma

Rhinoscleroma

- By Klebsiella rhinoscleromatis (Frisch bacillus)
- Aka HEBRA nose

- *Clinical features:* Purulent foul smelling discharge with crusting before development of nodule
- *HPE:* Mikulicz cells: Large foam cells with central nucleus, vacuolated cytoplasm containing causative bacilli
- *3 stages:* Atrophic, Granulomatous and Cicatricial

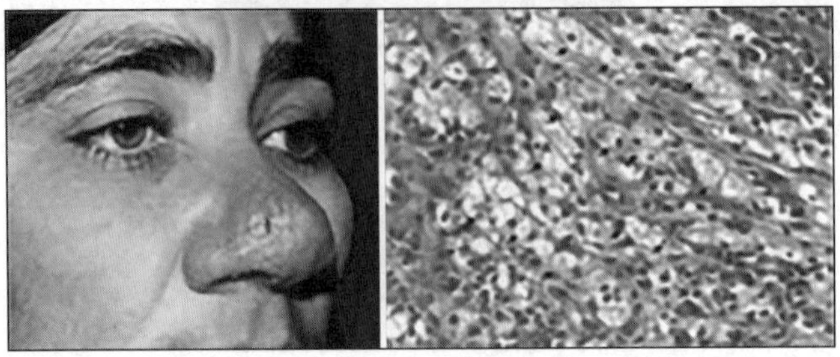

- *Treatment:* Streptomycin 1 g/day × 4–6
  Tetracycline 2 g/day × 4–6 weeks

If fibrosis present→ add steroids Surgical treatment: To manage airway and correct nasal deformity

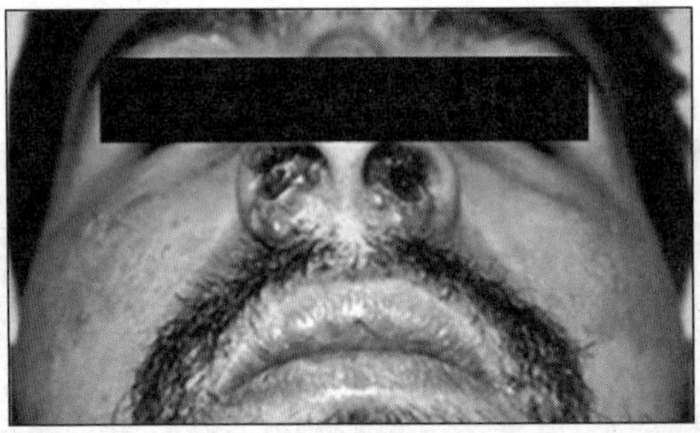

Rhinosporidiosis

- Caused by Rhinosporidium seeker I
- Males; age 15–40 years
- *Exposure history:* Ponds/stagnant water
- Granulomatous
- *Clinical features:* Nasal discharge, epistaxis, nasal obstruction by polyp
- *HPE:* sporangia, oval/round and filled with spores
- *Treatment:* Surgical excision of lesions

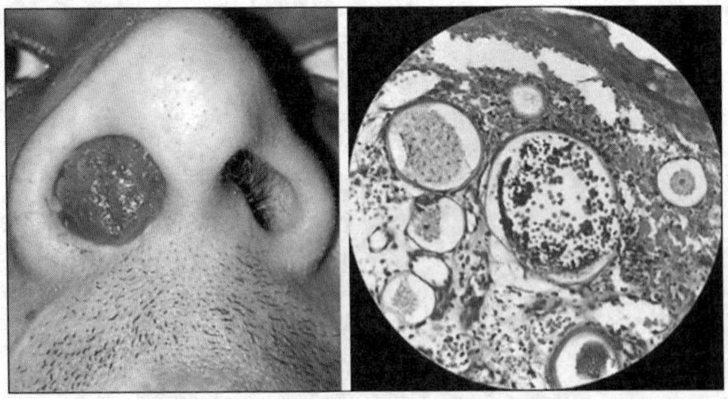

Nasopharyngeal Angiofibroma

- Adolescent males
- Vascular benign tumour
- Testosterone dependent tumour
- *Most common site:* Sphenopalatine fossa
- *Clinical features:* Recurrent epistaxis, nasal blockage
- Avoid debunking surgery and BIOPSY
- Approach—in toto
- Dumbbell shaped tumour

Note: Pterygopalatine fossa

- ❖ Maxillary artery ligation = Resistant bleeding
- ❖ Vidian Neurectomy = Vasomotor rhinitis

90. Identify the Bone shown in the image: *(NEET 2022)*

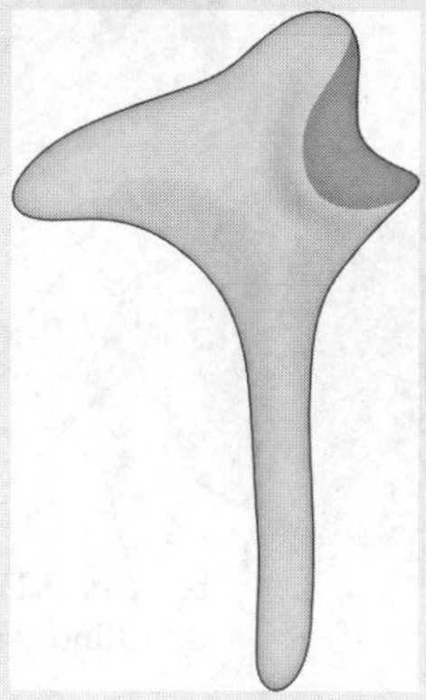

a. Malleus
b. Incus
c. Stapes
d. None of the above

Ans. is 'b' Incus

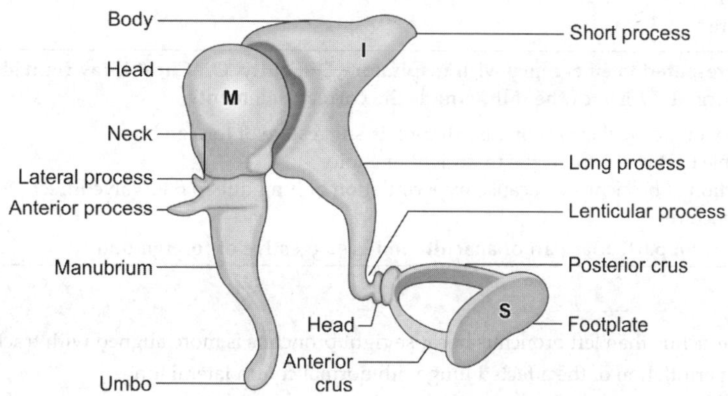

91. A patient with damage to basilar membrane presented with high frequency hearing loss. Where is the location of most likely lesion? *(NEET 2022)*

a. Modiolus
b. Stria Vascularis
c. Helicotrema
d. Oval Window

Ans. is 'd' Oval Window

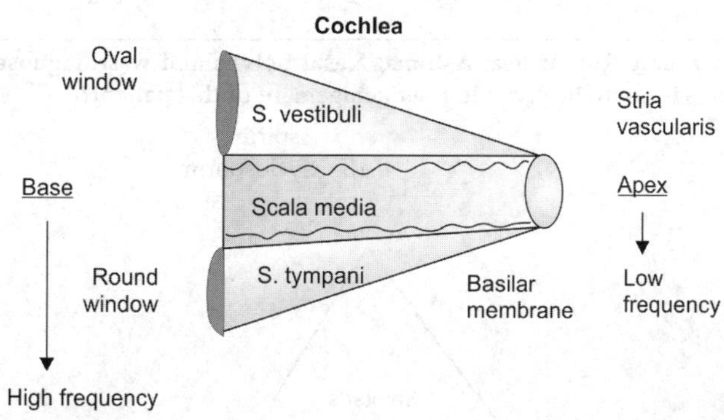

- ❖ Cochlea is spiralled around MODIOLUS
- ❖ *Scalia media:* ENDOLYMPH
- ❖ *Scalia tympani & scala vestibuli:* PERILYMPH

92. A young male while eating in a restaurant suddenly started experiencing shortness of breath as seen below. What will you do next for this patient? *(NEET 2022)*

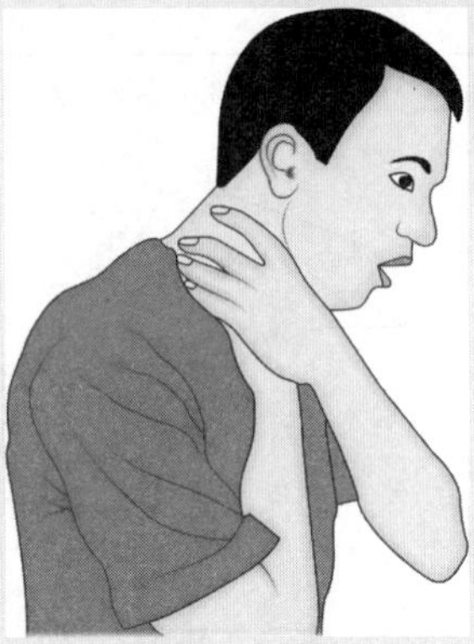

a. Chest thrust
b. Chest Thrust and Back Slaps
c. Heimlich Maneuver
d. Blindly sweep through the mouth to look for foreign body

Ans. is 'c' Heimlich Maneuver

Children:

❖ Chest thrust
❖ Chest thrust and back slaps

Adults: HEIMLICH manoeuvre

93. A 2 years old Child presented to emergency with respiratory Difficulty. On Chest X-ray right side shows hyperinflation of lung with Left side normal. Which of the following is the correct statement? *(NEET 2022)*

a. Decreased air entry on particular part of auscultation is suggestive of foreign body
b. Removal by Flexible bronchoscopy is the treatment of choice
c. Complete obstruction at bronchus can cause hyperinflation of lung due to Ball Valve Effect
d. Acute Tracheobronchitis

Ans. is 'a' Decreased air entry on particular part of auscultation is suggestive of foreign body

Foreign Body in Trachea

❖ More common in right bronchus than left bronchus because right bronchus is more aligned with trachea.
❖ U/L blockage leads to hyperinflation of the affected lung with normal contra lateral lung
❖ Removal by rigid Bronchoscope

Three Phases of Obstruction

❖ *First phase:* Air entry during inspiration present but no exit during expiration—hyper inflated lung present
❖ *Second phase:* Partial edema around the foreign body so, air entry stops but exit is present which leads to collapse of the lung. Ball valve effect is seen here.
❖ *Third phase:* Complete edema around the foreign body so complete air movement stops and atelectasis occurs. Ball valve effect STOPS.

94. A patient presented with Chronic Rhinorrhea, Asthma, Nasal polyps and was diagnosed to be having Samter's Triad. Which of the following drugs is not to be given in the management of this patient? *(NEET 2022)*

a. Amoxy-clav
b. Aspirin
c. Co-trimoxazole
d. Cyclosporin

Ans. is 'b' Aspirin

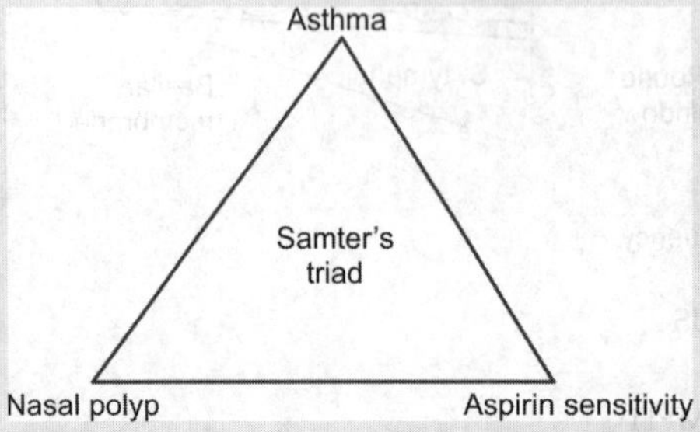

95. A Diabetic Patient previously treated for COVID-19 4 months ago presented with complaints of loosening of teeth, hemifacial pain. Which of the following tests is to be done on priority basis? *(NEET 2022)*

a. Nasal Swab for Mucor
b. Serum Ferritin
c. MRI Head
d. HbA1C

Ans. is 'c' MRI Head

Mucormycosis

Clinical features:

- Nasal blockage
- Blood tinged nasal discharge
- Headache
- Pain in Eye
- U/L Facial Pain/Swelling
- Double vision
- Swelling of eye & adnexa
- Toothache, Loosening Teeth, discomfort during CHEWING

Pathogenesis:

In diabetics, hyperglycaemia leads to:

- Polymorphonuclear dysfunction
- *Ketoacidosis:* Increase in free iron in serum which increases the virulence of mucorales.

Microscopy: Hyphae—thick, aseptate, broad, irregular branching

Acute lesions	*Chronic lesions*
Necrosis Angioinvasion Neutrophils Perineural invasion	Giant cells Eosinophilic material around hyphae

Investigations:

- Nasal biopsy
- MRI head or Cranial CT

96. A patient has stroke 2 days ago presented with slurred speech, difficulty in closing right eye, with deviation of angle of mouth to left side with drooling of saliva, Unable to puff the face. Which of the following Nerve is involved? *(NEET 2022)*

a. 3rd
b. 5th
c. 7th
d. 9th

Ans. is 'c' 7th

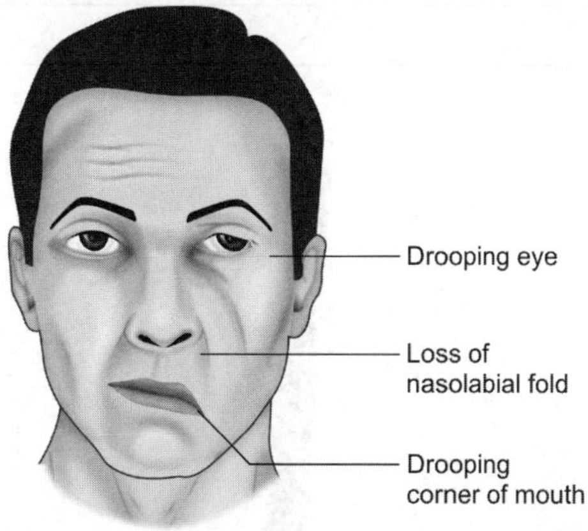

Treatment of BELL's Palsy

- Steroids: 1 mg/kg body weight
- Acyclovir
- B complex and physiotherapy (not in the first 3 days to avoid dyskinesia)

If no improvement occurs after 3 weeks, then → electrophysiological testing is done. If nerve compression is present, then surgical decompression is done.

PSM

97. Many children from a particular community coming to a hospital were detected as having ALL. The hospital said that it is due to a chemical in the water of that community. If a case control study has to be done to find whether that chemical and ALL are associated, children introduced to chemicals having ALL are taken as cases. Then what will be taken as controls? *(NEET 2022)*

a. Children in same community with ALL getting exposed to chemicals
b. Children in same community without ALL not getting exposed to chemicals
c. Children from hospital with ALL getting exposed to chemicals
d. Children from hospital without ALL not getting exposed to chemicals

Ans. is 'b' Children in same community without ALL not getting exposed to chemicals

- **Cases = both disease and exposure present**
- **Controls = both disease and exposure not present**

98. For Applied nutrition program, Seeds and manure supply under School health services has been done by: *(NEET 2022)*

a. WHO
b. UNICEF
c. CARE
d. UNDP

Ans. is 'b' UNICEF

Applied nutrition program was introduced in 1964, Punjab. Later this program extended through the whole country by the government of India. India signed a masterplan of operation with UNICEF, WHO & FAO; UNICEF assisted ANP with equipment and supplies. Hence, seeds, manure and water for school gardens were supplied by UNICEF.

99. For an Institutional delivery, ASHA worker motivated a woman in an Urban area of Madhya Pradesh. The ASHA worker and the Second gravida mother are given what amount (₹) under JSSK? *(NEET 2022)*

a. 1400 to mother and 1000 to ASHA
b. 1000 to mother and 400 to ASHA
c. 1400 to mother and 600 to ASHA
d. 700 to mother and 400 to ASHA

Ans. is 'b' 1000 to mother and 400 to ASHA

	Rural	*Rural*	*Urban*	*Urban*
CATEGORY	MOTHER'S PACKAGE	ASHA'S PACKAGE	MOTHER'S PACKAGE	ASHA'S PACKAGE
LPS	1400	600	1000	400
HPS	700	600	600	400

LPS = low performing states = Rajasthan, UP, Uttarakhand, MP, Jharkhand, Bihar, Chhattisgarh, Assam, Odisha, and Jammu & Kashmir.

100. Copper-T is contraindicated in: *(NEET 2022)*

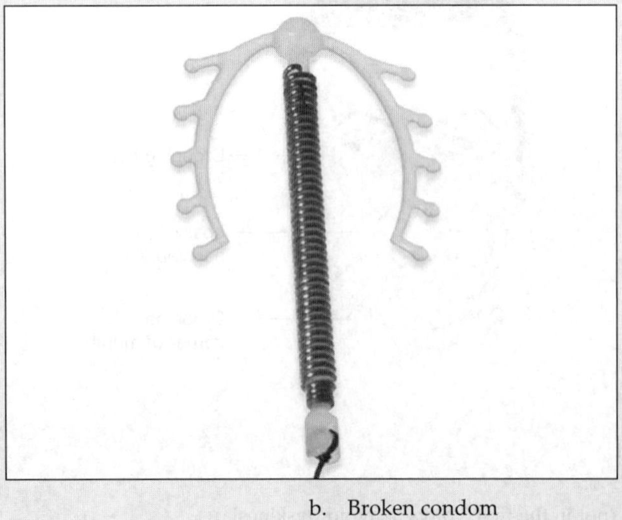

a. Menstruation
b. Broken condom
c. Trophoblastic disease
d. Post-partum immediately after delivery

Ans. is 'c' Trophoblastic disease

IUCD Contraindications

Absolute

- Pregnancy
- PID OR STI
- Puerperal sepsis
- Immediate post-septic abortion
- Severely distorted uterine cavity
- Unexplained vaginal bleeding
- Cervical or endometrial cancer
- Malignant trophoblastic disease
- Copper allergy (For copper IUDs)
- Breast cancer (For LNG-IUS)

101. Green color in Triage signifies: *(NEET 2022)*

a. Dead patients
b. High priority patients
c. Ambulatory patients
d. Moderate priority patients

Ans. is 'c' Ambulatory patients

For detail see explanation on page 460

102. Criteria for establishing Urban CHC to ensure facilities: *(NEET 2022)*

a. Where subdistrict or district hospital are not present
b. Referral centre for 2–3 Urban primary health centers
c. For city with 1–1.5 Lac population
d. 100 bedded in Metro cities

Ans. is 'd' 100 bedded in Metro cities

For detail see explanation on page 506

103. A Cohort study is undertaken to study association between Green tea intake and Diabetes mellitus. Relative risk was found to be '0.85'. Which of the following is correct regarding association between green tea and DM? *(NEET 2022)*

a. Green tea consumption increases the risk of DM
b. Green tea consumption decreases the risk of DM
c. Green tea consumption has no effect on the risk of DM
d. Cannot be determined

Ans. is 'b' Green tea consumption decreases the risk of DM

For detail see explanation on page 465

104. WHO stepwise approach include all, *except*: *(NEET 2022)*

a. Physical
b. Psychological
c. Behavioural
d. Therapeutic

Ans. is 'b' Psychological & 'd' Therapeutic

WHO stepwise approach is for two types:

1. NCD risk factor surveillance
2. STROKE surveillance

Three steps:

1. Behavioral measurements
2. Physical measurements
3. Biochemical measurements

105. A patient having cough 3 weeks was started on ATT under NTEP. IP and CP were completed and then he tested smear negative for AFB on two samples. What's the status of patient? *(NEET 2022)*

a. Treatment completed
b. Cured
c. Improper follow-up
d. Failure

Ans. is 'b' Cured

- IP & CP completed followed by sputum testing = cured
- IP & CP completed, not followed by sputum testing = treatment completed

106. Most logical and cost effective approach of controlling Rabies in Urban population: *(NEET 2022)*

a. Test all the dogs for Rabies
b. Remove Stray dogs and vaccinate the dog population
c. Administer Rabies vaccine to the entire human populations
d. Health education of people

Ans. is 'b' Remove Stray dogs and vaccinate the dog population

- Testing all dogs, administering rabies vaccine to entire population: Not cost effective ways
- Health education of people: Though cost effective but has limited approach.
- Best cost effective and wide approach = removing stray dogs and vaccinate the dog population

107. A 24 years old female with 18 months' baby on breast feed has heavy irregular bleeding on mensuration. What is best contraception advisable? *(NEET 2022)*

a. Mala N
b. Progestasert
c. cuT 380 A
d. Depot formulation

Ans. is 'b' Progestasert

For detail see explanation on pages 668–671

108. Things you will not do as a Medical officer of PHC when posted in Seismic areas? *(NEET 2022)*

a. Ensure funds and resources are available and can be mobilized at the time of disaster for quick evacuation
b. Preparedness to handle emergency
c. Disaster simulation practices and then check the response
d. Follow the announcements given on loudspeakers

Ans. is 'd' Follow the announcements given on loudspeakers

Ensuring funds and resources; preparedness; simulation practices are responsibility of a medical officer when posted in Seismic areas.

109. Life span of Japanese women is 84.3 years. As Japanese have longest life expectancy, their life expectancy statistics are used as a standard for measuring premature death in? *(NEET 2022)*

a. HALE
b. QALY
c. DELE
d. DALY

Ans. is 'd' DALY

For detail see explanation on pages 459–460

MEDICINE

110. CSF specimen of patient is shown below. Report shows Mononuclear cytosis with moderately low sugar with elevated protein values. Which of the following is the likely etiology? *(NEET 2022)*

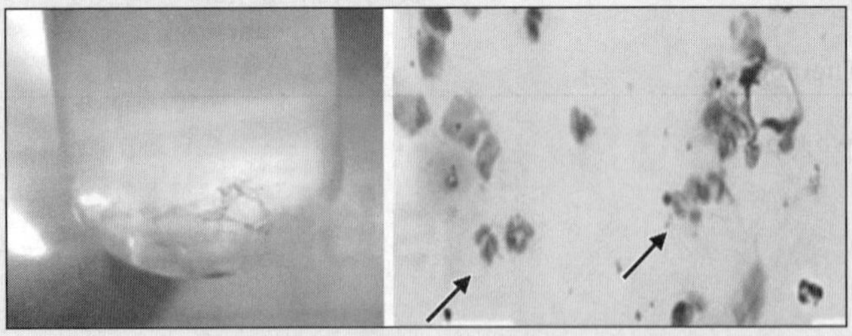

a. Pyogenic meningitis
b. Aseptic meningitis
c. Viral meningitis
d. Tubercular meningitis

Ans. is 'd' Tubercular meningitis

	Normal	Bacterial	Viral	Tuberculous	Fungal
Opening pressure	12–20	Raised	Normal/mildly raised	Raised	Raised
Appearance	Clear	Turbid, cloudy purulent	Clear	Clear or cloudy	Clear or cloudy
CSF WCC (cells/uL)	<5	Raised (typically >100)	Raised (typically 5–1000)	Raised (Typically 5–500)	Raised (typically 5–500)
Predominant cell type	n/a	Neutrophils	Lymphocytes	Lymphocytes	Lymphocytes

Contd...

Contd...

	Normal	*Bacterial*	*Viral*	*Tuberculous*	*Fungal*
CSF protein (g/L)	<0.4	Raised	Mildly raised	Markedly raised	Raised
CSF glucose (mmol)	2.6–4.5	Very low	Normal/slightly low	Very low	Low
CSF/plasma glucose ratio	> 0.66	Very low	Normal/slightly low	Very low	Low

CSF: cerebrospinal fluid; WCC: white cell count

111. An adult patient complains of palpitations and presents with irregularly irregular pulse. Pulse deficit is 20, HR = 120/min, BP = 110/70 mm Hg. Which of the following will be found in this patient? *(NEET 2022)*

a. Absent a wave
b. Canon a wave
c. Absent y
d. Prominent V wave

Ans. is 'a' Absent a wave

- ❖ This is a case of Atrial fibrillation (palpitations and irregularly irregular pulse).
- ❖ As the SA node is no longer the main generating node (ectopic foci takes its place and has a faster rate), P wave is absent in atrial fibrillation and hence, in JVP a wave is also present.

112. A 74-year-old patient with CAD presents with palpitations. ECG is shown below. BP = 120/84 mm Hg. Which of the following shall be the best treatment for this patient? *(NEET 2022)*

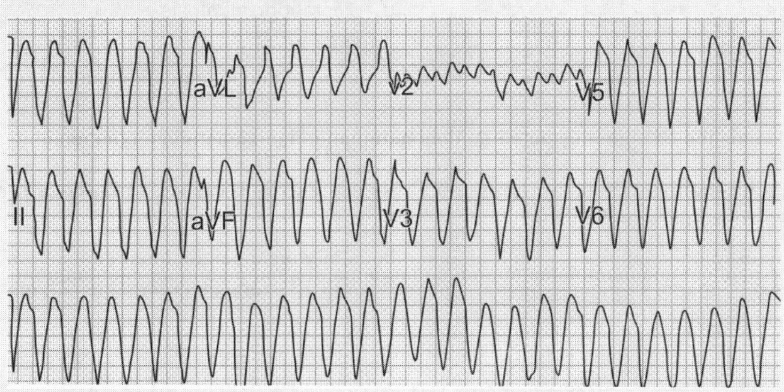

a. Oral metoprolol
b. IV metoprolol
c. IV amiodarone
d. Oral amiodarone

Ans. is 'c' IV amiodarone

This is a case of stable ventricular tachycardia.

Two causes:

1. With structural heart disease:
   Stable patient: Rx = IV amiodarone
   Unstable patients: Rx = DC Cardioversion
2. Without structural heart disease or young patients:
   Treatment: Beta blockers

113. A 25-year-old patient with dental caries is undergoing dental extraction. Which of the following does not need prophylaxis for endocarditis? *(NEET 2022)*

a. Previous history of endocarditis
b. Artificial heart valve
c. Untreated cyanotic heart disease
d. ASD

Ans. is 'd' ASD

Indications of prophylaxis required before dental procedures at high risk of endocarditis:

- ❖ Prosthetic heart valve
- ❖ Prior endocarditis
- ❖ Unrepaired congenital heart disease
- ❖ Completely repaired congenital heart disease (<6 months)
- ❖ Incomplete repaired congenital heart disease
- ❖ Valvulopathy after cardiac transplant

114. A female who is a known case of diabetes mellitus and noncompliant to medication is brought to ER with abdominal pain, vomiting episodes and recent onset confusion. On examination she is dehydrated with SBP = 90 mm Hg. Work up shows Urine ketones present with RBS = 598 mg%. Which of the following will be the next best step in management of this patient? *(NEET 2022)*

a. IVF
b. Insulin
c. IVF with regular insulin
d. Long-acting insulin

Ans. is 'c' IVF with regular insulin

Management of Diabetic keto Acidosis:

- IV fluids with regular insulin
  IV fluids: 0.9% NS; switch to 5% dextrose when
  RBS < 250 mg/dL; RLN not given
- $NaHCO_3$ to treat acidosis (if pH <7)
- KCL @20–40 meq/hr = If hypokalemia develops after resolving acidosis

115. An old age smoker presents with respiratory difficulty. ABG report: pH = 7.2, pO_2= 75 mm Hg, pCO_2= 84 mm Hg, HCO_3 = 35 mEq. Diagnosis: *(NEET 2022)*

a. Respiratory acidosis
b. Respiratory alkalosis
c. Metabolic acidosis
d. Metabolic alkalosis

Ans. is 'a' Respiratory acidosis

- pH has decreased = acidosis
- pCO_2 & HCO_3 have increased (the change is opposite of the change in pH) = respiratory acidosis

116. An 11-year-old child with manifestations of rheumatic fever is prescribed 0.6 MU i.m. Benzathine penicillin. Which of the following is correct for secondary prevention? *(NEET 2022)*

a. Lifelong every 3 weekly
b. Only once single dose
c. Till 5 years 3 weekly
d. Till 10 years 3 weekly or till 25 years of age

Ans. is 'c' Till 5 years 3 weekly

Category	*Duration from last attack*
RF without carditis	5 years or until 21 years of age (whichever is longer)
RF with carditis but no residual heart disease	10 years of until 21 years of age (whichever in longer)
RF with carditis + residual heart disease	10 years of until 40 years of age (whichever is longer), sometimes lifelong prophylaxis

117. Which of the following electrolyte imbalance will produce ECG findings of ST depression and U waves? *(NEET 2022)*

a. Hyperkalemia
b. Hypokalemia
c. Hypocalcemia
d. Hypercalcemia

Ans. is 'b' Hypokalemia

ECG Changes of Hypokalemia

- *T wave:* Depression/inversion/absence
- St depression
- Pseudo P pulmonale
- Prolongation of PR interval
- Prominent U waves
- Prolonged QU interval

118. A child born by normal vaginal delivery has repeats attacks of flexion of neck over the trunk jerks in hands. EEG shows hypsarrhythmia. What is the drug of choice? *(NEET 2022)*

a. Phenytoin
b. ACTH
c. Phenobarbitone
d. Levetiracetam

Ans. is 'b' ACTH

Infantile Spasms/Salaam Seizures/WEST Syndrome

- 4–8 months old infants
- Flexor contractions of head, trunk & extremities
- Symmetric contractions
- *EEG:* Generalised chaotic pattern of high voltage slow waves = HYPSARRYTHMIA

Etiology:

- Idiopathic/crypto genie
- *Secondary:* HIE, structural malformations, Down syndrome, tuberous sclerosis

Treatment:

- DOC = ACTH
- Infantile spasms + tuberous sclerosis: Rx = VIGABATRIN

119. A 10-year-old child has abdominal pain with melena. On examination palpable purpura is found on calves and buttocks. Which drug will be used? *(NEET 2022)*

a. Azathioprine
b. Methotrexate
c. Corticosteroids
d. Cyclosporine

Ans. is 'c' Corticosteroids

- *Diagnosis:* Henoch-Schonlein purpura
- *First line drug:* Steroids

120. Which fluid is shown below? *(NEET 2022)*

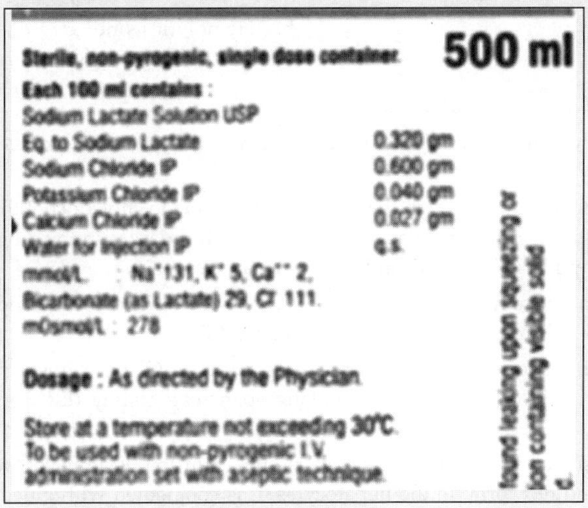

a. RL
b. Haemaccel
c. Isolyte-P
d. Isolyte-M

Ans. is 'a' RL

The given fluid is Ringer Lactate.

121. A patient who suffered from stroke previously has now presented with sudden onset flailing arm ballistic movement. Comment on site of lesion: *(NEET 2022)*

a. Subthalamic nucleus
b. Globus pallidus
c. Putamen
d. Substantia nigra

Ans. is 'a' Subthalamic nucleus

Movement disorder	*Lesion*
Athetosis	Globes pallidus
Chorea	Caudate nucleus
Hemiballismus	Subthalamic nucleus

122. A child presents with epigastric pain, vomiting for past 10 days with oliguria and features of dehydration. P. Smear shows Presence of lymphoblasts. What will be immediate management? *(NEET 2022)*

a. Hydration
b. Send for USG
c. Probenecid
d. Urgent chemotherapy

Ans. is 'a' Hydration

In patients having tumour lysis syndrome, there is increased risk of ATN which presents as oliguria and dehydration, which is treated by hydration therapy.

123. Which of the following is most likely to be seen due to rupture of saccular aneurysm in brain? *(NEET 2022)*

a. Subdural hemorrhage
b. Subarachnoid hemorrhage
c. Hydrocephalus
d. Intracerebral hemorrhage

Ans. is 'b' Subarachnoid hemorrhage

Causes of subarachnoid haemorrhage:

- MC cause of SAH = Trauma
- MC cause of spontaneous SAH = Saccular/berry aneurysm
- Arteriovenous malformation
- *Idiopathic:* Location @ perimesencephalic cistern; source—venous

124. Laboratory investigations of a patient being evaluated for jaundice show elevated bilirubin and alkaline phosphatase levels. Levels of the remaining liver enzymes are normal. What is the likely diagnosis? *(NEET 2022)*

a. Obstructive jaundice
b. Hemolytic jaundice
c. Hepatic jaundice
d. Prehepatic jaundice

Ans. is 'a' Obstructive jaundice

- The given laboratory reports showing elevated alkaline phosphatase and bilirubin points to a likely diagnosis of obstructive jaundice.
- Obstructive jaundice arises due to an obstruction in the biliary outflow due to choledocholithiasis, cholelithiasis, biliary strictures, etc. The patient presents with jaundice, right upper quadrant pain, pruritus, dark urine, and light-colored stools. The symptoms can be intermittent is cases of periampullary carcinoma and cholangiocarcinoma.
- Elevated conjugated bilirubin and alkaline phosphatase (ALP) are characteristic of the condition. An associated rise in gamma-glutamyl transpeptidase (GGT) levels confirms the hepatic origin of ALP.
- An ultrasound is done initially in suspected cases of obstructive jaundice. A CT or magnetic resonance cholangiopancreatography (MRCP) is recommended next. Endoscopic retrograde cholangiopancreatography (ERCP) is considered the gold standard for choledocholithiasis.
- Jaundice arises due to the deposition of bilirubin in the body tissues. Bilirubin is a breakdown product of heme that circulates in the blood in the unconjugated/indirect form. In the hepatocytes, it is conjugated with glucuronic acid to form conjugated/direct bilirubin. Direct and indirect bilirubin can be assessed using van den Bergh reaction.

125. A patient diagnosed to be retro-positive was started on highly active antiretroviral therapy (HAART). Which of the following can be used to monitor treatment efficacy?

a. CD4+ T cell count
b. Viral load
c. p24 antigen
d. Viral serotype

Ans. is 'b' Viral load

- The viral load can be assessed in a retro-positive patient started on HAART to monitor treatment efficacy.
- HAART or combination antiretroviral therapy is the mainstay in the management of retro-positive patients. It is initiated soon after diagnosis except in cases of cryptococcal or tuberculous meningitis.
- After initiation of therapy, a ten-fold reduction in plasma human immunodeficiency virus (HIV) RNA levels in 1–2 months can be expected. Within 6 months, a slower decline to < 50 copies/mL is anticipated. During the first month of therapy, a rise in CD4+ T cell count is also predicted. Out of these two parameters, viral load is the better choice to monitor treatment efficacy as it is more cost-effective.
- Plasma HIV RNA levels signify the rate of CD4+ T cell destruction and the magnitude of HIV replication. It should be monitored within 2–4 weeks of initiation of therapy and after any change in the treatment regimen. It should be repeated every 4–8 weeks till the RNA levels drop to < 200 copies/mL and then every 3–6 months subsequently.

SURGERY

126. A 35 years old female presented to OPD. Physical examination findings are given in the image. Which structure is affected in this condition? *(NEET 2022)*

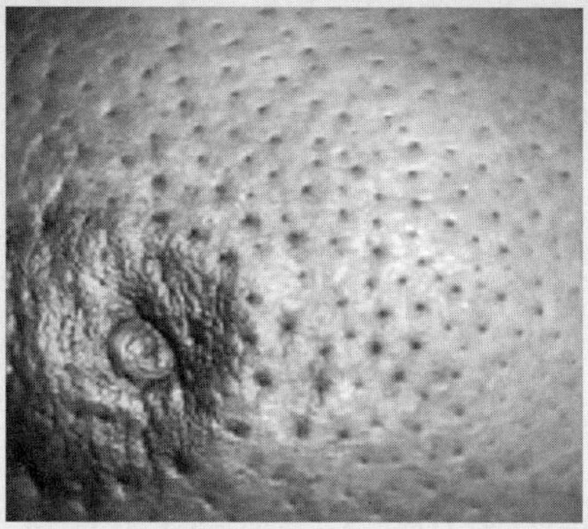

a. Involvement of chest wall
b. Involvement of subdermal lymphatics
c. Involvement of Cooper's ligaments
d. Involvement of connective tissue

Ans. is 'b' Involvement of subdermal lymphatics

- ❖ The physical examination findings show pitting and oedema resembling orange peel, case of peau d'orange. It is caused due to blockage of subdermal lymphatics.
- ❖ PDO is the most evident/conspicuous sign of breast cancer. PDO may also be seen with breast abscess, mastitis, benign conditions.

127. A young male presented with slow growing midline swelling in anterior part of neck. After 6 months, bilateral cervical lymphadenopathy developed. Histopathology slide is given below. All of the following are correct about this condition, *except*? *(NEET 2022)*

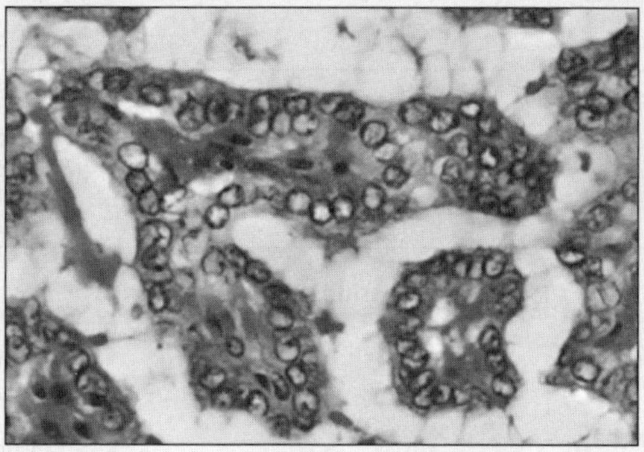

a. Lymphatic spread is seen
b. Specific nuclear pattern on histology
c. Has excellent prognosis
d. FNAC is not diagnostic

Ans. is 'd' FNAC is not diagnostic

This is a case of Papillary Carcinoma Salient features:

- ❖ Most common thyroid malignancy
- ❖ Seen in iodine sufficient areas
- ❖ *HPE:* Papillary projection, pseudo inclusion bodies, orphan Annie eye nuclei
- ❖ *Most common route of spread:* LYMPHATICS
- ❖ *Most common site of mets:* Lungs
- ❖ Excellent prognosis
- ❖ *Investigation of choice:* FNAC

128. A 45-year-old female underwent thyroidectomy. On 3rd day, she developed perioral numbness. Investigation involves: *(NEET 2022)*

a. Free T3, T4
b. Calcium, phosphate and PTH Levels
c. RAI scan
d. T3, T4, TSH

Ans. is 'b' Calcium, phosphate and PTH Levels

Complications of Thyroid Surgery

Immediate Complications

- Haemorrhage
- Infection
- Laryngeal nerve palsies
- Thyroid crises/storm
- Respiratory obstruction: Laryngeal edema, tension hematoma
- Parathyroid insufficiency

Late Complications

- Thyroid insufficiency
- Recurrent thyrotoxicosis
- Progressive exophthalmos
- Hypertrophic scar/keloid

1. HYPOPARATHYROIDISM
   Causes: Due to vascular insult (inferior thyroid artery)
   Clinical features: Early within 48–72 hours Perioral numbness
   Signs: Chvostek sign
   Trousseau sign
   Treatment: If Serum calcium
   >8 mg/dL= oral calcium & vitamin D_3
   <8 mg/dL= IV Calcium Gluconate+ oral calcium+oral vitamin D_3
2. Most common cause of post-operative laryngeal distress = laryngeal edema
3. If tension hematoma occurs→ open the sutures and evacuate hematoma
4. RLN injury most common @Berry's ligament
   B/L RLN injury is life threatening.

129. All of the following are the components of MEN-2b, *except*? *(NEET 2022)*

a. Parathyroid adenoma
b. Megacolon
c. Marfanoid habitus
d. Mucosal neuroma

Ans. is 'a' Parathyroid adenoma

Multiple endocrine neoplasia (MEN)

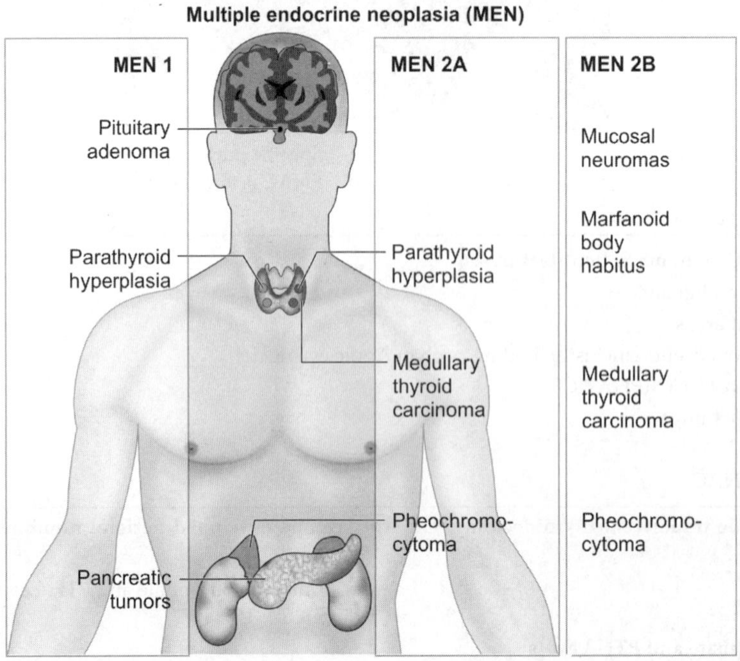

130. A 35-year-old patient presented with severe abdominal pain and vomiting. His vitals are stable. The radiograph is given below. What is the most effective way to treat this patient? *(NEET 2022)*

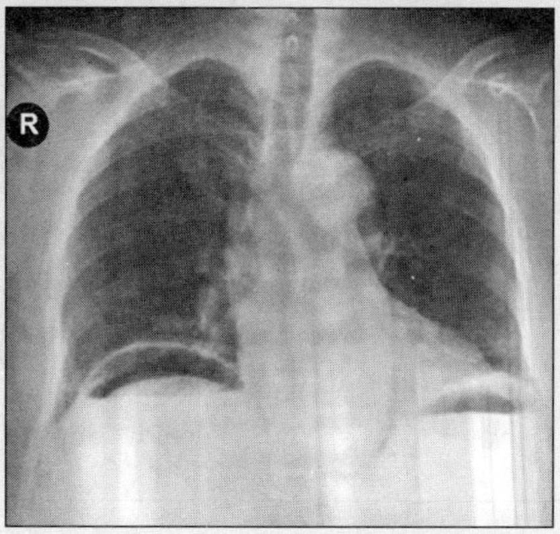

a. Gastric lavage with cold saline
b. Tracheostomy
c. Chest tube insertion
d. Resuscitation and laparotomy

Ans. is 'd' Resuscitation and laparotomy

- This is a case of pneumoperitoneum.
- Most effective way to treat this patient is by resuscitation and laparotomy to locally explore and repair the perforation.

131. An 11-month-old was brought to emergency with pain abdomen and multiple episodes of vomiting. On examination, mass was palpable in right lumbar region. Barium enema image is given below. What is the diagnosis? *(NEET 2022)*

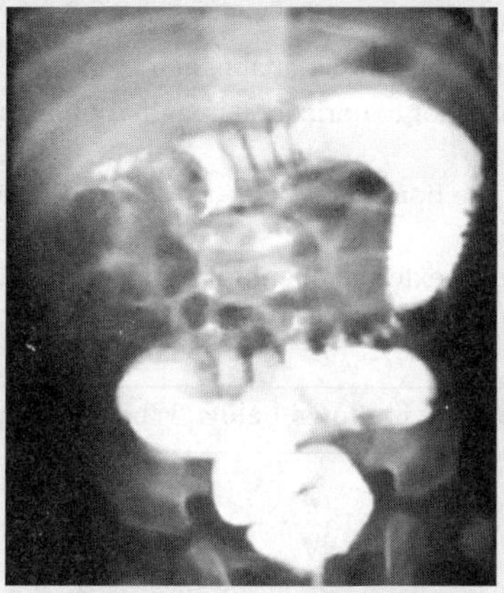

a. Intussusception
b. Volvulus
c. Malrotation
d. Duodenal atresia

Ans. is 'a' Intussusception

Intussusception

Intussusception occurs when one segment of bowel is pulled into itself or a neighboring loop of the bowel by peristalsis.

While the classic triad of intermittent abdominal pain, vomiting, and right upper quadrant mass, plus occult or gross blood on rectal examination has great positive predictive value for intussusception in children, these findings are seen in less than 20% of intussusception cases.

A contrast enema remains the gold standard, demonstrating the intussusception as an occluding mass prolapsing into the lumen, giving the "coiled spring" appearance (barium in the lumen of the intussusceptum and in the intraluminal space). The main absolute contraindication for an enema is a perforation, which needs to be treated surgically.

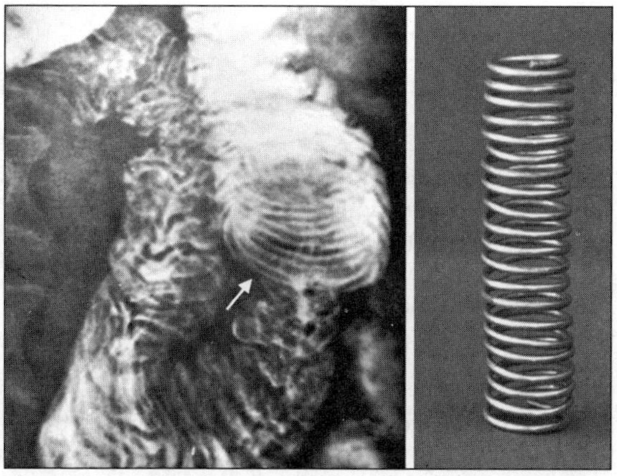

132. A 30 years old male presented with recurrent painful perianal nodules on buttocks with serous discharge. The image is given below. What is the most probable diagnosis? *(NEET 2022)*

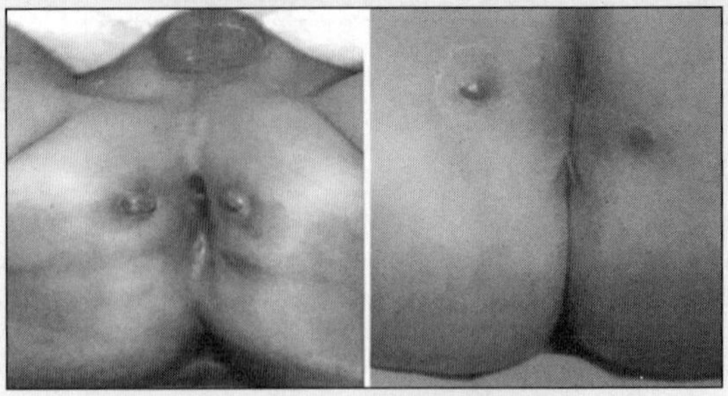

a. Perianal boils
b. Carbuncle
c. Fistula-in-ano
d. Pilonidal sinus

Ans. is 'c' Fistula-in-ano

Fistula in-ano

- Track, lined by granulation tissue, that connects internally in the anal canal or rectum and superficially on the skin around the anus
- Usually results from an anorectal abscess (cryptoglandular abscess). Other causes are Crohn's disease, malignancy, radiation, tuberculosis
- Two types—high and low, according to whether their internal openings is below or above the anorectal ring
- A low level can be treated by fistulotomy (opening the tract) without causing damage to the sphincter
- High level fistulas can be treated only by 'staged' operation as there is risk of incontinence.

Goodsall's Rule

- Is used to determine the location of internal opening of perianal fistula
- It states that Fistulas with external opening anterior to horizontal imaginary line drawn across the mid-point of anus, connect to the internal opening by short straight tract
- Fistulas with external opening posterior to the horizontal line—run a curvilinear course and open internally into the posterior midline
- Exceptions to this rule often occur if an anterior external opening is greater than 3 cm from the anal margin. Such fistulas track to the posterior midline. Also, when there is an anterior and also a posterior opening of the same fistula, the rule of posterior opening applies.

133. A delayed intravenous urogram of the patient is shown below. What is the most likely diagnosis? *(NEET 2022)*

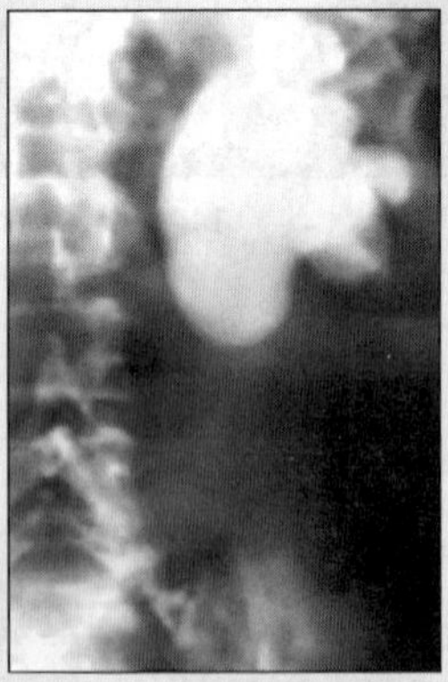

a. Putty kidney
b. Staghorn calculus
c. Pelviureteric junction obstruction
d. Renal cyst

Ans. is 'c' Pelviureteric junction obstruction

Pelviureteric Junction Obstruction

- Most common in boys
- Usually unilateral
- Most common cause of hydronephrosis found on prenatal USG (AP diameters: >7–7.5 mm in third trimester)
- Mostly asymptomatic after birth as other kidney is working; if symptomatic-palpable intraabdominal mass

- *Pyelogram:* Stricture @ PUJ, dilated clubbed calyces
- *IOC:* DTPA> IVP

Treatment of choice: Anderson Haynes dismembered pyeloplasty

134. A 6-year-old child presented with recurrent UTI. Micturating cystourethrogram image of the patient is given below. What is the most likely diagnosis? *(NEET 2022)*

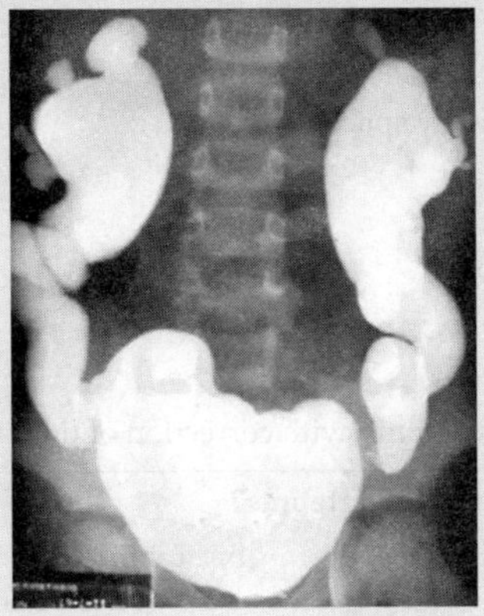

a. Vesicoureteric reflux
b. Vesicocolic fistula
c. Urinary bladder hernia
d. Urinary bladder diverticula

Ans. is 'a' Vesicoureteric reflux

Vesicoureteral Reflux

- Most common congenital abnormality of urogenital tract
- Most common in children
- Second most common cause of hydronephrosis
- Autosomal dominant condition

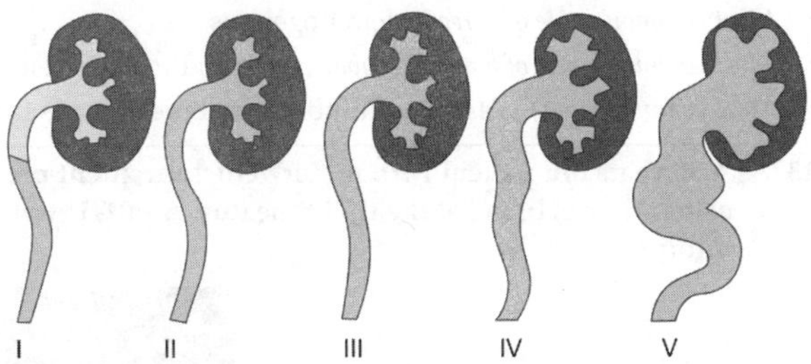

Grade	*Description*
I	Into a nondilated ureter
II	Into the pelvis and calyces without dilatation
III	Mild-to-moderate dilatation of the ureter, renal pelvis, and calyces with minimal blunting of the fornices
IV	Moderate ureteral tortuosity and dilatation of the pelvis and calyces
V	Gross dilatation of the ureter, pelvis, and calyces; loss of papillary impressions; and ureteral tortuosity

135. Identify the correct diagnosis on the basis of given image of newborn baby: *(NEET 2022)*

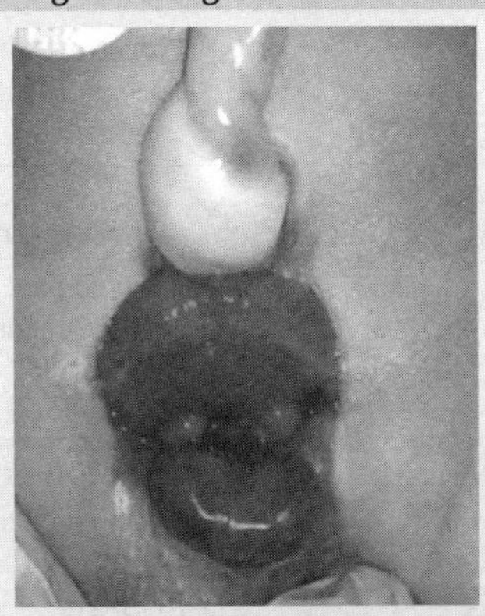

a. Gastroschisis
b. Omphalocele
c. Exstrophy bladder
d. Patent vitellointestinal duct

Ans. is 'c' Exstrophy bladder

Bladder Exstrophy

It is caused due to abnormal over development of urogenital sinus which leads to rupture of ventral walls infra umbilical region.

Characteristic features:

- Absence of infraumbilical abdominal wall
- *Widely separated pubic rami:* X-ray: Manta ray sign
- Absent ventral wall of urinary bladder with exposed posterior wall with urine dribbling from trigone
- *Males:* Epispadias with undescended testes with shallow scrotum
- *Females:* Epispadias with bifold clitoris with widely spaced labia
- Umbilical hernia
- Rectal prolapse
- Associated with increased risk of adenocarcinoma

Treatment:

- Augmentation enterocystoplasty
- Abdominal wall closure after post iliac bone osteotomy with correction of underlying defect.

136. Route of metastasis of prostate cancer to lumbar vertebrae? *(NEET 2022)*

a. Transcoelomic spread
b. Lymphatics
c. Prostatic venous plexus
d. Inferior vesical vein

Ans. is 'c' Prostatic venous plexus

Prostate Cancer

- *Most common route of spread:* Hematogenous
- *Most common route of mets to lumbar vertebrae:* Prostatic venous plexus
- *Most common site of mets:* Bone-lumbar vertebrae. It leads to osteoblastic secondaries.

137. A 30 years old patient with motor vehicle accident presented to the causality. His vitals are stable but he is unable to pass urine. He has blood at the tip of meatus. An RGU was performed as shown below. What is the most likely site of urethral injury? *(NEET 2022)*

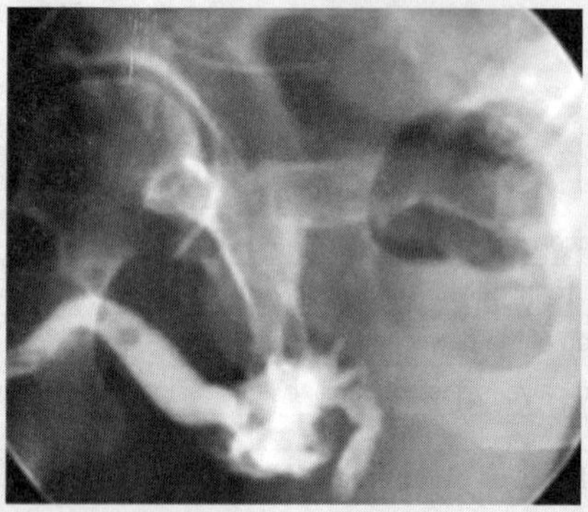

a. Membranous urethra
b. Penile urethra
c. Bulbar urethra
d. Spongy urethra

Ans. is 'a' Membranous urethra

Posterior urethral injury	*Anterior urethral injury*
Most common: Membranous *Urethra:* Bulbomembranous > prostatomembranous >Mc cause: RTA causing pelvic fracture >Associated with extraperitoneal bladder rupture	Mc injured part: Bulbar > penile *Causes:* Straddle injury, external below or kick to urethra
C/f: urinary retention + pelvic hematoma + blood@ meatus	*C/f:* Urinary retention+blood@meatus + superficial perineal hematoma
IOC: MCU *IVP:* PIE on SKY appearance	Hematoma-butterfly shape-involves shaft of penis, B/L scrotum
Treatment: • Suprapubic catheterization followed by delayed repair • Avoid emergency repair due to increased risk of urethral rupture, impotence, incontinence	*IOC:* RGU *Treatment:* Suprapubic catheterization followed by delayed repair

138. A 55 years patient presented to emergency with scrotal swelling, ecchymosis, fever and serous discharge. Image is given below. What is the most probable diagnosis? *(NEET 2022)*

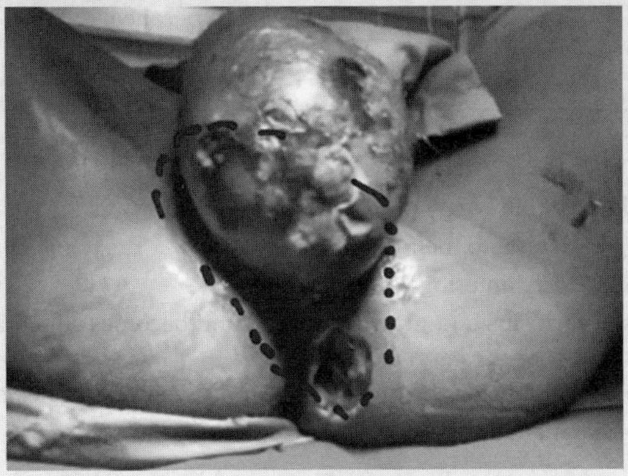

a. Fournier's gangrene
b. Epididymo-orchiditis
c. Torsion testis
d. Carcinoma testis

Ans. is 'a' Fournier's gangrene

Fournier's Gangrene

- Idiopathic scrotal gangrene
- Necrotising fasciitis of scrotal region
- Abrupt onset
- Polymicrobial leads to obliterative endarteritis which leads to necrosis of skin, superficial fascia, deep fascia
- Sparing of corpora cavernosa, corpora spongiest, urethra, testis, cord structures
- *Predisposing factors:* DM, anal infections, instrumentation, immunosuppressive
- *Discharge:* Dish water like discharge with FETID ODOUR
- Purple to blackish discolouration
- *Clinical features:* Pain, fever, marked systemic toxicity
- *Management:* IV fluids + IV antibiotics followed by extensive surgical debridement

139. A patient presented to emergency with claudication of calf muscle, numbness in thigh with impotence. Image showing gangrene of foot is given below. Which artery is involved? *(NEET 2022)*

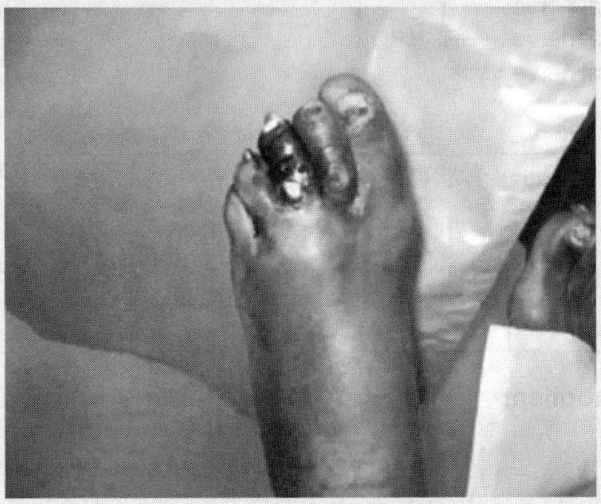

a. Aortic-iliac bifurcation
b. Internal iliac artery
c. Bilateral popliteal artery
d. Femoral artery

Ans. is 'a' Aortic-iliac bifurcation

Aorto-Iliac Obstruction

Buttock and hip claudication: Patients with aortoiliac disease may complain of buttock, hip, and, in some cases, thigh claudication. The pain is often described as aching in nature and may be associated with weakness of the hip or thigh with walking. Pulses in one or both groins are diminished. Bilateral aortoiliac PAD that is severe enough to cause lower extremity symptoms almost always causes erectile dysfunction in men. Leriche syndrome is the triad of claudication, absent or diminished femoral pulses, and erectile dysfunction.

140. Following surgery for varicose veins, patient started complaining of numbness along the medial aspect of leg. Which nerve is most commonly affected? *(NEET 2022)*

a. Superficial peroneal
b. Deep peroneal
c. Saphenous nerve
d. Sural nerve

Ans. is 'c' Saphenous nerve

Saphenous Nerve

- *Origin:* Posterior division of femoral nerve (L3, L4)
- Descends through the femoral triangle—lateral to the femoral artery
- Enters adductor canal, crosses femoral artery anteriorly to lie medial to it
- Pierces fascia Lata between tendons of sartorius and gracilis muscles and becomes subcutaneous—supplies skin over the anterior surface of the patella
- Descends down the medial aspect of leg, alongside the greater saphenous vein—supplies medial side of leg
- Terminates proximal to the tip of medial malleolus.

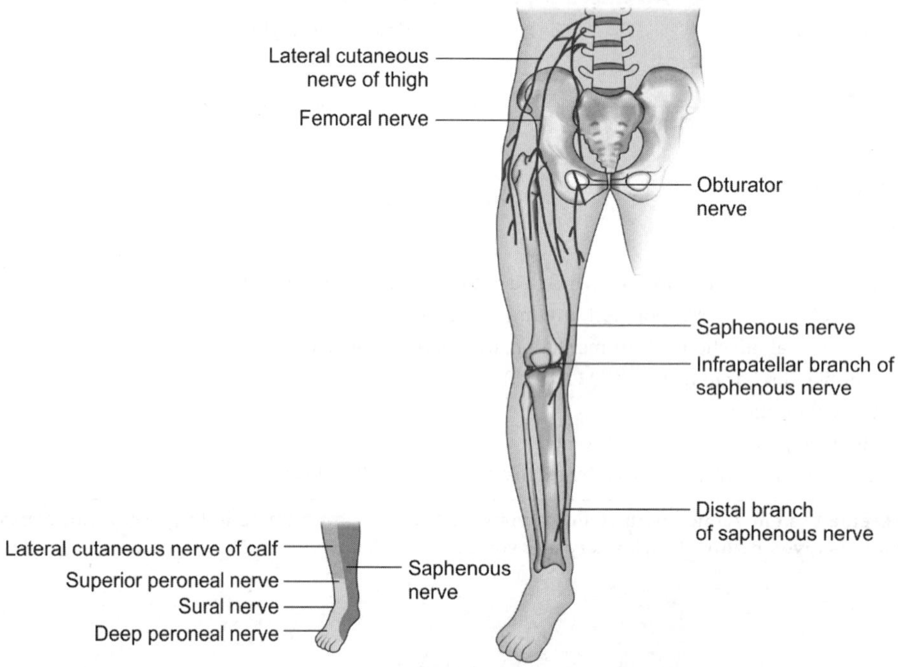

141. A 25 years old patient with history of massive RTA developed dyspnoea and petechial rashes after 3 days of trauma. What is the most likely cause? *(NEET 2022)*

a. Massive hemorrhage
b. Fat embolism
c. Thromboembolism
d. Air embolism

Ans. is 'b' Fat embolism

Gurd's Diagnostic Criteria for Fat Embolism

Major Criteria (4)

1. Axillary or subconjunctival petechia
2. PaO_2 below 60 mm Hg
3. CNS depression
4. Pulmonary edema

Minor Criteria (8)

1. Tachycardia
2. Pyrexia
3. Anemia
4. Thrombocytopenia

5. Fat globules present in sputum
6. Fat present in urine: GURD TEST
7. Increasing ESR
8. Emboli present in retina

1 Major + 4 Minor = Fat Embolism

Treatment of choice = oxygenation/IPPV

142. A 30 years old patient presented to the casualty after a motor vehicle accident. He has bruises on the chest. His pulse is 120 beats per minute. BP is 90/60 mm Hg and respiratory rate is 40/minute. A chest X-ray was performed and show below. What is the next most appropriate step in the management of this patient? *(NEET 2022)*

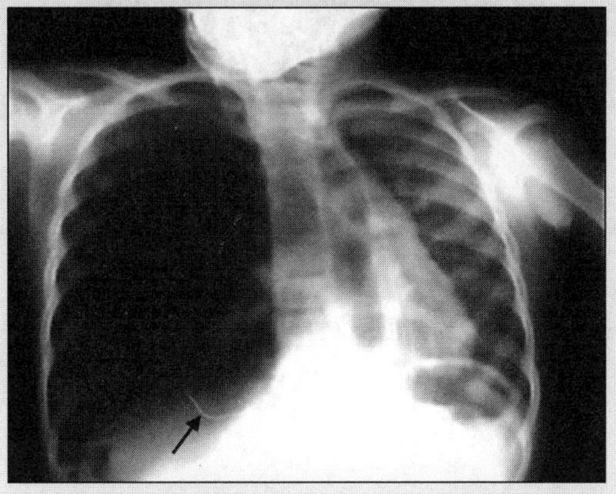

a. Immediate thoracotomy
b. Pericardiocentesis
c. Pleurodesis
d. Chest drain insertion and drainage

Ans. is 'd' Chest drain insertion and drainage

This is a case of tension Pneumothorax

Management:

- ❖ Chest drain insertion and drainage (Needle followed by tube)

Needle thoracocentesis:

- ❖ Adults: 5th intercostal space
- ❖ Children: 2 nd intercostal space @midclavicular line

* Simple pneumothorax management

- ❖ <25% of thoracic volume = observe
- ❖ >25% of thoracic volume = directly insert chest tube

143. A 9 years old child was brought to the hospital after burns. There was involvement of half of chest wall and abdomen towards left side, posterior arm and thigh. Calculate the burnt surface area? *(NEET 2022)*

a. 5–10%
b. 15–20%
c. 25–30%
d. 35–40%

Ans. is 'b' 15–20%

Adult body		Child body	
Part	*BSA*	*Part*	*BSA*
Arm	9%	Arm	9%
Head and neck	9%	Head and neck	18%
Leg	18%	Leg	14%
Anterior trunk	18%	Anterior trunk	18%
Posterior trunk	18%	Posterior trunk	18%
Perineum		1%	

144. A 65 years old patient presented with gradually increasing growth besides the nose near the medial canthus with ulceration. Histopathology image is shown below. What is the most likely diagnosis? *(NEET 2022)*

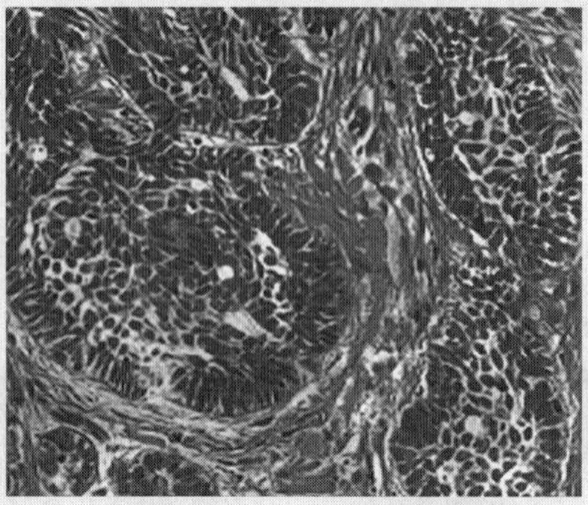

a. BCC
b. SCC
c. Melanoma
d. Nevus

Ans. is 'a' BCC

NEVUS

Pigmentation (benign/malignant), e.g., nevus of OTA, NEVUS of ITO.

Melanoma

Malignant cancer of skin.

Basal Cell Carcinoma

- Aka rodent ulcer
- *Lesion:* Central ulceration, rolled/pearly edges
- Sites face, nose, cheek except superficial type: @trunks and limbs
- No mets, no lymphatic spread
- Locally invasive: Slow

HPE: Islands of basal cells with artificial clefts

Treatment: Local excision with 5 mm margin except 2 cm margins removed in Morphic type MOH's microscopic surgery in >2 cm size.

Squamous Cell Carcinoma

- Occurs in pre-existing damaged skin- scars/photo damaged/leukoplakia
- Rapid growth
- Lymph node mets present
- Visceral mets uncommon
- *Site:* Anywhere in the body including mucosa
- *Lesion:* Fungating lesion—Cauliflower like with red base/induration

145. A 73 years old male was bed ridden for 15 years. The image of bed sore is given below. What is the grade of bed sore? *(NEET 2022)*

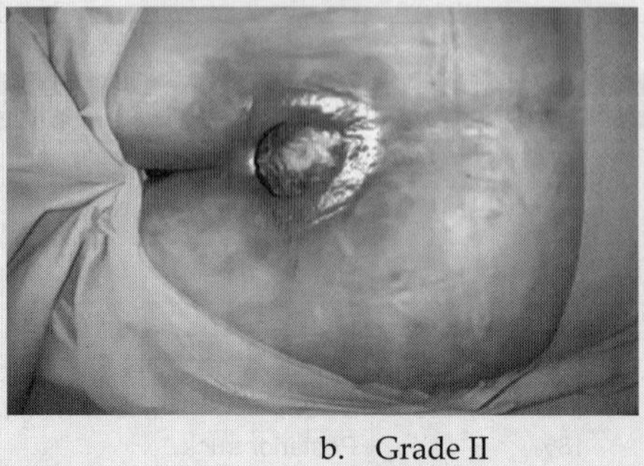

a. Grade I
b. Grade II
c. Grade III
d. Grade IV

Ans. is 'd' Grade IV

Grade description	
I	Non-blanchable erythema of intact skin
II	Partial-thickness skin loss involving epidermis, dermis or both
III	Full-thickness skin loss involving damage to or necrosis of subcutaneous tissue that may extend down to, but not through, underlying fascia
IV	Full-thickness skin loss with extensive destruction, tissue necrosis, or damage to muscle, bone or supporting structures

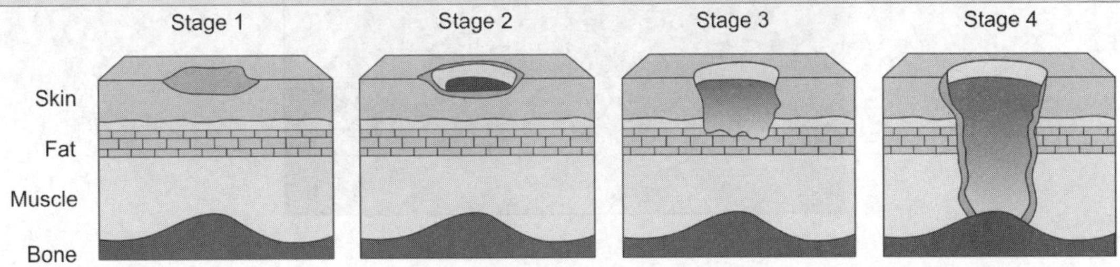

Pressure sores

146. A patient with history of chronic alcoholism presented to OPD with whitish patch, whose image is given below. What is the most probable diagnosis? *(NEET 2022)*

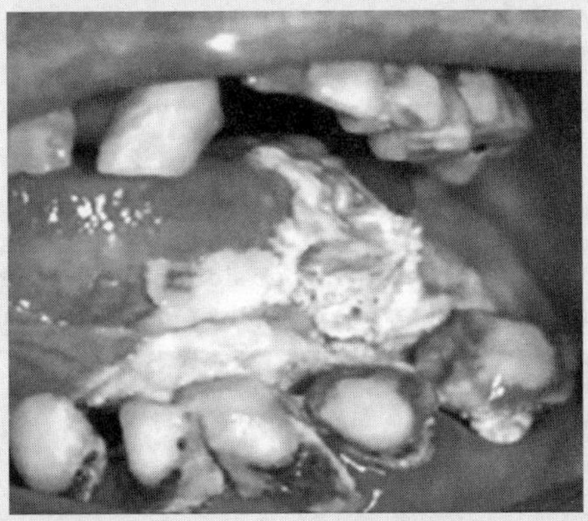

a. Leukoplakia
b. Submucosa fibrosis
c. Erythroplakia
d. Malakoplakia

Ans. is 'a' Leukoplakia

Submucous Fibrosis

- Scarring
- Grey lesions

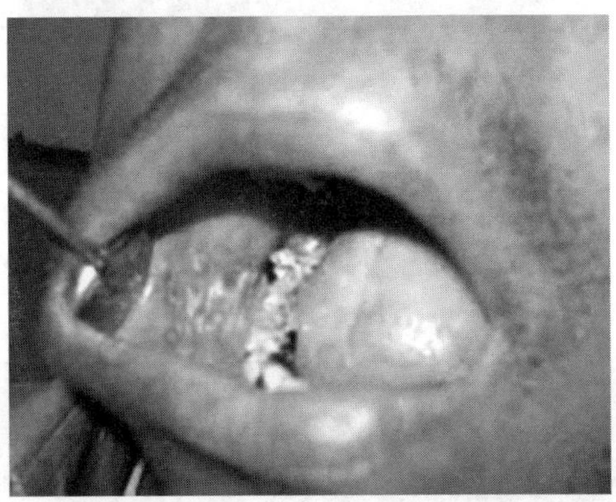

Erythroplakia

- Erythro = red
- *More premalignant*: Increases risk of malignancy by 6–9 times
- *Most aggressive:* Speckled erythroplakia

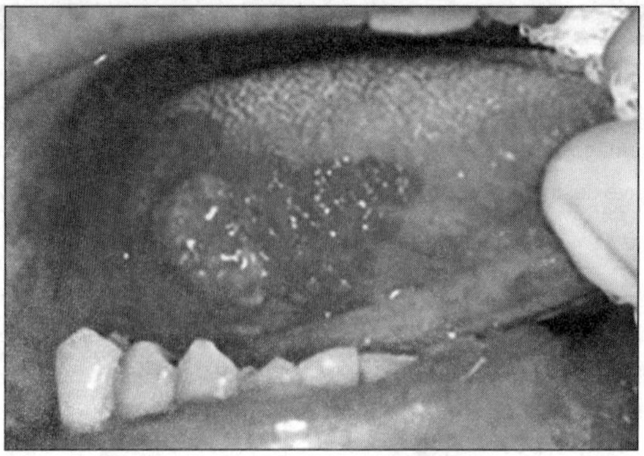

Malakoplakia

- ❖ Mainly affects: Genitourinary tract
- ❖ Yellow brown plaques with central umbilication

Leukoplakia

- ❖ More common
- ❖ Less malignant → ↑ risk by 5– 6 times
- ❖ Cannot be Rubbed off

∗ CANDIDIASIS → Hyperemia when Rubbed off

147. A 45 years old patient complaints of recurrent swelling in one side of the neck. She is afraid of eating food as it worsens the swelling. Imaging was performed and shown below. What is the most likely diagnosis? *(NEET 2022)*

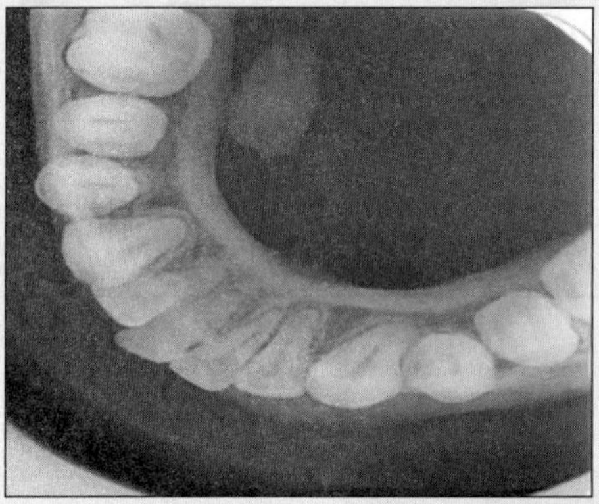

a. Sialolithiasis
b. Penetrating irregular foreign body
c. Isolated osteoma of floor of mouth
d. Cervical lymphadenopathy

Ans. is 'a' Sialolithiasis

Osteoma

- ❖ Bone in bone
- ❖ Associated with Gardner's syndrome

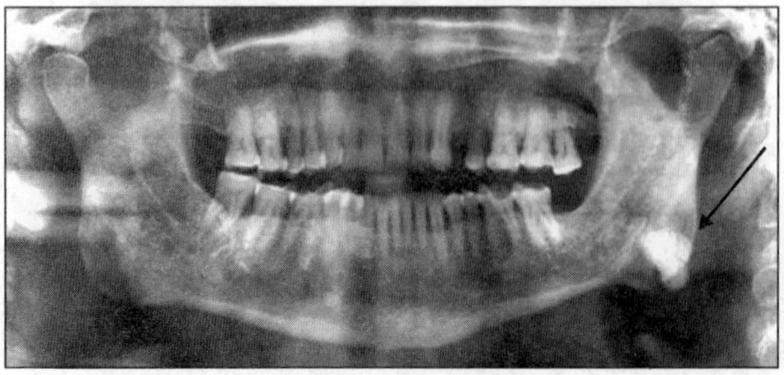

Submandibular Duct Abscess

Proximal duct dilatation but no radiopaque calculus or obstruction

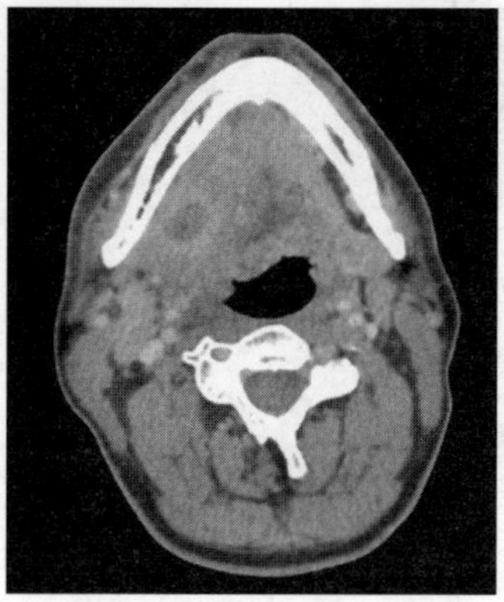

Foreign Body

Obstruction due to foreign body leads to sialoadenitis and calculus formation extremely rare condition

Sialolithiasis

Clinical features:

- Swelling of the affected salivary gland
- Difficulty in opening the mouth
- Difficulty in swallowing
- Gritty sensation

Investigation: X-ray

Treatment:

- Supportive treatment
- Minimally invasive p/m sialoendoscopy
- *Surgical:* Sialectomy

148. Patient came to OPD with erythematous neck swelling in supraclavicular region. Pulsations were present over the swelling. Image is given below. What is the next best step? *(NEET 2022)*

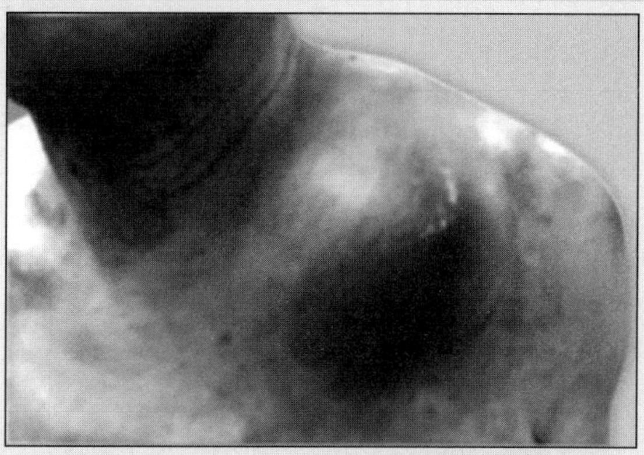

a. Needle biopsy
b. USG Doppler neck
c. CT Angio+Percutaneous
d. Oral antibiotics for 7 days

Ans. is 'b' USG Doppler neck

- Swelling is pulsatile, therefore, vascular in nature.
- In vascular swelling we avoid Biopsy and oral antibiotics may not be beneficial.
- *Next investigation:* USG Doppler
- CT Angiography would give better vascular imaging but next step of investing would be USG Doppler.

149. A patient with stab injury was brought to the emergency. Vitas were stable. Image is given below. What is next best step of management? *(NEET 2022)*

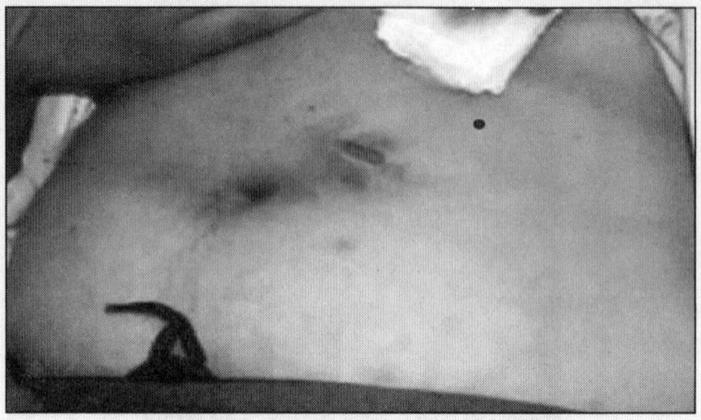

a. Further investigation
b. IV fluids
c. Wait and watch after dressing
d. Exploratory laparotomy

Ans. is 'a' Further investigation

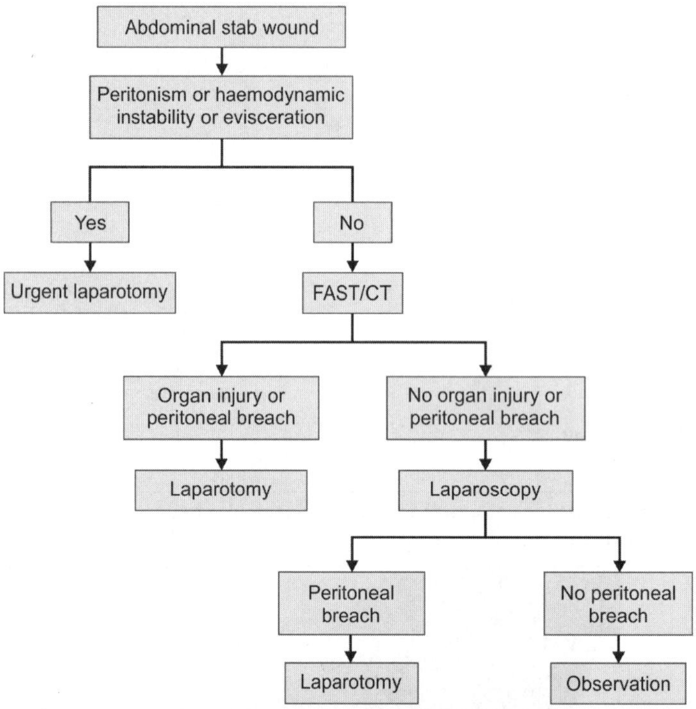

150. Known case of CLD with Ascites presents with abdominal pain and tenderness. Ascitic tap shows presence of 600 PNM cells/Cu. mm. Which of the following is the likely etiology? *(NEET 2022)*

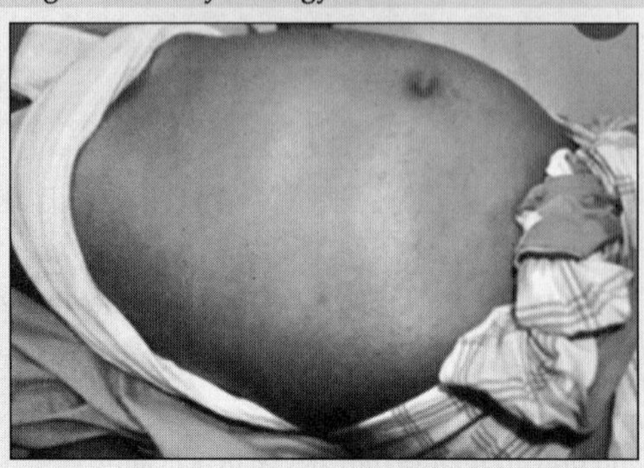

a. Tubercular ascites
b. Malignant ascites
c. Spontaneous bacterial peritonitis
d. Chylous ascites

Ans. is 'c' Spontaneous bacterial peritonitis

Spontaneous Bacterial Peritonitis

- *Prerequisite:* Ascites
- *Most common cause of ascites in adult:* Cirrhosis
- *Most common cause of ascites in children:* Nephrotic syndrome
- *Pathogenesis:* Bacteria in gut translocates to mesentric lymph node and reaches the ascites fluid
- SBP is monomicrobial infection
- *Most common organism:* E. coli > Klebsiella
- *Most common organism in children:* Group A Streptococci
- *Clinical features:* diffuse abdominal pain with tenderness, tachycardia, fever with rigor
- *Diagnosis:* monomicrobial growth with neutrophil >250 per cubic mm
- *Treatment:* IV antibiotic (cefotaxime) + albumin (as albumin decreases in Nephrotic syndrome and CLD)

PEDIATRICS

151. A mother reported that her baby did not pass urine on post-natal day 1. What will the next step? *(NEET 2022)*

a. Start IV hydration
b. Shift to NICU and investigate
c. Continue breastfeeding and observe
d. Start formula milk

Ans. is 'c' Continue breastfeeding and observe

Baby will pass urine within the first 48 hours so the patient needs to breast feed and observe her baby. If the baby does not pass urine after 48 hours, then the baby should be shifted to NICU and investigated.

152. Regarding High risk infants, which of the following are correct? *(NEET 2022)*

i. Weight 2.5 kg
ii. Birth order > 3
iii. Single parent
iv. Artificial feeding
v. Birth weight < 85 percentile

a. iii & iv
b. i and ii
c. i, ii and iii
d. ii, iv and v

Ans. is 'a' iii & iv

High Risk Infants

- Social factors = maternal age < 16 or >40 years, unmarked, physical stress
- Past medical history = DM, Hypertension, Genetic disorders
- *Previous pregnancy:* Intrauterine death, neonatal death, IUGR, congenital malformations
- *Present pregnancy:* Bleeding PV, PROM, multiple gestations, preeclampsia, abnormal USG findings
- *Labor and delivery:* Obstructed labor, Fetal distress, forceps delivery, meconium stained labor
- *Neonate:* Birthweight <2000 gm or >4000 gm, gestation <37 weeks or >42 weeks, SGA, RDS, Congenital malformation

153. Pentavalent vaccine and MR vaccine vials were open, and cold chain was maintained, and vaccines were not expired. What will you do with these opened vaccine vials? *(NEET 2022)*

a. Discard both
b. Discard pentavalent, use MR
c. Discard MR and use pentavalent
d. Use both MR and pentavalent

Ans. is 'c' Discard MR and use pentavalent

Open Vial Policy

Allows reuse of partially used multiple-dose vials in subsequent immunisation sessions (up to 4 weeks) provided:

- Expiry date not reached
- Cold chain maintained
- Date of opening vial mentioned
- Aseptic techniques used to withdraw vaccine
- Vaccine vial septum not submerged in water

OVP applicable	OVP not applicable
• DPT • TT • HEPATITIS B • PCV • PENTAVALENT • OPV • IPV	• MEASLES/MR • ROTAVIRUS • JE • BCG

154. A 6-year-old male with a history of recurrent blood transfusions presented with pain in hands and feet. Hb HPLC shows increased HbF, HbA2 and a peak is seen in the S window. What is the diagnosis? *(NEET 2022)*

a. Beta thalassemia
b. Autoimmune Hemolytic Anemia
c. Sickle Cell Anemia
d. Anemia of chronic disease

Ans. is 'c' Sickle Cell Anemia

Diagnosis of Sickle Cell Anemia

- *PBS:* Hemolysis, sickle cells, hotel jolly bodies
- *Spleen biopsy:* Gamma handy bodies
- *Hb electrophoresis:* HbS peak
- *Confirm:* Genetic defect confirmed = Glutamine replaced with valine at 6th position in beta chain

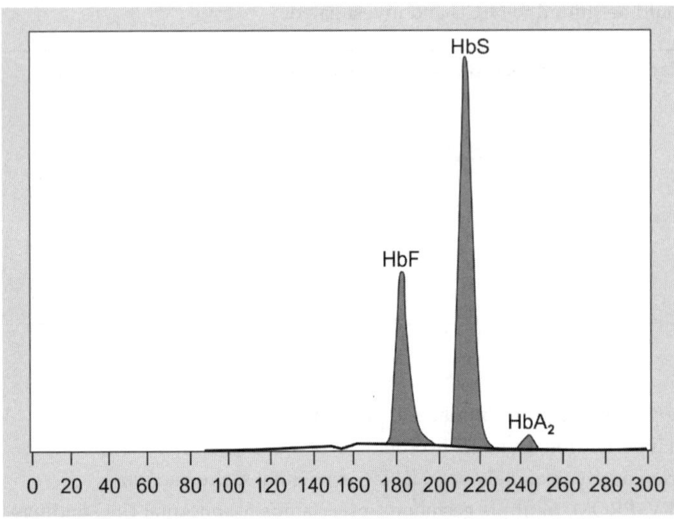

155. A neonate was found to have TSH > 100 U/L on day 4 of life. USG shows ectopic thyroid gland. What should be the next investigation? *(NEET 2022)*

a. Urinary iodine concentration
b. Thyroid receptor Antibody levels
c. Thyroid nuclear scan
d. T3 and T4 levels

Ans. is 'c' Thyroid nuclear scan

Diagnosis: Congenital Hypothyroidism

Next investigation done to detect the cause of
Congenital hypothyroidism = Ultrasound of thyroid gland followed by thyroid nuclear scan

156. A 12-year-old male presents with bloating, recurrent loose stools and features of malabsorption. His HLA DQ2 is positive. What should be the best management? *(NEET 2022)*

a. Low lactose diet
b. High lactose diet
c. Gluten free diet
d. Low protein diet

Ans. is 'c' Gluten free diet

Diagnosis: Celiac Disease

Cause: Hypersensitive to gliaden protein (present in gluten)

Site: Proximal Small intestine

Clinical features: Steatorrhea, bloating, malabsorption, dermatitis herpetiformis, type 1 DM, IgA deficiency

Serology

- Most specific antibody = anti-endomysial
- Most sensitive antibody = anti-tissue glutaminase antibody-ATTG
- If IgA deficiency = IgG antialiasing antibody

Treatment: Lifelong gluten free diet

157. A child presented to OPD with multiple episodes of loose stools repeated vomiting's. He was lethargic and not able to drink breast milk. Skin pinch was going back very slowly. Which grade of dehydration the child has? *(NEET 2022)*

a. Mild
b. Moderate
c. Severe
d. None of the above

Ans. is 'c' Severe

	Level of dehydration		
	Mild	***Moderate***	***Severe***
General appearance	Irritable thirsty	Irritable extremely thirsty	Drowsy or unconscious
Anterior fontanelle	Normal	Depressed	Strikingly depressed
Eyes	Normal	Sunken	Sunken
Tongue	Normal wet	Dry	Very dry, furred
Skin pinch	Goes back immediately	Goes back slowly	Goes back very slowly
Breathing	Normal	Rapid	May be very rapid
Pulse	Normal	Rapid and feeble	Weak and thready
Urine output	Normal	Deep color	Scanty
Weight loss	<5%	6–9%	≥10%

158. A 10-year-old boy with generalized edema and massive proteinuria. He was diagnosed as a case of minimal change disease. True about this disease is: *(NEET 2022)*

a. Light microscopy shows effacement of foot plates of podocytes
b. Good response to steroids
c. More common in adults
d. Non-selective proteinuria

Ans. is 'b' Good response to steroids

Minimal Change Disease

- MC nephrotic disease of childhood
- No findings on light microscopy and no
- Deposition of immune complex/antibody
- *Electron microscopy:* Effacement of foot plates of podocytes
- Good response to steroids present

OBSTETRICS AND GYNAECOLOGY

159. Which of the following is the correct calorie requirement in 12 weeks pregnant woman? *(NEET 2022)*

a. 400 in 1st trimester
b. 400 in 3rd trimester
c. 300 in 1st trimester
d. 300 in all trimesters

Ans. is 'b' 400 in 3rd trimester

Calorie requirement increases in pregnancy by

- *Second trimester:* + 350 kcal/day
- *Third trimester:* + 450 kcal/day
- *Lactation (0–6 m):* + 600 kcal/day
- *Lactation (6–12 m):* + 520 kcal/day

160. Identify the HSG image given below: *(NEET 2022)*

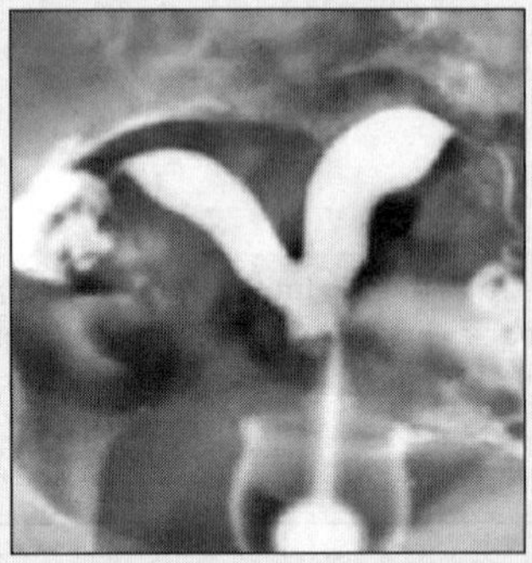

a. Didelphys uterus
b. Bicornuate uterus
c. Septate uterus
d. Unicornuate

Ans. is 'c' Septate uterus

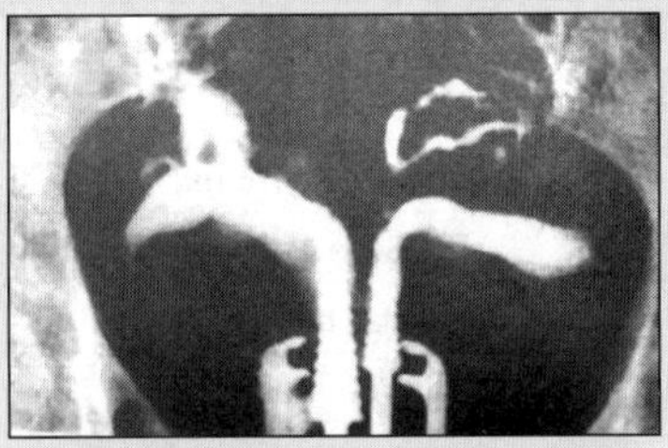	**Uterus didelphys** 2 cervix & 2 horns
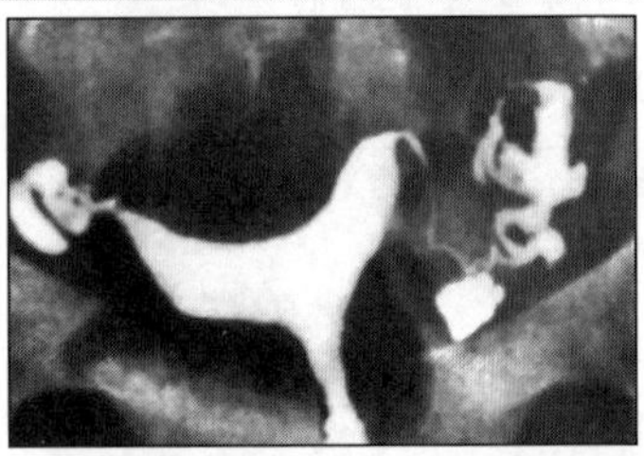	**Bicornuate uterus** 1 cervix and 2 horns Angle between the 2 horns > 105 degrees (obtuse angle)
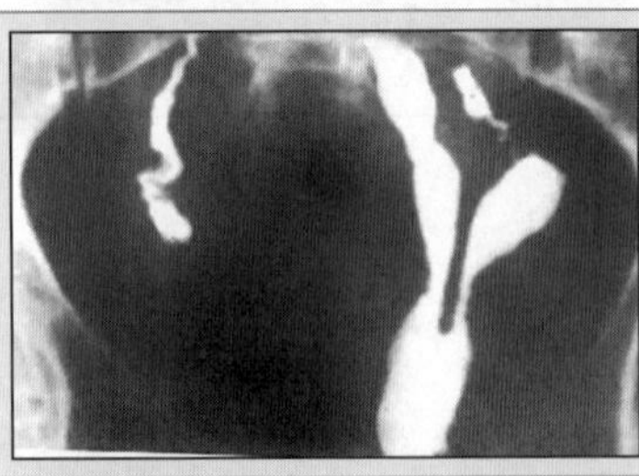	**Septate uterus** 1 cervix and 2 horns Angle between the horns <75 degrees (acute angle)
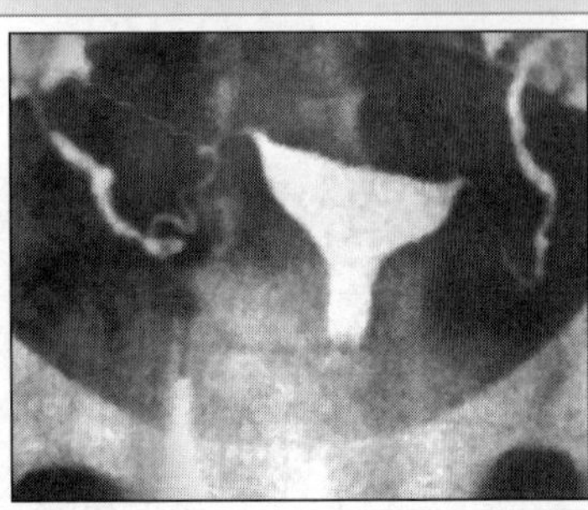	**Arcuate uterus**

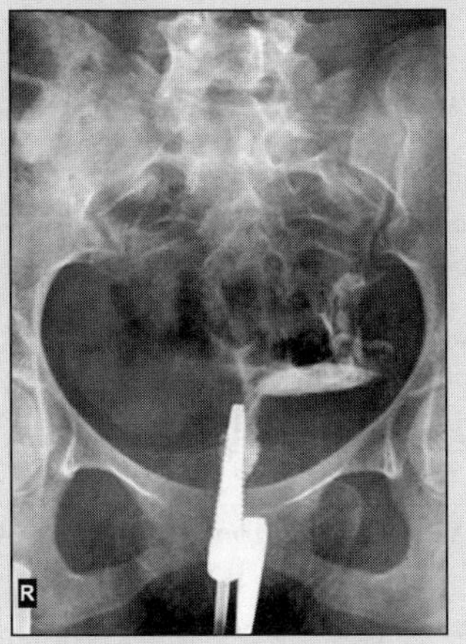	**Unicornuate uterus** 1 cervix and 1 horn

161. A Primigravida is brought home by her relatives just after 1 hour of a vaginal delivery of a full term health infant. The baby is doing well. On examination, the patient is hypotensive, hypoxic, and has disseminated intravascular coagulation. Which of the following is the most likely cause? *(NEET 2022)*

a. Vaginal bleeding
b. Albuminuria
c. Abdominal distension due to rupture uterus
d. Amniotic fluid embolism

Ans. is 'd' Amniotic fluid embolism

Amniotic Fluid Embolism

- Very rare condition
- Diagnosis of exclusion
- Diagnosed clinically

Two phases:

- *First phase:* Sudden onset of breathlessness with hypotension leads to cardiac arrest and coma. Most of the women die in first phase, those who survive follow the second phase.
- *Second phase:* Disseminated intravascular coagulation (DIC), characterised by bleeding from everywhere.

Ruptured uterus: Presents with either hemoperitoneum (complete rupture) or braid ligament hematoma (incomplete rupture)

162. Identify the area marked in Green: *(NEET 2022)*

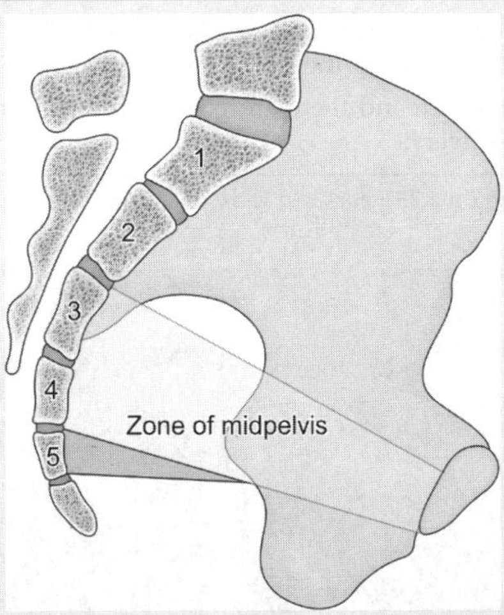

a. Pelvic outlet
b. Anatomical outlet
c. Midpelvis
d. Obstetric outlet

Ans. is 'c' Midpelvis

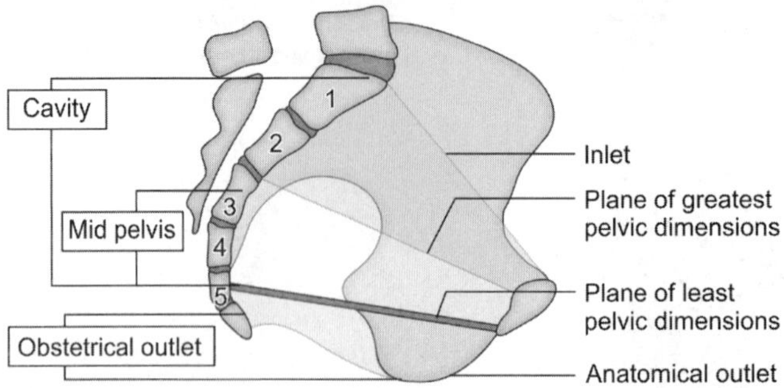

163. A 34-year-old female, previous classical C section, is now having breech presentation confirmed on USG at 34 weeks, insists of normal delivery, what will you do? *(NEET 2022)*

a. Wait for 36 weeks
b. Plan Cesarean Section at 37 weeks
c. Repeat USG after a week and decide
d. Do vaginal delivery

Ans. is 'b' Plan Cesarean Section at 37 weeks

Absolute indications of repeat CS:

- Previous classical CS
- Previous history of uterine/scar rupture
- More than three previous seasons
- History of surgery in which uterine cavity was opened, e.g., hysterotomy, myomectomy
- CPD in current pregnancy
- Any contraindication for vaginal delivery

Relative indications of caesarean section:

- With current Breech pregnancy
- Macrosomia
- Post-term pregnancy (>42 weeks POG)

164. A primigravida patient presented with soft tender abdomen, on examination fetus is on right occiput posterior (ROP) position, how will you deliver? *(NEET 2022)*

a. Vacuum assisted delivery
b. C section
c. Normal vaginal delivery
d. Forceps delivery

Ans. is 'c' Normal vaginal delivery

- Right occiput posterior is the most common occiput posterior position of the fetal head.
- OP is more commonly seen in primigravidas. In OP, engagement is delayed. Most common cause of OP is android pelvis. At the onset of labour about 20% babies are in OP position, as the labour progresses only 5% babies are in OP.
- When the pelvis is normal, baby is average size and there are good uterine contractions, then the baby will rotate all by itself therefore we will go for a normal vaginal delivery.

165. The following procedure is being done on a 25 years old lady in labor. The cord gets torn. What should be the best thing to do? *(NEET 2022)*

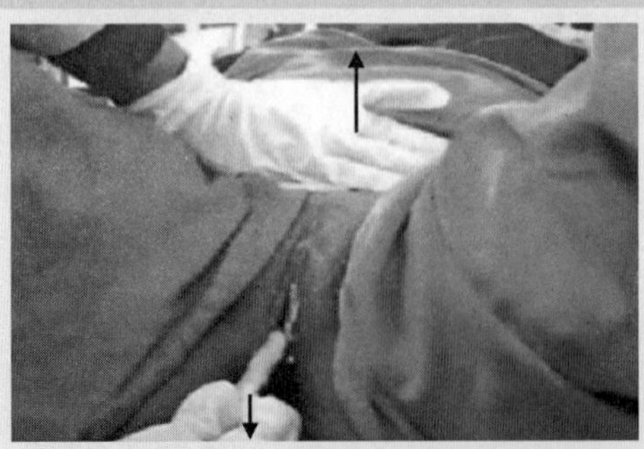

a. Uterine massage
b. Inj oxytocin
c. Manual removal
d. Arrange blood and remove placenta via Crede's method

Ans. is 'c' Manual removal

- Controlled cord traction is done by modified Brandt Andrews method as a component of active management of third stage of labour (AMTSL).
- With right hand we hold the cord, with left hand the fundus is pushed up.
- When the cord gets torn, we remove the placenta manually.

166. Uterine artery Doppler done at 14 weeks detects which of the following? *(NEET 2022)*

a. Late onset preeclampsia
b. Early onset preeclampsia
c. IUGR
d. All of the above

Ans. is 'b' Early onset preeclampsia

- Preeclampsia is generally diagnosed after 20 weeks of pregnancy.
- To detect early onset preeclampsia, USG Doppler is done at 12–14 weeks to see the presence of diastolic notch.
- These patients are again evaluated at 24 weeks as they are at higher risk of developing Hypertension and Preeclampsia.

167. A 25-year-old female with history of 2 weeks amenorrhea came in emergency department with c/o scantly vaginal bleeding. On examination no adnexal mass noted. In lab investigation hCG was 1400 mlU/mL, on USG, uterus was bulky, trilaminar endometrium was seen. Patient vitals stable, what is the net step to do? *(NEET 2022)*

a. Repeat hCG after 48 hrs
b. Give progesterone
c. Wait and watch
d. All of the above

Ans. is 'a' Repeat hCG after 48 hrs

- In the given case ectopic pregnancy should be ruled out. As the hCG level is less than 1500 IU/mL, so repeat beta hCG levels after 48 hours.
- If the increase in beta hCG levels is more than 66% then it is a case of intrauterine pregnancy
- If the increase is less than 66% then it's a case of ectopic pregnancy
- If there is fall in the hCG levels it is a case of abortion or non-viable pregnancy.
- If ectopic pregnancy is diagnosed, repeat hCG levels every 48 hours till reaching the critical tighter bracket open 1500 bracket close.

168. What is the position of uterus on postpartum day 2? *(NEET 2022)*

a. Two fingers below umbilicus
b. Four finger below umbilicus
c. Just above symphysis pubis
d. At the level of umbilicus

Ans. is 'b' Four finger below umbilicus

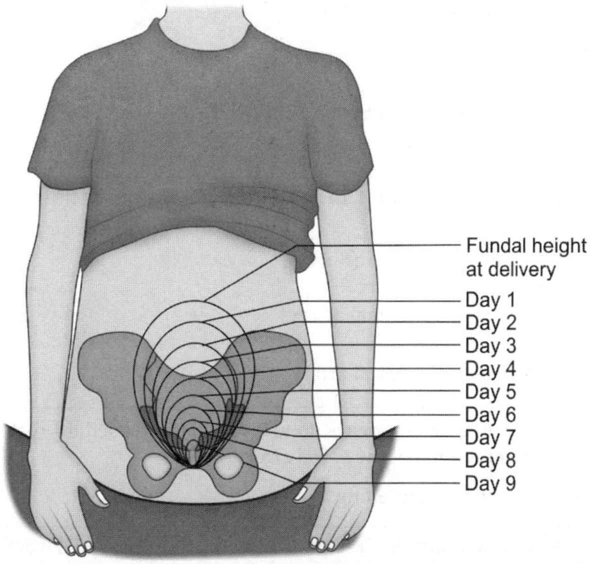

- After the delivery, the uterus is just below the umbilicus and by the end of 24 hours it its position is that of 20 weeks of POG-2 cm below the umbilicus.
- During the next few days, the fundus descends 1–2 cm (fingerbreadth) every 24 hours.
- On day 12 to 14 (about 2 weeks) after delivery the uterus becomes a pelvic organ again.

169. Which site of implantation will cause severe vaginal bleeding; no sign of rupture ectopic despite 22 weeks of gestation? *(NEET 2022)*

a. Internal os
b. Ovary
c. Tube
d. Abdominal

Ans. is 'd' Abdominal

- ❖ Abdominal ectopic pregnancies are diagnosed late, towards the term.
- ❖ Cervical, ovarian, tubal ectopics are diagnosed earlier than nominal ectopic pregnancy.

170. The fetus is at the level of ischia spine, ROT. Molding ++, caput++. What's the appropriate management? *(NEET 2022)*

a. Vacuum
b. Forceps
c. LSCS
d. Normal vaginal delivery

Ans. is 'c' LSCS

- ❖ Molding means overlapping of the skull bones. Caput means localised edema over the scalp
- ❖ ROT with caput and molding makes a diagnosis of Deep Transverse Arrest.
- ❖ Mode of delivery should be LSCS.

171. A preeclampsia patient presented with absent Bilateral plantar reflex. Lungs clear, RBS-200+, patellar reflex absent. What is the possible diagnosis? *(NEET 2022)*

a. Diabetes insipidus
b. Postpartum eclampsia
c. $MgsO_4$ toxicity
d. All of the above

Ans. is 'c' $MgsO_4$ toxicity

Monitoring for Magnesium Toxicity

- ❖ Urine output should be at least 30 mL/hr
- ❖ Deep tendon reflexes (Patellar reflex) should be present
- ❖ Respiration rate should be more than 14/min
- ❖ Pulse oximetry should be ≥ 96%.

172. What is the absolute contraindication of cervical cerclage? *(NEET 2022)*

a. Rupture of membrane
b. Bag of water in vagina
c. History of ectopic pregnancy
d. Previous miscarriage

Ans. is 'a' Rupture of membrane

Absolute contra indications of cervical Cerclage:

- ❖ If the membranes are ruptured
- ❖ Presence of gross congenital anomalies
- ❖ Presence of infections chorioamnionitis or any current pelvic infection

These are also the prerequisites before doing cervical cerclage.

173. A pregnant lady at 32 weeks gestation develop proteinuria and hypertension, doctor suspect a case of placental insufficiency. Due to: *(NEET 2022)*

a. Extravillous cytotrophoblast invasion in spiral artery
b. Villous cytotrophoblast invasion in spiral artery
c. Extravillous cytotrophoblast invasion in luminal artery
d. All of the above

Ans. is 'a' Extravillous cytotrophoblast invasion in spiral artery

In normal pregnancy, vascular remodelling of spiral arteries is done in the placental bed to create a permanent state of way so dilation. This is done by extravillous cytotrophoblast invasion of the spiral artery.

In preeclampsia, there is absence of vascular remodelling.

174. A pregnant lady with 34 weeks of amenorrhea has the following findings: LDH: 700 IU/L, platelets: 75,000/mm^3, serum bilirubin: 1.5 mg/dL, SGOT-200 U/L, SGPT-150 U/L, and BP: 140/96 mm Hg. Her coagulation profile and renal function tests are normal. What is the diagnosis? *(NEET 2022)*

a. HELLP syndrome
b. Acute fatty liver of pregnancy
c. Viral hepatitis
d. Intrahepatic cholestasis

Ans. is 'a' HELLP syndrome

The given clinical scenario with elevated liver enzymes and bilirubin, low platelet count, and hypertension indicates the diagnosis of HELLP syndrome.

HELLP is an acronym for hemolysis (H), elevated liver enzymes (EL), and low platelet count (LP). It usually occurs in patients with severe preeclampsia, the patients typically present with right upper quadrant pain, nausea, and vomiting. Hypertension and proteinuria are seen but may be absent in some cases.

In this condition, there is periportal necrosis of the liver causing an elevation in liver enzymes (AST, ALT, and LDH) and bilirubin. Tennessee criteria used to diagnose HELLP syndrome include:

- Platelet count → 1 lakh/mm^3
- ASD → 70 IU/L
- LDH → 600 IU/L
- Hemolysis

Prompt delivery is indicated for ≥ 34 weeks gestational age. Cesarean section is the common mode of delivery. Platelet transfusion is required counts are less than 50,000/mm^3. Magnesium sulfate is given as anti-seizure prophylaxis, and anti-hypertensives are given for severe hypertension.

Complications of HELLP include eclampsia, placental abruption, hepatic subcapsular hematoma, coagulopathy, stroke and pulmonary edema.

175. A Woman at 26 weeks of gestation presents for routine evaluation. On examination, fundal height corresponds to 24 weeks. Ultrasonography revealed decreased amniotic fluid. Which of the following conditions would have led to this presentation? *(NEET 2022)*

a. Renal agenesis
b. Tracheoesophageal fistula
c. Cardiac abnormalities
d. Ureteral stricture

Ans. is 'a' Renal agenesis

The given clinical scenario and decreased amniotic fluid on ultrasonography are suggestive of oligohydramnios. Among the given conditions, renal agenesis is the most likely cause.

Oligohydramnios is a condition where the amount of amniotic fluid is reduced. The major source of amniotic fluid in the second trimester is fetal urine. When the fetus has renal agenesis, urine production is affected. This leads to decreased amniotic fluid/ oligohydramnios.

A woman with oligohydramnios usually presents with decreased fundal height for gestational age and decreased fetal movements. On examination, fetal parts can be clearly felt because of less liquor. Fetal malpresentation and intrauterine growth retardation are seen in this condition. It is diagnosed with the help of ultrasonography when the deepest vertical pocket (DVP) of liquor is < 2 cm or when the amniotic fluid index (AFI) is < 5 cm at gestational age, from 28 to 40 weeks.

It can lead to abortion, deformities like wry neck, club foot, etc. fetal pulmonary hypoplasia, and cord compression. Adequate hydration and amnioinfusion can be used to manage this condition.

Polyhydramnios or hydramnios is a condition where the amount of amniotic fluid is abnormally increased. Ultrasonographic diagnosis is made when the DVP is > 8 cm or when the AFI is > 25 cm.

Other options:

Option D: Ureteral stricture usually arises secondary to trauma or iatrogenic interventions like surgery.

176. While discharging a patient who underwent a vesicovaginal fistula repair, which of the following would you recommend? *(NEET 2022)*

a. Sexual abstinence for 3 months and avoid pregnancy for a year
b. Sexual abstinence for 3 weeks and avoid pregnancy for 6 months
c. Sexual abstinence for 6 weeks and avoid pregnancy for a year
d. Sexual abstinence for 6 months and avoid pregnancy for 6 years

Ans. is 'a' Sexual abstinence for 3 months and avoid pregnancy for a year

While discharging a patient who underwent vesicovaginal fistula repair, sexual abstinence for 3 months and avoiding pregnancy for a year would be recommended.

Vesicovaginal fistula (VVF) is a type of urinary fistula which commonly arises due to obstetric trauma. Small fistulas due to difficult childbirth can heal spontaneously. Most established fistulas need to be repaired vaginally usually after 3 months to allow the inflammation to subside. Post-operatively, continuous bladder drainage for 14 days along with antibiotics is recommended. Vaginal or speculum examination and intercourse are not advised for 3 months. Avoiding pregnancy for a year is also recommended. A cesarean section is usually done for future pregnancies.

Presenting features of VVF include constant dribbling of urine/true incontinence. Excoriation of the vagina, vulva, and thighs can occur due to constant contact with urine. Few patients might develop bladder stones. Vaginal urine collection can be seen on retraction of the posterior vaginal wall with a speculum. A bimanual examination can be used to assess the fixity and scarring of the surrounding tissues. A cystourethroscopy can be used for localization and assessing bladder mucosa viability.

177. A primigravida presents to the labour room at 40 weeks of gestation with lower abdominal pain. She has been in labour for 3 hours. Which of the following will determine if she is in active labour? *(NEET 2022)*

a. Fetal head 5/5 palpable on abdominal examination
b. Two contractions lasting for 10 seconds in 10 minutes
c. More than 5 cm cervical dilatation with complete effacement
d. Rupture of membranes

Ans. is 'c' More than 5 cm cervical dilatation with complete effacement

This patient will have presented in active labour if she had more than 5 cm cervical dilatation with complete effacement.

The first stage of labour is characterized by dilatation and effacement of the cervix and can be divided into latent phase and active labour. The onset of latent labour is the point at which the mother perceives regular contractions. Cervical dilatation of >5 cm in the presence of uterine contractions can be taken to reliably represent the threshold for active labour.

The first symptom to appear is intermittent painful uterine contractions followed by the expulsion of blood- stained mucus (show) per vagina. In the late first stage, the contraction comes at intervals of 3–5 minutes and lasts 45 seconds.

The second stage of labour begins with complete cervical dilatation and ends with fetal delivery.

The third stage of labour is characterized by the delivery of the placenta.

The fourth stage is a stage of observation for at least an hour after the full expulsion of the placenta.

Fetal head 5/5 on abdominal examination, signifies the degree of descent in relation to the pelvic inlet and denotes the head is floating above the brim.

Rupture of membranes at or near term signifies the labour is likely to begin soon.

More than 12 uterine contractions in 1 hour may signify labour onset. partograph is charted every half an hour recording the number of contractions in 10 minutes and the duration of each contraction in seconds. Contractions can be classified as mild (contraction duration less than 20 seconds), moderate (between 20 and 40 seconds), and strong (more than 40 seconds).

178. A 20-year-old woman presented at 7 weeks of gestation, unwilling to continue the pregnancy. What are the drugs used for medical termination of pregnancy in this patient? *(NEET 2022)*

a. Misoprostol and Medroxyprogesterone
b. Misoprostol and Mifepristone
c. Mifepristone and Methotrexate
d. Mifepristone and Medroxyprogesterone

Ans. is 'b' Misoprostol and Mifepristone

The drugs used for medical termination of pregnancy (MTP) in this patient presenting at 7 weeks of gestation are misoprostol and mifepristone.

Mifepristone 200 mg is administered orally on day 1. The minimum recommended interval between mifepristone & misoprostol is 24 hours.

24-48 hours later, misoprostol 800 mcg is administered by the vaginal, sublingual, or buccal route. Clinical confirmation of MTP is done On day 14.

The various methods of termination of pregnancy are:

Timing	*Medical methods*	*Surgical methods*
1st trimester (up to 12 weeks)	• Mifepristone • Mifepristone and misoprostol • Methotrexate and misoprostol • Tamoxifen and misoprostol	• Menstrual regulation • Vacuum aspiration (MVA/EVA) • Suction evacuation and/or curettage • Dilatation and evacuation: – Rapid method – Slow method
2nd trimester (13–20 weeks)	• Misoprostol • Mifepristone and misoprostol • Dinoprostone • Carboprost	• Dilatation and evacuation • Intrauterine instillation of hyperosmotic solutions • Oxytocin infusion • Hysterotomy

179. Testosterone helps in the development of various organs in the fetus. Which of the following stimulates its production? *(NEET 2022)*

a. LH from maternal pituitary
b. hCG from placenta
c. Inhibin from corpus luteum
d. GnRH from fetal hypothalamus

Ans. is 'b' hCG from placenta

- Human chorionic gonadotropin (hCG) from placenta stimulates the production of testosterone in the male fetus.
- hCG released from the placenta is the initial stimulus for testosterone production in the male fetus. Later by the eighth week of gestation, fetal pituitary LH (luteinizing hormone) stimulates the leydig cells of the testes to produce testosterone.
- Sex differentiation of the embryo depends on the Y chromosome, which contains the testis- determining gene called the SRY (sex-determining region on Y) gene, in a genetically male embryo (46, XY), the gonad is converted into testis under the influence of this gene. Female development occurs in the absence of this gene.

- Testosterone released from the leydig cells acts on the wolffian duct to develop vas deferens, epididymis, and seminal vesicles. Testosterone is converted to dihydrotestosterone (DHT) with the help of 5-alpha-reductase which helps in the differentiation of male external genitalia.
- The sertoli cells of the seminiferous tubules of tests secrete antimullerian hormone (AMH)/Mullerian inhibiting substance (MIS) by 7 weeks of gestation. It causes regression of the mullerian duct and prevents the development of the uterus, fallopian tube, and upper vagina.

ORTHOPEDICS

180. MC complications of untreated radial head dislocation: *(NEET 2022)*

a. Cubitus varus
b. Cubitus valgus
c. Damage to ulnar nerve
d. Myositis ossificans

Ans. is 'b' Cubitus valgus

- Most common complication: nonunion—Cubitus Valgus
- Malunion (rare) if present leads to cubitus varus
- Nerve involvement in cubitus valgus leads to Tardy ulnar nerve palsy

181. A patient presented with multiple swelling in hand & wrist. Finger X-ray is given. Identify: *(NEET 2022)*

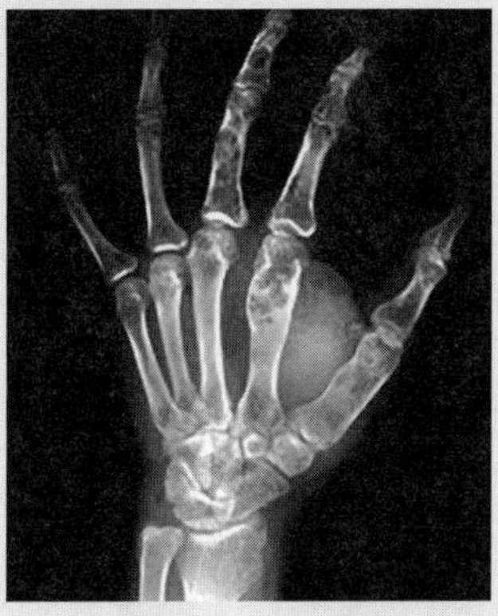

a. Multiple Endochromatosis
b. Multiple Brown Tumour
c. Multiple Osteophytic Growth
d. None of the above

Ans. is 'a' Multiple Endochromatosis

Enchondroma

- Medullary cavity tumour
- Metaphysical tumour
- Most common tumour of *bones* hand and feet
- 5% premalignant
- *Treatment:* Extended Curettage + bone grafting

OLLIERS: Multiple enchondromas all over the body

Maffucci

- Calcified superficial veins = phlebolith
- Enchondromas in bone
- Hemangiomas

182. Which will be the ideal treatment module for Fibular Fracture? *(NEET 2022)*

a. Analgesic-closed reduction-cast
b. Neurological assessment-analgesic
c. Neurological testing-CRIF
d. Neurological assessment-analgesic-cast

Ans. is 'd' Neurological assessment-analgesic-cast

Fibular fracture treated in the following sequence: Neurological assessment-analgesiccast @fibular neck—common peroneal nerve so associated with palsy fracture is stabilised with cast.

183. Given the radiograph of a 13-year-old child presented with fall on elbow. Which of the bone has a fracture? *(NEET 2022)*

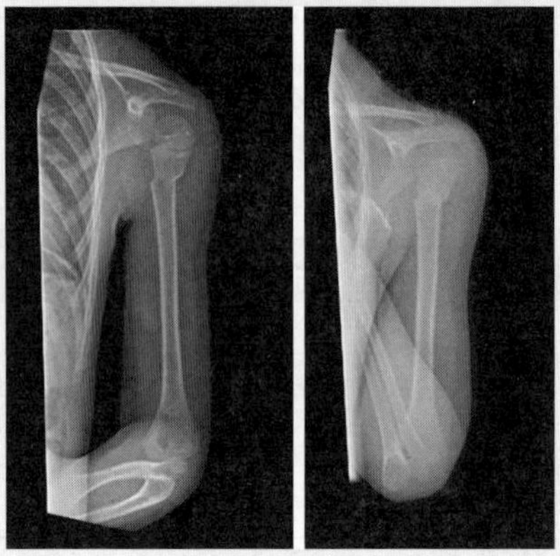

a. Humerus
b. Clavicle
c. Scapula
d. Ribs

Ans. is 'a' Humerus

The image shows fracture of the upper end of humerus.

184. Identify the condition and the instrument: *(NEET 2022)*

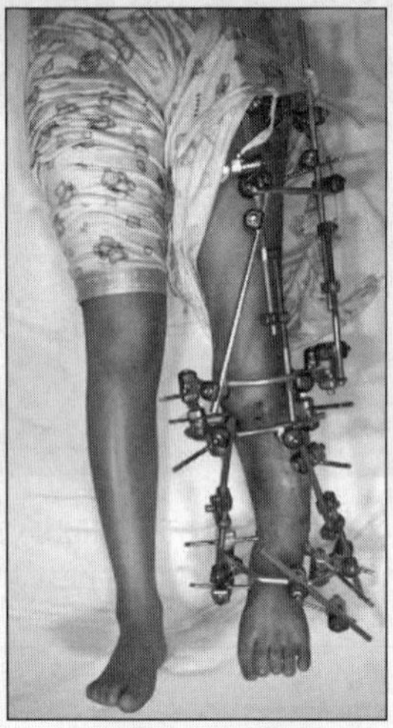

a. Tibia fracture, ilizarov fixator
b. Femoral fracture, spanning fixator
c. Tibia fracture, spanning fixator
d. Periarticular fracture of knee, spanning fixator

Ans. is 'd' Periarticular fracture of knee, spanning fixator

- *Rule of immobilisation:* Immobilise one joint above and 1 joint below the main target
- *Femur fracture:* Fixation at hip joint and knee joint
- *Tibia fracture:* Fixation at knee joint and ankle joint
- *Periarticular Knee fracture:* Fixation at hip joint and ankle joint

185. Which of the following condition will cause intermittent breaking of long bones in a child? *(NEET 2022)*

a. Achondroplasia
b. Marfan Syndrome
c. Osteogenesis Imperfecta
d. Cretinism

Ans. is 'c' Osteogenesis Imperfecta

Osteogenesis Imperfecta

- Autosomal dominant
- Most common cause of multiple fractures in childhood
- Aka Lobstein-Vrolik brittle bone disease
- *Cause:* Defect in type 1 collagen formation
- *Prenatal diagnosis:* Abnormal Pro a chain

- Skeleton—white crumpled-bone shaped not maintained
- *Clinical features:* Blue sclera, deafness, dentinogenesis imperfect
- SILLENCE classification
- *Treatment:* Gene therapy, SOFIELD MILLER surgery (SEEKH KEBAB surgery)

186. Patient check came in emergency department with #galeazzi. With sharp ends. Soft tissue swelling was seen on wrist on X-ray. Management in emergency? *(NEET 2022)*

a. Check vascularity, close reduce, check vascularity, pop cast
b. Check vascularity, close reduce, external fix
c. Check vascularity, close reduce, pop slab
d. Open reduce internal fix

Ans. is 'c' Check vascularity, close reduce, pop slab

Galeazzi Fracture

- Lower half of radius + dislocation of Radioulnar junction + Interosseous membrane damage + triangular fiber cartilage complex
- *Emergency management:* Check vascularity, close reduction and POP slab
- *Definitive management:* Open reduction and internal fixation along with stabilisation of distal radio-ulnar joint with K-wires

PSYCHIATRY

187. A patient consumed a large number of TCA pills during the depressive episode and presented with altered sensorium, hypotension and ECG showed wide QRS complexes. What is the next best step in the treatment? *(NEET 2022)*

a. DC Cardioversion
b. Start antiarrhythmic drug
c. $NAHCO_3$
d. None of the

Ans. is 'c' $NAHCO_3$

Side-effects of TCA pills;

- Anticholinergic effects
- Histamine receptor blocking
- Alpha adrenergic receptor blocking
- Seizures
- Arrhythmia
- Metabolic acidosis

Altered sensorium, hypotension and wide QRS complex are due to metabolic acidosis therefore treated with $NAHCO_3$.

188. After 5 days of normal vaginal delivery, a woman is brought to casualty by her husband. He reported that she has been crying all night. There's a history of loss of appetite, difficulty in sleeping and feeling low. General physical examination is unremarkable and there are no significant findings in the pelvic examination. Which of the following is the best term to describe her condition? *(NEET 2022)*

a. Postpartum blues
b. Postpartum depression
c. Postpartum anxiety
d. Postpartum psychosis

Ans. is 'a' Postpartum blues

Diagnosis	*Duration*	*Clinical features*	*Treatment*
Postpartum blues	<2 weeks	Tearfulness	Tearfulness No treatment required
PP depression	<4 weeks	Low mood >2 weeks Anhedonia Guilt Suicidal	Antidepressant + ECT
PP psychosis	<4 weeks	Depression + delusions/hallucinations Infanticide (risk)	Antidepressant + ECT + separation of baby from mother

189. A 16-year-old female was referred for irresistible urge to eat (cravings) following by episodes of self-induced vomiting. The patient is also on appetite suppressants. What's the most likely diagnosis? *(NEET 2022)*

a. Bulimia nervosa
b. Anorexia nervosa
c. Pica disorder
d. Binge eating disorder

Ans. is 'a' Bulimia nervosa

Key features of bulimia nervosa:

- Normal weight individual
- Binge eating followed by Post binge anguish followed by compensation by vomiting or purging
- No avoidance of food

Anorexia nervosa:

- Underweight individual
- Body image preoccupation
- Morbid fear of gaining weight

Binge eating disorder

Only binge eating, no compensation

RADIOLOGY

190. A middle aged male patient presented with acute onset pain in right limb. An investigation was performed. What is the name of the investigations? *(NEET 2022)*

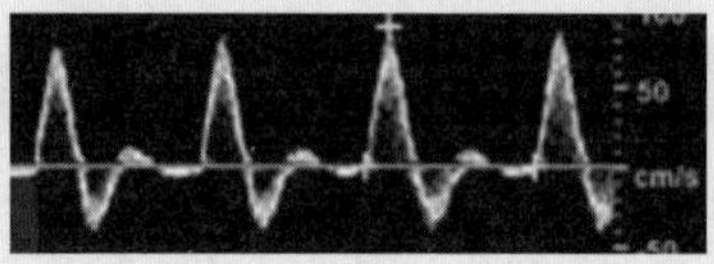

a. Digital subtraction angiography
b. Ultrasound Doppler
c. Plethysmography
d. MR Angiography

Ans. is 'b' Ultrasound Doppler

- Image given shows triphasic waveform = USG Doppler
- Indications of DOPPLER USG
  - DVT
  - Varicose veins
  - Portal hypertension
  - Carotid Doppler-screening atherosclerosis
  - Fetal Doppler
  - AV fistula for hemodialysis
  - Renal stenosis in young patients

Color Doppler:

- Color indicates direction (red = towards the transducer and BLUE = away from transducer/probe)
- Intensity indicates the speed

191. A 35-year-old female presented with fever, expectoration and difficulty breathing. HRCT of chest was performed and shown. What is the likely diagnosis? *(NEET 2022)*

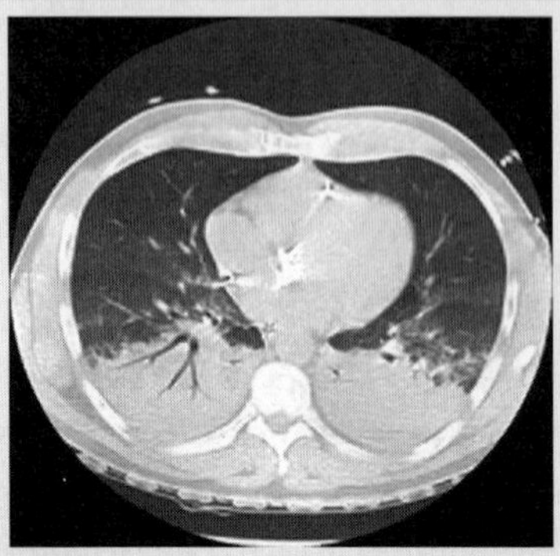

a. Mediastinal mass
b. Pleural effusion
c. Diaphragmatic hernia
d. Consolidation with air bronchogram

Ans. is 'd' Consolidation with air bronchogram

HRCT image of lungs is given in the question

White B/L consolidation with black – air bronchogram

192. Name the investigation shown: *(NEET 2022)*

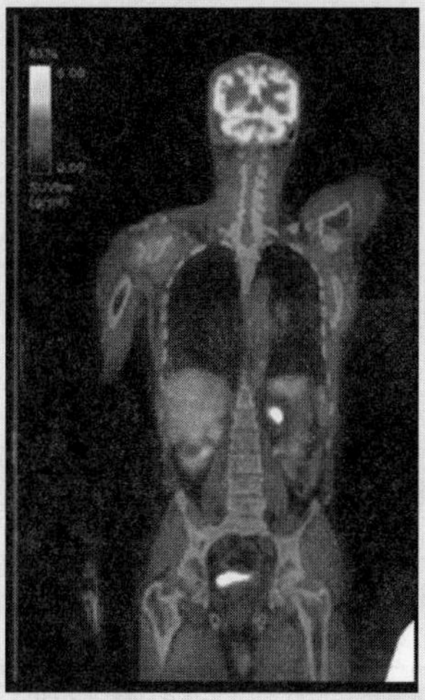

a. PET-CT

b. Technetium scan

c. Cerebral flow study

d. Tc sestamibi scan

Ans. is 'a' PET-CT

PET-CT

- *Radiotracer dye:* FDG 18-positron emitter
- *Principle:* Annihilation coincidence circuit
- *Physiological uptake:* Brain and urinary bladder

193. A 25-year-old patient presented with fever dry cough, breathlessness and night sweats. On chest X-ray, bilateral hilar lymphadenopathy was seen. What is the most likely cause? *(NEET 2022)*

a. Hypersensitive pneumonitis

b. Sarcoidosis

c. Lymphoma

d. Tuberculosis

Ans. is 'b' Sarcoidosis

- Panda sign @face
- Lambda sign @lungs

Lofgren Syndrome Triad

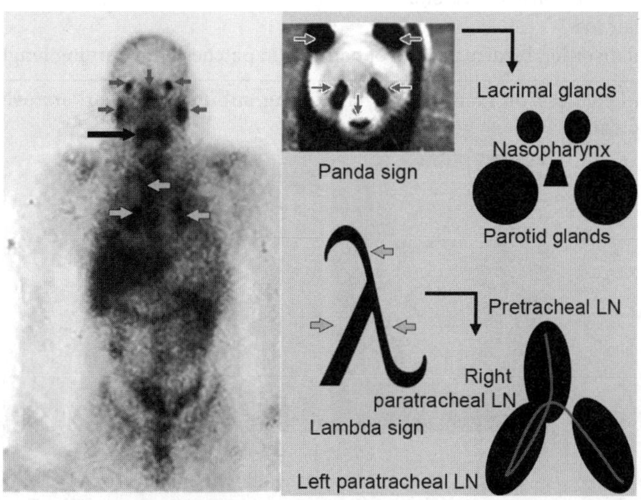

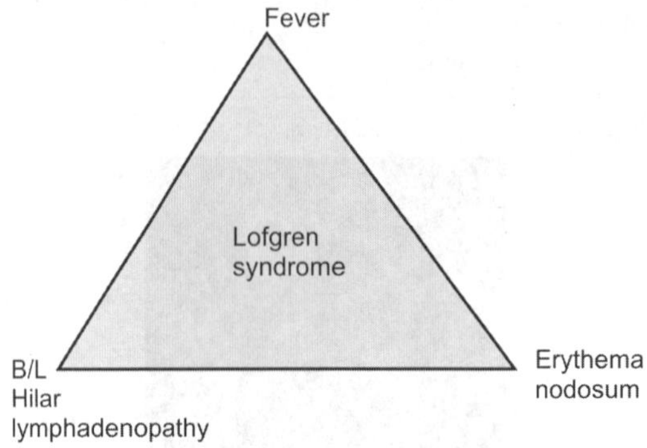

DERMATOLOGY

194. A female presented with hair loss since 1 month, given history of COVID 8 weeks back, what is the most likely diagnosis? *(NEET 2022)*

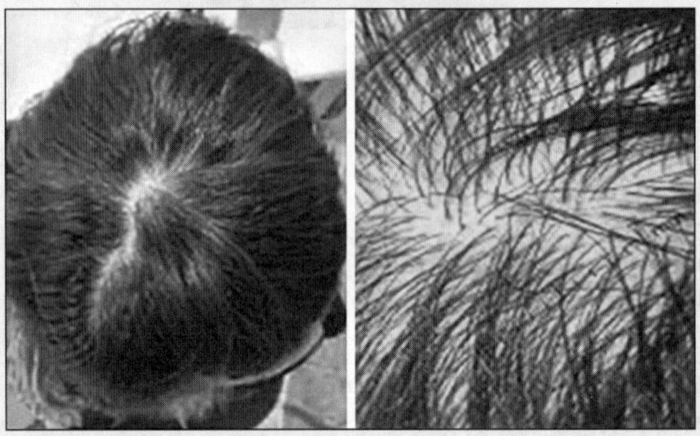

a. Telogen effluvium
b. Trichomania
c. Anagen effluvium
d. Androgenic alopecia female pattern

Ans. is 'a' Telogen effluvium

❖ *Anagen effluvium:* Seen in patients of Chemotherapy
❖ *Telogen effluvium:* Seen 3–4 months after pregnancy, major surgery, chronic illness, stress
❖ *Androgenic alopecia:*
  - Male pattern: Bilateral temporal hairline recession
  - Female pattern: Diffuse hair loss
  - Trichomania: Behavioural disorder; bizarre pattern of hair loss in patches with varying lengths.

195. A patient came in with nail changes, on examination nail pitting, subungual hyperkeratosis, and oil drop changes are seen, what is the probable diagnosis? *(NEET 2022)*

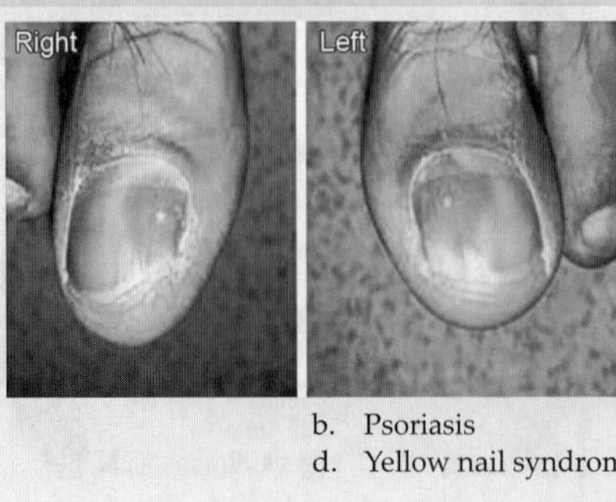

a. Lichen planus
b. Psoriasis
c. Onchomycosis
d. Yellow nail syndrome

Ans. is 'b' Psoriasis

Features of Nail Psoriasis

- Pitting@ proximal nail matrix
- *Salmon Patch/Oil Drop sign:* Pathognomonic
- Subungual hyperkeratosis
- Splinter haemorrhage
- Thinning & ridging

Yellow Nail Syndrome

Triad

- Yellow nail discolouration
- Pleural effusion
- Lower limb lymphoedema

196. The given skin condition is seen in which of the following disorder? *(NEET 2022)*

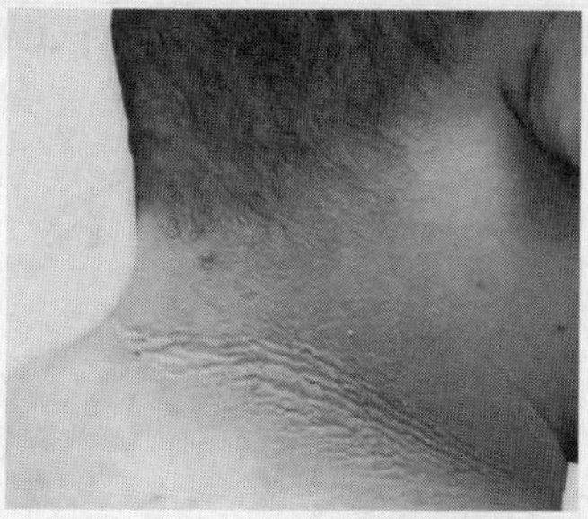

a. Addison's disease
b. Metabolic syndrome
c. Thyroid disorder
d. All of the above

Ans. is 'd.' All of the above

- The given image shows acanthosis nigricans which is associated with obesity and insulin resistance, e.g., metabolic syndrome.
- Acanthosis is diffuse epidermal hyperplasia (thickening of the skin).
- Implies increased thickness of the Malpighian layer (stratum basale and stratum spinosum).
- Occurs primarily in flexural areas as velvety hyperpigmentation.
- Commonly seen in axilla.
- May be a reflection of endocrinopathy such as acromegaly, Cushing's syndrome, polycystic ovarian syndrome and GIT malignancy.

197. A patient undergoing treatment of borderline tuberculoid leprosy presents with lesion on forehead, nose and extending to bilateral cheeks. What is the most common nerve affected in this patient? *(NEET 2022)*

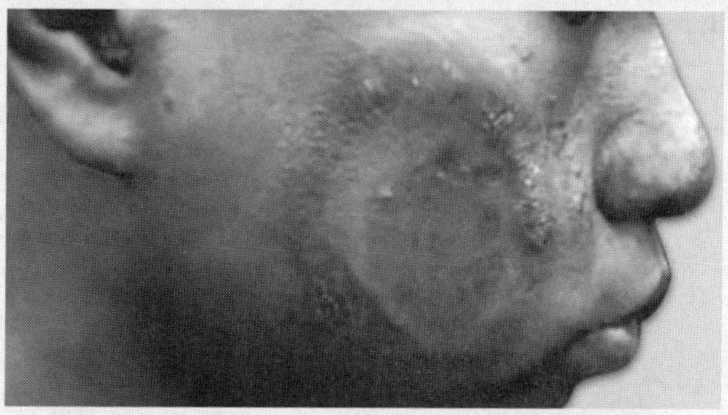

a. Trochlear nerve
b. Abducent nerve
c. Ulnar nerve
d. Trigeminal nerve

Ans. is 'd' Trigeminal nerve

Trochlear and abducting nerves supply the extra ocular muscles.

Ulnar nerve is an upper limb nerve.

The lesion defined as on the forehead, nose and extending to bilateral cheeks is along the course of the trigeminal nerve.

198. What is the causative agent of anogenital wart? *(NEET 2022)*

a. HPV 2
b. HPV 11
c. HPV 15
d. HPV 18

Ans. is 'b' HPV 11

HPV 6 and 11

- Condyloma accuminatum
- Sinonasal papilloma
- Squamous papilloma of larynx

HPV 16 and 18

- LSIL, HSIL, carcinoma Cervix
- Carcinoma anogenital region

HPV 16: Vulvar carcinoma, Bowen disease

ANESTHESIA

199. Identify the following equipment which is often used for COVID-19 patients: *(NEET 2022)*

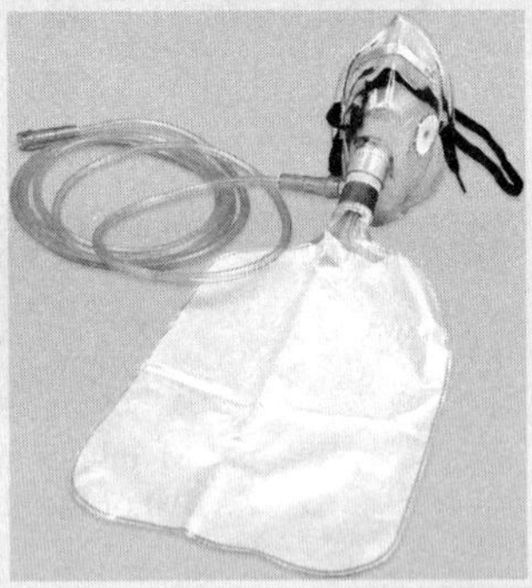

a. Venturi mask
b. Hudson mask
c. Nonrebreathing face mask
d. Nebulizer mask

Ans. is 'c' Nonrebreathing face mask

Oxygen therapy devices: High flow and Low flow

Low Flow

- Nasal cannula/prongs
- Simple Face mask/Hudson mask
- Non rebreathing facemask/Mask with reservoir bag

High Flow

- Venturi mask
- Ventilator
- CPAP
- Nebuliser
- Tracheostomy mask

Nasal Cannula

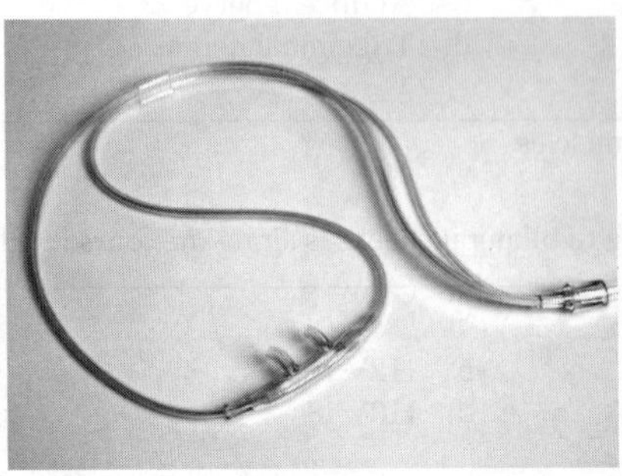

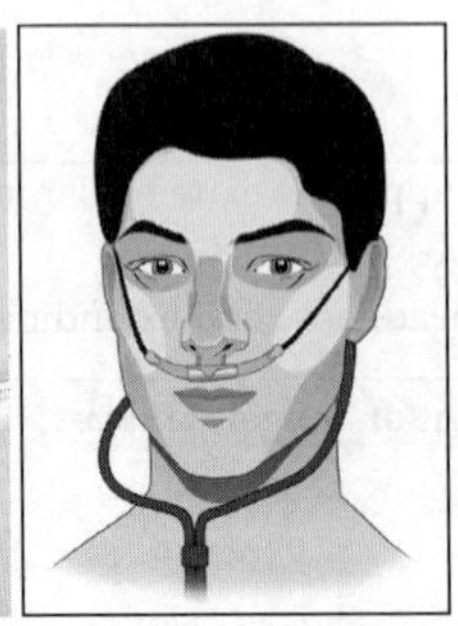

Non-Rebreather Mask

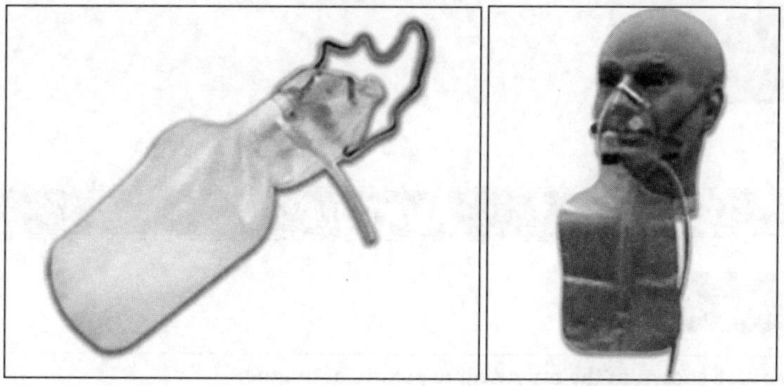

Simple Face Mask

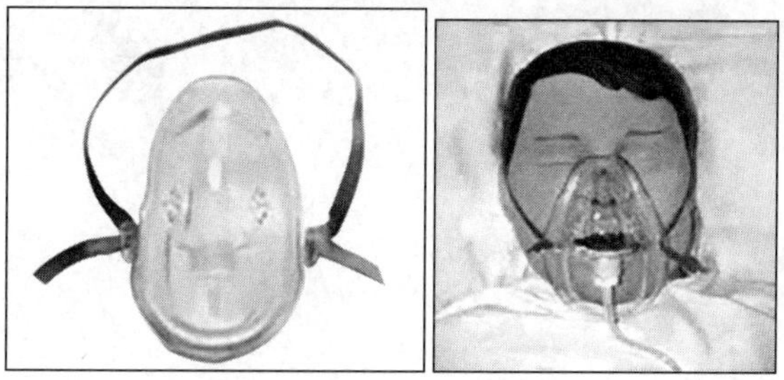

Venturi Mask

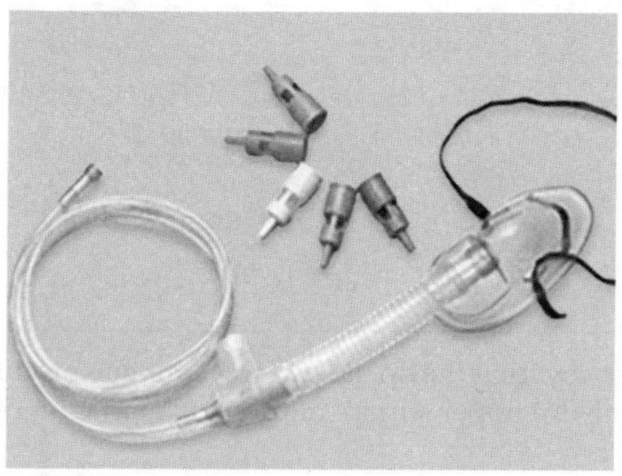

200. Identify the nerve being tested with the following monitoring procedure? *(NEET 2022)*

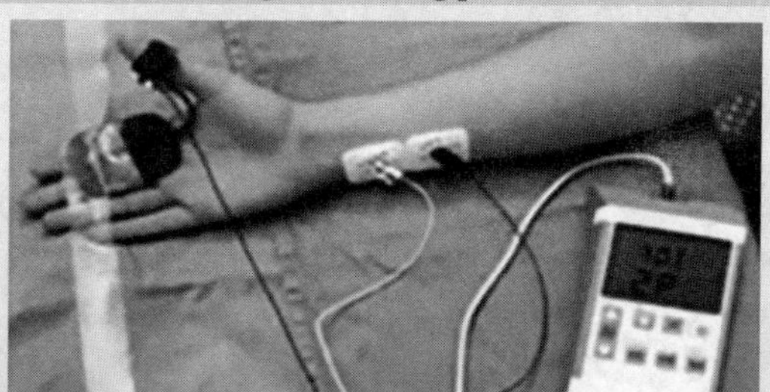

a. Ulnar
b. Radial
c. Median
d. Metacarpal

Ans. is 'a' Ulnar

- Ulnar nerve is tested for monitoring the neuromuscular block in anaesthetised patients. (TOF: train of four)
- 2 electrodes are placed over the skin area of ulnar nerve- 1 for stimulating the nerve and the other for recording it.

*Modified ALLEN's test is performed before cannulation of Radial Artery.

Recent NEET 2021

ANATOMY

NEET PG September 2021

1. Identify the type of papillae shown in the microscopic picture of tongue:

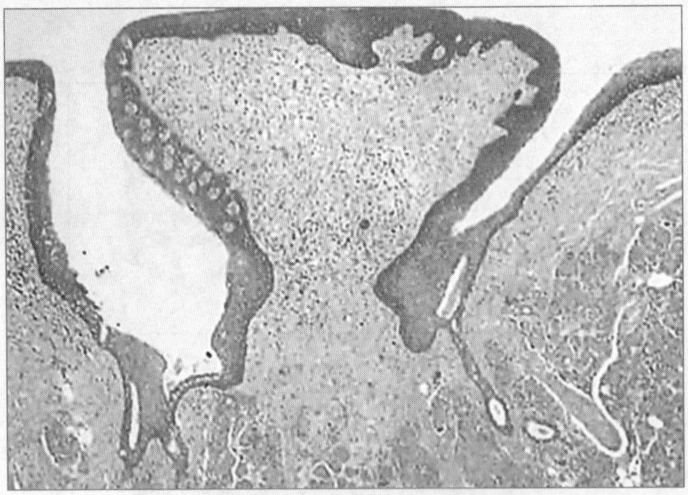

For colour version see Plate 1

a. Circumvallate
b. Fungiform
c. Filiform
d. Foliate

Ans. is 'a' Circumvallate

- Lingual papillae are projections of mucosa covering the dorsal surface of tongue producing roughness (friction) and increasing area of contact. They are limited to (present only in) upper surface of presulcal part (anterior 2/3rd) of tongue.

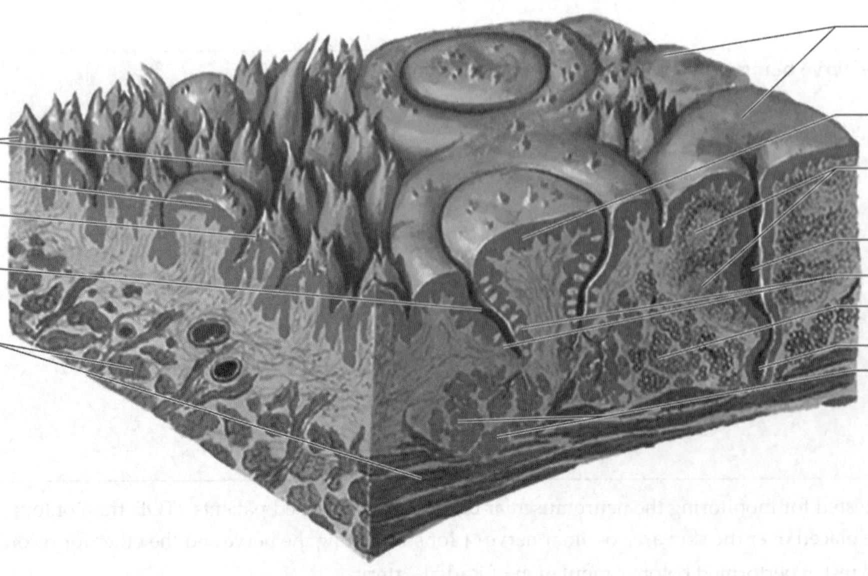

- Lingual papillae are of 4 types, named filiform, fungiform, foliate and circumvallate papillae, all except the filiform papillae bear the taste buds. All except circumvallate are innervated by chorda tympani (facial) nerve (for taste) and lingual nerve (general). Circumvallate papillae is innervated by glossopharyngeal nerve (both taste and general sensation). Foliate papillae are least developed in humans.
- Taste buds are numerous on all types of lingual papillae (except filiform papillae), particularly on their lateral aspects. However, tastes buds are not restricted to papillae and are scattered over almost the entire dorsal and lateral surfaces of tongue and rarely on epiglottis and soft palate (lingual aspect). Each taste bud (a paraneurone) is linked to one of three cranial nerve which carry taste i.e., facial glossopharyngeal or vagus.

2. A 30-year-old patient complaints of diminishing vision of right halves of both eyes. Where is the most probable lesion?

a. Right optic nerve
b. Optic chiasma
c. Left optic tract
d. Right occipital lobe

Ans. is 'c' Left optic tract

Functional and simulated visual loss

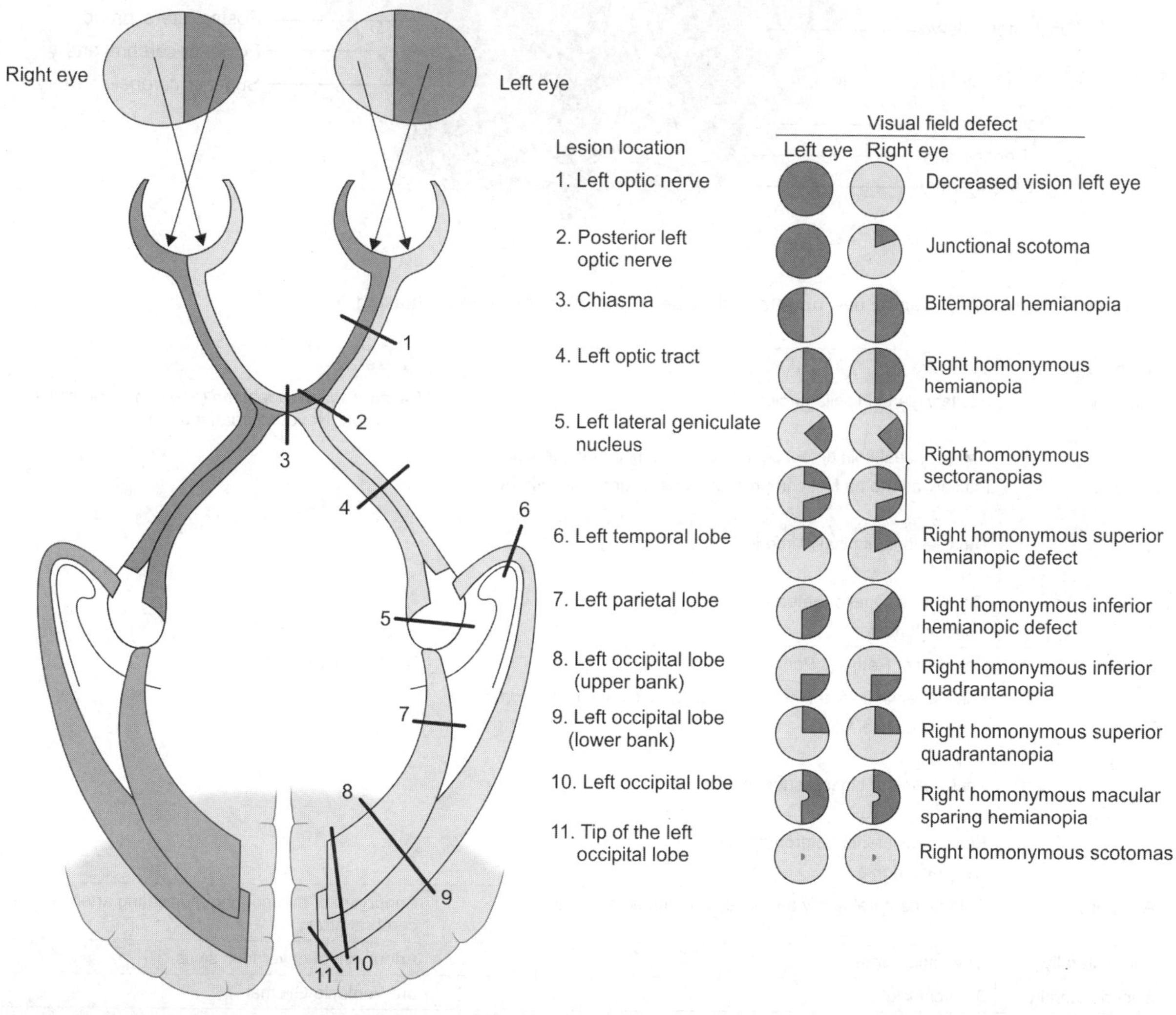

3. A patient presented with history of vision loss. On investigation an aneurysm was identified causing compression on the optic chiasma. Which of the following artery is most likely involved?

a. Anterior choroidal artery
b. Anterior communicating artery
c. Middle cerebral artery
d. Anterior cerebral artery

Ans. is 'b' Anterior communicating artery

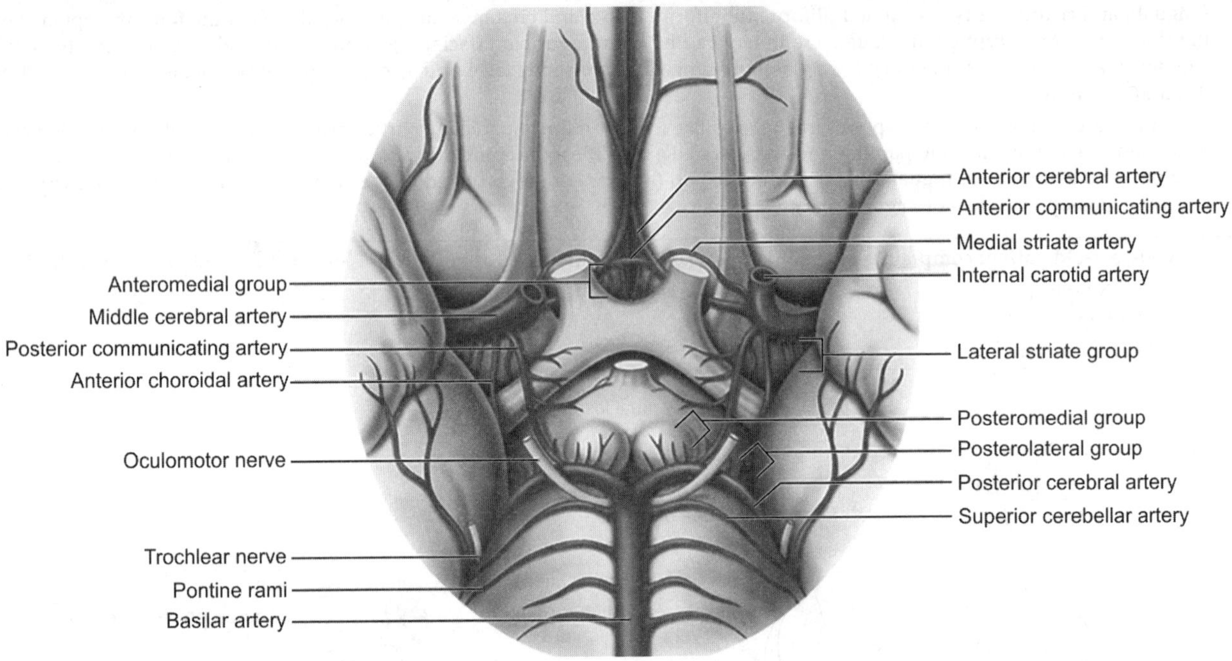

❖ **Bitemporal hemianopia:** Can be best understood by anatomic relations of optic chiasma

Relation	*Structure*	*Cause*
Inferiorly	Pituitary gland in sella turcica	Pituitary, macro adenoma (>10 mm) suprasellar extension (Never Microadenoma)
	Earliest visual field defect seen in cases of pituitary adenoma Pituitary adenoma first compresses the inferior binasal fibers ↓ Thus, lesions of binasal inferior fibres ↓ Bitemporal superior heteronymous Quadrantanopia	
Superiorly	Remnant of Rathke's Pouch	Craniopharyngioma
	Earliest visual field defect seen in cases of craniopharyngioma Superior binasal fibers ↓ Thus, lesion of binasal superior fibers ↓ Bitemporal inferior heteronymous Quadrantanopia	
Anteriorly	Anterior cerebral artery and anterior communicating artery	Aneurysm of anterior communicating artery > anterior cerebral artery
Inferolaterally	Cavernous sinus	Aneurysm of cavernous sinus
Superiolaterally	3rd Ventricle	3rd Ventricle Glioma

4. A patient has undergone submandibular gland excision and the Wharton's duct was ligated in the process. Which of the following nerve is most likely to be damaged during the process of ligating the duct?

a. Inferior alveolar nerve
b. Lingual nerve
c. Hypoglossal nerve
d. Marginal mandibular branch of facial nerve

Ans. is 'b' Lingual nerve

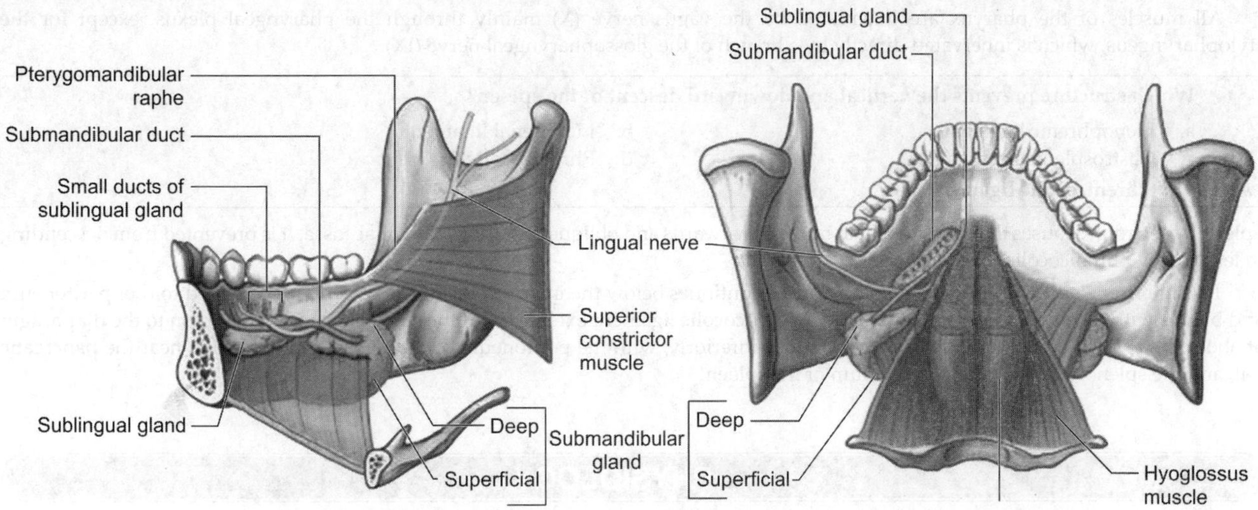

The **submandibular duct** emerges from the medial side of the deep part of the gland in the oral cavity and passes forward to open on the summit of a small **sublingual caruncle** (papilla) beside the base of frenulum of the tongue.

The lingual nerve loops under the submandibular duct, crossing first the lateral side and then the medial side of the duct, as the nerve descends anteromedially through the floor of the oral cavity and then ascends into the tongue.

5. A patient was admitted with skull base trauma and difficulty in swallowing. The doctor was touching the marked structure. Which of the following cranial nerve is being tested?

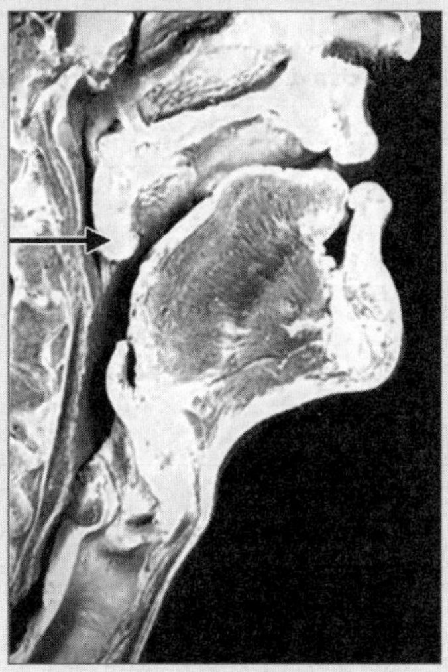

For colour version see Plate 1

a. X
b. IX
c. VII
d. V

Ans. is 'a' X

Motor and most sensory innervation (except for the nasal region) of the pharynx is mainly through branches of the vagus (X) and glossopharyngeal (IX) nerves, which form a plexus in the outer fascia of the pharyngeal wall.

The pharyngeal plexus is formed by:

- ❖ The pharyngeal branch of the vagus nerve (X);
- ❖ Branches from the external laryngeal nerve from the superior laryngeal branch of the vagus nerve (X);
- ❖ Pharyngeal branches of the glossopharyngeal nerve (IX).

The pharyngeal branch of the vagus nerve (X) originates from the upper part of its inferior ganglion above the origin of the superior laryngeal nerve and is the major motor nerve of the pharynx, in addition to carrying sensory information from the laryngopharynx.

All muscles of the pharynx are innervated by the vagus nerve (X) mainly through the pharyngeal plexus, except for the stylopharyngeus, which is innervated directly by a branch of the glossopharyngeal nerve (IX).

6. Which structure prevents the vertical and downward descent of the spleen?

a. Lienophrenic ligament
b. Lienorenal ligament
c. Gastrosplenic ligament
d. Phrenicocolic ligament

Ans. is 'd' Phrenicocolic ligament

Spleen hypertrophy causes the enlargement to move downwards and obliquely towards right iliac fossa. It is prevented from descending to left side by phrenicocolic ligament.

The anterior aspect of the gastrosplenic ligament continues below the inferior pole of the spleen as fan-shaped fold of peritoneum and blends with the phrenicocolic ligament. The phrenicocolic ligament extends from the splenic flexure of the colon to the diaphragm at about the level of the eleventh rib. It is continuous inferiorly, with the peritoneum of the transverse mesocolon near the pancreatic tail, and the splenorenal ligament at the hilum of the spleen.

PHYSIOLOGY

NEET PG September 2021

7. Following are the levels of various ions in a body fluid. Identify the fluid ~Na^+ = 10 mEq/L, K^+ = 140 mEq/L, Cl^- = 15 mEq/L, HCO_3^- = 12 mEq/L:

a. ICF
b. Plasma
c. Interstitial fluid
d. CSF

Ans. is 'a' ICF

Ion	*Cell (ICF) in mOsm/L*	*ISF in mOsm/L*	*Blood (ECF) in mOsm/L*
K^+	140 (max cation)	4	4.2
Na^+	14	139	145 (max cation)
Cl^-	4	108	108 (max anion)
HCO_3^-	10	28	24
HPO_4, H_2PO_4	11/max anion	2	2
Protein	4	0.2	1.2
Ca^{2+}	<0.0002	1.2	1.8
Mg^{2+}	20	0.7	1.5
Corrected osmolar activity (mOsm/L)	281	281	282
Total osmotic pressure at 37° C (mmHg)	5423	5423	5443

8. Tetany will result from which of the following disorder?

a. Metabolic acidosis
b. Respiratory alkalosis
c. Hyperoxemia
d. Hypercalcemia

Ans. is 'b' Respiratory alkalosis

Alkalosis, by promoting the binding of calcium to albumin, can reduce the fraction of ionized calcium in blood, causing tetany. Symptomatic hypocalcemia is more common with respiratory alkalosis than with metabolic alkalosis.

9. Cardiovascular findings in a patient were as follows: large 'a' wave on JVP, mid-diastolic murmur. Pedal edema+. The most probable diagnosis is:

a. MS
b. MR
c. TS
d. TR

Ans. is 'c' TS

Types

Name	Diagram	Causes
I. Systolic Murmurs		
1. Ejection Systolic/ Mid-systolic/ Crescendo-Murmurs	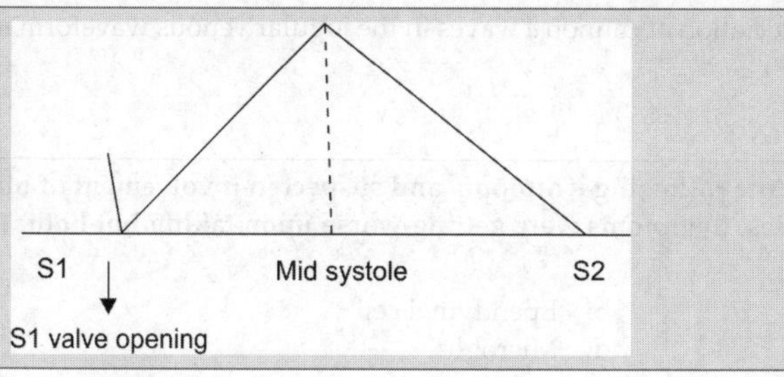	Turbulence during ejection phase ↓ AS, PS High CO states HOCM CoA
2. Pan systolic Murmur	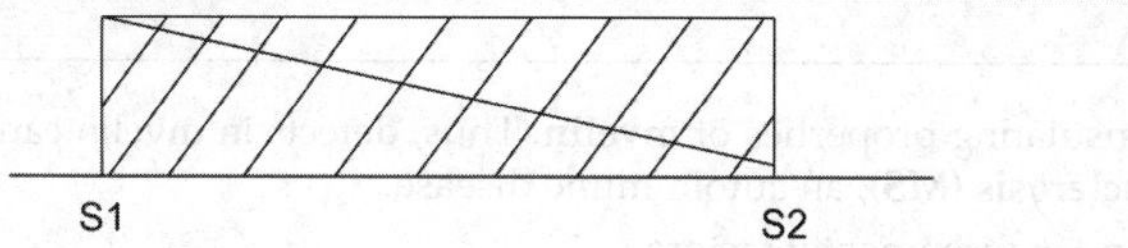	Ventricular septal defect (LV pressure >> RV pressure) Throughout systole • Chronic mitral regurgitation on LV pressure >> LA pressure throughout systole (cooing/seagull like) • Chronic TR to RV pressure >> RA pressure throughout systole. (intensified on inspiration – Carvallo sign)
3. Early systolic [Will stop ≤ Mid systole]	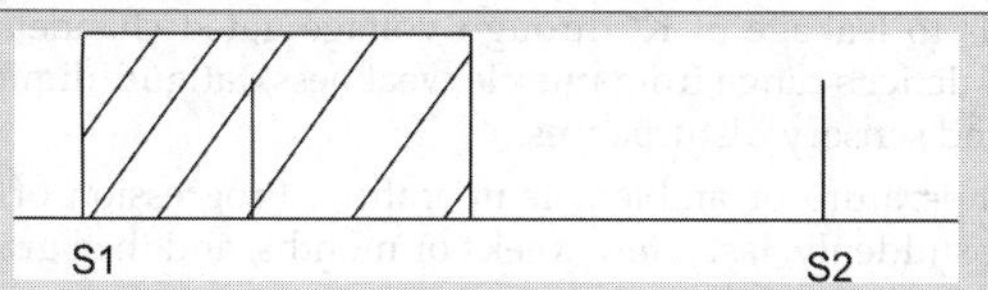 or 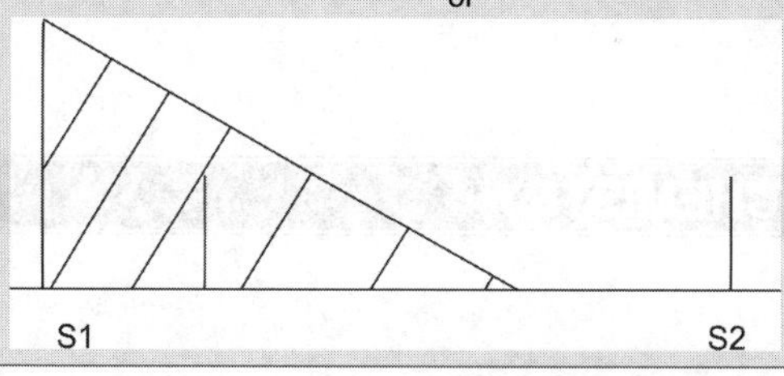	If defect closes ≤ mid systole • Small muscular VSD If pressure gradient becomes zero ≤ mid systole • Acute mitral regurgitation or acute TR (LA/RA not dilated) [Unlike chronic] During early systole → LV blood enters LA and LA pressure rises rapidly During mid systole → LA pressure = LV pressure [Murmur will stop]
4. Late systolic starts ≥ mid systole	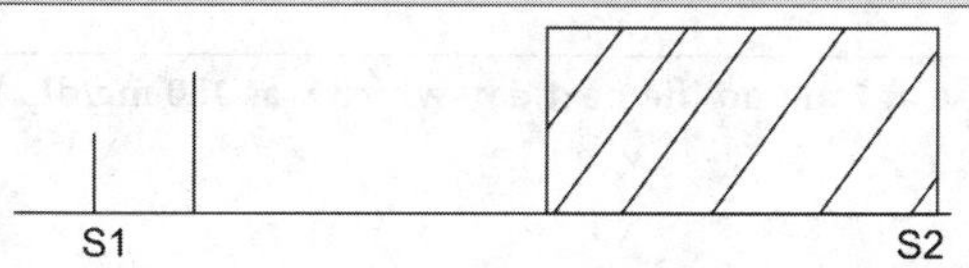	Mitral valve prolapsed [whooping/konking type heard best @apex]
II. Diastolic Murmurs		
1. Early Diastolic = decrescendo	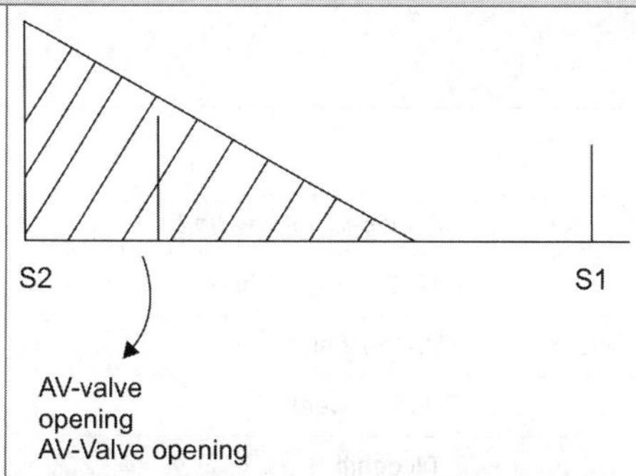 AV-Valve opening	Aortic regurgitation Pulmonary regurgitation
2. Mid Diastolic	Presystolic accentuation (atrial contraction) 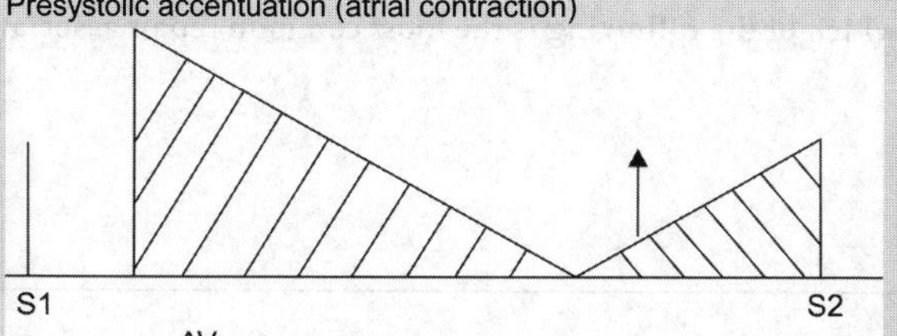	Turbulence of blood flow across AV valve ↓ MS, TS

The *a* wave reflects right atrial presystolic contraction and occurs just after the electrocardiographic P wave, preceding the first heart sound (S1).

A prominent *a* wave is seen in patients with reduced right ventricular compliance; a cannon *a* wave occurs with atrioventricular (AV) dissociation and right atrial contraction against a closed tricuspid valve.

In a patient with a wide complex tachycardia, the appreciation of cannon *a* waves in the jugular venous waveform identifies the rhythm as ventricular in origin.

The *a* wave is not present with atrial fibrillation.

10. Neurologic examination of a patient revealed the following ~ diplopia and suspected involvement of other cranial nerves, tingling and numbness in the lower extremities. Symptoms were getting worse upon taking hot both. Defect of which of the following cells is the most likely causes?

a. Oligodendrocyte
b. Ependymal cell
c. Astrocyte
d. Microglia

Ans. is 'a' Oligodendrocyte

Normal conduction of action potentials relies on the insulating properties of **myelin.** Thus, defects in myelin can have major adverse neurological consequences. One example is **multiple sclerosis (MS),** an autoimmune disease.

The cause of MS appears to include both genetic and environmental factors.

In MS, antibodies and white blood cells in the immune system attack myelin, causing inflammation and injury to the sheath and eventually the nerves that it surrounds. Loss of myelin leads to leakage of K^+ through voltage gated channels, hyperpolarization, and failure to conduct action potentials. Typical physiological deficits range from muscle weakness, fatigue, diminished coordination, slurred speech, blurred or hazy vision, bladder dysfunction, and sensory disturbances.

Symptoms are often exasperated by increased body temperature or ambient temperature. Progression of the disease is quite variable. In the most common form, transient episodes appear suddenly, last a few weeks or months, and then gradually disappear.

Oligodendrocytes and **Schwann cells** are involved in myelin formation around axons in the CNS and peripheral nervous system, respectively.

BIOCHEMISTRY

NEET PG September 2021

11. A person had a meal at 8 pm and records blood glucose at 7 am on the next day which was 180 mg/dL. What is the source of glucose in this patient?

a. Dietary glucose
b. Hepatic gluconeogenesis
c. Hepatic glycogenolysis
d. Muscle glycogenolysis

Ans. is 'c' Hepatic glycogenolysis

Compensatory mechanisms during starvation

Process	*Provides energy up to*
Glycogenolysis	12–24 (avg. 18 hrs)
Gluconeogenesis (from glutamine and alanine from skeletal muscles)	Up to 72 hrs
FA oxidation and KB synthesis	Up to 2 weeks
Proteolysis of structural proteins	Till death

12. A patient who is diagnosed case of HNPCC, which of the following is the most common repair associated with it?

a. Mismatch repair
b. Base excision repair
c. Nucleotide excision repair
d. Homologus recombinant repair

Ans. is 'a' Mismatch repair

For detail see explanation on page 124 Table

13. This multienzyme complex converts Pyruvate to Acetyl CoA. Identify E1 and E2:

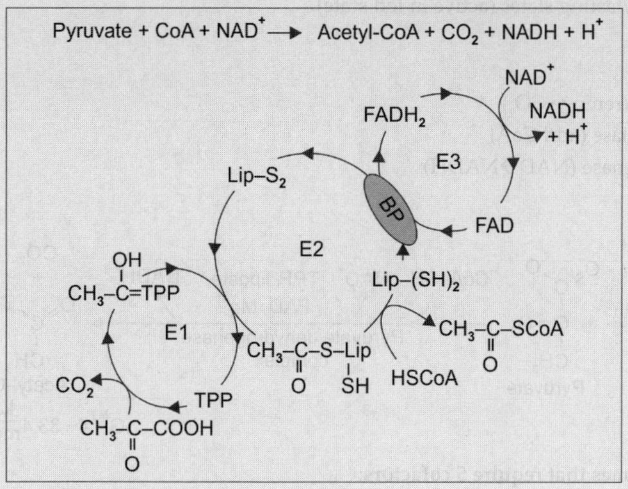

a. E1: Pyruvate dehydrogenase E2: Dihydrolipoyl transacetylase
b. E1: Pyruvate decarboxylase E2: Dihydrolipoyl dehydrogenase
c. E1: Pyruvate carboxylase E2: Dihydrolipoyl transacetylase
d. E1: Pyruvate dehydrogenase E2: Dihydrolipoyl dehydrogenase

Ans. is 'a' E1: Pyruvate dehydrogenase E2: Dihydrolipoyl transacetylase

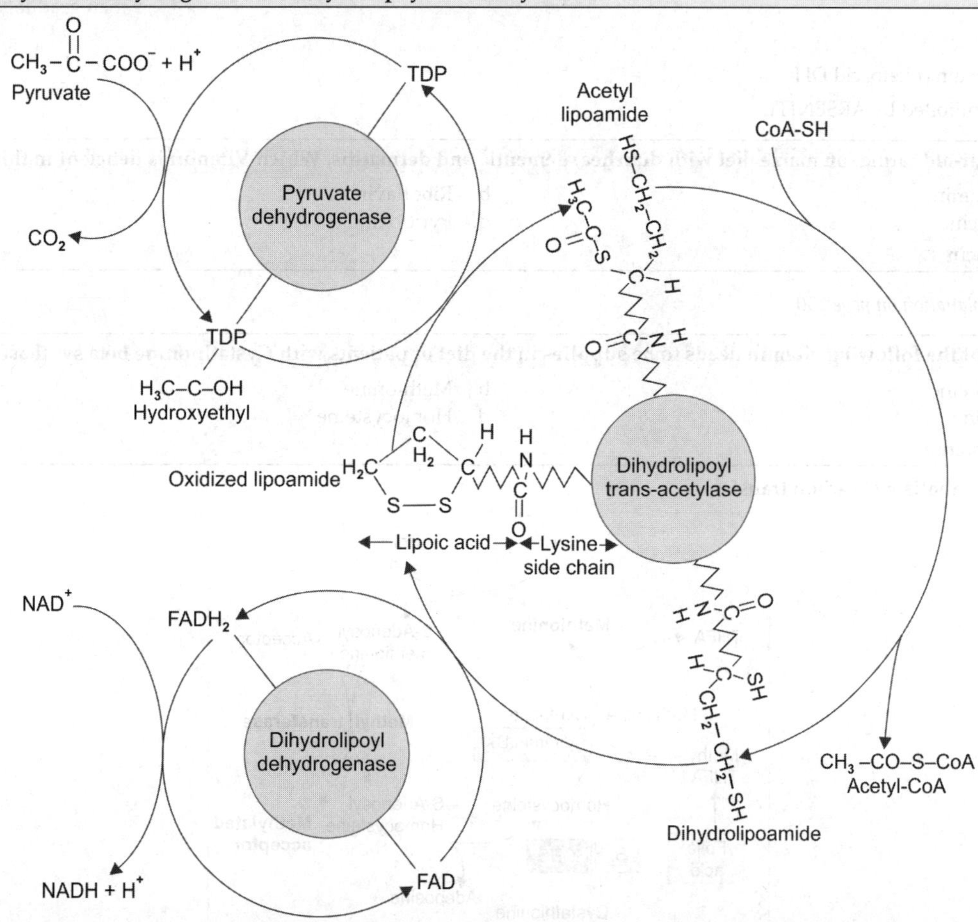

Oxidative decarboxylation of pyruvate by the pyruvate dehydrogenase complex. Lipoic acid is joined by amide link to a lysine residue of the transacetylase component of the enzyme complex. It forms a long flexible arm, allowing the lipoic acid prosthetic group to rotate sequentially between the active sites of each of the enzymes of the complex. (FAD, Flavin adenine dinucleotide; NAD^+, nicotinamide adenine dinucleotide; TDP, thiamin diphosphate)

PDH is Mitochondrial enzyme complex linking glycolysis and TCA cycle.

Differentially regulated in fed/fasting states (active in fed state).

Components

- Pyruvate dehydrogenase (remove CO_2)
- Dihydrolipoyl Transacetylase (add CoA)
- Dihydrolipoyl Dehydrogenase (NAD→NADH)

Reaction

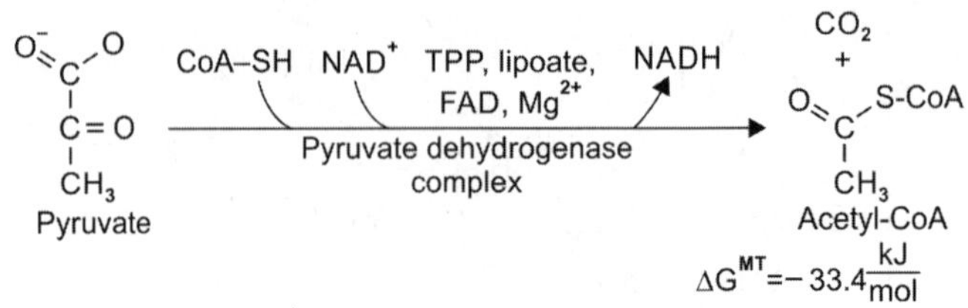

The complex contains 3 enzymes that require 5 cofactors:

- Thiamine pyrophosphate (B1)
- Lipoic acid
- CoA (B5, pantothenic acid)
- FAD (B2, riboflavin)
- NAD+ (B3, niacin)

Lipoic acid dependant enzymes:

- PDH
- αKG DH
- Branched chain α ketoacid DH

Lipoic acid → inhibited by ARSENITE

14. A 35-year-old farmer on maize diet with diarrhea, dementia and dermatitis. Which Vitamin is deficient in this patient?

a. Thiamine
b. Riboflavin
c. Niacin
d. Pyridoxine

Ans. is 'c' Niacin

For detail see explanation on page 130

15. Which of the following vitamin needs to be supplies in the diet of patients with Cystathionine beta synthase defect?

a. Cysteine
b. Methionine
c. Serine
d. Homocysteine

Ans. is 'a' Cysteine

Methionine metabolism (1 carbon transfer)

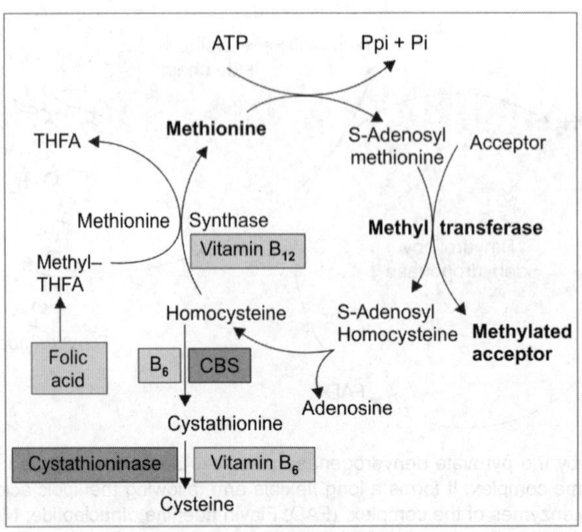

(CBS- cystathionine β synthase)

Disease	Defect/deficiency	Features
Homocysteinemia type 1	Cystathionine β synthase	• MR • Charlie Chaplin gait • Inferomedial ectopia lentis • IV thrombosis (due to thiolactone adducts)
Homocysteinemia type 2	Methyl THFA reductase	
Homocysteinemia type 3	Methionine synthase	
Homocysteinemia type 4	Dietary B12 deficiency	

16. A patient has multiple tendon xanthomas. Serum cholesterol (398 mg/dL) and LDL (220 mg/dL) were found to be raised. Statins were given to this patient. What is the diagnosis?

a. Lipoprotein lipase deficiency
b. Familial hypercholesterolemia
c. Tangier's disease
d. Huntington's disease

Ans. is 'b' Familial hypercholesterolemia

For detail see explanation on page 115 Table

17. A patient presented with weakness, anemia, bony pain and hepatosplenomegaly. Which of the following enzyme is deficient?

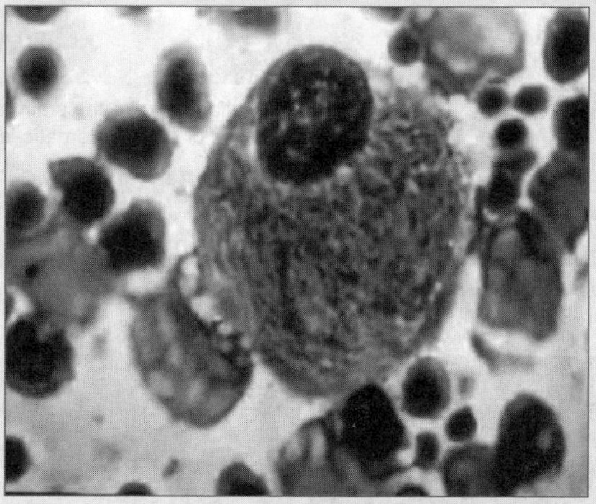

For colour version see Plate 1

a. Glucose 6 phosphatase
b. Gluco-cerebrosidase
c. Hexosaminidase A
d. Alpha galactosidase

Ans. is 'b' Gluco-cerebrosidase

Sphingolipidoses for lipid storage diseases

No	Disease	Enzyme defect	Lipid accumulating	Salient features
1.	Gaucher's disease	β-glucosidase	Glucocerebroside	3 types—adult, infantile, juvenile hepatosplenomegaly, erosion of bone, moderate anemia
2.	Niemann-Pick disease	Sphingomyelinase	Sphingomyelin	Severe CNS damage, mental retardation, hepatosplenomegaly, Cherry red spot in macula. Death occurs by 2 years of age
3.	Krabbes leukodystrophy	β-galactosidase	Galactocerebroside	Severe mental retardation. Total absence of myelin in CNS Globoid bodies in white matter
4.	Metachromatic leukodystrophy	Sulfatidesulfatase	Sulfogalactocerebroside	Accumulates in most tissues. Neurological deficit, difficult in speech and optic atrophy. Demyelination is also seen
5.	Fabry's disease	α-galactosidase	Ceramide trihexoside	Kidney is the site of accumulation. Progressive renal failure, death by 5 years of age. Purplish papules appear. 'X' linked inheritance
6.	Tay Sach's disease	Hexosaminidase A	Ganglioside (GM2)	Incidence 1 in 6000 births. Mental retardation. Cherry red spot in the macula. Progressive deterioration. Death by 3–4 years
7.	Generalized gangliosidoses	β-galactosidase	Ganglioside (GM1)	Mental retardation, hepatomegaly, skeletal deformities. Foam cells in bone marrow. Cherry red spot in the retina
8.	Lactosyl ceramidoses	β-galactosidase	Lactosyl ceramide	Mainly CNS and reticuloendothelia system affected
9.	Sandhoff's disease	Hexosaminidase A and B	Globoside	Neurological deficit, mental retardation

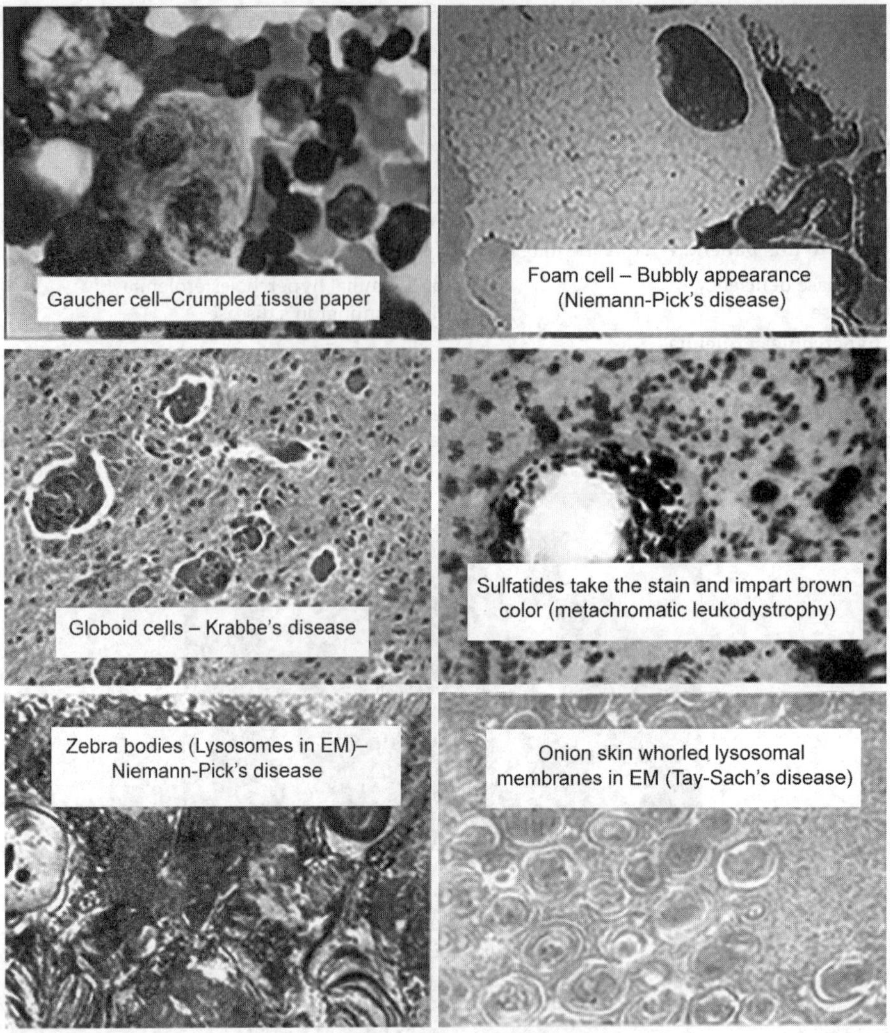

For colour version see Plate 2

18. Transparency of corneal endothelium is maintained by:

a. Heparan sulphate
b. Keratan sulphate
c. Chondroitin sulphate
d. Hyaluronic acid

Ans. is 'b' Keratan sulphate

Glycosaminoglycans

Proteoglycan	*Repeated units*	*Location*
Hyaluronic acid	Glucuronic acid + NAG	Only GAG that is NON-SULFATED Synovial fluid, vitreous Role in cell migration
Chondroitin sulfate	Glucuronic acid + NAGal	Commonest GAG Cartilages, tendons
Heparan sulfate	Glucuronic acid + sulfoglucosamine	ECM
Heparin	Iduronic acid + sulfoglucosamine	Only intracellular within organs and monocytes
Dermatan sulfate	Iduronic acid + NAGal	Skin, heart valves Blood vessels Sclera—gives shape to eye
Keratan sulfate	Galactose + NAG	Only GAG with NO URONIC ACID Type-1: Cornea, hair nails, horns, claws Type-2: Cartilage

19. Which vitamin deficiency causes this?

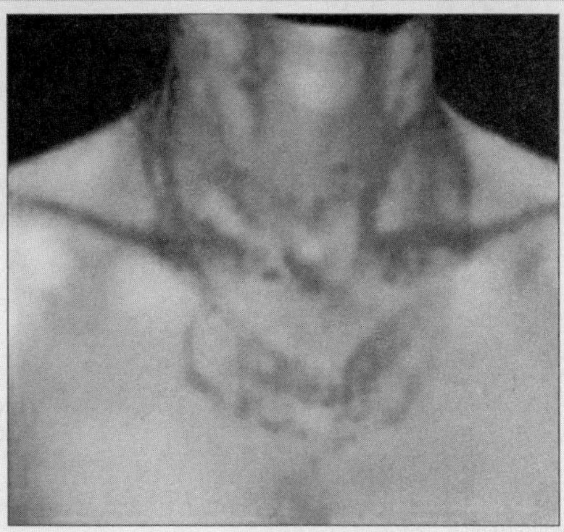

a. Thiamine
b. Niacin
c. Zinc
d. Pyridoxine

Ans. is 'b' Niacin

For detail see explanation on page 130

20. A 25-year-old patient presented with dark urine, which further blackens on exposure to air. What is the enzyme defect in this case?

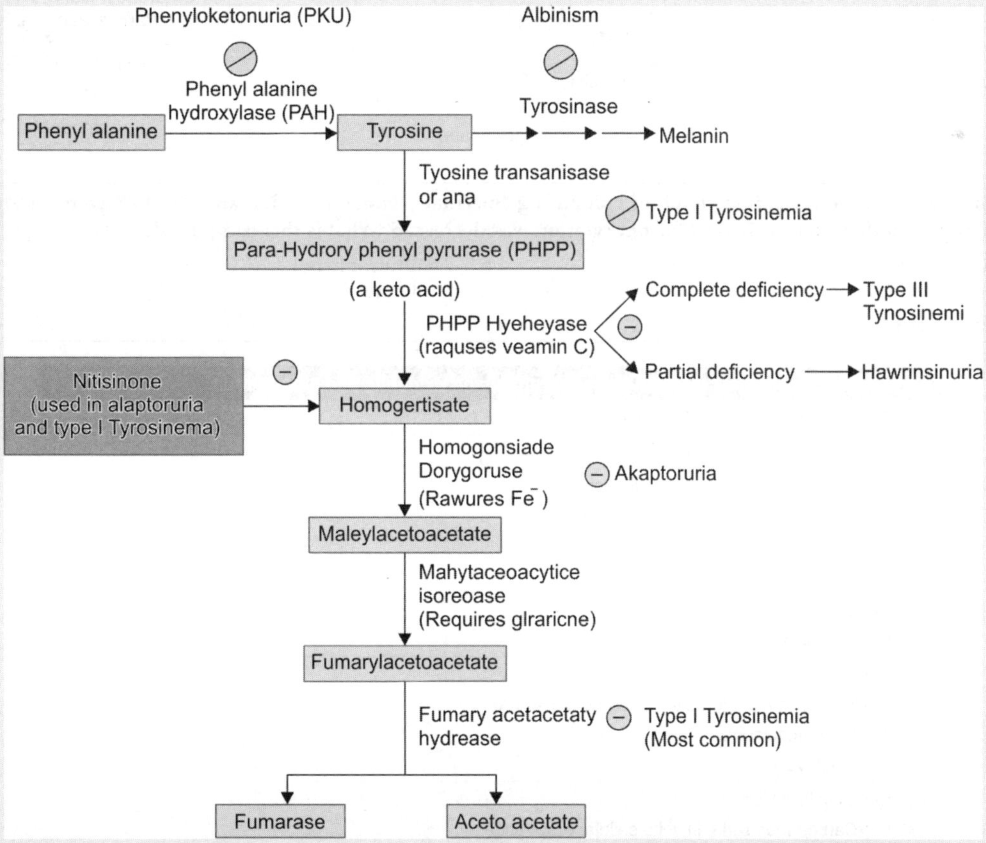

a. Fumaryl acetoacetate hydrolase
b. Dihydroxy phenyl acetate dioxygenase
c. Homogentisate dehydrogenase
d. Phenyl alanine hydroxylase

Ans. is 'b' Dihydroxy phenyl acetate dioxygenase

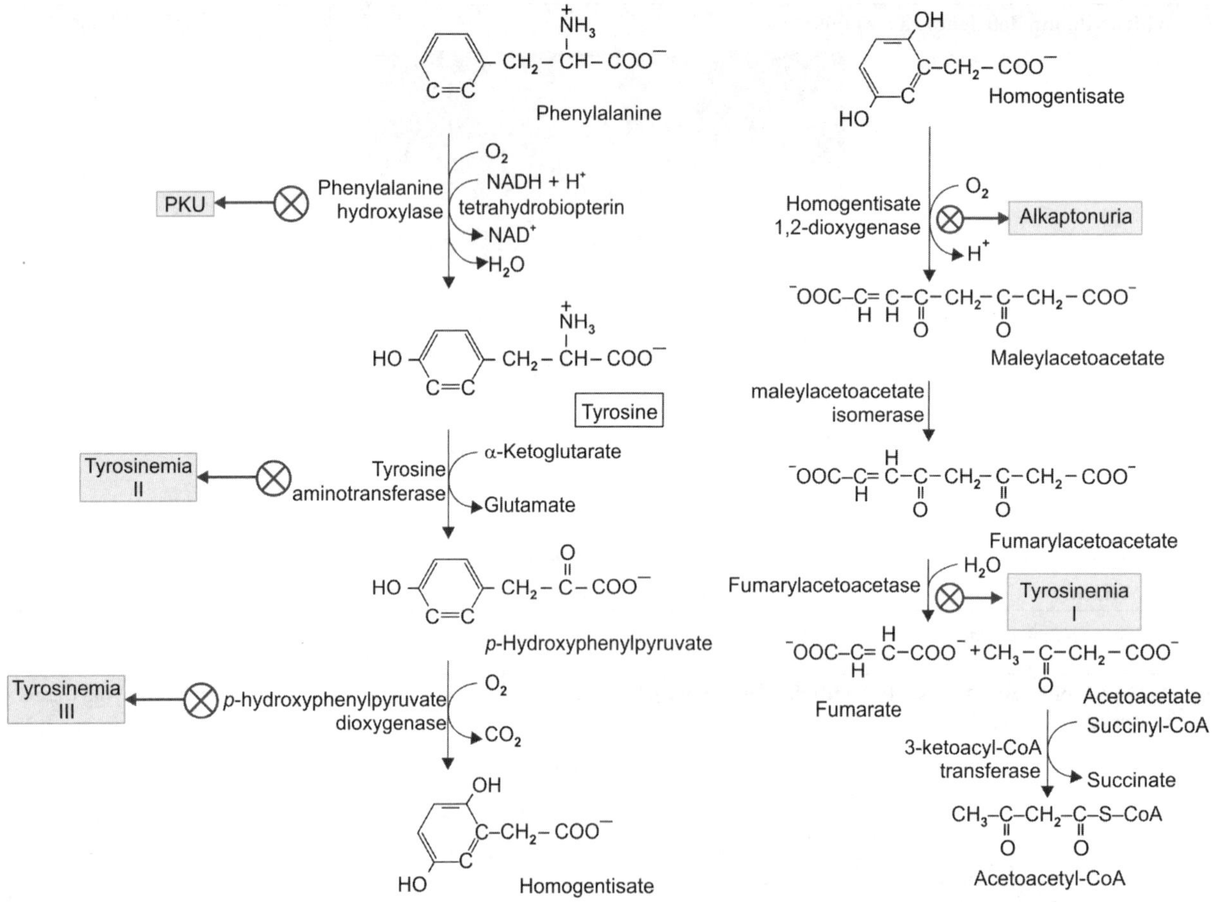

21. In an isolated mitochondria, in a medium containing Succinate, Fumarate, ADP and Pi, ATP were produced. Later a compound was added, and oxidative phosphorylation was decreased. What is that compound?

a. **Oligomycin**
b. 2,4 dinitrophenol
c. Antimycin
d. Rotenone

Ans. is 'a' Oligomycin

Compounds which affect electron transport chain and oxidative phosphorylation	
1.	Complex I to Co-Q specific inhibitors
	i. Alkylguanides (guanethide), hypotensive drug ii. Rotenone, insecticide and fish poison iii. Barbiturates (amobarbital), sedative iv. Chlorpromazine, tranquilizer v. Piericidin, antibiotic
2.	Complex II to Co-Q I. Carboxin
3.	Complex II to cytochrome c inhibitors i. Bal (British anti-lewisite), antidote of war gas ii. Naphthoquinone iii. Antimycin
4.	Complex IV inhibitors i. Carbon monoxide, inhibits cellular respiration ii. Cyanide (CN^-) iii. Azide (N_3^-) iv. Hydrogen sulfide (H_2S)

Contd...

Contd…

	Compounds which affect electron transport chain and oxidative phosphorylation
5.	Site between succinate dehydrogenase and Co-Q i. Carboxin, inhibits transfer of ions from $FADH_2$ ii. Malonate, competitive inhibitor of succinate DH
6.	Inhibitors of oxidative phosphorylation i. Atractyloside, inhibits translocase ii. Oligomycin, inhibits flow of protons through Fo iii. Ionophores, e.g. valinomycin
7.	Uncouplers i 2, 4-dinitrophenol (2, 4-DNP) ii. 2, 4-dinitrocresol (2, 4-DNC) iii. CCCP (chlorocarbonylcyanidephenyl hydrazone)
8.	Physiological uncouplers i. Thyroxine, in high doses ii. Thermogenin in brown adipose tissue

22. Night blindness history, corneal drying and patient has Bitot's spots. Which of the following is found in this patient?

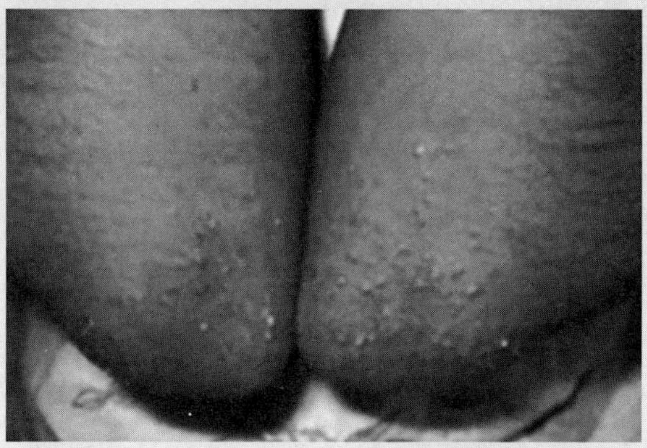

a. Keratosis pilaris rubra
b. Eczema
c. Phrynoderma
d. Icthyosis

Ans. is 'c' Phrynoderma

For detail see explanation on page 128

23. A 4-year-old boy presented with developmental delay, recurrent chest infections and worsening bony pain. Serum PTH was normal. Calcium was normal and phosphate was low. There is no response to Vitamin D. The probable diagnosis is:

a. Nutritional rickets
b. X-linked hypophosphatemia rickets
c. Vitamin D dependent rickets type I
d. Vitamin D dependent rickets type II

Ans. is 'b' X-linked hypophosphatemia rickets

	Biochemical criteria	*Clinical signs/symptoms*	*Treatment effect*	*Radiologic signs of rickets*
Nutritional rickets	(ab)25 *(OH) D available*: 25(OH)D < 125 nmol/L or 25(OH)D: 12.5-25 nmol/L and at least one of the following: • ↑ALP (c) • ↑PTH (d) • ↓Ca (e) No 25(OH)D measures: At least one of the following: • ↑ALP • ↑PTH • ↓Ca	*Infants and young children* At least one of the following: • Craniotabes • Rachitic rosary • Harrison groove • Enlargement of the wrists, knees or ankles • Bowing of weight bearing extremities • Hypocalcemic seizures *Adolescents:* • At least one of following: Enlargement of the wrists, knees or ankles; bowing of legs • Muscles weakness • Pain of the lower limbs or in the back • Hypocalcemic seizures	Heals on vitamin D treatment	Widening of the growth plates with irregularity and cupping of their metaphyseal borders

	Biochemical criteria	Clinical signs/symptoms	Treatment effect	Radiologic signs of rickets
Vitamin D Resistant rickets	All of the following: • ↑ALP • ↑PTH • ↓↔Ca • ↓PO_4(f) • 1,25(OH)2D(g)<15 pmol/L • 25(OH)D: 50–178 nmol/L			
Hypophosphatemic rickets	All of the following: • ↑ALP • ↔PHT • ↓PO_4 • ↔Ca	At least one of the following: • Rachitic rosary • Harrison groove • Enlargement of the wrist, knees or ankles Bowing of weight bearing extremities Pain of the lower limbs	Refractory to vitamin D	

(a) Definition of stages of vitamin D insufficiency (124):
- 25(OH)D <50 nmol/L: Vitamin D insufficiency
- 25(OH) D: 12.5-25 nmol/L vitamin D deficiency
- 25(OH)D <12.5 nmol/L: Severe vitamin D deficiency

(b) 25 (OH)D: 25-hydroxy vitamin D
(c) ALP; Alkaline phosphatase
(d) PTH: Parathyroid hormone
(e) Ca: Calcium
(f) PO_4 Phosphate
(g) 1,25 $(OH)_2$ D: 1.25-dihydroxy vitamin D

24. A child is presented with multiple times loose stools. He is managed with ORS. Glucose in ORS is absorbed via which transporter in GIT?

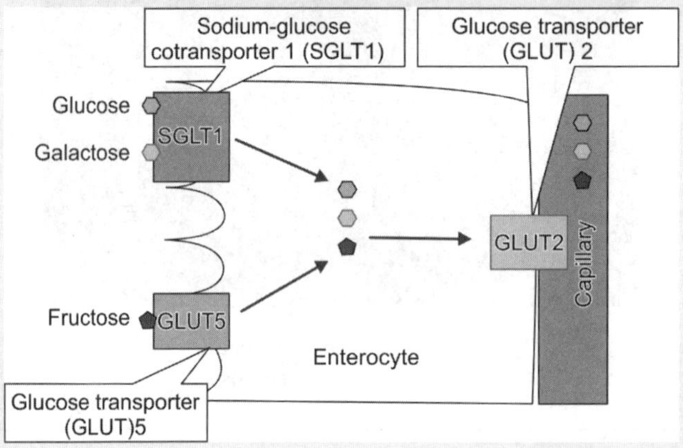

a. **SGLT-1**
b. SGLT-2
c. GLUT-4
d. GLUT-2

Ans. is 'a' SGLT-1

For detail see explanation on page 110

PATHOLOGY

NEET PG September 2021

25. A patient with squamous cell carcinoma of lung has undergone pulmonectomy. During the procedure blackish hilar lymph node of 1 cm is seen. Identify the cause of pigmentation:

a. Anthracotic pigment
b. Hemosiderosis
c. Lipofusion
d. Melanin

Ans. is 'a' Anthracotic pigment

The most common exogenous pigment is *carbon*, a ubiquitous air pollutant of urban life. When inhaled, it is phagocytosed by alveolar macrophages and transported through lymphatic channels to the regional tracheobronchial lymph nodes. Aggregates of the pigment blacken the draining lymph nodes and pulmonary parenchyma (*anthracosis*)

26. A chronic alcoholic patient presented with increasing abdominal grith and decreased liver span. Liver biopsy featuring hepatocytes with reddish inclusions. What is in the content of the inclusions?

a. Actin
b. Intermediate filaments
c. Microtubules
d. Fibronectin

Ans. is 'b' Intermediate filaments

See detail explanation on page 214

27. A 56-year-old man was working in a benzene factory for a long time. He got retired 5 years before. What would be the possible complication in this patient?

a. Bladder cancer
b. Blood cancer
c. Lung cancer
d. Skin cancer

Ans. is 'b' Blood cancer

Chemical Carcinogens

Carcinogen	*Means of exposure/sources*	*Associated cancer*
Aflatoxin (from Aspergillus)	Ingestion of maize of peanuts grown in hot/humid climates	Hepatocellular carcinoma in association with hepatitis B virus
Alkylating agents	Oncology chemotherapy	Malignant lymphoma
Arsenic	Herbicides (common in vineyard workers), fungicides, animal dips; metal smelting; intentional/accidental poisoning	Squamous cell carcinoma of skin, lung cancer, liver angiosarcoma
Azo dyes	Used in paints, printing inks, varnishes, leather products, carpets, food products	Hepatocellular carcinoma
Asbestos	Roofing material (roofers with over 20 years of experience have had contact with this); insulation for pipes in ships in shipyards, old homes; old cars with brake liners	Bronchogenic carcinoma (most common), pleural mesothelioma
Benzene	Component of light oil; used in printing industry, dry cleaning, paint, adhesives and coatings	Acute leukemia, Hodgkin lymphoma
Beryllium	Used in the space industry (missile fuel and space vehicles; metal alloys in aerospace appliances and nuclear reactors)	Bronchogenic carcinoma
Cadmium	Industrial industries where one is being smelted; electroplating; welders who have welded on cadmium-containing alloys or worked with silver solders; found in some batteries	Prostate and lung cancer
Cyclophosphamide	Chemotherapy agent	Transitional cell carcinoma of urinary bladder
Diethylstilbesterol	Once used to treat women with threatened abortions	Daughters exposed to mothers who took DES may develop clear cell carcinoma of vagina/cervix
B-Naphthylamine (aniline dyes) and aromatic amines	Workers in the rubber, chemical, leather, textile, metal, and printing industries	Transitional cell carcinoma of urinary bladder
Nickel	Nickel plating, by product of stainless steel welding, ceramics, batteries, spark plugs	Bronchogenic carcinoma, nasal cavity cancer
Oral contraceptives	Birth control pill	Breast and cervical cancer, hepatic adenoma
Polycyclic hydrocarbons	These are formed when coal, soot (chimney sweeper), wood, gasoline, oil, tobacco, or other organic material are burned'; also formed in food when fish or meats are charbroiled on an open flame	Squamous cell carcinoma; skin (scrotum with soot in chimney sweeper), oral cavity midesophagus, larynx, lung Adenocarcioma; distal esophagus, pancreas, kidney Transitional cell carcinoma; urinary bladder renal pelvis
Polyvinyl chloride	Found in plastic piping material, adhesive plastics, refrigerant	Liver angiosarcoma
Radon and decay products	By-product of decay of uranium, hazard in quarries and underground mines	Bronchogenic carcinoma
Silica	Chemical of silicon dioxide, rock quarries, sandblasting	Bronchogenic carcinoma

28. A 30-year-old women on pap smear having disorganized growth of the cells with hyperchromatic nuclei. What phenomenon is occurring here?

a. Dysplasia
b. Metaplasia
c. Hypertrophy
d. Carcinoma

Ans. is 'a' Dysplasia

For detail explanation see on page 162

29. In a patient of iron deficiency anemia, all of the following increases except:

a. TIBC
b. RBC protoporphyrin
c. Transferrin saturation
d. Transferrin receptor

Ans. is 'c' Transferrin saturation

Iron stores Erythron iron	Normal	Negative iron balance	Iron-deficient erythropoiesis	Iron-deficiency anemia
Marrow iron stores	1–3+	0–1+	0	0
Serum ferritin (μg/L)	50–200	<20	<15	<15
TIBC (μg/L)	300–360	>360	>380	>400
SI (μg/L)	50–150	NL	<50	<30
Saturation (%)	30–50	NL	<20	<10
Marrow sideroblasts (%)	40–60	NL	<10	<10
RBC protoporphyrin (μg/L)	30–50	NL	>100	>200
RBC morphology	NL	NL	NL	Microcytic/hypochromic

30. A 12 year patient with history of recurrent infection and bleeding gums. On investigations the patient had pancytopenia and the peripheral smear showed macrocytes. The bone marrow biopsy showed no megakaryocytes and filled with fat globules. What is your diagnosis?

a. Myelodysplasia
b. Aplastic anemia
c. ITP
d. PNH

Ans. is 'b' Aplastic anemia

Aplastic Anemia

- **Aplastic anemia refers to a syndrome of chronic primary hematopoietic failure and attendant** ***pancytopenia*** (anemia, neutropenia, and thrombocytopenia).
- In the majority of patients autoimmune mechanisms are suspected, but inherited or acquired abnormalities of hematopoietic stem cells also seem to contribute in at least a subset of patients.
- **The markedly hypocellular bone marrow is largely devoid of hematopoietic cells; often only fat cells, fibrous stroma, and scattered lymphocytes and plasma cells remain. Marrow aspirates often yield little material (a "dry tap"); hence, aplasia is best appreciated in marrow biopsies.**
- **Initial manifestations vary somewhat, depending on which cell line is predominantly affected, but pancytopenia ultimately appears, with the expected consequences. Anemia can cause progressive weakness, pallor, and dyspnea; thrombocytopenia is heralded by petechiae and ecchymoses; and neutropenia manifests as frequent and persistent minor infections or the sudden onset of chills, fever, and prostration.**
- **Splenomegaly is characteristically absent; if it is present, the diagnosis of aplastic anemia should be seriously questioned.**
- **The red cells are usually slightly macrocytic and normochromic.**
- **Reticulocytopenia is the rule.**
- The prognosis is variable. Bone marrow transplantation is the treatment of choice in those with a suitable donor and provides a 5-year survival of more than 75%. Older patients or those without suitable donors often respond well to immunosuppressive therapy.

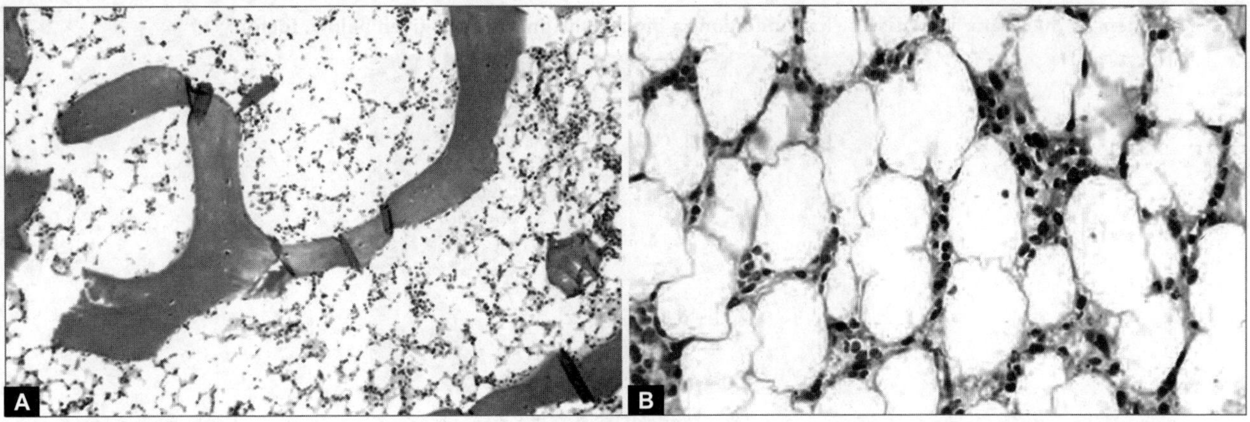

Aplastic anemia (bone marrow biopsy). Markedly hypocellular marrow contains mainly fat cells. (A) Low power; (B) High power.
(For colour version see Plate 2)
Courtesty: Dr. Steven Kroft, Department of Pathology, University of Texas Southwestern Medical School, Dallas, Texas)

31. A patient who has been eating junk food regularly for few months and avoid fruits and vegetables. His Hb is 9 g/dL MCV is >125 fL. What is the deficiency she would likely having?

a. Folate deficiency
b. Cyanocobalamin deficiency
c. Sideroblastic anemia
d. Acute blood loss

Ans. is 'a' Folate deficiency

For detail explanation see on page 178 Table

32. A 20-year-old female presented with webbed neck and shielded chest, which of the following investigation and finding is most likely in this patient?

a. Streak ovaries on ultrasonography
b. Cardiomegaly on chest X-ray
c. May be a risk of mitral valve prolapse
d. Subluxation of lens

Ans. is 'a' Streak ovaries on ultrasonography

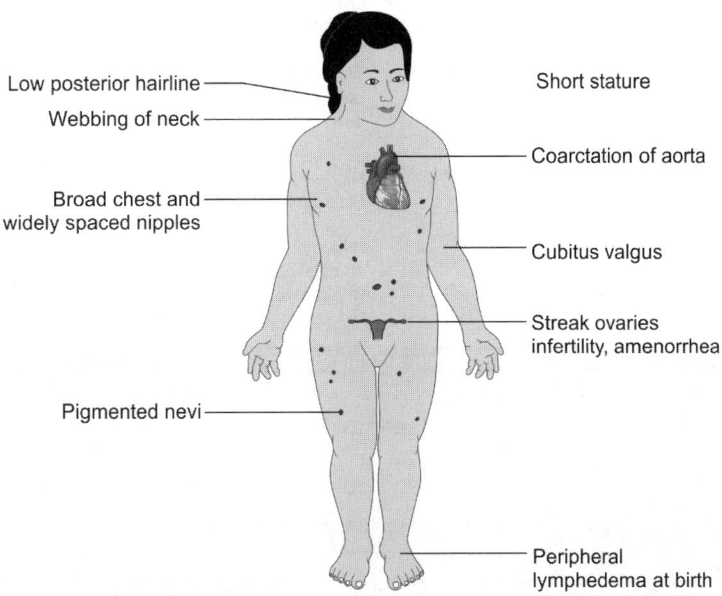

Clinical features and karyotypes of Turner syndrome

33. A patient of rheumatic heart disease has undergone a biopsy, the findings are given below. Identify:

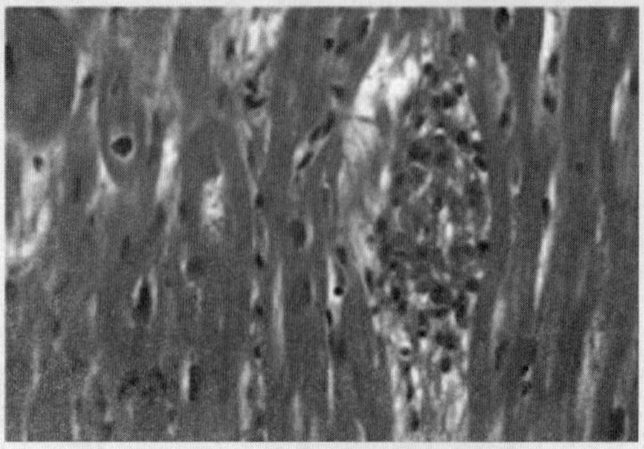

For colour version see Plate 3

a. Aschoff bodies
b. Granuloma annular
c. Epithelioid granuloma
d. Granulomatous vasculitis

Ans. is 'a' Aschoff bodies

For detail see explanation on page 193.

34. A 55-year-old male who is a diagnosed case of multiple myeloma has camp up for follow-up. Which of the following is a poor prognostic factor?

a. Beta 2 microglobulin
b. Creatine
c. Albumin
d. Anemia

Ans. is 'a' Beta 2 microglobulin

For detail see explanation on page 178

Prognostic Factors for Multiple Myeloma

Recognized prognostic factors	
Factor	***Significance***
Clinical • Age • Performance status	 • Younger — better • Low levels — poor
Routine laboratory testing • β_2-microglobulin • Serum albumin • Serum creatinine • LDH level • C-reactive protein • Hemoglobin • Platelet count	 • Higher — poor • Lower — poor • Elevated — poor • Elevated — poor • Elevated — poor • Low — poor • Low — poor
Specialized tests • Plasma cell labeling index • Plasma cell morphology • Bone marrow cytogenetic - Standard cytogenetic - Fish analysis (Chromosome 13) - Microarray techniques - Whole-body FDG/PET scan	 • HIgh — poor • Plasmablastic — poor • • Hypodiploidy/deletion 13 — poor • 13 deletion — poor • Differential patterns • Extramedullary — disease poor

International myeloma working group staging system
Proposed IPI[b] staging ststem
Stage I
β_2 M <3.5; S. Alb <3.5
Stage II
β_2 M <3.5: S. Alb >3.5
or β_2 M 3.5–5.5.
Stage III
β_2 M >5.5

[b]Greipp PR et al. Development of an international prognostic index (IPI) or myeloma: Report of the international Myeloma working Group. Haematol. 2003;4(Suppl 1): P7.S42-S45

35. A patient with lymphoma with CD10 and Bcl2 marker is likely to be diagnosed with which of the following?

a. Follicular lymphoma
b. Burkitt's lymphoma
c. Mycosis fungoides
d. Non-Hodgkin lymphoma

Ans. is 'a' Follicular lymphoma

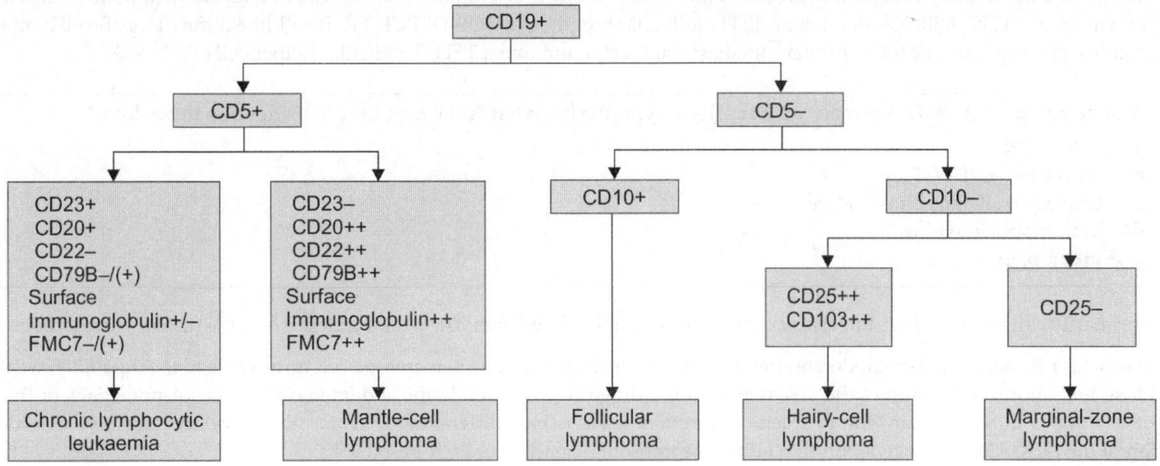

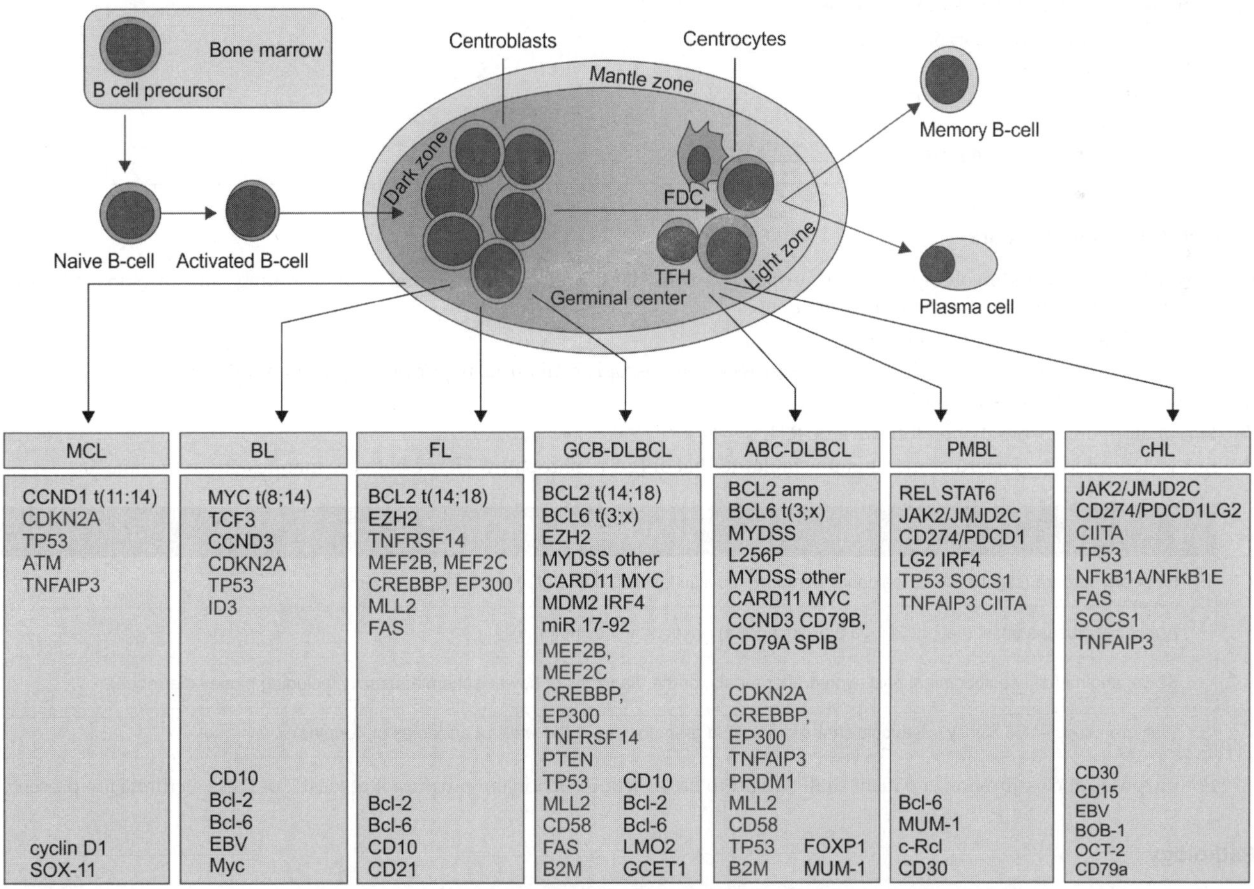

For colour version see Plate 3

Schematic representation of B-cell development and summary of molecular and immunophenotypic biomarkers in B-cell non-Hodgkin lymphomas and Hodgkin lymphomas. The GC is an important structure during B-cell differentiation (black arrows direct the B-cell development). Most types of B-cell lymphoma are proposed to be derived from GC or post-GC B cells (purple arrows indicate the proposed cellular origin of B-cell lymphomas). FL, BL, and GCB-DLBCL are of GC origin, whereas ABC-DLBCL, PMBL, and cHL are inferred to be post-GC origin. MCL is thought to be derived from the mantle zone. Certain molecular features are relatively specific for given type of lymphoma and have diagnostic or prognostic potential. Recurrent gain of function (red) and loss of function (blue) molecular biomarkers of common types of B-cell lymphoma and HLs are summarized. Immunohistochemical biomarkers (green) that are of diagnostic value in B-cell lymphomas are also shown. ABC-DLBCL, activated B-cell-DLBCL; BL, Burkitt lymphoma; cHL, classical Hodgkin lymphoma; FDC, follicular dendritic cell; FL, follicular lymphoma; GCB-DLBCL, GC B-cell-like diffuse large B-cell lymphoma; MCL, mantle cell lymphoma; PMBCL, primary mediastinal B-cell lymphoma; TFH, T follicular helper cell.

36. A male patient with splenomegaly with myeloid hyperplasia. What is the next best investigation to be done?

a. FISH, PCR
b. Whole body PET CT
c. Leucocyte alkaline phosphatase
d. Immunophenotyping

Ans. is 'a' FISH, PCR

CML is primarily a disease of adults but also occurs in children and adolescents. The peak incidence is in the fifth to sixth decades of life.

The onset is insidious. Mild-to-moderate anemia and hypermetabolism due to increased cell turnover lead to fatigability, weakness, weight loss, and anorexia. Sometimes the first symptom is a dragging sensation in the abdomen caused by splenomegaly, or the acute onset of left upper quadrant pain due to splenic infarction. CML is best differentiated from other myeloproliferative disorders by detection of the *BCR-ABL* fusion gene through either chromosomal analysis or PCR-based tests.

37. A 25-year-old man patient presenting with palpable purpura with B/L knee joint involvement upon urinalysis is RBC and protein is noted. What is the diagnosis?

a. Idiopathic thrombocytic purpura
b. Chikungunya
c. Henoch Schonlein purpura
d. Dengue

Ans. is 'c' Henoch Schonlein purpura

Henoch-Schönlein Purpura

- Purpuric skin lesions involving extensor surfaces of arms, legs, buttocks; abdominal pain, vomiting, and intestinal bleeding; nonmigratory arthralgia; and renal abnormalities.
- Children 3-8 yrs, also occurs in adults
- Renal manifestations occur in 1/3 of patients—gross or microscopic hematuria, nephritic , nephrotic syndrome
- A few, mostly adults, develop RPGN
- H/o of atopy in 1/3, onset often follows an URTI.
- IgA is deposited in glomerular mesangium similar to that of IgA nephropathy. Hence both are manifestations of same d/s

ACR criteria
• Palpable purpura (slightly raised 'palpable' hemorrhagic skin lesions, not related to thrombocytopenia)
• Age 20 at disease onset (patient 20 years or younger at onset of first symptoms)
• Bowel angina (diffuse abdominal pain, worse after meals, or the diagnosis of bowel ischemia, usually including bloody diarrhoea)
• Wall granulocytes on biopsy (histologic changes showing granulocytes in the walls of arterioles or venules)

For purposes of classification, a patient shall be said to have Henoch-Schonlein purpura if at least 2 of these 4 criteria are present.

Pathology

- Renal lesions vary from mild focal to diffuse mesangial proliferation and/or endocapillary to crescentic glomerulonephritis.
- If—deposition of IgA, sometimes with IgG and C3, in mesangial region
- Skin lesions consist of subepidermal hemorrhages, necrotizing vasculitis involving small vessels of dermis with IgA deposits
- Vasculitis also occurs in other organs

38. A patient underwent Radical cysto-prostatectomy and the specimen is given below. Identify:

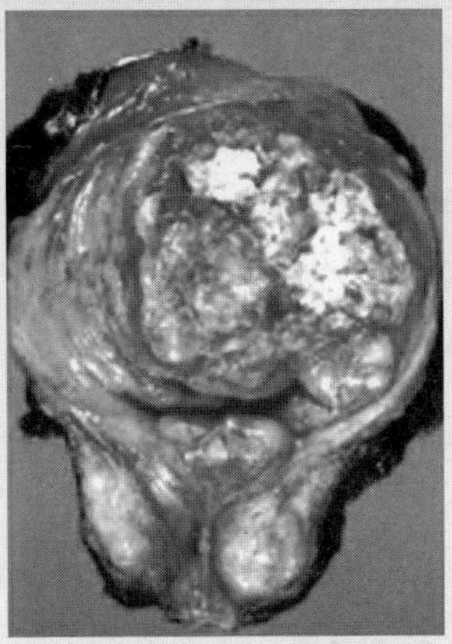

For colour version see Plate 4

a. Bladder cancer
b. Schistosomiasis
c. Prostatic cancer
d. Malakoplakia

Ans. is 'a' Bladder cancer

Invasive urothelial cancer may be associated with papillary urothelial cancer, usually high-grade, or adjacent CIS. The extent of the invasion into the muscularis mucosae is of prognostic significance, and understaging on biopsy is significant problem. **The extent of spread (staging) at the time of initial diagnosis is the most important factor in determining the outlook for a patient**. Almost all infiltrating urothelial carcinomas are high-grade, and as a result grading of the infiltrating component is not critical, as opposed to the importance of grading noninvasive papillary urothelial carcinoma.

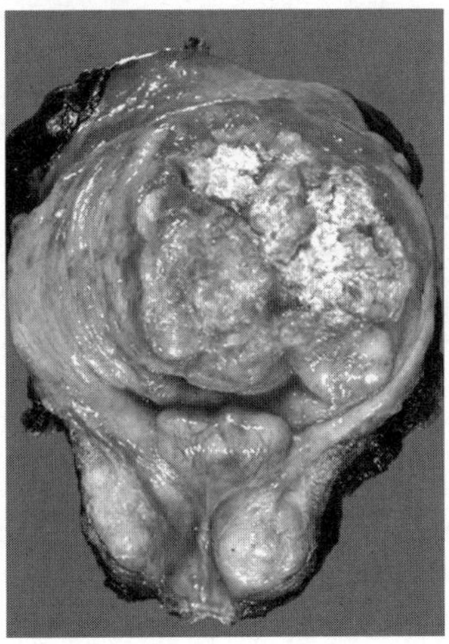

Opened bladder showing a high-grade invasive transitional cell carcinoma at an advanced stage. The aggressive multinodular neoplasm has fungated into the bladder lumen and spread over a wide area. The white areas represent areas of ulceration and necrosis.

Pathologic T (Primary tumor) staging of bladder carcinoma	
Depth of invasion	***AJCC/UICC***
Ta	Noninvasive, papillary
Tis	Carcinoma in situ (noninvasive, flat)
T1	Lamina propria invasion
T2	Muscularis propria invasion
T3a	Microscopic extravesicle invasion
T3B	Grossly apparent extravesicle invasion
T4	Invades adjacent structures

jAJCC/UICC, American Joint Commission on Cancer/Union Internationale Contre le Cancer

PHARMACOLOGY

NEET PG September 2021

39. As an Indian medical intern, which of the following is the correct format for prescription of alprazolam?

a. Tablet alprazolam 0.5 mg once a day before bed time for 7 days
b. Tablet alprazolam 0.5 mg HS for 7 days
c. Tablet alprazolam 500 mcg one tablet OD for 7 days
d. Tablet alprazolam ½ mg tablet HS daily

Ans. is 'a' Tablet alprazolam 0.5 mg once a day before bed time for 7 days

Prescription Writing

The prescription consists of the *superscription*, the *inscription*, the *subscription*, the *signa*, and the *name and signature of the prescriber*, all contained on a single form (Figure). The *superscription* includes the date the prescription order is written; the name, address, weight, and age of the patient; and the Rx (*Take*). The body of the prescription, or *inscription*, contains the name and amount or strength of the drug to be dispensed or the name and strength of each ingredient to be compounded.

The *subscription* is the instruction to the pharmacist, usually consisting of a short sentence, such as "dispense 30 tablets." The *signa* or "Sig" is the instruction for the patient regarding how to take the prescription, interpreted and transposed onto the prescription label by the pharmacist.

The patient's name and address are needed on the prescription order to ensure that the correct medication goes to the proper patient and also for identification and recordkeeping. For medications whose dosage involves a calculation, a patient's pertinent factors, such as weight, age, or body surface area, also should be listed on the prescription; both the calculated dose and the dosage formula used, such as "240 mg every 8 h (40 mg/ kg/d)," should be included to allow another healthcare professional to double check the prescribed dosage.

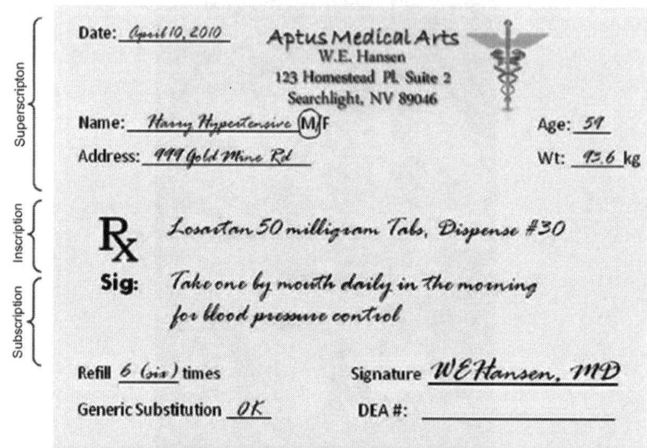

The prescription: The prescription must be accurately and legibly prepared to identify the patient, the medication to be dispensed, and the mode of drug administration. Avoid abbreviations and Latin; they lead to dispensing error. Include the therapeutic purpose in the subscription (e.g., "for control of blood pressure') to prevent errors in dispensing. For example, the use of losaran *for the treatment of hypertension* may require 100 mg/d (1.4 mg/kg/d), whereas *for treatment of congestive heart failure*, the dose of this angiotensin II receptor antagonist generally should not exceed 50 mg/d. Including the therapeutic purpose of the prescription also can assist patients in organizing and understanding their medications. Including the patient's weight on the prescription can be useful in avoiding dosing errors, particularly when drugs are administered to children.

40. Rate of administration of a drug is equal to rate of elimination. How will you calculate the dosing rate of the drug to maintain steady state concentration?

a. Dosing rate = Vd x target plasma concentration
b. Dosing rate = CL x target plasma concentration
c. Dosing rate = Vd/target plasma concentration
d. Dosing rate = CL/target plasma concentration

Ans. is 'b' Dosing rate = CL x target plasma concentration

Repeated Drug Administration

When a drug is repeated at relatively short intervals, it accumulates in the body until elimination balances input and a *steady state* plasma concentration (*Cpss*) is attained:

$$Cpss = \frac{\text{Dose rate}}{\text{CL}}$$

From this equation it is implied that doubling the dose rate would double the average *Cpss* and so on. Further, if the therapeutic plasma concentration of the drug has been worked out and its *CL* is known, the dose rate needed to achieve the target *Cpss* can be determined

Dose rate = Target Cpss × CL

The dose rate-*Cpss* relationship is linear only in case of drugs eliminated by first order kinetics. For drugs (e.g. phenytoin) which follow Michaelis Menten kinetics, elimination changes from first order to zero order kinetics over the therapeutic range. Increase in their dose beyond saturation levels causes an increase in *Cpss* which is out of proportion to the change in dose rate.

41. A patient with bronchial asthma presents with raised intraocular pressure. Treatment of open angle glaucoma in this patient is:

a. Latanoprost
b. Alprostadil
c. Gemeprost
d. Carboprost

Ans. is 'a' Latanoprost

For detail see on page 249 Table

42. A 45-year-old patient being treated with low dose aspirin since 6 months presented with rectal bleeding. Inhibition of which of the following substance is likely to responsible for the bleeding?

a. TXA_2
b. LT
c. Bradykinin
d. PGI_2

Ans. is 'a' TXA_2

NSAIDs inhibit synthesis of both proaggregatory (TXA_2) and antiaggregatory (PGI_2) prostanoids, but effect on platelet TXA_2 (COX-1 generated) predominates. Therapeutic doses of most NSAIDs inhibit platelet aggregation: bleeding time is prolonged. Aspirin is highly active; acetylates platelet COX irreversibly in the portal circulation before it is deacetylated by first pass metabolism in liver. Small doses are therefore able to exert antithrombotic effect for several days. Risk of surgical and anticoagulant associated bleeding is enhanced.

43. A 34-week pregnant female with polyhydramnios presents with labour pain. She was treated with indomethacin earlier. Which of the following can be likely outcome in the baby if delivery occurs at this time?

a. Patent ductus arteriosus
b. Premature closure of ductus arteriosus
c. Patent ductus venosus
d. Premature closure of ductus venosus

Ans. is 'b' Premature closure of ductus arteriosus

Human teratogenic drugs

Drug	*Abnormality*
Anticancer drugs (methotrexate)	Cleft palate, hydrocephalus, multiple defects, foetal death
Androgens	Virilization; limb, esophageal, cardiac defects
Progestins	Virilization of female foetus
Stilboestrol	Vaginal carcinoma in teenage female offspring
Alcohol	Low IQ baby, growth retardation, foetal alcohol syndrome
Indomethacin/aspirin	Premature closure of ductus arteriosus
Isotretinoin	Craniofacial, heart and CNS defects, hydrocephalus

44. A 60-year-old female with renal disease was admitted for pyelolithotomy. Postoperative analgesic of choice in this patient is:

a. Diclofenac
b. Indomethacin
c. Naproxen
d. Acetaminophen

Ans. is 'd' Acetaminophen

Dose to dose ACETAMINOPHEN is equally efficacious as aspirin for noninflammatory conditions. It is much safer than aspirin in terms of gastric irritation, ulceration and bleeding (can be given to ulcer patients), does not prolong bleeding time. Hypersensitivity reactions are rare; no metabolic effects or acid-base disturbances; can be used in all age groups (infants to elderly), pregnant/lactating women, in presence of other disease states and in patients in whom other NSAIDs are contraindicated. It does not have significant drug interactions. Thus, it may be preferred over other NSAIDs for most minor conditions.

45. A 45-year-old patient presented with the symptoms shown in image below. Patient is a known hypertensive and was taking some antihypertensive drug. Which of the following drug is the likely cause of this condition?

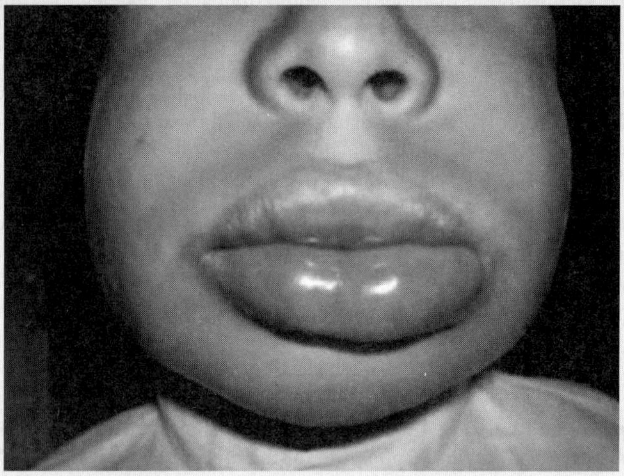

a. Lisinopril
b. Clonidine
c. Nifedipine
d. Timolol

Ans. is 'a' Lisinopril

The given image is suggestive of angioedema which is a potential side effect of ACE inhibitors. Side effects of ACEIs can be summarised as below:

Captopril

- Cough/C1 esterase deficiency *contraindication*
- Angioedema/Agranulocytosis
- Proteinuria/Potassium excess (hyperkalemia)
- Taste change
- Orthostatic hypotension
- Pregnancy *contraindication* (fetal renal damage)
- Renal artery stenosis *contraindication*
- Increases renin Leukopenia/Liver toxicity

46. Tocilizumab is an immunosuppressive drug used for Rheumatoid arthritis. It is a monoclonal antibody against:

a. IL-6
b. IL-12
c. IL-2
d. IL-3

Ans. is 'a' IL-6

For detail see explanation on page 252

47. A patient on digoxin therapy and had a level of 1 ng/mL. He was receiving several other drugs and presented 2 months later with flattening of T waves in ECG. Now the plasma level of digoxin is 3.8 ng/mL. Which of the following drug is likely to be responsible?

a. Triamterene
b. Atenolol
c. Clarithromycin
d. KCl

Ans. is 'c' Clarithromycin

Drug Interactions of Digoxin

- *Diuretics*: Cause hypokalemia which increases the risk of digitalis arrhythmias; potassium supplements should be given prophylactically.
- *Calcium*: Synergises with digitalis → precipitates toxicity.
- Drugs inhibiting p-glycoprotein (*Quinidine, Verapamil, diltiazem, captopril, propafenone,macrolides* and *amiodarone*): Reduces binding of digoxin to tissue proteins as well as its renal and biliary clearance by inhibiting efflux transporter P-glycoprotein → plasma concentration of digoxin is doubled → toxicity can occur.
- *Adrenergic drugs*: Can induce arrhythmias in digitalized patients; both increase ectopic automaticity.

- Digoxin absorption may be reduced by *metoclopramide, sucralfate, antacids, neomycin, sulfasalazine.* Absorption of digoxin is increased by atropinic drugs, including tricyclic antidepressants.
- *Propranolol, verapamil, diltiazem and disopyramide:* May additively depress A-V conduction and oppose positive inotropic action.
- *Succinylcholine*: Can induce arrhythmias in digitalized patients.

48. A hypertensive patient presented with chronic renal insufficiency and pedal edema. On investigations, serum creatinine was found to be 1.9 mg/dL. Which of the following drug should be used for management of hypertension in this patient?

a. Prazosin
b. Aliskiren
c. Chlorthalidone
d. Metoprolol

Ans. is 'c' Chlorthalidone

Desirable properties of thiazide diuretics as antihypertensives are:

- Once a day dosing and flat dose-response curve permitting simple standardized regimens.
- No fluid retention, no tolerance.
- Low incidence of postural hypotension and relative freedom from side effects, especially CNS, compared to sympatholytics.
- Effective in isolated systolic hypertension (ISH).
- Lessened risk of hip fracture in the elderly due to hypocalciuric action of thiazides.
- Low cost.

49. A 26-year-old female came to hospital for pre-conceptional counselling. Patient is a known hypertensive compliant to drug therapy. Which of the following drugs will you advise to stop?

a. Methyl dopa
b. Labetalol
c. Lisinopril
d. Nifedipine

Ans. is 'c; Lisinopril

ACEI are known to be teratogenic and should be avoided if pregnancy is under consideration.

Safe Anti-Hypertensives in Pregnancy

- **Better**: **B**eta blockers (Cardioselective and Labetalol)
- **Mother**: **M**ethyl dopa
- **Care**: **C**lonidine
- **During**: **D**ihydropyridine CCB (sustained release nifedipine, amlodipine)
- **Hypertensive**: **H**ydralazine
- **Pregnancy**: **P**razosin (and other alpha blockers)

50. A 36-week pregnant female was taking warfarin for prosthetic heart valves and has INR value of 3. Next step in the management is:

a. Stop warfarin and start heparin
b. Stop warfarin and start heparin plus aspirin
c. Continue warfarin and add heparin
d. Switch to aspirin

Ans. is 'a' Stop warfarin and start heparin

Oral anticoagulants should not be used during pregnancy. Warfarin given in early pregnancy increases birth defects, especially skeletal abnormalities. It can produce *foetal warfarin syndrome*—hypoplasia of nose, eye socket, hand bones, and growth retardation. Given later in pregnancy, it can cause CNS defects, foetal haemorrhage, foetal death and accentuates neonatal hypoprothrombinemia.

51. A female taking oral contraceptives acquired tuberculosis. After prescribing anti-tubercular therapy, physician advised the patient for alternative contraception. What is the probable reason of this advise?

a. Rifampicin causes teratogenicity
b. Isoniazid is teratogenic
c. Rifampicin increases the metabolism of oral contraceptives
d. Oral contraceptives decrease the efficacy of anti-tubercular therapy

Ans. is 'c' Rifampicin increases the metabolism of oral contraceptives

Rifampin is a microsomal enzyme inducer—increases several CYP450 isoenzymes, including CYP3A4, CYP2D6, CYP1A2 and CYP2C subfamily. It thus enhances its own metabolism (area under the plasma concentration-time curve is reduced by ~35%) as well as that of many drugs including warfarin, oral contraceptives, corticosteroids, sulfonylureas, steroids, HIV protease inhibitors, nonnucleoside reverse transcriptase inhibitors (NNRTIs), theophylline, metoprolol, fluconazole, ketoconazole, clarithromycin, phenytoin, etc. Contraceptive failures have occurred. It is advisable to switch over to an oral contraceptive containing higher dose (50 µg) of estrogen or use alternative method of contraception.

52. Metronidazole is used for treatment of various anaerobic infections as well as bacterial vaginosis. Patient is instructed to avoid taking which of the following substance after metronidazole prescription to avoid possible adverse effects?

a. Grapefruit juice
b. Milk
c. Alcohol
d. Orange juice

Ans. is 'c' Alcohol

A disulfiram-like intolerance to alcohol occurs in some patients taking metronidazole. Alcohol-metronidazole interaction occurs only in some individuals, while majority of those taking it can consume alcohol without any reaction. There is no convincing evidence of disulfiram-like action of metronidazole, but manufactures advise caution in drinking during metronidazole therapy.

Drugs that cause disulfiram like effects:

- Metronidazole (azole drugs; similar action like fomepizole)
- Cefoperazone,cefamandole, cefotetan
- Procarbazine
- Chlorpropamide, glimiperide
- Griseofulvin

53. A 20-year-old boy presented with slow growing mass on the medial side of thigh. Investigations revealed it to be osteosarcoma and patient was started on methotrexate. Mechanism of action of methotrexate as an anticancer drug is:

a. Inhibition of dihydrofolate reductase
b. Inhibition of N5 tetrahydrofolate reductase
c. Inhibition of tyrosine kinase
d. Inhibition of purine metabolism

Ans. is 'a' Inhibition of dihydrofolate reductase

Methotrexate

MOA: Inhibit DHF reductase

- To ↓ toxicity— Leucovorin
- S/E : B.M Suppression, Mucositis, crystalluria
  : hepatoxicity, pneumonitis
- Tx. of toxicity—dialysis/Glucarpidase (methotrexate cleaving enzyme)
- **Uses of methotrexate:**

C	Choriocarcinoma (DOC)
O	Osteosarcoma
M	Malignant leukemia
B	Breast cancer
My	Mycosis fungoides
All	ALL
Hair	H&N cancer
Or	Organ transplant
People	Psoriasis
Will	Wegners
S	Sarcoidosis
C	Crohn's disease
R	RA (DMARD of choice)
E	Ectopic pregnancy
A	Abortion
M	Multiple sclerosis

MICROBIOLOGY

NEET PG September 2021

54. A child presented with abdominal pain, fever and blood in stool. Which enrichment media should be used to isolate the organism from the stool sample?

a. Selenite F broth
b. Alkaline Peptone water
c. Robertson cooked media
d. BHI

Ans. is 'a' Selenite F broth

For detail see explanation on page 289

The given clinical scenario is s/o dysentery. Dysentery is characterized by diarrhea with increased blood and mucus, often associated with fever, abdominal pain. and tenesmus (a feeling of incomplete defecation).

Shigella is the most common cause of dysentery. Enrichment media used for shigella is selenite F broth.

55. A patient admitted with 50% burns, develops an infection of the burnt site. The swab is cultured and the isolate is an obligate aerobe and the test shown in the figure is positive. Which of the following is the likely etiology?

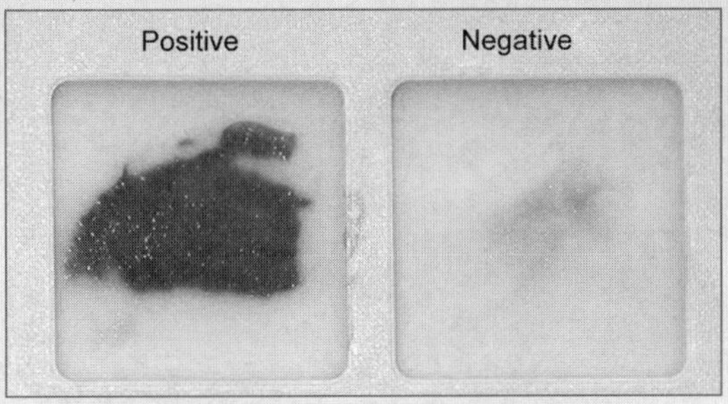

For colour version see Plate 4

a. Staphylococcus epidermidis
b. Klebsiella species
c. Pseudomonas aeruginosa
d. Staphylococcus aureus

Ans. is 'c' Pseudomonas aeruginosa

Pseudomonas Aeruginosa

- Obligate aerobe; motile → polar flagella; noncapsulated; nonsporing
- Part of normal intestinal flora → oxidase +ve. Does not Ferment lactose
- Selective media → Cetrimide agar
- Pigments – Pyocyanin [blue green], pyorubin [red], pyomelanin [brown-black], pyoverdin (fluorescin) [greenish yellow]
- Pyocyanin – only by P. aeruginosa
- Grape like odour
- **Virulence factors:**
  - Endotoxin → Fever and shock
  - Exotoxin A – inhibit protein synthesis by inhibiting EF-2
  - Alginate coat/slime layer
- **Clinical features:**
  - Pneumonia – ventilator associated pneumonia
  - Sepsis
  - Malignant otitis externa, Swimmer's ear
  - Hot tub folliculitis – Jacuzzi syndrome
  - UTI – in catheterized patients
  - Shanghai fever
  - Osteomyelitis e.g.: puncture wounds
  - Green nail syndrome
  - **Ecthyma gangrenosum:** Rapidly progressive necrotic cutaneous lesion caused by pseudomonas bacteremia in immunocompromised patients
- Most common cause of infection in burns.
- Chronic pneumonia in cystic fibrosis patients → Mucoid polysaccharide capsule, Biofilm formation

Treatment: DOC→Aminoglycoside + penicillin; except in:

- UTI→ Ciprofloxacin
- CNS infection → ceftazidine +/– Aminoglycoside
- Malignant otitis externa→cephalosporins/carbapenem

56. An HIV positive patient presented with fever, chills and productive cough. His CD4 count is less than 55. On examination findings of consolidation in right infrascapular area with X-ray showing right lower lobe consolidation are noted. Most probable diagnosis of the infection is:

a. *S. aureus* b. *Pneumococcus*
c. *Pseudomonas aeruginosa* d. *P. jiroveci*

Ans. is 'b' *Pneumococcus*

For detail see explanation on page 303

57. An unimmunized 2-year-old child presented to emergency department with history of 4-day fever, coryza, conjunctivitis and on examination, white lesions seen on buccal mucosa. A day later, maculopapular rash appeared on face and neck. What is the nature of the causative virus?

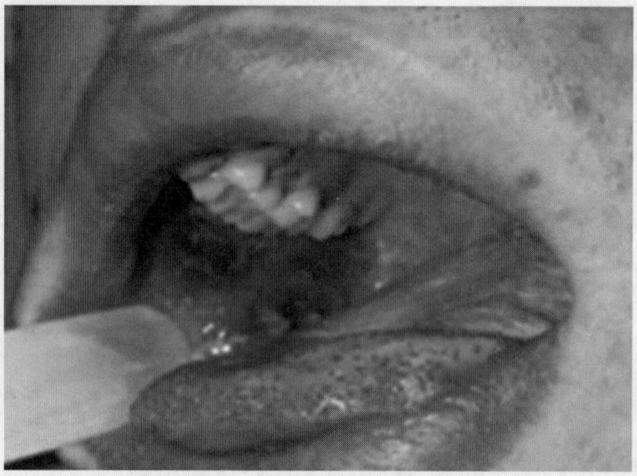

a. SS RNA b. DS RNA
c. SS DNA d. DS DNA

Ans. is 'a' SS RNA

The clinical scenario is suggestive of measles infection and image shows Koplik spots, characteristic of measles. Measles virus belongs to paramyxovirus family which are SS-RNA viruses.

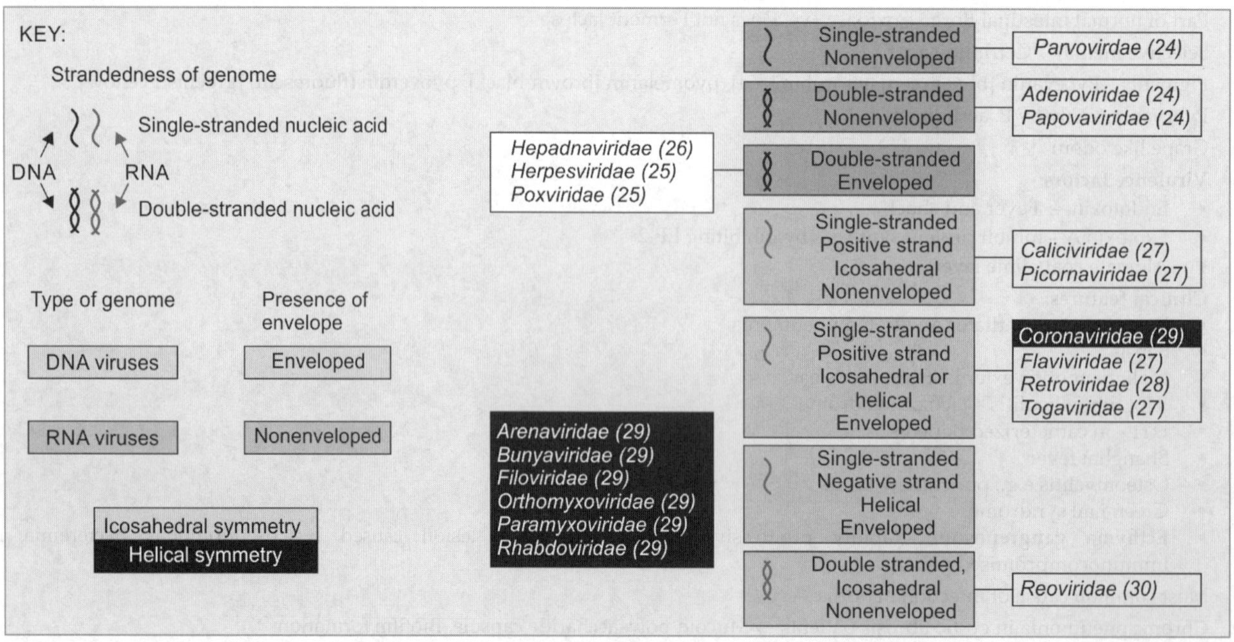

58. A group of 20 friends had a late night party at a restaurant. Next morning one started to vomit followed by another. Both of them had stopped back to eat pastry from a roadside vendor. Which of the following is the likely etiology?

a. Vero toxin of E.coli
b. Bacillus cereus emetic toxin
c. Staph aureus enterotoxin
d. Shiga toxin of S. dysentery

Ans. is 'c' Staph aureus enterotoxin

For detail see explanation on page 313

59. Child is presented with history of Pharyngitis. Swab was taken and sent for microscopy. After preparing the smear, swab material should be discarded in:

a. Yellow bag
b. Red bag
c. White box
d. None of these

Ans. is 'a' Yellow bag

For detail see explanation on page 352 Table

60. A patient is suspected of suffering from acute brucellosis. His serum sample is put on standard agglutination test but it comes out to be negative. However, on doing the test after serial dilutions of the serum, the test comes out positive. Which of the following is responsible for initial negative test?

a. Post zone
b. Pro zone
c. Complement inactivation
d Incomplete antibodies

Ans. is 'b' Pro zone

Standard Agglutination Test (SAT)

It remains the gold standard test against which other serological tests are compared.

- **Procedure:** It is a tube agglutination test. The equal volumes of serial dilutions of patient's sera are mixed with the killed smooth suspension of a standard strain of B. abortus and incubated at 37°C for 48 hours.
- Results: Significant titer is:
  - Titer of more than 1:160 is considered as significant in nonendemic areas.
  - In an endemica area, demonstration of rising titer by repeatiting the test after 2-4 weeks is more reliable.
- **Interpretation:**
  - SAT detects antibodies against antigens or smooth LPS. Use of *B. abortus* can detect antibodies against *B. melitensis, B. abortus* and *B. suis* but not *B. canis* (as it lacks smooth LPS).
  - In acute infection, lgM antibodies appear early and are followed by lgG and lgA antibodies. The SAT measures the total quantity of agglutinating antibodies but does not differentiate between immunoglobulin isotypes.
  - As the disease progresses, lgM levels decline, and the avidity and subclass distribution of IgG and lgA change. Thus, SAT may become negative.
- **False-negative SAT** may occur due to:
  - Prozone phenomenon (due to excess of antibodies in patient's sera): This may be obviated by performing the test in serially diluted patient's sera.
  - Presence of 'blocking' or nonagglutinating lgG or lgA antibodies: This can be removed by:
    - Prior healing of serum at 55°C for 30 min
    - Using 4% saline to dilute patient's sera
  - Detecting 'incomplete' antibodies by Coombs antiglobulin test (most reliable)
- **False-positive SAT** may occur due to antigenic cross reactions with some other gram-negative bacteria having similar O chains, such as *Escherichia coli* 0157, *Francisella tularensis, Salmonella enterica* group *N, Stenotropphonomas maltophilia* and *Vibrio cholerae.*

61. While shifting a patient receiving an emergency blood transfusion, there is an accidental Blood spill in the ambulance. Which of the following should be used to disinfect the blood spill?

a. Ethyl alcohol
b. Chlorhexidine
c. Formaldehyde
d. Sodium hypochlorite

Ans. is 'd' Sodium hypochlorite

- Sodium hypochlorite (household bleach – 5 to 6%) is the disinfectant of choice for blood spills.
- Spill < 10 mL → 1:100 dilution is used (0.05%)
- Spill > 10 mL → 1:10 dilution is used (0.5%)

Guidelines for Management of Infectious Spills

- Block off area of spill
- Put on non-sterile disposable gloves and PPE as applicable
- Use tongs or a pan and brush to sweep up the broken glass as possible. Discard the broken glass in a sharps container

- Wipe up spill using paper towels and place it in a plastic garbage bag
- Gently pour on all contaminated areas, sodium hypochlorite.
- Let bleach solution remain on the contaminated area for 20 minutes
- Wipe up the bleach solution with paper towels and place in the plastic garbage bag
- Remove gloves and place in plastic garbage bag with all soiled cleaning materials
- Double bag and securely tie up plastic garbage bags and discard
- Clean as usual with detergents and water
- Thoroughly wash hands with soap and water.

62. Wedge-shaped perforations in the hair shaft is seen in:

a. *T. rubrum* b. *T. mentagrophytes*
c. *M. audouinii* d. *E. flocossum*

Ans. is 'b' *T. mentagrophytes*

Hair perforation rest: *It* is positive for *Trichophyton mentagrophytes* and *Microsporum canis.* the test is performed by inoculating a colony into a petri dish containing water, yeast extract, and hair. Fungi pierce the hair producing wedge-shaped perforations.

Dermatophytes

Organism	Involves
Microsporum	Skin, hair
Epidermophyton	Skin, nails
Trichophyton	Skin, hair and nails

General	Microconidia	Macroconidia
Trichophyton	Abundant microconidia, arranged in clusters along hyphae	Relatively scanty, elongated with blunt ends (Pencil shaped), thin walled
Microsporum	Rare, Single microconidia (multicellular)	Numerous, Single macroconidia (multicellular) spindle shaped, thick walled, rough
Epidermophyton	No microconidia	Club-shaped or boat shape

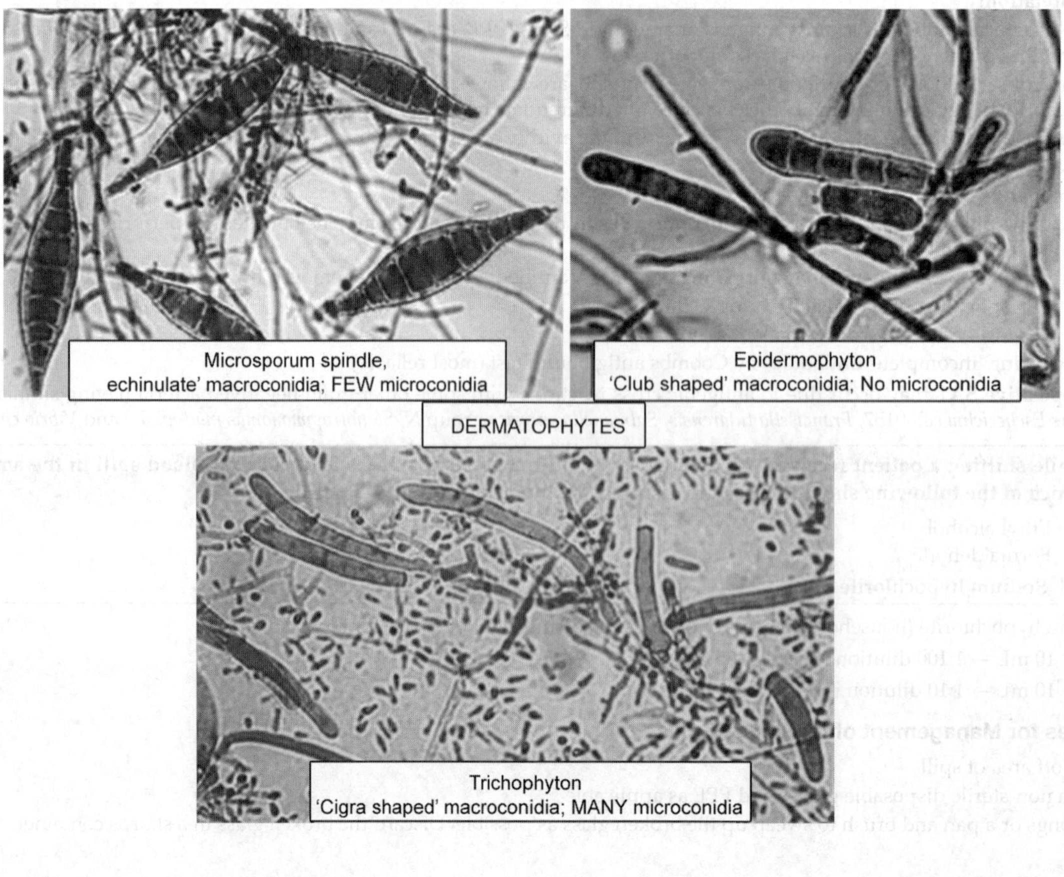

DERMATOPHYTES

63. A 35-year-old male presents to the OPD with complain of progressive swelling of left thigh region. Peripheral blood smear was taken and stained with Giemsa. Smear showed microfilariae have a sheath with no nucleus seen at the end/tail. Which is the most likely agent?

a. Brugia malayi
b. W. bancrofti
c. Mansonella perstans
d. O. volvulus

Ans. is 'b' W. bancrofti

Filarial Worms

Viviparous → microfilariae larvae

- Lymphatic — *W. Bancrofti, B. malayi*
- Subcutaneous — Loa loa, onchocerca volvulus, mansonella streptocerca
- Serous cavity — Mansonella ozardi

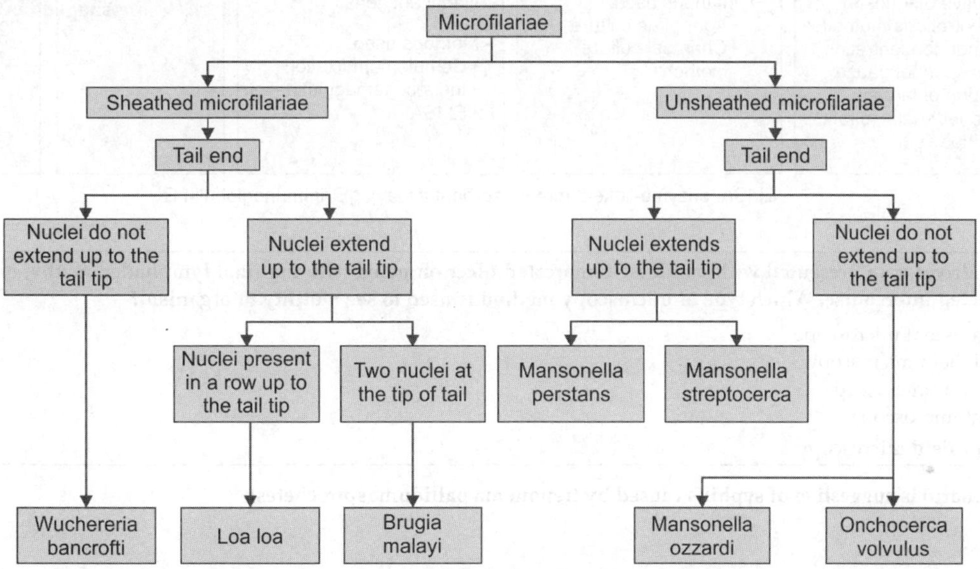

Differentiating features of various microfilariae on the basis of nuclei in tail end

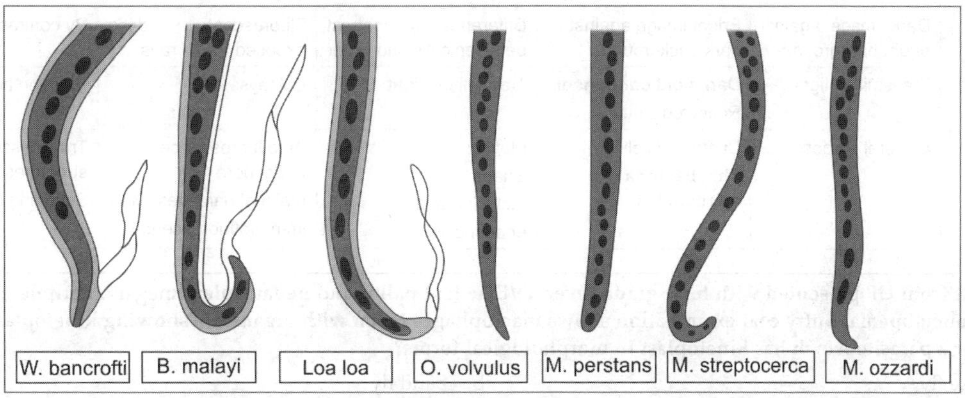

64. A patient was on steroids for chronic urticaria for 2 years. Now he has presented to emergency with acute worsening of respiratory symptoms. He was having nocturnal cough for last several weeks. Hemogram showed marked eosinophilia. Bronchoscopy was done and BAL collected showed small larvae. Most likely cause:

a. Ancyclostoma caninum
b. Stongyloides stercoralis
c. Enterobius vermicularis
d. Capillaria philippinensis

Ans. is 'b' Stongyloides stercoralis

Detection of larval forms in BAL aspirate is suggestive of lung migration of the parasite in their life cycles.

Parasites undergoing lung migration in their life cycles are:

- **Ascaris**
- **Hookworms**
- **Strongyloides**

Laboratory diagnosis of *Strongyloides stercoralis*

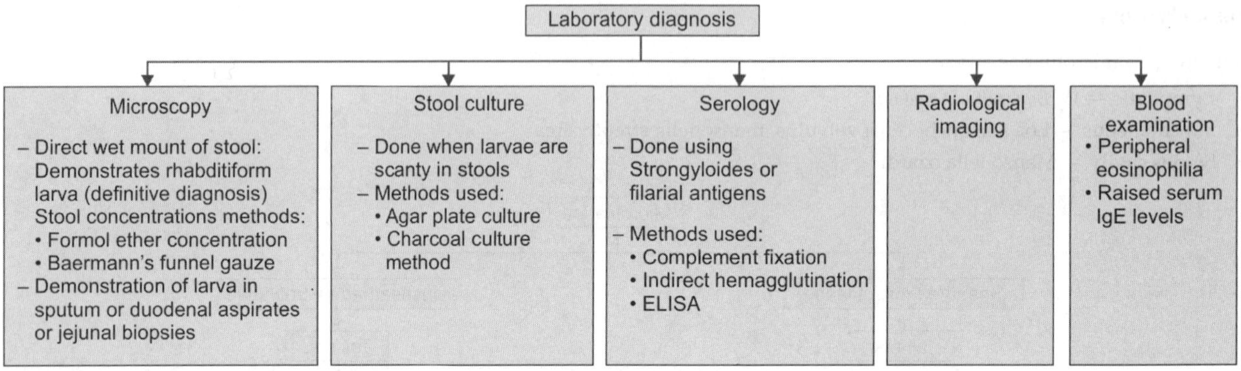

ELISA, enzyme-linked immunosorbent assay; IgE, immunoglobulin E

65. A truck driver man presented with painless, demarcated ulcer on penis with inguinal lymphadenopathy, one week after unprotected intercourse. Which type of microscopy method is used to see motility of organism?

a. Fluorescent microscope
b. Dark field microscopy
c. Electron microscope
d. Light microscope

Ans. is 'b' Dark field microscopy

The clinical scenario is suggestive of syphilis caused by treponema pallidum (spirochetes).

Microscopy

Feature	*Light*	*Dark field*	*Phase contrast*	*Fluorescence*	*Electron*
Resolution	0.2 μm				0.5 nm
Principle	Dark image against bright background	Bright image against dark background	Difference in contrast between cells and water	Fluorescent dyes exposed to UV rays	By contrast difference
Type of light used	Transmitted light	**Dark field condenser** Reflected light	Transmitted light	UV rays	Electron beam
Application	General purpose	Unstained cells **Thin bacteria like spirochetes**	Motility Shape Inclusion bodies endospores	Autofluorescence – cyclospora Malarial parasites, M.tb immunofluorescence	Transmission EM – internal structures Scanning EM—surfaces

66. A patient from UP presented with high-grade fever. O/E he had pallor and hepatosplenomegaly. Peripheral blood smear shows pancytopenia. Buffy coat examination shows macrophages laden with organisms showing kinetoplast. What is the vector for a parasite which has kinetoplast in morphological forms?

a. Tsetse fly
b. Sand fly
c. Anopheles mosquito
d. Triatomine bug

Ans. is 'b' Sand fly

For detail see explanation on page 347

Morphology of Leishmania: The parasite exists in two forms:

1. *Amastigote form:* In humans and other mammals.
2. *Promastigote form:* In the sandfly and in artificial culture.

Amastigote: The amastigote form (LD body) is an ovoid or rounded cell, about 2-4 μm in size.

It is typically intracellular, being found inside macrophages, monocytes, neutrophils, or endothelial cells. They are also known as *LD bodies.*

The large oval nucleus is stained red. Lying at the right angles to nucleus, is the red or purple-stained *kinetoplast*. In well-stained preparations, the kinetoplast can be seen consisting of a *parabasal body* and a dot-like *blepharoplast with* a delicate thread connecting the two. The axoneme arising from the blepharoplast extends to the anterior tip of the cell.

Promastigote: It is a flagellar stage and is present in insect vector, sandfly and in cultures.

The promastigotes, which are initially short, oval or pear-shaped forms, subsequently become long spindle-shaped cells, 15- 25 μm in length and 1.5-3.5 μm in breadth. A single nucleus is situated at the center. The kinetoplast lies transversely near the anterior end. The flagellum is single, delicate and measures 15-28 μm.

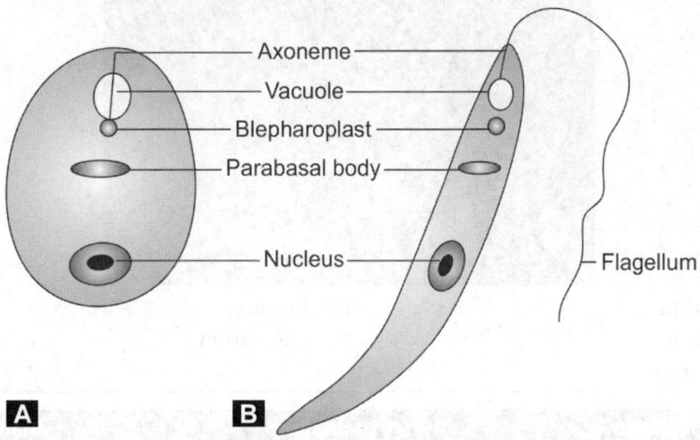

Morphology of Leishmania donovani. (A) Amastigote (LD body); (B) Promastigote

67. A 25-year-old man presented with urethral discharge one week after an unprotected intercourse as shown in figure, what can be the cause?

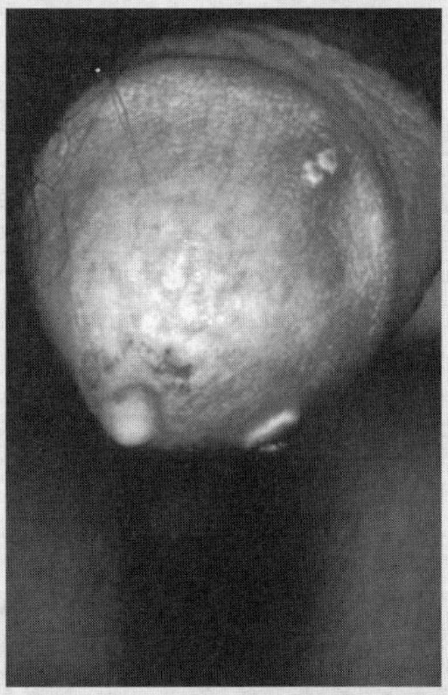

a. Gonococcus
b. Herpes
c. Trichomonas
d. Ureaplasma

Ans. 'a' Gonococcus

The given image shows purulent urethral discharge. The most likely organism in the clinical setting of young male developing complains after sexual intercourse is Neisseria gonorrhea.

❖ **Causes of non-gonococcal urethritis:**
- MCC – Chlamydia trachomatis
- Ureaplasma urealyticum
- Mycoplasma hominis
- Viruses – herpes, CMV
- Fungi – candida albicans
- Parasite – T. vaginalis

FORENSIC MEDICINE

NEET PG September 2021

68. Identify the injury:

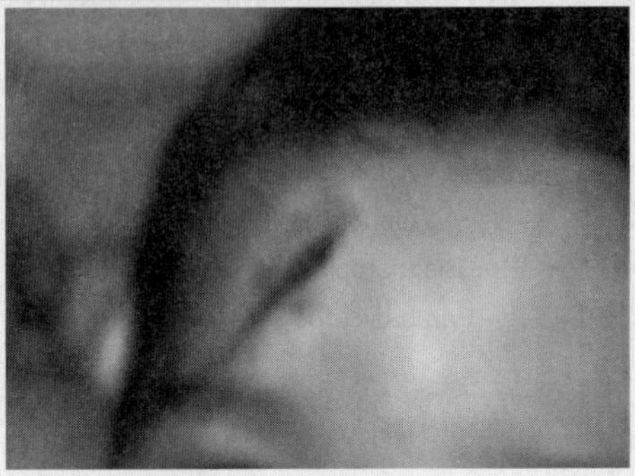

a. Incised looking laceration
b. Incision
c. Laceration looking incision
d. Laceration

Ans. is 'a' Incised looking laceration

Features	Incision	Laceration	Stab wound
Mode of injury	By sharp objects or weapons	By blunt objects or weapons	By pointed sharp or blunt weapons
Site	Anywhere in the body	Usually over bony prominences	Anywhere in the body; usually in the trunk
Margins	Smooth, clean cut and everted edges	Irregular and undermined edges	Clean-cut, parallel edges Irregular edges if blunt weapon is used
Surrounding abrasions and bruising	Absent	Usually present	Absent
Shape	Linear	Usually irregular	Linear or irregular
Dimensions	Usually longer than deep; often gaping	Usually longer than deep	Depth greater than length and breadth
Depth of wound	Structures cleanly cut to the depth of wound	Small strands of tissue at the bottom bridge across margins	Structures cleanly cut
Hemorrhage	Usually profuse and external spurting of blood may be seen	Slight except scalp and external	Varies; usually internal
Hair bulbs	Cleanly cut	Crushed or torn	Usually clean cut
Bones	May be cut	May be fractured	May be punctured
Foreign bodies	Absent	Present	Absent
Clothes	May be cut	May be torn	May be cut

69. Which of the following is true regarding the above change?

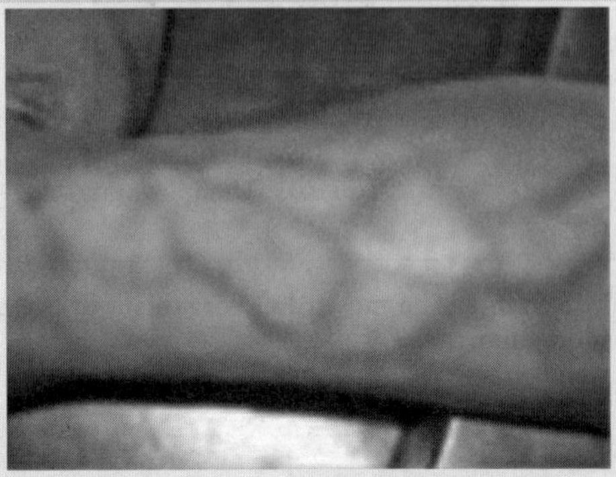

For colour version see Plate 4

a. Seen in 24 hours
b. Due to sulfhemoglobin
c. Due to non-bacterial cause
d. Due to asepsis

Ans. is 'b.' Due to sulfhemoglobin

Marbling of Skin: The superficial veins especially over the roots of the limb, thighs, sides of the abdomen, shoulders, chest and neck are stained greenish-brown or purplish-red depending on the total amount of sulphhaemoglobin formation within the affected vessels (linear branching pattern) due to the haemolysis of red cells, which stains the wall of the vessel and infiltrates into the tissue, giving a marbled appearance (red, then greenish pattern in skin resembling the branches of a tree). This starts in 24 hours, but is prominent in 36 to 48 hours.

The bacteria that largely originate from the intestines get infested in the venous system, the blood acting as nutrient for them. The blood in the vessels is haemolysed, which stains the vessel walls and the adjacent tissues, giving rise to **marbled appearance**.

70. While recording evidence in the court of law, the lawyer asked the witness 'Did A killed B?' Witness said 'Yes'. The type of question is permitted in:

a. Examination in chief
b. Direct examination
c. Re-direct examination
d. Cross examination

Ans. is 'd' Cross examination

A leading question is one which suggests to the witness the answer desired, or which includes a material fact, and admits of a conclusive answer by a simple "Yes" or "No" (S.141, I:E.A.). "Was this injury caused by a sharp weapon?" Was the length of cut 3 cm?". "Was it on the front of the abdomen?". They are all leading questions, as they suggest the answer "Yes" or "No". The proper questions should be: "What type of weapon would cause this injury?" What was the length of the cut? Where was it seen"?

Leading questions are permissible during cross-examination (S.143, I.E.A.).

71. The active principle of this poison is:

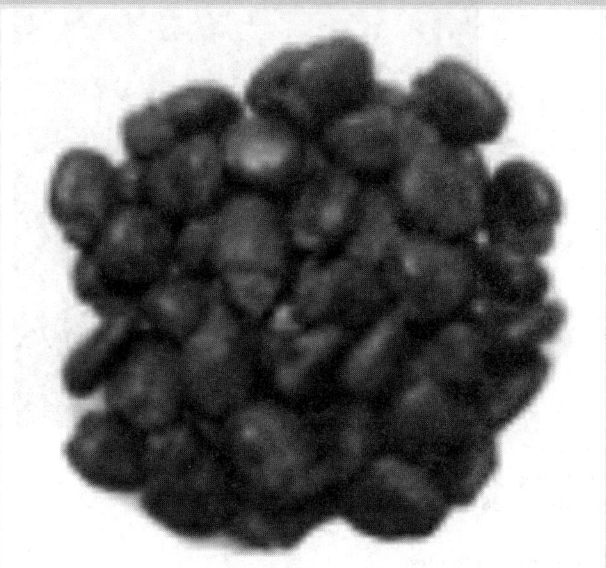

a. Abrin
b. Ricin
c. Crotin
d. Bhilawanol

Ans. is 'd' Bhilawanol

Semecarpus Anacardium (Marking Nut)

The fruit of this plant is known as *Bhilawan* or the marking nut because its juice is used by washermen as marking ink on clothes. The main active principles contained in fruit juice are semecarpol and bhilawanol.

Fatal Dose and Fatal Period

The fatal dose is usually 5–10 gm and the fatal period may be 12–24 hours.

Medicolegal Aspects

Accidental poisoning may result from the administration of juice internally by quacks. The juice may be used criminally as an abortifacient by application to the os uteri by means of an abortion stick. It may be applied to the genitals as a punishment for adultery. It may be used by malingerers to produce an artificial bruise to support a false charge. Its presence, however, can be detected by chemical analysis of the blister fluid.

Differentiating features of artificial and true bruise		
Features	***Artificial bruise***	***True bruise***
Cause	Chemical	Trauma
Situation	Accessible parts	Anywhere
Appearance	Blister formation	No blister formation
Fingers	May show marks due to scratching	Not so
Itching	Present	Not so
Color changes	Nil	Characteristic
Contents	Acrid serum	Extravasated blood
Analysis	Chemical detectable in the blister fluid	Not so

72. The above phenomenon is due to:

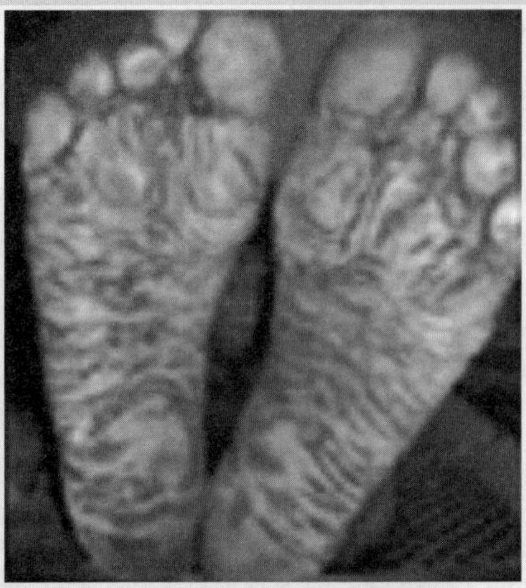

a. Case of torture in hot water
b. Case of post-mortem hanging
c. Case of immersion in water for 36 hours
d. Case of falanga

Ans. is 'c' Case of immersion in water for 36 hours

Maceration of the Skin (Washerwoman's Hands)

Submersion causes progressive maceration of the skin, particularly the hands and feet and the areas exposed to friction.

Hence, the areas usually involved are finger tips, palms, back of the hands and the soles. **After prolonged submersion**, wide areas of the skin present the similar appearance, such as extensor surfaces of the knees and elbows. The skin at these areas becomes whitened, swollen, sodden, wrinkled and corrugated. Later on, the epidermis gets loosened followed by the nails and from the hands and feet, it can be detached in 'glove and stocking' fashion. Hands showing these changes have often been termed as **'washerwoman's hands'** because the changes are similar to those as produced in women after prolonged washing of clothes. The change has nothing to do with the antemortem or postmortem nature of drowning and simply speaks of the duration of submersion of the body in water. The change is attributed to the imbibition of water into the outer layers of the skin. It is first seen in finger tips usually by 3–4 hours and the entire hand may get involved by 24 hours.

73. A child was playing with a fruit and ate it. He was having irritability, not passing urine, agitation & constipation. Choose the poison and antidote?

a. Datura & physostigmine
b. Yellow oleander & physostigmine
c. Datura & digibind
d. Yellow oleander & digibind

Ans. is 'a' Datura & physostigmine

THE most likely poison in this case is DHATURA.

Accidental cases may occur in children and adults who eat the raw fruit or seeds mistaking them for edible fruits or capsicum seeds.

The important signs and symptoms can be summarised under the **Ds**, viz.:

- Dryness of the mouth and throat
- Difficulty in talking
- Dysphagia
- Dilatation of cutaneous blood vessels
- Dilatation of pupils
- Dry hot skin
- Dysuria
- Drunken gait
- Delirium and
- Drowsiness leading to coma.

Antidote: Physostigmine one mg., IV or IM, at hourly intervals. In many cases a single dose is sufficient.

74. A man was working in fields, collapsed in a hot summer afternoon. Which of the following symptoms least likely to be seen?

a. Sweating b. Hot Skin
c. Hypotension d. Temperature 105.2°F

Ans. is 'a' Sweating

The given case is that of a heat stroke.

Heat cramps/miner's cramps/stoker's cramps	***Health exhaustion/heat prostration/heat collapse***	***Heat stroke/sun stroke/heat hyperpyrexia/thermic fever***
Painful spasm of voluntary muscles, especially those of the extremities and the abdominal wall. Usually occurs in persons who do heavy muscular work in high temperature and humidity	Prodromal symptoms usually comprise of increasing thirst, nausea, vomiting, headache, irritability with feeling of exhaustion. Usually occurs in person after several days of hard work in closed environment and under moderately high temperature.	Often rapid in onset. May be preceded by headache, nausea, weakness, myalgia, confusion, disorientation, locomotor disturbances, etc. Usually occurs in persons undergoing strenuous work in the open fields under conditions of high temperature with lack of acclimatisation.
	• Skin is moist and clammy • Pale face • Pulse is thready • Low blood pressure • Breathing is sighing • Temperature normal or sub-normal • Fainting and manifestations of peripheral vascular collapse may ensure.	• Skin is dry and hot • Flushed face • Pulse is fast, theady • Hypotension • Breathing is rapid, deep • Very high fever (may reach 105°–107°F • Varying manifestations of cerebral deficit usually constitute an important feature
Cause is stated to be loss of sodium and chlorides from the body	Cause is stated to be water and /or salt loss from excessive sweating that is inadequately replaced. May be similar in presentation to insulin shock, alcohol/drug abuse or hypovolemia from occult blood loss	Cause is stated to be failure of thermo-regulatory systems resulting in severe hyperthermia and multisystem damage in the form of neurological deficit, DIC, rhabdomyolysis, renal and hepatic failure, etc. First 24 hours are most critical, Autopsy findings lack specificity. Postmortem caloricity may be a distinct feature. Rigor mortis appears early and passes off quickly. Increased body temperature causes diminished peripheral resistance leading to increased venous return, and thus triggering high output cardiac failure. However, ultimate manifestations attending death are considered to be deprivation of oxygen to the tissues rather than the direct effect of increased heat load.
Management consists in maintaining an adequate salt intake in food or in saline drinks. Sources needs be removed.	Management consists in making the patient lie in cool area. Fluids and salt need be replenished. If needed, intravenous fluid may be administered.	Management consists in shifting the patient to the cooler place and hospitalization. Maintaining always and circulation. Intravenous fluids and electrolyte therapy.

75. A guy was sitting in balcony, which was overlooking park. He was sitting naked for sexual gratification. This condition is:

a. Voyeurism
b. Masochism
c. Exhibitionism
d. Fetichism

Ans. is 'c'. Exhibitionism

Paraphilia DSM-IV diagnosis	*Paraphilic disorder DMS-5 diagnosis*	*Summary definitions*
Exhibitionism	Exhibitionistic disorder	Exposing ones' genitals to an unsuspecting person or performing sexual acts that can be watched by others
Frotteurism	Frotteuristic disorder	Touch or rubbing against a non-consenting person
voyeurism	Voyeuristic disorder	Urges to observe an unsuspecting person who is naked, undressing or engaging in sexual activities, or in activities deemed to be of a private nature
Fetishism	Fetishistic disorder	Use of inanimate objects of gain sexual excitement
Paedophilia	Pedophilic disorder	Sexual preference for prepubescent children
Sexual masochism	Sexual masochism disorder	Wanting to be humiliated, beaten, bound or otherwise made to suffer for sexual pleasure
Sexual sadism	Sexual sadism disorder	In which pain or humiliation of a person is sexually pleasing
Transvestic fetishism	Transvestic fetishism	Arousal from clothing associated with members of the opposite sex
Not otherwise specified	Other specified paraphilic disorder	These include a variety of paraphilic behaviours such as: partialism; zoophilia; necrophilia; klismaphilia; coprophilia; urophilia; infantilism; telephone scatologia

76. A woman gave birth to twins. The father thought the children does not belong to him. DNA fingerprinting was done and it was found that one child belong to him. It is a________?

a. Case of superfecundation
b. Case of suppositious child
c. Case of atavism
d. Case of superfetation

Ans. is 'a' Case of superfecundation

Superfoetation and Superfecundation

Superfoetation means the fertilisation of an ovum from a subsequent ovulation in a woman who is already pregnant, and the consequence is the birth of two children at the same time, one of whom may be mature and the other immature. They may however be born at full term, one few weeks ahead of the other. The condition, though not impossible, is difficult to prove. Pregnancy does not close the cervical or tubal orifices immediately. The ovulation usually stops with the onset of pregnancy, but should it occur after the onset of pregnancy as ovulation may take place particularly during first trimester of pregnancy until the decidua vera comes into apposition with decidua reflexa and the decidual cavity gets obliterated, fertilisation of the newly released ovum may take place following coitus.

Superfecundation means multiple pregnancy resulting from the fertilisation of two or more ova liberated in the same menstrual cycle by spermatozoa introduced during successive acts of coitus. The condition is possible but difficult to prove since both fertilised ova develop as twins and go to full term at about the same period. If the mother has had sexual relation with two men of different race and two children are born at term, having different racial characters, it is substantial indication of superfecundation.

77. Not suggestive of Cocaine poisoning:

a. Agitation
b. Hyperthermia
c. Bradycardia
d. Myocardial infarction

Ans. is 'c' Bradycardia

Signs and Symptoms of Cocaine Poisoning

- **Stage of Excitement:** There is bitter taste, dryness in the mouth, dysphagia, feeling of well-being and loss of depression and fatigue. The patient may be excited, restless and talkative, but this passes into a calm, dull condition. The pulse is rapid, respirations rapid and deep, pupils dilated, headache, pallor of the skin, cyanosis, sweating, and the temperature is raised. It produces hypertension like amphetamine which may lead to cerebral bleeding. The reflexes are exaggerated, and there may be tremors or convulsions. Occasionally, the patients may have hallucinations and become maniacal. There is often a feeling of tingling or numbness in the hands and feet, and a numb feeling at the place where the drug has touched, e.g. nose and back of throat, when it has been sniffed. With spinal anaesthesia there is an occasional case of post-anaesthetic myelitis, which leads to permanent symptoms of cord degeneration.
- **Stage of Depression:** Within an hour or even less, respirations become feeble, profuse perspiration, collapse, convulsions and death occurs. Death is due to respiratory failure, cardiac failure, or vascular collapse. Sudden death may occur following IV injection, and smoking than snorting, due to cardiac arrhythmias due to direct action on myocardium, and cardiopulmonary arrest.

ORTHOPEDICS

NEET PG September 2021

78. A 20 years old male complains of gradual swelling around wrist for 3 months, X-ray is given below. What is the most likely diagnosis?

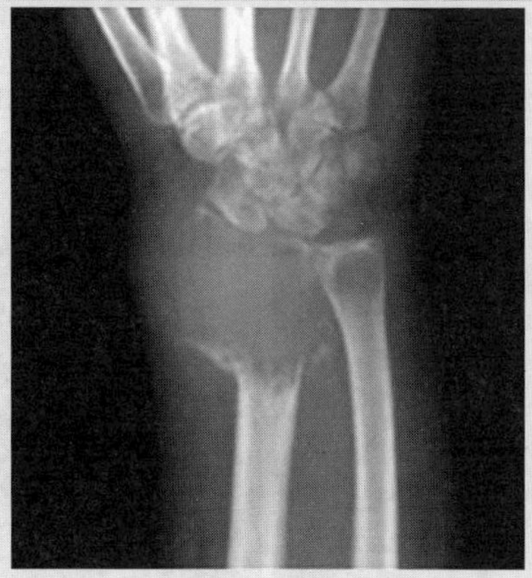

a. Giant cell tumor
b. Osteoid osteoma
c. Osteosarcoma
d. Ewing's sarcoma

Ans. is 'a' Giant cell tumor

For detail see explanation on page 389

79. A 20-year-old patient presenting with chronic low back pain and early morning stiffness since last 2 years associated with bilateral heel pains. What is the most likely diagnosis?

a. TB spine
b. Ankylosing spondylitis
c. Mechanical back pain
d. Prolapsed intervertebral disc

Ans. is 'b' Ankylosing spondylitis

For detail see explanation on page 407

80. A 26-year-old male with back ache, morning stiffness and reddening of eyes. X- ray of the patient is given below. Identify the diagnosis of this patient:

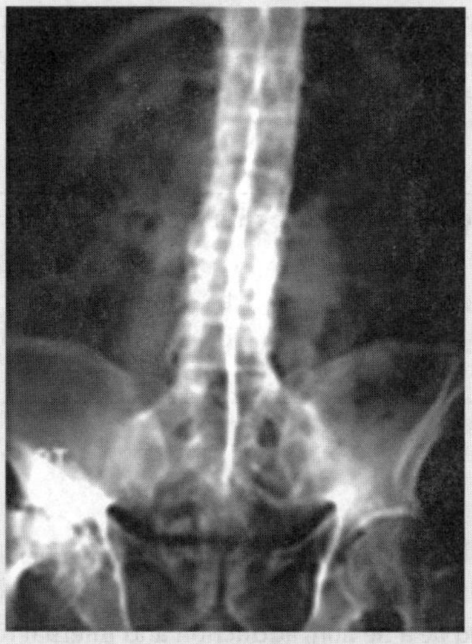

a. Rheumatoid arthritis
b. Psoriatic arthritis
c. Ankylosing spondylitis
d. Paget's disease

Ans. is 'c' Ankylosing spondylitis

For detail see explanation on page 407

81. A post-menopausal women with previous history of Colle's fracture is complaining of backache. Which of the following statement is false? Page 405 explanation done

a. Teriparatide should be given before supplementing bisphosphonates one at a time
b. Bisphosphonates are not given for more than one year
c. Calcium requirement is 1200 mg per day
d. Oral Vit D3 given along with oral calcium

Ans. is 'b' Bisphosphonates are not given for more than one year

For detail see explanation on page 405

82. A 10-year-old child with normal bone mineral density. X-ray is given below. Identify the diagnosis:

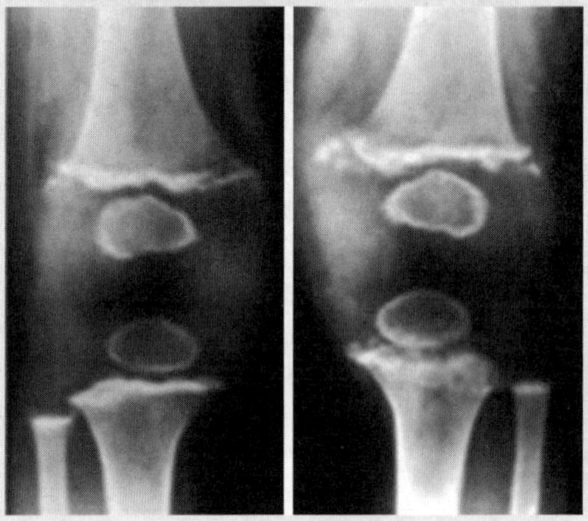

a. Rickets
b. Scurvy
c. Osteopetrosis
d. Metaphyseal dysplasia

Ans. is 'b' Scurvy

Radiological Features (sclerosed margins of epiphysis)

Osteopenia (ground glass appearance) (1st sign) with thinning of cortex (pencil thin cortex).

- Metaphysis maybe deformed or fractured.
- Frankel's line (zone of provisional calcification increases in width and opacity) due to failure of resorption of calcified cartilage and stands out compared to the severely osteopenic metaphysis.

Scurvy line or scorbutic zone (Trummerfeld zone) is radiolucent transverse band adjacent to the dense provisional zone.

- Margins of the epiphysis appears relatively sclerotic, termed ringing of epiphyses or Wimberger's sign (Ring sign)—most important.
- Lateral metaphyseal spur (Pelkan spur) at ends of metaphysis is produced by outward projection of zone of provisional calcification and periosteal reaction.
- Corner or angle sign is peripheral metaphyseal cleft.
- Subperiosteal hemorrhage

83. A patient fell down riding a bicycle, he started having pain around hip, shortening of limb, attitude of limb was Flexion, Adduction and internal rotation.

a. Anterior dislocation
b. Posterior dislocation
c. Inter-trochanteric fracture
d. Fracture neck of femur

Ans. is 'b' Posterior dislocation

Posterior Dislocation of Hip

- It is more common (90%)
- **Mechanism of injury**: Dashboard injury—occur with axial load applied on a flexed knee placed in adduction—seen as one sits in the front seat of the car.
- The typical attitude of the lower limb would be a flexion, adduction and internal rotation.
- Complications include AVN of femoral head, sciatic nerve injury, associated fractures of femoral head and acetabulum and also associated knee injuries
- Imaging
- Findings: Dislocation is usually seen on AP view; in a few cases, lateral view may be needed to establish the diagnosis.

- Treatment
  - More the deformity is a sign that probably there is no associated fracture of acetabulum or femoral head/neck. These cases can undergo closed reduction under some sedation.
  - Reduction under general anesthesia (GA).
- Complication: Avascular necrosis

Anterior Dislocation of Hip

- It is less common than posterior dislocation
- It is divided into various types: Type I: Pubic (femoral head lies superiorly); – Type II: Obturator (femoral head lies inferiorly).
- Clinical Features
  - Patient assumes externally rotated, abducted and slightly flexed posture at the affected hip, with restriction of movement.
  - Head of femur is often felt either anteriorly (superior type) or in the groin (inferior type).
- Imaging
- Findings: Dislocation is usually seen on AP view; in a few cases, lateral view may be needed to establish the diagnosis.
- Treatment: Reduction under general anesthesia (GA).
- Complication: Avascular necrosis

84. Identify the nerve involved in this test:

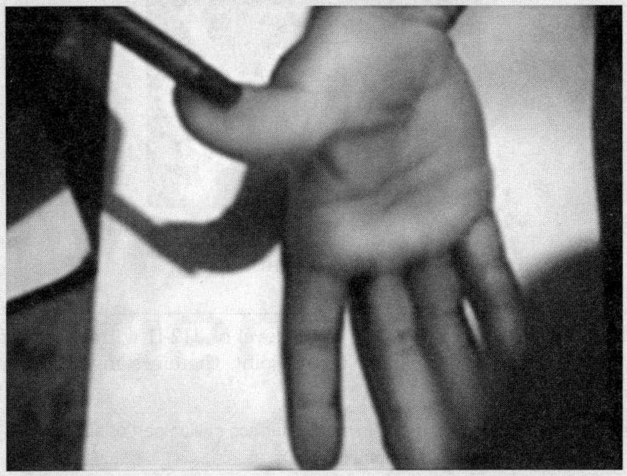

a. Median nerve
b. Ulnar nerve
c. Posterior interosseous nerve
d. Musculocutaneous nerve

Ans. is 'a' Median nerve

Special Tests for Median Nerve Injury

Pen Test

Test: Patient keeps his/her hand flat on the table and at the same time, examiner brings a pen above the thumb.

Interpretation: Patient tries to touch the pen by abduction the thumb and examiner feels the tendon of abductor pollicis brevis (APB) at the wrist. Patient fails to touch in APB paralysis and examiner will not be able to palpate the tendon.

Note: Median nerve invariably and exclusively supply APB.

Pointing Index Sign/Ochsner's Clasping/ Benediction Test

Test: Patient clasps his both hand together.

Interpretation: The index finger fails to flex in median nerve injury and it points outward as pointing index.

Note: It occur in high median nerve palsy where flexor digitorum superficialis and lateral half of flexor digitorum profundus gets involved.

85. A patient presenting with multiple humeral shaft fracture following which he had difficulty in flexion elbow and supination of forearm. He also complaints of loss of sensation over lateral-side of forearm:

a. Median nerve
b. Musculocutaneous nerve
c. Axillary nerve
d. Radial nerve

Ans. is 'b' Musculocutaneous nerve

Musculocutaneous Nerve (C5, 6, 7)

- ❖ Is one of the two terminal branches of the lateral cord, the other being the lateral root of the median nerve.
- ❖ Is supplies coracobrachialis, both heads of biceps brachii and most of branchialis, and continues as the lateral cutaneous nerve of forearm, running down the lateral aspect of the forearm.
- ❖ Injury to the musculocutaneous nerve results in weakness of supination (biceps) and flexion (biceps, brachialis, and coracobrachialis) of the forearm and loss of sensation on the lateral side of the forearm.

86. A 24-year-old male with history of intermittent evening rise of temperature and weight loss has presented with a flexion deformity of the right hip. He had occasional low back ache and on examination there was hyperreflex on knee jerk. Identify the marked structure responsible to be involved in this pathology:

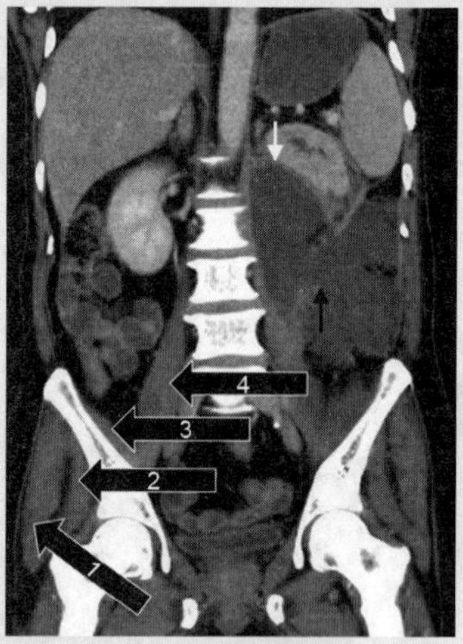

a. 1 b. 2
c. 3 d. 4

Ans. is 'd' 4

This could be a case of tuberculosis of the spine most probably at the level of d12-l1 with psoas abscess. Iliopsoas muscle is the main flexor of the hip and is attached to the lesser trochanter distal to the hip joint. Therefore any irritation to the same can lead to formation of flexion deformity at the hip.

1	Gluteus medius taking origin from medial surface of iliac part of hip bone. It lies deep and anterior to gluteus maximus
2	Gluteus maximus taking origin from lateral surface of iliac part of hip bone.
3	Iliacus muscles taking origin from medial surface of iliac part of hip bone.
4	Psoas major muscle

OPHTHALMOLOGY

NEET PG September 2021

87. A 15-year-old female with myopic astigmatism refuses to wear glasses; what would be the ideal management?

a. LASIK b. Femto LASIK
c. ICL d. Spherical equivalent glasses

Ans. is 'd' Spherical equivalent glasses

Patient selection criteria for any refractive surgeries are:

- ❖ Patients above 20 years of age.
- ❖ Stable refraction for at least 12 months.
- ❖ Motivated patient.
- ❖ Absence of corneal pathology.
- ❖ Presence of ectasia or any other corneal pathology and a corneal thickness less than 450 µm is an *absolute contraindication* for LASIK. Since the age of the patient given in question is 15 years, options a, b, c are eliminated.

88. A child with whitish pupillary reflex has undergone enucleation and shows bright round blue cells with Flexner—Wintersteiner rosettes. What is the diagnosis?

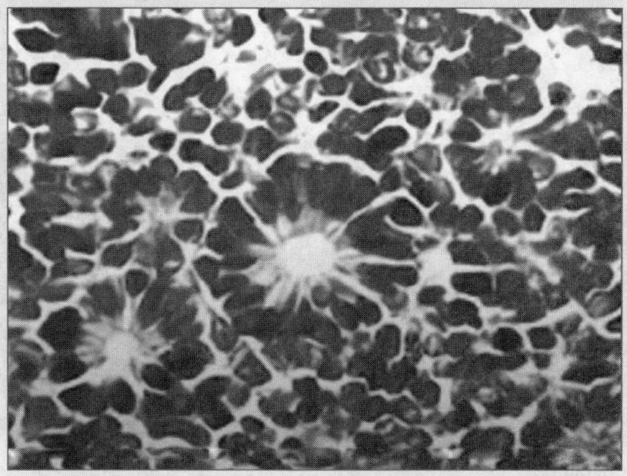

For colour version see Plate 4

a. Retinoblastoma
b. Rhabdomyosarcoma
c. Medulloblastoma
d. Astrocytoma

Ans. is 'a' Retinoblastoma

Retinoblastoma/Masquarade Syndrome

- Most common primary intraocular malignancy of childhood.
- Genetics and inheritance:
  - RB gene – tumor suppressor gene – chr 13q14
  - Sporadic cases – 60% - U/L
  - Heritable cases – 40% - AD inheritance – B/L
  - Trilateral Rb – 10% - B/L Rb + pinealoblastoma
  - MC 2nd malignancy in Rb – osteosarcoma
  - Genetic mutations – by Knudson's 2 hit hypothesis.
- Clinical presentation:
  - MC – leucocoria – white papillary reflex
  - 2nd MC – strabismus
  - Preseptal cellulitis
  - Secondary glaucoma
  - Psuedohypopion – tumor cells deposit in AC
  - Lens dislocation
  - Phthisis bulbi
- Types:
  - Intraretinal—homogeneous, dome-shaped white lesion that becomes irregular, often with white flecks of calcification.
  - Endophytic—tumour projects into the vitreous as a white mass that may 'seed' into the gel
  - Exophytic—tumour forms multilobular subretinal white masses and causes overlying retinal detachment
- Diagnosis:
  - Imaging—USG B scan, IOC - MRI
  - Elevated aqueous humor levels of LDH, PGI, NSE, synaptophysin.
  - Histopathology—Flexner Wintersteiner rosettes, Homer Wright rosettes, pseudorosettes
- Classification and management:

International classification		Description	Treatment
I	Group A	<3 mm	Peripheral—cryotherapy Central – photocoagulation
	Group B	3–6 mm	Chemotherapy V- vincristine E- etoposide C- carboplatin Intravitreal melphalan
	Group C	>6 mm Asso.with SRF or focal vitreous seeds	
	Group D	Diffuse vitreous seeds	
	Group E	Large tumor filling >1/2 of eyeball	Enucleation with optic nerve stump of at least 15 mm

Contd...

Contd...

International classification		Description	Treatment
II	–	Spread to optic nerve	Postoperative RT to optic nerve
III	–	Orbital spread	Exenteration
IV	–	Distant mets	palliative

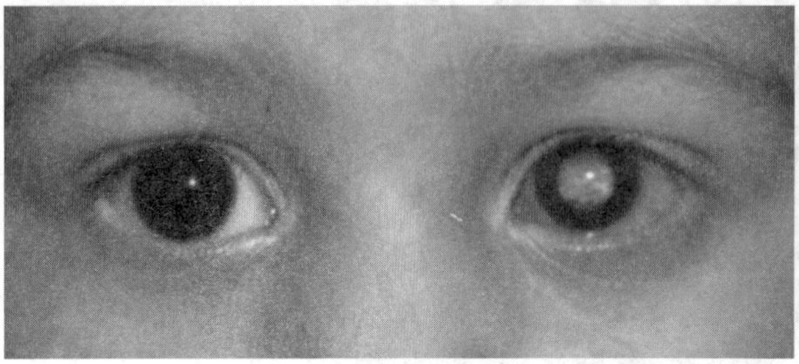

Leukocoria

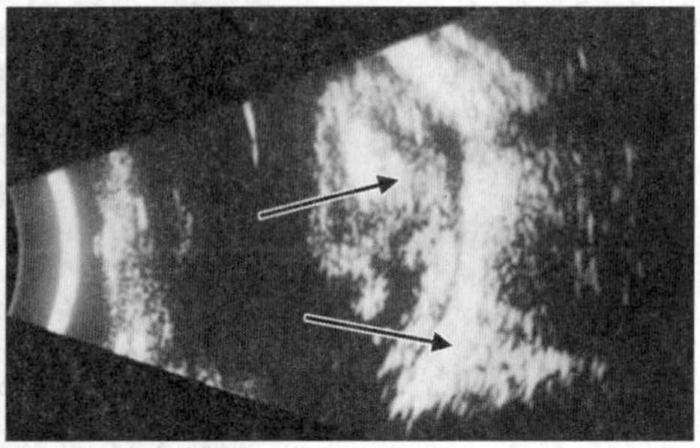

B-scan USG of retinoblastoma showing solid, posterior intraocular mass contains strong particulate reflections attributable to intralesional calcification

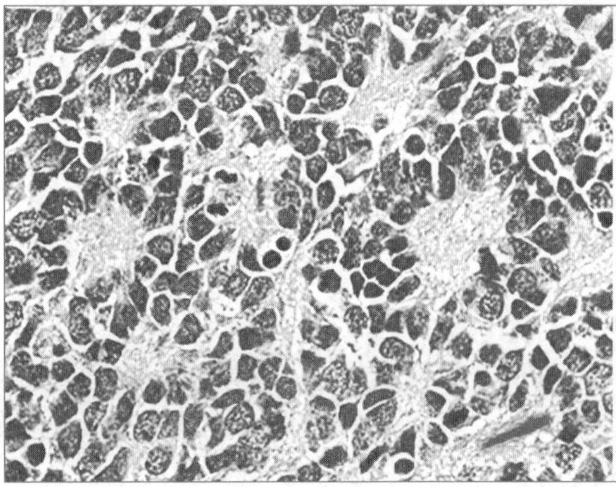

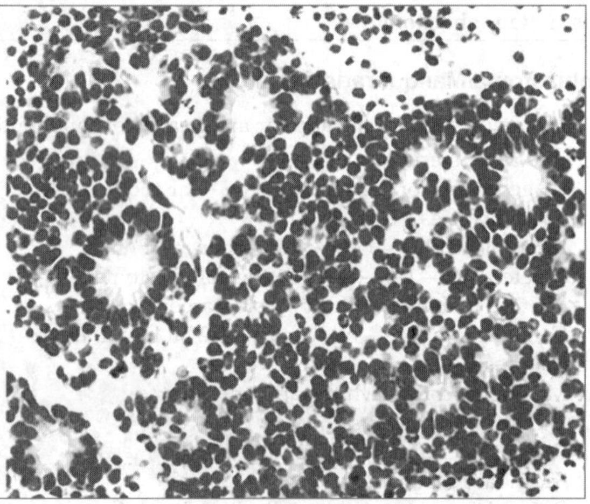

For colour version see Plate 4

89. A 1-month-old baby comes with watering eyes and a cloudy cornea. Identify the diagnosis:

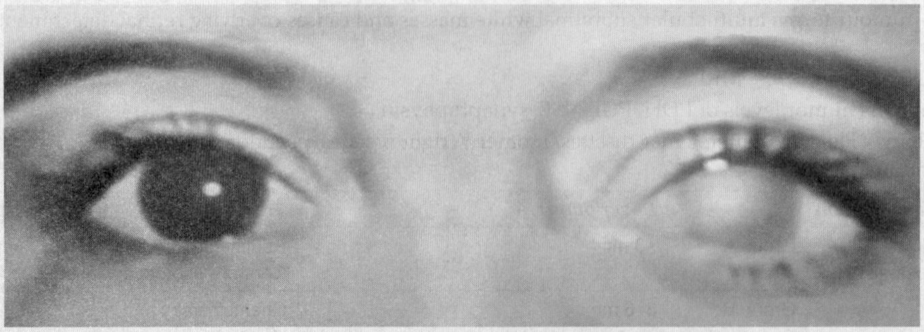

a. Cataract
b. Congenital glaucoma
c. Ophthalmia neonatorum
d. Mucopolysaccharidosis

Ans. is 'b' Congenital glaucoma

For detail see explanation on page 429

90. A female comes with a 2-year-old history of contact lens presents with eye pain, irritation and foreign body sensation. Sport the diagnosis:

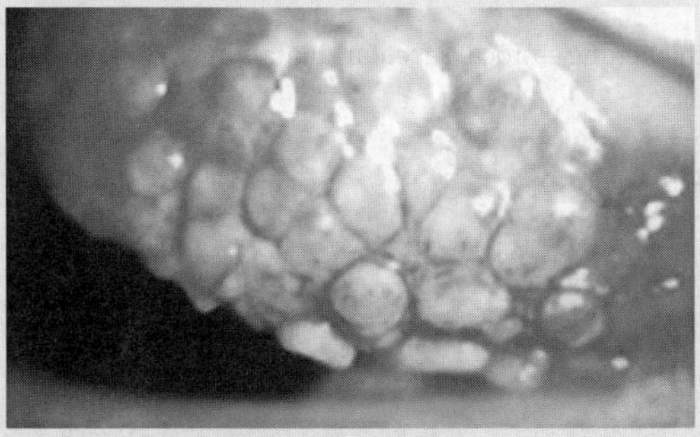

For colour version see Plate 5

a. Trachoma
b. Giant papillary conjunctivitis
c. Spring catarrh
d. Acute follicular conjunctivitis

Ans. is 'b' Giant papillary conjunctivitis

Giant Papillary Conjunctivitis (GPC)

GPC is the inflammation of conjunctiva with formation of very large sized papillae.

Etiology

GPC, also known as mechanically-induced papillary conjunctivitis, is a localised allergic response to a physically rough or deposited surface (contact lens, prosthesis, exposed nylon sutures and scleral buckle).
Probably, it is a sensitivity reaction to components of the plastic leached out by the action of tears.

Clinical Features

Symptoms: Itching, stringy discharge and reduced wearing time of contact lens or prosthetic shell.

Signs: Papillary hypertrophy (0.5 mm to 1 mm in diameter) of the upper tarsal conjunctiva, similar to that seen in palpebral form of VKC with hyperaemia are the main signs.

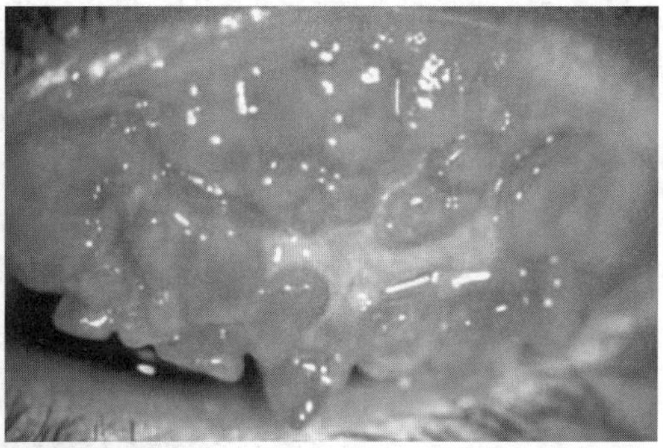

Treatment

- *The offending cause should be removed.* After discontinuation of contact lens or artificial eye or removal of nylon sutures, the papillae resolve over a period of one month.
- *Mast cell stabilizer* such as sodium cromoglycate
- Steroids – in resistant cases

91. An elderly female presents with gradual painless vision loss. The fundus picture is given below. What is the diagnosis?

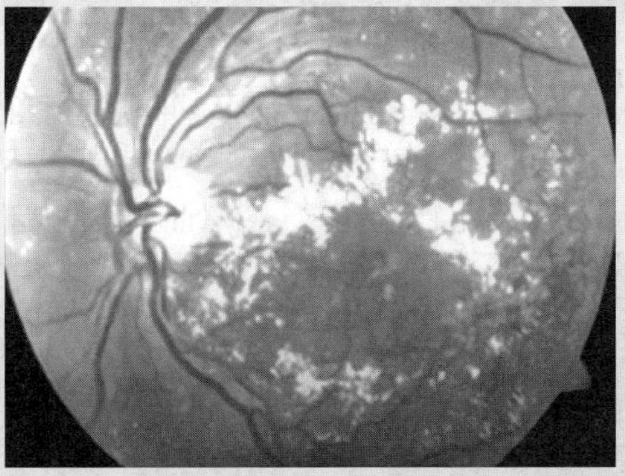

For colour version see Plate 5

a. Hard exudates in DM
b. Flame-shaped haemorrhage in hypertension
c. Soft exudates in hypertension
d. CRVO

Ans. is 'a' Hard exudates in DM

Ophthalmologic Signs of Diabetic Retinopathy

- **Microaneurysms**
  - Earliest sign of DR
  - Loss of pericytes → vessel wall thickening → focal saccular dilatation
  - Site → inner nuclear layer

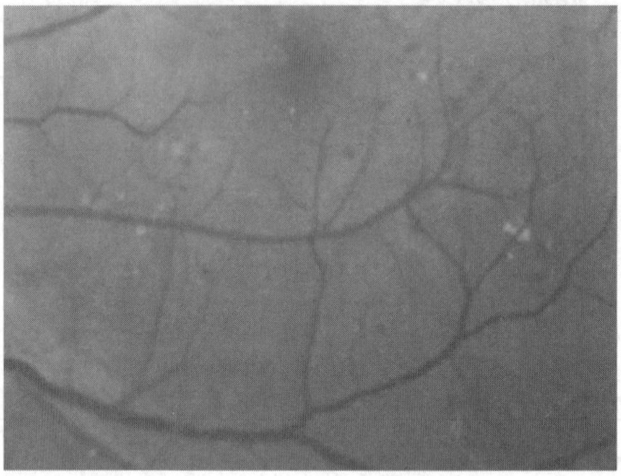

- **Retinal haemorrhages**
  - Superficial hemorrhage – flame-shaped, located in nerve fibre layer.
  - Deep hemorrhage – dot/blot hemorrhages, located in inner nuclear layer
  - Deep dark hemorrhage – hemorrhagic retinal infarcts in inner nuclear layer.
- **Exudates**
  - Hard exudates – composed of lipoproteins and lipid laden macrophages in outer plexiform layer
  - Soft exudates – cotton wool spots – neuronal debris within nerve fibre layer

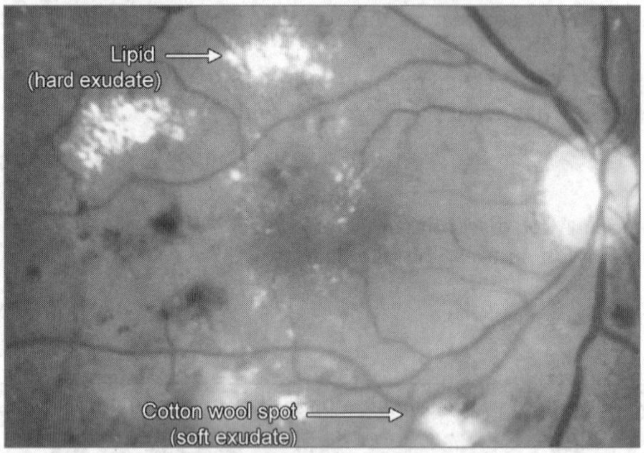

- **Neovascularization – hallmark of PDR**
  - New vessels at the disc (NVD) describes neovascularization on or within one disc diameter of the optic nerve head
  - New vessels elsewhere (NVE) describes neovascularization further away from the disc; it may be associated with fibrosis if long-standing.
  - New vessels on the iris (NVI), also known as rubeosis iridis, carry a high likelihood of progression to neovascular glaucoma.

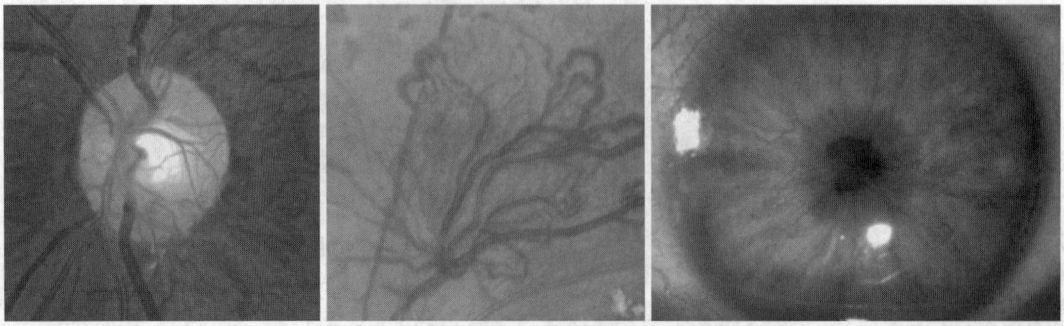

92. A patient presenting with diminishing vision in dim light with dry eyes and roughening of corneal surface. Which of the following deficiencies can be associated with it?

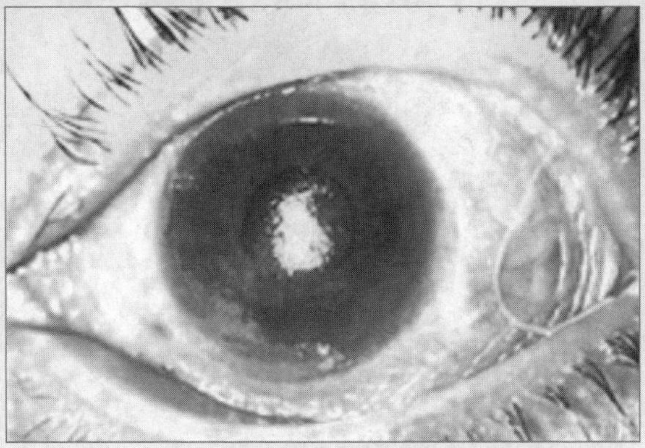

For colour version see Plate 5

a. Iron
b. Protein
c. Retinoic acid
d. Niacin

Ans. is 'c' Retinoic acid

Ocular Manifestations of Nutritional Deficiencies

- *Deficiency of vitamin A.* Ocular manifestations of vitamin A deficiency are referred to as xerophthalmia.
- *Deficiency of vitamin B1 (thiamine).* It can cause corneal anaesthesia, conjunctival and corneal dystrophy and acute retrobulbar neuritis.
- *Deficiency of vitamin B2 (riboflavin).* It can produce photophobia and burning sensation in the eyes due to conjunctival irritation and vascularisation of the cornea.
- *Deficiency of vitamin C.* It may be associated with haemorrhages in the conjunctiva, lids, anterior chamber, retina and orbit. It also delays wound healing.
- *Deficiency of vitamin D.* It may be associated with zonular cataract, papilloedema and increased lacrimation.

Xerophthalmia

- **Etiology**

  It occurs either due to *dietary deficiency* of vitamin A or its *defective absorption* from the gut.

- **WHO Classification (1982)**
  - The new xerophthalmia classification (modification of original 1976 classification) is as follows:
    - XN Night blindness
    - X1A Conjunctival xerosis
    - X1B Bitot's spots
    - X2 Corneal xerosis
    - X3A Corneal ulceration/keratomalacia affecting less than one-third corneal surface
    - X3B Corneal ulceration/keratomalacia affecting more than one-third corneal surface
    - XS Corneal scar due to xerophthalmia
    - XF Xerophthalmic fundus.

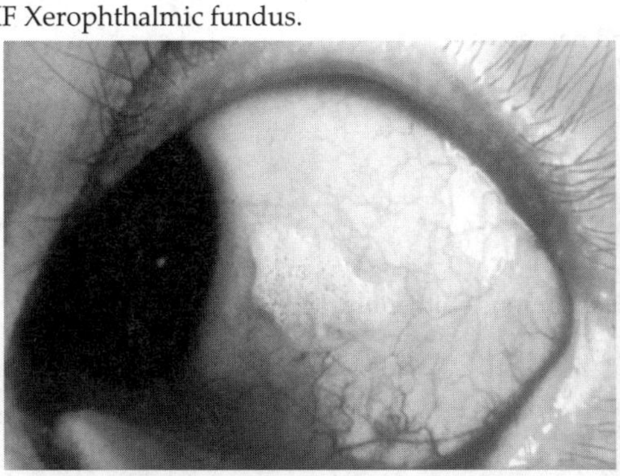

Xerophthalmia, stage X1B: Bitot spots

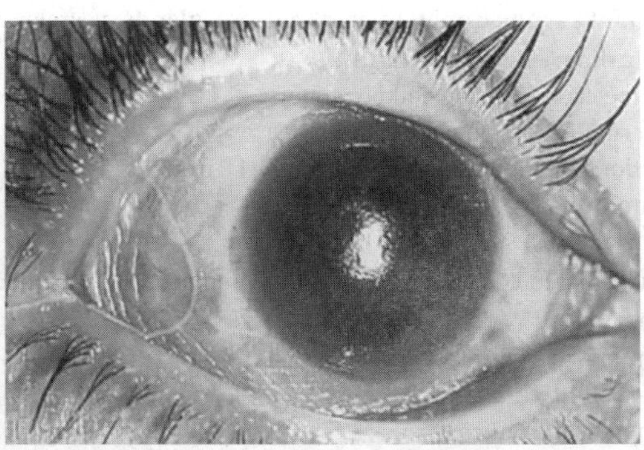

Xerophthalmia, stage X2: Corneal xerosis

93. A patient presents with the following finding. What is the most likely complication associated with it?

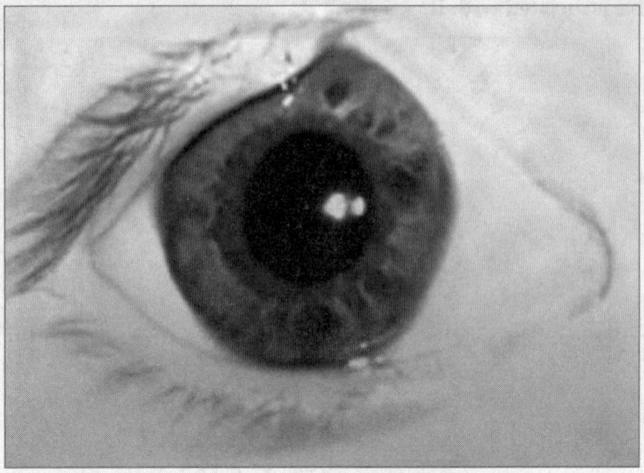

a. Cataract
b. Exposure keratitis
c. Difficulty in ocular movements
d. Glaucoma

Ans. is 'b' Exposure keratitis

Congenital Coloboma

- It is a rare condition characterised by a full thickness triangular gap in the tissues of the lids.
- The anomaly usually occurs near the nasal side and involves the upper lid more frequently than the lower lid.
- There are often other congenital defects of the eye or other parts of the body such as coloboma of the iris or accessory auricles.
- Some cases are due to incomplete closure of the embryonic facial cleft, others probably to the pressure of amniotic bands.
- Occasionally there is a notch at the outer part of the lower lid, associated with maldevelopment of the first visceral arch (mandibulofacial dysostosis, Goldenhar syndrome).
- It leads to incompelete closure of eyelid and so can result in exposure keratitis
- *Treatment* consists of plastic repair of the defect.

ENT

NEET PG September 2021

94. A patient presented with Roomy nasal cavity with foul smelling, yellow discharge. What is the diagnosis?

a. Atrophic rhinitis
b. Nasal mass
c. Nasal polyp
d. GDM

Ans. is 'a' Atrophic rhinitis

Atrophic Rhinitis/Ozaena

- Chronic rhinitis with atrophy of nasal mucosa, glands, vessels and nerves.
- **Causes** of primary atrophic rhinitis:
  - Infective cause → Klebsiella ozanae
  - Endocrinal → oestrogen deficiency
  - Nutritional → deficiency of vitamin A, D, iron
  - Autoimmune
  - Hereditary
- **Pathology**: Ciliated columnar epithelium→ replaced by stratified squamous epithelium.
- Females @ puberty
  - Anosmia – merciful/ blissful anosmia
  - Foul smelling discharge.
  - Roomy nasal cavities
  - Nasal obstruction due to crusting.

❖ **Treatment:**
- Warm nasal alkaline solution → loosen and remove crust.
- 25% glucose in glycerin → hygroscopic → moisture mucosa.
- Local antibiotic:
  - Kimecetine antiozaena solution
  - Chloramphenicol
  - Estradiol
  - Vitamin D_2
- Propylene glycol

❖ **Surgery**: ↓ size of nasal cavity
- Young operation – close both nostrils × 6 months.
- Modified Young's – close both nostril PARTIALLY × 2 years
- Lautenslagers operation – medialization of lateral wall of nose by insertion of Teflon/cartilage.

95. Topical application of 400 mcg/mL mitomycin C is used for:

a. Subglottic stenosis
b. Tympanoplasty
c. Rhinocerebral mucormycosis
d. Nasopharyngeal bleeding

Ans. is 'a' Subglottic stenosis

Mitomycin C is used following surgical interventions in the airway, either open or endoscopic, to prevent re-scarring and stenosis. It is used by topical application in a dose of 400 mcg/mL. Although it is still used by paediatric airway surgeons, there is limited high-quality evidence to support its use.

96. A 9-year-old male baby was brought to emergency by the mother with difficulty in swallowing for past few hours and a history of playing unsupervised. X-ray was taken. Identify the location of foreign body:

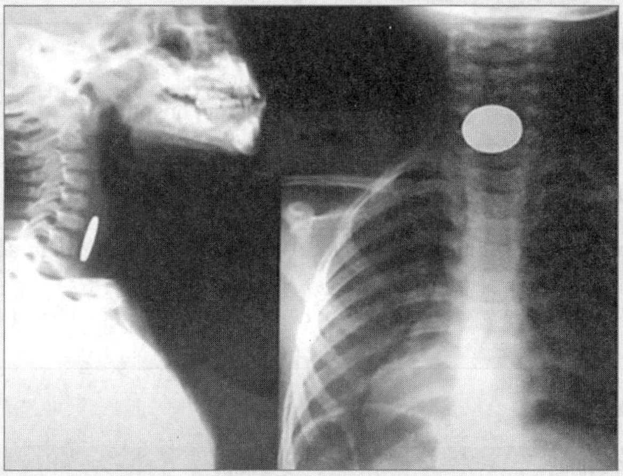

a. Oesophagus
b. Trachea
c. Soft tissue of neck
d. Artifact of X-ray

Ans. is 'a' Oesophagus

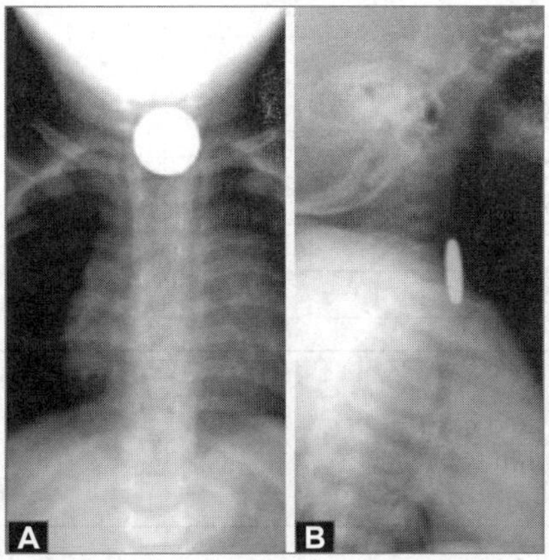

Esophagus
- PA view will show flat surface of coin
- Lateral view will show sagittal plane

Trachea
- Lateral view will show flat surface of coin
- PA view will show sagittal plane

Radiographs of a coin in the esophagus. When foreign body lodge in the esophagus, the flat surface of the object is seen in the anteroposterior view (A) and the edge is seen in the lateral view (B). The reverse is true for objects in the trachea

97. A 40-year-old female presented with nasal bleeding. Initial nasal packing was done and stoppage of bleeding was expected. However once the pack was removed the clinician noticed repeated bleed. An ENT referral was given. What would be the next step that the ENT surgeon would do?

a. ICA ligation
b. ECA ligation
c. Endoscopic sphenopalatine artery ligation
d. Maxillary artery ligation

Ans. is 'c' Endoscopic sphenopalatine artery ligation

Ligation is reserved for intractable bleeding where the source cannot be located or controlled by the conservative management. Knowledge of the blood supply of the nasal cavity and the likely sources of epistaxis will inform the choice of ligation technique. Ligation should be performed as close as possible to the likely bleeding point, thus the hierarchy of ligation is:

- Sphenopalatine artery
- Internal maxillary artery
- External carotid artery
- Anterior/posterior ethmoidal artery

The sphenopalatine artery is the main supply of the nasal cavity and thus the most logical target for ligation. Modern endoscopic techniques have seen an increase in popularity of this procedure and it has now largely replaced all other ligations as the procedure of choice. The operation has been performed with an operating microscope but much more commonly using modern endoscopic techniques. A mucosal flap is raised to identify the vessel and is cauterized or ligated.

PSM

NEET PG September 2021

98. School health is the responsibility of:

a. Sub-centre
b. PHC
c. Sub-district hospital
d. District hospital

Ans. is 'b' PHC

School health services are provided at the level of PHC and CHC.

99. Which of the following vaccines can be administered to a 10 years old boy attending a school?

a. BCG
b. IPV
c. TT/Td
d. Typhoid

Ans. is 'c' TT/Td

Upper Age Limit for Vaccination

Vaccine	*Age limit*
BCG	1 year
OPV	5 years
IPV	1 year
Hep-B	1 year
Pentavalent	1 year
Rotavirus	1 year
Measles	5 years
DPT	7 years
JE	15 years
TT	No age limit

100. Culture plate is disposed in which BMW bag?

a. White container
b. Red bag
c. Yellow bag
d. Blue bag

Ans. is 'c' Yellow bag

For detail see explanation on page 501

101. A study conducted in 30,000 women where Researcher wanted to find out if there is any relationship between CRP levels and risk of MI/stroke. The study subjects were divided into five groups of 6000 subjects each. RR of MI/Stroke was plotted against CRP levels. See the image given below and interpret your findings:

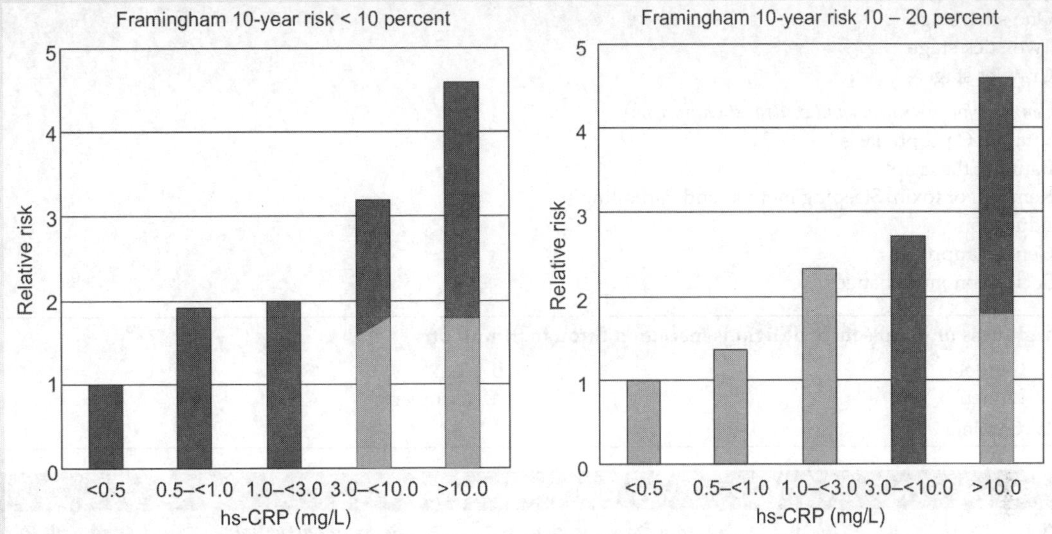

a. CRP has no relation to MI/Stroke risk
b. Increase in CRP decreases MI/Stroke risk
c. Increase in CRP levels increases MI/Stroke risk
d. Decrease in CRP levels increases MI/Stroke risk

Ans. is 'c' Increase in CRP levels increases MI/Stroke risk

Interpretation of Relative Risk

			Example	
RR	***Interpretation***[Q]		***Risk factor***	***Disease***
RR > 1	$I_{exp} > I_{nonexp}$	So many times chances/incidence of disease development is more among exposed as compared to non-exposed **(Positive Association)**	Smoking	Lung cancer
RR = 1	$I_{exp} = I_{nonexp}$	Chances/incidence of disease development is same among exposed as compared to non-exposed **(No Association)**	Smoking	HIV/AIDS
RR < 1	$I_{exp} < I_{nonexp}$	Chances/incidence of disease development is less among exposed as compared to non-exposed **(Negative Association)**	Vitamin-A intake	Epithelial cancers

102. A 55-year-old farmer from the state of Chhattisgarh presented with complaints of progressive muscle weakness, stiffness and pain in both legs. On examination, pure motor paresis is present. What further history would you take?

a. History of fever
b. History of vaccination
c. History of diet
d. History of similar events in the past

Ans. is 'c' History of diet

Lathyrism

It is a neurodegenerative disorder, caused by the consumption of a pulse called 'lathyrus sativus' over a long period of time, clinically characterized by progressive, permanent, spastic paraplegia (upper motor neurone type of paralysis of both lower limbs), resulting in crippling deformity.

❖ *Lathyrism is of two types:*
- *Neurolathyrism*: In human beings
- *Osteolathyrism (Odoratism)*: In animals

*Neurolathyrism is caused by eating the pulse 'Khesari Dal (Lathyrus sativus)'. Diets containing over 30% of this dal consumed over a period of 2–6 months result in neurolathyrism.

* Lathyrism affects 15–45 years of age.

- *Toxin*: Present in lathyrus seeds is 'Beta oxalyl amino alanine (BOAA)'[Q]
- *It manifests as following stages*:
    - Latent stage
    - No-stick stage
    - One-stick stage
    - Two-stick stage
    - Crawler stage
- *Interventions for prevention and control of Lathyrism*:
    - Vitamin C prophylaxis[Q]
    - Banning the crop
    - Removal of toxin: Steeping method and Parboiling[Q]
    - Education
    - Genetic approach
    - Socio-economic changes.

103. Brightness of point source of light is measured through SI unit of:

a. Candela
b. Lux
c. Lumen
d. Lambert

Ans. is 'a' Candela

Light measurement units			
Description	***Quantity measured name***	***Recommended unit****	***Other units***
Brightness of point source	Luminous intensity	Candela	Candle power
Flow of light	Luminous flux	Lumen	
Amount of light reaching surface	Illumination, illuminance	Lux (Phot)	Foot candle Lumen/cm^2
Amount of light re-emitted by surface	Brightness, luminance	Lambert	Foot lamber Candles/cm^2
*Recommended by the International Organization for Standardization			

104. For analysis of functioning of a health centre with respect to evaluation, which of the following is the most important for assessing clinical management?

a. Input
b. Output
c. Process
d. Structure

Ans. is 'c' Process

105. Post flood in Pathanamthitta district of Kerala fever syndrome is being reported. Health authorities distribute Doxycycline along with a chemical poison spray. Identify the chemical:

a. Lindane
b. Paris green
c. Zinc phosphide
d. Malathion

Ans. is 'b' Paris green

Paris green or copper acetoarsenite is an emerald green, micro-crystalline powder practically insoluble in water. A good sample of paris green must contain 50 per cent arsenious oxide. Paris green is a stomach poison and to be effective it must be ingested by the larvae. Paris green kills mainly the *Anopheles* larvae because they are surface-feeders. Bottom-feeding larvae are also killed when paris green is applied as a special granular formulation.. Paris green is applied as 2 per cent dust which is prepared by mixing 2 kg of paris green and 98 kg of a diluent such as soapstone powder or slaked lime in a "rotary mixer". The resulting mixture must be fine with the size of the particles ranging from 20–25 microns. The dusting is accomplished by hand blowers or rotary blowers. The recommended dose is 1 kg of actual paris green per hectare of water surface. In the dosage applied, paris green does not harm fish, man or domestic animals.

106. Acute encephalitis syndrome cases are being reported from Gorakhpur, Uttar Pradesh. The Health team decides for mass vaccination which comes under Universal Immunization Program. Identify the vaccine type and route:

a. Live attenuated intramuscular
b. Killed subcutaneous
c. Killed intramuscular
d. Live attenuated subcutaneous

Ans. is 'd' Liver attenuated subcutaneous

The case scenario in question is suggestive of Japanese encephalitis. SA 14-14-2 is the commonly used vaccine for JE in India. SA 14-14-2 is live attenuated vaccine given by SC route.

Differences between live JE vaccine and killed JE vaccine		
	Live JE vaccine	***Killed JE vaccine***
Nature	Lyophilized using SA 14-14-2 strain of JE virus grown on vero cells (or primary Hamster kidney cells)	Lyophillized or liquid vaccine prepared from Nakayama strain (mouse brain inactivated vaccine)
Presentation	Single or five dose vial supplied with diluents	Single or ten dose vaccine
Primary course	Single dose 0.5 mL	Two doses of 1.0 mL (0.5 mL for < 5 yrs) with 1-4 weeks interval
Route	Subcutaneously in (L) upper arm	Subcutaneously or intramuscularly
Booster dose	Not necessary	First booster dose after one year. Repeated booster doses are required
Schedule	Ideal at 9th month along with measles vaccine	Commence at 12th month of age
Manufacture	In China Used in India	In Korea, Taiwan, Thailand and Vietnam. Stopped in Kasauli (HP) India and in Japan
Use	To be used within one hour of reconstitution	To be used within 6 hours of reconstitution
Safety and efficacy	Safe and effective 1-3% develop pain 5-10% develop transient fever 95% effective	Less safe and effective 20% develop local reaction 1 in 1000 develop allergic reaction 80% effective
Storage temperature	2–8°C	2–8°C

107. New Delhi reported the following Air Quality Index during November month last year (as given below):

20 Nov AQI-370
21 Nov AQI-320
22 Nov AQI-360
23 Nov AQI-380
24 Nov AQI-470

Which type of air quality was reported on 24 November?

a. Moderate
b. Poor
c. Very poor
d. Severe

Ans. is 'd' Severe

108. Which is a 'conditioning factor' for Malnutrition—a man-made disease?

a. Infectious disease
b. Socio-economic factors
c. Child rearing habits
d. Food habits

Ans. is 'a' Infectious disease

In the 1970s, it was widely held that PEM was due to protein deficiency. Over the years, the concept of "protein gap" has given place to the concept of "food gap". That is, PEM is primarily due to (a) an inadequate intake of food {food gap) both in quantity and quality, and (b) infections, notably diarrhoea, respiratory infections, measles and intestinal worms which increase requirements for calories, protein and other nutrients, while decreasing their absorption and utilization. It is a vicious circle-infection contributing to malnutrition and malnutrition contributing to infection, both acting synergistically.

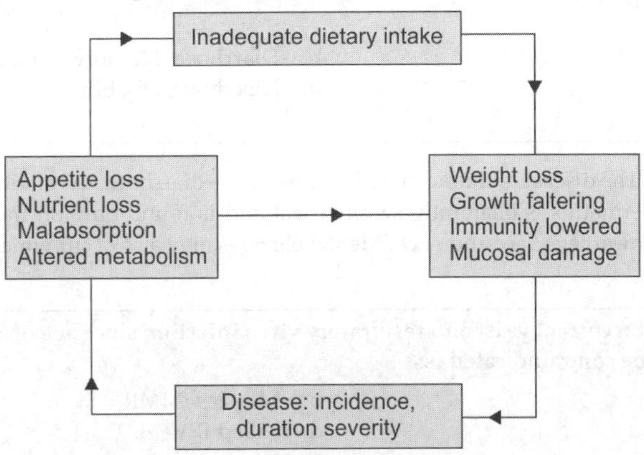

Malnutrition/infection cycle

109. Instrument to measure Low wind velocity measurement and cooling power:

a. Silvered thermometer
b. Wet globe thermometer
c. Kata thermometer
d. Globe thermometer

Ans. is 'c' Kata thermometer

Instrument	*Uses*
Ice liner refrigerator	Cold chain temperature maintenance
Dial thermometer	Cold chain temperature monitoring
Horrock's apparatus	Chlorine demand estimation
Chloronome	Regulating the dose of chlorine
Chloroscope	Measuring residual chlorine
Kata thermometer	Currently- air velocity assessment
Globe thermometer	Mean radiant temperature
Anemometer	Assess wind/air velocity
Sling psychrometer	Air humidity
Assman psychrometer	Air humidity
Salter's scale	Field instrument for LBW
Infantometer	Length of infant
Stadiometer	Height of adults
Shakir's tape	Mid arm circumference

110. A 34-year-old patient presented to OPD with lesion around the neck (see image). Which other manifestations do you expect?

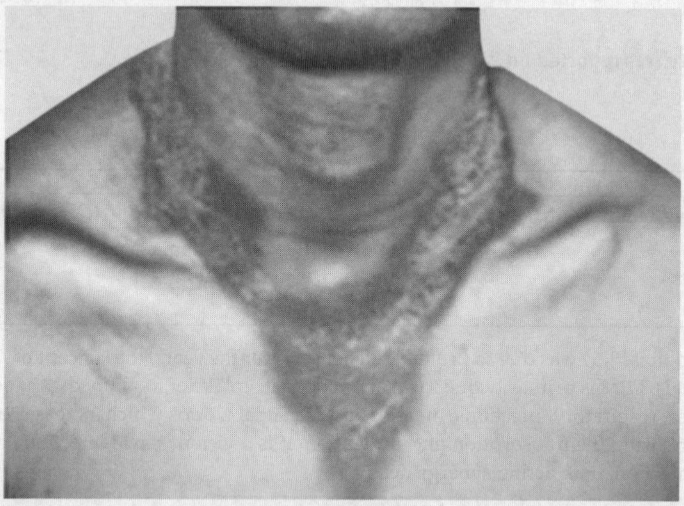

a. Diarrhoea, Dementia
b. Diarrhoea, Memory impairment
c. Diarrhoea, Arthritis
d. Diarrhoea, Disability

Ans. is 'a' Diarrhoea, Dementia

Niacin deficiency results in pellagra. The disease is characterized by three D's - diarrhoea, dermatitis and dementia. In addition glossitis and stomatitis usually occur. The dermatitis is bilaterally symmetrical and is found only on those surfaces of the body exposed to sunlight, such as back of the hands, lower legs, face and neck. Mental changes may also occur which include depression, irritability and delirium.

111. A female child has history of recurrent yeast and respiratory virus infection since age of 3 months. Immunity status studies are being undertaken. Vaccine contraindicated is:

a. TT/Td
b. Measles /MMR
c. DPT
d. Killed IPV

Ans. is 'b' Measles/MMR

Contradiction	*Vaccine*
Pregnancy	All live vaccines EXCEPT YELLOW FEVER
Fever	Typhoid vaccines
Asymptomatic HIV	None
Symptomatic HIV	All live vaccines except BCG
Immunosuppresion/steroids therapy	All live vaccines
C/I together	Yellow fever and cholera vaccine
Preterm < 2 kg BW	Hepatitis B
Infants	Yellow fever Pneumococcal Meningococcal
Age < 2 years	Typhoid vaccine
Age > 2 years	Pertussis vaccine
Progressive neurologic disease	Pertussis vaccine

112. International Food Policy Research Institute calculated global hunger index for a country with given parameters:

1. Proportion of undernourished population 27%
2. Prevalence of underweight children 25%
3. Mortality rate of under -5 children 29%
4. Infant mortality rate 20%

Which of the following will not be used in calculation?

a.. IMR
b. Child mortality
c.. Child undernourishment
d. Child underweight

Ans. is 'a' IMR

GHI combines three equally weighted indicators into one index:

1. *Undernourishment:* The proportion of undernourished people as a percentage of the population (reflecting the share of the population with insufficient calorie intake);
2. *Child underweight:* The proportion of children under the age of five who are underweight (that is, have low weight for their age, reflecting wasting, stunted growth, or both), which is one indicator of child undernutrition; and
3. *Child mortality:* The mortality rate of children under the age of five (partially reflecting the fatal synergy of inadequate food intake and unhealthy environments).

113. A 25 years old woman has been taking OCPs gave a history of 4 missed pills on different days over last 7 days. Next line of management is:

a. Take next pill as soon as possible and consider barrier method/emergency contraception if had intercourse in last 72 hours
b. Take 4 pills as soon as possible and consider barrier method/emergency contraception if had intercourse in last 72 hours
c. Adopt another method of contraception
d. Disregard the current pack and start a new cycle of pack

Ans. is 'a' Take next pill as soon as possible and consider barrier method/emergency contraception if had intercourse in last 72 hours

Missed Pills

Pills should be taken every day to be most effective. If not taken correctly there will be a risk of becoming pregnant. Most common mistake is missing the pill or starting new packets late.

- *Missed 1 pill*: She should take it as soon as she remembers and take the rest as usual.
- Missed 2 pills or more, in the first two rows (i.e. the first 14 pills) **(See figure below)**. She should take one pill as soon as she remembers and the rest as usual. Meanwhile, she must also use another method such as condoms or spermicides for 7 days or avoid sex for 1 week.
- *Missed 2 pills or more in the third row:* She should take the pill as soon as she remembers and takes a rest as usual meanwhile she must also use another method such as condoms for 7 days or avoid sex for one week and she should start a new pack the next day after the completion of 3rd row. She should throw the last row of this pack away.
- *Missed any pill in the fourth row:* She should throw the missed pill away and take the rest as usual. Start a new packet as usual on the next day. Thus, forgetting to take placebos, she is still protected from pregnancy.

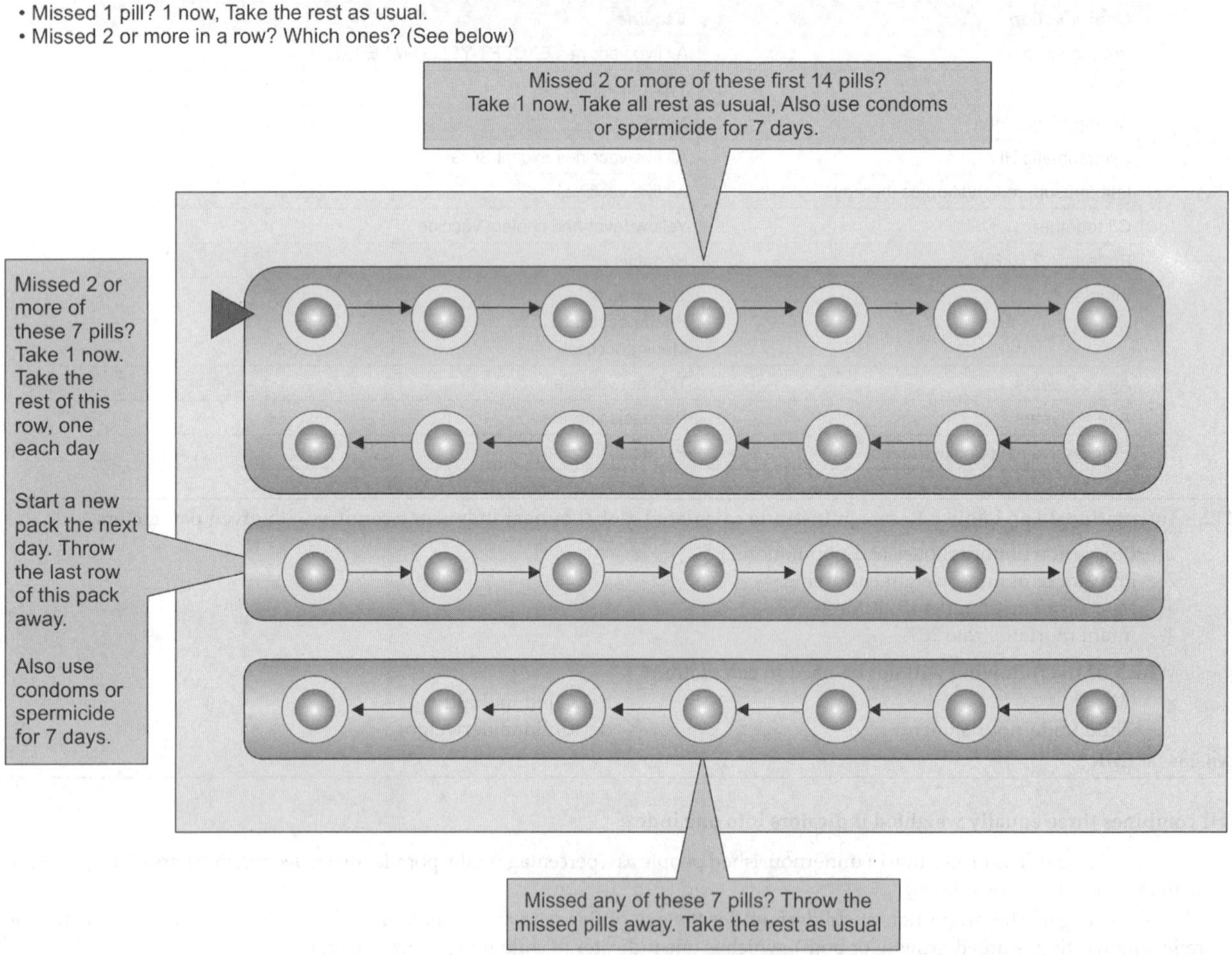

114. A patient is known case of inguinal buboes. He now presents with multiple buboes in axilla and groin. Identify the vector:

a. Sandfly
b. Phlebotamus bug
c. Triatominae bug
d. Xenopsylla cheopsis

Ans. is 'd' Xenopsylla cheopsis

The given case scenario is suggestive of bubonic plague—primary vector is rat flea (xenopsylla cheopsis)

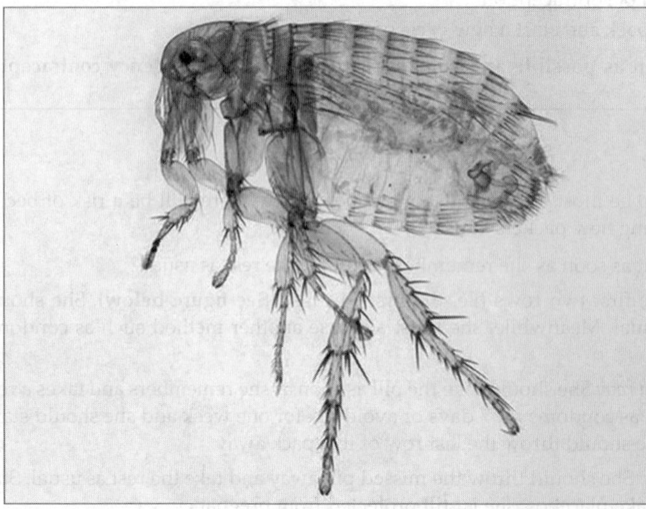

Vector	Disease(s) transmitted
Housefly (Musca domestica)	Diarrhoeal and dysentrical diseases, Poliomyelitis, Yaws, Anthrax, Trachoma
Sandfly (Phlebotamus argentipes)	Kala azar (Visceral Leishmaniasis), Oriental sore (Cutaneous Leishmaniasis), Sandfly fever, Oroya fever
Tse-Tse fly (Glossina palpalis)	Sleeping sickness of Africa (African Trypanosomiasis)
Reduviid bug (Triatominae)	Chagas disease (Sleeping sickness of America—American Trypanosomiasis)
Black fly (Simulum)	Onchocerciasis (River Blindness)
Soft tick	Relapsing fever, Q fever, KFD (outside India)
Hard tick	Tularemia, Babesiosis, KFD (India), Tick paralysis, Tick encephalitis, Tick hemorrhagic fever, Indian Tick Typhus, RMSF
Louse	Epidemic typhus, Trench fever, Relapsing fever
Mite	Scrub typhus, Rickettsial pox
Flea	Plague, Murine typhus
Anopheles mosquito	Malaria, Filaria (outside India)
Culex mosquito	Bancroftian Filariasis, Japanese Encephalitis, West Nile fever, Viral arthritis
Aedes mosquito	Yellow fever, Dengue, DHF, Chikungunya, Rift Valley fever, Filariasis (Outside India)
Mansonoides mosquito	Malayan (Brugian) filariasis, Chikungunya

MEDICINE

NEET PG September 2021

115. A 56-year-old patient with history of recurrent retrosternal chest pain, each episode lasting 3–5 min and subsiding with sublingual nitrate. Now he presented to emergency with excruciating chest pain. He is a k/c/o HTN, DM, hypercholesterolemia. He is already on Lovastatin, aspirin, statins, and 50 mg metformin. ECG shows LVH with ST-T changes with T wave flattening. Trop I is normal. What is next step in management?

a. Increase beta blocker dose
b. LMWH subcutaneous
c. IV NTG drip
d. Add tab clopidogrel

Ans. is 'b' LMWH subcutaneous

Patient has presented with acute chest pain and there is past history of anginal pain. Since there is ST-T changes with T wave flattening, it suggests patient is suffering from unstable angina. NSTEMI is ruled out as the troponin is normal. The immediate and most important treatment for unstable angina is anticoagulants hence the answer is LMWH.

116. A 30-year-old man with weight of 70 kg is admitted due to multiple episodes of seizures. On work up his Serum sodium —120 mEq/L. Calculate total sodium deficit:

a. 420 mEq
b. 840 mEq
c. 1400 mEq
d. 280 mEq

Ans. is 'b' 840 mEq

The formula to calculate sodium deficit is:

Sodium deficit: TBW* (Desired Na = patients Na)

In a male TBW is 0.6* weight as 60 % of body weight is water in a male. (in a female TBW = 0.5* weight)
So putting the values: Sodium deficit: 70*0.6 (140–120) = 840

The reason why 140 has been considered as desired sodium is question is simply asking deficit and not how much correction has to be given in 24 hours.

Now earlier many books (CMDT 2019, API textbook of medicine etc.) used to use various desired sodium values and in many the idea was to under correct sodium in order to avoid rapid correction and osmotic demyelination. Most new editions of those books have removed that under correction calculation as now regardless of the total sodium deficit calculated, it has been established that in chronic hyponatremia one should restrict sodium correction to 6–8 mM in a day. This is to prevent rapid correction of sodium. In acute hyponatremia as there is no risk of osmotic demyelination with rapid correction there is no such restriction and full correction of sodium can be achieved in a day.

117. A female patient with hysteria was hyperventilating. She subsequently developed carpopedal spasm. On work up, ABG value of pH = 7.53, pCO_2 = 20 mm Hg, HCO_3 = 26 meq/L is seen. The clinical diagnosis is:

a. Respiratory acidosis
b. Respiratory alkalosis
c. Metabolic acidosis
d. Metabolic alkalosis

Ans. is 'b' Respiratory alkalosis

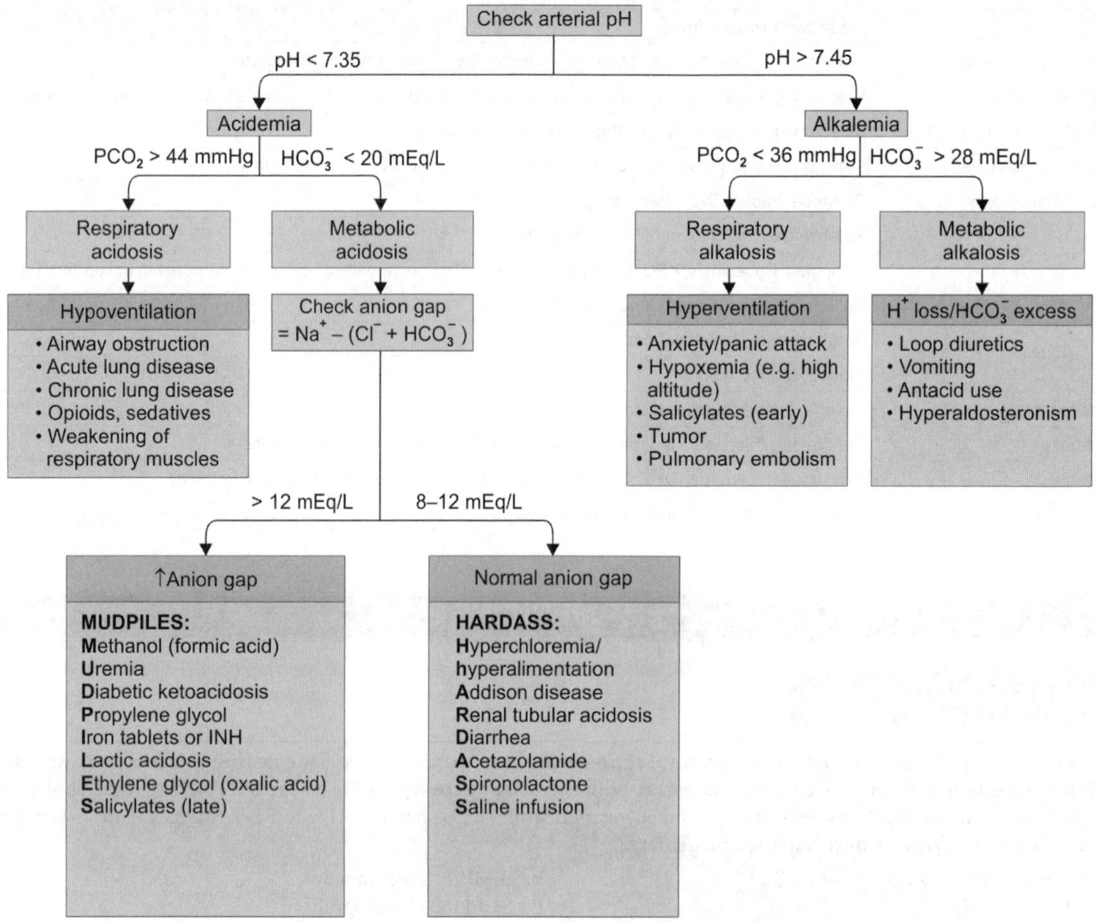

118. A patient is experiencing respiratory alkalosis. What is the most classic sign seen?

a. Bradypnea
b. Chvostek sign
c. Bradycardia
d. Hoover sign

Ans. is 'b' Chvostek sign

Acute respiratory alkalosis causes intracellular shifts of Na^+, K^+, and PO_4 and reduces free [Ca^{2+}] by increasing the protein-bound fraction. Hypocalcemia can present as Chvostek sign.

119. A 30-year-old patient was behaving strangely and developed an episode of seizure on presentation to ER. On work up of patient, urine osmolality 1000 and plasma osmolality 200. Which of the following is most probable dyselectrolytemia present in this case?

a. Hypernatremia
b. Hypokalemia
c. Hyperkalemia
d. Hyponatremia

Ans. is 'd' Hyponatremia

The main electrolyte that has an impact on osmolarity is sodium. And since in this question patients plasma Osm has reduced from 285 to 200, patient has hyponatremia.

120. A child is born with congenital hydrocephalus and VP shunt was put. He developed an obstruction in shunt 4 months back that shunt was successfully replaced. Now he has developed irritability, tiredness, and fever which on evaluation with rectal thermometer showed a value of 38.4°C. Which is next best step in management of this patient?

a. Blood culture from peripheral blood and CSF sample by LP
b. Blood culture from peripheral blood and CSF sample by tap of VP shunt reservoir
c. Do radionuclide scan for functioning of VP shunt
d. Acetaminophen whenever fever Spikes with Spiking TLC

Ans. is 'b' Blood culture from peripheral blood and CSF sample by tap of VP shunt reservoir

In this child the blockage and presence of fever with irritability indicate child has developed an infection in the shunt and is at risk of going into sepsis. So to treat the source blood cultures and CSF tap from the reservoir would be the next step.

121. A 30-year-old lady had moderate headache thrice in a week following which she was using medication for last three consecutive years. She says that in the recent six months she stopped using medication and her headache has decreased. Which of the following is most probable diagnosis?

a. Migraine
b. Tension type headache
c. Cluster headache
d. Medication overuse headache

Ans. is 'd' Medication overuse headache

If a patient develops headache more than/equal to 4 headaches per month patient should be started on prophylactic medication. If prophylactic medication is not started and patient takes frequent analgesics each time headache occurs then the consequence is medication overuse headache (MOH). In MOH despite taking analgesics the headaches keep getting more worse and do not respond to them. The treatment for this condition is stop all medications and start the patient on prophylactic medications.

Criteria for MOH is:

Medication Overuse Headache

- Headache present on >15 d/month
- Regular overuse for >3 month of one or more acute medications
- Headache has developed or markedly worsened during medication overuse

122. An elderly diabetic female has presented with multiple episodes of vomiting after few hours of consuming food from outside. On admission BP is low and ABG shows pH = 7.5, pCO_2 = 45 mm Hg and HCO_3= 30 mEq. Na = 130, K = 3.5 and Chloride = 90 meq/L. Comment on the etiology of these findings:

a. Renal tubular acidosis
b. Diabetic ketoacidosis
c. Protracted vomiting
d. Septic shock

Ans. is 'c' Protracted vomiting

Since patient has metabolic alkalosis with decreased electrolytes protracted vomiting is the answer. DKA, RTA and sepsis usually present with acidosis.

123. A 50-year-old patient presents with nocturnal cough, breathlessness and wheezing episodes. Absolute eosinophil count is 5000 (n = 40–400 cells/cu mm) and miliary pattern is noticed on CXR. The clinical diagnosis is:

a. Miliary TB
b. Tropical pulmonary eosinophilia
c. Bronchial asthma
d. Hypersensitivity pneumonitis

Ans. is 'b' Tropical pulmonary eosinophilia

Since patient has nocturnal cough eosinophilia and Milliary infiltrates on X-ray the diagnosis is tropical pulmonary eosinophila. The criteria to diagnose TPE is given below.

Diagnostic criteria of tropical pulmonary eosinophilia
• Living in or visited an endemic area
• Paroxysmal nocturnal cough and breathlessness
• Pulmonary infiltrations on chest radiograph
• Absolute eosinophil count >3000/mm^3
• Elevated serum IgE levels
• Elevated serum antifilarial antibodies (IgE or IgG)
• Clinical improvement with diethylcarbamazine

The typical X-ray in TPE showing milliary infiltrates is shown below:

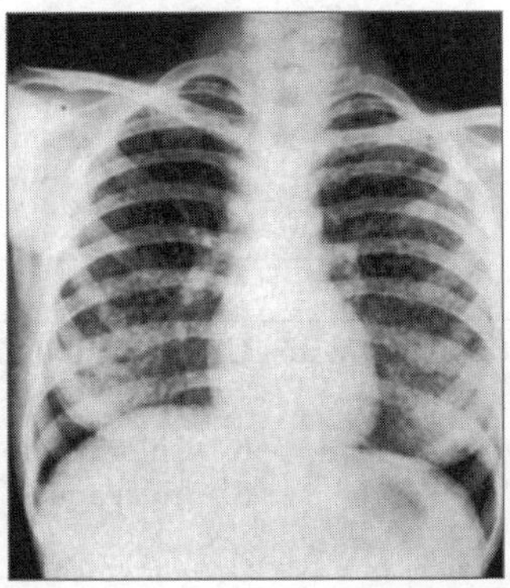

124. A 25-year-old patient with mitral stenosis with irregularly irregular pulse has presented to OPD. Pulse deficit 10. Echo is normal and shows no thrombi. What is the best way to prevent thrombosis in this patient?

a. Dabigatran
b. Aspirin plus clopidogrel
c. Warfarin
d. LMWH

Ans. is 'c' Warfarin

The major options for anticoagulation are the antithrombin inhibitor dabigatran, factor Xa inhibitors rivaroxaban, apixaban, and edoxaban, the vitamin K antagonist warfarin. Antiplatelet agents alone are generally not sufficient. In non-valvular AF, warfarin reduces the annual risk of stroke by 64% compared to placebo and by 37% compared to antiplatelet therapy. Patients with AF with an increased risk of stroke also have an increased risk of venous thromboembolism, which appears to be lower with oral anticoagulation.

The antiplatelet agents aspirin and clopidogrel are inferior to warfarin for stroke prevention in AF and do not have less risk of bleeding. Clopidogrel combined with aspirin is better than aspirin alone for stroke prevention, but is inferior to warfarin and has a greater bleeding risk than aspirin alone.

125. CKD patient lands in uremic encephalopathy. Which ABG report will be seen?

a. pH = 7.15, PCO_2 = 23 mm Hg and HCO_3 = 9
b. pH = 7.46, PCO_2 = 45 mm Hg and HCO_3 = 30
c. pH = 7.15, PCO_2 = 60 mm Hg and HCO_3 = 26
d. pH = 7.46, PCO_2 = 30 mm Hg and HCO_3 = 20

Ans. is 'a' pH = 7.15, PCO_2 = 23 mm Hg and HCO_3 = 9

Uremia results in high anion gap metabolic acidosis. ABG report corresponding to metabolic acidosis is option a.

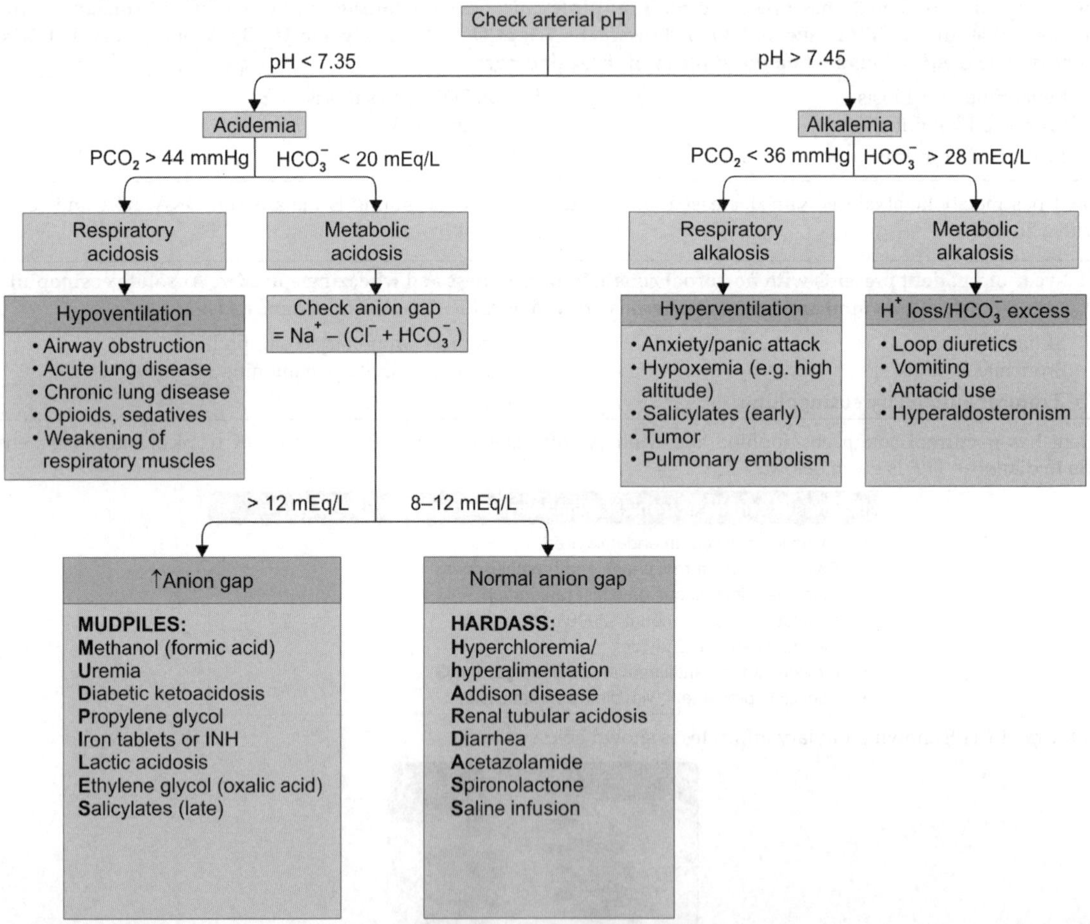

126. A hypertensive patient presents with Grade 4 CKD with eGFR < 30 mL/min. Doctor wants to prescribe a thiazide diuretic. Which of the following will be best for the patient?

a. Hydrochlorothiazide
b. Chlorthalidone
c. Metolazone
d. Indapamide

Ans. is 'c' Metolazone

Metolazone: In common with loop diuretics, it is able to evoke a clinically useful response even in severe renal failure (GFR ~15 mL/min), and has marked additive action when combined with furosemide. An additional proximal tubular action has been demonstrated; PO_4 reabsorption that occurs in PT, is inhibited. It is excreted unchanged in urine.

127. A patient has history of vomiting and doctor gave anti-emetic. Patient developed motor symptoms. What would be given?

a. Levodopa
b. Benzhexol
c. Hyoscine
d. Cyproheptadine

Ans. is 'b' Benzhexol

The anti-emetic most probably administered in this case is a neuroleptic agent. The patient has developed drug induced parkinsonism features.

Centrally acting Anticholinergics like benzhexol are the only drugs effective in drug (phenothiazine) induced parkinsonism.

128. A 65-year-old male presents with excessive tiredness towards the fag end of the day and symptoms reduce with rest. On examination ptosis and difficulty in mastication is noted on sustained use of muscles. The clinical diagnosis is:

a. Lambert syndrome
b. M. Gravis
c. SMA
d. Channelopathy

Ans. is 'b' M. Gravis

For detail see explanation on page 561-562

129. A 35-year-old lady has temporal headache with arm claudication. On examination weak femoral pulses are noted. Fundus shows retina hemorrhages. Diagnosis is:

a. PAN
b. TAO
c. Takayasu arteritis
d. MPA

Ans. is 'c' Takayasu arteritis

Takayasu arteritis affects the aorta and its major branches. In contrast to atherosclerosis, which is characterized by focal irregular lesions, the lesions of Takayasu arteritis are long, smooth, tapered stenoses.

The most commonly involved arteries are the subclavian and innominate arteries. Takayasu arteritis has been termed "pulseless disease" because of its ability to obliterate peripheral pulses (particularly in the upper extremities).

The pulmonary circulation is involved in approximately 50% of cases of Takayasu arteritis.

Patients with severe narrowing of the aortic arch vessels supplying the head may develop Takayasu retinopathy, a hypotensive retinopathy leading to neovascularization.

Takayasu arteritis involvement of the ascending aorta may lead to aortic dilation, aortic regurgitation, aneurysm formation, and aortic rupture.

Pathologic characteristics of selected forms of vasculitis

	Takayasu arteritis	*Polyarteritis nodosa*	*Granulomatosis with polyangiitis (Wegener granulomatosis)*	*Churg-Strauss syndrome*	*Henoch-Schonlein purpura*	*Cutaneous leukocytoclastic angiitis*
Vessels involved	Elastic (large) or muscle (medium-sized) arteries	Medium-sized and small muscle arteries	Small arteries and veins; sometimes medium-sized vessels	Small arteries and veins; sometimes medium-sized vessels	Capillaries, venules, and arterioles	Capillaries, venules, and arterioles
Organ involvement	Aorta, aortic arch and major branches, and pulmonary arteries	Skin, peripheral nerves, gastroin-testinal tract, and other viscera	Upper respiratory tract, lungs, kidneys, skin, eyes	Upper respiratory tract, lungs, heart, peripheral nerves	Skin, joints, gastrointestinal tract, kidneys	Skin, joints
Type of vasculitis and inflammatory cells	Granulomatous with some giant cells; fibrosis in chronic stages	Necrotizing, with mixed cellular infiltrate	Necrotizing or granulomatous (or both); mixed cellular infiltrate plus occasional eosinophils	Necrotizing or granulomatous (or both); prominent eosinophils and other mixed infiltrate	Leukocytoclastic, with some lymphocytes and variable eosinophils; IgA deposits in affected tissues	Leukocytoclastic, with occasional eosinophils

130. A 50-year-old chronic alcoholic with drinking history of 20 years came with jaundice/yellow sclera abdominal distention and decreased urine output. What is the next best step in management of this patient?

a. Octreotide plus albumin
b. Torsemide
c. Saline infusion
d. Propranolol

Ans. is 'a' Octreotide plus albumin

Hepatorenal Syndrome (HRS)

HRS is a form of functional renal failure without renal pathology that occurs in about 10% of patients with advanced cirrhosis or acute liver failure.

The diagnosis is made usually in the presence of a large amount of ascites in patients who have a stepwise progressive increase in creatinine.

Type 1 HRS is characterized by a progressive impairment in renal function and a significant reduction in creatinine clearance within 1–2 weeks of presentation.

Type 2 HRS is characterized by a reduction in glomerular filtration rate with an elevation of serum creatinine level, but it is fairly stable and is associated with a better outcome than that of type 1 HRS.

HRS is often seen in patients with refractory ascites and requires exclusion of other causes of acute renal failure.

Currently, patients are treated with midodrine, an α-agonist, along with octreotide and intravenous albumin.

The best therapy for HRS is liver transplantation; recovery of renal function is typical in this setting.

131. A 10-year-old child with recurrent pulmonary infections now presents with bulky stools with fat > 10 g. Which of the following is true?

a. Serum shows hypernatremia
b. Child has protein losing enteropathy
c. Rectal prolapse may occur
d. Patient has distal intestinal obstruction at this age

Ans. is d' Patient has distal intestinal obstruction at this age

The given scenario is consistent with diagnosis of cystic fibrosis.

Clinical Manifestions of Cystic Fibrosis

Infancy	Childhood	Adolescence/adulthood
Sinopulmonary		
• Infection	• ABPA • Sinusitis • Polyposis	• ABPA • Haemoptysis, pneumothorax • Respiratory failure • Sinusitis, polyposis, anosmia
Gastrointestinal		
• Fetal echogenic bowel • Meconium ileus • Pancreatic insufficiency • Rectal prolapse	• DIOS • Intussusception • Hepatic steatosis, biliary fibrosis • Rectal prolapse	• DIOS • Intussusception • Biliary fibrosis, cirrhosis • Digestive tract cancer (adenocarcinoma)
Renal, endocrine, other		
• Dehydration • Hyponatraemic hypochloraemic metabolic alkalosis	• Renal calculi • Hyponatraemic hypochloraemic metabolic alkalosis	• Delayed puberty, osteoporosis, CFRD • Renal calculi, renal failure • CBAVD, HPOA • Arthritis, vasculitis • Hyponatraemic hypochloraemic metabolic alkalosis

132. A male patient is noted to have weak femoral pulses with upper limb BP of 180/90 mm Hg. On examination increased pulsations of intercostal arteries is noted. Diagnosis is:

a. Takayasu arteritis
b. Coarctation of aorta
c. Aortic dissection
d. PAN

Ans. is 'b' Coarctation of aorta

The classic sign of coarctation of the aorta is a disparity in pulsation and BP in the arms and legs. The femoral, popliteal, posterior tibial, and dorsalis pedis pulses are weak (or absent in up to 40% of patients), in contrast to the bounding pulses of the arms and carotid vessels. The radial and femoral pulses should always be palpated simultaneously for the presence of a **radial-femoral delay**.

Normally, the femoral pulse occurs slightly before the radial pulse. A radiofemoral delay occurs when blood flow to the descending aorta is dependent on collaterals, in which case the femoral pulse is felt after the radial pulse.

In normal persons (except neonates), systolic BP in the legs obtained by the cuff method is 10-20 mm Hg higher than that in the arms. In coarctation of the aorta, BP in the legs is lower than that in the arms; frequently, it is difficult to obtain.

This differential in BPs is common in patients with coarctation who are older than 1 yr, approximately 90% of whom have systolic hypertension in an upper extremity >95th percentile for age. It is important to determine the BP in each arm; a BP higher in the right than the left arm suggests involvement of the left subclavian artery in the area of coarctation.

The precordial impulse and heart sounds are usually normal; the presence of a systolic ejection click or thrill in the suprasternal notch suggests a bicuspid aortic valve (present in 70% of cases). A short systolic murmur is often heard along the left sternal border at the 3rd and 4th intercostal spaces. The murmur is well transmitted to the left infrascapular area and occasionally to the neck. Often, the typical murmur of mild aortic stenosis can be heard in the 3rd right intercostal space.

In older patients with well-developed collateral blood flow, systolic or continuous murmurs may be heard over the left and right sides of the chest laterally and posteriorly. In these patients, a palpable thrill can occasionally be appreciated in the intercostal spaces on the back.

133. CKD patient is having ECG findings of tall T waves. Which of the following derangement is likely to be found in this patient?

a. Hypokalemia
b. Hyperkalemia
c. Hypernatremia
d. Hypophosphatemia

Ans. is 'b' Hyperkalemia

The presence of tall T waves are classical ECG finding in a patient of hyperkalemia. Other important cause of tall T waves is acute MI. The difference between the conditions is that in hyperkalemia the T waves are pointed whereas the T waves of MI are more blunt and not pointed at the peak.

Different causes of tall T waves

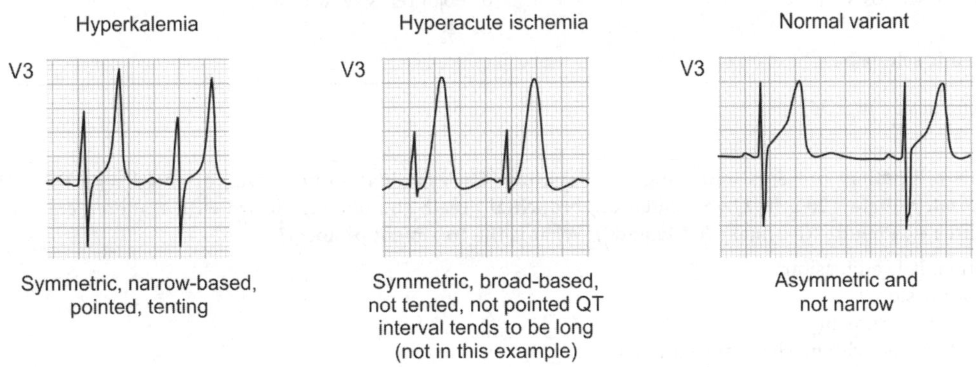

134. A 10-year-old girl has myoclonic jerks all through the day since last one month. The class teacher has complained to parents about lack of concentration and poor performance. Past medical history is significant for viral exanthema at 2 years of age. EEG shows burst suppression pattern. What is the next investigation to be scheduled for the child?

a. Anti GM1 Ab in CSF
b. Anti GQ1 Ab in CSF
c. Anti MOG Ab in CSF
d. Anti-Measles Ig Ab in CSF

Ans. is 'd' Anti- Measles Ig Ab in CSF

Subacute Sclerosing Panencephalitis (SSPE)

SSPE is a rare, chronic, progressive demyelinating disease of the CNS associated with a chronic nonpermissive infection of brain tissue with measles virus.

The incidence has declined dramatically since the introduction of a measles vaccine. Most patients give a history of primary measles infection at an early age (2 years), which is followed after a latent interval of 6–8 years by the development of a progressive neurologic disorder.

Initial manifestations include poor school performance and mood and personality changes. Typical signs of a CNS viral infection, including fever and headache, do not occur. As the disease progresses, patients develop progressive intellectual deterioration, focal and/or generalized seizures, myoclonus, ataxia, and visual disturbances. In the late stage of the illness, patients are unresponsive, quadriparetic, and spastic, with hyperactive tendon reflexes and extensor plantar responses.

Diagnosis

MRI—areas of increased T2 signal develop in the white matter of the brain and brainstem as disease progresses.

EEG—may initially show only nonspecific slowing, but with disease progression, patients develop a characteristic periodic pattern with bursts of high-voltage, sharp, slow waves every 3–8 s, followed by periods of attenuated ("flat") background.

The CSF is acellular with a normal or mildly elevated protein concentration and a markedly elevated gamma globulin level (>20% of total CSF protein). CSF antimeasles antibody levels are invariably elevated, and oligoclonal antimeasles antibodies are often present.

135. A 50-year-old male presents to the hospital with complaint of chest pain. Angiogram revealed left circumflex artery occlusion. Stenting is done and patient was started on aspirin 75 mg, atorvastatin 20 mg and metoprolol 50 mg. Which of the following statement is correct regarding further management of this patient?

a. Add a P2Y12 receptor blocker
b. Increase dose of aspirin
c. Increase dose of metoprolol to 100 mg
d. Add nifedipine

Ans. is 'a' Add a P2Y12 receptor blocker

Patients undergoing stenting with primary PCI for acute MI will usually be on a drug eluting stent. These patients should be on dual antiplatelet therapy for a year, post-procedure as per the current AHA guidelines. Since patient is already on aspirin, one more antiplatelet drug needs to be added preferably from the P2Y12 inhibitor group like clopidogrel.

136. Patient presents with numbness and color changes in fingertips with shiny face and facial skin tightness. ANA is positive and IF shows nucleolar pattern. Which of the following is correct diagnosis?

a. Systemic sclerosis
b. Sjogren's syndrome
c. SLE
d. RA

Ans. is 'a' Systemic sclerosis

For detail see explanation on page 541

137. A 68-years-old patient presents with cough and sputum. On examination he is well oriented with BP = 110/80 mm Hg and Respiratory Rate = 20/min. On auscultation, bronchial breath sounds were heard with scattered crackles. Lab reports showed urea—44 mg/dL. (Normal = 5–20 mg/dL). What is the treatment protocol?

a. Inpatient ICU admission
b. ICU admission
c. Outpatient treatment
d. ICU admission with mechanical ventilation

Ans. is 'a' Inpatient ICU admission

The CURB-65 criteria include five variables: Confusion (C); urea > 7 mmol/L (U); respiratory rate ≥ 30/min (R); blood pressure, systolic ≤ 90 mmHg or diastolic ≤ 60 mmHg (B); and age ≥ 65 years. Patients with a score of 0, among whom the 30-day mortality rate is 1.5%, can be treated outside the hospital. With a score of 1 or 2, the patient should be hospitalized unless the score is entirely or in part attributable to an age of ≥65 years. In such cases, hospitalization may not be necessary. Among patients with scores of ≥3, mortality rates are 22% overall; these patients may require ICU admission.

138. A patient with giant cell arteritis presents with history of headache, Jaw claudication and polymyalgia rheumatica. What will be the first line treatment?

a. Steroids
b. Tocilizumab
c. Tofacitinib
d. Etanercept

Ans. is 'a' Steroids

The goals of treatment in giant cell arteritis are to reduce symptoms and, most importantly, to prevent visual loss. The treatment approach for cranial and large-vessel disease in giant cell arteritis is currently the same. Giant cell arteritis and its associated symptoms are exquisitely sensitive to glucocorticoid therapy. Treatment should begin with prednisone, 40–60 mg/d for ~1 month, followed by a gradual tapering. When ocular signs and symptoms occur, consideration should be given for the use of methylprednisolone 1000 mg daily for 3 days to protect remaining vision. Although the optimal duration of glucocorticoid therapy has not been established, most series have found that patients require treatment for ≥2 years.

SURGERY

NEET PG September 2021

139. A 55-year-old woman undergone modified radical mastectomy 3 months back for breast cancer, which was located in the upper outer quadrant of left breast. Now, she developed painless swelling in the left upper limb, whose image is given below. What is the most probable cause?

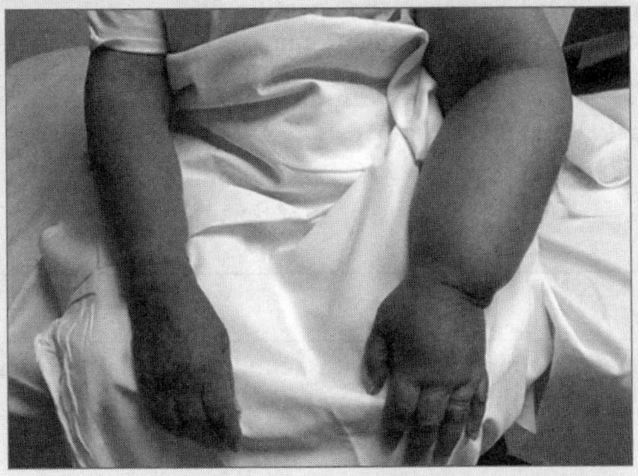

a. Lymphedema
b. Lymphangiosarcoma
c. Axillary vein thrombosis
d. Cellulitis

Ans. is 'a' Lymphedema

For detail see explanation on page 620

140. After total thyroidectomy under GA, anesthetist tried to extubate the patient but he was unable to extubate. What is the most probable reason?

a. Unilateral recurrent laryngeal nerve damage
b. Bilateral recurrent laryngeal nerve damage
c. Hemorrhage
d. Superior laryngeal nerve damage

Ans. is 'b' Bilateral recurrent laryngeal nerve damage

Bilateral vocal cord paralysis from injuries to both RLNs is a rare (0.4% of cases) but devastating complication of total thyroidectomy that occurs most commonly with reoperations. Bilateral vocal cord paralysis is usually recognized immediately after surgery when the patient develops dyspnea and stridor upon extubation. Immediate reintubation is usually possible, but a tracheostomy may be required if the patient cannot be orotracheally reintubated.

Hypoparathyroidism: Hypoparathyroidism is the most frequent complication of total or near-total thyroidectomy. Transient hypoparathyroidism occurs in up to 20% of patients after surgery for thyroid cancer. The hallmark of acute hypocalcemia is tetany, which is characterized by neuromuscular irritability. The symptoms of tetany may be mild (peri-oral numbness, paresthesias of the hands and feet, muscle cramps) or severe (carpopedal spasm, laryngospasm, and focal or generalized seizures).

141. All of the following statements are true about management of pheochromocytoma patient *except*:

a. Propranolol is the initial drug to be started
b. Surgery is the treatment of choice
c. VMA and catecholamines are the diagnostic tests
d. None of the above

Ans. is 'a' Propranolol is the initial drug to be started

After adequate alpha-adrenergic blockade has been achieved, beta-adrenergic blockade is initiated, which typically occurs two to three days preoperatively. The beta-adrenergic blocker should never be started first, because blockade of vasodilatory peripheral beta-adrenergic receptors with unopposed alpha-adrenergic receptor stimulation can lead to a further elevation in blood pressure.

The diagnosis of pheochromocytoma is typically made by measurements of urinary and plasma fractionated metanephrines and catecholamines. Once a pheochromocytoma is diagnosed, all patients should undergo a resection of the pheochromocytoma following appropriate medical preparation.

142. A 50-year-old male presented to the hospital with colicky abdominal pain and bilious vomiting. On evaluation, air was present in the CBD. What is the most probable diagnosis?

a. Adhesions
b. Gastroenteritis
c. Outlet obstruction
d. Gallstone ileus

Ans. is 'd' Gallstone ileus

Post-cholecystectomy syndrome: Postcholecystectomy syndrome (PCS) is a complex of heterogeneous symptoms, including persistent abdominal pain and dyspepsia, that recur and persist after cholecystectomy. PCS is defined as "early" if it occurs in the postoperative period and "late" if it occurs months or years after surgery. The symptoms of pain and dyspepsia referred to as PCS can be caused by a wide spectrum of conditions, both biliary and extra biliary.

Biliary causes of PCS include:

- Early PCS can be due to biliary injury, retained cystic duct, or common bile duct stones
- Late PCS can be due to recurrent CBD stones, bile duct strictures, an inflamed cystic duct or gallbladder remnant, papillary stenosis, or biliary dyskinesia. Biliary dyskinesia refers to motor forms of sphincter of Oddi dysfunction. Sphincter of Oddi dysfunction can be evaluated with sphincter of Oddi manometry.

Extra biliary causes of PCS include:

- Gastrointestinal causes such as irritable bowel syndrome, pancreatitis etc.
- Extraintestinal causes such as intercostal neuritis, wound neuroma, coronary artery disease, or psychosomatic disorders.

143. A 45-year-old female patient presented to hospital with obstructive jaundice and CBD stone. Patient has the history of cholecystectomy, done 2 years back. What is the type of stone seen in CBD?

a. Primary
b. Secondary
c. Retained
d. Recurrent

Ans. is 'c' Retained

For detail see explanation on page 603

144. A 40-year-old male patient presented to emergency with acute abdominal pain and distention. A fluid filled lesion is present in the epigastric region. Which of the following parameter will be raised?

a. Bilirubin
b. GGT
c. Lipase
d. CEA

Ans. is 'c' Lipase

For detail see explanation on page 603

145. A 60-year-old male patient presented to the hospital with gastric outlet obstruction. On evaluation, there was antral gastric carcinoma extending to head of pancreas with multiple metastasis to right lobe of liver. What is the most appropriate management?

a. Right lobe hepatectomy with radical gastrectomy
b. Whipple operation
c. Palliative gastrojejunostomy with chemotherapy
d. Radical gastrectomy with chemotherapy

Ans. is 'c' Palliative gastrojejunostomy with chemotherapy

For detail see explanation on page 629

146. An 18-month-old male child was brought to the hospital with multiple episodes of non-bilious vomiting and poor feeding. The child was passing dry pellets like stools. Which of the following findings will be seen?

a. Hypochloremic hypokalemic metabolic alkalosis
b. Hypochloremic hypokalemic metabolic acidosis
c. Hypochloremic hyperkalemic metabolic alkalosis
d. Hypochloremic hyperkalemic metabolic acidosis

Ans. is 'a' Hypochloremic hypokalemic metabolic alkalosis

For detail see explanation on page 611

147. A patient presented to emergency with pain abdomen and fever for 3 days and dehydrated face. Abdominal X-ray images are shown below. What is the most probable diagnosis?

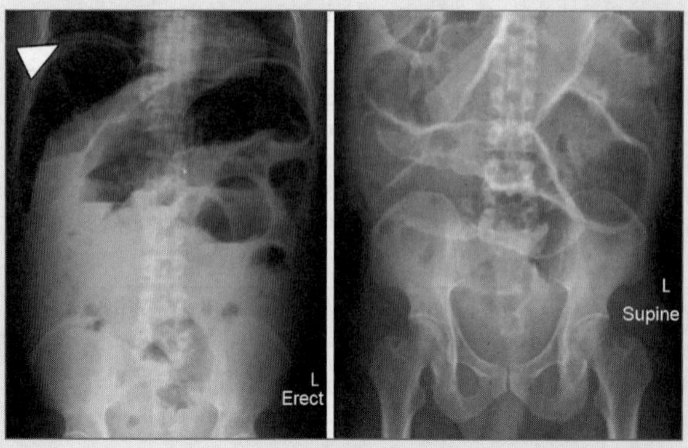

a. Liver abscess
b. Gastric volvulus
c. Empyema thoracis
d. Hollow viscus perforation

Ans. is 'd' Hollow viscus perforation

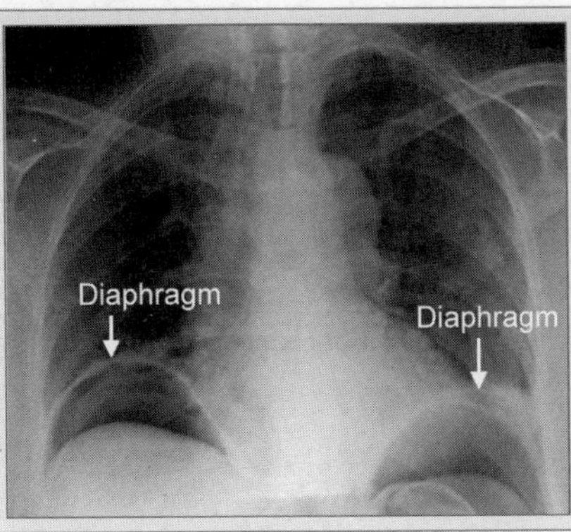	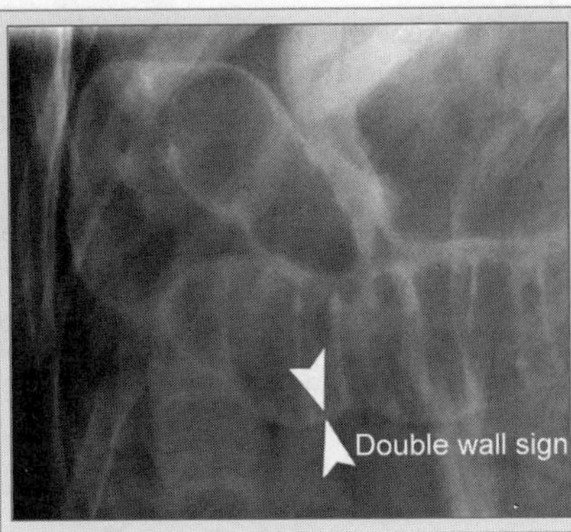	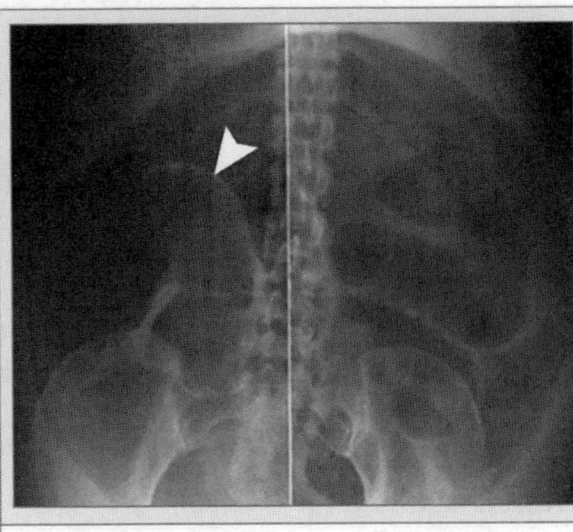
Air/gas under the diaphragm If perforation is suspected you must look very closely. In this patient, only a very thin crescent has formed under only the right hemidiaphragm. Pneumoperitoneum due to insufflation of gas at laparoscopy has identical.	Rigler's/double wall sign: The double wall sign (Rigler's sign) is visible. Gas separates bowel segments and forms sharp angles and triangles.	Football sign - example • Two radiographs were required to completely cover the abdomen in this large patient • A large volume of free gas has risen to the front of the peritoneal cavity resulting in a large round black area - 'football sign' • The double wall sign (Rigler's) is also visible (arrowhead).

148. A 55-year-old patient underwent hysterectomy 2 years back, now presented with colicky abdominal pain and bilious vomiting. On examination, abdomen was tender with exaggerated bowel sounds. On investigations, multiple air fluid levels were seen in the abdomen. What is the most probable diagnosis?

a. Adhesive small bowel obstruction
b. Gastroenteritis
c. Ischemic enterocolitis
d. Gallstone ileus

Ans. is 'a' Adhesive small bowel obstruction

The most common cause of mechanical small bowel obstruction is intraperitoneal adhesions. Prior abdominal or pelvic surgery is the main risk factor for adhesion formation. Other causes of obstruction include tumors and complicated hernias, Crohn disease, infections, volvulus and intussusception.

149. A 45-years-old male patient with paralysis operated for rectal prolapse as shown in the image. Which of the following procedure is done?

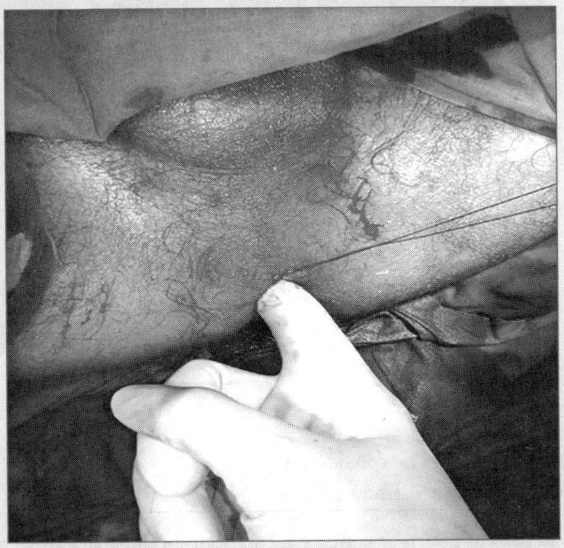

a. Stapled hemorrhoidopexy
b. Well's procedure
c. Thiersch wiring
d. Altemeier repair

Ans. is Ans. 'c' Thiersch wiring

For detail see explanation on page 624

150. A 54-year-old male presented with right groin swelling, located below inguinal ligament, medial to inferior epigastric artery. Cough impulse was present. What is the type of hernia and its management?

a. Direct hernia and Bassini repair
b. Direct hernia and Lichtenstein repairs
c. Indirect hernia and Bassini repair
d. Indirect hernia and Lichtenstein repair

Ans. is 'b' Direct hernia and Lichtenstein repairs

For detail see explanation on page 610

151. A patient of RTA was brought to the hospital with left flank bruise associated with hematuria. Patient was hemodynamically stable. Which of the following investigation should be done for hematuria?

a. CECT
b. DPL
c. RGU
d. MCU

Ans. is 'a' CECT

For detail see explanation on page 612

152. What is the preferred treatment option for an 85-year-old patient, known case of prostate cancer with Gleason score 6, having 2 x 3 cm nodule in prostate and level of PSA is 8 ng/mL?

a. Brachytherapy
b. Palliative external beam radiotherapy
c. Active surveillance
d. Radical prostatectomy

Ans. is 'c' Active surveillance

For detail see explanation on page 611.

153. A 10-years-old boy skids while cycling. The child was stable and abdominal examination was normal. Blood was noticed at the tip of meatus. What is the next best step?

a. Nephrostomy
b. Suprapubic cystostomy
c. Foley's catheterization
d. Bilateral ureteric diversion

Ans. is 'b' Suprapubic cystostomy

For detail see explanation on page 607

154. A 26-year-old male was operated for redness over the perineal area. Postoperative day 5 image is given below. Which of the following statement is correct about this condition?

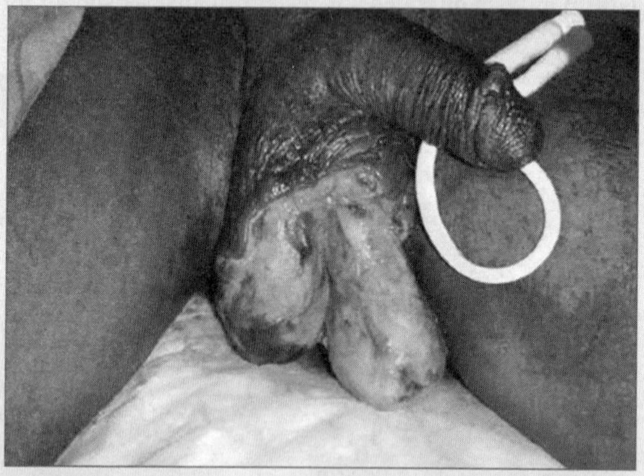

a. Caused by mixed aerobic anaerobic infection
b. Urinary diversion is required in this patient
c. Bilateral orchidectomy should be done
d. Anti-gas gangrene serum should always be considered

Ans. is 'a' Caused by mixed aerobic anaerobic infection

Necrotizing fasciitis of the perineum, known as Fournier gangrene, can occur because of a breach in the integrity of the gastrointestinal or urethral mucosa. Fournier gangrene is a form of polymicrobial (type I) infection. Fournier gangrene typically begins abruptly with severe pain and may spread rapidly to the anterior abdominal wall and the gluteal muscles. Men are more commonly affected than women. Involvement in men may include the scrotum and penis.

Typically, at least one anaerobic species (most commonly *Bacteroides, Clostridium,* or *Peptostreptococcus*) is isolated in combination with Enterobacteriaceae (e.g., *Escherichia coli, Enterobacter, Klebsiella, Proteus*) and one or more facultative anaerobic streptococci.

155. A 35-year-old HIV positive female on ART had a severe migraine headache for which she was given multiple doses of ergotamine 2 days ago. Now, she presented with claudication of right thigh with some numbness and tingling in the right lower limb and peripheral pulses were feeble. Angiography image is given below. What will be the next step of management?

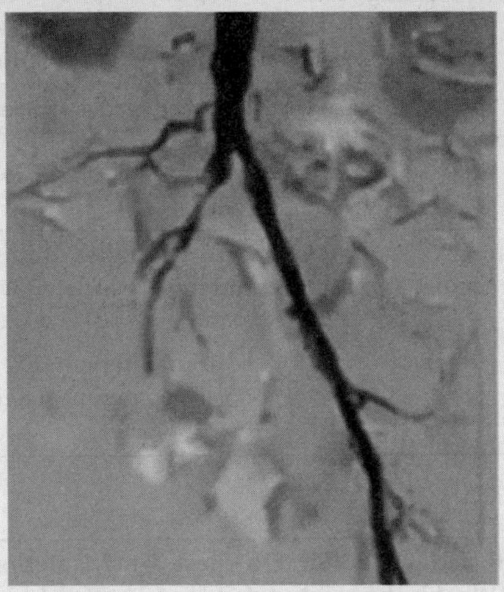

a. Aortofemoral bypass
b. Aortoiliac bypass
c. Iliofemoral bypass
d. PTA with stenting

Ans. is 'd' PTA with stenting

156. A 45-year-old male patient presents to the hospital with asymptomatic varicose veins, whose image is given below. Which CEAP classification does the patient fall under?

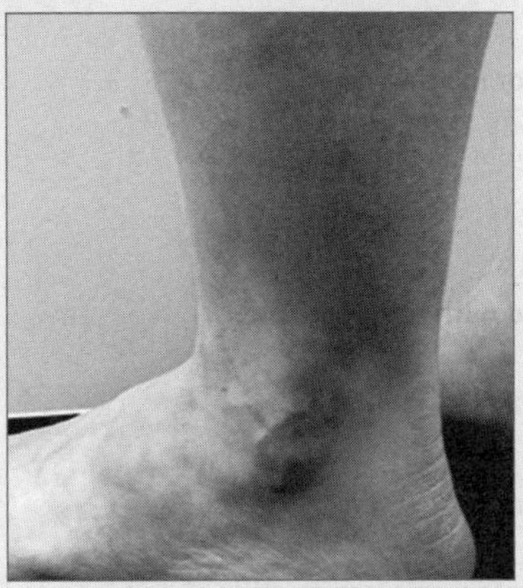

a. 2a
b. 2b
c. 3a
d. 3b

Ans. is 'a' 2a

Basic CEAP classification of chronic venous disease*		
Clinical		
CO	:	No visible or palpable signs of venous disease
C1	:	Telangiectasias or reticular veins
C2	:	Varicose veins
C3	:	Edema
C4a	:	Pigmentation or eczema
C4b	:	Lipodermatosclerosis or atrophie blanche
C5	:	Healed venous ulcer
C6	:	Active venous ulcer

Each clinical class is further characterised by a subscript 's' for 'symptomatic' or a subscript 'a' for 'asymptomatic'. Symptoms encompass aching, pain, tightness, skin irritation, heaviness, muscle cramps and other complaints attributable to venous disease.

Etiology		Anatomy		Pathophysiology	
Ec	Congenital	As	Superficial veins	Pr	Reflux
Ep	Primary	Ap	Perforating veins	Po	Obstruction
Es	Secondary	Ad	Deep veins	Pr, o	Reflux and obstruction
En	No venous cause identified	An	No venous location identified	Pn	No venous pathophysiology identifiable

*The advanced CEAP classification comprises the basic classification and 18 named venous segments that are used as locators for venous pathology.
CEAP = Clinical, Etiology, Anatomy, Pathophysiology.
Source: Adapted from Eklöf et al (2004)

157. A 64-year-old male patient underwent CABG, for which graft was taken from great saphenous vein. The patient is now complaining of lack of sensation over medial aspect of leg and foot, associated with heel pain. What is the most likely nerve affected in this scenario?

a. Saphenous nerve
b. Sural nerve
c. Superficial peroneal nerve
d. Deep peroneal nerve

Ans. is 'a' Saphenous nerve

For detail see explanation on page 621

158. An 80-year-old female presented with fatigue, pallor. On chest X-ray, anterior mediastinal mass was seen. Patient was diagnosed with pure red cell aplasia. What is the most probable cause of aplasia?

a. Thymic neoplasia
b. Non-Hodgkin's lymphoma
c. Bronchogenic carcinoma
d. Germ cell tumor

Ans. is 'a' Thymic neoplasia

The most common lesions that you will see in the anterior mediastinum will either be of thymic or lymph node origin. Even the germ cell tumors arise from the pluripotent cells of the thymus. Before you want to biopsy an anterior mediastinal mass, do not forget that some of these lesions can be vascular in origin.

The four T's make up the mnemonic for anterior mediastinal masses:

1. Thymus
2. Teratoma (germ cell)
3. Thyroid
4. Terrible lymphoma

Important paraneoplastic syndromes associated with thymoma are:

- Myasthenia gravis
- Pure Red cell aplasia
- Immunodeficiency
- Thymoma-associated multiorgan autoimmunity

159. A 25-year-old male patient presented to the emergency with history of road traffic accident. On examination, the patient had subcutaneous emphysema, absence of air entry on the right side and hypotension. Which of the following will be the next step of management?

a. Needle decompression in 5th intercostal space
b. Fluid resuscitation with wide bore needle
c. Plan for intubation
d. Positive pressure ventilation

Ans. is 'a' Needle decompression in 5th intercostal space

For detail see explanation on page 614

160. A 25-years-old male patient with alleged history of road traffic accident sustained injury over chest and abdomen. At the time of presentation, systolic BP was 70 mm Hg and pulse rate was 110/minute. Which of the following is the next step?

a. FAST
b. CECT
c. Chest X-ray
d. MRI

Ans. is 'a' FAST

For detail see explanation on page 612

OBSTETRICS AND GYNECOLOGY (OBG)

NEET PG September 2021

161. A pregnant lady has a history of delivering twins. If she is pregnant for the second time now, which of the following is her obstetric score?

a. G2P1L2
b. G2P2L2
c. G3P1L2
d. G3P2L2

Ans. is 'a' G2P1L2

For detail see explanation on page 653

162. A lady presents with history of recurrent abortions at 8 weeks, 11 weeks and 22 weeks. She also had preeclampsia in the last pregnancy. Cardiac activity of all the three pregnancies were normal. Which of the following is the most probable cause?

a. Syphilis
b. Antiphospholipid antibody syndrome
c. TORCH
d. GDM

Ans. is 'b' Antiphospholipid antibody syndrome

For detail see explanation on page 663

163. A 28-year-old married female, anxious about conception with complaints of profuse white discharge with no h/o itching presented on 12th day of LMP. Which of the following is the most probable diagnosis?

a. Candida
b. Trichomonas
c. Bacterial vaginosis
d. Physiological

Ans. is 'd' Physiological

For detail see explanation on page 668

In the given case, the patient presents with whitish, non foul smelling discharge without associated complaints. As she is presenting in peri-ovulational period, the cause is likely to be physiological.

164. A 18 years old girl with Partial transverse vaginal septum presents with hospital with dysmenorrhea and chronic pelvic pain. Which of the following is the most common complication?

a. Endometriosis
b. Tubo-ovarian abscess
c. Dermoid cyst
d. Theca luteal cyst

Ans. is 'a' Endometriosis

Transverse vaginal septa are a rare type of mullerian anomaly that results from failed fusion or canalization of the vaginal plate and the caudal end of the mullerian ducts. Septa are most commonly imperforate and manifest as primary amenorrhea, abdominal pain, and hematocolpos in adolescence. Perforate septa have a more variable presentation, usually associated with the foreshortened vagina and can present in adolescence or young adulthood. Proper diagnosis is made with clinical exam and imaging, usually Magnetic Resonance Imaging (MRI). Surgical management is highly dependent on the thickness and location of the septum and includes vaginal and abdominoperineal procedures. The patients' age, developmental level, and ability to perform postoperative dilation should be considered when exploring surgical options, since prolonged dilation is often indicated in the postoperative period. Long-term complications include vaginal stenosis and re-obstruction, which may require repeat surgery. The risk of endometriosis increases with imperforate septa that are located higher in the vagina. There is limited data available on reproductive outcomes, but vaginal births have been reported.

165. Which of the following is least common in Didelphys uterus?

a. Preterm labour
b. Transverse lie
c. Endometriosis
d. Abortions

Ans. is 'c' Endometriosis

Uterine Didelphys (Class III)

This müllerian anomaly arises from a complete lack of fusion that results in two entirely separate hemiuteri, cervices, and usually two vaginas. Most women have a double vagina or a longitudinal vaginal septum.

Uterine didelphys may be isolated. Or, it may compose a triad with an obstructed hemivagina and with ipsilateral renal agenesis (OHVIRA), also known as Herlyn-Werner-Wunderlich syndrome.

These anomalies are suspected on pelvic examination by identification of a longitudinal vaginal septum and two cervices. During HSG for fertility evaluation, contrast shows two separate endocervical canals. These open into separate noncommunicating fusiform endometrial cavities that each ends with a solitary fallopian tube.

In women without fertility issues, 2- or 3-D TVS is a logical initial imaging tool, and separate divergent uterine horns with a large intervening fundal cleft are seen. Endometrial cavities are uniformly separate. MR imaging may be valuable in cases without classic findings. Adverse obstetrical outcomes associated with uterine didelphys are similar but less frequent than those seen with unicornuate uterus. Increased risks include miscarriage, preterm birth, and malpresentation.

Metroplasty for either uterine didelphys or bicornuate uterus involves resection of intervening myometrium and fundal recombination. These rarely performed surgeries are chosen for highly selected patients with otherwise unexplained miscarriages. Moreover, no evidence-based data confirm the efficacy of such surgical repair.

166. A 32 years old pregnant female with infraumbilical flattening fetal heart rate heard in the left flank. Which of the following will be the most probable presentation?

a. Right dorsoanterior
b. Occipitoposterior
c. Brow
d. Occipitoanterior

Ans. is 'b' Occipitoposterior

Diagnosis of Occipitoposterior Position

Abdominal Examination

Inspection: The abdomen looks flat, below the umbilicus

Umbilical grip: The findings are: (1) The fetal limbs are more easily felt near the midline on either side. (2) The fetal back is felt far away from the midline on the flank and often difficult to outline clearly. (3) The anterior shoulder lies far away from the midline.

Pelvic grips: The findings are: (1) The head is not engaged. (2) The cephalic prominence (sinciput) is not felt so prominent as found in well-flexed occipitoanterior. **In direct occipitoposterior, the small sinciput is confused with breech.**

Auscultation: The maximum intensity of the fetal heart sounds is heard on the flank and often difficult to locate especially in LOP. However, in direct occipitoposterior, the FHS is distinctly felt in the midline.

167. A 28-years-old pregnant female patient at 36 weeks POG with painful reddish vesicular lesions in the vulva. What is the management?

a. Acyclovir and elective cesarean section
b. Induction of labor
c. Acyclovir and allow spontaneous progression of labor pregnancy
d. Antibiotics and pain medication

Ans. is 'a' Acyclovir and elective cesarean section

Herpes Simplex (DNA) Virus (HSV) Infection in Pregnancy

Genital tract infection is due to HSV-2. Infection may be primary, nonprimary, first episode and recurrent.

It is transmitted by sexual contact.

Primary infection may occur during pregnancy. Reactivation or recurrent infection occurs resulting in virus shedding with or without symptomatic lesions. HSV-1 infection is usually herpes simplex labialis.

Effect on pregnancy: Increased risk of miscarriage is inconclusive. If the primary infection is acquired in the last trimester there is chance of premature labor or IUGR. Transplacental infection is not usual. The fetus becomes affected by virus shed from the cervix or lower genital tract during vaginal delivery. The baby may be affected *in utero* from the contaminated liquor following rupture of the membranes. **Risk of fetal infection is high in primary genital HSV at term due to high virus shedding compared to a recurrent infection. Cesarean delivery is indicated (ACOG) in an active primary genital HSV infection** where the membranes are intact or recently ruptured. Acyclovir 400 mg three times daily for five days is the drug of choice when virus culture is positive.

Neonatal infection may be disseminated (fatal) or localized or it may be asymptomatic. **Diagnosis** is made by detection of the viral DNA by PCR. It is manifested as chorioretinitis, microcephaly, mental retardation, seizures and deaths. Neonatal HSV infection is treated with intravenous acyclovir. Neonatal mortality is high.

Prophylactic acyclovir (400 mg twice daily) or valacyclovir (1 gm twice daily) can reduce HSV shedding, neonatal transmission and cesarean delivery. **Breastfeeding** is allowed provided the mother avoids any contact between her lesions, her hands and the baby.

168. A 32-years-old female presents to the hospital with cannon ball appearance on the chest X-ray. Patient had a history of molar evacuation. Which of the following is the best management?

a. Hysterectomy
b. EMACO regimen
c. Single agent chemotherapy like methotrexate
d. Radiotherapy

Ans. is 'c' Single agent chemotherapy like methotrexate

GTN is staged clinically using the system of the International Federation of Gynecology and Obstetrics (FIGO) (2009). This includes a modification of the World Health Organization (WHO) (1983) prognostic index score, with which scores of 0 to 4 are given for each of the categories shown in Table.

Women with WHO scores of 0 to 6 are considered to have low-risk disease, whereas those with a score ≥7 are considered in the high-risk group.

Anatomical staging				
Stage I	Disease confined to the uterus			
Stage II	GTN extends outside of the uterus but is limited to the genital structures (adnexa, vagina, broad ligament)			
Stage III	GTN extends to the lungs without known genital tract involvement			
Stage IV	All other metastatic sites			
Modified World Health Organization (WHO) prognostic scoring system[a]				
Scores[b]	0	1	2	4
Age (years)	<40	≥ 40	—	—
Antecedent pregnancy	Mole	Abortion	Term	—
Interval after index pregnancy (mo)	<4	4–6	7–12	>12
Pretreatment serum β-hCG (mIU/mL)	10^3	10^3 to 10^4	10^4 to 10^5	≥10^5
Largest tumor size (including uterus)	< 3 cm	3–4 cm	≥ 5 cm	–
Site of metastases		Spleen, kidney	GI	Liver, brain
Number of metastases	–	1–4	5–8	>8
Previous failed chemotherapy drugs	–	–	1	≥2

Treatment

Single-agent chemotherapy protocols are usually sufficient for nonmetastatic or low-risk metastatic neoplasia (Lawrie, 2016). Monotherapy protocols with either methotrexate or actinomycin D were equally effective compared with a regimen containing both. In general, methotrexate is less toxic than actinomycin D (Chan, 2006; Seckl, 2010). Regimens are repeated until serum β-hCG levels are undetectable.

Combination chemotherapy is given for high-risk disease, and reported cure rates approximate 90 percent (Lurain, 2010). Several regimens have been used with success. One is EMA-CO, which includes etoposide, methotrexate, actinomycin D, cyclophosphamide, and Oncovin (vincristine). In selected cases, adjuvant surgical and radiotherapy may also be employed (Hanna, 2010).

Frequent causes of death include hemorrhage from metastatic sites, respiratory failure, sepsis, and multiorgan failure due to widespread chemoresistant disease (Lybol, 2012; Neubauer, 2015).

169. A 25 years old primigravida female after giving birth to a child have continuous bleed from uterus. The patient was taken to OT and planned for uterine devascularization. Which of the following is the correct order of devascularization?

a. Uterine artery, Pudendal artery, Vaginal artery
b. Uterine artery, Internal iliac artery, Obturator artery
c. Uterine artery, Ovarian artery, Internal iliac artery
d. Uterine artery, Ovarian artery, External iliac artery

Ans. is 'c' Uterine artery, Ovarian artery, Internal iliac artery

Surgical Methods to Control PPH

An outline of stepwise uterine devascularization procedures are given below:

(a) **B-Lynch compression suture (1997) and multiple square sutures:** Both these surgical methods work by tamponade (like bimanual compression) of the uterus. Success rate is about 80% and it can avoid hysterectomy.
(b) **Ligation of uterine arteries**—the ascending branch of the uterine artery is ligated at the lateral border between upper and lower uterine segment. The suture (No. 1 chromic) is passed into the myometrium 2 cm medial to the artery. In atonic hemorrhage, bilateral ligation is effective in about 75% of cases.
(c) **Ligation of the ovarian and uterine artery anastomosis,** if bleeding continues, is done just below the ovarian ligament .
(d) **Ligation of anterior division of internal iliac artery** (unilateral or bilateral)—reduces the distal blood flow. It helps stable clot formation by reducing the pulse pressure up to 85%. Bilateral ligation (not division) can avoid hysterectomy in about 50% of the cases.

(e) **Angiographic selective arterial embolization** (bleeding vessel) under fluoroscopy (interventional radiology) can be done using gel foam. Success rate is more than 90% and it avoids hysterectomy.

(f) **Hysterectomy**—rarely uterus fails to contract and bleeding continues in spite of the above measures. Hysterectomy has to be considered involving a second consultant. Decision of hysterectomy should be taken earlier in a parous woman. Depending on the case, it may be subtotal or total.

170. A 34-years-old lady using OCP since 5 months presents with amenorrhea since 6 weeks. Which of the following is best to calculate gestational age in this case?

a. 280 days from LMP
b. 256 days from LMP
c. CRL by USG
d. Abdominal girth

Ans. is 'c' CRL by USG

Ultrasonography: Intradecidual gestational sac (GS) is identified as early as 29 to 35 days of gestation.

Fetal viability and gestational age is determined by detecting the following structures by **transvaginal ultrasonography.** *Gestational sac and yolk sac* by 5 menstrual weeks; *Fetal pole and cardiac activity* — 6 weeks; *Embryonic movements* by 7 weeks. Fetal gestational age is best determined by measuring the CRL between 7 and 12 weeks (variation ± 5 days). **Doppler effect of ultrasound can pick up the fetal heart rate reliably by 10th week.** The instrument is small, handy and cheap.

171. A 25-years-old female with primary infertility came to the hospital with USG finding of uterine anomaly. Which of the following is used to confirm the diagnosis?

a. TVS
b. Hysteroscopy and laparoscopy
c. Laparoscopy
d. HSG

Ans. is 'b' Hysteroscopy and laparoscopy

For detail see explanation on page 649

Diagnosis of Mullerian Anomalies

Combined hysteroscopy and laparoscopy help to differentiate between bicornuate uterus and septate uterus. The presence of the uterine fundus suggests a septate uterus. It is Gold std – because it is diagnostic and curative.

Ultrasonography—septate uterus appears as two cavities without sagittal notching and the intercornual distance <4.0 cm. Diagnosis of bicornuate uterus is favoured, if the fundal midpoint indentation is >5 mm above the inter-ostial line.

Hysterosalpingography (HSG)—cannot reliably differentiate between septate and a bicornuate/arcuate uterus. If the angle of divergence between the two uterine cavities is <75°, the defect is most likely to be septate uterus. If the angle of divergence is >75° but <105° a diagnosis cannot be made.

Magnetic resonance imaging (MRI)—it is an accurate and noninvasive investigation to make a diagnosis of septate uterus. If the septum extends to >30% of the septal cavity, surgical resection is indicated.

172. A 25-years-old female present to the hospital with midline septum in uterus. Which of the following is the management of this condition?

a. Laparoscopic metroplasty
b. Hysteroscopic septoplasty
c. Uterine metroplasty
d. Septoplasty

Ans. is 'b' Hysteroscopic septoplasty

For detail see explanation on page 650

173. A 55-years-old multigravida with history of frequently micturating due to coughing laughing & sneezing .... diagnosis?

a. Urge incontinence
b. Stress incontinence
c. Neurogenic bladder
d. Urinary Tract Infection

Ans. is 'b' Stress incontinence

Stress Urinary Incontinence (SUI)

The common type of stress incontinence is associated with cystocele and genital prolapse when the woman voids a small quantity of urine involuntarily while sneezing, coughing or laughing. The condition also develops during pregnancy and soon after delivery.

❖ Cause
- Bladder neck descent (70–80%) – loss of integrity of fibromuscular tissue that support bladder neck and urethra.
- Intrinsic sphincter defect

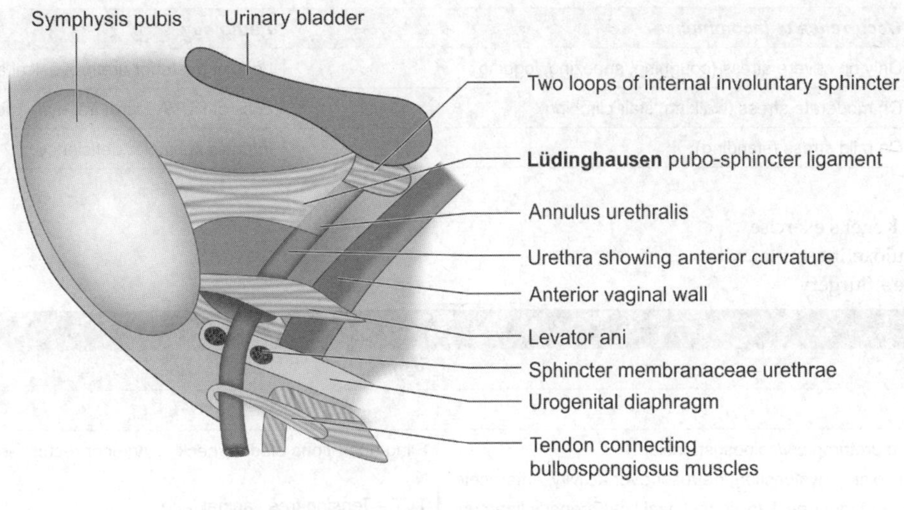

Normal support of internal sphincter

- C/F – no urgency, frequency, nocturia or dysuria (+nt in urge incontinence)
- Tests
  - Bonney's test – insert 2 fingers in paraurethral region → bladder neck lifted → SUI get corrected. (indicate bladder neck descent)
  - Marchetti test –similar to Bonney's test – uses Allis forceps
  - Q tip test – sterile cotton swab introduced into the level of bladder neck – patient asked to strain. Elevation >30° indicates urethra hypermobility

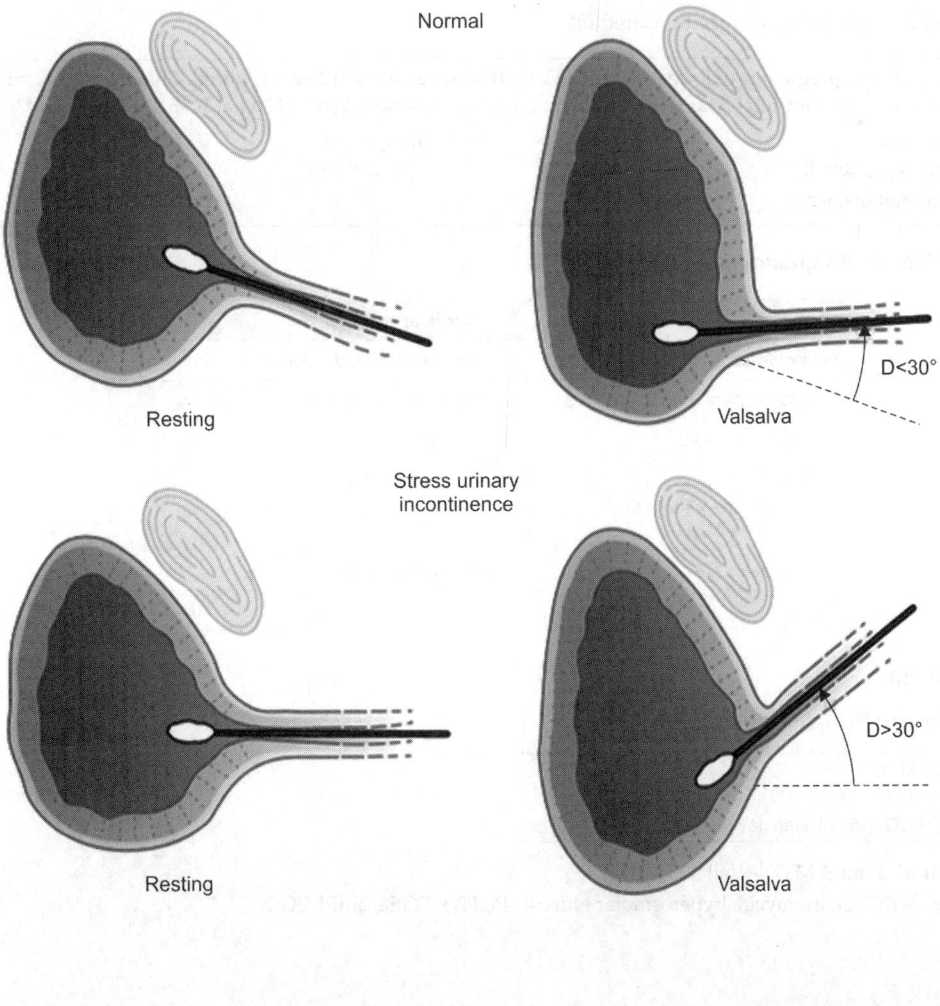

❖ Grades of SUI

Grade	Occurrence of incontinence	Pathology
1	Only on severe stress (coughing, sneezing, jogging)	Loss of posterior urethrovesical angle
2	On moderate stress (walking, stair climbing)	Loss of PUVA + urethral hypermobility
3	On mild stress (standing)	Intrinsic sphincter deficiency

❖ Management
- 1st line – Kegel's exercise
- DOC – duloxetine/venlafaxine
- Definitive – Surgery

Sx	
Abdominal	*Vaginal*
↓	↓
• Retropubic urethropexy/colposuspension • Problems voiding dysfunction; detrusor over activity, enterocele – Burch → bladder neck to iliopectineal line/Cooper's ligament – Marshall Marchettikrantz→ attach to pubic symphysis. No longer used because → osteitis pubis	Sling operations bladder neck → anterior rectus fascia ↓ TVT – Tension free vaginal tape TOT- Trans obturator tape TVT – highest success rate M.C. Complication of TVT → bladder perforation. "Most serious" → bowel/vascular injury Overall – TOT > TVT (due to less complications)

Other Procedures

❖ Kelly's plication – in elderly women unfit for Sx

❖ Periurethral bulking agents: Inj collagen transurethral

174. A lady presents with pregnancy of 6 weeks. On USG a left adnexal mass of 3 cms is noted. This mass has a small gestational sac and a fetal pole but not fetal heart action is seen. β-hCG levels were 2800 IU. What is the management?

a. Wait and watch
b. Salpingectomy
c. Medical management
d. Salpingostomy

Ans. is 'c' Medical management

Management of Ectopic Pregnancy

Medical	*Surgical*
Pre-requisites	*Indication: Failed medical*
• Stable patient	MTX cannot be given
• hCG < 5000 IU/L	Unstable
• Size of Gestational sac – < 3.5 cm → if CA (+) – 4 cm → if CA (–)	Ruptured ectopic
• Pref absent CA	Family complete
	ART

Medical Management

❖ Drugs: Methotrexate: 50 mg/m^2 in single dose therapy

Day 1: inj MTX
Day 4: β hCG
Day 7: β hCG - 15% ↓ than day 4

- Failed medical: 3 times MTX → fall < 15%
- Other drugs – KCl, actinomycin, hyperosmolar glucose, PGF2α, PGE2, anti-hCG

Surgical Management

- Laparoscopy > laparotomy: except unstable patient
- Unstable patient - laparotomy
- Salpingostomy > salpingectomy→ no suturing done, opening done and conceptus removed → ↓ adhesion rate

Indications of Salpingectomy

- Ruptured ectopic
- Family complete
- Sac size > 5 cm
- Hemostasis cannot be achieved
  - Family complete = total
  - Family not complete = partial

Expectant M_X→ monitor vitals and follow-up hCG

- Stable
- Sac < 3 cm
- No CA
- hCG < 2000 and falling trend

175. A lady with primary infertility was diagnosed to have 2 uterine fibroids in the cornual region. Right side is 7 x 5 cms and left side is 5 x 4 cms. On HSG both the tubes are found to be blocked. What is your management if you are told that the woman is ovulating and the semen analysis of her partner is normal?

a. Myomectomy
b. ART
c. Hysterectomy
d. Hysteroscopic cannulation of tubes

Ans. is 'a' Myomectomy

Fibroids do not necessarily cause infertility. Infertility is either due to associated PID, endometriosis or anovulatory cycles, or due to distortion of the uterine cavity causing obstruction to sperm ascent, poor nidation or cornual tubal block. A fibroid bigger than 4 cm in size can cause infertility.

Submucous myoma is responsible for infertility and recurrent pregnancy loss in 20% cases.

Indications for treatment in an asymptomatic fibroid are as follows:

- Infertility caused by a cornual fibroid blocking the tube and habitual abortions due to a submucous fibroid. Other causes of infertility and abortions should be ruled out before myomectomy is undertaken.
- A fibroid more than 12 weeks size and a pedunculated fibroid which can cause torsion.
- An asymptomatic fibroid causing pressure on the ureter, that is broad ligament fibroid and pressure on the bladder, leaving residual urine and causing urinary infection.
- Rapidly growing fibromyoma in a menopausal woman implying impending malignancy and requiring surgery.
- When the nature of the tumour cannot be ascertained clinically (laparotomy is needed in this occasion).
- All symptomatic fibroids.

Managment of uterine fibromyoma

Asymptomatic	*Symptomatic*	*Cervical 1%*
• Observation with regular follow-up - Size < 12 weeks - Uncomplicated pregnancy with fibroid • Surgery - Size > 12 weeks - Cornual fibroid causing inferetility - Pedunculated cornual fibroid - Pregnancy with torsion of pedunculated fibroid	• Medical - Hormones to shrink the fibroid —surgery - Uterine artery embolization - Myomectomy - Lap myomectomy - Lap myolysis • MRI guided ablation - Total/subtotal abdominal hysterectomy - Vaginal hysterectomy - Total laparoscopic hysterectomy	• Vaginal polypectomy or myomectomy • Myomectomy • Lap myomectomy • MRI guided myolysis - Vaginal hysterectomy - Total abdominal hysterectomy

DERMATOLOGY

NEET PG September 2021

176. A 25-year-old female with paronychia on little finger and with the given finding. What is the suitable antibiotic for this case?

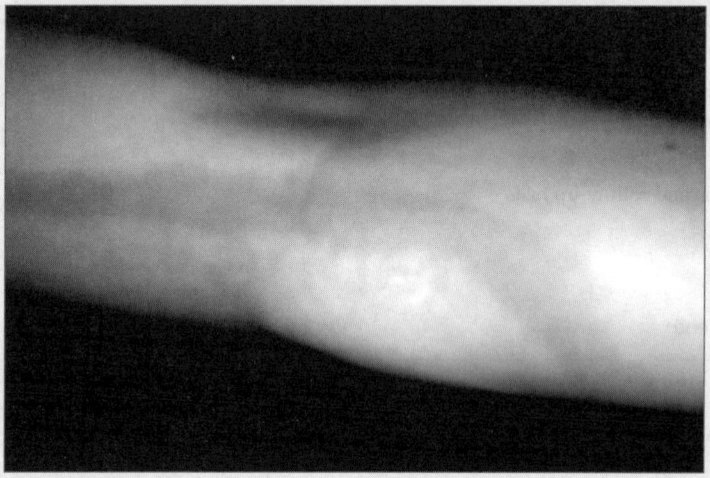

a. Amoxiclav
b. Amikacin
c. Norfloxacin
d. Metronidazole

Ans. is 'a' Amoxiclav

The given image is suggestive of ascending lymphangitis in a case of paronychia. Antibiotic of choice for this condiiton is amoxyclav.

177. A patient of 30 years came with flaccid bullae with crusting on her skin which are easy to rupture. Biopsy revealed suprabasal split. Identify the diagnosis:

a. Pemphigus vegetans
b. P. Vulgaris
c. Erythema multiforme
d. P. foliaceus

Ans. is 'b' P. Vulgaris

For detail see explanation on page 709

178. A patient is on MBMDT therapy and presented with inflammation and edema over pre-existing lesion and nerve involvement. What is your next line of management?

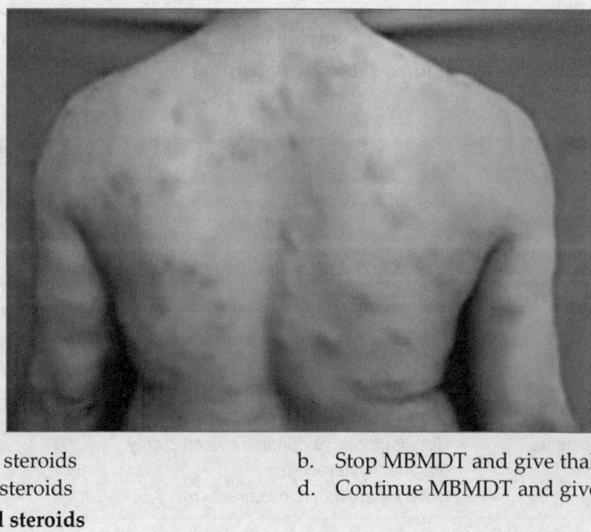

a. Stop MBMDT and Start steroids
b. Stop MBMDT and give thalidomide
c. Continue MBMDT and steroids
d. Continue MBMDT and give thalidomide

Ans. is 'c' Continue MBMDT and steroids

Lepra Reactions

Type I	Type II/erythema nodosum leprosum
• Occurs in borderline leprosy • Cause: It is due to alteration in host's CMI • Type IV HS	• Occurs in LL and sometimes BL leprosy • Cause: Immune complex reaction • Type III HS
• Upgrading reaction/reversal reaction – CMI improves (BL→ BB→ BT) • Downgrading reaction. – CMI worsens (BT→ BB→ BL) – Seen during natural course of disease and pregnancy	
• Manifestations – Erythema, edema and scaling of preexisting lesions – Appearance of new lesions – Neuritis—nerve tenderness – New area of sensory and motor deficits appear	• Manifestations – ENL- appearance of several tender, evanescent erythematous nodules on face, flexures legs – Neuritis – Arthralgia – Orchitis, iridocyclitis – Fever

Treatment: Do not stop antileprosy drugs

	Type I	Type II
Mild	NSAIDs.	NSAIDs
Moderate	NSAIDs; oral steroids	NSAIDs; Thalidomide Clofazimine: Chloroquine
Severe	NSAIDs; oral steroids	Thalidomide, oral steroids

Treatment of Recurrent ENL

Steroids + clofazimine for 3 months → tapering Steroids + clofazimine for 3 months → stop Steroids , only clofazimine for 3 months

179. A male child with mild painful swelling in scalp for 3 months. The patient has a dog pet at house:

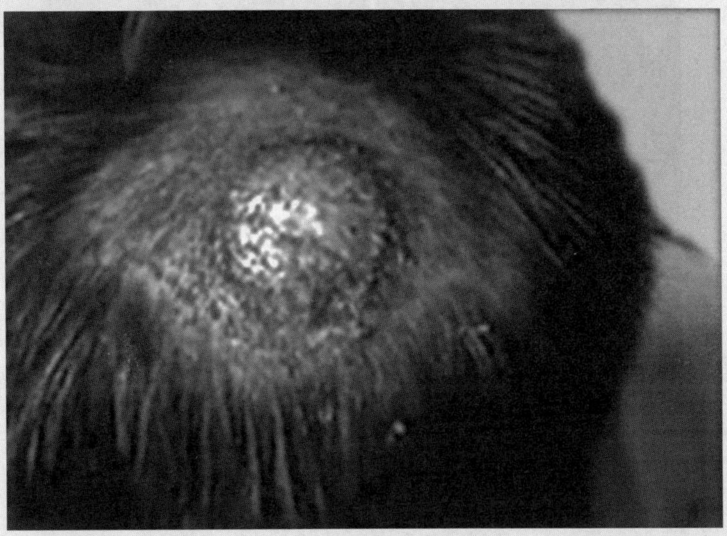

a. Folliculitis
b. Abscess
c. Kerion
d. Sebaceous cyst

Ans. is 'c' Kerion

Tinea Capitis

- Invariably a child.
- Morphology: Discoid patch of partial alopecia from which hair can be easily and painless be plucked.
    - Non-inflammatory
    - Inflammatory (kerion)
    - Favus.
- Wood's lamp—blue green fluorescence

Non-inflammatory

- Caused by anthropophilic organism: T. verrucosum
- Human to human spread
- Black dot (endothrix) – T. tonsurans, T. violaceum
- Gray patch (ectothrix) – M. canis
- Broken hair—gray/black dots.

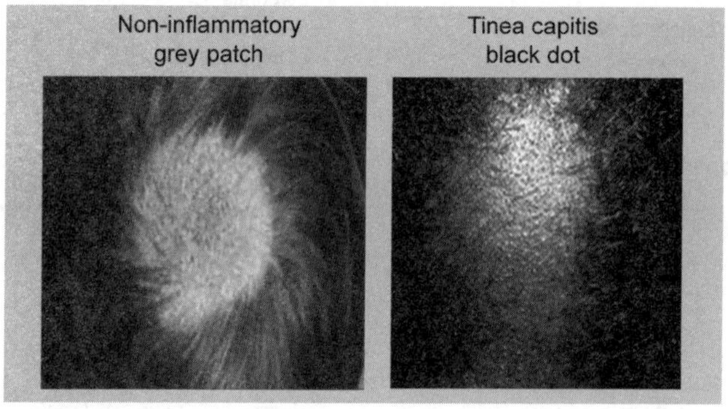

Kerion (Inflammatory)

- Zoophilic organism: M. canis, T. mentagrophytes.
- Boggy swelling of scalp with easy pluckable hair.
- Lymphadenopathy

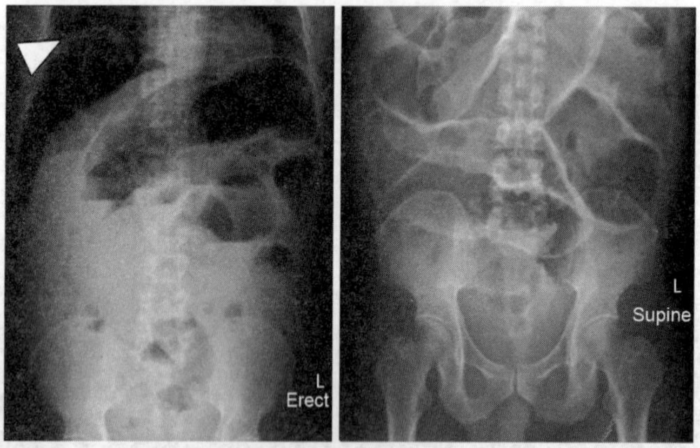

Favus

- Foul swelling yellowish cup-shaped crusts (SCUTULA) entangling scalp hair.
- Results in cicatricial alopecia
- Causative agent: T. schoenleinii

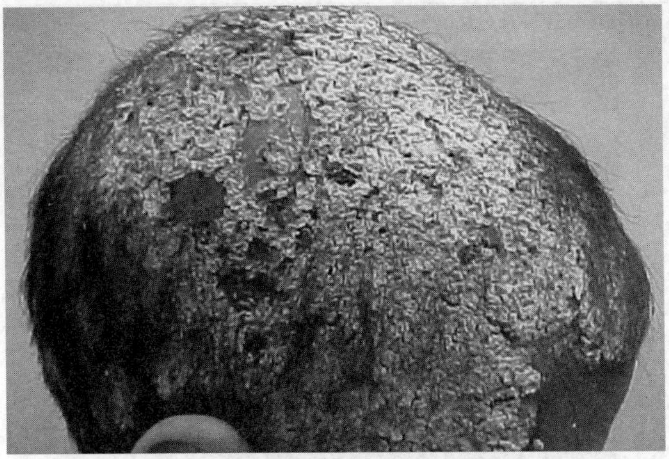

ANESTHESIA

NEET PG September 2021

180. Endotracheal intubation was done for a patient. Which of the following will you do to confirm the placement of ET tube?

a. $ETCO_2$
b. Chest auscultation
c. Chest X-ray
d. Oxygen saturation

Ans. is 'a' $ETCO_2$

After intubation, the chest and epigastrium are immediately auscultated, and a capnographic tracing (the definitive test) is monitored to ensure intratracheal location. If there is doubt as to whether the tube is in the esophagus or trachea, repeat the laryngoscopy to confirm placement.

End-tidal CO_2 will not be produced if there is no cardiac output. FOB through the tube and visualization of the tracheal rings and carina will likewise confirm correct placement. Otherwise, the tube is taped or tied to secure its position.

Although the persistent detection of CO_2 by a capnograph is the best confirmation of tracheal placement of a TT, it cannot exclude bronchial intubation. The earliest evidence of bronchial intubation often is an increase in peak inspiratory pressure.

181. A patient is undergoing a surgery where anesthesia is maintained on Halothane. The patient developed muscled rigidity and hyperthermia. Which of the following agent would have also contributed to this condition?

a. Succinyl choline
b. D-tubocurarine
c. Rocuronium
d. Atracurium

Ans. is 'a' Succinyl choline

Malignant hyperthermia (IMP TOPIC)

- **Triggering drugs**:
  - Halothane, fluranes
  - Succinylcholine
  - Lignocaine
- Protective
  - Thiopentone
  - Pancuronium
- Safe
  - Propofol
  - Ketamine
  - Etomidate
  - N_2O
  - Opioids

182. Which of the following maneuver is being done?

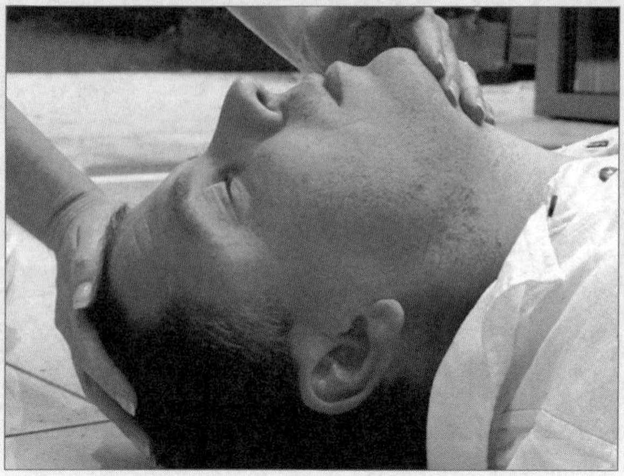

a. Head extension
b. Head tilt-chin lift
c. Jaw thrust
d. Manual inline stabilization

Ans. is 'b' Head tilt-chin lift

Head Tilt vs Jaw Thrust

Head tilt, chin-lift is used to open airway of an unconscious person	Jaw thrust opens the airway when a spinal injury is suspected
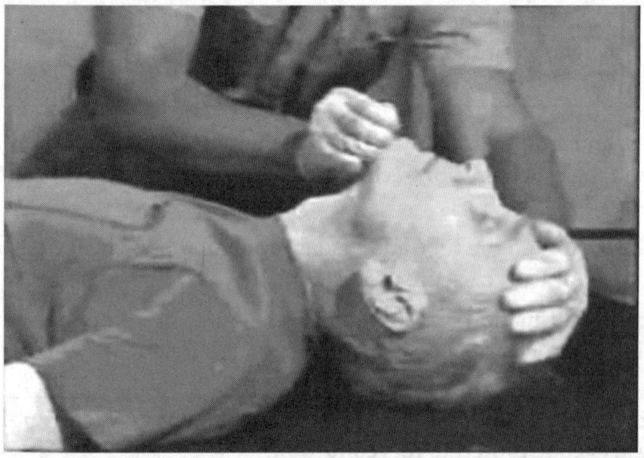	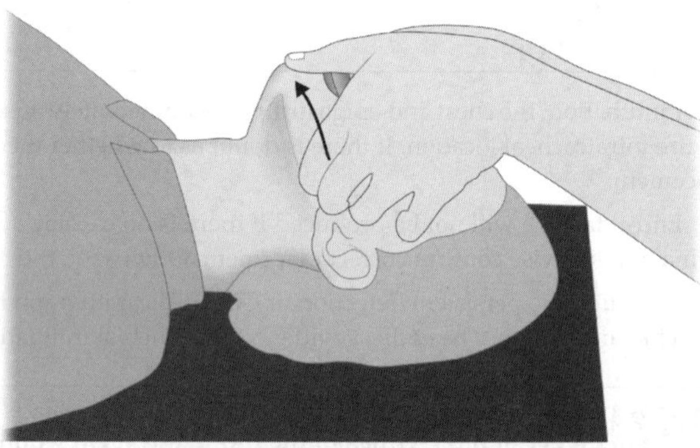

183. An anesthetist was doing shoulder block with 0.25% bupivacaine, the patient become unresponsive and pulse become unreportable. The best management in this patient would be:

a. CPR with 20% intralipid emulsion
b. CPR with dobutamine
c. CPR with calcium
d. CPR with sodium bicarbonate

Ans. is 'a' CPR with 20% intralipid emulsion

Local Anaesthetic Systemic Toxicity (LAST)

- Increased by:
  - Hypercapnia
  - Hypoxia
  - Acidosis
  - Extremes of age
  - HF/RF/LF
- Toxicities
  - CNS—circumoral numbness (MC), paraesthesia, dizziness, light headedness, restlessness, agitation, twitching, slurred speech, resp. depression
  - Methemoglobinemia—treatment – methylene blue
  - Allergy/anaphylaxis
  - CVS – arrhythmias, cardiac arrest

- Treatment of LA toxicity
  - $NaHCO_3$—for acidosis
  - BZD—for seizures
  - CPR + 20% intralipid IV – for cardiac arrest
  - Amiodarone – for arrhythmia

The most potent local anesthetics—bupivacaine, etidocaine, and to a lesser degree, ropivacaine—seem to have the most potent effects on the heart, particularly on Purkinje fibers and ventricular muscle. Bupivacaine binds open or inactivated sodium channels and dissociates from them slowly. It can cause profound sinus bradycardia and sinus node arrest and malignant ventricular arrhythmias; furthermore, it can depress left ventricular contractility. Twenty percent lipid emulsions have been used to treat local anesthetic cardiac toxicity. The mechanisms of action of this therapy are unclear, although possibilities include serving as a lipid reservoir and decreasing lipophilic toxic local anesthetics in the myocardium.

184. The last layer to be pierced to enter lumbar cisternae is:

a. Duramater
b. Arachnoid mater
c. Ligamentum flavum
d. Supraspinous ligament

Ans. is 'b' Arachnoid mater

Structures pierced during spinal anesthesia: Skin→ s/c tissue → supraspinous lig. → interspinous lig. → lig. flavum → duramater → arachnoid matter → SAS

RADIOLOGY

NEET PG September 2021

185. A patient presenting with abdominal pain and distension. Multiple air fluid levels are seen. Dilated loops are?

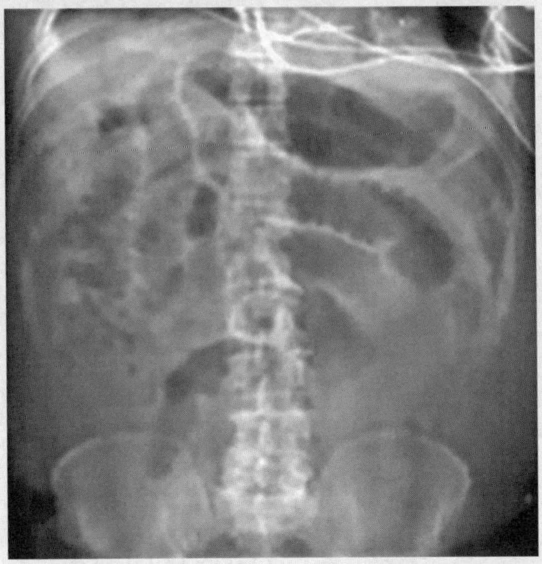

a. Jejunum
b. Duodenum
c. Ileum
d. Transverse colon

Ans. is 'a' Jejunum

Large bowel	*Small bowel*
• Peripheral • Presence of haustration, diameter > 8 cm • Distended caecum—a rounded gas shadow in the right iliac fossa >10 cm diameter	• Central • Jejunum—valvulae conniventes • Ileum—featureless • Diameter >5 cm • No gas is seen in the colon

Large bowel	Small bowel
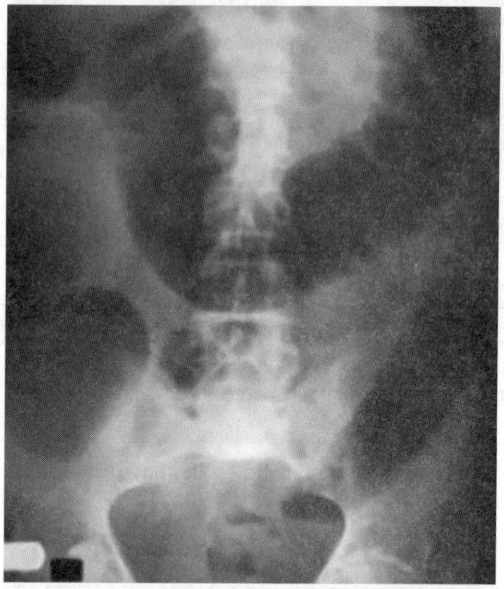	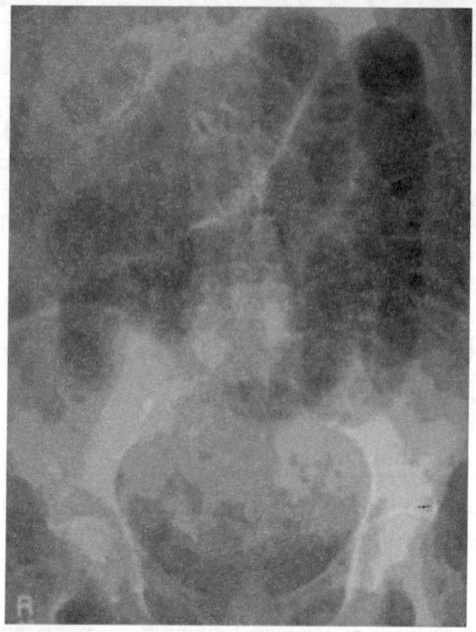

186. A 30-year-old female presenting with sterile pyuria. Radiograph is shown. Identify the diagnosis:

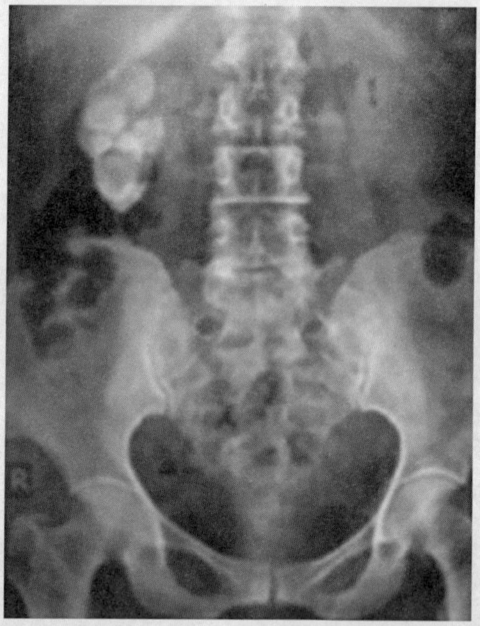

a. Nephrocalcinosis
b. Putty kidney
c. Staghorn calculus
d. Psoas calcification

Ans. is 'b' Putty kidney

A putty kidney refers to a pattern of renal calcification associated with renal tuberculosis conventionally described on plain radiography. The calcification is characteristically very homogeneous and ground glass-like, representing calcified caseous tissue.

187. A child undergoes prophylactic irradiation as a preparation for bone marrow transplant for treatment of ALL. Which of the following is affected least?

a. Spermatogonia
b. Intestinal epithelial cells
c. Neurons
d. Bone marrow

Ans. is 'c' Neurons

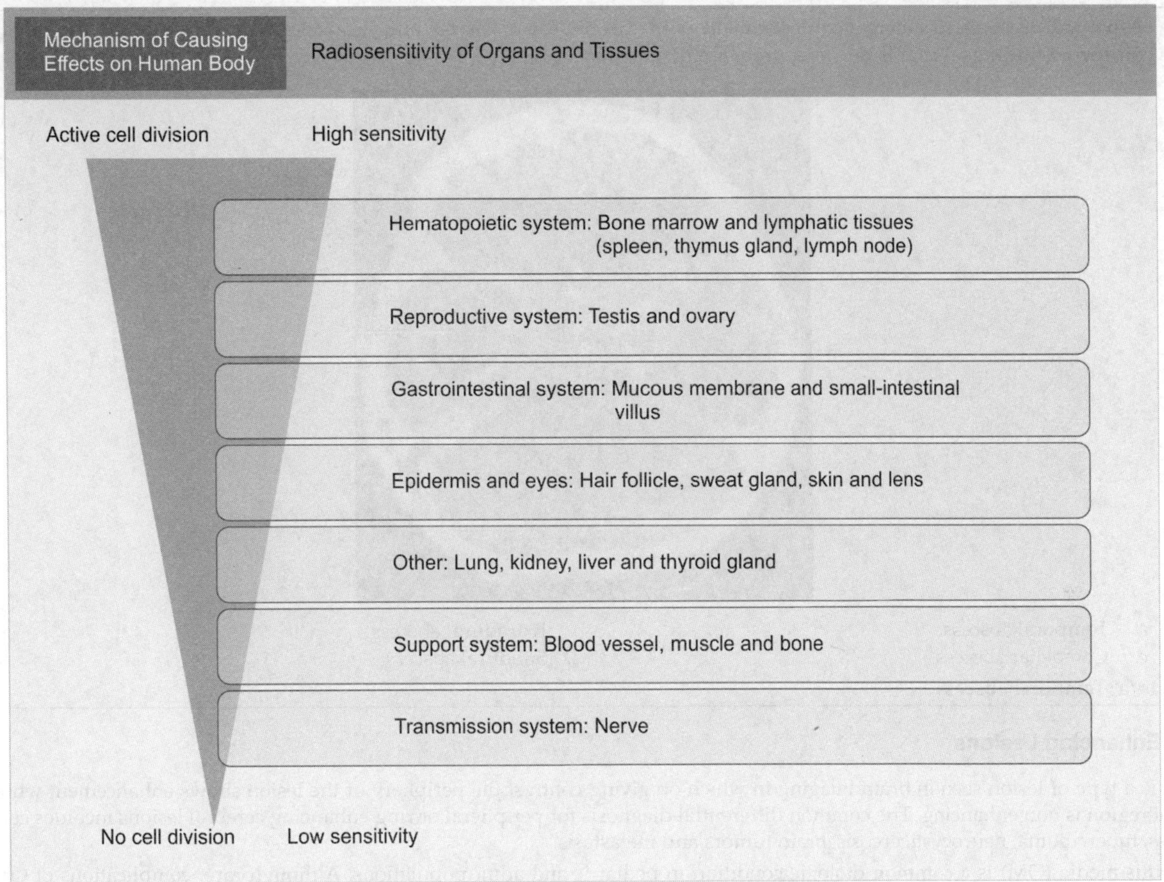

188. A child presents with cyanosis. X-ray of the patient is given below. Identify the diagnosis:

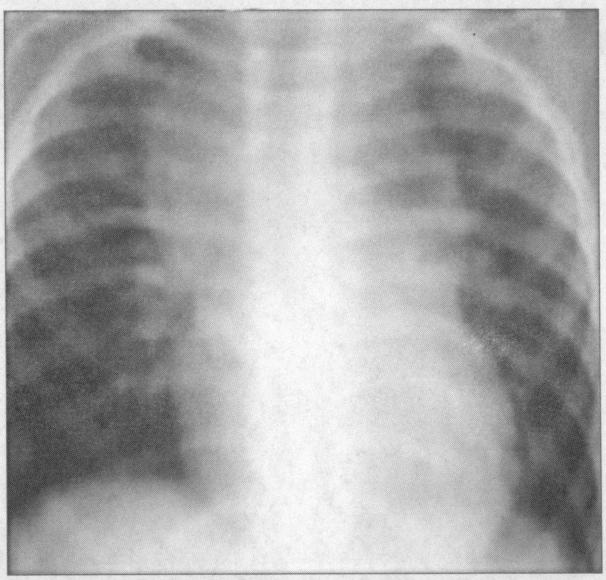

a. Cottage loaf, truncus arteriosus
b. Snowman sign, Supracardiac TAPVC
c. Egg on side, TGA
d. Boot shaped heart, TOF

Ans. is 'b' Snowman sign, Supracardiac TAPVC

For detail see explanation in page 732.

189. A patient presents to emergency department with chronic ear discharge and headache with ear pain. CT Revealed the following findings. What is the most probable diagnosis?

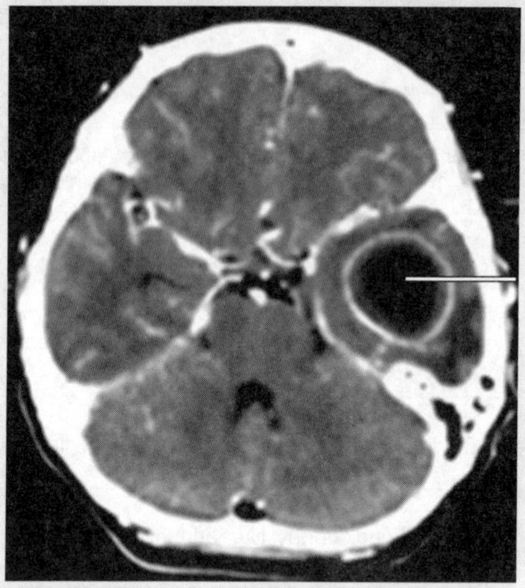

a. Temporal abscess
b. Extradural abscess
c. Cerebellar abscess
d. Subdural abscess

Ans. is 'a' Temporal abscess

Ring Enhancing Lesions

These is a type of lesion seen in brain imaging in which on giving contrast the periphery of the lesion shows enhancement while the central region is non enhancing. The common differential diagnosis for peripheral or ring enhancing cerebral lesions includes cerebral abscess, tuberculoma, neurocysticercosis, brain tumors and metastasis.

Otitis media (OM) is a common otologic condition in pediatric and adult populations. Although rare, complications of OM are commonly encountered given its high prevalence. Complications of OM are classified as extracranial or intracranial. Autogenic brain abscess are considered the second most common intracranial complication of OM after meningitis and are usually seen in the temporal lobe (60%) and cerebellum (30%).

190. Identify the investigation:

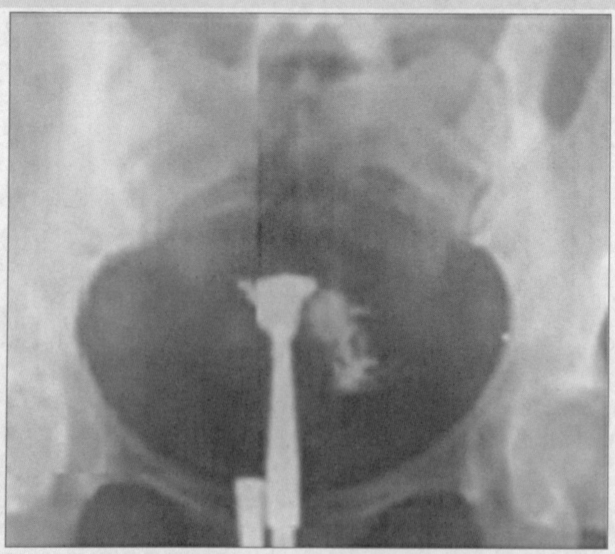

a. Hysterosalpingography
b. Laparoscopy
c. Hysteroscopy
d. Saline infusion hysterography

Ans. is 'a' Hysterosalpingography

For detail see explanation on page 739

191. A 35-year-old male working with hammer and chisel had an accident and a foreign body enters the eye. Which of these investigations will be detrimental?

a. X-ray
b. CT
c. USG
d. MRI

Ans. is 'd' MRI

Magnetic resonance imaging (MRI) is contraindicated in the detection of suspected metallic IOFBs because the associated electromagnetic field can cause foreign body migration, potentially damaging intraocular tissues.

PSYCHIATRY

NEET PG September 2021

192. During the course of psychotherapy, the therapist had mixed conscious and unconscious feeling towards the patient, this phenomenon is known as:

a. **Countertransference**
b. **Dissociation**
c. **Transference**
d. **Preoccupation**

Ans. is 'a' Countertransference

Psychoanalysis

Transference[Q] is the feeling that patient develops for the doctors and countertransference[Q] is a feeling that the clinician develops for the patients.

Freud published 'The Interpretation of Dreams'[Q] in 1900[Q] and proposed 'Topographical theory of mind'[Q]. According to this theory the mind can be divided into three regions: the conscious, the preconscious and the unconscious.

- The conscious is the part of the mind which is accessible to us
- The preconscious can be recalled or brought into our awareness by focused attention. The preconscious mind has a barrier call repression.
- The unconscious is not accessible and it contains the instinct dual drives. The unconscious mind is characterized by 'primary process thinking'[Q] which is a logical and contradictory.

Later on, Freud replaced the topographical theory of mind with another theory called 'The structural theory of mind'. There are three components of Mind according to this theory: Id, Ego and Superego.

- Id works on pleasure principle and completely determined by the unconscious domain of mind.
- Ego works on reality principle and has both conscious and unconscious components.
- Superego follows the moral principles and is mostly unconscious.

According to Freud, unconscious conflicts[Q] among the components of mind leads to psychiatric disorders.

Psychosexual Stages of Development

Sigmund Freud[Q] said that the sexuality develops in multiple stages:

- Oral Stage (0–1.5 yrs)
- Anal Stage (1.5–3 yrs): OCD patients are said to be fixated at this stage[Q].
- Phallic Stage (3–5 yrs): Associated with Oedipus complex[Q] and Castration anxiety[Q] in male child and Electra Complex[Q] in female child. Neurotic illness develops due to fixation at phallic stage[Q].
- Latent Stage (5–12 yrs)
- Genital Stage (>12 yrs)

193. A chronic alcoholic patient decides to get abstinent, after 3 days he presents with confusion, disorientation, agitation and visual hallucinations. What is the diagnosis?

a. Delirium tremens
b. Wernicke's encephalopathy
c. Korsakoff psychosis
d. Alcohol withdrawal seizure

Ans. is 'a' Delirium tremens

For detail see explanation on page 754

194. Which of the following is a formal thought disorder?
- a. Derailment
- b. Obsession
- c. Delusion
- d. Thought insertion

Ans. is 'a' Derailment

Classification of Thought Disorders

Type	*Examples*
Form disorders	• Derailment (loosening of asssociation) • Neologisms
Content disorders	• Delusion • Obscession
Possession disorders	• Thought insertion • Thought withdrawal • Thought forecast
Flow disorders	• Flight of ideas • Slowing of thoughts • Perseveration • Thought block

195. A 16-year-old female patient was brought by family members. On evaluation she had symptoms of overfamiliarity, flight of ideas, elevated mood, increased sexual desire. What is the likely diagnosis?
- a. Mania
- b. Schizomania
- c. Hypomania
- d. Cyclothymia

Ans. is 'a' Mania

Bipolar Disorder/Mania Depressive Psychosis

Characterized by unpredictable swings in mood from mania (or hypomania) to depression at different times and in the intervening period, patient may be normal.

Bipolar I: Characterized by clinical course of ≥1 manic (severe) episodes and sometimes major depressive (severe) episodes (recurrent manic episodes with or w/o depression).

Bipolar II

Characterized by episodes of major (severe) depression and hypomania (Not requiring hospital admission)

- ❖ Manic episode—abnormal and persistently elevated, expansive or irritable mood for at least 1 week or less if patient must be hospitalized.
- ❖ Hypomanic episode—last at least 4 days. Similar to manic episode except that it is NOT severe enough to cause impairment in social or occupational functioning and NO psychotic features are present.
- ❖ Both mania and hypomania are associated with—inflated self-esteem, decreased need for sleep, distractibility, great physical and mental activity and over involvement in pleasurable behavior.
- ❖ Mixed episodes are a period of at least 1 week in which both a manic episode and a depressive episode occur almost daily.
- ❖ Rapid cyclers → > 4 episodes in a year
- ❖ Ultra-rapid cyclers → Switching from one phase to other occurs in hour or days.

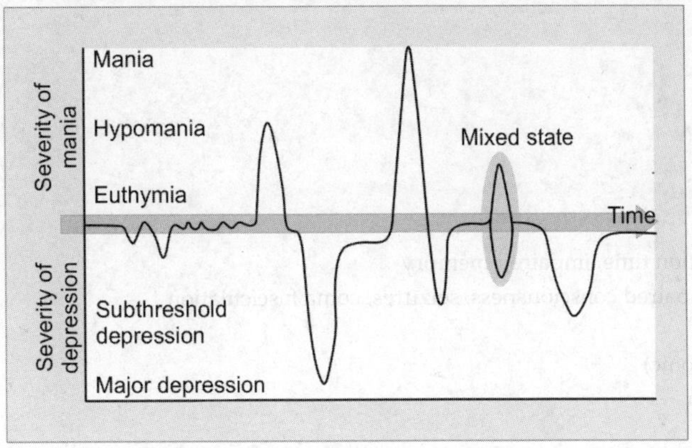

Prognostic Factors

Good	Bad
• Acute onset • Severe depression • Typical symptoms • Good response • Well-adjusted premorbid personality	• Double depression • Marked hypochondriac features • Poor compliance to treatment • Comorbid disorders, alcohol dependence • Catastrophic stress

Treatment

a. **Treating acute mania (or hypomania)**

i. **Lithium or valproate – DOC**

Lithium	*Valproate*
Toxic to kidney • Pre-Lithium → S. creatinine • TSH (Hypothyroidism) • Pregnancy test – Ebstein anomaly 1/10,000 • ECG → T wave changes – Fine tremors – Hypothyroid – Polyuria, polydipsia thirst Toxicity < Neuro – coarse tremor; Nephrology - DI Nephrology - DI	Toxic to liver • SGDT, SGPT if x 3 times → C/I • Pregnancy test → Neural tube defect (1-4%) Much more Teratogenic **Common S/E** → Nausea, vomiting, weight gain, PCOD, Alopecia. Rare S/E → Fulminant hepatotoxicity (Infant) Hyperammonemia—Contraindicated in G6PD patient's SIADH, pancreatitis, Thrombocytopenia

Lithium Therapeutic range 0.6 – 1.2 mg/L

0.6 – 0.8 Maintenance

0.8 – 1.2 Acute mania

> 1.5 – Toxicity starts

>2 – Toxicity severe

>4 – Hemodialysis

Valproate 50–150 mg/mL – Therapeutic range

ii. Response takes 7–14 days → So antipsychotic is often required helps to control acute manic symptoms

iii. High potency Benzodiazepine e.g. Clonazepam and Lorazepam used temporarily to treat hyperactivity, agitation, panic and insomnia can also be given with antipsychotics to lower its dose.

iv. Mania with impaired judgment, loss of insight, hyperactively and diminished behavior require hospitalization.

v. ECT used for

Severe case

- Refractory mania
- Patient with medical complication as well as extreme exhaustion (malignant hyperthermia or lethal catatonia)

Mood Stabilizers

i. Lithium

- Onset slow
- Dose should be titrated
- Adverse effect:
  - Neurological
    - Postural tremors
    - Dysphoria, slow reaction time, impaired memory
    - Ataxia, dysarthria, impaired consciousness, seizures, coma fasciculation
  - Endocrine
    - Hypothyroidism (chronic)
    - Hyperparathyroidism
  - CVS
    - T wave inversion
    - Sinus dysrhythmia, heart block
  - Renal
    - Polyuria, polydipsia (chronic)
- Prominent depressive symptoms, rapid cycling disorder and psychotic features predict poorer response to Lithium

ii. Valproate

- Indicate for acute mania
- Onset is sooner
- Effective in patient with prominent dysphoric symptoms and rapid cycling well-tolerated.

iii. Carbamazepine and Oxcarbazepine

- Slow onset of action
- Slow upward titration required

iv. Other agents – Lamotrigine

- NOT for acute mania
- But prevent recurrence

v. Atypical antipsychotics

- Olanzapine, risperidone
- NOT used for maintenance
- Advantage over atypical antipsychotics
  - Lesser liability for excitatory post synaptic potential
  - No tardive dyskinesia
  - No prolactin increases
- **Side effects**
  - Weight gain
  - Insulin resistance, diabetes mellitus
  - Hyperlipidemia, Hypercholesterolemia
  - Cardiovascular impairmentPediatrics

PEDIATRICS

NEET PG September 2021

196. An anganwadi worker takes weight & height of a 4-year-old and finds out that her height for age is <-2 SD. The likely cause is:

a. Chronic under-nutrition b. Acute malnutrition
c. Wasting d. Recent infections

Ans. is 'a' Chronic under-nutrition

For detail see explanation on page 771.

197. A 16-month-old boy whose weight is 8 kg was brought to the clinic by his mother. Image of growth chart given (weight for age):

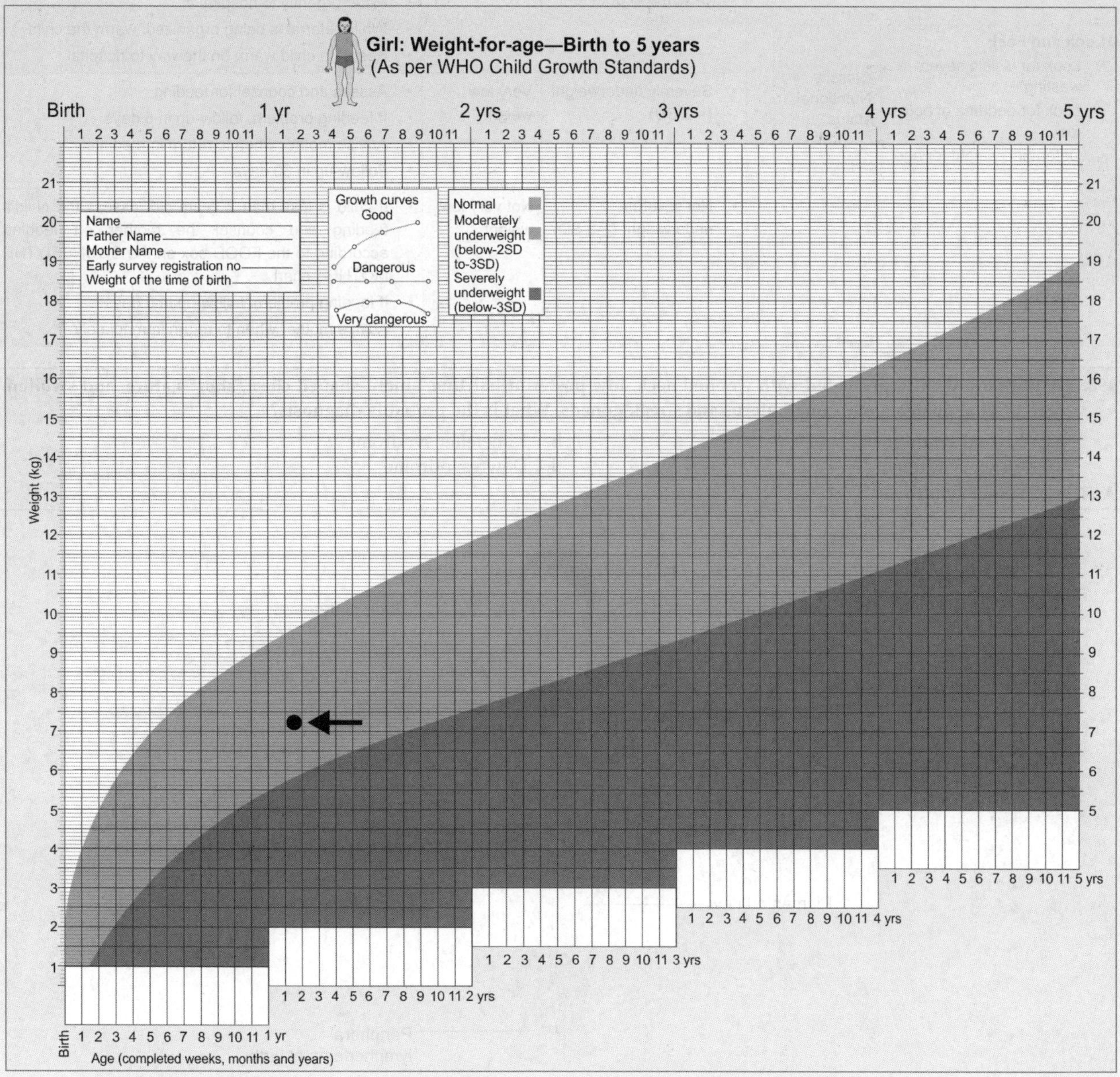

For colour version see Plate 6

What should be the next step?

a. Child is healthy, no advice
b. Severely malnourished child, refer to nutritional rehabilitation centre
c. Severely malnourished, advice mother for home-based care
d. Moderately malnourished, advice mother to feed calorie dense food

Ans. is 'd' Moderately malnourished, advice mother to feed calorie dense food

Then check for malnutrition **Look and Feel:** • Look for visible severe wasting • Look for oedema of both feet • Determine weight for age	Classify Nutritional status	• Visible severe wasting or • Oedema of both feet	Severe malnutrition	• Give single dose of Vitamin A • Prevent low blood sugar • Refer urgently to hospital # • While referral is being organized, warm the child • Keep the child warm on the way to hospital
		• Severely underweight (<-3 SD)	Very low weight	• Assess and counsel for feeding • If feeding problem, follow-up in 5 days • Advise mother when to return immediately • Follow-up in 30 days
		• Not severely underweight ($\geq$-3 SD)	Not very low weight	• If child is less than 2 years old, assess the child's feeding and counsel the mother on feeding according to the FOOD box on the COUNSEL THE MOTHER chart. • If feeding problem, follow-up in 5 days • Advise mother when to return immediately

198. A 10-year-old child presented with webbed neck, low posterior hairline, shield-shaped chest, short stature, and swollen feet. USG abdomen shows small uterus and streak gonads. What is the probable diagnosis?

a. Edward syndrome
b. Klinefelter syndrome
c. Turner syndrome
d. Down syndrome

Ans. is 'c' Turner syndrome

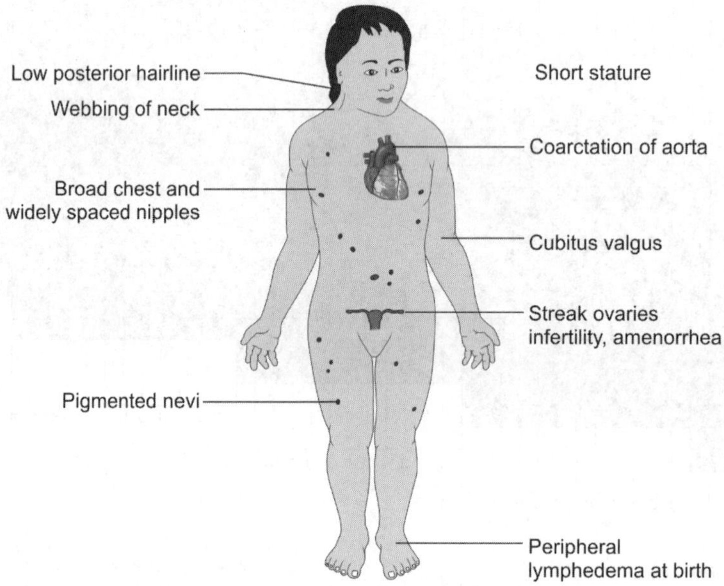

199. Which of the vessels carries deoxygenated blood back to placenta in fetal circulation?

a. Umbilical vein
b. Umbilical artery
c. Descending aorta
d. Pulmonary artery

Ans. is 'b' Umbilical artery

For detail see explanation on page 759

200. A 10-year-old child presented with generalized edema. On investigation, his serum cholesterol level was 238 mg/dL, Urine protein was 3+ and stool microscopy revealed oval fat bodies. What is the probable diagnosis?

a. Goodpasture syndrome
b. Urine infection
c. Nephrotic syndrome
d. Nephritic syndrome

Ans. is 'c' Nephrotic syndrome

Nephrotic syndrome is the clinical manifestation of glomerular diseases associated with heavy (nephrotic-range) proteinuria. Nephrotic-range proteinuria is defined as proteinuria > 3.5 g/24 hr or a urine protein:creatinine ratio > 2. The triad of clinical findings associated with nephrotic syndrome arising from the large urinary losses of protein are hypoalbuminemia (≤2.5 g/dL), edema, and hyperlipidemia (cholesterol > 200 mg/dL).

Summary of primary renal diseases that manifest as idiopathic nephrotic syndrome

Features	*Minimal change nephrotic syndrome*	*Focal segmental glomerulosclerosis*	*Membranous nephropathy*	*Membranous glomerulus* *Type-1*
Demographics				
Age (yr)	2–6, some adults	2–10, some adults	40–50	5–15
Sex (male:female)	2:1	1.3:1	2:1	1:1
Clinical manifestations				
Nephrotic syndrome	100%	90%	80%	60%
Asymptomatic porteinuria	0	10%	20%	40%
Hematuria (microscopic or gross)	10–20%	60–80%	60%	80%
Hypertension	10%	20% early	Infrequent	35%
Rate of progression to renal failure	Does not progress	10 year	50% in 10–20 year	10–20 year
Associated conditions	Usually none	HIV, heroin use, sickle cell disease, reflux nephropathy	Renal vein thromb osis, medications; SLE; hepatitides B,C; lymphoma; tumors	None
Genetics				
	None except in congenital nephrotic syndrome	Podocin, α-actinin 4, TRPC6 channel, INF-2, MYH-9	None	None
Laboratory findings				
	Manifestations of nephrotic syndrome ↑ BUN in 15–30% Normal complement levels	Manifestations of nephrotic syndrome ↑ BUN in 20–40% Normal complement levels	Manifestations of nephrotic syndrome Normal complement levels	Low complement levels—C1, C4, C3-C9
Renal pathology				
Light microscopy	Normal	Focal sclerotic lesions	Thickened GBM, spikes	Thickened GBM, proliferation
Immunofluorescence	Negative	IgM, C3 in lesions	Fine granular IgG, C3	Granular IgG, C3
Electron microscopy	Foot process fusion	Foot process fusion	Subepithelial deposits	Mesangial and subendothelial deposits
Remission achieved after 8 weeks of oral corticosteroid therapy				
	90%	15–20%	Resistant	Not established/resistant

COLOUR PLATES

Plate 1

Latest NEET 2022

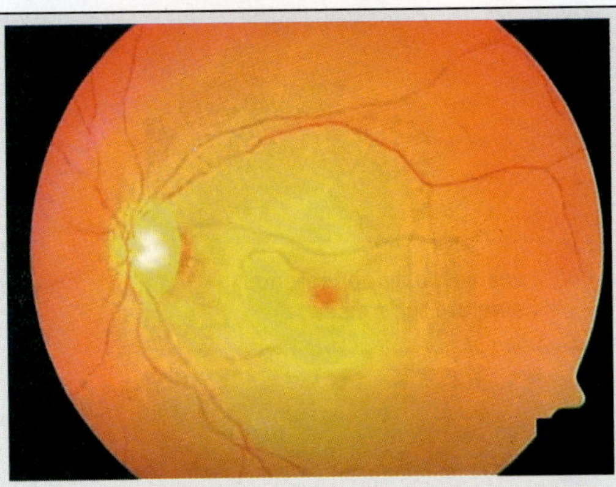

Biochemistry Question 18 *(Page p8)*

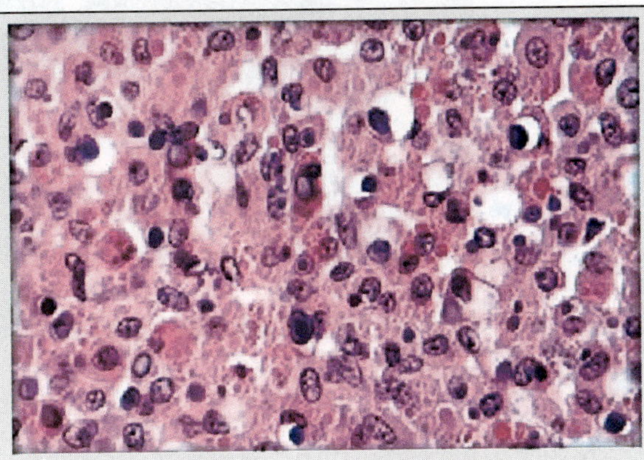

Pathology Question 31 *(Page p13)*

Recent NEET 2021

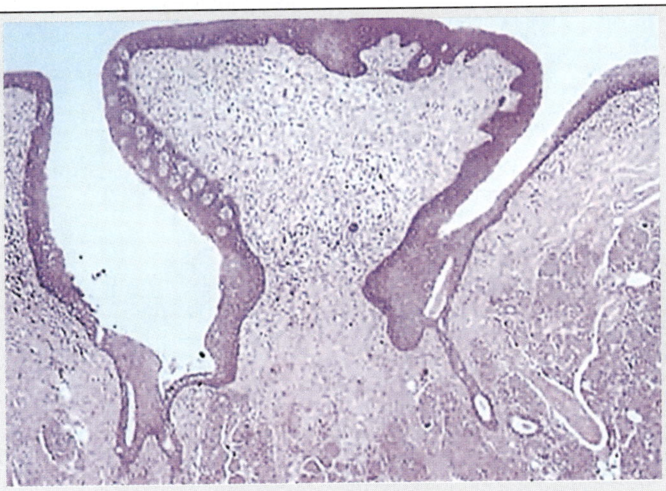

Anatomy Question 1 *(Page p76)*

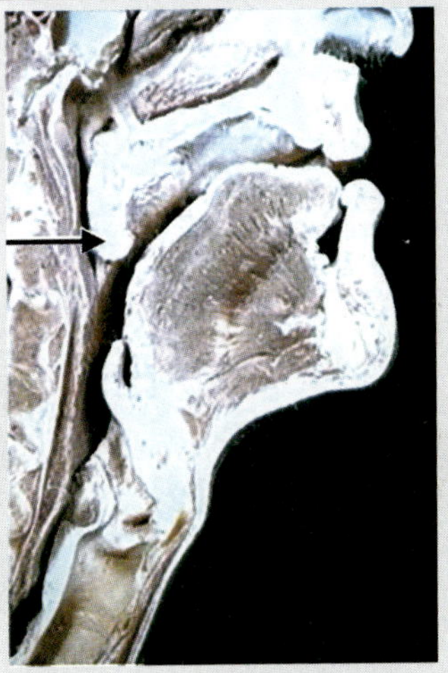

Anatomy Question 5 *(Page p79)*

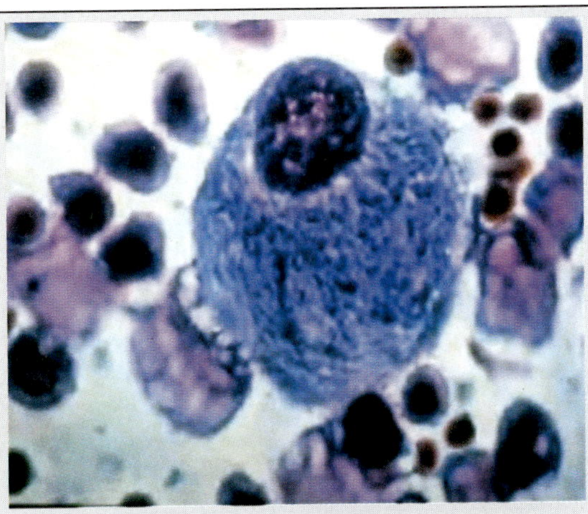

Biochemistry Question 17 *(Page p85)*

Plate 2

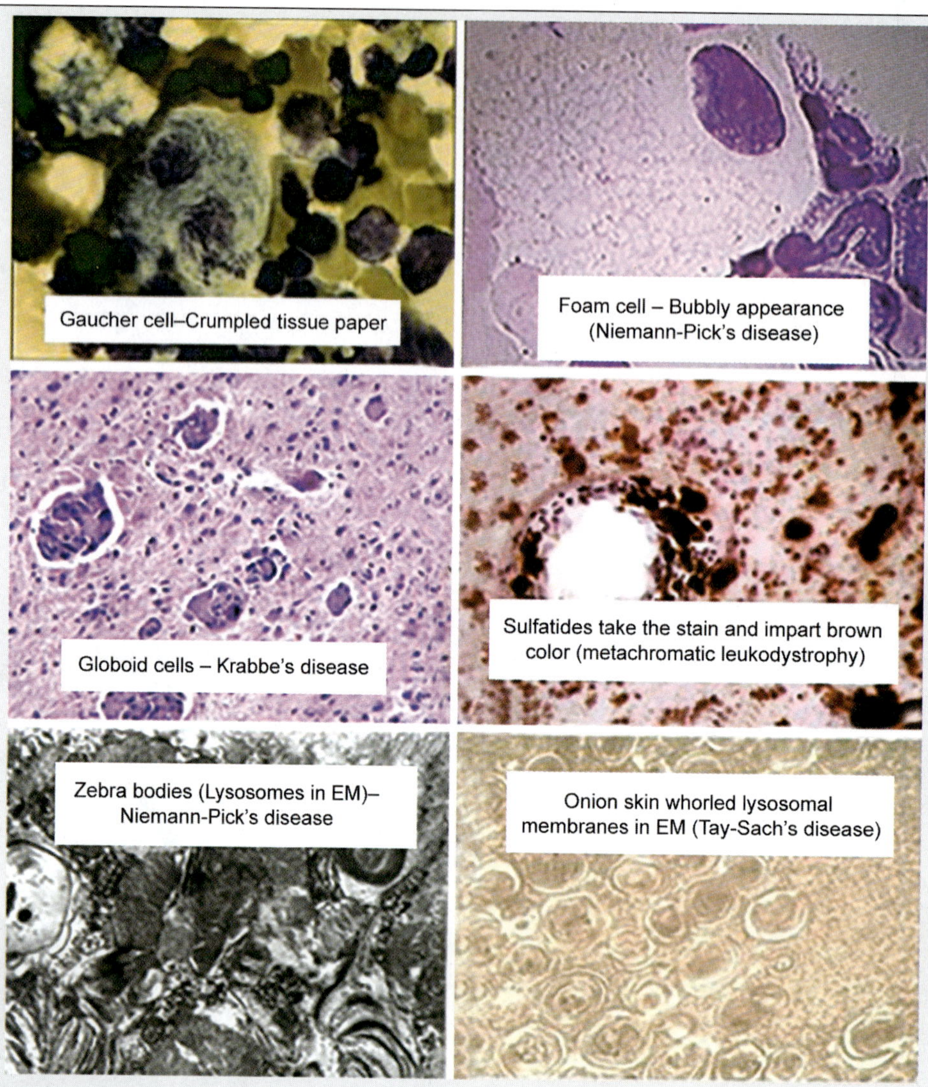

Biochemistry Explanation 17 *(Page p86)*

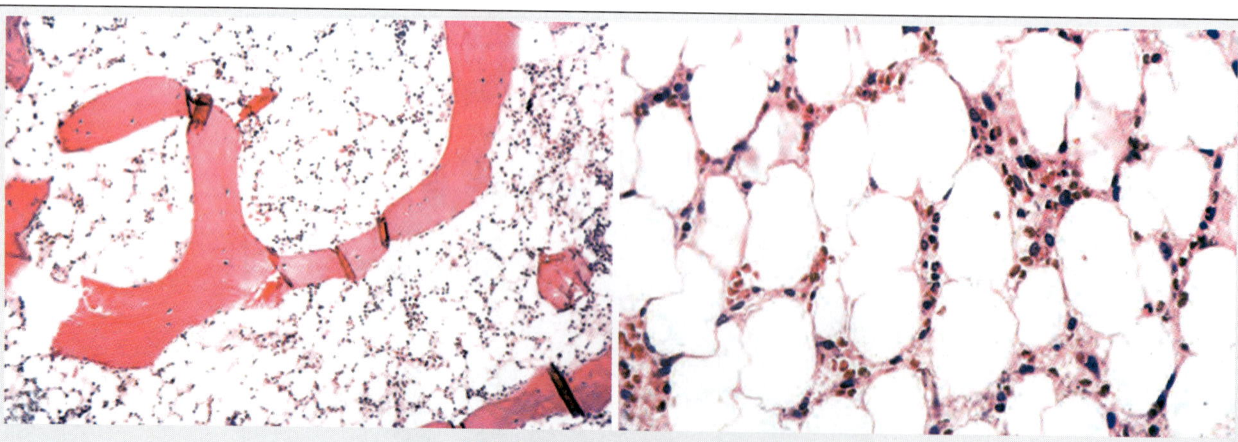

Pathology Explanation 30 *(Page p93)*

Plate 3

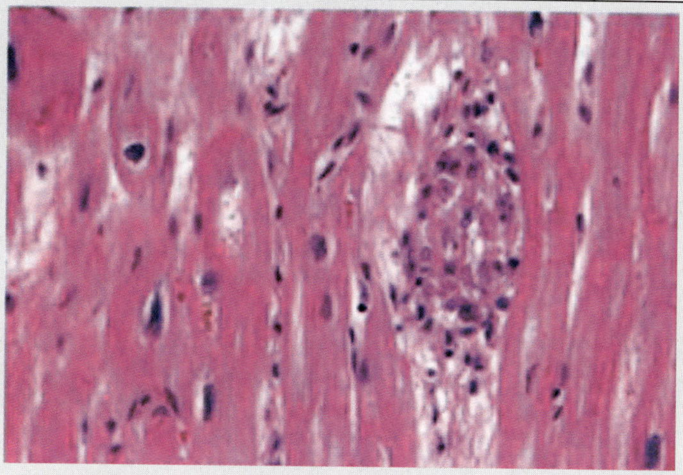

Pathology Question 33 *(Page p94)*

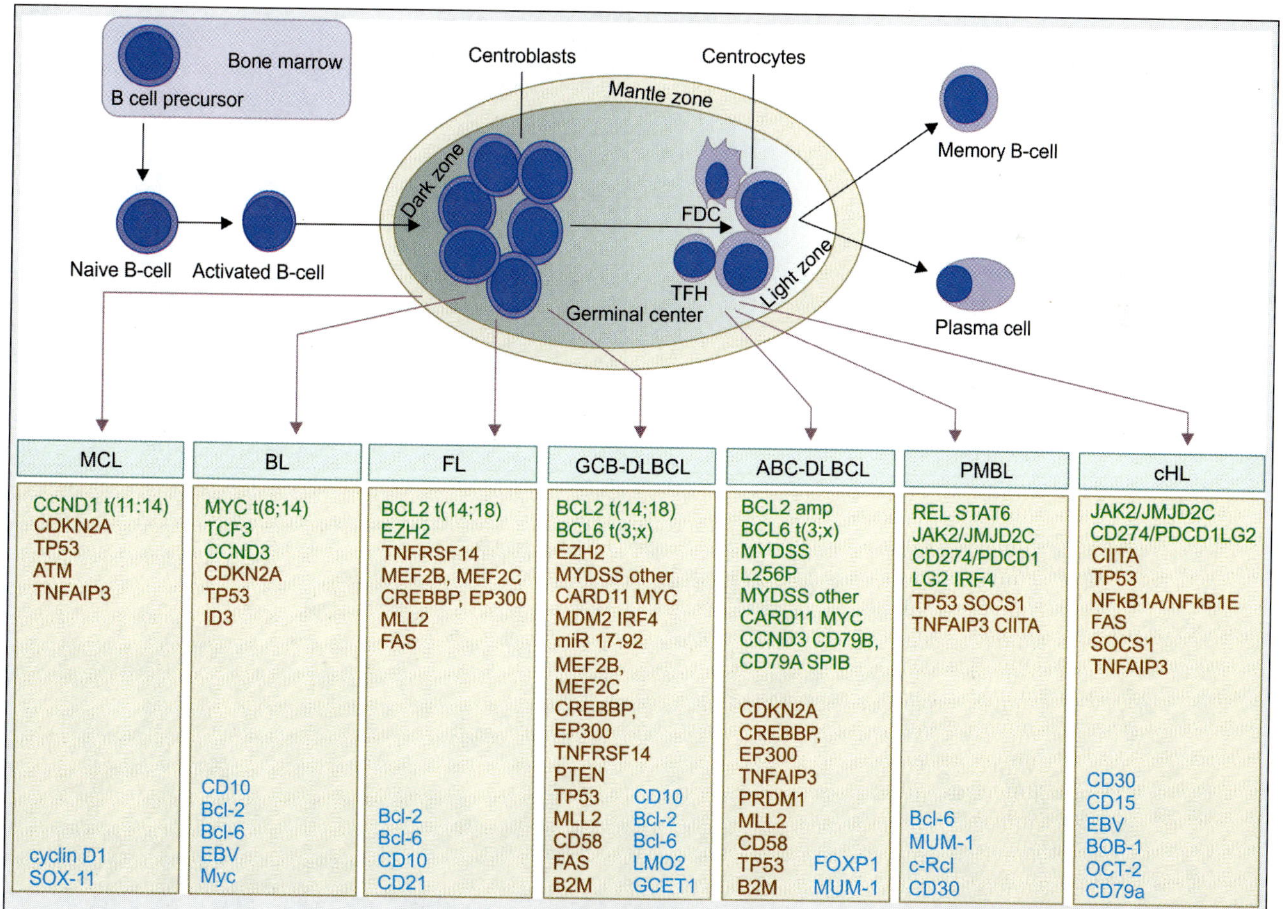

Pathology Explanation 35 *(Page p95)*

Plate 4

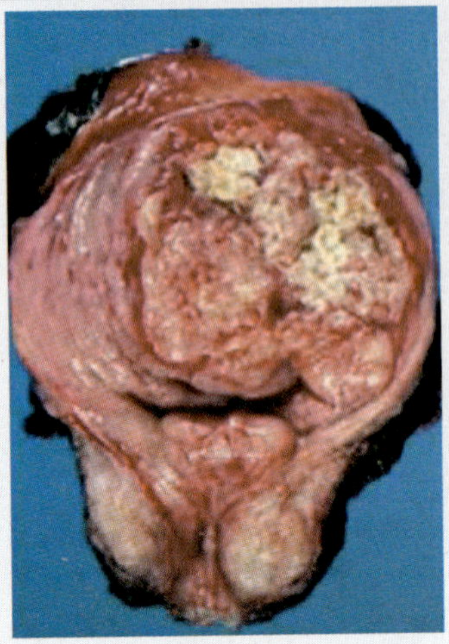

Pathology Question 38 *(Page p97)*

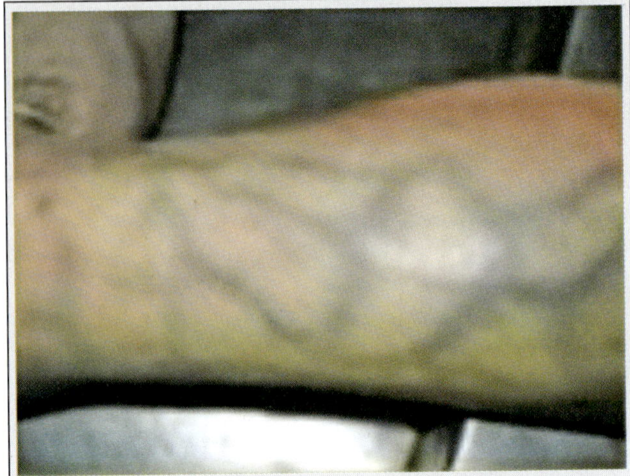

Forensic Medicine Question 69 *(Page p110)*

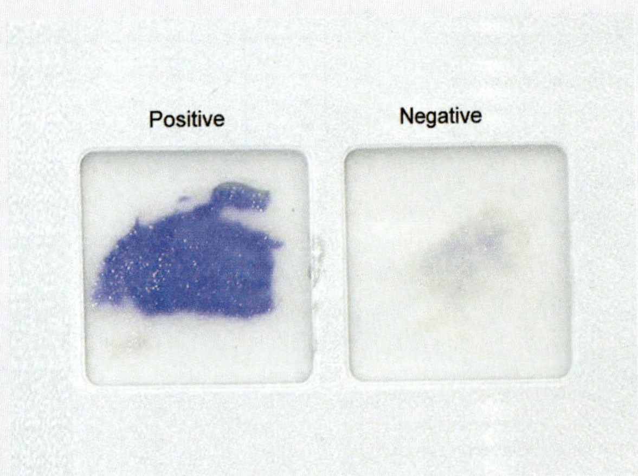

Microbiology Question 55 *(Page p103)*

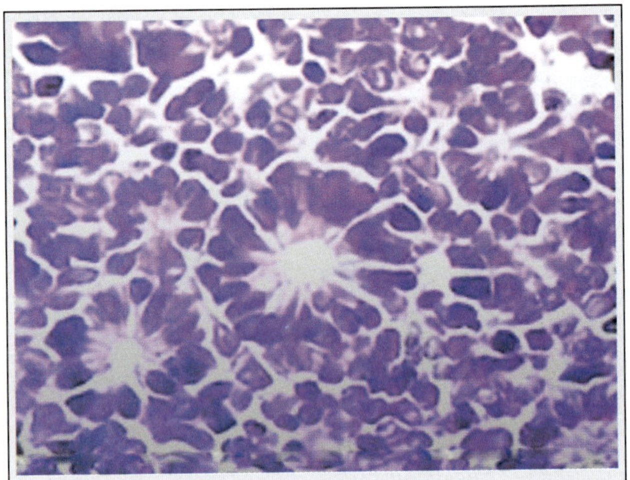

Ophthalmology Question 88 *(Page p119)*

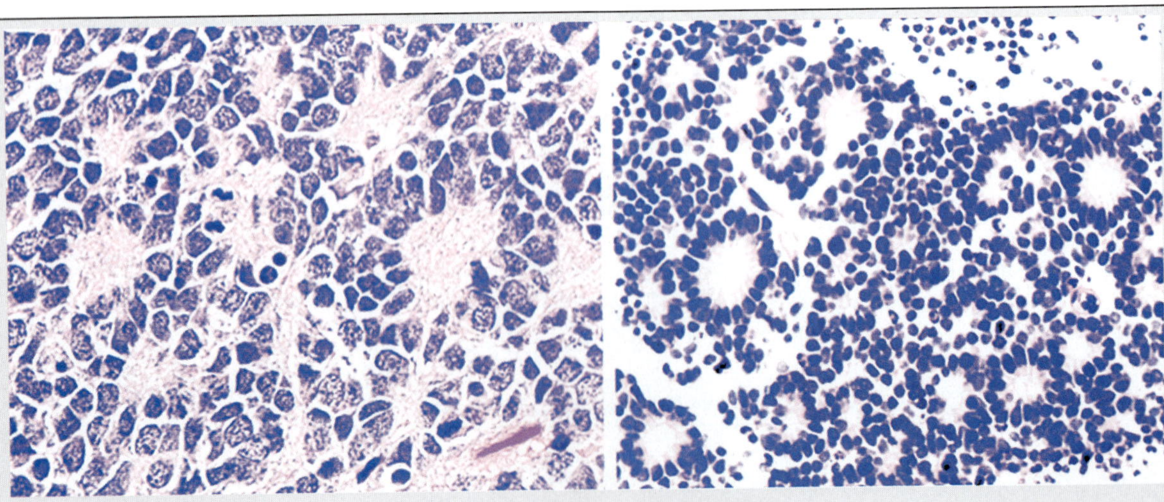

Ophthalmology Explanation 88 *(Page p120)*

Plate 5

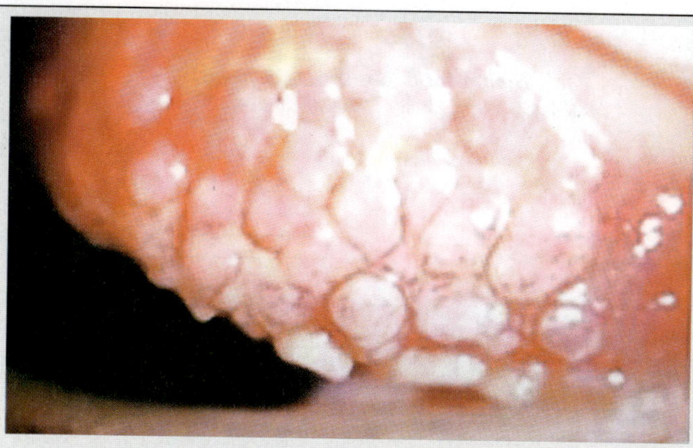

Ophthalmology Question 90 *(Page p121)*

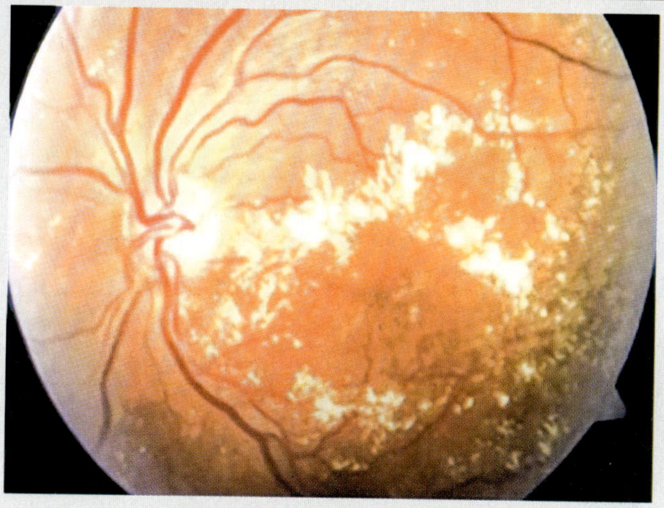

Ophthalmology Question 91 *(Page p121)*

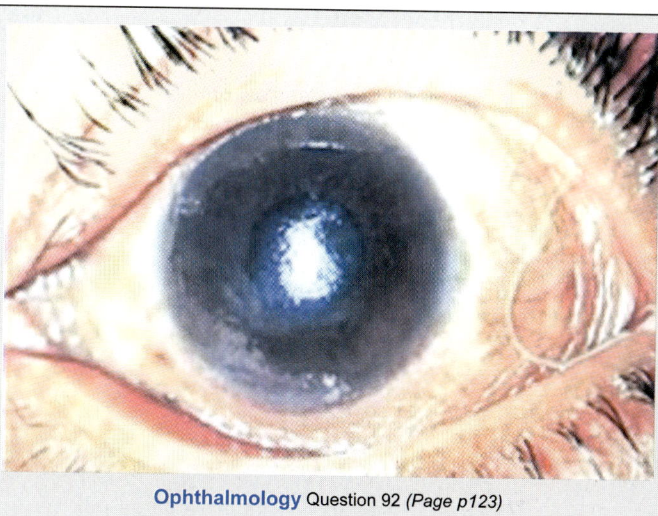

Ophthalmology Question 92 *(Page p123)*

Plate 6

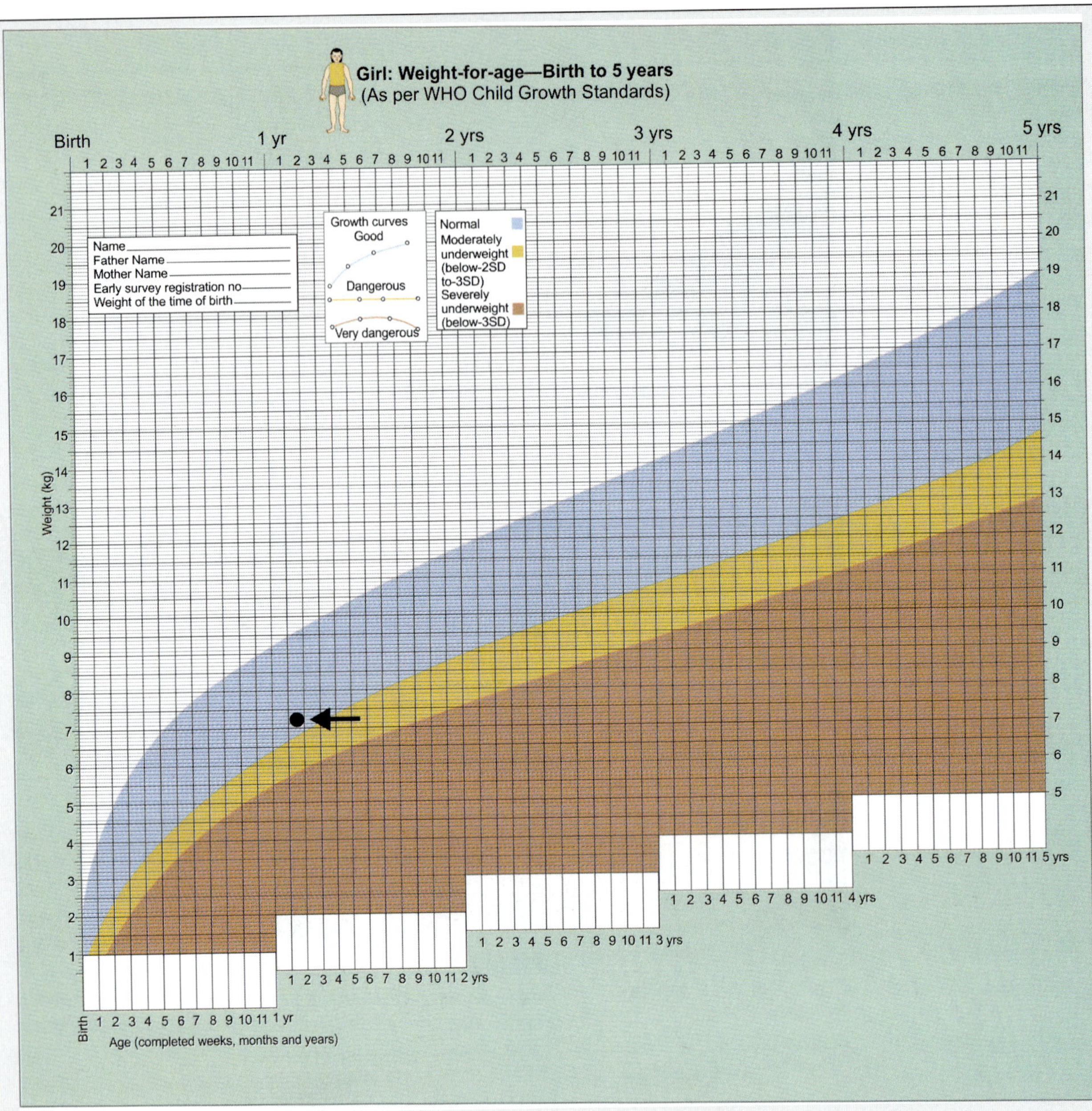

Pediatrics Question 197 *(Page p167)*

CHAPTER 1 Anatomy

GENERAL ANATOMY

SKELETAL MUSCLE—ARRANGEMENT OF FASCICLES

The individual muscle fibres may be arranged either parallel or oblique to the long axis of the belly of the muscle.

Parallel arrangement: Fasciculi are parallel to the line of pull and have greater degree of movement.

- They are further classified based upon the shape:
  - *Quadrilateral:* Thyrohyoid
  - *Strap-like:* Sternohyoid and Sartorius
  - *Strap-like with tendinous intersections:* Rectus abdominis
  - *Fusiform:* Biceps brachii, digastric

Oblique arrangement: Fasciculi are arranged oblique to the line of pull. This increases the power of the muscle, but reduces the range of movement.

- They are further classified into:
  - *Triangular:* Temporalis, adductor longus, trapezius
  - *Spiral or Twisted:* **Pectoralis major**, latissimus dorsi, trapezius
  - *Cruciate muscle (superficial and deep fibres arranged in crossed fashion):* Sternocleidomastoid, masseter, adductor magnus
  - *Unipennate:* Flexor pollicis longus, extensor digitorum longus
  - *Bipennate:* Rectus femoris, flexor hallucis longus
  - *Multipennate:* Tibialis anterior, subscapularis, deltoid (acromian fibers)

1. What is the feature of the muscle shown in the image below? *(NEET 2018)*

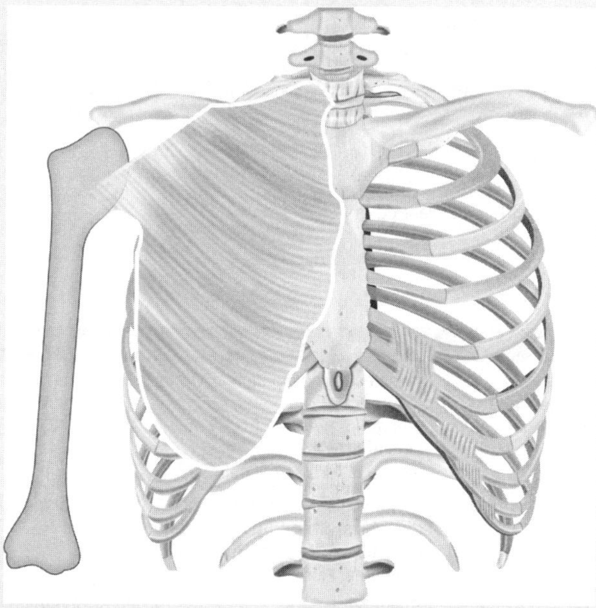

a. Cruciate
b. Multipennate
c. Spiral
d. Unipennate

Ans. is 'c' Spiral

HYBRID/COMPOSITE MUSCLES

- Muscles which have more than one set of fibers but perform the same function and are usually supplied by different nerves for different set of fibers

Composite muscle	Nerve supply
Digastric	*Anterior belly*: Nerve to mylohyoid (branch of mandibular nerve) *Posterior belly*: Facial nerve
Flexor digitorum profundus	*Medial half*: Ulnar nerve *Lateral half*: Anterior interosseous (branch of median nerve)
Adductor magnus	*Adductor part:* Obturator nerve *Hamstring part*: Tibial nerve
Biceps femoris	*Long head*: Tibial nerve *Short head*: Common peroneal nerve
Pectineus	*Anterior fibres*: Femoral nerve *Posterior fibres*: Obturator nerve
Brachialis	*Proprioceptive*: Radial nerve *Motor*: Musculocutaneous
Flexor pollicis brevis	*Superficial head*: Median nerve *Deep head*: Deep branch of ulnar nerve
Pectoraiis majorand minor	Medial and lateral pectoral nerves
Subscapularis	Upper and lower subscapsular nerves

2. Which muscle acting on the thumb has dual nerve supply? *(NEET 2016)*

a. Flexor pollicis longus
b. Flexor pollicis brevis
c. Adductor pollicis
d. Opponens pollicis

Ans. is 'b' Flexor pollicis brevis

EMBRYOLOGY

PHARYNGEAL APPARATUS

- Key embryonic structure for head and neck development

Three components

- Pharyngeal arches
- Pharyngeal clefts
- Pharyngeal pouches

Pharyngeal arches

- Pharyngeal arch cartilage–derived from Neural crest cells
- Core of mesenchyme
- Artery–forms Aortic Arches
- 5th arch involutes in humans

Pharyngeal arch	Bones	Muscles	Nerve	Artery
1st (Mandibular arch)	Maxilla, Zygomatic bone, Mandible, Meckel's cartilage (forms Incus and Malleus)	Muscles of mastication (Temporalis, masseter, pterygoids), Anterior belly of digastric, Mylohyoid, Tensor tympani, Tensor veli palatini	Trigeminal nerve (Maxillary and Mandibular divisions; V2 and V3)	Portion of Maxillary artery
2nd (Hyoid arch)	Derived from 'Reichert's cartilage'-Stapes, Styloid process, Lesser horn of hyoid bone	Stylohyoid, Posterior belly of digastrics, **Stapedius**, Muscles of facial expression, Buccinator, Platysma, Auricular muscles	Facial nerve (VII)	Stapedial artery (usually involutes)
3rd	Hyoid bone **(Body and greater horn)**	Stylopharyngeus	Glossopharyngeal nerve (IX)	Common carotid and Internal carotid
4th	Laryngeal cartilages (Thyroid, epiglottis, Cuneiform, Cricoid, Corniculate)	Cricothyroid, all intrinsic muscles of soft palate (levator palatini), pharyngeal constrictors	Vagus nerve (X)–Superior Laryngeal nerve	*Left*: Aortic arch *Right*: Proximal right subclavian artery
6th (Pulmonary arch)	Arytenoid cartilage	All intrinsic muscles of larynx (except cricothyroid)	Vagus nerve (X)–Recurrent Laryngeal nerve	*Left*: Proximal pulmonary artery, ductus arteriosus Right proximal pulmonary artery

Pharyngeal Pouches

- Four pharyngeal pouches
- Composed of Endoderm

Pouch	Adult derivatives
1st	Epithelial lining of auditory tube and middle ear cavity, contributes to tympanic membrane
2nd	Epithelial lining of crypts of palatine tonsil; **including crypta magna**
3rd	Thymus, Left and right inferior parathyroid glands
4th	Superior parathyroid glands, ultimobranchial body (Derived from neural crest cells; forms C-cells of thyroid)

Pharyngeal Clefts

- Four pharyngeal clefts
- Lined by ectoderm

Cleft	Adult derivatives
1st	External auditory meatus, contributes to tympanic membrane
2nd–4th	Cervical sinus–Obliterates in development May persist as Brachial cyst/sinus

Treacher-Collins Syndrome

- First arch syndrome
- Failure of neural crest migration
- Micrognathia, microtia, glossoptosis (retraction of tongue)—may cause airway obstruction

DiGeorge Syndrome

- Failure of development of 3rd and 4th pharyngeal pouches
- Congenital thymic aplasia and absence of parathyroid glands
- Presents with hypoparathyroidism, recurrent infections, nasal cleft, cardiac anomalies and thyroid hypoplasia.

3. Structure derived from first pharyngeal pouch: *(NEET 2019)*

a. Levator palatini
b. Buccinator
c. Stylohyoid
d. Anterior belly of digastric

Ans. is 'd' Anterior belly of digastric

4. Failure of development of 3rd pharyngeal pouch leads to: *(NEET 2016)*

a. Treacher-Collins syndrome
b. DiGeorge syndrome
c. Pierre Robin syndrome
d. Branchial fistula

Ans. is 'b' DiGeorge syndrome

5. Nerve of the 2nd branchial arch is: *(NEET 2016)*

a. Mandibular nerve
b. Maxillary nerve
c. Facial nerve
d. Vagus

Ans. is 'c' Facial nerve

6. Crypta magna develops from which pouch? *(NEET 2016)*

a. 1st
b. 2nd
c. 3rd
d. 4th

Ans. is 'b' 2nd

DEVELOPMENT OF TONGUE

Development of Tongue	
Epithelium	
Anterior 2/3rd	Lingual swellings of 1st arch and tuberculum impar
Posterior 1/3rd	Large dorsal part of hypobranchial eminence; 3rd arch
Posterior most part	Small dorsal part of hypobranchial eminence; 4th arch
Muscles	Occipital myotomes (except Palatoglossus derived from 6th arch)

7. Tongue develops from all of the following *except*: *(NEET 2016)*

a. Lingual swellings of 1st arch
b. Occipital myotomes
c. Small dorsal part of hypobranchial eminence
d. 5th pharyngeal arch

Ans. is 'd' 5th pharyngeal arch

8. Posterior part of the tongue develops from: *(NEET 2016)*

a. Lingual swelling
b. Tuberculum impar
c. Hypobranchial eminence
d. Tongue bud

Ans. is 'c' Hypobranchial eminence

NOTOCHORD

The notochord represents the earliest foetal axial skeleton, and extends from the Rathke's pouch to the coccyx. It is a primitive cell line around which the skull base and the vertebral column develop. The nucleus pulposus of the intervertebral discs represent residual notochord.

Vestigial non-neoplastic notochordal remnants are seen in up to 2% of cadavers, usually in the midline. They are located:

- Spheno-occipital synchondrosis
- Sacrococcygeal regions
- Smaller scattered foci in the spine (especially C2 and lumbar spine)

Chordoma is a tumor that arises from remnants of notochord; found in midline cranial and sacral regions.

9. Nasopharyngeal chordoma arises from: *(NEET 2018)*

a. Notochord
b. Mesoderm
c. Endoderm
d. Rathke's pouch

Ans. is 'a' Notochord

DEVELOPMENT OF KIDNEY AND GENITAL DUCTS

Kidneys

- Kidneys derive from mesoderm
- Three embryonic renal structures in utero
  - *Pronephros*: Degenerates in week 4
  - *Mesonephros*: Interim kidney in 1st trimester; Associated duct–Mesonephric duct
  - Metanephros
    - Forms definitive kidney
    - Appears around 5th week
    - Becomes functional (urine formation) by 12th week
    - Develops into kidney through weeks 32–36
    - Metanephric blastema—forms excretory unit of kidney (glomerulus, PCT, loops of henle, DCT)
- *Ureteric bud (from mesonephric duct)*: Forms collecting unit of kidney (pelvis, major and minor calyces, collecting ducts) and ureter; stimulates metanephros to form kidney

Genital Duct System

- Two pairs of genital ducts in embryo
  - Mesonephric duct (Wolffian duct): Main genital duct in males
  - Paramesonephric duct (Mullerian duct): Main genital duct in females

Mesonephric duct derivatives	Paramesonephric duct derivatives
Males	***Males***
Ductus deferens, Ejaculatory duct Epididymis, Seminal vesicles Posterior wall of proximal prostatic urethra Peripheral prostate gland	Prostatic utricle Appendix of testis
Females	***Females***
Epoophoron Paroophoron Gartner's duct	Fallopian tubes Uterus Upper 2/3rd vagina
Both male and female	
Trigone of urinary bladder Ureteric bud derivatives	

Anatomy

Urogenital sinus (endoderm)–forms **urinary bladder** (except trigone), male urethra (anterior wall of prostatic urethra, membranous urethra and penile urethra upto glans), **female urethra** and lower 1/3rd vagina.

10. Ureteric bud develops from: *(NEET 2018)*

a. Metanephros
b. Mesonephros
c. Mesonephric duct
d. Genital sinus

Ans. is 'c' Mesonephric duct

11. Trigone of the bladder is derived from: *(NEET 2018)*

a. Mesonephric duct
b. Paramesonephric duct
c. Urogenital folds
d. Mullerian tubercle

Ans. is 'a' Mesonephric duct

12. Human renal system is functional at what age? *(NEET 2018)*

a. 10–12 weeks of intrauterine life
b. 15–17 weeks of intrauterine life
c. 20–22 weeks of intrauterine life
d. 25–27 weeks of intrauterine life

Ans. is 'a' 10–12 weeks of intrauterine life

13. Female urethra develops from: *(NEET 2016)*

a. Urogenital sinus
b. Mesonephric duct
c. Ureteric bud
d. Metanephric blastema

Ans. is 'a' Urogenital sinus

14. Kidney parenchyma is derived from: *(NEET 2016)*

a. Ureteric bud
b. Mesonephros
c. Metanephros
d. Paramesonephros

Ans. is 'c' Metanephros

GONADAL DEVELOPMENT

Indifferent Gonad

- Gonadal ridges (mesodermal) form about 7 weeks
- Germ cells derived from epiblast invade gonadal ridges

Default Genital Development is Female

Male Gonad Differentiation

- Testicular morphogenesis is dependent on SRY **gene on short arm of chromosome Y**
- Codes for Testis Determining Factor (TDF)
- Produces special factors required for male differentiation:
    - **Mullerian Inhibiting Substance (MIS)–from Sertoli cells**
    - Testosterone–from Leydig cells
    - Dihydrotestosterone (DHT)–conversion of testosterone

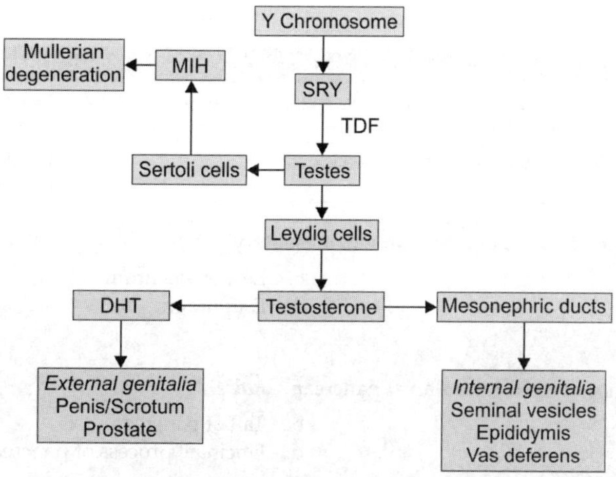

Male differentiation

15. Secretion of Mullerian inhibiting Substance is controlled by gene present on: *(NEET 2019)*

a. Long arm of chromosome X
b. Short arm of chromosome Y
c. Long arm of chromosome Y
d. Short arm of chromosome 21

Ans. is 'b' Short arm of chromosome Y

16. Meiosis occurs in which of the following organs in an adult? *(NEET 2020)*

a. Adrenal
b. Adult ovaries
c. Prepubertal testis
d. Posterior pituitary

Ans. is 'b' Adult ovaries

Explanation: Meiosis occurs during formation of gametes, the number of chromosomes is reduced to half and returned to full amount when the two gametes fuse during fertilization.

DEVELOPMENT OF GUT

- Gut is endodermal in origin and derived from yolk sac

Portion of developing gut	Artery	Derived part of gut
Foregut	Celiac trunk	Mouth to ampulla of Vater
Midgut	**SMA**	Ampulla of Vater to proximal 2/3 transverse colon
Hindgut	IMA	Distal transverse colon to rectum

Distal part of rectum and upper part of anal canal are derived from endodermal cloaca.

Derivatives of Mesentery

- Double layer of peritoneum that suspends abdominal organs from cavity walls
- *Dorsal mesentery*: Covers most organs
- *Ventral mesentery*: Only present around foregut; Liver grows into ventral mesentery

Ventral mesentery derivatives	Dorsal mesentery derivatives
Lesser omentum (Hepatogastric and Hepatoduodenal ligament)	Greater omentum
Falciform ligament	Gastrosplenic ligament
Triangular ligament of liver	Lienorenal ligament
Coronary ligament of liver	Gastrophrenic ligament
	Mesentery of small intestine and mesoappendix
	Transverse and sigmoid mesocolon

Development of Pancreas

- Develops from two pancreatic buds which subsequently undergo rotation and fuse

Pancreatic bud	Mesentery	Derived parts of pancreas
Dorsal pancreatic bud	Dorsal	Most of head, Neck, Body, Tail
Ventral pancreatic bud	Ventral	Uncinate process

Pancreatic duct	Derived from	Opening into duodenum
Main pancreatic duct (Duct of Wirsung)	Duct of ventral bud communicating with distal part of dorsal pancreatic duct	Major duodenal papilla (in 2nd part of duodenum)
Accessory pancreatic duct (Duct of Santorini)	Proximal part of dorsal pancreatic duct	Minor duodenal papilla (2 cm cranial to major papilla, **in 2nd part of duodenum)**

17. Which of the following structure develops from dorsal mesentery? *(NEET 2018)*

a. Greater omentum
b. Lesser omentum
c. Liver
d. Diaphragm

Ans. is 'a' Greater omentum

18. Which of the following is not derived from dorsal pancreatic bud?

a. Head of pancreas
b. Tail of pancreas
c. Body of pancreas
d. Uncinate process of pancreas

Ans. is 'd' Uncinate process of pancreas

19. Which of the following is not derived from the gut, up to the level of dorsal pancreatic bud?

a. Liver
b. Pancreas
c. Small intestine
d. Stomach

Ans. is 'c' Small intestine

Explanation: Dorsal pancreatic bud is at the level of ampulla of Vater. So, the question is asking structure that is not derived from foregut.

20. Which of the following is not a derivative of primitive dorsal mesentery?

a. Lienorenal ligament
b. Gastrosplenic ligament
c. Hepatoduodenal ligament
d. Greater omentum

Ans. is 'c' Hepatoduodenal ligament

UMBILICAL CORD

Connection between embryo and placenta

Contents

- *2 umbilical arteries*: Deoxygenated fetal blood to placenta
- *1 umbilical vein*: Oxygenated blood from placenta to fetus
- Wharton's Jelly
  - Mesenchymal core
  - Contains mucopolysaccharides
- Remnant of yolk sac and allanto-enteric diverticulum

Fetal Circulation

- High resistance to flow in lungs
- Oxygenated blood in umbilical veins–80% saturated
- Travels directly to right atrium
  - Bypasses liver by ductus arteriosus
- Bypasses lungs via foramen ovale
- Some blood goes to right ventricle
  - Bypasses lungs via ductus arteriosus (left PA to aorta)

Single Umbilical Artery

- Abnormal variant
- Identified on prenatal ultrasound
- **Associated with fetal anomalies**–aneuploidy, congenital malformations (renal, cardiovascular, musculoskeletal)

21. True about umbilical cord is: *(NEET 2018)*

a. Has 2 veins and 1 artery
b. Umbilical artery takes blood to fetal circulation
c. Contains special connective tissue called Wharton's jelly
d. Absence of umbilical vein suggests fetal anomaly

Ans. is 'c' Contains special connective tissue called Wharton's jelly

Fetal–postnatal derivatives	
Fetal structure	***Postnatal derivative***
Urachus	**Median umbilical ligament**
Ductus arteriosus	Ligamentum arteriosum
Ductus venosus	Ligamentum venosum
Foramen ovale	Fossa ovalis
Notochord	Nucleosus pulposus
Umbilical arteries	***Proximal part*: Superior vesical artery** ***Distal part*: Medial umbilical ligament**
Umbilical vein	Ligamentum teres

22. Which of the following is remnant of distal umbilical artery? *(NEET 2016)*

a. Ligamentum teres
b. Superior vesical artery
c. Medial umbilical ligament
d. Ligamentum arteriosum

Ans. is 'c' Medial umbilical ligament

VENTRAL WALL DEFECTS

Developmental defects due to failure of rostral fold closure (e.g. sternal defects like ectopia cordis), lateral fold closure (e.g. omphalocele, gastroschisis) or caudal fold closure (e.g. bladder exstrophy)

Gastroschisis	Omphalocele
Extrusion of abdominal contents through abdominal folds (typically right of umbilicus)	Failure of lateral walls to migrate at umbilical ring → persistent midline herniation of abdominal contents into umbilical cord
Not covered by peritoneum or amnion	Surrounded by peritoneum (shiny sac)
Not associated with chromosome abnormalities	Associated with congenital anomalies (e.g. trisomies 13 and 18, Beckwith–Wiedemann syndrome) and other structural abnormalities (e.g. cardiac, GU, neural tube)

23. A child presented with herniation of loops of intestine just from the right of umbilicus. What is the diagnosis? *(NEET 2020)*

a. Omphalocele
b. Gastroschisis
c. Malrotation
d. Physiological hernia

Ans. is 'b' Gastroschisis

GERM LAYER DERIVATIVES

Ectoderm	Mesoderm	Endoderm
Surface ectoderm	Muscles	**Epithelial lining of GIT, Respiratory and genitourinary system**
Epidermis, hair, nails	Blood, lymph, cardiovascular organs	Liver
Anterior pituitary	Serous membranes	Pancreas
Parotid gland	Bone and cartilage	Submandibular and sublingual glands
Corneal epithelium, lens of eye	Urogenital system	Follicles of thyroid gland
Enamel of teeth	Connective tissue	
Inner ear	Adrenal cortex	
Neuroectoderm	Spleen	
CNS		
Retina		
Posterior pituitary		
Pineal gland		
Macroglia (Astrocytes, Oligodendrocytes, ependymal cells)		

Neural crest cell derivatives
Adrenal medulla
Sensory and autonomic ganglia
Melanocytes
Schwann cells
Pharyngeal arch cartilage
Cranial nerves
Corneal endothelium, stroma, Descemet's membrane
Parafollicular (C) cells
Aorticopulmonary septum, Endocardial cushions
Meninges–Pia and arachnoid mater
Odontoblasts

24. Nerves supplying pharyngeal arches are developed from: *(NEET 2018)*

a. Mesoderm
b. Neural crest
c. Endoderm
d. Notochord

Ans. is 'b' Neural crest

25. Which of the following parts of the eye are derived from neural crest cells? *(NEET 2016)*

a. Descemet's membrane
b. Extraocular muscles
c. VItreous
d. Choroid

Ans. is 'a' Descemet's membrane

26. Astrocytes are derived from which germ layer? *(NEET 2016)*

a. Mesoderm
b. Neuroectoderm
c. Endoderm
d. None

Ans. is 'b' Neuroectoderm

27. Epithelium of urinary bladder is derived from: *(NEET 2016)*

a. Ectoderm
b. Mesoderm
c. Endoderm
d. Neuroectoderm

Ans. is 'c' Endoderm

NEURAL TUBE DERIVATIVES

Neurons develop in Mantle layer of neural tube. Mantle layer divides into two parts

- **Basal lamina**—gives rise to structures that are **motor** in function
- **Alar lamina**—gives rise to structures that are **sensory** in function

	Alar lamina derivatives	Basal lamina derivatives
Midbrain	Colliculi **Substantia nigra** Mesencephalic nucleus of trigeminal nerve	Occulomotor nucleus **Edinger westphal nucleus** Trochlear nucleus
Pons	**Pontine and vestibular nuclei** Nucleus of spinal tract of trigeminal nerve Nucleus of tractus solitarius	Motor nuclei of trigeminal and facial nerves Abducent nucleus Superior salivatory and Lacrimatory nuclei
Medulla	Inferior olivary nucleus	Inferior salivatory nucleus Nucleus ambiguus Hypoglossal nucleus
Spinal cord	Dorsal gray column	Ventral gray column

28. Which of the following is derived from basal lamina of neural tube? *(NEET 2016)*

a. Substantia nigra
b. Edinger Westphal nucleus
c. Pontine nuclei
d. Vestibular nucleus

Ans. is 'b' Edinger Westphal nucleus

FATE OF EMBRYONIC VENOUS STRUCTURES

Embryonic structure	Adult derivatives
Vitelline veins	
Right and left	Hepatic vein and sinusoids, ductus venosus, inferior hepatic part of IVC, portal vein, superior and inferior mesenteric vein, splenic vein Most portion of left vitelline vein disappears
Umbilical veins	
Right	Regresses early in development
Left	Ductus venosus; Ligamentum teres
Cardinal veins	Internal jugular vein, SVC, part of IVC, common iliac veins, renal veins, gonadal veins, intercostal veins, hemiazygos and azygos vein

Inferior Vena Cava is formed by (caudal to cranial)

- **Posterior intercardinal anastomosis**
- Caudal portion of right supracardinal vein
- Anastomosis between supracardinal and subcardinal veins
- **Segment of right subcardinal vein**
- Anastomosis between right subcardinal and right vitelline veins
- **Terminal portion of right vitelline vein**

29. All of the following help in formation of IVC *except*: *(NEET 2016)*

a. Posterior intercardinal anastomosis
b. Terminal portion of right vitelline vein
c. Segment of right cardinal vein
d. Subcardinal sinus

Ans. is 'd' Subcardinal sinus

FETAL CIRCULATION

- Blood in umbilical vein has a PO_2 of ~ 30 mm Hg and is ~ 80% saturated with O_2. Umbilical arteries have low O_2 saturation.
- Three important shunts
  - Blood entering fetus through the umbilical vein is conducted via the **ductus venosus** into the IVC, bypassing hepatic circulation.
  - Most of the highly Oxygenated blood reaching the heart via the IVC is directed through the **Foramen Ovale** and pumped into the aorta to supply the head and body.
  - Deoxygenated blood from the SVC passes through the RA → RV → main pulmonary artery → **Ductus arteriosus** → Descending aorta; shunt is due to high fetal pulmonary artery resistance (due partly to low O_2 tension).

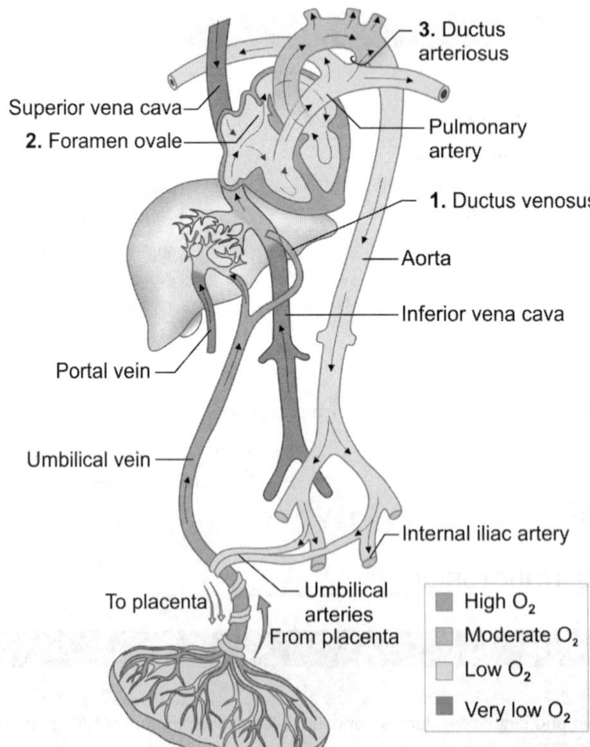

30. In fetal circulation, maximum oxygen saturation is seen in: *(NEET 2020)*

a. SVC
b. IVC
c. Ascending aorta
d. Right ventricle

Ans. is 'b' IVC

HISTOLOGY

TYPES OF EPITHELIUM

Type of epithelium	Tissue
Simple squamous	Lung alveoli Mesothelium Endothelium Loop of Henle Resting thyroid follicle
Keratinized stratified squamous	Epidermis Duct of sebaceous gland **Hard palate (with minor mucous salivary glands)**
Non-keratinized stratified squamous	Tongue Tonsil Pharynx **Esophagus** Cornea Vagina Ectocervix (lower cervix) Vocal cords
Simple columnar epithelium	Large intestine lining Stomach lining Endocervix (upper cervix) Active thyroid follicle
Columnar epithelium with striated border (regularly arranged microvilli)	Small intestine lining
Columnar epithelium with brush border (irregularly placed microvilli)	Gallbladder
Ciliated columnar epithelium	**Uterus and fallopian tubes** **Eustachian tube** Central canal of spinal cord and ventricles of brain Respiratory epithelium
Secretory columnar epithelium (goblet cells) Pseudostratified columnar epithelium	Stomach and intestines Trachea and bronchi Olfactory epithelium Trachea, Eustachian tube Vas deferens Urethra
Simple cuboidal epithelium	Proximal and distal convoluted tubule Thyroid follicles Ovarian surface epithelium
Transitional epithelium (Urothelium)	Renal pelvis, calyces Ureter Urinary bladder Part of urethra

31. Lining epithelium of hard palate is: *(NEET 2018)*

a. Keratinized with no salivary glands
b. Non-keratinized with no salivary glands
c. Keratinized with minor salivary glands
d. Non-keratinized with minor salivary glands

Ans. is 'c' Keratinized with minor salivary glands

32. Ciliated columnar epithelium is seen all *except*:

a. Uterine cavity
b. Eustachian tube
c. Fallopian tube
d. Cervical canal

Ans. is 'd' Cervical canal

STRUCTURE OF KIDNEY

Excretory System

Each uriniferous tubule consists of Nephron and Collecting tubule.

- Nephron–Renal corpuscle and Renal tubule (PCT → Loop of Henle → DCT)
- Collecting (Junctional) tubule–Between terminal part of distal convoluted tubule and collecting duct

Collecting System

- Collecting ducts → **Papillary Ducts of Bellini** → Minor calyx [at apex (papilla) of renal pyramid] → Major calyces → Pelvis → Ureter

33. Ducts of Bellini are present in: *(NEET 2019)*

a. Pancreas b. Kidney
c. Liver d. Salivary gland

Ans. is 'b' Kidney

LIVER ARCHITECTURE

Liver is covered by **Glisson's capsule**

Hepatic Blood Supply

- Portal vein (75%)–supplies nutrients
- Hepatic artery (25%)–supplies oxygen

Three Dimensional Arrangement of Hepatocytes

- Arranged in plates
- Apical surface facing sinusoids
- Basal surface forms biliary canaliculi
- Bile canaliculi → **Canals of Hering** → Interlobular bile ducts
- Lateral surfaces are in contact with other hepatocytes

Hepatic Sinusoids

- Blood from both portal vein and hepatic artery enter into sinusoids
- Sinusoids are distensible vascular channels lined by fenestrated endothelium bounded circumferentially by hepatocytes

Space of Disse

- Space between hepatocytes and sinusoids
- As blood flows through sinusoids, plasma is filtered into space of Disse; providing a major fraction of body's lymph
- **Hepatic Stellate cell of Ito**–Present in Space of Disse; Helps in storage of Vitamin A

Direction of Blood Flow in Liver

Portal vein and Hepatic artery → Sinusoids → Central vein → Hepatic vein → Systemic circulation

Portal Triad

- Hepatic artery
- Portal vein
- Bile duct

HEPATIC LOBULES/ACINI

Classic Lobule

- **Hexagonal**
- Central vein at centre; Portal triads at periphery

Portal Lobule

- Triangular
- Portal triad in centre; 3 central veins at periphery

Hepatic Acinus

- ❖ Widely accepted
- ❖ Depends upon blood carried by branches of hepatic artery and portal veins
- ❖ At sides–Central vein on one side; portal triad on other side diagonally
- ❖ Zones of ischemia or toxic injury
  - *Zone 1*: Highly oxygenated; more affected by toxins
  - *Zone 2*: Less oxygenated; less affected by toxins
  - *Zone 3*: Least oxygenated; least affected by toxins

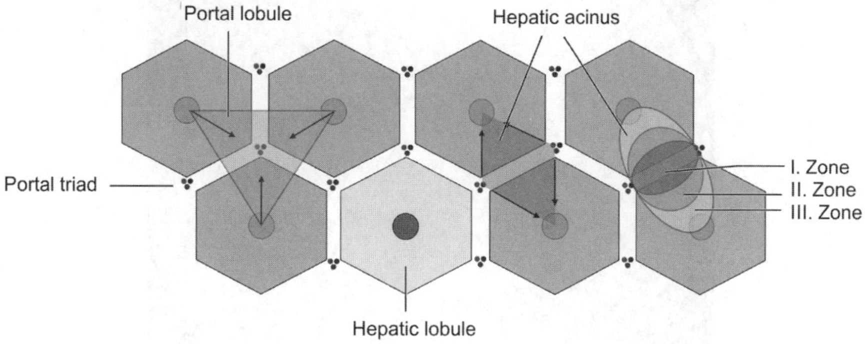

34. Space of Disse is seen in:	*(NEET 2019)*
a. Spleen	b. Liver
c. Bone	d. None

Ans. is 'b' Liver

HISTOLOGY OF THYMUS

- ❖ **Cortical portion is mainly composed of lymphocytes** supported by trabeculae
- ❖ Medullae of adjacent lobules are continuous
- ❖ **Hassall's corpuscles** are seen in medullary portion. These are composed of a central mass, consisting of one or more granular cells, and a capsule formed by epithelial cells.
- ❖ Thymus is largest and most active during the neonatal and pre-adolescent periods. By the early teens, the thymus begins to atrophy and stroma is replaced by adipose (fat) tissue.

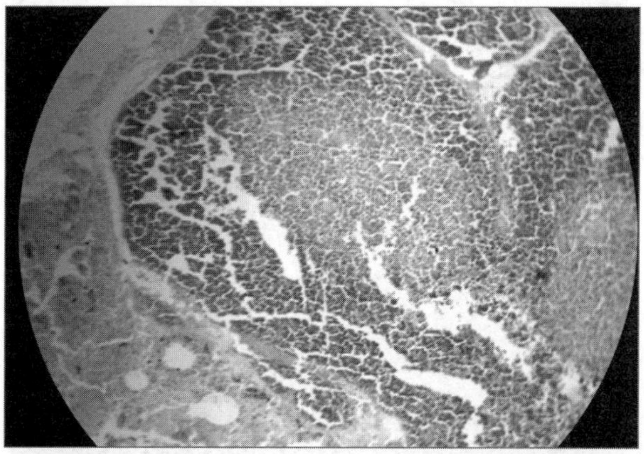

35. All of the following are true about thymus *(NEET 2016)*

a. The cortical portion is mainly composed of lymphocytes
b. The medulla contains Hassall's corpuscles
c. It is derived from the fourth Pharyngeal pouch
d. It undergoes atrophy puberty onwards

Ans. is 'c' It is derived from the fourth Pharyngeal pouch

Explanation: Thymus is derived from third pharyngeal pouch.

TYPES OF CARTILAGE

Elastic Cartilage

- Highly flexible due to elastic fibres
- Locations, Auricle, Auditory tube, Corniculate laryngeal cartilage, Cuneiform laryngeal cartilage, External auditory meatus (lateral part), Epiglottis, Apex of arytenoid cartilage, Inlet of larynx
- Microscopic features–perichondrium is seen; short elastic fibres, single chondrocyte in each lacuna.

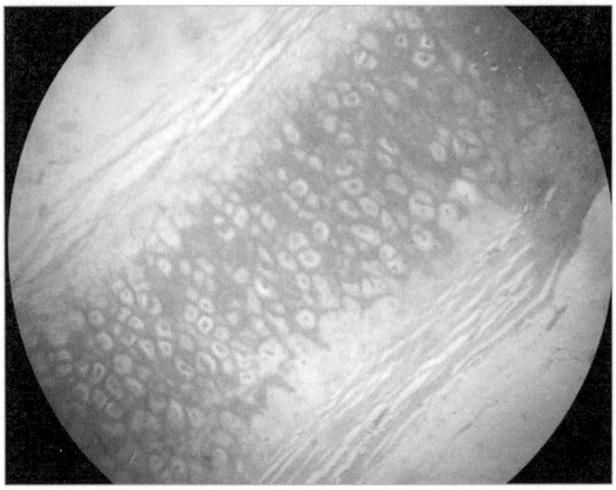

Fibrocartilage

- Made of type I collagen fibres to withstand stress
- *Locations*: Articular disc, Symphysis pubis, Glenoid labrum (shoulder joint), Acetabular labrum (hip joint), Menisci), Sternoclavicular joint, Temporomandibular joint, Inferior radio-ulnar joint
- Microscopic features—Collagen fibres in bundles, with a few chondrocytes in between; no perichondrium; feathery appearance.

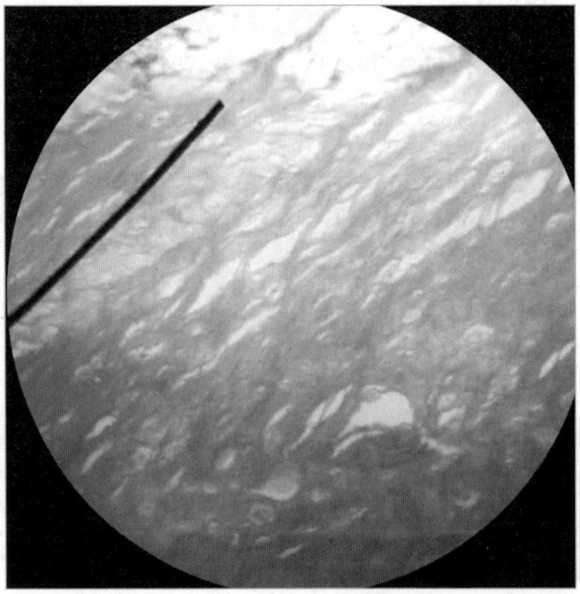

Hyaline Cartilage

- Most abundant cartilage
- Tendency to calcify in old age (except articular cartilage)
- All hyaline cartilages are covered by perichondrium except articular cartilages
- *Locations*: Arytenoid, Articular cartilage (most synovial joints), Larynx (arytenoid lower end and cricoid cartilage), Costal cartilage, Thyroid cartilage, Tracheobronchial cartilage, Nose (septum and lateral wall), Epiphyseal plate
- *Microscopic features*: Perichondrium is present; homogenous glassy appearance; 2–4 chondrocytes in each lacuna.

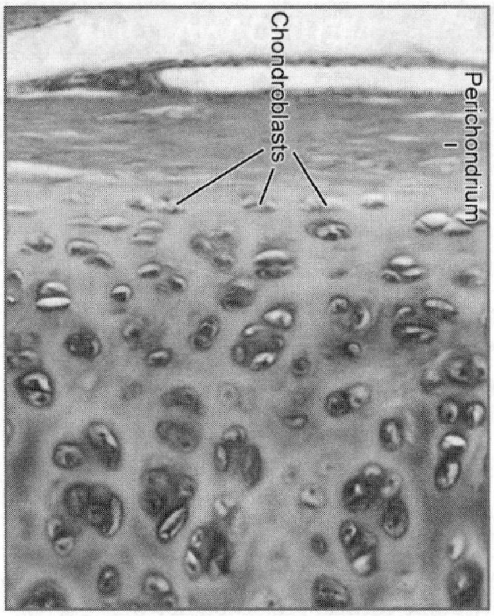

36. Which is the most abundant cartilage? *(NEET 2016)*

a. Hyaline cartilage
b. Elastic cartilage
c. Fibrocartilage
d. None of the above

Ans. is 'a' Hyaline cartilage

37. Identify the type of cartilage from the histology. *(NEET 2020)*

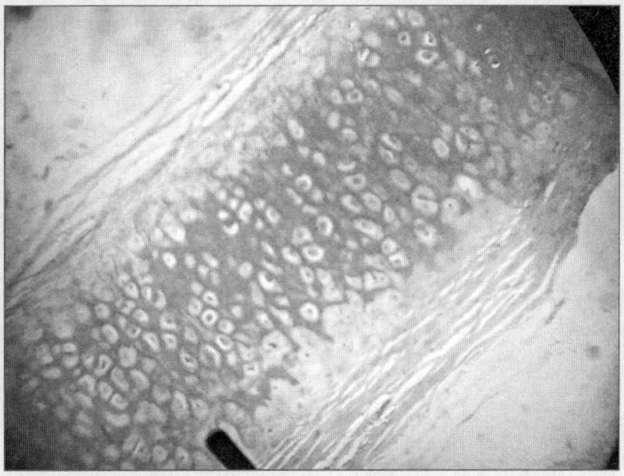

a. Articular cartilage
b. Synovial cartilage
c. Elastic cartilage
d. Fibrocartilage

Ans. is 'c' Elastic cartilage

DISTRIBUTION OF COLLAGEN FIBRES IN CONNECTIVE TISSUE

Type I: Connective tissue of skin, bone, tendon, ligaments, fibrocartilage, dentin, sclera, fascia, and organ capsules.

Type II: **Cartilage (hyaline and elastic),** notochord, and inter vertebral disc

Type III: Loose connective tissue and organs (uterus, liver, spleen, kidney, lung, etc.), blood vessels and fetal skin. It forms reticular fibers.

Type IV: Basal laminae of epithelia and lens capsule. Provides support and filtration barrier

38. Type of collagen in hyaline cartilage: *(NEET 2016)*

a. Type I
b. Type II
c. Type III
d. Type IV

Ans. is 'b' Type II

NEUROANATOMY

CEREBRAL WHITE MATTER

Three types of fibres in cerebral white matter

1. **Association fibres**: Link different cortical areas in the same hemisphere
    - Short association (arcuate or 'U') fibres–link adjacent gyri
    - Long association fibres–link widely separated gyri
        - Uncinate fasciculus (Broca's area with temporal pole cortex)
        - Cingulum (lies deep to cingulate gyrus)
        - Superior longitudinal fasciculus (Largest of association fasciculi)
        - Inferior longitudinal fasciculus
2. **Commissural fibres**: Link corresponding cortical areas in the two hemispheres
    - *Corpus callosum*: Four parts (anterior to posterior)–rostrum, genu, body/trunk and splenium
    - *Anterior commissure*: Crosses anterior to columns of fornix
3. **Projection fibres**: Connect the cerebral cortex with the corpus striatum, diencephalon, brain stem and the spinal cord
    - **Internal capsule** contains the majority of the cortical projection fibres

Parts of Internal Capsule

- **Anterior limb** of the internal capsule contains frontopontine fibres, which arise from the cortex in the frontal lobe.
- **The genu** of the internal capsule contains corticobulbar fibres which terminate mostly in the contralateral motor nuclei of cranial nerves.
- **Posterior limb** of the internal capsule includes the corticospinal tract.
- **The retrolenticular part of** the internal capsule contains parietopontine, occipitopontine, and occipitotectal fibres.
- **The sublenticular part** of the internal capsule contains temporopontine and auditory radiation from the medial geniculate body to the superior temporal gyrus.

BRAIN SECTIONS

Coronal Section

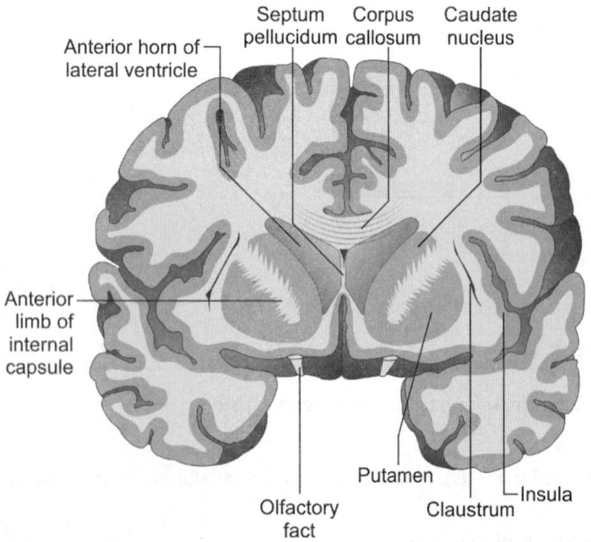

Axial Section

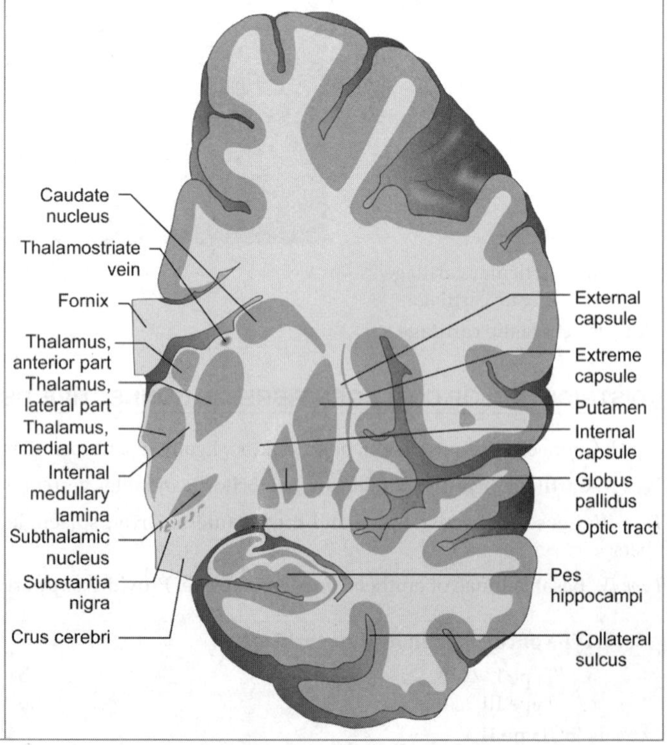

Sagittal Section

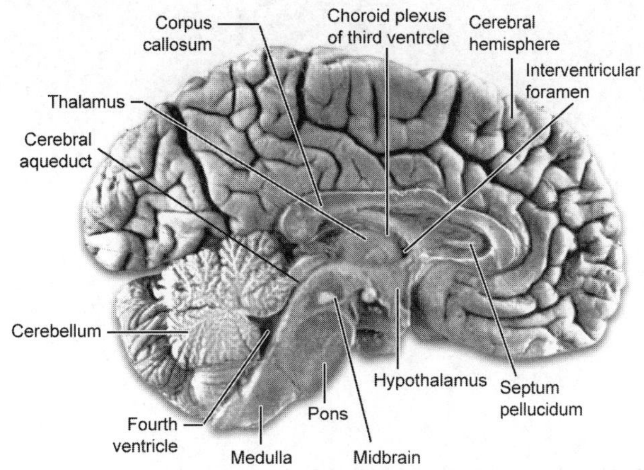

39. Identify the type of fibre marked in the image: *(NEET 2019)*

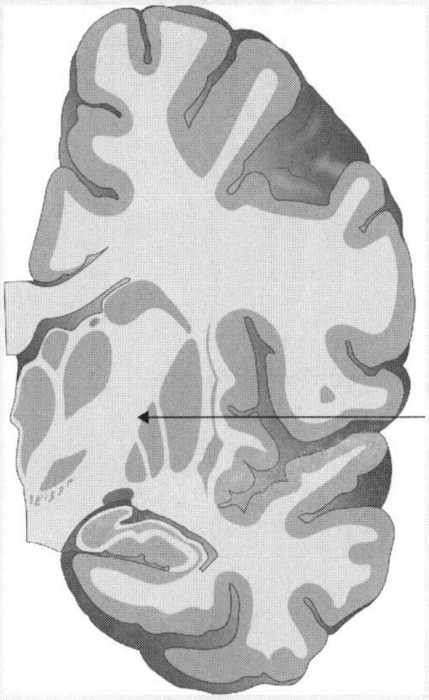

a. Projection fibres
b. Short association fibres
c. Long association fibres
d. Commissural fibres

Ans. is 'a' Projection fibres

40. Identify the structure marked in the image. *(NEET 2019)*

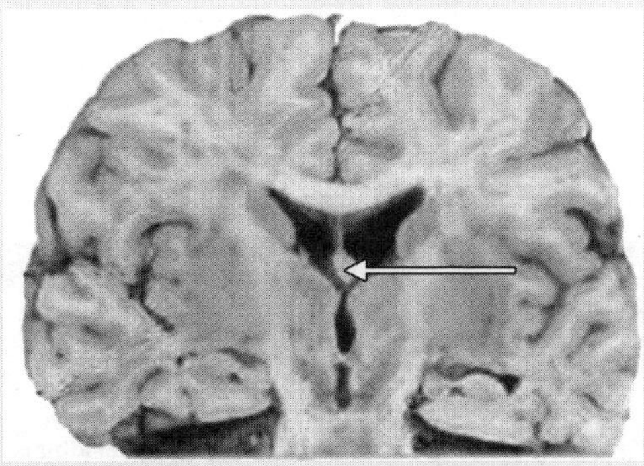

a. Great vein of Galen
b. Pineal gland
c. Fornix
d. Falx cerebri

Ans. is 'c' Fornix

41. Identify the marked structure. *(NEET 2019)*

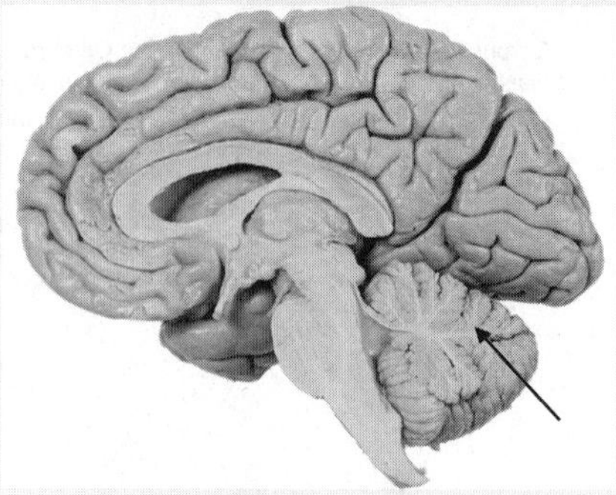

a. Cerebrum
b. Brain stem
c. Corpus callosum
d. Cerebellum

Ans. is 'd' Cerebellum

42. All of the following are parts of internal capsule *(NEET 2016)*

a. Anterior limb
b. Sublentiform part
c. Retrolentiform
d. Prelentiform

Ans. is 'd' Prelentiform

GLIAL CELLS IN CNS

Two Types

1. **Macroglia**
   - Astrocytes
     - Important for support of neurons
     - Remove excess neurotransmitter
     - Repair, scar formation (Gliosis)
     - Glial Fibrillary Acidic Protein (GFAP)–Marker for astrocytes
   - Oligodendrocytes
     - Myelinate CNS axons
     - Each cell myelinates multiple axons
     - Most common glial cell in white matter
     - Destroyed in multiple sclerosis
   - Ependyma
     - Ventricular lining
2. **Microglia**
   - CNS macrophages
   - Proliferate in response to injury
   - HIV can persist in brain via microglia
   - **Gitter Cells–Lipid-laden macrophages** after phagocytosis of degenerated myelin and cellular debris

43. What are Gitter cells? *(NEET 2019)*

a. Macroglia
b. Modified macrophages in CNS
c. Astrocytes
d. Oligodendrocytes

Ans. is 'b' Modified macrophages in CNS

BRODMANN AREAS

Brodmann areas of cerebral cortex

Area	Name	Location	Lesion
1, 2, 3	Primary sensory cortex	Post-central gyrus	Impairment of all somatic sensations in contralateral side of body
4	Primary motor cortex	Pre-central gyrus	Spastic paresis of contralateral side of body
5, 39, 40	Somatosensory association cortex	**Part of parietal cortex (superior parietal lobule, supramarginal gyrus, angular gyrus)**	Apraxia and astereognosis
6	Premotor cortex and supplementary motor cortex (Secondary Motor Cortex)	Part of the frontal cortex, situated just anterior to primary motor cortex (BA4)	Apraxia

Contd...

Contd...

Area	Name	Location	Lesion
8	Frontal eye fields	Situated just anterior to premotor cortex	Contralateral horizontal gaze palsy
17	Primary visual cortex	Lies in **calcarine fissure of occipital pole**	Unilateral lesion; contralateral homonymous hemianopia with macular sparing Bilateral lesion; cortical blindness with intact pupillary light reflex
22	Wernicke's speech area (includes part of 39 and 40 also)	Lies in the posterior part of superior temporal lobe	Sensory or fluent or receptive aphasia
44, 45	Broca's speech area	Lies in the posterior part of **inferior frontal gyrus**	Aphasia and agraphia
27	Piriform cortex	Rostral part of the parahippocampal gyrus	Impaired olfaction
41, 42	Primary auditory cortex	Lies on cephalic border of superior temporal gyrus in depths of lateral fissure	Unilateral lesion: Contralateral slight hearing loss and difficulty ¡n localizing sounds Bilateral lesion: Deafness

44. Broca's area is located in which lobe of brain? *(NEET 2018)*

a. Inferior temporal
b. Inferior parietal
c. Inferior frontal
d. Inferior occipital

Ans. is 'c' Inferior frontal

45. Location of visual cortex: *(NEET 2016)*

a. Precentral gyrus
b. Postcentral gyrus
c. Sylvian fissure
d. Calcarine sulcus

Ans. is 'd' Calcarine sulcus

46. Supramarginal gyrus is a part of: *(NEET 2016)*

a. Parietal lobe
b. Frontal lobe
c. Temporal lobe
d. Occipital lobe

Ans. is 'a' Parietal lobe

Aphasia

	Comprehension	Repetition of spoken language	Naming	Fluency
Wernicke's	Impaired	Impaired	Impaired	Preserved or increased
Broca's	Preserved (except grammar)	Impaired	Impaired	Decreased
Global	Impaired	Impaired	Impaired	Decreased
Conduction	Preserved	Impaired	Impaired	Preserved
Nonfluent (motor) transcortical	Preserved	Preserved	Impaired	Impaired
Fluent (sensory) transcortical	Impaired	Preserved	Impaired	Preserved
Isolation	Impaired	Echolalia	Impaired	No purposeful speech
Anomic	Preserved	Preserved	Impaired	Preserved except for word-finding pauses
Pure word deafness	Impaired only for spoken language	Impaired	Preserved	Preserved
Pure alexia	Impaired only for reading	Preserved	Preserved	Preserved

Aphasia	Area affected in left (dominant) hemisphere
Broca's aphasia	Inferior frontal gyrus
Wernicke's aphasia	Superior temporal gyrus
Conduction aphasia	Arcuate fasciculus
Global aphasia	Arcuate fasciculus, Broca and Wernicke areas Stroke in entire left MCA distribution Associated right hemiplegia and visual loss
Pure word deafness	Superior temporal gyrus; Left MCA infarct

47. Injury to the posterior and superior part of superior temporal gyrus leads to: *(NEET 2020)*

a. Fluent aphasia
b. Nonfluent aphasia
c. Conduction aphasia
d. Mixed aphasia

Ans. is 'a' Fluent aphasia

48. Area involved in injury to inferior frontal gyrus is: *(NEET 2020)*

a. Broca's area
b. Wernicke's area
c. Prefrontal area
d. Primary motor area

Ans. is 'a' Broca's area

LAYERS OF CEREBELLUM

The cerebellar cortex has three layers–Molecular layer, Purkinje cell layer and Granule cell layer

Purkinje Cells

- Purkinje cells are a class of GABAergic neurons located in the cerebellum, and send inhibitory projections to the deep cerebellar nuclei, and constitute the sole output of all motor coordination in the cerebellar cortex.
- These cells are 2nd largest neurons in the human brain. *Note*: Betz cells (giant pyramidal cells located within the fifth layer of the grey matter in the primary motor cortex) are the largest.
- They have an intricately elaborate dendritic arbor, characterized by many dendritic spines.
- The parallel fibers from deeper layers make relatively weaker excitatory (glutamatergic) synapses to spines in the Purkinje cell dendrite whereas **climbing fibers originating from the inferior olivary nucleus in the medulla provide very powerful excitatory input to the proximal dendrites and cell soma.**
- Both basket and stellate cells (found in the cerebellar molecular layer) provide inhibitory (GABAergic) input to the Purkinje cell.

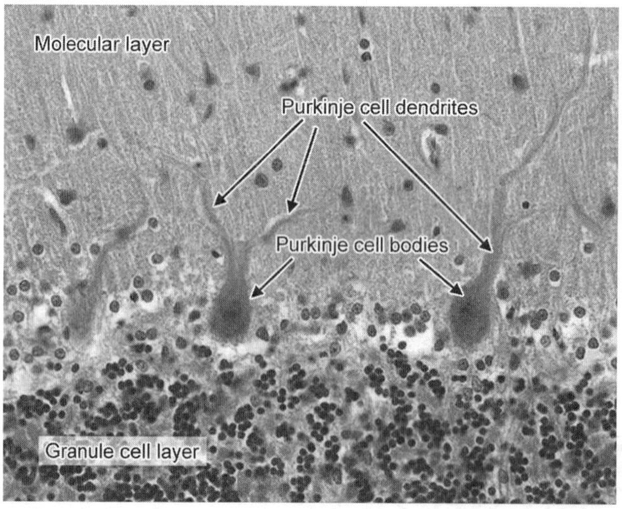

49. Identify the cells marked in the slide of cerebellum: *(NEET 2020)*

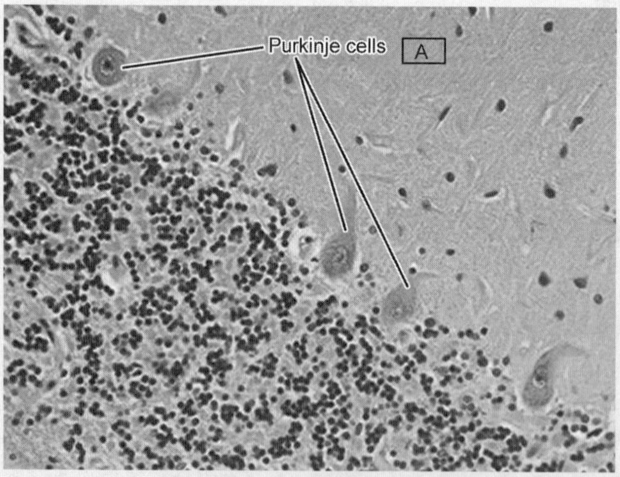

a. Basket cells
b. Golgi cells
c. Granule cells
d. Purkinje cells

Ans. is 'd' Purkinje cells

50. Climbing fibres arise from: *(NEET 2016)*

a. Inferior olivary nucleus
b. Red nucleus
c. Caudate nucleus
d. Putamen

Ans. is 'a' Inferior olivary nucleus

CRANIAL AND PERIPHERAL NERVES

CRANIAL NERVES

CN	Modalities and function	Exit from skull
CN I (olfactory)	**Special somatic afferent**: Smell	Cribriform plate of the ethmoid bone
CN II (optic)	**Special somatic afferent**: Sight	Optic canal
CN III (oculomotor)	**General somatic efferent**: **Levator palpebrae superioris muscle**; superior, medial, and inferior rectus muscle; inferior oblique muscle **General visceral efferent**: Sphincter pupillae muscle (pupil constriction), and ciliary muscle (lens accommodation): Edinger Westphal Nucleus through ciliary ganglion	Superior orbital fissure
CN IV (trochlear)	**General somatic efferent**: superior oblique muscle	Superior orbital fissure
CN V (trigeminal)	**General somatic afferent** (Main sensory nucleus, Spinal nucleus and Mesencephalic nucleus): CN V-1: Obit and forehead CN V-2: Maxillary region CN V-3: Mandibular region, tongue **Special visceral efferent** (Motor nucleus of Trigeminal): CN V-3: Muscles of mastication, mylohyoid, anterior digastric, tensor tympani, and tensor veli palatini muscle	CN V-1: Superior orbital fissure CN V-2: Foramen rotundum CN V-3: Foramen ovale
CN VI (abducens)	**General somatic efferent**: lateral rectus muscle	Superior orbital fissure
CN VII (facial)	**General somatic afferent**: External acoustic meatus and auricle **Special visceral afferent** (Nucleus tractus solitarius): anterior two-thirds of tongue (taste) **Special visceral efferent** (Nucleus of facial nerve): Muscles of facial expression and stylohyoid, posterior digastric, stapedius muscle **General visceral efferent**: Lacrimal, nasal and palatal glands (Lacrimatory nucleus through pterygopalatine ganglion) Submandibular, sublingual glands (Superior salivatory nucleus through submandibular ganglion)	Internal acoustic meatus
CN VIII (vestibulocochlear)	**Special somatic afferent**: Hearing, balance, and equilibrium	Internal acoustic meatus
CN IX (glossopharyngeal)	**General visceral afferent**: Posterior third of tongue, oropharynx, tympanic membrane, middle ear, and auditory tube **Special visceral afferent** (Nucleus tractus solitarius): Taste from posterior one-third of tongue **General visceral afferent** (Nucleus tractus solitarius): Carotid sinus (baroreceptor) and carotid body (chemoreceptor) **Special visceral efferent** (Nucleus ambiguus): Stylopharyngeus muscle **General visceral efferent**: Parotid gland (Inferior salivatory nucleus through otic ganglion)	Jugular foramen
CN X (vagus)	**General somatic afferent**: Skin of the posterior ear and external acoustic meatus **General visceral afferent** (Nucleus tractus solitarius): aortic and carotid bodies (chemoreceptors) and aortic arch (baroreceptor), pharynx, larynx, trachea **Special visceral efferent** (Nucleus ambiguus): Palatal muscles (except tensor tympani); pharyngeal muscles (except stylopharyngeus muscle) and laryngeal muscle **General visceral efferent** (Dorsal nucleus of Vagus): Heart, smooth muscle, and glands of the respiratory tract, gastrointestinal tube, and viscera of the foregut and midgut	Jugular foramen
CN XI (spinal accessory)	**Special visceral efferent** (Nucleus ambiguus): Trapezius and sternocleidomastoid m.	Jugular foramen
CN XII (hypoglossal)	**General somatic efferent**: Tongue m. (except palatoglossus muscle)	Hypoglossal canal

Location of cranial nerve nuclei	
III	Superior colliculus (Midbrain)
IV	Inferior colliculus (Midbrain)
V-VIII	Pons
IX-XII	Medulla

	Cranial nerve nuclei
General somatic efferent (somatic motor; voluntary)	Oculomotor nucleus Trochlear nucleus Abducent nucleus Hypoglossal nucleus
Special visceral efferent (Motor to branchial arch muscles; voluntary)	Motor nucleus of trigeminal Nucleus of facial nerve Nucleus ambiguus
General visceral efferent (Involuntary)	Edinger-Westphal nucleus Superior salivatory nucleus Inferior salivatory nucleus Lacrimatory nucleus Dorsal nucleus of vagus

Contd…

Contd...

	Cranial nerve nuclei
General and special visceral afferent	Nucleus tractus solitaries
General somatic afferent	Main sensory nucleus of trigeminal Spinal nucleus of trigeminal Mesencephalic nucleus of trigeminal
Special somatic afferent	Vestibulo-cochlear nuclei

Facts about cranial nerves	
Longest intracranial course	Trochlear nerve
Longest course overall and most widely distributed	Vagus
Smallest (thinnest) cranial nerve	Trochlear nerve
Largest (thickest) cranial nerve	Trigeminal nerve
Only cranial nerve arising from dorsal aspect	Trochlear nerve
Only cranial nerve decussating before emerging	Trochlear nerve
Cranial nerve most commonly involved in raised ICP	Abducent nerve
Cranial nerve most commonly involved in intracranial aneurysm	Oculomotor nerve

51. Which of the following belongs to special visceral efferent nuclei? *(NEET 2018)*

a. Nucleus of tractus solitarius
b. Nucleus ambiguus
c. Edinger-Westphal nucleus
d. Mesencephalic nucleus of trigeminal

Ans. is 'b' Nucleus ambiguus

52. Thickest cranial nerve is: *(NEET 2016)*

a. Trochlear nerve
b. Vagus
c. Facial nerve
d. Trigeminal nerve

Ans. is 'd' Trigeminal nerve

POSTERIOR CIRCULATION STROKES

Medial medullary syndrome	Lateral medullary syndrome (Wallenberg syndrome)
Corticospinal tract–Contralateral hemiparesis	Vestibular nuclei–Nystagmus, vertigo
Medial lemniscus–Contralateral loss of proprioception/vibration	Sympathetic tract–Horner's syndrome
CNXII–Flaccid paralysis of tongue	Spinothalamic tract–Contralateral pain/temp loss
	Spinal V nucleus–Ipsilateral face pain/temp loss
	Nucleus ambiguus (IX, X)–Hoarseness, dysphagia
	Inferior cerebellar peduncle–Ipsilateral ataxia, dysmetria
Anterior spinal artery stroke	Posterior inferior cerebellar artery stroke

Lateral Pontine Syndrome

- Secondary to anterior inferior cerebellar artery stroke
- Facial nucleus–Paralysis of face (lower motor neuron lesion), loss of lacrimation and salivation, loss of taste from anterior 2/3 of tongue
- Vestibular nuclei–Nystagmus, vertigo
- Spinothalamic tract–Contralateral pain/temp loss
- Spinal V nucleus–Ipsilateral face pain/temp loss
- Sympathetic tract–Horner's syndrome
- Middle and inferior cerebellar peduncles–Ipsilateral ataxia, dysmetria

53. A patient presents with dysarthria, dysphagia, ataxia and loss of sensory supply of left limb. Which part is likely to be affected? *(NEET 2020)*

a. Lateral pons
b. Medial pons
c. Medial medulla
d. Lateral medulla

Ans. is 'd' Lateral medulla

54. A patient presents with right facial paralysis along with loss of sensations on face on right side and left upper and lower limbs. Which artery is likely to be involved? *(NEET 2020)*

a. AICA
b. PICA
c. Posterior cerebral artery
d. Anterior cerebral artery

Ans. is 'a' AICA

Explanation: Facial nucleus effects are specific to AICA lesions

DERMATOMES

Specific segment of skin supplied by a single spinal nerve

Nerve	Dermatome
C2	Occipital protuberance
C3	Supraclavicular fossa
C4	Acromioclavicular joint
C5	Lateral antecubital fossa
C6	Thumb
C7	Middle finger
C8	Little finger
T1	Medial antecubital fossa
T2	Apex of axilla
T3	Third intercostal space
T4	Fourth intercostal space (level of nipples)
T5	Fifth intercostal space (midway between level of the nipples and xiphoid process)
T6	Xiphoid process
T10	Umbilicus
T12	Inguinal ligament
L2	Mid anterior thigh
L3	Medial femoral condyle
L4	Medial malleolus
L5	Dorsum of third metatarsophalangeal joint
S1	Lateral aspect of calcaneus
S2	Popliteal fossa
S3	Ischial tuberosity
S4, S5	Perianal area

55. Umbilicus is supplied by which dermatome? *(NEET 2019)*

a. T8
b. T9
c. T10
d. T11

Ans. is 'c' T10

HEAD AND NECK

PARASYMPATHETIC NERVE SUPPLY OF HEAD AND NECK

Structure	Cranial nerve nucleus	Preganglionic parasympathetic	Ganglion	Postganglionic parasympathetic
Pupillary and ciliary muscles	Edinger westphal nucleus	CN III	Ciliary ganglion	Nasociliary nerve
Lacrimal gland, nasal and Palatal glands	Superior salivatory nucleus	CN VII (greater petrosal nerve, nerve of pterygoid canal)	Pterygopalatine ganglion	Maxillary nerve (Zygomaticotemporal nerve), Ophthalmic nerve (Lacrimal nerve)
Sublingual and submandibular glands	Superior salivatory nucleus	CN VII (Chorda tympani), Lingual nerve	Submandibular ganglion	Lingual nerve
Parotid gland	Inferior salivatory nucleus	CN IX (Tympanic branch, lesser petrosal nerve)	Otic ganglion	Mandibular nerve (Auriculotemporal nerve)

Vidian Nerve (Nerve of Pterygoid canal): Contains

- Parasympathetic preganglionic fibers from the greater petrosal nerve which synapse in pterygopalatine ganglion
- Sympathetic postganglionic fibers from the deep petrosal nerve which do not synapse in pterygopalatine ganglion.

56. What is the nerve supply of submandibular gland? *(NEET 2019)*

a. Auriculotemporal nerve
b. Lingual nerve
c. Glossopharyngeal nerve
d. Inferior alveolar nerve

Ans. is 'b' Lingual nerve

FORAMINA OF SKULL

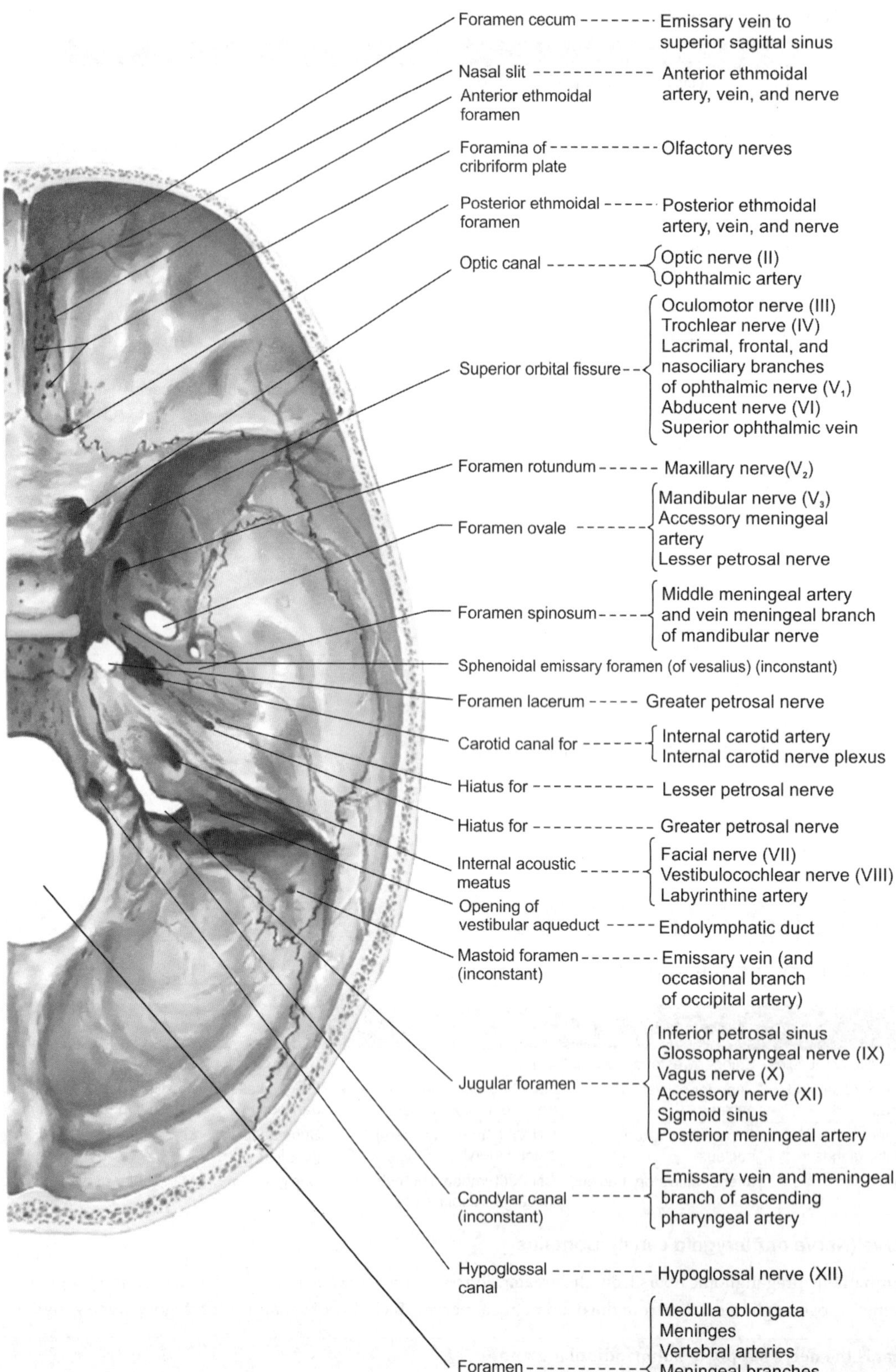

Anatomy

Mandibular Foramen

- Opening on the internal surface of the ramus of the mandible
- **Inferior alveolar nerve (branch of the mandibular nerve) and artery** pass through
- Enter the foramen traveling through the body in the mandibular canal and exit at the mental foramen on the anterior mandible at which point the nerve is known as the mental nerve.
- These nerves provide sensory innervation to the lower teeth, as well as the lower lip and skin on the lower face.

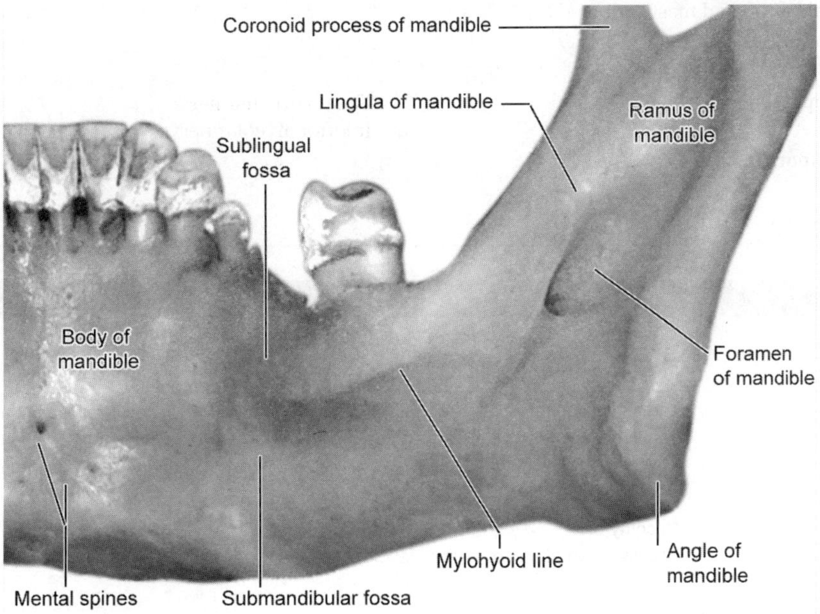

57. Which nerve passes through marked foramen? *(NEET 2019)*

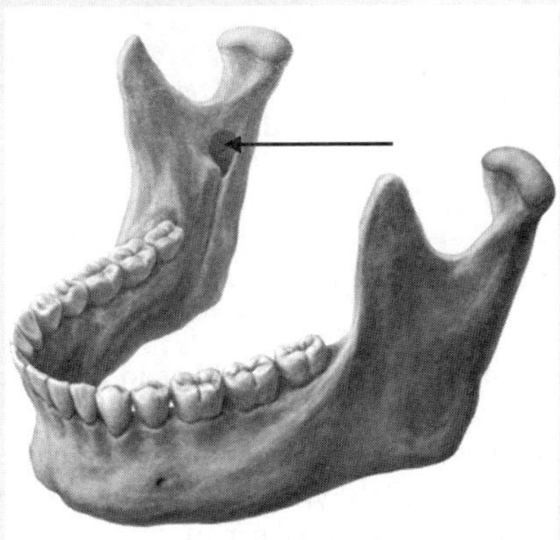

a. Lingual nerve
b. Mandibular nerve
c. Chorda tympani nerve
d. Inferior alveolar nerve

Ans. is 'd' Inferior alveolar nerve

58. Which structure doesn't pass through foramen ovale? *(NEET 2016)*

a. Middle meningeal artery
b. Lesser petrosal nerve
c. Mandibular nerve
d. Accessory meningeal artery

Ans. is 'a' Middle meningeal artery

59. Which of the following passes through foramen spinosum? *(NEET 2016)*

a. Middle meningeal artery
b. Lesser petrosal nerve
c. Mandibular nerve
d. Accessory meningeal artery

Ans. is 'a' Middle meningeal artery

FREY'S SYNDROME

- Rare disorder resulting from **damage to Auriculotemporal nerve often from surgery**
- **Symptoms:** Excessive sweating and flushing of the cheek in response to food–'gustatory sweating'
- **Cause:** Auriculotemporal nerve carries postganglionic parasympathetic fibres from cranial nerve IX to parotid gland and sympathetic fibres to sweat glands. Following injury, there is aberrant reinnervation of these postganglionic parasympathetic fibres to nearby denervated sweat glands and cutaneous blood vessels. This results in sweating and flushing of skin in response to parasympathetic activation during salivation and mastication.

60. Nerve injured in Frey's syndrome is: *(NEET 2019)*

a. Auriculotemporal nerve
b. Great auricular nerve
c. Lingual nerve
d. Inferior alveolar nerve

Ans. is 'a' Auriculotemporal nerve

LARYNGEAL MUSCLES

	Muscles	Nerve supply
Action on vocal cords		
Abductors (open glottis)	Posterior cricoarytenoid	Recurrent laryngeal nerve
Adductors (close glottis)	Lateral cricoarytenoid Transverse arytenoid (Interarytenoid) Thyroarytenoid Cricothyroid	Recurrent laryngeal nerve Recurrent laryngeal nerve Recurrent laryngeal nerve External branch of superior laryngeal nerve
Tensors	Cricothyroid Vocalis (internal part of thyroarytenoid)	Recurrent laryngeal nerve
Action on laryngeal inlet		
Openers	Thyro-epiglottic (part of thyroarytenoid)	Recurrent laryngeal nerve
Closers	Oblique arytenoid (Interarytenoid)	Recurrent laryngeal nerve

61. Tensor of vocal cord is: *(NEET 2018)*

a. Posterior cricoarytenoid
b. Transverse arytenoid
c. Lateral arytenoid
d. Cricothyroid

Ans. is 'd' Cricothyroid

RECURRENT LARYNGEAL NERVE

- Branch of Vagus nerve
- **Right RLN winds around first part of right subclavian artery and lies in the Tracheoesophageal groove**. It may be anterior or posterior to inferior thyroid artery.
- Left RLN winds around the arch of aorta and **lies in the Tracheoesophageal groove.** It is posterior to inferior thyroid artery.
- RLN supplies all intrinsic muscles of larynx (except cricothyroid) and sensory supply to mucous membrane of larynx below vocal fold (Above vocal fold, sensory supply is by Internal Laryngeal nerve).
- During thyroidectomy, Inferior thyroid artery is ligated away from gland to avoid RLN injury.

62. Right recurrent laryngeal nerve loops around: *(NEET 2016)*

a. Right subclavian artery
b. Right axillary artery
c. Right external carotid artery
d. Right superior thyroid artery

Ans. is 'a' Right subclavian artery

63. Left recurrent laryngeal nerve has a longer course compared to right due to persistence of: *(NEET 2020)*

a. 3rd arch
b. 4th arch
c. 5th arch
d. 6th arch

Ans. is 'd' 6th arch

Explanation: The left RLN has a longer course because it courses under the arch of aorta at the ligamentum arteriosum (which develops due to persistence of left 6th arch

64. Left recurrent laryngeal passes between: *(NEET 2016)*

a. Trachea and larynx
b. Trachea and esophagus
c. Esophagus and bronchi
d. Esophagus and aorta

Ans. is 'b' Trachea and esophagus

LYMPHATIC DRAINAGE OF LARYNX

Part of larynx	Lymphatics
Supraglottis	Lymphatics along superior laryngeal vein and adjacent to thyrohyoid membrane
Infraglottis	Pretracheal and Prelaryngeal nodes
Vocal cord	Devoid of lymphatic supply

65. Larynx below the vocal cords drain into: *(NEET 2018)*

a. Pretracheal lymph nodes
b. Occipital lymph nodes
c. Mediastinal nodes
d. Lymphatics along the superior laryngeal vein

Ans. is 'a' Pretracheal lymph nodes

NASMYTH'S MEMBRANE

- Also known as Primary Enamel Cuticle
- Thin membrane that covers a newly erupted tooth; produced by ameloblast
- Secretes desmolytic enzymes for elimination of dental sac; allows eruption of tooth without bleeding
- Also protects enamel from resorption by cells of dental sac

66. Newly erupted tooth is covered by: *(NEET 2018)*

a. Perikymata
b. Nasmyth's membrane
c. Fibrous tissue
d. Mucopolysaccharide

Ans. is 'b' Nasmyth's membrane

Nerve supply of tongue		
Part of tongue	***Taste***	***General***
Anterior 2/3rd (except vallate papilla)	**Chorda tympani (branch of facial nerve)**	Lingual nerve (branch of mandibular nerve)
Posterior 1/3rd (including vallate papilla)	Glossopharyngeal nerve	Glossopharyngeal nerve
Posterior most or vallecula	Internal laryngeal branch of vagus	Internal laryngeal branch of vagus

67. Taste sensation from anterior 2/3rd of tongue is carried by: *(NEET 2016)*

a. Glossopharyngeal nerve
b. Facial nerve
c. Vagus nerve
d. Hypoglossal nerve

Ans. is 'b' Facial nerve

LYMPHATIC DRAINAGE OF FACE

Area of the face	Nodal supply
Forehead, Lateral half of eyelids, lateral part of cheek, parotid area	Pre-auricular (Superficial Parotid) nodes
Central forehead, External nose, Upper lip, Lateral lower lip, Medial half of eyelids, Medial part of cheek, Lower jaw	Submandibular nodes
Central lower lip, Chin	Submental nodes

68. Submandibular lymph nodes drain the following areas of the face: *(NEET 2016)*

a. Medial half of eyelids
b. Central part of lower lip
c. Medial part of cheek
d. Central part of fore head

Ans. is 'b' Central part of lower lip

EXTERNAL AUDITORY CANAL

- 'S' shaped canal with a length of 24 mm

Cartilaginous part	Bony part
Outer 1/3 (8 mm) of EAC	Inner 2/3 (16 mm) of EAC
Fissures of Santorini–in anterior part; Parotid infection can spread into EAC and vice versa	**Foramen of Huschke**: Antero-inferior deficiency in children < 4 years of age; Spread infection to and from parotid
Skin: Thick; ceruminous glands and hair +nt	**Skin**: Thin; ceruminous glands and hair -nt
Furuncles occur (due to presence of hair)	Furuncles cannot occur

- *Isthmus*: Narrowest portion of bony canal 5 mm lateral to tympanic membrane. Foreign bodies lodged in isthmus are difficult to remove.

69. Fissures of santorini are seen in: *(NEET 2016)*

a. Stomach
b. Rectum
c. Thyroid gland
d. External auditory meatus

Ans. is 'd' External auditory meatus

DANGER SPACE OF NECK

- Potential space located behind true retropharyngeal space, which connects deep cervical spaces to mediastinum.
- **Boundaries**:
  - *Anteriorly*: Alar fascia
  - *Posteriorly*: Prevertebral layer of deep cervical fascia
  - *Superiorly*: Clivus
  - *Inferiorly*: Ends at the level of diaphragm
- It is clinically indistinguishable from retropharyngeal space and visible only when distended by fluid or pus. The retropharyngeal space, however, ends at the level of T1-T6.
- It is called the danger space because infections involving this space can spread all the way down to the mediastinum. It is a median space without a midline raphe and infection can spread easily to either side.

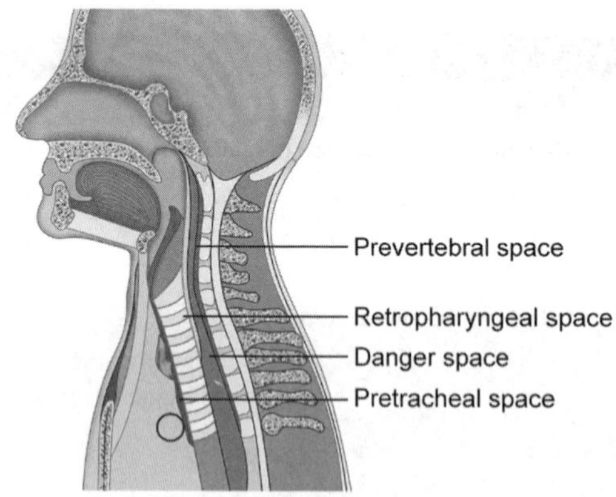

70. Danger space in the neck is found between: *(NEET 2016)*

a. Buccopharyngeal fascia and alar fascia
b. Prevertebral fascia and alar fascia
c. Buccopharyngeal fascia and prevertebral fascia
d. None

Ans. is 'b' Prevertebral fascia and alar fascia

THYROID GLAND

Gross Anatomy and Relations

- Anterior in the neck below and lateral to thyroid cartilage
- Two lateral lobes with an isthmus that connects the two lobes
- The thyroid gland is unsheathed by the visceral fascia, a division of the middle layer of deep cervical fascia, which attaches it firmly to the laryngoskeleton.

Anatomy

- The posteromedial aspect of the gland is attached to the side of the cricoid cartilage, first and second tracheal ring, by the posterior suspensory ligament (i.e. Berry ligament).
- The lateral surface of the thyroid is covered by the sternothyroid muscle, and its attachment to the oblique line of the thyroid cartilage prevents the superior pole from extending superiorly under the thyrohyoid muscle.
- More anteriorly are the sternohyoid and superior belly of the omohyoid muscle, overlapped inferiorly by the anterior border of the sternocleidomastoid muscle.

Vasculature

- *Arterial supply*: Superior thyroid artery (first branch of external carotid artery), Inferior thyroid artery (branch of thyrocervical trunk which arises from first part of subclavian artery). Occasionally, a thyroid ima artery arises from aortic arch or brachiocephalic trunk.
- *Venous drainage*: Superior and middle thyroid veins drain into internal jugular vein; Inferior thyroid vein empties into brachiocephalic vein
- *Lymphatic drainage*: Paratracheal nodes and deep cervical nodes inferior to omohyoid muscle along internal jugular vein

71. Superior extension of the thyroid gland is limited by which structure? *(NEET 2020)*

a. Pretracheal fascia
b. Ligament of berry
c. Sternothyroid muscle
d. Thyrohyoid membrane

Ans. is 'c' Sternothyroid muscle

MUSCLES OF MASTICATION

Muscle	Origin	Insertion	Nerve supply	Actions
Masseter	Zygomatic arch and maxillary process of zygomatic bone	Lateral surface of mandibular ramus	**Masseteric nerve**: Branch of anterior division of Mandibular nerve	Elevation of mandible; Small effect in side-to-side movements, protraction and retraction
Temporalis	Temporal fossa and deep surface of the temporalis fascia	Coronoid process of mandible and anterior border of mandibular ramus	**Deep temporal nerve**: Branch of anterior division of Mandibular nerve	Elevation and retraction of mandible
Medial pterygoid	Deep head arises from medial surface of lateral pterygoid plate of sphenoid bone Superficial head arises from maxillary tuberosity and pyramidal process of palatine bone	Medial surface of ramus and angle of mandible	**Medial pterygoid nerve**: Branch of main trunk of Mandibular nerve	Elevation, protrusion and side-to-side movement of mandible
Lateral pterygoid	Upper head arises from roof of infratemporal fossa Lower head arises from lateral surface of lateral pterygoid plate	**Capsule of temporomandibular joint in region of attachment to articular disc** and pterygoid fovea on the neck of the mandible	**Lateral pterygoid nerve**: Branch of anterior division of Mandibular nerve	Depression, **protrusion** and side-to-side movement of mandible

Most important muscle for protrusion is lateral pterygoid. Depression of mandible is carried out by digastrics, geniohyoid and mylohyoid muscles along with lateral pterygoids.

72. Which muscle is attached to the disc of the temporomandibular joint? *(NEET 2016)*

a. Buccinator
b. Lateral pterygoid
c. Masseter
d. Temporalis

Ans. is 'b' Lateral pterygoid

LAYERS OF SCALP

- Soft tissue which covers the calvaria of skull.
- It consists of five layers (mnemonic–SCALP)
  a. Skin
  b. Close network of connective tissue (superficial fascia)–contains large blood vessels and nerves of scalp
  c. Aponeurosis (galea aponeurotica) with occipitofrontalis muscles
  d. Loose areolar (subaponeurotic) tissue–Dangerous area of scalp because emissary veins can spread infection to intracranial venous sinuses
  e. Pericranium (outer periosteum of skull)

73. Which layer of the scalp is vascular? *(NEET 2016)*

a. Pericranium
b. Superficial fascia
c. Skin
d. Aponeurosis

Ans. is 'b' Superficial fascia

Gaps between pharyngeal muscles and traversing structures	
Between base of skull and superior constrictor **(Sinus of Morgagni)**	**Levator veli palatini** **Eustachian tube** **Ascending palatine artery**
Between superior and middle constrictors	Stylopharyngeus muscle Glossopharyngeal nerve
Between middle and inferior constrictors	Internal laryngeal nerve Superior laryngeal vessels
Between lower border of inferior constrictor and esophagus	Recurrent laryngeal nerve Inferior laryngeal vessels

74. All of the following pass through the sinus of Morgagni *except:* *(NEET 2016)*

a. Auditory type
b. Levator veli palatine
c. Ascending palatine artery
d. Stylopharyngeus

Ans. is 'd' Stylopharyngeus

BACK AND SPINAL CORD

ASCENDING TRACTS IN SPINAL TRACT

Tract	Origin	Termination	Function
Lateral spinothalamic tract	Posterior horn cell of opposite side	Ventral posterolateral nucleus of thalamus	Pain and temperature–Opposite side
Anterior spinothalamic tract	Posterior horn cell of opposite side	Ventral posterolateral nucleus of thalamus	Crude touch, pressure–Opposite side
Spinocerebellar tracts	Posterior horn cell of opposite side	Cerebellum	Unconscious proprioception–Opposite side
Fasciculus gracilis and Fasciculus cuneatus	Dorsal root ganglion of spinal nerve of same side	Nucleus gracilis and nucleus cuneatus in medulla of same side	Conscious proprioception, vibration, Fine touch, Two-point discrimination, stereognosis–Same side

75. Contralateral loss of pain and temperature is seen due to injury of: *(NEET 2019)*

a. Anterior spinothalamic tract
b. Lateral spinothalamic tract
c. Fasciculus gracilis
d. Fasciculus cuneatus

Ans. is 'b' Lateral spinothalamic tract

ILIOLUMBAR LIGAMENT

- **Extends from transverse process of 5th (occasionally, 4th) lumbar vertebra to inner lip of posterior part of iliac crest**
- Two parts:
  - Upper part–attached to iliac crest and **continuous above with anterior layer of thoracolumbar fascia**
  - Lower part–**blends with anterior sacroiliac ligament**
- Function:
  - **Stabilizes anterior sacroiliac joints**
  - **Stabilizes lumbosacral joint by limiting trunk side flexion (lateral bending)**
  - May contribute to low back pain

76. Regarding iliolumbar ligament, what is not true? *(NEET 2018)*

a. The stem is attached to transverse process of L4 lumbar vertebra
b. Lower slip blends with anterior sacroiliac ligament
c. Upper part is continuous with anterior layer of thoracolumbar fascia
d. Provides stability and support to posterior sacroiliac joint

Ans. is 'd' Provides stability and support to posterior sacroiliac joint

VERTEBRAL MORPHOLOGY

Feature	Cervical	Thoracic	Lumbar
Body	Small; broad from side to side	Medium size; heart shaped	Large; kidney shaped
Vertebral foramen	Large and triangular	Small and circular	Triangular
Spinous process	Small; bifid	**Long**	Short, flat and projected backwards
Transverse process	Have foramen transversarium (vertebral artery)	Possess costal facets	Long
Superior articular facets face	Backwards and upwards	Backwards and laterally	Medially
Inferior articular facets face (opposite of superior)	Forwards and downwards	Forwards and medially	Laterally

77. Long spinous process is seen in: *(NEET 2016)*

a. Cervical vertebrae
b. Thoracic vertebrae
c. Lumbar vertebrae
d. Sacrum

Ans. is 'b' Thoracic vertebrae

ARTERIAL SUPPLY OF SPINAL CORD

Artery	Branch of	Territory of supply
Anterior spinal artery (1)	4th part of verterbral artery	Ventral 2/3rd cross section of spinal cord
Posterior spinal arteries (2)	4th part of vertebral artery, sometimes from posterior, inferior cerebellar artery	Posterior 1/3rd of the cross section of spinal cord
Segmental spinal branches from a. Vertebral artery (2nd part) b. Deep cervical artery c. **Ascending cervical artery** d. Posterior intercostal arteries e. Lumbar arteries	 Subclavian artery Subclavian artery Thyrocervical trunk Thoracic aorta Abdominal aorta	Reinforce blood supply from spinal arteries

78. Spinal segmental artery is a branch of: *(NEET 2016)*

a. Ascending cervical artery
b. Basilar artery
c. Posterior spinal artery
d. Anterior spinal artery

Ans. is 'a' Ascending cervical artery

SPINAL MENINGES

Structure	Extends up to
Adult spinal cord	***Lower border of L1/upper border of L2 vertebra***
Infant spinal cord	Upper border of L1 vertebra
Dural sheath / Dural sac	S2
Arachnoid mater	S2
Subarachnoid space	S2
Filum terminale (continuation of Pia mater)	Tip of coccyx

79. What is the extent of spinal cord in an adult? *(NEET 2016)*

a. Lower border of L1
b. Tip of Coccyx
c. Upper border of L3
d. S2

Ans. is 'a' Lower border of L1

UPPER LIMB

BRACHIAL PLEXUS BRANCHES

Terminal nerves of brachial plexus	
Musculocutaneous nerve (C5-C6)	All muscles of anterior compartment of arm
Median nerve (C5-T1)	Anterior compartment of forearm (except flexor carpi ulnaris and ulnar half of flexor digitorum profundus) Thenar muscles 1st and 2nd Lumbricals
Ulnar nerve (C8-T1)	Flexor carpi ulnaris and ulnar half of flexor digitorum profundus) Hypothenar muscles 3rd and 4th Lumbricals Palmar and dorsal interossei Adductor pollicis
Axillary nerve (C5-C6)	Deltoid, teres minor
Radial nerve (C5-T1)	Posterior compartment muscles of arm and forearm

Collateral nerves of brachial plexus	
Dorsal scapular nerve	Rhomboids, Levator scapulae
Long thoracic nerve	Serratus anterior
Suprascapular nerve	Supraspinatus and Infraspinatus
Lateral pectoral nerve	Pectoralis major
Medial pectoral nerve	Pectoralis major and minor
Upper subscapular nerve	Subscapularis
Thoracodorsal nerve	Latissimus dorsi
Lower subscapular nerve	Subscapularis and teres major

80. What is the nerve supply of the muscle marked? *(NEET 2020)*

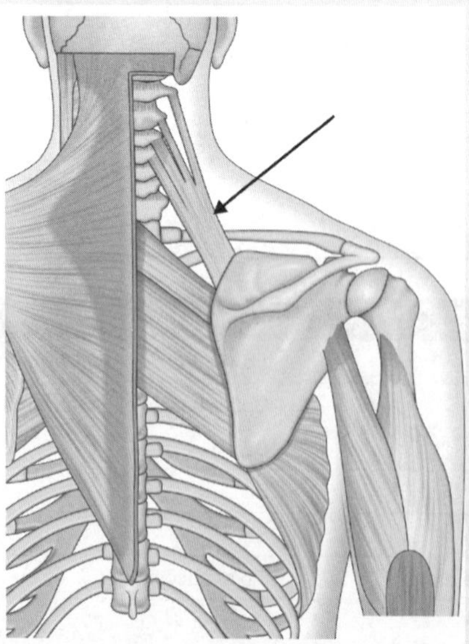

a. Dorsal scapular nerve
b. Dorsal rami of C1
c. Suprascapular nerve
d. Subscapular nerve

Ans. is 'a' Dorsal scapular nerve

Explanation: Arrow points to levator scapulae muscle. It is innervated by Anterior rami of the nerves C3 and C4 and Dorsal scapular nerve.

Anatomy

Muscles of posterior compartment of forearm		
Muscle	***Nerve supply***	***Function***
Superficial muscles		
Brachioradialis	Radial nerve	Flexes forearm in mid-pronation
Extensor carpi radialis longus	Radial nerve	Extends and abducts wrist joint
Extensor carpi radialis brevis	Deep branch of radial nerve	Extends and abducts wrist joint
Extensor digitorum	Posterior interosseous nerve	Extends fingers at metacarpophalangeal joints
Extensor digiti minimi	Posterior interosseous nerve	Extends fifth finger at metacarpophalangeal joint
Extensor carpi ulnaris	Posterior interosseous nerve	Extends and adducts wrist joint
Deep muscles		
Supinator	Deep branch of Radial nerve	Supinates forearm
Extensor indicis	Posterior interosseous nerve	Extends second finger
Abductor pollicis longus	Posterior interosseous nerve	Abducts thumb; extends thumb at carpometacarpal joint
Extensor pollicis longus	Posterior interosseous nerve	Extends thumb at carpometacarpal, metacarpophalangeal and Interphalangeal joints
Extensor pollicis brevis	Posterior interosseous nerve	Extends thumb at carpometacarpal and metacarpophalangeal joints

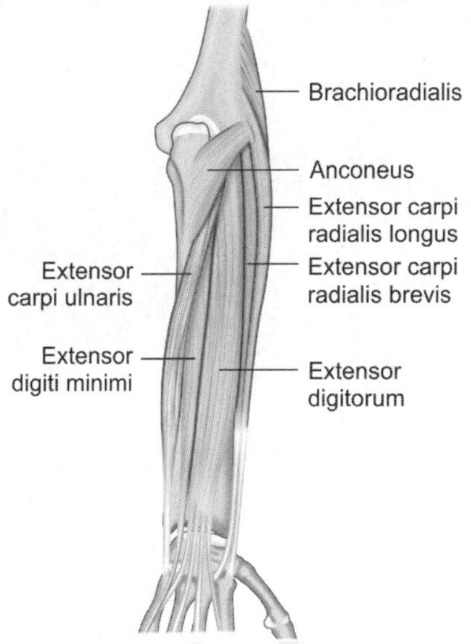

Superficial muscles of posterior compartment of forearm

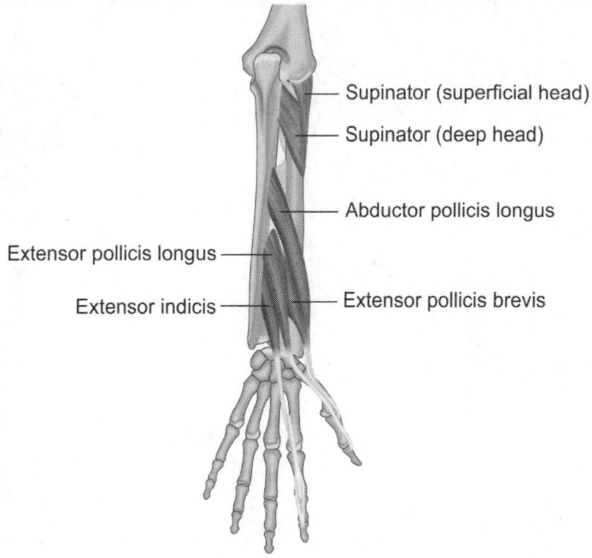

Deep muscles of posterior compartment of forearm

Muscles of anterior compartment of forearm		
Muscle	***Nerve supply***	***Function***
Superficial muscles		
Flexor carpi ulnaris Palmaris longus Flexor carpi radialis Pronator teres	Ulnar nerve Median nerve Median nerve Median nerve	Flexes and adducts wrist joint Flexes wrist joint Flexes and abducts wrist joint Pronates forearm
Intermediate muscle		
Flexor digitorum superficialis	Median nerve	Flexes MCP and proximal interphalangeal joints
Deep muscles		
Flexor digitorum profundus Flexor pollicis longus Pronator quadratus	Ulnar nerve–Medial half Anterior interosseous nerve–Lateral half Anterior interosseous nerve (Branch of median nerve) Anterior interosseous nerve	Flexes distal interphalangeal joints Flexes metacarpophalangeal and interphalangeal joints of thumb Pronates forearm

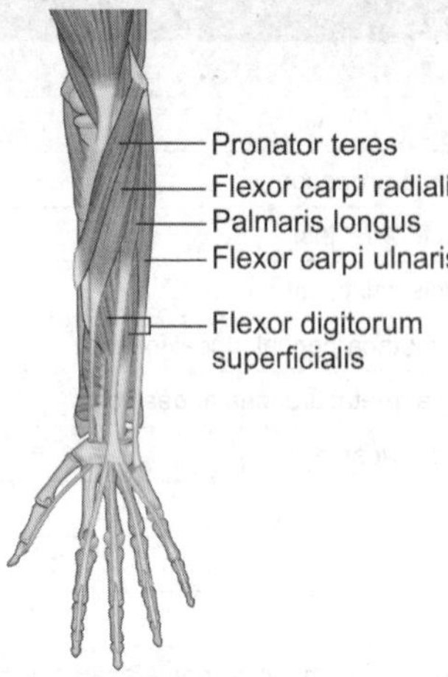

Superficial Muscles of Anterior Compartment of Forearm

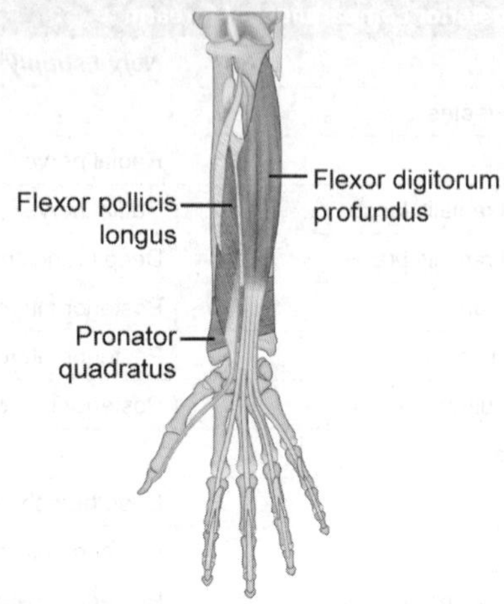

Deep Muscles of Anterior Compartment of Forearm

81. Identify the muscle shown in the diagram. *(NEET 2019)*

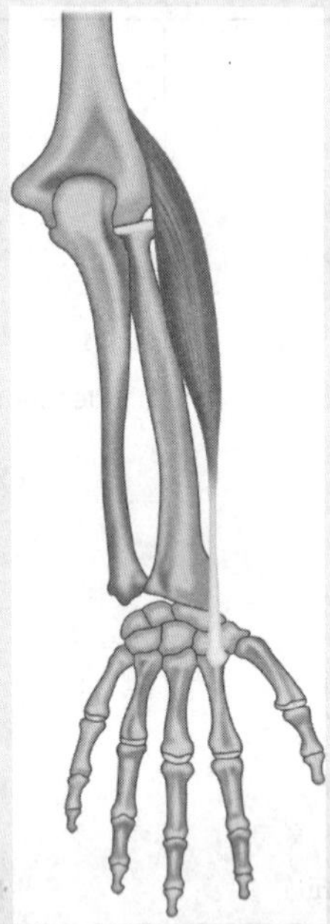

a. Brachioradialis
b. Extensor carpi radialis longus
c. Flexor carpi radialis
d. Extensor carpi ulnaris

Ans. is 'b' Extensor carpi radialis longus

82. Median nerve supplies all of the following muscles *except:* *(NEET 2016)*

a. Flexor carpi ulnaris
b. Flexor digitorum superfacialis
c. Pronator teres
d. Flexor Pollicis Longus

Ans. is 'a' Flexor carpi ulnaris

83. A 41-year-old male presents with a weak flexor pollicis longus and flexor digitorum profundus of the index finger. The nerve involved could be: *(NEET 2016)*

a. Ulnar nerve
b. Median nerve
c. Posterior interosseus nerve
d. Radial nerve

Ans. is 'b' Median nerve

Intrinsic muscles of hand		
Muscle	***Nerve supply***	***Function***
Thenar muscles		
Abductor pollicis brevis Flexor pollicis brevis Opponens pollicis Adductor pollicis	Median nerve Median nerve–Superficial head Deep branch of ulnar nerve –Deep head Median nerve Deep branch of Ulnar nerve	Abducts thumb Flexes thumb Opposes thumb to other digits Adducts thumb
Hypothenar muscles		
Palmaris brevis	Superficial branch of Ulnar N.	Wrinkles skin on medial side of palm
Abductor digiti minimi Flexor digiti minimi brevis Opponens digiti minimi	Deep branch of ulnar nerve Deep branch of ulnar nerve Deep branch of ulnar nerve	Abducts little finger Flexes little finger Opposes little finger to thumb
Central muscles		
Lumbricals (4) 1st and 2nd–Unipennate 3rd and 4th–Bipennate	**Median nerve–First and Second** Deep branch of ulnar nerve–Third and fourth	**Flex Metacapophalangeal joints and extend Interphalangeal joints of fingers**
Palmar interossei (4) All are unipennate	Deep branch of ulnar nerve	Adducts digits, flex metacarpophalangeal joints and extend Intephalangeal joints
Dorsal interossei (4) All are bipennate	Deep branch of ulnar nerve	Abducts digits, flex metacarpophalangeal joints and extend intephalangeal joints

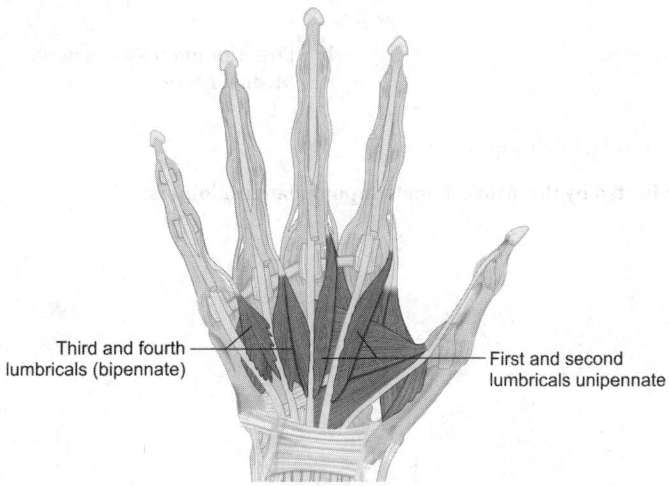

Lumbricals

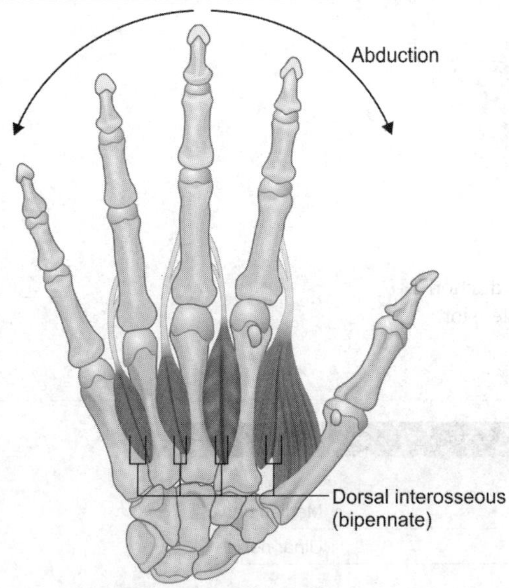

Dorsal interossei

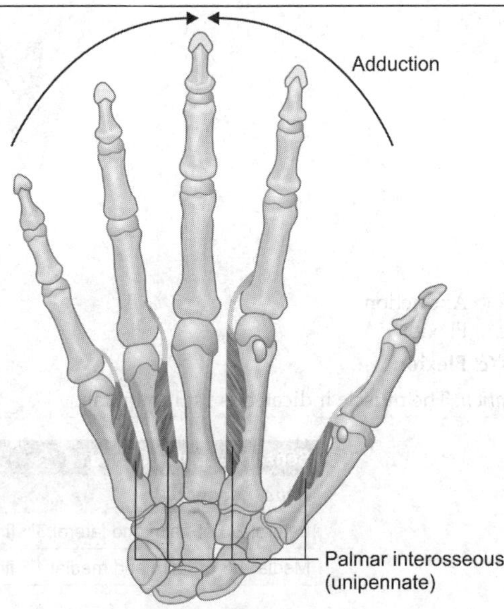

Palmar interossei

84. What is the nerve supply of the marked muscle? *(NEET 2019)*

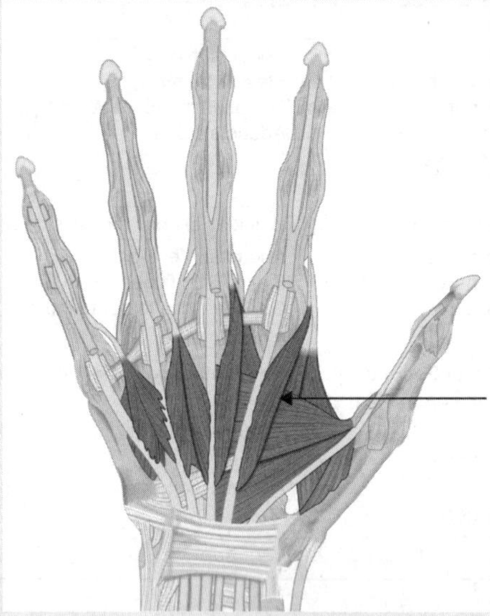

a. Anterior interosseous nerve
b. Posterior interosseous nerve
c. Ulnar nerve
d. Median nerve

Ans. is 'd' Median nerve

Explanation: The muscle indicated is 1st lumbrical.

85. Action of the muscle, indicated by the arrow, at metacarpophalangeal joint is: *(NEET 2018)*

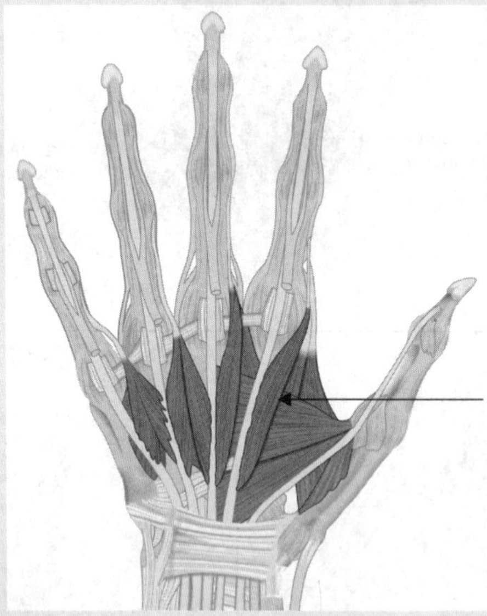

a. Abduction
b. Adduction
c. Flexion
d. Extension

Ans. is 'c' Flexion

Explanation: The muscle indicated is 1st lumbrical.

Sensory supply of hand	
Palmar aspect	
Lateral 2/3 of palm and lateral $3^{1/2}$ fingers	Median nerve
Medial 1/3 of palm and medial $1^{1/2}$ fingers	Ulnar nerve

Contd...

Contd...

Dorsal aspect	
Lateral 2/3 of dorsum of hand	Radial nerve
Medial 1/3 of dorsum of hand and medial $1^{1/2}$ fingers	Ulnar nerve
Dorsum of lateral $3^{1/2}$ fingers over proximal and middle phalanx	Radial nerve
Distal phalanx of lateral $3^{1/2}$ fingers	Median nerve

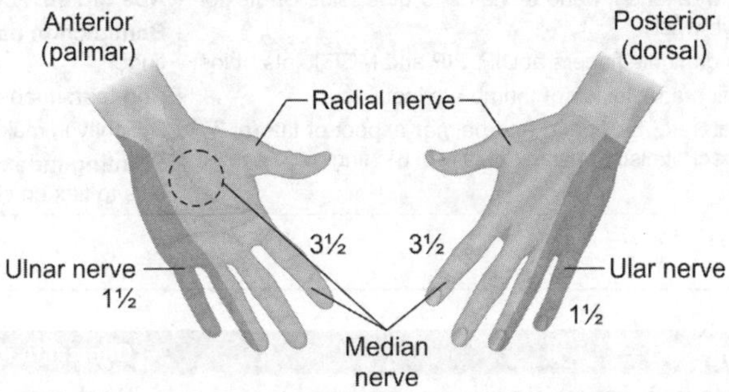

86. Which nerve supplies the marked area of hand? *(NEET 2019)*

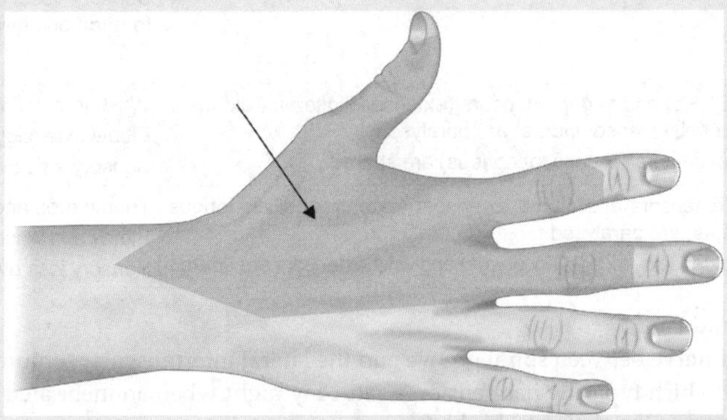

a. Ulnar nerve
b. Median nerve
c. Radial nerve
d. Posterior interosseous nerve

Ans. is 'c' Radial nerve

87. Sensory region of the ulnar nerve is: *(NEET 2016)*

a. Tip of little finger
b. Tip of index finger
c. 1st web space
d. Lateral upper aspect of arm

Ans. is 'a' Tip of little finger

UPPER LIMB NERVES

Nerves of the upper limb associated with various spaces	
Guyon canal	Ulnar nerve
Carpal tunnel	Median nerve
Spiral groove	Radial nerve
Quadrangular space	Axillary nerve
Triangular space	Radial nerve
Cubital tunnel	Ulnar nerve

88. Guyon's canal contains which of the following nerve? *(NEET 2016)*

a. Ulnar nerve
b. Radial nerve
c. Median nerve
d. Anterior interosseous nerve

Ans. is 'a' Ulnar nerve

UPPER LIMB NERVE INJURIES

Nerve	Loss of function	Clinical impairment
Long thoracic nerve	Abduction of arm > 90 degrees	Push against a wall causing Winging of Scapula
Axillary nerve	Abduction of arm 15-90 degrees Sensory loss on lateral side of upper arm **(Regimental Badge sign)**	Patient not able to hold arm at 90 degrees abduction
Median nerve	Flexion of wrist is weakened, hand deviates to ulnar side on flexion (Only if injury above wrist) Flexion of index and middle fingers at DIP, PIP and MCP joints at lost Abduction, opposition and flexion of thumb are lost Sensory loss on lateral 2/3 of palm and palmar aspect of lateral $3^{1/2}$ fingers; dorsal aspect of distal phalanx of lateral $3^{1/2}$ fingers	**Ape thumb**: adducted and laterally rotated thumb **Benediction hand:** unable to flex the index and middle finger **Pen test:** unable to touch the pen, held above the thumb Difficulty in making an 'O' with thumb and index finger **Pointing index or oschsner's clasp test**: index finger fails to flex on clasping hand

RADIAL NERVE INJURY

Level of injury	Muscles affected	Clinical features
High–Above spiral groove	All muscles supplied by radial nerve are paralysed	Wrist drop, thumb drop and finger drop–loss of extension at MCP joint (can extend interphalangeal joints due to action of lumbricals and interossei) Sensory loss over posterior surface of arm and forearm and lower lateral half of forearm
Low–Below spiral groove		
I–Between spiral groove and elbow joint	Wrist (ECRL) and finger extensors (extensor digitorum, extensor digiti minimi, extensor indicis) are paralysed Elbow extensors (Triceps, anconeus) are spared	Wrist drop, thumb drop and finger drop Elbow extension is preserved Sensory loss over the dorsum of first web space
II–Below elbow joint	Finger extensors and thumb extensors (extensor pollicis longus and brevis) are paralysed Elbow extensors (triceps, anconeus) and wrist extensors are spared	Thumb drop and finger drop Elbow and wrist extension is preserved Sensory loss over the dorsum of first web space

- **Saturday Night Palsy (Weekend Palsy)**
  - Compression of the **radial nerve** between spiral groove and the lateral intermuscular septum
  - It is named after an event which typically happens on a saturday night when an inebriated person slumps with his mid-arm compressed between the arm of the chair and his body.

ULNAR NERVE INJURY

Level of injury	Motor loss	Sensory loss
Wrist (low lesion)	• Claw hand deformity (more pronounced) • Hypothenar and interosseous wasting • Loss of abduction and adduction of fingers (card test positive) • Loss of adduction of thumb (Froment sign positive)	Over palmar and dorsal surface of medial 1/3 of hand and medial $1^{1/2}$ fingers No sensory loss over medial aspect of dorsum of hand (dorsal cutaneous branch is spared)
Elbow (high lesion)	• Claw-hand deformity • Hypothenar and interosseous wasting • Loss of abduction and adduction of fingers (**card test positive**) • Loss of adduction of thumb (**Froment sign positive**) • Loss of flexion of MCP joints • Weakness of wrist flexion, hand deviates to radial side on flexion) • Inability to adduct the small finger in against the ring finger—**Wartenberg's sign**	Over palmar and dorsal surface of medial 1/3 of hand and medial $1^{1/2}$ fingers

	Ulnar claw hand	Median claw hand
Nerve involved	Ulnar nerve at wrist	Median nerve at elbow or wrist
Typical presentation	Appears in long-standing cases of nerve damage	Appears when the patient attempts to make a first
Fingers affected	Little and ring fingers	Middle and index fingers
Muscles paralyzed	Medial half of flexor digitorum profundus Medial two lumbricals	Lateral half of flexor digitorum profundus Lateral two lumbricals
Movements involved	Overextension at MCP joints Unopposed flexion at IP joints	Inability to perform flexion at MCP and IP joints of middle and index fingers

Ulnar Paradox

- Claw-hand deformity is more pronounced in low ulnar nerve injury as compared to high ulnar nerve injury due to sparing of Flexor digitorum profundus causing marked flexion of DIP joints

89. Injury to the radial nerve at elbow spares: *(NEET 2016)*

a. Wrist extension
b. Finger extension
c. Thumb extension
d. Sensations in 1st web space

Ans. is 'a' Wrist extension

90. Wrist drop is due which palsy? *(NEET 2016)*

a. Radial nerve palsy
b. Posterior interosseous nerve injury
c. Ulnar nerve palsy
d. Carpal tunnel syndrome

Ans. is 'a' Radial nerve palsy

91. Which of the following is seen in median nerve injury? *(NEET 2016)*

a. Pointing index
b. Wrist drop
c. Wartenberg's sign
d. Regimental badge sign

Ans. is 'a' Pointing index

92. Winging of the scapula is seen in injury to which nerve? *(NEET 2016)*

a. Long thoracic nerve of bell
b. Ulnar nerve
c. Lower subscapular nerve
d. Thoracodorsal nerve

Ans. is 'a' Long thoracic nerve of bell

SHOULDER ABDUCTION

Degree of Abduction	Muscles involved	Nerve
Initiation (up to 15°)	Supraspinatus	Suprascapular
15–90°	**Deltoid (Middle fibres)**	**Axillary**
Overhead (>90°)	Trapezius, Serratus anterior	Accessory, long thoracic

- In abduction, out of total 180 degrees elevation, humerus moves 120 degrees at the shoulder joint and the remaining 60 degrees is done by rotation of scapula.

93. Which of the following muscles carries out shoulder abduction from 15° to 90°? *(NEET 2016)*

a. Supraspinatus
b. Trapezius
c. Deltoid
d. Serratus Anterior

Ans. is 'c' Deltoid

AXILLARY ARTERY

- Begins at the level of outer border of first rib as a continuation of subclavian artery
- Ends at the level of lower border of teres major to continue as brachial artery
- Pectoralis minor lies anterior to Axillary artery and divides it into three parts.

Part	Location	Branches
First part	Proximal to upper border of pectoralis minor	Superior thoracic artery
Second part	Behind pectoralis minor	Thoracoacromial artery Lateral thoracic artery
Third part	Distal to lower border of pectoralis minor	Subscapular artery Anterior and posterior circumflex Humeral artery

94. Which muscle divides the axillary artery into three parts? *(NEET 2016)*

a. Pectoralis minor
b. Pectoralis major
c. Serratus anterior
d. Scalenus anticus

Ans. is 'a' Pectoralis minor

Cubital fossa	
Lateral boundary	**Brochioradialis**
Medial boundary	Pronator teres
Base	Line joining the two epicondyles of humerus
Apex	Point joining lateral and medial boundaries
Floor	Brachialis, Supinator
Roof	Skin, superficial fascia (containing median cubital vein, lateral and medial cutaneous nerve of forearm), deep fascia, bicipital aponeurosis
Contents (Lateral to Medial)	Radial nerve, Biceps brachii tendon, Brachial artery bifurcating into radial and ulnar artery, Median nerve

95. Lateral border of the cubital fossa is: *(NEET 2016)*

a. Brachioradialis
b. Pronator teres
c. Flexor carpi radialis
d. Triceps

Ans. is 'a' Brachioradialis

LOWER LIMB

Myotomes of important muscles	
Muscle	***Myotome***
Extensor hallucis longus	**L5**
Tibilais anterior	L4
Flexor hallucis longus	S1
Gastrocnemius	S1
Gluteus medius and minimus	L5
Gluteus maximus	S1
Quadriceps femoris	L3

96. Weakness of Extensor Hallucis Longus is due to which nerve root mainly? *(NEET 2016)*

a. L5
b. L4
c. S1
d. S2

Ans. is 'a' L5

ARCHES OF FOOT

Medial longitudinal arch: Most important; primarily affected in pes planus and pes cavus.

- Formed by calcaneus, talus, navicular, three cuneiforms and medial three metatarsals
- *Dynamic supports*: Tibialis posterior, tibialis anterior, flexor hallucis longus, fibularis longus, intrinsic plantar muscles
- *Passive supports*: **Plantar fascia (acts as a tie beam),** Spring ligament, Plantar calcaneonavicular ligament, Short and Long plantar ligament

Lateral longitudinal arch

- Formed by calcaneum, cuboid, 4th and 5th metatarsals
- **Plantar fascia acts as a tie beam**
- Peroneus longus, peroneus brevis and peroneus tertius support this arch

Posterior transverse arch: Formed by three cuneiforms and cuboid

Anterior transverse arch: Formed by the heads of five metatarsals

97. Which of the following is common between the medial and lateral plantar arch? *(NEET 2016)*

a. Flexor digitorum brevis
b. Plantar fascia
c. Spring ligament
d. Deltoid ligament

Ans. is 'b' Plantar fascia

Branches of lumbosacral plexus		
Nerve	***Motor supply***	***Sensory supply***
Iliohypogastric nerve (L1)	Anterior abdominal wall muscles	Skin over lower anterior abdominal wall and buttock
Ilio-inguinal (L1)	Anterior abdominal wall muscles	Skin of upper medial aspect of thigh; root of penis and scrotum in male; mons pubis and labia majora in female
Genitofemoral (L1, L2)	**Cremaster muscle in scrotum**	Skin of anterior upper thigh and anterior perineum
Femoral (L2, L3, L4)	Muscles of anterior compartment of thigh; Iliacus and pectineus	**Skin of anterior and medial thigh**, anteromedial knee, medial leg, medial foot
Obturator (L2, L3, L4)	Muscles of medial compartment of thigh (except pectineus and ischial part of adductor magnus), obturator externus	**Skin of upper medial thigh**
Sciatic (L4-S3)	Muscles of posterior compartment of thigh; Ischial part of adductor magnus; all muscles in leg and foot	Skin of lateral leg and foot, sole and dorsal foot
Superior gluteal (L4, L5, S1)	**Gluteus medius, Gluteus minimus, Tensor fasciae latae**	No sensory supply
Inferior gluteal (L5, S1, S2)	**Gluteus maximus**	No sensory supply
Lateral cutaneous nerve of the thigh (L2, L3)	No motor supply	Skin of **anterolateral thigh**
Posterior cutaneous nerve of thigh (S1, S2, S3)	No motor supply	Skin over gluteal fold and upper medial aspect of thigh, posterior thigh, upper posterior leg
Nerve to quadratus femoris (L4, L5, S1)	Quadratus femoris, Gemellus inferior	No sensory supply
Nerve to obturator internus (L5, S1, S2)	Obturator internus, Gemellus superior	No sensory supply

98. Cremaster muscle is supplied by: *(NEET 2016)*

a. Iliohypogastric nerve
b. Genitofemoral nerve
c. Obdurator nerve
d. Femoral nerve

Ans. is 'b' Genitofemoral nerve

99. Superior gluteal nerve supplies all of the following *(NEET 2016)*

a. Gluteus medius
b. Gluteus maximus
c. Gluteus minimus
d. Tensor fascia lata

Ans. is 'b' Gluteus maximus

100. Medial side of the thigh is supplied by: *(NEET 2016)*

a. Iliohypogastric nerve
b. Genitofemoral nerve
c. Obturator nerve
d. Femoral nerve

Ans. is 'd' Femoral nerve

Explanation: Most of the medial part of thigh is supplied by femoral nerve through medial cutaneous nerve of thigh. A small portion superiorly is supplied by obturator nerve.

KNEE MENISCI

Medial meniscus	Lateral meniscus
• Semilunar in shape (Less circular) • Larger in diameter but narrower in body • Anterior horn is small while posterior horn is large • Entire periphery of the meniscus is attached to the joint capsule • Attached to the medial collateral ligament • Less mobile • **More prone to injury** (due to reduced mobility)	• **Semicircular** in shape (C shaped; more circular) • **Smaller in diameter** but wider in body • Anterior horn and posterior horn are uniform in size • Area where the popliteus tendon crosses the joint through the popliteus hiatus is not attached to joint capsule • Not attached to the lateral collateral ligament • **More mobile** • **Less prone to injury** (due to increased mobility)

101. All are true about lateral meniscus *(NEET 2016)*

a. Smaller in diameter than medial meniscus
b. Semicircular in shape
c. More mobile
d. More prone to injury

Ans. is 'd' More prone to injury

MUSCLES OF LEG

Muscle	Action	Nerve supply
Anterior compartment of Leg		
Tibialis anterior	Dorsiflexion of foot at ankle joint; inversion of foot	Deep fibular nerve (L4, L5)
Extensor digitorum longus	Extension of lateral digits 2–5 and dorsiflexion of foot	Deep fibular nerve (L5, S1)
Extensor hallucis longus	Extension of great toe and dorsiflexion of foot	Deep fibular nerve (L5, S1)
Fibularis (peroneus) tertius	Dorsiflexion and eversion of foot	Deep fibular nerve (L5, S1)
Lateral compartment of Leg		
Fibularis (peroneus) longus	Eversion and plantar flexion of foot	Superficial fibular nerve (L5, S1, S2)
Fibularis (peroneus) brevis	Eversion and plantar flexion of foot	Superficial fibular nerve (L5, S1, S2)
Posterior compartment of Leg (Superficial group)		
Gastrocnemius	Plantar flexes foot and flexes knee	Tibial nerve (S1, S2)
Plantaris	Plantar flexes foot and flexes knee	Tibial nerve (S1, S2)
Soleus	Plantar flexes the foot	Tibial nerve (S1, S2)
Posterior compartment of Leg (Deep group)		
Popliteus	**Unlocks knee joint; laterally rotates femur on fixed tibia**	Tibial nerve (L4, L5, S1)
Flexor hallucis longus	Flexes great toe	Tibial nerve (S2, S3)
Flexor digitorum longus	Flexes digits 2–5	Tibial nerve (S2, S3)
Tibialis posterior	Inversion and plantar flexion of foot; support of medial arch of foot during walking	Tibial nerve (L4, L5)

102. Action of popliteus is: *(NEET 2016)*

a. Locking of knee joint
b. Unlocking of knee joint
c. Medial rotation of femur on tibia
d. None

Ans. is 'b' Unlocking of knee joint

THORAX

ARTERIAL SUPPLY OF HEART

Coronary Arteries

- Arise from aortic sinuses in aortic root
- Three sinuses
  - **Anterior (Right):** Gives rise to right coronary artery
  - **Left Posterior (Left):** Gives rise to left coronary artery
  - **Right posterior (Non-coronary):** No coronary artery arises

Right Coronary Artery (RCA) Branches

- SA nodal artery, AV nodal artery and posterior interventricular artery

Left Coronary Artery (LCA) Branches

- Left anterior descending (LAD) and left circumflex (LCX)

Coronary artery territories	
Territory	***Artery***
Interventricular septum	
Posterior 1/3rd	Posterior interventricular artery
Anterior 2/3rd	Left anterior descending artery
Left ventricle	
Anterior wall, Apex	Left anterior descending artery
Posterior wall, Inferior wall	Posterior interventricular artery
Lateral wall	Left circumflex artery

Contd...

Anatomy

Contd...

Coronary artery territories	
Conducting system	
Proximal (SA node, AV node) Distal (AV Bundle of His, right and left bundle branches)	Right coronary artery **Left coronary artery (via left anterior descending)**

Cardiac Dominance

- Decided by posterior interventricular artery
  - Right cardiac dominance (Branch of RCA)–65%
  - Left cardiac dominance (Branch of LCX)–10%
  - Co-dominance–25%

103. Right coronary artery arises from: *(NEET 2019)*

a. Anterior aortic sinus
b. Left posterior aortic sinus
c. Right posterior aortic sinus
d. Non-coronary aortic sinus

Ans. is 'a' Anterior aortic sinus

104. Blood supply of the right bundle branch is by: *(NEET 2016)*

a. Right coronary artery
b. Left coronary artery
c. Coronary sinus
d. Left circumflex artery

Ans. is 'b' Left coronary artery

BORDERS AND SURFACES OF HEART

Borders	
Right border Left border (Obtuse margin) Inferior border (Acute margin) Upper border Apex	Right atrium Left ventricle, Left auricle (upper most part) Right ventricle, Left ventricle (near apex) Left atrium, Right atrium (where SVC enters) Left ventricle
Surfaces	
Anterior (Sternocostal) Inferior (Diaphragmatic) **Base (Posterior)** Right surface Left surface	Right ventricle, right auricle Left ventricle (left 2/3), Right ventricle (right 1/3) **Left atrium** Right atrium Left ventricle, left auricle

105. Base of the heart is formed by: *(NEET 2016)*

a. Left ventricle
b. Right ventricle
c. Right atrium
d. Left atrium

Ans. is 'd' Left atrium

SUPRAPLEURAL MEMBRANE

- **Sibson's fascia** or Diaphragm of superior thoracic aperture
- Tent-shaped (triangular) dense fascial sheath enclosing thoracic inlet
- Morpholgically, represents degenerated tendon of **scalenus minimus (pleuralis) muscle**
- **Attachments**
  - *Apex*: Transverse process of C7 vertebra
  - *Base*: Inner border of 1st rib
- **Relations**
  - *Superiorly*: Subclavian vessels
  - *Inferiorly*: Cervical pleura covering lung apex

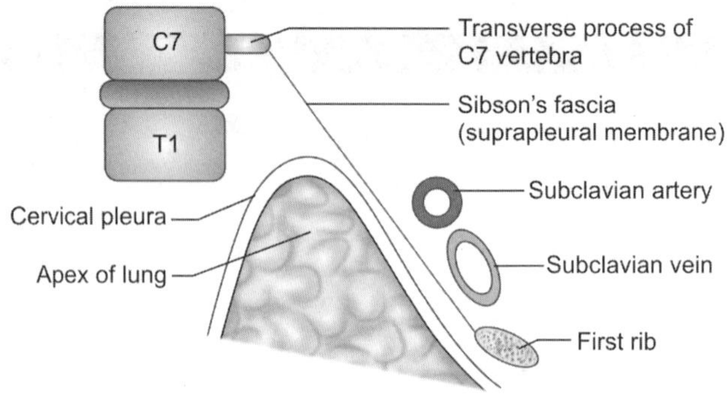

Suprapleural Membrane: Relations

106. True about Sibson's fascia/suprapleural membrane are all *except*: *(NEET 2018)*

a. Subclavian vessels arch over it
b. Attached to transverse process of C7
c. Develops from scalenus anterior
d. Attached to inner border of 1st rib

Ans. is 'c' Develops from scalenus anterior

DIAPHRAGM OPENINGS

Opening	Vertebral level	Location	Structures passing
Vena caval hiatus	T8	Central tendon of diaphragm	Inferior vena cava Right phrenic nerve
Oesophageal hiatus	T10	Muscular part of right crus of diaphragm	Oesophagus Gastric/Vagus nerve Esophageal branch of left gastric artery
Aortic hiatus	T12	Osseoaponeurotic between right and left crus	Aorta Thoracic duct Azygous vein

Nerve supply of Diaphragm

- *Motor*: Phrenic nerve (C3,C4,C5)
- *Sensory*: Centrally by Phrenic nerve; Peripherally by lower six intercostals nerves

107. Which of the following does not pass through aortic opening of diaphragm? *(NEET 2018)*

a. Aorta
b. Phrenic nerve
c. Thoracic duct
d. Azygous vein

Ans. is 'b' Phrenic nerve

108. Diaphragm is supplied by: *(NEET 2016)*

a. Phrenic nerve
b. C2, C3, C4 Roots
c. Thoracodorsal nerve
d. Long thoracic nerve

Ans. is 'a' Phrenic nerve

ESOPHAGUS

- Length of 25 cm
- Begins as a continuation of laryngopharynx at the level of lower border of cricoid cartilage at C6 vertebral level and ends at T11 level by opening into cardiac orifice of stomach
- Within the abdominal portion (1-2 cm) of esophagus, the abdominal part of LES is located. Another 1-2 cm of LES lies above the diaphragm in mediastinum, i.e. thoracic part of LES. Thus, **total length of LES is 3-4 cm.**

Esophagus part	Arterial supply	Venous drainage	Lymphatic drainage
Cervical (4 cm)	**Inferior thyroid artery**	Inferior thyroid veins	Deep cervical nodes
Thoracic (20 cm)	Esophageal branches of descending thoracic aorta	Azygos vein	Posterior mediastinal nodes
Abdominal (1-2 cm)	Left gastric artery and left inferior phrenic artery	Left gastric vein	Left gastric nodes

Anatomy

Esophageal constrictions			
Number	***Distance from incisor***	***Bony level***	***Anatomical landmark***
1st	15 cm (6 inches)	C6	At its beginning
2nd	22.5 cm (9 inches)	T4	**Crossing of aortic arch**
3rd	27.5 cm (11 inches)	T6	Crossing of left main bronchus
4th	37.5-40 cm (15-16 inches)	T10	Piercing diaphragm **(at lower esophageal sphincter)**

109. Which of the following structures is related to the esophagus 22.5 cm from the incisor teeth? *(NEET 2016)*

a. Arch of aorta
b. Right principal broncus
c. Thoracic duct
d. Azygos vein

Ans. is 'a' Arch of aorta

110. All are true about the esophagus *except*: *(NEET 2016)*

a. It is around 25 cm long
b. Abdominal part of esophagus is supplied by the left gastric artery
c. It is lined by ciliated columnar epithelium
d. Cervical part of esophagus is supplied by inferior thyroid artery

Ans. is 'c' It is lined by ciliated columnar epithelium

Explanation: Esophagus is lined by stratified squamous non-keratinized epithelium.

THORACIC DUCT

- Largest lymphatic duct in body
- Beaded appearance due to presence of many valves
- Begins as cisterna chyli near lower border of T12 vertebra → enters thorax through the aortic opening of diaphragm at T12 → Ascends in posterior mediastinum → **Crosses from right to left side at T5 level → Opens into junction of left subclavian and internal jugular veins**
- **Rupture of thoracic duct can cause chylothorax**
- **Thoracic duct drains both halves of the body below the diaphragm and the left half above the diaphragm. Its tributaries are– Right and left lumbar trunk, Left jugular trunk and left bronchomediastinal trunk in neck.**
- **Right lymphatic duct drains right side of body above the diaphragm into junction of right subclavian and internal jugular vein**

111. Thoracic duct opens into systemic circulation at: *(NEET 2016)*

a. Junction of SVC and left branchicephalic vein
b. Junction of left internal jugular and left subclavian vein
c. Directly into coronary sinus
d. Into azygos vein

Ans. is 'b' Junction of left internal jugular and left subclavian vein

112. All of the following are tributaries of the thoracic duct *expect*: *(NEET 2016)*

a. Left lumbar trunk
b. Right lumbar trunk
c. Left jugular trunk
d. Right jugular trunk

Ans. is 'd' Right jugular trunk

Explanation: Right jugular trunk drains into right bronchomediastinal lymphatic trunk.

HILUM OF THE LUNG

Relations of the hilum of the lung			
Anterior	***Posterior***	***Superior***	***Inferior***
Common on both sides • Phrenic nerve • Pericardiophrenic vessels • Anterior pulmonary plexus *On right side* • SVC • Part of right atrium	*Common on both sides* • Vagus nerve • Posterior pulmonary plexus *On left side* • Descending thoracic aorta	*On right side* • Terminal part of azygous vein *On left side* • Arch of aorta	• Pulmonary ligament

Arrangement of structures at lung hilum (superior to inferior)	
Right side	***Left side***
Epi-arterial bronchus Pulmonary artery Hyparterial bronchus Inferior pulmonary vein	Pulmonary artery Left main bronchus Inferior pulmonary vein

❖ Bronchus and bronchial arteries are the posterior most structures at the hila of both lungs.

113. Which of the following passes posterior to the hilum of the lung? *(NEET 2016)*

a. Vagus
b. Phrenic nerve
c. SVC
d. Right atrium

Ans. is 'a' Vagus

MEDIASTINUM

Mediastinum	Contents
Superior	• Trachea, esophagus, thymus, thoracic duct • Nerves: Vagus, phrenic, left recurrent laryngeal nerve • Arteries: Arch of aorta, brachiocephalic artery, left common carotid artery left subclavian artery • Veins: Brachiocephalic veins, upper half of SVC, left superior intercostal vein
Anterior	• Inferior part of thymus, areolar tissue.
Middle	• Heart with pericardium, tracheal carina, right and left principal bronchi • Arteries: Ascending aorta, pulmonary trunk, two pulmonary arteries. • Veins: Lower part of SVC, terminal part of azygos vein, right and left pulmonary veins. • Nerves: Phrenic nerve
Posterior	• Esophagus, thoracic duct • Arteries: Descending thoracic aorta and its branches (bronchial, esophageal and posterior intercostals) • Veins: Azygos, hemiazygos • Nerves: Vagus

114. Arch of aorta lies in which mediastinum? *(NEET 2016)*

a. Superior mediastinum
b. Posterior mediastinum
c. Middle mediastinum
d. Anterior mediastinum

Ans. is 'a' Superior mediastinum

Surface anatomy and auscultatory areas of cardiac valves		
Valve	***Surface marking***	***Auscultatory area***
Pulmonary	Sternal end of left 3rd costal cartilage (upper border)	Left 2nd intercostal space near sternum
Aortic	Sternal end of left 3rd costal cartilage (lower border)	Right 2nd intercostal space near sternum
Mitral	Sternal end of left 4th costal cartilage	Cardiac apex (just medial to midclavicular line in left 5th intercostal space)
Tricuspid	Right half of sternum along 4th, 5th intercostal space	Right lower end of sternum

115. What is the surface marking of the pulmonary valve? *(NEET 2016)*

a. 3rd intercostal space
b. 4th costal cartilage
c. 3rd costal cartilage
d. 2nd intercostal space

Ans. is 'c' 3rd costal cartilage

ABDOMEN

CALOT'S TRIANGLE

Oriented with its apex directed at the liver.

Borders

❖ *Medial*: Common hepatic duct
❖ *Inferior*: Cystic duct
❖ *Superior*: Inferior surface of liver

Contents

- ❖ Right hepatic artery
- ❖ Cystic artery
- ❖ Lymph node of Lund (first lymph node of gallbladder)

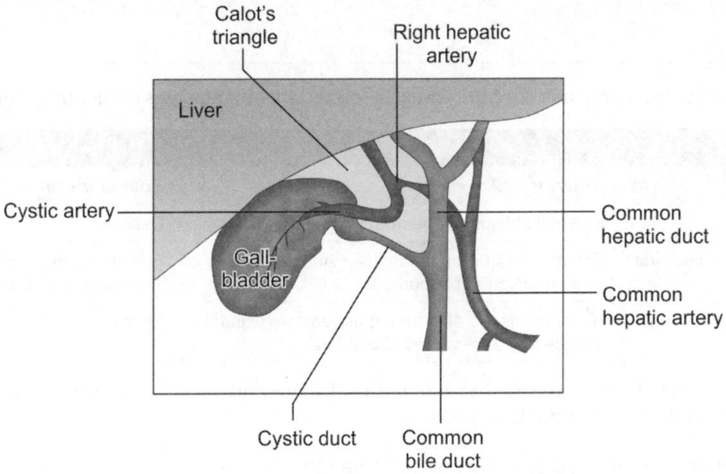

Calot's Triangle

116. Which of the following is not a boundary of Calot's triangle? *(NEET 2019)*

a. Common hepatic duct
b. Cystic duct
c. Inferior surface of liver
d. Gallbladder

Ans. is 'd' Gallbladder

EXTERNAL OBLIQUE MUSCLE AND APONEUROSIS

External oblique muscle is the largest and the outermost of the three flat muscles of the lateral anterior abdomen (Internal oblique and Transversus abdominis are other two muscles)

Ligaments derived from external oblique aponeurosis

- ❖ **Inguinal ligament (Poupart's ligament)** is the folded lower border of external oblique aponeurosis.
- ❖ **Lacunar ligament (Gimbernat ligament)** is the crescent shaped expansion from the medial end of inguinal ligament attached to pectineal line of pubis.
- ❖ **Pectineal ligament (Cooper's ligament)** is strong fibrous band extending laterally from the lacunar ligament along pectineal line of pubis.

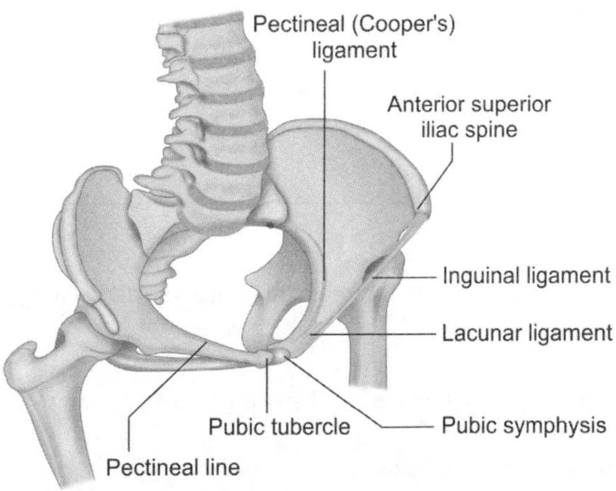

Linea semilunaris (also called the Spigelian line) corresponds to the lateral border of the rectus abdominis formed by the aponeurosis of the internal oblique at its line of division and strengthened anteriorly by the external oblique and posteriorly by the transverses abdominis. A hernia through this region is called a Spigelian hernia.

117. Which of the following structures is not derived from external oblique muscle? *(NEET 2019)*

a. Inguinal ligament
b. Lacunar ligament
c. Cooper ligament
d. Linea semilunaris

Ans. is 'd' Linea semilunaris

RECTUS SHEATH

❖ It is an aponeurotic sheath enclosing rectus abdominis muscle formed by aponeuroses of the three flat abdominal muscles.

Walls of rectus sheath		
	Anterior wall	***Posterior wall***
Above costal margin	External oblique aponeurosis	Deficient
Between costal margin and arcuate line	External oblique aponeurosis + Anterior lamina of internal oblique aponeurosis	Posterior lamina of Internal oblique aponeurosis + Transversus abdominis aponeurosis
Below arcuate line	Aponeurosis of all three muscles (ext. and int. oblique and transverses abdominis)	Deficient

Linea alba: Three aponeurotic layers forming rectus sheath of both sides interlace with each other to form a midline tendinous raphe, Linea alba. It extends from xiphoid process to pubic symphysis.

118. Anterior Rectus Sheath just above pubic symphysis is formed by: *(NEET 2016)*

a. External oblique aponeurosis
b. Aponeurosis of three muscle including external oblique, internal oblique and transversus abdominis
c. Linea alba
d. Internal oblique only

Ans. is 'b' Aponeurosis of three muscle including external oblique, internal oblique and transversus abdominis

ADRENAL GLAND

Arterial supply	Superior suprarenal artery (branch of inferior phrenic artery)
	Middle suprarenal artery (branch of abdominal aorta)
	Inferior suprarenal artery (branch of renal artery)
Venous supply	**Right suprarenal (adrenal) vein drains into IVC**
	Left suprarenal vein drains into the left renal vein and then into IVC
Lymphatics	Lateral aortic (para-aortic) nodes

119. Right suprarenal veins drain into: *(NEET 2016)*

a. Inferior vena cava
b. Right renal vein
c. Left renal vein
d. Accessory Hemiazygos vein

Ans. is 'a' Inferior vena cava

HERNIAS IN INGUINAL REGION

Indirect Inguinal Hernia

❖ "Indirectly" through abdominal wall via inguinal canal through internal and external inguinal rings
❖ Origin lateral to inferior epigastric vessels
❖ Follows path of descent of testes
❖ Covered by all layers of spermatic fascia: Contrast with direct hernias (outer layer only)
❖ Congenital defect
  • Bowel protrudes through patent processus vaginalis
❖ Most common type of inguinal hernia
❖ More common in men
❖ Commonly extend into scrotum
❖ Usually occurs in adults with risk factors (heavy lifting, constipation)

Direct Inguinal Hernia

- Bowel bulges "directly" through abdominal wall
- Protrudes through Hesselbach's triangle
- Origin is medial to inferior epigastric vessels
- Through external ring (not deep/internal)
- Covered by external spermatic fascia only
- Should never bulge into scrotum
- Usually occurs in older men due to transversalis fascia breakdown (acquired)

Hesselbach's triangle: The site of direct inguinal hernia.

- *Medial border*: Linea semilunaris (lateral margin of the rectus sheath)
- *Superolateral border*: Inferior epigastric vessels
- *Inferior border*: Inguinal ligament (Pouparts ligament)

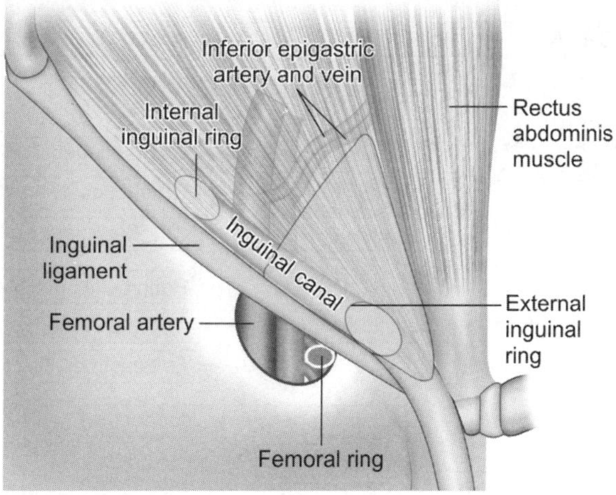

Femoral Hernia

- *Hernia through femoral ring*: Medial to femoral vessels
- *Bowel protrudes below inguinal ligament*: Differentiates from both types of inguinal hernias
- *Below and Lateral to pubic tubercle (Vs Inguinal hernias*: Above and medial to pubic tubercle)
- *More common in women than men*: But indirect most common type for both genders
- *High risk of incarceration*: Femoral ring is small opening

120. Which hernia occurs below and lateral to the pubic tubercle? *(NEET 2016)*

a. Femoral hernia
b. Inguinal hernia
c. Morgagnian hernia
d. Sliding hernia

Ans. is 'a' Femoral hernia

GREATER OMENTUM

- Large 4 layered peritoneal fold hanging down like an apron from greater curvature of stomach
- Develops from dorsal mesogastrium
- Anterior two layers fold upon themselves to form posterior two layers, i.e. first layer becomes the fourth layer and second layer becomes third layer
- Lesser sac between 2 and 3rd layers gets obliterated, except for about 2.5 cm below the greater curvature of stomach
- Contains the anastomosis of right and left gastroepiploic vessels
- *'Policeman of Abdomen'*: adheres to areas of inflammation, localizes infections, prevents diffuse peritonitis

121. How many layers are present in the greater omentum? *(NEET 2016)*

a. 1
b. 2
c. 3
d. 4

Ans. is 'd' 4

LYMPHATIC DRAINAGE OF STOMACH

Nodal group	Drainage area
Left gastric arterial group	Lesser curvature
Short gastric and Left gastroepiploic group	Left half of greater curvature
Right gastroepiploic group	Right half of greater curvature
Pyloric nodes	Pylorus

All nodal groups drain into celiac nodes → Intestinal lymph trunks → Cisterna chyli

122. Stomach wall is mainly drained by all lymph nodes *except*: *(NEET 2016)*

a. Pyloric nodes
b. Short gastric vessel nodal group
c. Right gastroepiploic nodes
d. Inguinal nodes

Ans. is 'd' Inguinal nodes

BRANCHES OF ABDOMINAL AORTA

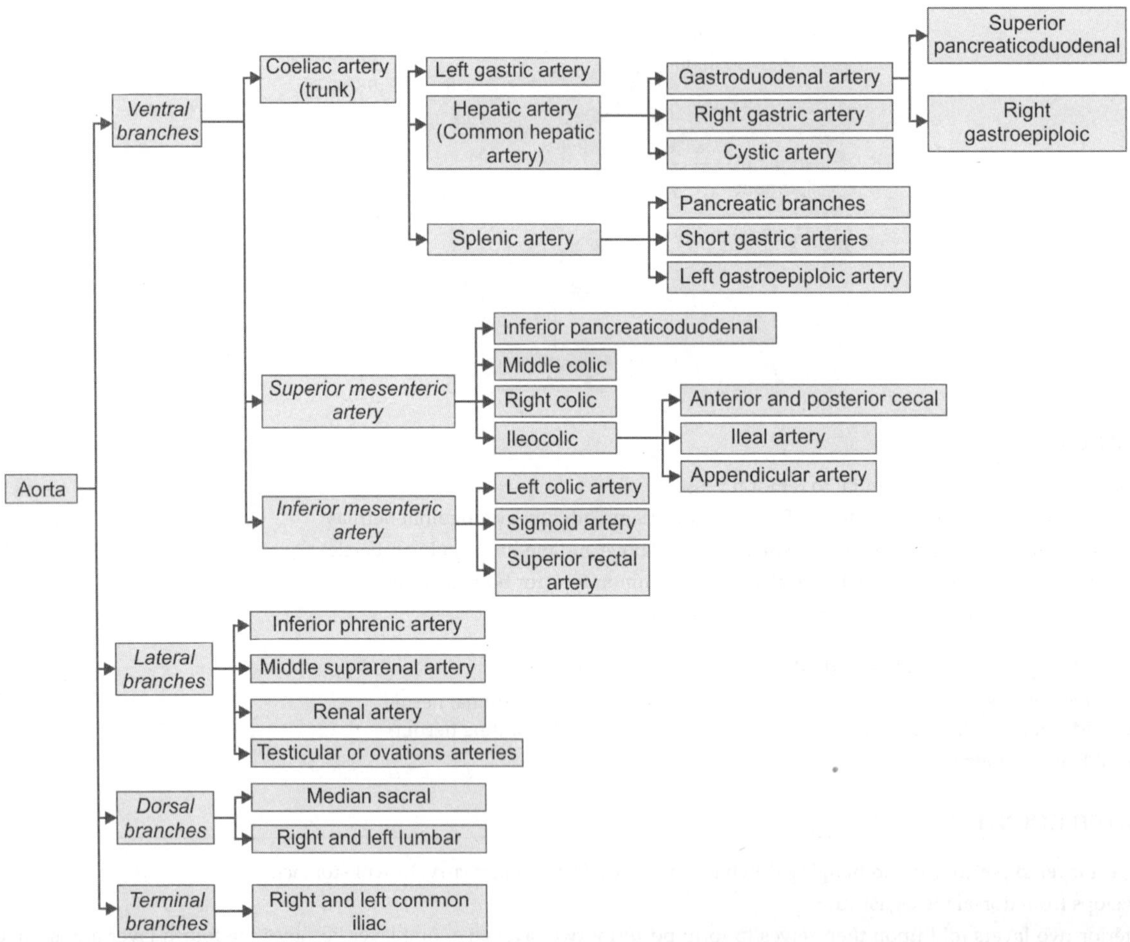

123. Gastroduodenal artery is a branch of: *(NEET 2016)*

a. Common hepatic artery
b. Superior mesenteric artery
c. Abdominal aorta
d. Splenic artery

Ans. is 'a' Common hepatic artery

124. Which of the following is a branch of the inferior mesenteric artery? *(NEET 2016)*

a. Sigmoid artery
b. Middle colic artery
c. Renal artery
d. Right colic artery

Ans. is 'a' Sigmoid artery

125. In ligation of common hepatic artery, blood supply of stomach is disturbed due to involvement of which pair of vessels? *(NEET 2016)*

a. Right and left gastric artery
b. Right and left gastroepiploic artery
c. Right gastric and right gastroepiploic artery
d. Right gastric and short gastric artery

Ans. is 'c' Right gastric and right gastroepiploic artery

EPIPLOIC FORAMEN

- Space which connects the greater sac and lesser sac in abdomen.

Boundaries

- **Anterior**: Right free border of the lesser omentum containing bile duct, vertical part of the hepatic artery , and portal vein, remember duct and artery are anterior to the vein with the duct being to the right of the artery (The duct is dexter, which means to the right)
- **Posterior**: Inferior vena cava and right suprarenal gland
- **Superior**: Caudate lobe of the liver
- **Inferior:** First part of the duodenum and horizontal part of the hepatic artery

126. Superior border of epiploic foramen formed by: *(NEET 2016)*

a. Caudate lobe
b. Hepatic artery
c. Bile duct
d. IVC

Ans. is 'a' Caudate lobe

PANCREAS

The pancreas horizontally crosses the posterior abdominal wall at approximately the level of transpyloric plane. The gland consists of 4 parts:

1. Head of the pancreas rests within the C-shaped area formed by the duodenum and is traversed by the common bile duct. It includes the uncinate process which is crossed by superior mesenteric vessels.
2. Posterior to the neck is the site of formation of hepatic portal vein.
3. Body passes to the left and passes anterior to aorta and left kidney. The splenic artery undulates along superior border of the body of pancreas with the splenic vein coursing posterior to the body.
4. Tail of the pancreas enters the splenorenal ligament to reach the hilum of spleen. Tail is the only part of pancreas that is intraperitoneal.

The main pancreatic duct courses through the body and tail of pancreas to reach head of pancreas, where it joins with the common bile duct to form the hepatopancreatic ampulla.

The head of the pancreas receives its blood supply from superior and inferior pancreatoduodenal branches of the gastroduodenal and superior mesenteric arteries, respectively. This region is important for collateral circulation because there are anastomoses between these branches of the celiac trunk and superior mesenteric artery.

The neck, body and tail of the pancreas receive their blood supply from the splenic artery.

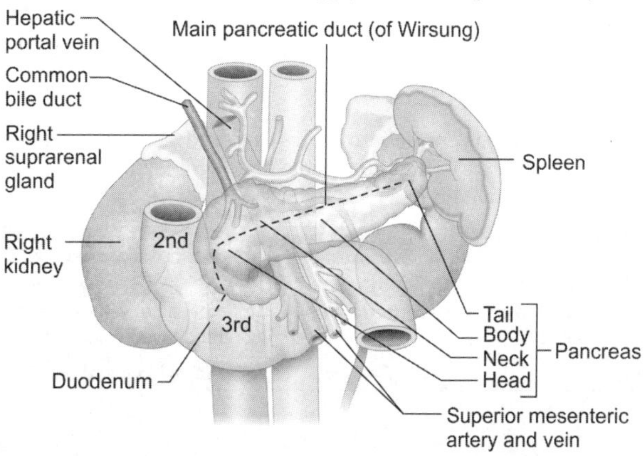

Adult Pancreas

127. Which vessel is compressed by tumor in uncinate process of pancreas? *(NEET 2020)*

a. SMA
b. IMA
c. Portal vein
d. Common hepatic artery

Ans. is 'a' SMA

PELVIS

UTERINE SUPPORTS

Supports of uterus	
Primary supports	
Muscular (Main) supports	• Pelvic diaphragm (levator ani) • Urogenital diaphragm • Perineal body
Fibromuscular/Mechanical supports	• Uterine axis • Pubocervical ligament • Transverse cervical ligament of Mackenrodt • Uterosacral ligament • Round ligament of uterus (weak support)
Secondary supports (Peritoneal folds)	• Broad ligament • Uterovesical fold of peritoneum • Rectovaginal fold of peritoneum

Normal uterine axis

- *Anteversion*: Long axis of uterus is bent forward on long axis of vagina
- *Anteflexion*: Long axis of body of uterus is bent forward at the level of internal os with long axis of cervix
  Anteversion is maintained by:
  - Forward pull on uterine fundus by **round ligament**
  - **Backward pull on cervix by uterosacral ligament**

128. Ligaments holding the uterus in anteversion are: *(NEET 2018)*

a. Round ligament and transverse cervical ligament
b. Round ligament and uterosacral ligament
c. Uterosacral ligament and transverse cervical ligament
d. Uterosacral ligament and broad ligament

Ans. is 'b' Round ligament and uterosacral ligament

ANAL CANAL

- Anal canal begins at anorectal junction and ends at anal verge
- *Length*: 4 cm in adults
- Anal canal has 3 parts:

1. **Upper third**
   - 15 mm long and insensitive to pain
   - Lined by simple columnar epithelium and has anal columns of Morgagni, anal valves, anal sinus and anal papilla.
2. **Middle third (Transitional zone)**
   - 15 mm long and sensitive to pain
   - Lined by non-keratinized stratified squamous epithelium without sweat and sebaceous glands
3. **Lower third**
   - 8 mm long and sensitive to pain
   - Lined by non-keratinized stratified squamous epithelium with sweat and sebaceous glands
   - Upper and middle-thirds are separated by the dentate/pectinate line, while white line of Hilton separates lower third from the middle third. Anal glands open at the dentate line.

	Above pectinate line	Below pectinate line
Arterial supply	Superior rectal artery	Inferior rectal artery (branch of pudendal artery)
Venous supply	**Superior rectal vein → inferior mesenteric vein →** Splenic vein → Portal vein	Inferior rectal vein →internal pudendal vein → Internal iliac vein → Common iliac vein → IVC
Lymphatics	Internal iliac LN	Superficial inguinal LN

Anal Sphincters

	Internal anal sphincter	External anal sphincter
Muscle	Circular muscles of lower rectum	Striated muscle
Control	Involuntary (resting tone)	Voluntary sphincter
Location	Surrounds upper 3/4th anal canal	Surrounds entire length of anal canal
Innervation	Sympathetic fibres from superior hypogastric plexus; Parasympathetic fibres from pelvic splanchnic nerves (S2, S3, S4)	Inferior rectal nerve (S2, S3, S4) and Perineal branch of S4

129. Internal anal sphincter is formed by: *(NEET 2016)*

a. Puborectalis
b. Circular muscles from lower rectum
c. Longitudinal iinvoluntary muscle
d. None

Ans. is 'b' Circular muscles from lower rectum

130. Superior rectal vein opens into: *(NEET 2016)*

a. Inferior mesenteric vein
b. Superior mesenteric vein
c. Internal iliac vein
d. Circumflex iliac vein

Ans. is 'a' Inferior mesenteric vein

PERINEAL BODY

- An important landmark of the urogenital triangle is the perineal body.
- This ill-defined, fibromuscular mass is located in the middle of the interischial line, between the urogenital and anal triangles.
- Many muscles get attachment at the perineal body. It has posterior communications with the external anal sphincter and anterior relations with bulbospongiosus and the deep and superficial transverse perinei. The perineal body also extends superiorly into the rectoprostatic (rectovaginal) septum of the pelvis.

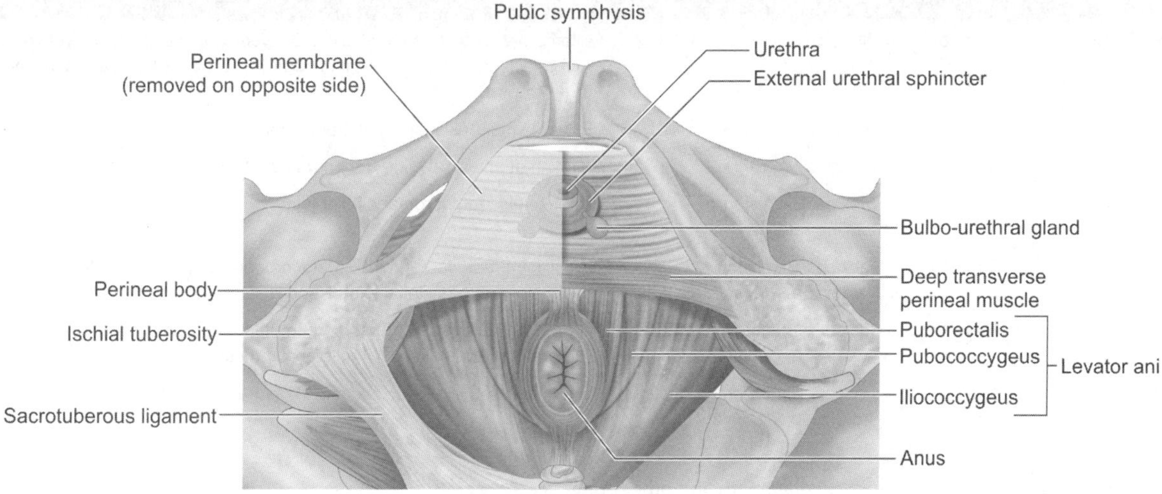

Deep perineal pouch in men

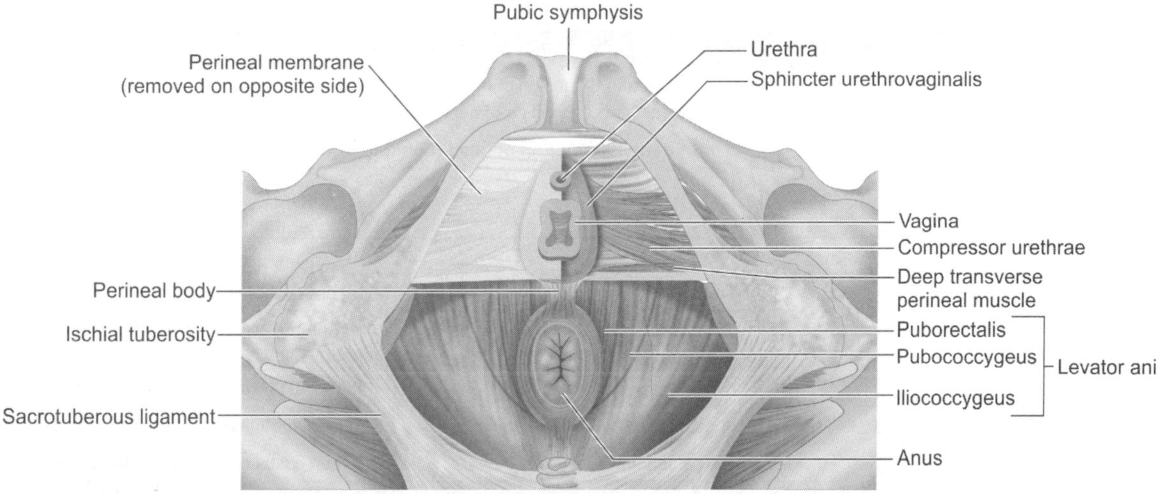

Deep perineal pouch in women

131. During posterior episiotomy, the structure damaged just posterior to perineal body is: *(NEET 2020)*

a. Urethral sphincter
b. External anal sphincter
c. Ischiococcygeus
d. Bulbospongiosis

Ans. is 'b' External anal sphincter

OSTEOLOGY

TYPES OF JOINTS

1. **Fibrous Joints**
   - *Sutures*: Skull bones
   - *Gomphosis*: Dentoalveolar joint
   - *Syndesmosis*: Interosseous middle radio-ulnar joint
2. **Cartilaginous Joints**
   - *Synchondrosis (Primary cartilaginous joint)*: Epiphyseo-diaphyseal joint; Costochondral junction, Xiphisternal joint
   - *Symphysis (Secondary cartilaginous joint)*: Midline joints; Sacro-coccygeal joint, Pubic symphysis, Manubriosternal
3. **Synovial Joints**

Type of synovial joint	Axis	Movements	Examples
Plane/Gliding joint	Uniaxial	Gliding	Intercarpal joints, Intertarsal joints, Between articular processes of vertebrae, Acromioclavicular joint, **Interchondral joint (Between costal cartilages of 6th–9th ribs)**
Hinge joints	Uniaxial	Flexion, Extension	Elbow joints, Ankle joints, Interphalangeal joints
Pivot joints	Uniaxial	Rotation	Median atlantoaxial joint, Superior and inferior radioulnar joints
Condylar joints	Biaxial	Flexion, Extension, Limited rotation	Knee joints, Temporomandibular joint
Ellipsoid joints	Biaxial	Flexion, Extension, Abduction, Adduction, Circumduction	Wrist joint(radiocarpal joint), Metacarpophalangeal joint, Atlantoaxial joints (lateral); Atlanto-occipital joint (Head NODDING)
Saddle joints	Biaxial	Flexion, Extension, Abduction, Adduction, Conjunct rotation	Sternoclavicular joint, First carpometacarpal joint, Calcaneocuboid joint (Lateral longitudinal arch), Malleus and Incus
Ball and socket joints	Multiaxial	Flexion, Extension, Abduction, Adduction, Circumduction, Rotation	Shoulder joint, Hip joint, Talocalcaneonavicular joint

Hyoid bone: Only bone that does not articulate with any other bone

Craniovertebral Junction Joints

Joint	Movements permitted
Atlanto-Occipital joint	Flexion and Extension of head (Nodding) Lateral flexion (Bending of neck)
Atlanto-Axial joint	**Side-to-side rotation of head (Looking towards left or right)**

JOINTS OF THORACIC WALL

Intervertebral	Symphysis	Adjacent vertebral bodies bound together by IV disc
Costovertebral • Joint of head of rib • Costotransverse	Synovial Plane/Gliding joint	Head of rib with superior and inferior facets of vertebral body Tubercle of rib with transverse process of vertebra
Costochondral	Synchondrosis	Cartilage and bone bound together by periosteum
Interchondral	Synovial plane joint	Between costal cartilages of 6th-9th ribs
Sternocostal	1st–Synchondrosis 2nd–7th–Synovial plane joint	Articulation of costal cartilages with sternum
Sternoclavicular	Saddle type of synovial joint	
Manubriosternal	Symphysis	
Xiphisternal	Synchondrosis	

132. Identify the type of joint shown below: *(NEET 2020)*

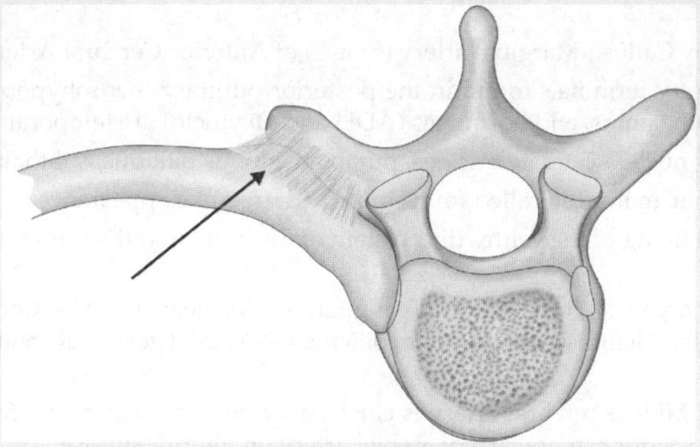

a. Synovial
b. Fibrous
c. Syndesmosis
d. Symphysis

Ans. is 'a' Synovial

Explanation: Arrow points to costotransverse joint–type of synovial plane joint.

133. Joint involved in movement of head from left to right is: *(NEET 2019)*

a. Atlanto-axial
b. Atlanto-occipital
c. C2-C3 joint
d. C3-C4 joint

Ans. is "a' Atlanto-axial

134. Costal cartilage of 8th and 9th ribs articulate with each other by which type of joint? *(NEET 2018)*

a. Fibrous joint
b. Primary cartilaginous joint
c. Secondary cartilaginous joint
d. Synovial joint

Ans. is 'd' Synovial joint

135. Movement occurring at atlantoaxial joint is: *(NEET 2016)*

a. Flexion
b. Bending
c. Rotation
d. Nodding

Ans. is 'c' Rotation

Types of epiphysis	
Pressure	Head of femur, head of humerus, **lower end of radius, tibial condyles**
Traction	Greater and lesser trochanters of femur, **mastoid process**, medial and lateral tubercles of humerus
Atavistic	**Coracoid process**, os trigonum
Aberrant	Head of 1st metacarpal, Base of other metacarpals

136. Which of the following is a traction epiphysis? *(NEET 2016)*

a. Distal radius
b. Mastoid process
c. Tibial condyles
d. Coracoid process

Ans. is 'b' Mastoid process

Previously Asked Facts

- Zona pellucida is a glycoprotein layer surrounding plasma membrane of oocyte. This layer binds spermatozoa and is required to initiate acrosome reaction.
- Spermatogenesis
  - Spermatogonia → *Mitosis* → Primary spermatocytes → *Meiosis* → Secondary spermatocytes → *Mitosis* → Spermatids → *Spermiogenesis (maturation)* → Sperms
- Stages of meiosis
  - Prophase (Leptotene → Zygotene → Pachytene → Diplotene → Diakinesis)
  - Metaphase
  - Anaphase
  - Telophase

- Blaschko's lines are lines of normal cell development in the skin. These are invisible lines along which certain skin diseases develop.
- Paracentral lobule is supplied by Calloso-Marginal artery (branch of Anterior Cerebral Artery)
- Herring bodies are neurosecretory terminals found in the posterior pituitary (neurohypophysis). They represent the terminal end of the axons from the hypothalamus, and hormones (ADH and Oxytocin) are temporarily stored in these locations.
- Basal ganglia include following nuclei - caudate nucleus, putamen, globus pallidus, subthalamic nucleus and substantia nigra.
- Arbor vitae is the cerebellar white matter, so called for its branched, tree-like appearance.
- Ependyma is the thin epithelial lining of the ventricular system of the brain and the central canal of the spinal cord, made up of ciliated simple columnar cells.
- *Auditory pathway*: Hair cells of organ of corti → Spiral ganglion → Cochlear nerve → Cochlear nuclei → Trapezoid body → Superior olivary complex → Lateral lemniscus → Inferior colliculus → Medial geniculate body → Auditory radiation → Superior temporal gyrus
- *Arterial supply of cerebral cortex*: Middle cerebral artery is chief artery on superolateral surface; Anterior cerebral artery is chief artery on medial surface and Posterior cerebral artery is chief artery on inferior surface.
- There are four extensions (recesses) of third ventricle: Suprapineal recess, Pineal recess, Infundibular recess and Optic recess.
- Chorda Tympani is a branch of facial nerve carrying taste sensations from anterior 2/3rd of the tongue and preganglionic parasympathetic fibers to the submandibular ganglion, providing secretomotor innervation to the submandibular and sublingual glands.
- Yoke extraocular muscles (contralateral synergists): Pair of muscles (one from each eye) which contract simultaneously during version movements. For example, right lateral rectus and left medial rectus act as yoke muscles for extroversion movements.
- Skin over the angle of jaw is supplied by Great auricular nerve.
- Skin on tip of nose is supplied by External nasal branch of Ophthalmic division of Trigeminal nerve.
- Parotid duct (Stenson's duct) pierces buccal fat pad, buccopharyngeal fascia and buccinator muscle and opens on the mucous membrane of cheek opposite to second upper molar tooth. It does not pierce deep cervical fascia.

Branches of external carotid artery	
From medial side	Ascending pharyngeal
From front	• Superior thyroid artery • Lingual artery • Facial artery
From behind	• Occipital artery • Posterior auricular artery
Terminal branches	• Superficial temporal artery • Maxillary artery

Branches of internal carotid artery	
Parts	***Branches***
Cervical	No branches
Petrous	• Caroticotympanic arteries, Artery of pterygoid canal
Lacerum	No branches
Cavernous	• Capsular branches (supply cavernous sinus wall) • Meningohypophyseal trunk
Cerebral	• Ophthalmic • Anterior cerebral • Middle cerebral • Posterior communicating • Anterior choroidal

- Laryngocele refers to dilatation of the laryngeal ventricular saccule located in paraglottic space of supraglottic.
- The sacral hiatus corresponds to the posterior caudal opening at the end of the sacral canal, which usually occurs at S5 vertebra. The fifth sacral nerve root exits via the sacral hiatus. It is covered posteriorly by the sacrococcygeal ligament, subcutaneous fatty layer and the skin.
- There are 31 pairs of spinal nerves (8 cervical, 12 thoracic, 5 lumbar, 5 sacral and 1 coccygeal). Spinal nerves are mixed nerves containing both sensory and motor fibres.
- Radiocarpal joint is formed by four bones – **Radius, Scaphoid, Lunate, Triquetrum**

- ❖ Axillary nerve is closely related to the inferior part of the shoulder joint capsule.

Nerve	Root value
Axillary nerve	C5,C6
Radial nerve	C5-8, T1
Median nerve	C5-8, T1
Ulnar nerve	C8,T1
Musculocutaneous nerve	C5, C6, C7

Some important nerves of upper limb and supplied muscles	
Dorsal scapular nerve (C5)	Rhomboid minor, Rhomboid major, Levator scapulae
Long thoracic nerve ((3, 6, 7)	Serratus anterior muscle
Supracapular nerve (C5, 6)	Supraspinatus and infraspinatus muscles
Nerve to subclavius (C5, 6)	Subclavius
Lateral pectoral nerve ((3, 6, 7)	Pectoralis major muscle
Musculocutaneous nerve (C5, 6, 7)	Coracobrachialis, Biceps brachii, Brachialis
Upper subcapsular nerve (C5, 6)	Subcapsularis
Thoracodorsal nerve (C6, 7, 8)	Latissimus dorsi
Lower subcapsular nerve (C5, 6)	Subscapsularis, Teres major
Axillary nerve (C5, 6)	Deltoid, Teres minor

- ❖ Anconeus assists in extension of elbow.
- ❖ Rotator cuff (Musculotendinous cuff) of shoulder is formed by blending of tendons of supraspinatus (superiorly), infraspinatus and teres minor (posteriorly) and subscapularis (anteriorly).
- ❖ Tennis elbow or lateral epicondylitis is a type of repetitive strain injury resulting from tendon overuse and failed healing of the tendon. The extensor carpi radialis brevis muscle plays a key role. Medial epicondylitis is also known as Golfer's elbow.
- ❖ Coracoclavicular ligament has two parts, conoid (medial) and trapezoid (lateral). The weight of the upper limb is transmitted to the clavicle through the coraco-clavicular ligament.
- ❖ The subclavius protects the underlying brachial plexus and subclavian vessels from a broken clavicle.
- ❖ The axillary sheath, derived from deep cervical fascia, is a fibrous sheath that encloses the first portion of the axillary artery, together with the brachial plexus
- ❖ Vastus medialis stabilizes patella and prevents its lateral dislocation by providing a medial tether.
- ❖ Sciatic nerve is the thickest in the body. Saphenous nerve is the longest cutaneous nerve in the body.
- ❖ Oblique popliteal ligament is an expansion from the tendon of semimembranosus attachment to intercondylar line of femur.
- ❖ Peroneus longus tendon is lodged in the groove on posterior surface of lateral malleolus.
- ❖ Sural nerve carries sensory supply of lateral border of the foot, 5th toe and posterolateral corner of foot. Saphenous nerve carries sensory supply of anterior and medial portion of leg and medial border of foot.
- ❖ The aortic valve is a semilunar valve with three cusps which include **left, right and posterior**.
- ❖ Heart receives parasympathetic supply from Vagus; sympathetic supply from T1-T5 spinal cord segments and pain sensation arising due to ischemia is conveyed by afferents which pass through sympathetic cardiac fibers and reach the T1 to T5 cord segments on left side. Pain gets referred to medial side of left arm, forearm and upper part of front of chest.
- ❖ Left Anterior Descending (LAD) artery is known as 'Widow's artery' in Myocardial infarction.
- ❖ Serosa is absent in esophagus.
- ❖ The lower limit of the inferior border of the lung is 2 ribs above the pleural reflection.

	Inferior margin of pleural reflection	Lower border of lung
Midclavicular line	8th rib	6th rib
Midaxillary line	10th rib	8th rib
Lateral border of erector spinae	12th rib	10th rib

- ❖ Inferior angle of scapula is at T7 level. Spine of scapula is at T4 level.
- ❖ The primary muscle of the upper esophageal sphincter is the cricopharyngeal part of the inferior pharyngeal constrictor.
- ❖ Latissimus Dorsi is also known as 'Tree climbing muscle'. Climbing of tree is helped by - Latissimus Dorsi and Pectoralis major.

- Only 3 to 6 intercostal nerves are typical intercostal nerves. Lower six intercostals nerves supply both thoracic and anterior abdominal walls and upper two intercostals also supply the upper limbs.
- Right bronchus is shorter and wider than left bronchus.
- The gallbladder lies on the inferior surface of the liver closely related to segment IV or the quadrate lobe.
- Caudate lobe or Segment I of liver (anatomical part of right lobe) belongs physiologically to both right and left lobes because it receives blood from right and left hepatic arteries; right and left branches of portal vein; and drains bile into both right and left hepatic duct.
- Characteristic features of large intestine are—3 longitudinal bands formed by longitudinal muscle coat called Taeniae coli; sacculations or haustrations, fat filled peritoneal pouches called appendices epiploicae (not found in appendix, caecum and rectum). Greater part is fixed except for appendix, transverse colon and sigmoid colon. Peyer's patches (seen in small intestine) are not present.
- Visceral surface of spleen is related to fundus of stomach (gastric impression), left kidney (renal impression), splenic flexure of colon (colic impression) and tail of pancreas (pancreatic impression).
- A posterior gastric ulcer may perforate into the lesser sac (omental bursa). The leaking fluid passes out through epiploic foramen to reach the hepatorenal pouch (greater sac).
- Dieulafoy's lesion is a characterized by a dilated tortuous submucosal artery most commonly in the stomach wall, that erodes overlying mucosa and bleeds.
- The prepyloric vein of mayo is a tributary of the right gastric vein and is the external landmark of the gastroduodenal junction.
- Cervix drains into Iliac nodes.
- The correct order of arterial supply of uterus is – Uterine artery + Ovarian artery → Arcuate artery anastomosis → Radial artery → Spiral and Basal arteries
- Transverse cervical ligament of Mackenrodt connects lateral aspect of cervix and upper vaginal wall to lateral pelvic wall.
- Narrowest part of male urethra is membranous urethra.
- Waldeyer's fascia connects rectum to sacrum.
- Pudendal canal (Alcock's canal) is a fascial canal in the lateral wall of ischiorectal fossa, enclosing pudendal nerve and internal pudendal vessels (artery and vein).
- Middle rectal artery is a branch of internal iliac artery. It is distributed to the rectum, anastomosing with the superior rectal artery and inferior rectal artery.
- The layers of scrotum from outside to inside are:
  - Skin
  - Dartos muscle (smooth muscle layer) continuous with Colle's fascia of perineum posteriorly and Scarpa's fascia and Camper's fascia anteriorly
  - The external spermatic fascia, extension from external oblique
  - The cremasteric muscle, continuous with fascia from internal oblique
  - The internal spermatic fascia, continuous with fascia from fascia transversalis

CHAPTER 2

Physiology

BODY FLUIDS

BODY FLUID COMPOSITION

The distribution of water in various compartments of the body is summarized in the following diagram:

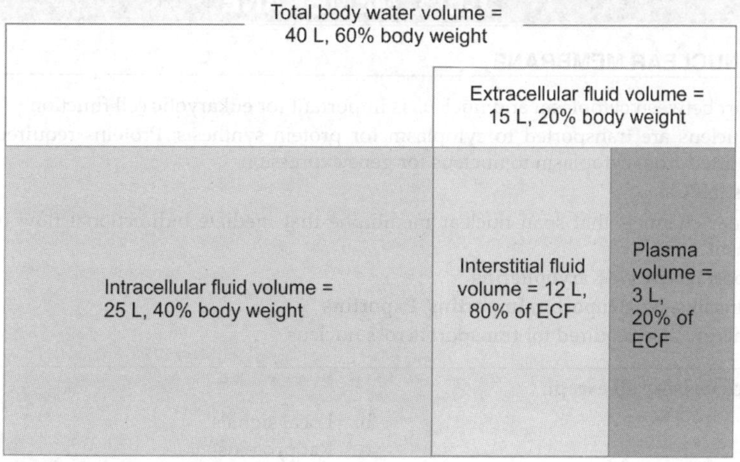

- Approximately 60% of total body weight in adults is composed of water.
- Most of the fluid volumes are calculated directly from dilution methods, except for ICF and interstitial fluid. Both of these are calculated indirectly by calculating other body fluids.
  - ICF = Total body water volume – ECF volume
  - Interstitial fluid = ECF volume – Plasma volume

Indicators used for fluid compartment volume estimation	
Total body water volume	Deuterium oxide, Tritium oxide, Aminopyrine, Antipyrine
Extracellular fluid volume	Inulin (most accurate) 22Na, 125I-iothalamate, thiosulfate
Plasma volume	Evans blue, Serum albumin labeled with I-125
Blood volume	51Cr-labeled RBCs

Body Fat Estimation

- Total body water constitutes 72–73% of fat free mass of body and is relatively a constant proportion.
- Thus, fat free mass of the body can be calculated from total body water using formula:
  - Fat free mass (kg) = Total body water (kg) / 0.732
- Total body fat (kg) = Body weight (kg)–Fat free mass (kg)

1. Estimation of total body fat can be done by measuring: *(NEET 2016)*

a. Waist-Hip ratio
b. Total body water
c. Body mass index
d. Total body calcium

Ans. is 'b' Total body water

POTASSIUM HOMEOSTASIS

Shifting K+ into cells	Shifting K+ out of cells
Insulin	Insulin deficiency
Aldosterone	Aldosterone deficiency
Beta adrenergic agonists	Beta adrenergic blockade
Alkalosis	Acidosis Cell lysis Strenuous exercise Increased ECF osmolarity

- ***Insulin***: It shifts the potassium from outside to inside, hence K^+ **influx.**
- ***Plasma osmolarity***: Increased extracellular fluid osmolarity causes osmotic flow of water out of the cells. The cellular dehydration increases intracellular potassium concentration, thereby promoting diffusion of potassium out of the cells.
- **Aldosterone** affects the renal handling of potassium via the principal cells of the DCT and Collecting ducts.
- **Epinephrine** increases the action of the sodium-potassium pump, thereby causing a change in the potassium concentration.

2. Hormone which affects K+ ion concentration: *(NEET 2016)*

a. GH
b. Thyroxine
c. Insulin
d. Oxytocin

Ans. is 'c' Insulin

CELL MEMBRANE

TRANSPORT ACROSS NUCLEAR MEMBRANE

- Macromolecular transport between cytoplasm and nucleus is important for eukaryotic cell function
- RNAs synthesized in nucleus are transported to cytoplasm for protein synthesis; Proteins required for nuclear function (like transcription) are transported from cytoplasm to nucleus for gene expression
- **Nuclear pore complexes (NPCs)**
  - Large macromolecular channels that span nuclear membrane that mediate bidirectional flow of macromolecules between nucleus and cytoplasm
  - Regulated by transport receptors–**Karyopherins**
  - Composed of proteins like–**Nucleoportin, Importins, Exportins**
  - Complex local signals are also required for transport across nucleus

3. Transport across nucleus is by all except: *(NEET 2018)*

a. Karyopherins
b. Local signals
c. Importins
d. Rat proteins

Ans. is 'd' Rat proteins

RAFTS AND CAVEOLAE

- **Lipid rafts are regions in plasma membrane** that are rich in cholesterol and sphingolipids
- They are thought to be involved in the regulation of signal transduction and in transcytosis
- Currently two basic types of lipid rafts have been identified:
  - Planar lipid rafts (noncaveolar or glycolipid rafts) - Continuous with plane of cell membrane (they do not invaginate)
  - Caveolae–Flask-shaped membrane depressions; caveolin protein is present in these regions

4. Lipid rafts are seen in: *(NEET 2016)*

a. Ribosomes
b. Mitochondria
c. Plasma membrane
d. ER

Ans. is 'c' Plasma membrane

RESTING MEMBRANE POTENTIAL

Resting membrane potential (RMP) is principally due to concentration difference of K^+ in ECF and ICF. In neurons, the resting membrane potential is usually about -70 mV, which is close to the equilibrium potential for K^+; but the value of RMP is exactly same as equilibrium potential of Cl^-. It is because other ions also diffuse through membrane, though their effect is very little.

Effects of ion concentration change on membrane potential

- *Hypokalemia*: Gradient more favourable for K^+ to diffuse out of the cell → membrane potential is reduced and the neuron is hyperpolarized
- *Hyperkalemia* : Has major effect on RMP; moves the resting potential closer to the threshold for eliciting an action potential
- *Hypercalcemia*: Stabilize the membrane by decreasing excitability
- *Hypocalcemia*: **Increases the excitability of nerve** by decreasing the amount of depolarization necessary to produce the action potential
- *Hyponatremia*: Has no effect on resting membrane potential; mainly it decreases the size of action potential

5. Excitability of cells is maximally affected by change in concentration of which ion? *(NEET 2016)*

a. K^+
b. Na^+
c. Cl^-
d. Ca^{+2}

Ans. is 'd' Ca^{+2}

EQUILIBRIUM POTENTIAL

Equilibrium potential is the membrane potential at which equilibrium exists between influx and efflux of ions.

The Nernst equation can be used to calculate the potential of an ion of charge z across a membrane. This potential is determined using the concentration of the ion both inside and outside the cell:

$$E = \frac{RT \ln [\text{ion outside the cell}]}{ZF [\text{ion inside the cell}]} = -\frac{2.3026\, RT \log 10 [\text{ion outside the cell}]}{ZF [\text{ion inside the cell}]}$$

When the membrane is in thermodynamic equilibrium (i.e. no net flux of ions), the membrane potential must be equal to the Nernst potential.

- E_m = The membrane potential
- R = The ideal gas constant
- T = The temperature in kelvin
- F = Faraday's constant (coulombs per mole)
- Z is the number of moles of electrons transferred in the cell reaction.

6. True about Nernst equation: *(NEET 2016)*

a. Used to calculate equilibrium potential
b. Calculated for non-ionic solution
c. Nernst potential for Cl^- is –90 mv
d. All are correct

Ans. is 'a' Used to calculate equilibrium potential

GIBBS-DONNAN EFFECT

- Behaviour of charged particles near a **semi-permeable membrane** that fail to distribute evenly across the two sides of membrane
- Cause is the **presence of a differently charged substance that is unable to pass through** the membrane and thus creates an uneven electrical charge
- **Gibbs-Donnan equilibrium** is established which satisfies two conditions -
  - Both the compartments must be electroneutral
  - The product of diffusible ions (anions and cations) must be equal in both compartments
- At Gibbs-Donnan equilibrium; following **disparities** are seen:
  - Concentration of total ions is greater in compartment that has non-diffusible anion
  - Total concentration of diffusible cation is greater in compartment that has non-diffusible anion
  - Total concentration of diffusible anion is greater in the opposite compartment
- ***Physiological role***: Intracellular fluid contains non-diffusible anions like proteins and organic phosphate where as K^+ and Cl^- are diffusible cation and anion. Due to Gibbs Donnan equilibrium:
  - Concentration of K^+ is greater in ICF than ECF
  - Concentration of Cl^- is greater in ECF than ICF
  - Total number of ions is greater in ICF than ECF
  - All these effects help to maintain the shape and volume of cells

7. Due to Donnan-Gibbs effect: *(NEET 2016)*

a. Concentration of K^+ is greater in ECF
b. Concentration of Cl^- is greater in ECF
c. Total ions are more in ICF
d. All are true

Ans. is 'c' Total ions are more in ICF

Types of transport across cell membrane

	Carrier protein involved	*Energy required*	*Concentration gradient*
Simple diffusion	No	No	Along
Facilitated diffusion	Yes	No	Along
Active transport	Yes	Yes	Against
Exocytosis	No	Yes	—
Endocytosis • Pinocytosis and phagocytosis • Receptor mediated endocytosis	 No Yes	 Yes Yes	 — —

Physiology

8. True about facilitated diffusion: *(NEET 2016)*

a. Active
b. Requires carrier
c. Require ATP
d. Against concentration gradient

Ans. is 'b' Requires carrier

NERVE-MUSCLE PHYSIOLOGY

CARDIAC MYOCYTE ACTION POTENTIAL

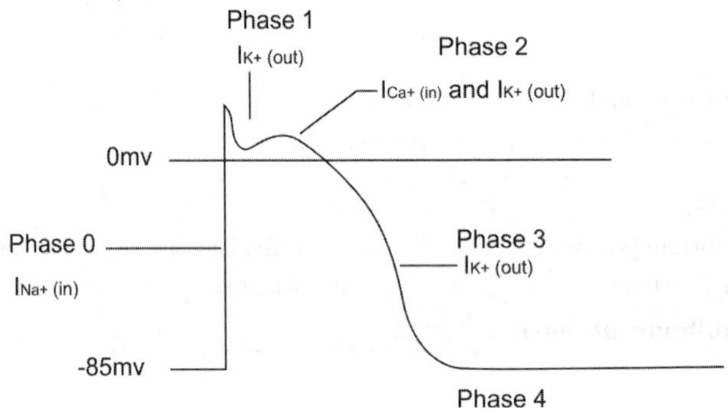

Phase 0	Phase of rapid depolarization	Opening of fast sodium channels with Na^+ influx
Phase 1	Initial phase of rapid repolarization	Closure of fast sodium channels and opening of K^+ channels
Phase 2	Plateau phase	Opening of voltage gated slow Ca^{++} channels with calcium influx
Phase 3	Final repolarization	Opening of K^+ channels with K^+ efflux
Phase 4	Resting membrane potential (-90 mV)	Constant K^+ efflux

9. Action potential in cardiac muscles is due to which ions? *(NEET 2016)*

a. K^+
b. Na^+
c. Cs^{+2}
d. Cl^-

Ans. is 'b' Na^+

MYOFIBRILS

- Each muscle fiber contains several hundred to several thousands myofibrils. Each myofibril is composed of about 1500 adjacent myosin filaments and 3000 actin filaments, which are large polymerized protein molecules that are responsible for the actual muscle contraction.
- The thick filaments are myosin, and the thin filaments are actin. The myosin and actin filaments partially interdigitate and thus cause the myofibrils to have alternate light and dark bands.
- The light bands contain only actin filaments and are called **I bands** because they are isotropic to polarized light. The dark bands contain myosin filaments, as well as the ends of the actin filaments where they overlap the myosin, and are called **A bands** because they are anisotropic to polarized light.
- The portion of the A band where the actin and myosin filaments do not overlap is called **H zone**. The line passing through the centre of A band is called the **M line**. The ends of the actin filaments are attached to a so-called **Z disc.**
- These bands give skeletal and cardiac muscle their striated appearance.
- The portion of the myofibril that lies between two successive Z discs is called a **sarcomere**.

Other Proteins in Muscle Fibres

- Troponin T binds the troponin components to tropomyosin.
- Troponin I inhibits the interaction of myosin with actin.
- Troponin C contains the binding sites for the Ca^{2+} that helps initiate contraction.
- Actinin binds actin to the Z lines

- **Titin connects the Z lines to the M lines** and provides scaffolding for the sarcomere.
- Desmin adds structure to the Z lines in part by binding the Z lines to the plasma membrane.

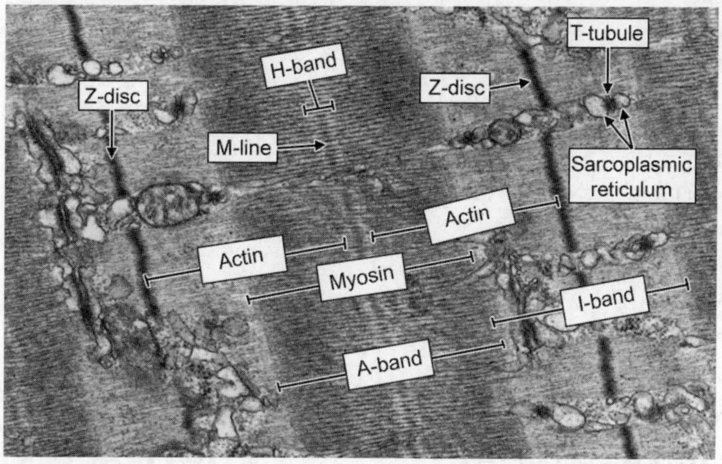

10. Protein connecting Z-lines to M-lines: *(NEET 2016)*

a. Kinin
b. Desmin
c. Titin
d. Actin

Ans. is 'c' Titin

MUSCLE CONTRACTION (OVERVIEW)

Thin Filament

- Initiated with calcium
- Tropomyosin blocks "binding groove" for myosin on actin
- Calcium binds troponin
- Ca-Troponin → removal of tropomyosin block (conformational change in tropomyosin)

Thick Filament

- Myosin binds ATP at rest
- Hydrolyzes to ADP and Pi–**via ATPase activity**
- Assumes "cocked" position (ready for contraction)

Contraction

- Tropomyosin block removed → myosin binding
- Myosin binds to actin
- Moves along actin filament → "Power stroke"
- Myosin binds new ATP

11. True about myosin: *(NEET 2016)*

a. Thin filament
b. Covers active site of action
c. Has ATPase activity
d. Ca^{+2} binding protein

Ans. is 'c' Has ATPase activity

SLOW AND FAST TWITCH MUSCLE FIBRES

Slow-twitch Fibers

- Time to peak tension = Slow
- Also called red fibers (deep red color)
- Color from amount of myoglobin (binds O_2)

- Extra myoglobin resists fatigue
- More mitochondria = More oxidative phosphorylation
- More fatty acid metabolism
- Moderate glycolytic activity
- **Postural muscles (spine)** = More slow twitch fibres for sustained tone

Fast-twitch Fibers

- Time to peak tension = Fast
- Also called white (pale color)
- Primarily metabolize glucose and glycogen
- More glycogen storage
- Increased glycolytic activity
- Few mitochondria = Less oxidative phosphorylation
- **Eyes and hand muscles** = Many fast twitch fibers

Most muscles have a mixture of fast/slow fibers

12. White fibers are present in which muscle? *(NEET 2016)*

a. Calf muscle
b. Back muscles
c. Gluteal muscles
d. Hand muscles

Ans. is 'd' Hand muscles

POST-SYNAPTIC POTENTIALS

- *Excitatory postsynaptic potential (EPSP)*: Neurotransmitter triggers the opening of **ligand-gated Na^+ channels** → influx of Na^+ and depolarization of postsynaptic membrane. The excitably of post-synaptic neuron is increased as RMP comes closer to threshold (firing) level.
- *Inhibitory postsynaptic potential (IPSP)*: Neurotransmitter triggers opening of **ligand-gated Cl channels** → influx of Cl^- and hyperpolarization of post synaptic membrane. The excitability of postsynaptic neuron is reduced, as RMP moves away from firing (threshold) level. IPSP can also be produced by opening of ligand-gated K^+ channels which causes efflux of K^+ and hyperpolarization.

13. EPSP is due to: *(NEET 2016)*

a. K^+ influx
b. Na^+ efflux
c. Na^+ influx
d. Ca^{++} influx

Ans. is 'c' Na^+ influx

CARDIOVASCULAR PHYSIOLOGY

BLOOD GROUPS

- Defined by RBC antigens

ABO Blood Group System

	Group A	Group B	Group AB	Group O
Antibodies in plasma	Anti-B	Anti-A	None	Anti-A and Anti-B
Antigens in RBC	A antigen	B antigen	A and B antigen	None

- Rh System
  - Rh positive: D antigen +ve
  - Rh negative: D antigen –ve

Blood Group Testing

- Patient RBCs plus antibodies–Anti-A, Anti-B, Anti-D
- Agglutination indicates presence of antigen

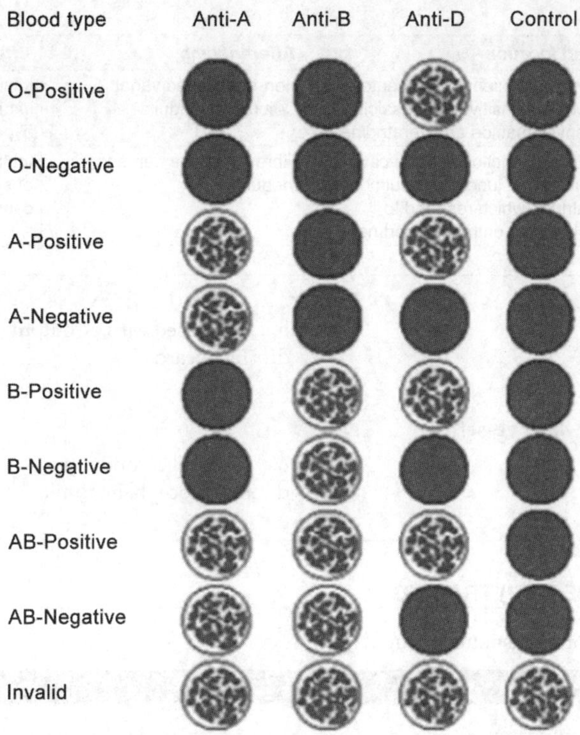

14. Which blood group does the given slide signify? *(NEET 2019)*

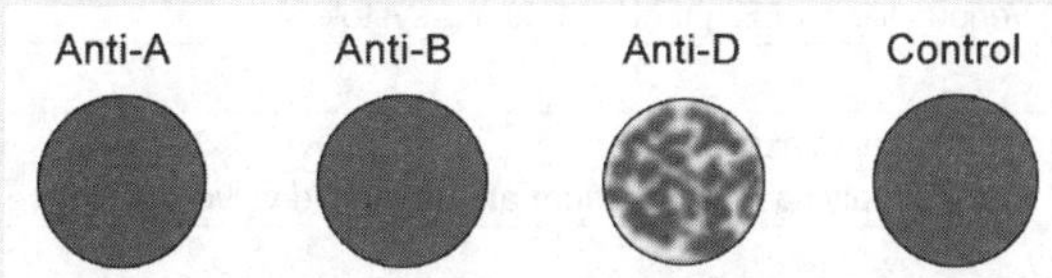

a. AB -ve
b. AB +ve
c. O -ve
d. O +ve

Ans. is 'd' O +ve

HEART SOUNDS

Feature	S1	S2	S3	S4
Character	Low pitched; slightly prolonged "lub"	Shorter high pitched "dup"	Soft low pitched weak rumbling	Atrial kick
Cause	Closure of mitral and tricuspid valves	Closure of aortic and pulmonary valves	Rapid early ventricular filling d/t high atrial pressure	Late ventricular filling d/t atrial contraction
Timing	Start of ventricular systole	Just after end of ventricular systole	Early diastole	Immediately before 1st heart sound (presystolic)
Causes	Normal	Normal	Normal in young patients and pregnancy; Acute heart failure	Hypertension, Hypertrophic cardiomyopathy

15. Heart sound occurring just before closure of AV: *(NEET 2016)*

A. S1
b. S2
c. S3
d. S4

Ans. is 'd' S4

Major cardiovascular reflexes			
Reflex	***Receptors and location***	***Afferent limb***	***Efferent limb and response***
Arterial baroreceptor reflex	Stretch receptors in vessel wall of carotid sinus **(Internal Carotid artery)** and aortic arch, which respond to changes in arterial blood pressure	Fibres in glossopharyngeal (carotid sinus) and vagus (aortic sinus) nerves to medulla	Homeostatic control of arterial blood pressure via changes in cardiac output and systemic vascular resistance mediated by autonomic nervous system

Contd...

Contd…

Reflex	*Receptors and location*	*Afferent limb*	*Efferent limb and response*
Bezold-Jarisch reflex (Coronary chemoreflex)	Mechanical and chemosensitive receptors in ventricular walls, sensitive to capsaicin, serotonin, phenylbiguanide and veratridine	Non-myelinated vagal C-fibres to medulla	Inhibition of sympathetic outflow resulting in bradycardia, peripheral vasodilation and hypotension
Bainbridge reflex	Stretch receptors at junction of vena cava and right atrium and at junction of pulmonary vein and left atrium, which respond to changes in volume in central compartment	Fibres in vagus nerve to medulla	Inhibition of vagal outflow and enhancement of sympathetic outflow to sinoatrial node causing tachycardia

16. Bainbridge reflex causes: *(NEET 2019)*

a. Bradycardia
b. Decreased cardiac output
c. Decreased venous return
d. Tachycardia

Ans. is 'd' Tachycardia

17. Baroreceptors are related to which vessel? *(NEET 2016)*

a. Internal carotid artery
b. External carotid artery
c. Subclavian artery
d. Brachiocephalic trunk

Ans. is 'a' Internal carotid artery

JUGULAR VENOUS PRESSURE (JVP) TRACING

❖ Right atrial pressure variations are transmitted to jugular veins

Jugular venous pressure	
Positive waves	
a-wave	Right atrial contraction
c-wave	Bulging of tricuspid valve into right atrium during **isovolumetric RV contraction**
v-wave	Venous filling of Right atrium during systole
Negative waves/Descents	
x-descent	Right atrial relaxation
y-descent	Rapid emptying of right atrium after tricuspid valve opening

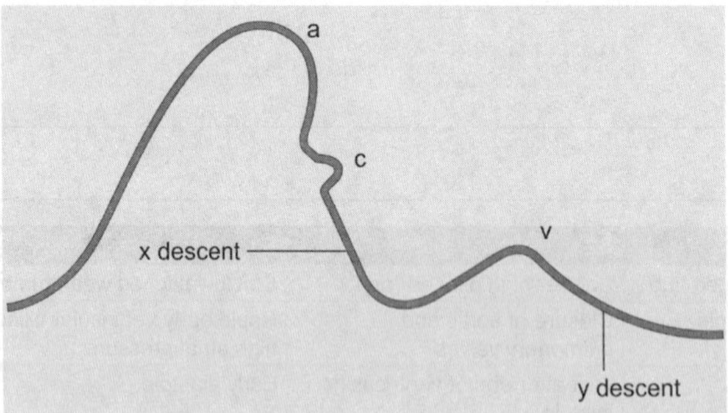

18. c-wave in jugular venous pressure corresponds to: *(NEET 2018)*

a. Atrial contraction
b. Atrial relaxation
c. Isovolumetric ventricular relaxation
d. Isovolumetric ventricular contraction

Ans. is 'd' Isovolumetric ventricular contraction

19. 'v' Wave in JVP is due to: *(NEET 2016)*

a. Right atrial contraction
b. Right atrial relaxation
c. Closure of tricuspid valve
d. Isovolumetric relaxation

Ans. is 'c' Closure of tricuspid valve

20. C wave in JVP is seen due to: *(NEET 2020)*

a. Atrial systole
b. Closure of tricuspid valve during isovolumetric contraction
c. Venous filling
d. Right ventricular outflow

Ans. is 'b' Closure of tricuspid valve during isovolumetric contraction

STRESS RESPONSE

Two Phases–Ebb phase and Flow phase

Ebb phase	Flow phase
Hypometabolic phase	Hypermetabolic/Catabolic phase
Begins immediately after injury	Begins after 36–48 hours
Lasts for 36–48 hours	Lasts for 10–12 days
Decreased body temperature	Increased body temperature
Decreased O_2 consumption	Increased O_2 cosumption
↑Lactate	Normal Lactate
Hyperglycemia, Insulin resistance	Hyperglycemia, Insulin resistance
↓Insulin levels	Normal Insulin levels
Immune activation	Immunosuppression
↓Cardiac output, ↓plasma volume	↑Cardiac output, ↑plasma volume

21. Ebb phase and flow phase are seen in: *(NEET 2018)*

a. Normal cardiac cycle
b. Normal respiratory cycle
c. Stress response
d. Muscle contraction during exercise

Ans. is 'c' Stress response

RESPIRATORY PHYSIOLOGY

CHANGES IN RESPIRATORY SYSTEM WITH AGING

Changes with aging	
Air space size	Increased
Chest wall compliance	Decreased
Lung compliance	**Increased**
Total respiratory system compliance	Decreased
FEV_1	Decreased
Vital capacity	Decreased
Residual volume	**Increased**
Total lung capacity	Unchanged
Dead space ventilation	Increased
Neutrophils% in bronchial fluid	Increased
CD4:CD8 ratio in bronchial fluid	Increased
Anti-oxidants in bronchial fluid	Decreased
Mucociliary clearance	**Decreased**
Fibrotic interstitial tissue	**Increased**

22. With aging, what is true for lungs? *(NEET 2019)*

a. Pulmonary compliance increases
b. Residual volume decreases
c. Mucociliary clearance increases
d. Fibrosis of intestitium decreases

Ans. is 'a' Pulmonary compliance increases

LUNG VOLUMES AND CAPACITIES

Lung volumes		Lung capacities	
Tidal volume (TV): Air that moves into the lung with each normal inspiration or volume of air that moves out of lung with each expiration	500 mL	***Inspiratory capacity: IC = TV + IRV*** - Total amount of air that can be breathed in.	3800 mL
Inspiratory reserve volume (IRV): Air inspired with a maximal Inspiratory effort in excess of tidal volume.	3300 mL	***Vital capacity: VC = TV + IRV + ERV*** - Maximal amount of air that can be expelled out forcefully after a **maximal (deep) inspiration.**	4800 mL
Expiratory reserve volume (ERV): Air expelled with a maximal expiratory effort in excess of tidal volume.	1000 mL	***Functional residual capacity: FRC = ERV + RV*** - Volume of air remaining in the lung after **normal expiration.**	2200 mL
Residual volume (RV): Amount of air remaining in the lungs even after **forced expiration.**	1200 mL	***Total lung capacity: TLC = TV + IRV + ERV + RV*** - Amount of air present In the lung after a maximal inspiration. This is maximum volume to which the lungs can be expanded.	6000 mL

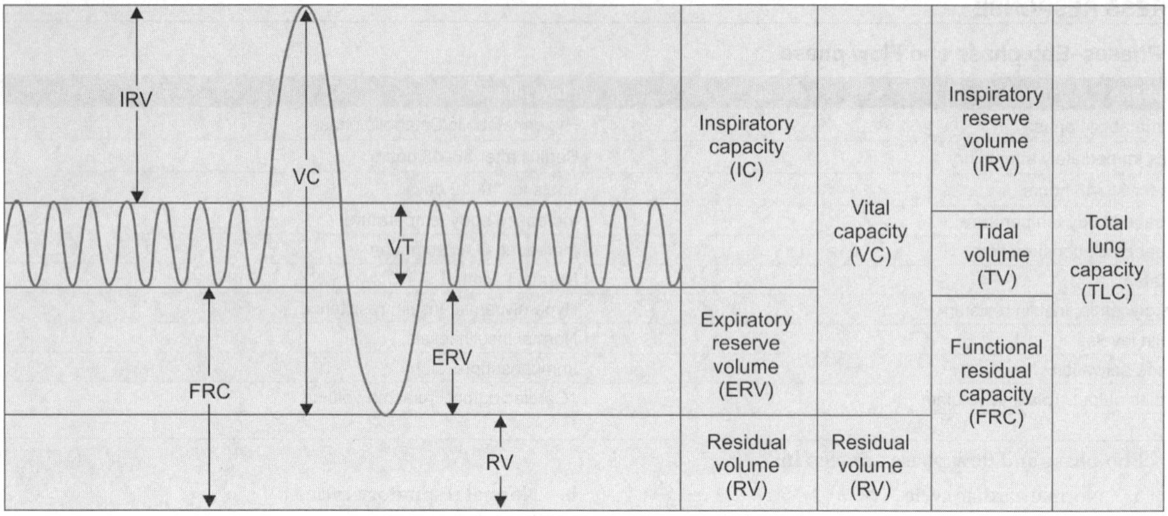

Closing Volume

- **Closing volume is the lung volume above residual volume at which airway in the lower, dependent parts of the lungs begin to close off.**
- *Example*: Suppose on forceful expiration, dynamic compression of airways closes smaller airways in lower dependent parts of lungs when lung volume is 1800 mL; then the closing volume is 600 mL (1800 - residual volume of 1200 mL).
- Closing capacity = Closing volume + residual volume.

The FEV1/FVC ratio: Used in the diagnosis of obstructive and restrictive lung disease.

- Represents the proportion of a person's vital capacity that they are able to expire in the first second of forced expiration to the full vital capacity.
- **Normal values are approximately 80%.**
- **It is decreased in obstructive lung disease and normal or increased in restrictive lung disease** (as the FEV_1 and FVC are equally reduced)

Pulmonary function measurement	Obstructive pulmonary disease	Restrictive pulmonary disease
FVC	Decrease/Normal	Decrease
FEV_1	Decrease	Decrease/Normal
FEV_1/FVC	Decrease	Normal/Increase

23. Functional residual capacity is lung volume: *(NEET 2019)*

a. After normal inspiration
b. After normal expiration
c. After forceful inspiration
d. After forceful expiration

Ans. is 'b' After normal expiration

24. In a pulmonary function test, values of FEV1 = 1.3 L and FVC = 3.9 L; signify: *(NEET 2019)*

a. Normal lung function
b. Obstructive lung disease
c. Restrictive lung disease
d. Both c and d

Ans. is 'b' Obstructive lung disease

Explanation: FEV_1/FVC = 1.3/3.9 = 33.3% (Normal value is approximately 80%)

25. Which of the following defines vital capacity? *(NEET 2016)*

a. Air in lung after normal expiration
b. Maximum air that can be expired after normal inspiration
c. Maximum air that can be expired after maximum inspiration
d. Maximum air in lung after end of maximal inspiration

Ans. is 'c' Maximum air that can be expired after maximum inspiration

26. True about residual volume: *(NEET 2016)*

a. Volume of air in lung normal inspiration
b. Volume of air in lung after maximum inspiration
c. Volume of air in lung after normal inspiration
d. Volume of air in lung after maximum expiration

Ans. is 'd' Volume of air in lung after maximum expiration

REGULATION OF RESPIRATION

Various brainstem centres are involved in regulation of respiration.

Dorsal respiratory group (DRG): It fires rhythmically during inspiration and hence is primarily responsible for maintaining inspiration. It also serves as initial processing centre for afferent inputs from peripheral chemoreceptors and baroreceptors.

Ventral respiratory group (VRG): It remains inactive during normal breathing and is primarily responsible for **active expiration during forceful breathing.**

Pre-Botzinger complex: Pacemaker for initiating spontaneous rhythmic respiration

Pneumotaxic center: It is located in the pons and is active during inspiration. It may play a role in switching between inspiration and expiration, because lesion involving this region results in apneusis (prolonged inspiration)

Apneustic center: It is located in the lower pons. It stimulates inspiration producing deep and prolonged inspiratory gasp.

Effect on respiration by transection at different levels of brain

Level of transection	*Effect on respiration*
Above pons	No effect on respiration
Mid-pontine (Pneumotaxic centre)	
• Vagi intact (inhibition of apneustic centre intact)	Deep and slow breathing; no change in rhythm
• B/l vagotomy (no inhibition of apneustic cenre)	Apneusis (sustained gasping inspiration)
Pontomedullary junction	Slightly irregular respiration
Below medulla	Respiration is stopped completely
B/l vagotomy (no brain lesion)	Deep and slow breathing

27. In forceful expiration, which of these neurons get fired? *(NEET 2019)*

a. Ventral respiratory group
b. Dorsal respiratory group
c. Pneumotaxic centre
d. Chemoreceptors

Ans. is 'a' Ventral respiratory group

28. Apneusis occurs when there is damage to: *(NEET 2016)*

a. Apneustic center with intact vagi
b. Apneustic center with bilateral vagotomy
c. Pneumotaxic center with intact vagi
d. Pneumotaxic center with bilateral vagotomy

Ans. is 'd' Pneumotaxic center with bilateral vagotomy

PERIPHERAL CHEMORECEPTORS

- Carotid body (in common carotid artery) and Aortic body (in aortic arch) detect change in blood-borne chemical concentrations
- Maintain homeostasis in cardiorespiratory system in response **to hypoxia and hypercapnia**
- **Glomus cells**
    - Contain variety of neurotransmitters (dopamine)
    - Transduce signals from bloodstream
    - Innervated by afferent nerve fibres from glossopharyngeal (carotid body) and vagus (aortic body) nerves
- Signal transduction
    - **Membrane depolarization is caused by inhibition of Potassium channels**–Most accepted theory
    - Neurotransmitter released from vesicles in Glomus cells
- Peripheral chemoreceptors convey information to the DRG neurons in medulla → Increase in the rate and depth of breathing
- Cause tachycardia vasoconstriction and increase in BP, along with hyperventilation
- Play a role in ventilation during exercise

29. Peripheral chemoreceptors respond to hypoxia using which channel? *(NEET 2019)*

a. Calcium channel
b. Sodium channel
c. Potassium channel
d. Chloride channel

Ans. is 'c' Potassium channel

CENTRAL CHEMORECEPTORS

- Located in a chemosensitive area on the ventral surface of the medulla near the exit of the ninth and tenth cranial nerves.
- The primary stimulus for the central chemoreceptors is an increase in the hydrogen ion concentration → excitation of the respiratory neurons → increase in the rate and depth of respiration.
- Hydrogen ions cannot cross blood-brain barrier. On the other hand, CO_2 being lipid soluble can easily cross blood brain barrier and is hydrated to give H^+ and HCO_3 ions. Now these H directly stimulate the central chemoreceptors.

- **Thus, central chemoreceptors are directly stimulated by an increase in H^+ concentration in CSF and brain interstitial tissue, which is brought about by change in arterial PCO_2 ($PaCO_2$).**
- Central chemoreceptors are not stimulated by hypoxia; rather like any other cells, they are depressed by hypoxia.

30. Central chemoreceptors are not stimulated by: (NEET 2016)

a. $\uparrow PCO_2$ b. $\uparrow H^+$ in CSF
c. Hypoxia d. All stimulate

Ans. is 'c' Hypoxia

VENTILATION–PERFUSION RATIO (V/Q RATIO)

- Considering normal value of cardiac output is 5 L/min and alveolar ventilation is 4.2 L/min; overall ventilation:perfusion ratio (V/Q ratio) = 0.8
- Apical alveoli are both underventilated and underperfused as compared to basal alveoli. However, effect of gravity is much more on perfusion. Thus, V/Q ratio is maximum at apex (about 3) and least at base (0.6) even in normal lungs.
- **Ventilation-Perfusion mismatch** - Due to less perfusion, partial pressures at apices are close to inspired air (high PaO_2 and low $PaCO_2$). Due to better perfusion, partial pressures at lung bases are close to pulmonary artery (low PaO_2 and high $PaCO_2$).
- V/Q ratio = Infinity
    - Means perfusion is zero
    - **Absolute dead space–No gas exchange (PO_2 is same as PO_2 in atmosphere)**
- V/Q ratio = Zero
    - Means there is no ventilation
    - Absolute shunt (Alveolar PO_2 is same as PO_2 in blood because O_2 diffuses from blood into alveoli and remains there due to absent ventilation)

31. True about infinite ventilation perfusion ratio: (NEET 2018)

a. Partial pressure of oxygen in alveoli is same as in blood b. Partial pressure of oxygen in alveoli is same as in atmosphere
c. There is absolute shunt d. There is relative dead space

Ans. is 'b' Partial pressure of oxygen in alveoli is same as in atmosphere

32. When V/Q ratio becomes infinity, what is true? (NEET 2020)

a. Partial pressures of oxygen and CO_2 becomes equal
b. Oxygen pressure is around 159 mm and CO_2 pressure is about 40 mm
c. Oxygen doesn't diffuse to blood and CO_2 doesn't diffuse into alveoli
d. Partial pressures of oxygen and CO_2 become equal to air in dead space

Ans. is 'c' Oxygen doesn't diffuse to blood and CO_2 doesn't diffuse into alveoli

SURFACTANT

- Major function: **Reduces the surface tension** of fluid lining the alveoli to avoid collapse
- Water molecules lining the alveoli produce an elastic contractile force due to surface tension which causes the alveoli to collapse.
- Surfactant is a mixture of phospholipids, proteins and ions, most important phospholipid of which is dipalmitoyl phosphatidyl choline (DPCC)
- **Secreted by type II alveolar epithelial cells**
- The phospholipid molecules have a hydrophilic head and two parallel hydrophobic 'tails'. Thus only head part of the molecule dissolves in the fluid lining the alveolar surface and the hydrophobic tails face the alveolar lumen. This new surface thus formed of the surfactant has a significantly reduced surface tension than the water molecules.
- **Deficiency of surfactant occurs in cigarette smokers.**
- **Infant Respiratory Distress Syndrome or Hyaline Membrane Disease** - Seen in premature infants not secreting adequate amounts of pulmonary surfactant. Therefore, surfactant is used therapeutically in HMD. Glucocorticoids administered to a pregnant woman cross the placenta to promote accelerated fetal lung maturation and production of surfactant.

33. Function of surfactant is: (NEET 2016)

a. Increases O_2 diffusion b. Decreases airway resistance
c. Prevents overexpansion of lung d. Reduction in surface tension

Ans. is 'd' Reduction in surface tension

34. Pulmonary surfactants is secreted by:

a. Type I pneumocytes b. Type II pneumocytes
c. Clara cells d. Bronchial epithelial cells

Ans. is 'b' Type II pneumocytes

OXYGEN-HEMOGLOBIN DISSOCIATION CURVE

- Plotting the amount of oxygen in association with hemoglobin (oxyhemoglobin) against the PO_2 of blood gives the oxygen-hemoglobin dissociation curve.
- **Sigmoid or S-shaped curve**
  - Four heme groups do not undergo simultaneous oxygenation
  - First O_2 molecule that binds INCREASES affinity of hemoglobin for 2nd molecule–**Co-operativity**
  - Co-operativity is a positive Allosteric effect (change in affinity of multi-subunit proteins for binding when influenced by other (smaller) molecules)
- Approximate saturation at 10 mm Hg is 10%, at 15 mm Hg is 20%, at 40 mm Hg is 75%, and at 60 mm Hg is 90%
- **Hb-O_2 curve shifts**
  - Right shift–Easier to release O_2
    - ↑–CO_2, 2,3-BPG, Temp, H+
    - **High altitude acclimatization** (rise in 2,3-BPG levels)
  - Left shift–Harder to release O_2
    - ↓–CO_2, 2,3-BPG, Temp, H+
    - **Fetal Hemoglobin (Higher O_2 affinity)**
    - Carboxy-hemoglobin
- 2,3-BPG levels
  - ↑2,3-BPG–Hypoxia, **alkalosis**, pregnancy, exercise
  - ↓2,3-BPG - **Acidosis**, Stored blood

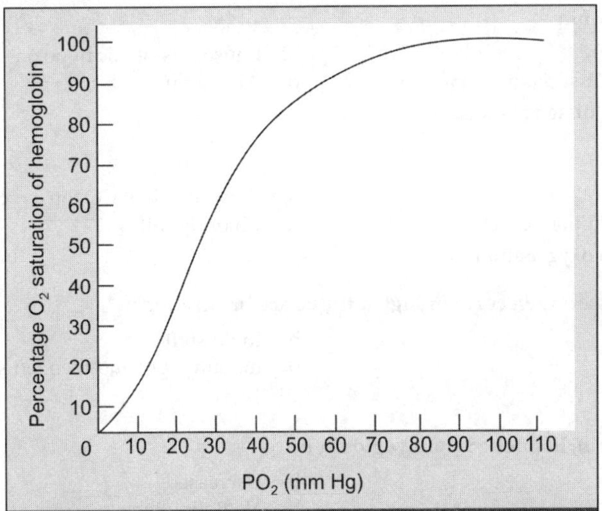

Oxygen-hemoglobin dissociation curve

Bohr Effect

- Increase in PCO_2 decreases the O_2 affinity to hemoglobin and shifts the oxygen dissociation curve to right
- Effect of CO_2 is mediated by increase in H^+ ions
- H^+ binds to globin chains (not heme) → Converts Hb to taut form which releases O_2 → shifts O_2 curve to right

Haldane Effect

- **Binding of O_2 to hemoglobin reduces its affinity for CO_2**
- In low O_2 environment, Hb is more likely to bind CO_2 to form Carbaminohemoglobin

Carbon Monoxide

- Toxic because it reacts with hemoglobin (at the same point as O_2) to form **Carboxyhemoglobin (COHb)**
- 240x the affinity of oxygen for Hb. So, CO-Hb dissociation curve is almost identical to O_2-Hb dissociation curve except that partial pressures are at a level of 1/250 as compared to O_2
- Blocks O_2 binding sites → Decreased O_2 carrying capacity of blood → **Anemic hypoxia**
- Other binding sites cannot offload O_2 → **Shift dissociation curve to Left**

Physiology

Gas Exchange in Tissue Vs Lungs

Tissues	Lungs
Low O_2 (consumption)	High O_2 (air)
High CO_2 (metabolism)	Low CO_2 (air)
High H^+	Low H^+
Favors O_2 unloading (Bohr effect)	Favors O_2 loading (Bohr effect)
Favors CO_2 loading (Haldane effect)	Favors CO_2 unloading (Haldane effect)

Myoglobin

- Myoglobin is a single polypeptide chain.
- One molecule of myoglobin can combine with one molecule of oxygen.
- Myoglobin has higher affinity to oxygen than that of Hb.
- **Bohr effect, Co-operativity and 2, 3-biphosphoglycerate effect are absent.**

35. Not true about Bohr effect: *(NEET 2016)*

a. Decrease affinity of O_2 by increase in PCO_2
b. Left shift of Hb-O_2 dissociation curve
c. It is due to H^+
d. All are true

Ans. is 'b' Left shift of Hb-O_2 dissociation curve

36. True about carboxyhemoglobin: *(NEET 2016)*

a. Take up O_2 very quickly
b. Causes histotoxic hypoxia
c. Causes left shift Hb-O_2 dissociation curve
d. All are true

Ans. is 'c' Causes left shift Hb-O_2 dissociation curve

37. Haldane effect: *(NEET 2016)*

a. Effect of 2, 3–BPG
b. Dissociation of CO_2 on oxygenation
c. Dissociation of O_2 on addition of CO_2
d. Chloride shift

Ans. is 'b' Dissociation of CO_2 on oxygenation

38. What happens to O_2-Hb dissociation curve in high altitude acclimatization? *(NEET 2016)*

a. No change
b. Right shift
c. Left shift
d. Initially right and then left shift

Ans. is 'b' Right shift

39. In comparison to hemoglobin, Bohr effect on myoglobin is: *(NEET 2016)*

a. Increased
b. Decreased
c. Same
d. No Bohr effect

Ans. is 'd' No Bohr effect

CHLORIDE SHIFT

- **Helps in transport of CO_2**
- RBCs convert CO_2 to HCO_3 - via **carbonic anhydrase**
- Bicarbonate inside RBCs leaves cell into plasma
- Chloride ions enter cell to maintain electrical neutrality–**Chloride shift**
- RBCs have high osmolality in venous blood → Water enters the RBC through osmosis. RBCs in venous blood are larger than normal. Hence, the hematocrit of venous blood is normally 3% greater than that of arterial blood

Note: Carbonic anhydrase is present in renal tubular cells (especially PCT), gastric mucosa, exocrine pancreas, cilia body of eye, erythrocytes and brain.

40. Function of chloride shift in RBCs:

a. Right shift of Hb-O_2 curve
b. Left shift of Hb-O_2 curve
c. Transport of CO_2
d. Diffusion of O_2 in alveoli

Ans. is 'c' Transport of CO_2

Physiology

HYPOXIA

Hypoxia is O_2 deficiency at the tissue level. Types of hypoxia:

Hypoxemia (Hypoxic Hypoxia)

- PO_2 of the arterial blood is reduced
- Causes–**Hypoventilation (COPD)**, high altitude, right to left shunt
- **Oxygen therapy useful**

Anemic Hypoxia

- Arterial PO_2 is normal but the amount of hemoglobin available to carry O_2 is reduced.
- Causes–Anemia, **Carbon monoxide poisoning**

Ischemic or Stagnant Hypoxia

- Blood flow to a tissue is so low that adequate O_2 is not delivered to it despite a normal PO_2 and hemoglobin concentration
- Causes–Shock, CHF

Histotoxic Hypoxia

- Amount of O_2 delivered to a tissue is adequate but, because of the action of a toxic agent, the tissue cells cannot make use of the O_2 supplied to them
- Cyanide poisoning

Hypoxia	Arterial O_2 (PaO_2)	Venous O_2 (PVO_2)
Hypoxic	↓	↓
Anemic	↓	↓
Histoxic	Normal	↑
Stagnant	Normal	↓

- Maximum A-V O_2 difference → Stagnant hypoxia
- Minimum A-V O_2 difference → Histotoxic hypoxia (Cyanide poisoning)

41. Oxygen therapy is useful in: *(NEET 2016)*

a. Anemic hypoxia
b. CO poisoning
c. Cyanide poisoning
d. COPD

Ans. is 'd' COPD

ALTITUDE ILLNESS

Acute Mountain Sickness (AMS) and High-Altitude Cerebral Edema (HACE)

- AMS is a neurologic syndrome characterized by non-specific symptoms (headache, nausea, fatigue and dizziness) with a paucity of physical findings, developing 6–12 hours after ascent to a high altitude.
- HACE is an encephalopathy whose hallmarks are ataxia and altered consciousness with diffuse cerebral involvement but generally without focal neurological deficits. Papilledema and retinal hemorrhages may develop.
- Risk factors–Rapid rate of ascent, prior history of altitude illness.
- Hypobaric hypoxia is the main trigger for altitude illness

High-Altitude Pulmonary Edema (HAPE)

- HAPE develops within 2–4 days after arrival at high altitude.
- *Risk factors:* Rapid rate of ascent, history of HAPE, respiratory tract infections and cold temperatures
- Non-cardiogenic pulmonary edema. Characterized by patchy pulmonary hypoxic vasoconstriction that leads to overperfusion in some areas
- *Manifestations:* Reduced exercise tolerance, cough, tachypnea and tachycardia. Crackles on auscultation

Prevention of Altitude Illness: Gradual ascent, with adequate time for acclimatization, is the best method for prevention of altitude illness. Another protective factor is high-altitude exposure during the preceding 2 months

Management of Altitude Illness

- Immediate descent
- Administration of oxygen
- Treatment with acetazolamide and/or dexamethasone
- Hyperbaric therapy if descent is not possible (to simulate descent)
- Adjunctive therapy with nifedipine for HAPE

42. A man develops dyspnea and palpitatitons after rapid ascent to 3000 m altitude. Which of the following should not be done? *(NEET 2020)*

a. Acetazolamide
b. Rapid descent
c. Oxygen supplementation
d. IV digoxin

Ans. is 'd' IV digoxin

DIFFUSING CAPACITY OF CARBON MONOXIDE (DLCO)

- Measures ability of lungs to transfer gas to RBCs
- DLCO is measured as an index of diffusing capacity because its uptake is diffusion limited
- O_2 diffusion is flow limited and therefore measuring the amount of oxygen transferred will underestimate the true diffusion capacity
- Patient inhales small amount (not dangerous) of CO → Amount taken up ≈ diffusion function lungs
- To convert carbon monoxide diffusing capacity to oxygen diffusing capacity, the value is multiplied factor of 1.23 because the diffusion coefficient for oxygen is 1.23 times that for carbon monoxide
- *Low DLCO conditions*: Interstitial lung disease, Emphysema, Abnormal vasculature (Pulmonary hypertension, Pulmonary embolism), Prior lung resection, Anemia
- *High DLCO conditions*: **Polycythemia, Alveolar hemorrhage**

43. Diffusion capacity is measured by: *(NEET 2016)*

a. O_2
b. CO_2
c. CO
d. N_2O

Ans. is 'c' CO

CNS PHYSIOLOGY

GOLGI TENDON ORGAN

- It is an encapsulated receptor, located within the tendon of a muscle.
- Each Golgi tendon organ is connected to 10–15 muscle fibers.
- Golgi tendon organ functions as a transducer in a feedback circuit that regulates muscle force in a fashion analogous to the spindle feedback circuit that regulates muscle length.
- Unlike muscle spindles, Golgi tendon organs are in series with the muscle fibers, so they are stimulated by both passive stretch and active contraction of muscle.
- **It is important to note that spindle detects muscle length and changes in muscle length, whereas Golgi tendon detects muscle tension.**
- So it is stimulated when muscle fiber is tensed by contracting or stretching muscle.
- **Stretch reflex through muscle spindle is Monosynaptic whereas Golgi Tendon reflex (Inverse stretch reflex) is Bisynaptic**

44. Golgi tendon organ is responsible for regulating: *(NEET 2019)*

a. Muscle tension
b. Muscle length
c. Pressure
d. Proprioception

Ans. is 'a' Muscle tension

TYPES OF NERVE FIBRES

Type	*Sensory function*	*Motor function*	*Diameter (microns)*	*Myelination*	*Conduction Velocity (m/s)*	*Sensitivity to nerve block*
Aα	Proprioception **Ia:** Muscle spindle (annulospiral ending) **Ib:** Golgi tendon organ	Motor supply to skeletal muscles (extrafusal fibres)	12–20	Heavy	70–120	+
Aβ	Touch, pressure **II:** Muscle spindle (Flowerspray ending)	No motor	5–12	Heavy	30–70	++
Aγ	No sensory	Motor to intrafusal fibres of muscle spindle	3–6	Heavy	15–30	++
Aδ	**III:** Pain (Fast pain for localizing site), **temperature**, touch, pressure	No motor	2–5	Heavy	12–30	+++
B Preganglionic autonomic	No sensory	No motor	<3	Light	3–5	++++
C Postganglionic autonomic	**IV: Pain (Slow pain; dull visceral pain)**	No motor	0.3–1	None	0.5–2	++++

Local anesthetics depress transmission in group C fibers before they affect group A touch fibers. Conversely, pressure on a nerve can cause loss of conduction in large-diameter motor, touch and pressure fibers while pain sensation remains relatively intact. Patterns of this type are sometimes seen in individuals who sleep with their arms under their heads for long periods, causing compression of nerves in arms (Saturday night palsy).

45. A female while watching movie at home sleeps with her hand under her head. Which nerve fibres are most susceptible to injury? *(NEET 2020)*

a. A
b. B
c. C
d. Sympathetic

Ans. is 'a' A

46. Slow conduction velocity is seen in which of the following fibres? *(NEET 2019)*

a. Preganglionic autonomic nerve fibres
b. Postganglionic autonomic nerve fibres
c. Motor nerves
d. Proprioceptive fibres

Ans. is 'b' Postganglionic autonomic nerve fibres

47. Dull visceral pain is carried by which type of neurons? *(NEET 2016)*

a. A gamma
b. A alpha
c. C fibres
d. B

Ans. is 'c' C fibres

48. Motor supply to muscle spindle is through:

a. Alpha
b. Beta
c. Gamma
d. Delta

Ans. is 'c' Gamma

Explanation: Afferent supply of intrafusal fibres of muscle spindles–**A**α, **A**β; Motor supply of intrafusal fibres of muscle spindles–**A**γ

ABNORMAL POSTURING

- Involuntary flexion or extension of limbs indicating severe brain injury
- Used in Glasgow Coma Scale to measure the severity of brain injury

Types

Decorticate rigidity	*Decerebrate rigidity*
Arms flexed over chest, legs extended	Arms extended at the sides, legs extended
Hypertonia is less pronounced	Intense hypertonia (rigidity)
Score of 3 in motor section in GCS	Score of 2 in motor section in GCS
Damage to cerebral hemispheres, internal capsule or thalamus (rubrospinal tract facilitation)	Damage to brainstem (below level of red nucleus)
Indicates less severe brain damage	Indicates more severe brain damage

49. True about decorticate rigidity: *(NEET 2019)*

a. Removal of cerebral cortex and basal ganglia
b. Flexion of lower limbs and extension of upper limbs
c. Rigidity is less pronounced than decerebrate rigidity
d. Indicates more severe brain damage than decorticate rigidity

Ans. is 'c' Rigidity is less pronounced than decerebrate rigidity

SLEEP STAGES

Sleep stage (% of total sleep time)	Description	EEG waveforms
Awake (eyes open)	Alert, active concentration	Beta (highest frequency >14 Hz, lowest amplitude)
Awake (eyes closed)	At rest, relaxed	Alpha (8–13 Hz)
Non-REM sleep		
Stage N1 (5%)	Light sleep	Theta (4–7 Hz)
Stage N2 (45%)	Deeper sleep; bruxism occurs	Sleep spindles (Sudden increased frequency) and K complexes (sudden increased amplitude)
Stage N3 (25%)	Deepest non-REM sleep; sleep-walking, night terrors, bed-wetting occurs	Delta (Lowest frequency 3–5 Hz, highest amplitude)
REM sleep (25%) **(Paradoxical sleep)**	Rapid eye movements, loss of motor tone, dreaming, nightmares, penile tumescence	Beta (Saw-toothed; low voltage pattern)

EEG recordings during sleep

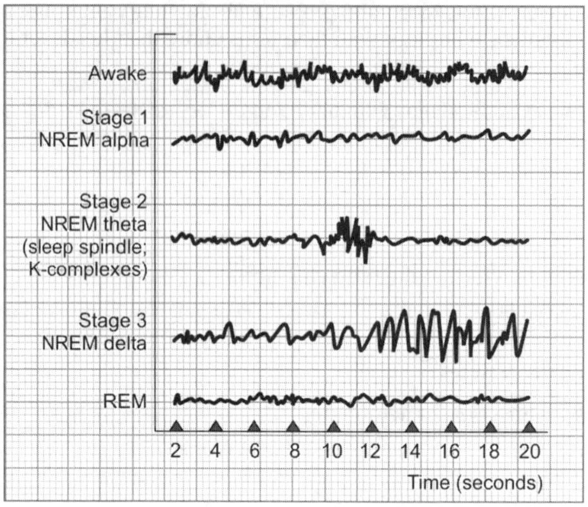

50. Identify the shown phase of EEG. *(NEET 2020)*

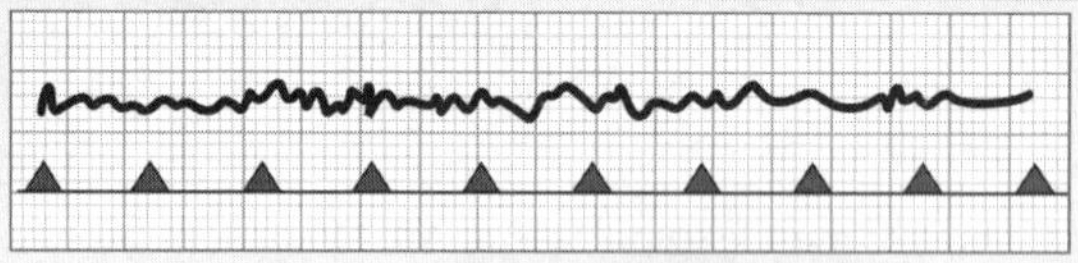

a. Stage 1 NREM
b. Stage 2 NREM
c. Stage 3 NREM
d. REM sleep

Ans. is 'd' REM sleep

51. Alpha waves are seen during: *(NEET 2018)*

a. Sleep
b. REM movements
c. Relaxed state
d. Active state

Ans. is 'c' Relaxed state

52. K-complex is seen in which stage of sleep cycle? *(NEET 2016)*

a. REM
b. Stage 1 NREM
c. Stage 2 NREM
d. Stage 3 NREM

Ans. is 'c' Stage 2 NREM

NISSL BODIES (NISSL GRANULE OR TIGROID BODY)

- Nissl bodies are large granular body found in neuron. **They are present all over the soma (body), except axon hillock** and they extend to some extent in the dendrites, but not within the axon. These granules are **rough endoplasmic reticulum** with free ribosomes and are the site of protein synthesis. They are thought to be involved in the synthesis of neurotransmitter such as acetylcholine.
- Chromatolysis (Disappearance of Nissl bodies) is an important histological sign of neuronal injury.

Functionally, neuron can be divided into four zones:

- Dendrites and Soma (cell body)→ Receptor zone
- **Axon hillock of body and initial segment of axon → Generator area (Nerve impulse is generated)**
- Axon → Transmitter zone (Transmits nerve impulse)
- Nerve terminals (Terminal knobs or buttons) → Release zone (Release neurotransmitters).

53. Nissl's granules are found in which part of nerve cell? *(NEET 2016)*

a. Axon hillock
b. Axons
c. Node of Ranvier
d. Body

Ans. is 'd' Body

HAIR CELLS

- Hair cells are the sensory receptors of hearing.
- Hair cells have a common structure—The tallest cilium is called as Kinocilium and the progressively shorter cilia are called as **Stereocilia.**
- In the inner ear, stereocilia are the mechanosensing organelle of hair cells.

Physiology

- Steraocilia exist in auditory and vestibular systems.
- Convert mechanical stimuli to electric stimuli
  - When the entire hair cells bend towards the tallest one, these channels open leading to influx of potassium (mainly). This causes depolarization and activation. Hair cells in inner ear are unique in the sense that their depolarization is due to potassium ion.
  - When all the hair cells bend away from the tallest one, these channels close leading to inhibition.

54. Steraocilia are present in: *(NEET 2016)*

a. Taste buds
b. Hair cells
c. Retina
d. Nose

Ans. is 'b' Hair cells

Note: Stereocilia are found in three places → Hair cells of inner ear, epididymis and ductus deferens

KEY CNS NEUROTRANSMITTERS

Norepinephrine

- Stress/Panic hormone
- Increased levels in anxiety
- Decreased levels in depression
- Main source of NE in brain–Locus ceruleus (posterior pons)

Dopamine

- Synthesized in:
  - Ventral tegmentum (midbrain)
  - Substantia nigra (midbrain)
- Increased levels in schizophrenia
- Decreased levels in Parkinson's
- Decreased levels in depression

γ-Aminobutyric Acid (GABA)

- **Largely inhibitory**
- Causes pre-synaptic inhibition
- Synthesized in nucleus accumbens (subcortex)
- Decreased levels in anxiety
- Decreased levels in Huntington's disease

Serotonin

- Various functions
- Synthesized in raphe nucleus (pons)
- Decreased levels in anxiety
- Decreased levels in depression

Acetylcholine

- Synthesized in basal nucleus of Meynert (subcortex)
- Increased levels in REM sleep
- Decreased levels in Alzheimer's
- Decreased levels in Huntington's disease

Glutamate

- Major excitatory neurotransmitter
- N-methyl-D-aspartate (NMDA) receptor is target
- **Causes pre-synaptic facilitation**
- Huntington's: neuronal death from glutamate toxicity

55. Major inhibitory neurotransmitter in nervous system: *(NEET 2016)*

a. Glutamate
b. Aspartate
c. Gamma-amino butyric acid
d. Taurine

Ans. is 'c' Gamma-amino butyric acid

56. Facilitatory presynaptic neurotransmitter is:	*(NEET 2016)*
a. GABA	b. Glycine
c. Glutamate	d. Aspartate

Ans. is 'c' Glutamate

PAPEZ CIRCUIT

- The Papez circuit is a component of the limbic system.
- It is a closed neural circuitry that starts and ends in the hippocampus. It is also known as the medial limbic circuit.
- Structures including:
  - Hippocampus and adjacent cortex (entorhinal cortex)
  - Fornix
  - Mammillary body
  - Anterior nucleus of thalamus
  - Cingulum

Information from cortical association areas passes to the hippocampus via the cingulum. Signals are transferred to the hypothalamus (mammillary body) via the fornix. Completion of the circuit and feedback to the cortex is accomplished through mammillothalamic fibers, relaying information from the hypothalamus to the anterior nucleus of the thalamus. The anterior nucleus of the thalamus projects fibers to the cingulum back to the hippocampus.

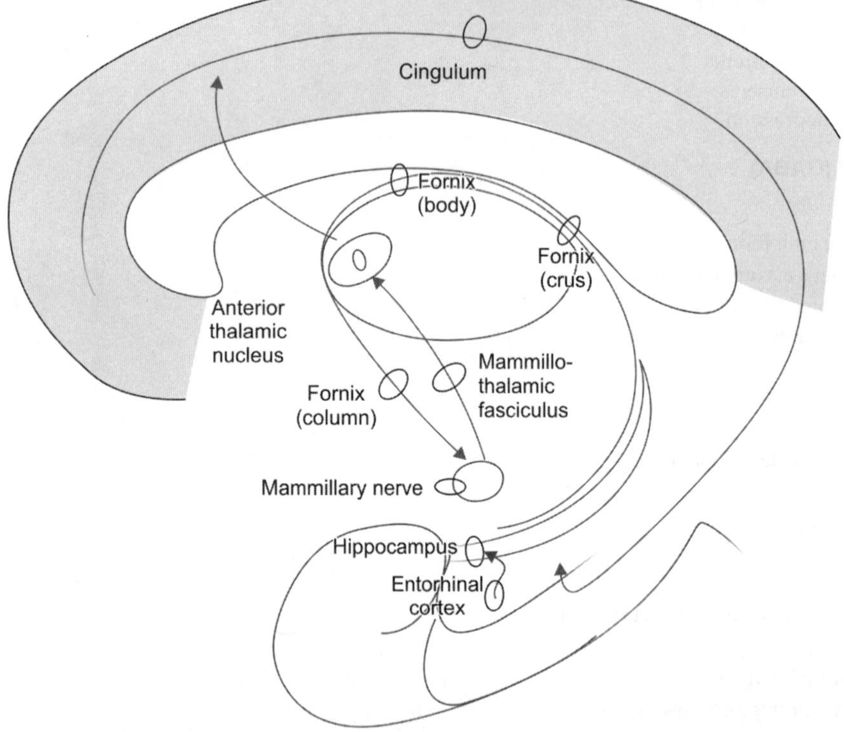

57. Which is not involved in Papez circuit?	*(NEET 2016)*
a. Hippocampus	b. Mamillary bodies
c. Cigulate gyrus	d. Posterior thalamic nuclei

Ans. is 'd' Posterior thalamic nuclei

TACTILE RECEPTORS

- *Superficial receptors*: Merkel's discs (Slowly adapting) and Meissner's corpuscles (Rapidly adapting)
- *Deep receptors*: Ruffini's end organ (Slowly adapting) and Pacinian corpuscle (Rapidly adapting).

Meissner's Corpuscles

- Touch receptors located near surface of skin **(Superficial touch)–Deep touch is detected by Ruffini's end organ**
- Concentrated in sensitive areas like fingers–Glabrous hairless skin
- Deformed by pressure → Nerve stimulation
- A-alpha (Large, myelinated) fibers

Pacinian Corpuscles

- **Vibration receptors**
- Located in deep skin, joints, ligaments
- Egg-shaped structure: Layers of tissue around free nerve ending
- Deformed by pressure → Nerve stimulation
- A-alpha (Large, myelinated) fibers

Merkel's Discs

- **Two-point discrimination**
- Many locations, but especially hair follicles
- A-alpha (Large, myelinated) fibers
- Sustained response to pressure
- 'Slowly adapting' - Provide continuous information
- Contrast with Meissner's and Pacinian corpuscles which are 'Rapidly adapting' Respond mostly to changes

Tactile (touch) sensation can be divided into:

- **Superficial touch**: Detected by Meissner's corpuscle (Detect texture of surface, i.e. rough or smooth) and Merkel's disc (Detect two point discrimination)
- **Deep**: (i) Pressure (Deep touch)—Detected by Ruffini's end organ; (ii) Vibrations—Detected by Pacinian corpuscle

58. Receptors for vibration sense: *(NEET 2016)*

a. Merkel's disc
b. Ruffin's end organ
c. Pacinian corpuscle
d. Meissner's corpuscle

Ans. is 'c' Pacinian corpuscle

59. Two point discrimination is mainly a function of which touch receptors? *(NEET 2016)*

a. Merkel's disc
b. Ruffini's end organ
c. Paccinian corpuscle
d. Meissner's corpuscle

Ans. is 'a' Merkel's disc

RENAL PHYSIOLOGY

TUBULAR FUNCTIONS OF NEPHRON

Proximal Tubule

- Active transport of many substances occurs–100% glucose and amino acids; about 67% of water, bicarbonate, NaCl, potassium and phosphate.
- Fluid remains Iso-osmotic due to permeability to water via Aquaporin-1.

Thin Descending Limb of Loop of Henle

- Impermeable to ions
- Permeable to water due to Aquaporin-1
- Water leaves lumen; drawn out by hypertonicity of medulla
- Fluid becomes hypertonic

Counter-current Mechanism

The descending and ascending limbs of loop of Henle lie close to each other with fluid flowing through them in opposite direction. Due to this **counter-current mechanism**, there is a graded increase in the osmolality of the interstitium of the pyramids in humans: The osmolality at the tips of the papillae can reach about 1200 mOsm/kg of H_2O, approximately four times that of plasma. Most important cause of high medullary osmolarity is co-transport of various ions with Na+ ions out of the thick ascending limb of loop of Henle into the medullary interstitium.

Thin Descending Limb of Loop of Henle and Early Segment of Distal Convoluted Tubule (DCT)

- Impermeable to water
- **Carrier (Na^+ K^+ $2Cl^-$ transporter)** transports one Na^+, one K^+, and two Cl^- ions from the lumen into the tubular cells (example of secondary active transport)
- **Fluid becomes hypotonic**

Late Segment of Distal Convoluted Tubule (DCT) and Collecting Ducts

- Aldosterone and Vasopressin (ADH) regulate collecting duct function
- *Vasopressin*
  - Promotes free water retention
  - Released by posterior pituitary
  - Acts via V2 receptors on principal cells in collecting duct
  - **Leads to Aquaporin-2 insertion into cell membrane- ↑water retention**
- *Aldosterone*
  - Increases Na channels (ENaC) of principal cells
  - Promotes K secretion principal cells
  - Promotes H^+ secretion intercalated cells
- In the presence of ADH, water moves out of the hypotonic fluid and the tubular fluid becomes isotonic.

60. Vasopressin acts through which channels in collecting duct? *(NEET 2019)*

a. Aquaporin-1 b. Aquaporin-2
c. GLUT-3 d. GLUT-4

Ans. is 'b' Aquaporin-2

61. Components responsible for counter-current mechanism in kidney are all except: *(NEET 2018)*

a. Sodium outflow in thick ascending limb
b. Water outflow in thin descending limb
c. Sodium outflow in thin descending limb
d. Flow of tubular fluid from PCT to DCT

Ans. is 'c' Sodium outflow in thin descending limb

62. Thick ascending limb of loop of Henle has which channels? *(NEET 2016)*

a. Na^+ Cl^+ cotransporter b. Na^+ $-2Cl^-$ $-K^+$ cotransporter
c. ENaC channel d. Na+ -aminoacid cotransporter

Ans. is 'b' Na^+ $-2Cl^-$ $-K^+$ cotransporter

63. Diluting segment of a nephron: *(NEET 2016)*

a. Proximal convoluted tubule b. Distal convoluted tubule
c. Descending limb of loop of Henle d. Ascending limb of loop of Henle

Ans. is 'd' Ascending limb of loop of Henle

VASOPRESSIN RECEPTORS

Receptor	Action
V1a receptor	Vasoconstriction
V2b (V3) receptor	Release of ACTH from anterior pituitary
V2 receptor	Collecting duct of kidney–Water retention Vasodilatation Release of vWF and factor VIII from endothelium

64. All are true about arginine vasopressin *except*: *(NEET 2016)*

a. Major action on kidney is through V1 receptor
b. Causes vasoconstriction
c. Causes release of vWF
d. Causes vasodilation

Ans. is 'a' Major action on kidney is through V1 receptor

ALDOSTERONE

- Steroid (Mineralocorticoid) hormone secreted by adrenal cortex (Zona Glomerulosa layer)
- Major controller of K^+ homeostasis
- Acts primarily on collecting ducts of nephron
  - Increases Na^+ channels (ENaC) in principal cells
  - Increases Na^+/K^+ ATPase pumps
  - Promotes K^+ secretion in principal cells
  - Promotes H^+ secretion in Intercalated cells
- Overall effect
  - ↑sodium/water reabsorption (↑effective circulating volume)
  - ↑K^+ excretion
  - ↑H^+ excretion
- Aldosterone release stimulated by (In order of reducing efficacy)
  - Hyperkalemia
  - **Angiotensin-II** (in hypovolemia)
  - ACTH (Not an important physiological regulator of aldosterone levels)
  - Hyponatremia

65. Aldosterone secretion is stimulated by: *(NEET 2018)*

a. Low potassium
b. Angiotensin II
c. High sodium
d. FSH

Ans. is 'b' Angiotensin II

JUXTAGLOMERULAR APPARATUS (JGA)

- JGA is a specialized region of a nephron where the afferent arteriole and distal convoluted tubule (DCT) come in direct contact with each other.
  - **Juxtaglomerular cells** (JG) (modified smooth muscle cells of afferent arteriole)
    - Synthesizes and stores renin
    - Function as mechanoreceptors to sense blood pressure
  - **Macula densa cells (Na^+ sensors) of distal convoluted tubule (DCT)**
    - Function as chemoreceptors to sense changes in the solute concentration and flow rate of filtrate
  - **Juxtaglomerular/Extraglomerular mesangial cells (Lacis cells)**
    - Allow for selective vasoconstriction/vasodilation of the renal afferent and efferent arterioles with mesangial cell contraction

66. Function of Lacis cells in nephrons: *(NEET 2016)*

a. H^+ secretion
b. Na^+ reabsorption
c. Renin secretion
d. Regulation of vasoconstriction / vasodilation of arterioles

Ans. is 'd' Regulation of vasoconstriction / vasodilation of arterioles

STIMULATION OF RENIN RELEASE

Secreted by JG cells (Modified smooth muscle of afferent arteriole); part of Renin-Angiotensin-Aldosterone system (RAAS)

- Low perfusion pressure
  - Low blood pressure or low circulating volume
  - Sensed by afferent arteriole → JG cell renin release
- Low NaCl delivery
  - Sensed by macula densa → JG cell renin release
  - Also constricts afferent arteriole–"Tubuloglomerular feedback"
- Sympathetic activation
  - β1 receptors
  - Also constricts (α receptor) afferent/efferent arterioles
  - Decreases GFR to limit sodium/water excretion
- **Prostacyclin (PGI_2)** stimulates renin secretion through a direct action

67. Renin secretion is decreased by:

a. Sympathetic stimulation
b. Prostacyclin (PGI_2)
c. NaCl in distal tubules
d. Hypotension

Ans. is 'c' NaCl in distal tubules

RENAL AUTOREGULATION

Maintains a constant glomerular filtration rate (GFR)/renal blood flow (RBF) over a range of blood pressures.
Primarily due to changes in resistance of afferent arterioles.

Two mechanisms

1. Myogenic response: Intrinsic property of smooth muscle is to contract when stretched–leads to afferent arteriole constriction
2. **Tubuloglomerular feedback**
   - Increased mean arterial pressure (MAP) leads to increase in RBF and GFR
   - High delivery of sodium ions to macula densa (part of nephron where thick ascending limb of loop of Henle connects with beginning of distal tubule) → Adenosine and ATP secretion → vasoconstriction of afferent arteriole → decreases renal blood and GFR

- Decreased delivery of sodium to macula dense dilates the arteriole and leads to increase in GFR

68. Tubuloglomerular feedback is useful for which of the following? *(NEET 2019)*

a. GFR
b. Plasma sodium
c. Plasma volume
d. Tubular secretion

Ans. is 'a' GFR

RENAL TRANSPORT MAXIMUM (Tm OR T_{max})

- Refers to the point at which increases in tubular concentration of a substance does not result in an increase in tubular reabsorption due to saturation of ion channels.
- **Renal threshold for glucose** is the plasma level at which the glucose first appears in the urine in more than the normal minute amounts. One would predict that the renal threshold would be about 300 mg/dL, that is, 375 mg/min (TmG) divided by 125 mL/min (GFR). **However, the actual renal threshold is about 200 mg/dL of arterial plasma, which corresponds to a venous level of about 180 mg/dL (filtered load of 250 mg/min).**
- The reason for the difference between threshold and transport maximum is that not all nephron have same transport maximum for glucose, and some of the nephron therefore begin to excrete glucose before others have reached their transport maximum.

69. Renal threshold for serum glucose level: *(NEET 2016)*

a. 100 mg/dL
b. 200 mg/dL
c. 300 mg/dL
d. 400 mg/dL

Ans. is 'b' 200 mg/dL

GLOMERULAR FILTRATION RATE

GFR = K_f * (Capillary hydrostatic pressure – glomerular hydrostatic pressure + glomerular oncotic pressure – capillary oncotic pressure)

Factors that increase GFR

- Increased gromerular capillary hydrostatic pressure - Increased arteriole pressure, afferent arteriole dilatation
- Decreased glomerular capillary oncotic pressure - Hypoproteinemia or increased renal blood flow.

Factors that Decrease GFR

- Decreased glomerular capillary hydrostatic pressure—Afferent arteriole constriction or efferent arteriole dilatation, decreased arterial pressure
- Increase glomerular capillary oncotic pressure—Dehydration or decreased renal blood flow
- Increased Bowman's capsule hydrostatic pressure—Tubular obstruction
- Decrease in KF - Diabetes mellitus or contraction of mesangial cells

	Renal plasma flow	Glomerular filtration rate	Filtration fraction
Afferent dilation	↑	↑	--
Efferent constriction	↓	↑	↑
↑Plasma proteins	--	↓	↓
Ureter obstruction	--	↓	↓

70. True about GFR: *(NEET 2016)*

a. Increase by afferent anteriole constriction
b. Increased by decreased renal blood flow
c. Increased in Hypotension
d. Increased in hypoproteinemia

Ans. is 'd' Increased in hypoproteinemia

GLOMERULAR FILTRATION BARRIER

Responsible for filtration of plasma according to size and charge selectivity.

Composed of:

- Fenestrated capillary endothelium
- Basement membrane with type IV collagen chains and heparan sulfate
- Visceral epithelial layer consisting of podocyte foot processes

Charge barrier: All 3 layers contain negatively charged glycoproteins that prevent entry of negatively charged molecules (e.g., albumin)

Size barrier: Fenestrated capillary endothelium (prevents entry of > 100 nm molecules/blood cells); podocyte foot processes interpose with basement membrane; slit diaphragm (prevents entry of molecules > 50–60 nm)

71. Which GAG is present in glomerular basement membrane? *(NEET 2020)*

a. Heparan sulfate
b. Chondroitin sulfate
c. Keratan sulfate 1
d. Keratan sulfate 2

Ans. is 'a' Heparan sulfate

RENAL FUNCTION MEASUREMENTS

Glomerular Filtration Rate (GFR)

- **Inulin clearance** used to determine GFR
- Inulin neither secreted or reabsorbed - All inulin filtered goes out
- Thus, amount of blood 'cleared' of inulin is amount of blood filtered by glomerulus; i.e. **Clearance of inulin (liters/min) = GFR**
- **Creatinine -** Breakdown product muscle metabolism
  - **Closest naturally occurring substance to inulin**
  - Creatinine - All filtered goes out + small amount secretion
  - Thus, creatinine slightly overestimates GFR
- Clearance is equal to the concentration of substance in urine (U) times the urine flow per unit of time (V) divided by the arterial plasma level of substance(P), or **UV/P**

Renal Plasma Flow (RPF)

- Use **para-aminohippuric acid (PAH)** to estimate RPF
- PAH is filtered and secreted → 100% of PAH that enters kidney leaves blood in urine
- Clearance PAH (l/min) = Renal Plasma Flow (l/min)

72. Plasma inulin of a person is 4 mg/mL and urine flow rate is 20 mL/min. What will be GFR if urine inulin is 50 mg/mL? *(NEET 2016)*

a. 125 mL/min
b. 250 mL/min
c. 500 mL/min
d. 1000 mL/min

Ans. is 'b' 250 mL/min

Explanation: Inulin Clearance = UV/P = 50 × 20/4 = 250 mL/min = GFR.

GIT PHYSIOLOGY

IRON ABSORPTION

Iron is absorbed from upper small intestine, mainly **duodenum.** Iron is absorbed in ferrous form.

Ion import protein **DMT-1 facilitates uptake of ferrous (Fe^{2+}) iron from intestinal lumen**.

Fraction of absorbed iron is delivered to plasma transferring; most of the iron is stored in enterocytes as **ferritin.**

Iron absorption is regulated by **Hepcidin** (synthesized by liver). It binds to ferroportin, thus inhibiting iron transfer from enterocyte to plasma. In iron deficiency, level of hepcidin falls.

Iron absorption from the intestine is summarized in the following diagram:

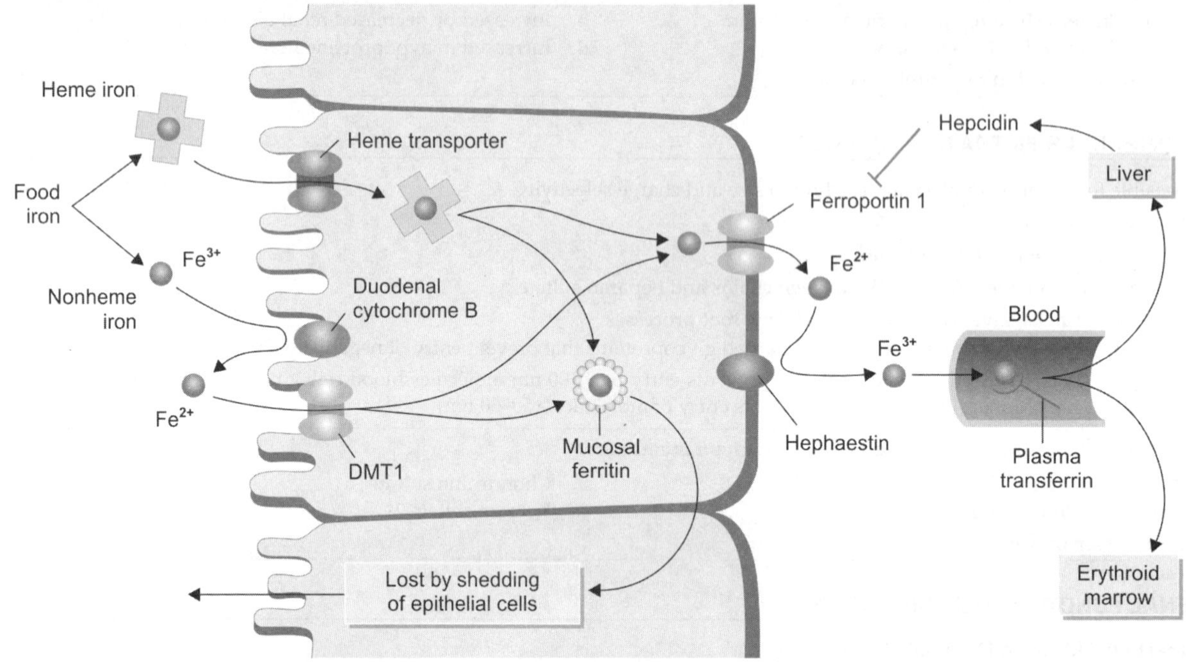

Factors affecting iron absorption	
Decreasing absorption	
Forming chelate with iron	Phytate, phosphate, milk, tetracycline
Opposing reduction of ferric to ferrous form	Antacids, alkalis, pancreatic secretions
Increasing absorption	
Causing reduction of ferric to ferrous form	Ascorbic acid, Gastric acid, Citric acid

73. Iron absorption in intestine occurs via: *(NEET 2018)*

a. Intrinsic factor
b. DMT-1
c. DMT-2
d. Hemopexin

Ans. is 'b' DMT-1

74. Major site for absorption of iron in GIT: *(NEET 2016)*

a. Duodenum
b. Ileum
c. Jejunum
d. Colon

Ans. is 'a' Duodenum

GLUCOSE ENTRY INTO CELLS

- Na independent entry
  - Facilitated diffusion via GLUT transporters
  - Varies by tissues
    - Insulin independent
      - GLUT-1: Brain, RBCs (Uptake when glucose high), **Placenta**
      - GLUT-2: Bidirectional glucose transporter; intestine (Glucose OUT of epithelial cells into blood), liver, kidney, **pancreas (B-cell glucose sensor)**
      - GLUT-3: Placenta, brain
    - Insulin dependent
      - GLUT-4: Fat tissue, skeletal muscle
- Na dependent entry
  - Secondary active transport (cotransport) with Na^+
    - **Intestinal epithelium (absorbed from lumen into epithelial cell)**–Carrier protein for co-transport is SGLT-1
    - Renal tubules–SGLT-1, SGLT-2

Physiology

Mechanism of absorption of nutrients from GIT	
Glucose, galactose	***Secondary active transport***
Fructose	Facilitated diffusion (GLUT 5)
Lipids	Passive diffusion
Amino acids	Facilitated diffusion

75. Glucose is absorbed from intestinal lumen by: *(NEET 2019)*

a. Secondary active transport
b. Facilitated diffusion
c. Simple diffusion
d. Primary active transport

Ans. is 'a' Secondary active transport

76. GLUT-1 is present in: *(NEET 2016)*

a. Skeletal muscle
b. Adipose tissue
c. Jejunum
d. Placenta

Ans. is 'd' Placenta

77. Glucose transporter affected on diabetes mellitus: *(NEET 2016)*

a. GLUT-2
b. GLUT-5
c. GLUT-4
d. SGLT-2

Ans. is 'c' GLUT-4

GIT HORMONES

	Gastrin	*Cholecystokinin*	*Secretin*
Secreted by	G cell in antral and duodenal mucosa	I cells in mucosa of duodenum and jejunum	S cells in duodenal mucosa
Stimulated by	• Amino acids in stomach • Distension of stomach • Vagal neurotransmitter GRP	• Peptides and amino acids in small intestine • Fatty acids and monoglycerides in duodenum	• H^+ in duodenum • Fatty acids in duodenum
Inhibited by	• Low pH • Somatostatin		
Effects	• Stimulates H^+ secretion by parietal cells in gastric body • Trophic effects on gastric mucosa • ↑gastric motility	• Gallbladder contraction • Pancreatic enzyme secretion • Relaxation of sphincter of Oddi • Inhibits gastric emptying	• Increases Pancreatic HCO_3- secretion • Potentiates action of CCK on pancreas • Inhibits gastric acid secretion; inhibits gastrin secretion • Increases bile production • Promotes pancreatic flow • Delays gastric emptying

78. True about function of secretin: *(NEET 2016)*

a. Antagonizes the action of CCK
b. Stimulates gastrin secretion
c. Delays gastric emptying
d. All of the above

Ans. is 'c' Delays gastric emptying

79. Most important site for gastrin producing cells: *(NEET 2016)*

a. Body of stomach
b. Funds
c. Pylorus/Antrum
d. All of the above

Ans. is 'c' Pylorus/Antrum

ENTERIC NERVOUS SYSTEM

Composed of two plexuses

- **Myenteric plexus or Auerbach's plexus:**
  - Outer plexus
  - Between the longitudinal and circular muscle layer
  - Controls mainly **gastrointestinal motility (peristalsis)**
- **Submucosal plexus or Meissner's plexus:**
  - Inner plexus
  - In submucosa
  - Controls mainly **gastrointestinal secretion and local blood flow**

80. Myenteric plexus in GIT controls: *(NEET 2016)*

a. GI secretions
b. Local blood flow
c. GI motility
d. All of the above

Ans. is 'c' GI motility

GIT REFLEXES

Movement and secretion are regulated by long reflexes from the central nervous system (CNS), short reflexes from the enteric nervous system (ENS), and reflexes from the gastrointestinal system (GI) peptides that work in harmony with each other.

Three main types of gastrointestinal reflexes

1. *Enterogastric reflex*: The enterogastric reflex is stimulated by the presence of acid levels in the duodenum at a pH of 3–4 or in the stomach at a pH of 1.5. When this reflex is stimulated, the release of gastrin from G- cells in the antrum of the stomach is shut off. In turn, this inhibits gastric motility and the secretion of gastric acid (HCl). Enterogastric reflex activation causes decreased motility.
2. *Gastrocolic reflex*: The gastrocolic reflex is the physiological reflex that controls the motility, or peristalsis, of the gastrointestinal tract. It involves an increase in motility of the colon in response to stretch in the stomach and the byproducts of digestion in the small intestine. Thus, this reflex is responsible for the urge to defecate following a meal. The small intestine also shows a similar motility response. The gastrocolic reflex also helps make room for food in the stomach.
3. *Gastroileal reflex*: The gastroileal reflex is a third type of gastrointestinal reflex. It works with the gastrocolic reflex to stimulate the urge to defecate. This urge is stimulated by the opening of the ileocecal valve and the movement of the digested contents from the ileum of the small intestine into the colon for compaction.

81. Decrease in gastric scretions due to presence of acidic chyme in intestine is mediated by: *(NEET 2020)*

a. Enterohepatic reflex
b. Enterogastric reflex
c. Gastrocolic reflex
d. Gastroileal reflex

Ans. is 'b' Enterogastric reflex

GHRELIN

- Ghrelin is a peptide secreted by oxyntic cells in gastric fundus
- **Ghrelin promotes food intake, i.e. stimulates appetite (orexigenic)**
- Ghrelin secretion increases with anorexia.
- Ghrelin is released from the stomach in fasting state. It increases hunger by inhibiting the ventromedial hypothalamus (Satiety center)

Note: **Satiety center is ventromedial nucleus of hypothalamus. Feeding center is Lateral nucleus of hypothalamus.**

- **Leptin:** Protein hormone produced by fat cells. It acts on hypothalamus to **reduce food intake**, decrease lipogenesis and increase lipolysis, thereby reducing the body fat stores. Plasma leptin levels are proportional to the amount of body fat and are therefore higher in women and obese individuals.

82. Function of Ghrelin: *(NEET 2016)*

a. Stimulate water absorption
b. Increase appetite
c. Regulation of temperature
d. Stimulate lipogenesis

Ans. is 'b' Increase appetite

MIGRATING MOTOR COMPLEX

- During fasting between periods of digestion, the pattern of electrical and motor activity in gastrointestinal smooth muscle becomes modified so that cycles of motor activity migrate from the stomach to the distal ileum - MMC.
- Each cycle starts with a quiescent period (phase I), continues with a period of irregular electrical and mechanical activity (phase II), and ends with a burst of regular activity (phase III).
- The MMCs are initiated by motilin. The circulating level of this hormone increases at **intervals of approximately 100 min** in the interdigestive state, coordinated with the contractile phases of the MMC.
- The contractions migrate aborally at a rate of about 5 cm/min, and also occur at intervals of approximately 100 min.
- Gastric secretion, bile flow, and pancreatic secretion increase during each MMC. They likely serve to clear the stomach and small intestine of luminal contents in preparation for the next meal.

83. Frequency of migratory moter complex:

a. 1 every 30 minutes
b. 1 every 45 minutes
c. 1 every 60 minutes
d. 1 every 90 minutes

Ans. is 'd' 1 every 90 minutes

BASIC ELECTRICAL RHYTHM

- **Except in the esophagus and the proximal portion of the stomach**, the smooth muscle of the gastrointestinal tract has spontaneous rhythmic fluctuations in membrane potential between about **–65 and –45 mV** - Basic electrical rhythm (BER), also known as slow wave potentials.
- BER is **initiated by the interstitial cells of Cajal**, stellate mesenchymal pacemaker cells.
- In the stomach and small intestine, there is a **descending gradient in pacemaker frequency**.
- BER itself rarely causes muscle contraction, but spike potentials superimposed on the most depolarizing portions of the BER waves do increase muscle tension.
- The depolarizing portion of each spike is due to Ca^{2+} influx, and the repolarizing portion is due to K^+ efflux.
- Many polypeptides and neurotransmitters affect the BER. For example, **acetylcholine increases the number of spikes and the tension of the smooth muscle, whereas epinephrine decreases the number of spikes and the tension.**
- The rate of the BER is about 4/min in the stomach. It is about 12/min in the duodenum and falls to about 8/min in the distal ileum. In the colon, the BER rate rises from about 2/min at the cecum to about 6/min at the sigmoid.
- The function of BER is to coordinate peristaltic and other motor activity, such as setting the rhythm of segmentation; contractions can occur only during the depolarizing part of the waves. After vagotomy or transection of the stomach wall, e.g. peristalsis in the stomach becomes irregular and chaotic.

84. True about basic electrical rhythm of GIT: *(NEET 2016)*

a. Fluctuate between – 65 and – 45 mV
b. Initiated by zymogen cells
c. Pacemaker cell are present in proximal stomach
d. All of the above

Ans. is 'a' Fluctuate between –65 and –45 mV

ENDOCRINE PHYSIOLOGY

TYPES OF HORMONAL RECEPTORS

Bind to intracellular receptor	Bind to cell surface receptor; acting via second messenger			
	c-AMP	*c-GMP*	*Ca^{2+}/phosphatidyl inositol (IP3-DAG)*	*Kinase/phosphatase*
Cytoplasmic receptors Glucocorticoids Mineralocorticoids Androgens, Estrogen and progestins Vitamin D3 (1,25-$(OH)_2$ D3) ***Nuclear receptors*** Thyroid hormones	Calcitonin Glucagon LH and FSH hCG ADH (V2 receptor) CRH PTH TSH ACTH GHRH Histamine (H_2-receptor)	ANF **NO**	α1 adrenergic receptor Angiotensin II **Oxytocin** GnRH Gastrin Muscarinic (acetylcholine) TRH **Endothelin** ADH (V1 receptor) Histamine (H_1-receptor)	***Receptor TK*** Insulin PDGF EGF, FGF ***Non-receptor TK*** GH IGF I and II Erythropoietin Prolactin

Endothelin

- Potent vasoconstrictor peptide produced by vascular endothelium
- Usually acts as paracrine regulator
- Causes vasoconstriction, bronchoconstriction, cardiac stimulation, release of aldosterone and ANP
- Role in ductus arteriosus closure at birth.

Nitric Oxide

- Also known as endothelium-derived-relaxing factor (EDRF)
- Formed from arginine by action of cytosolic enzyme No synthase
- Acts through cGMP as second messenger

85. Which hormone acts via tyrosine kinase receptors? *(NEET 2020)*

a. Insulin
b. TRH
c. TSH
d. MSH

Ans. is 'a' Insulin

86. Nitric oxide produces its action via: *(NEET 2018)*

a. cAMP
b. cGMP
c. IP3-DAG
d. Transcription factor

Ans. is 'b' cGMP

Physiology

87. Endothelin acts through: *(NEET 2018)*

a. Tyrosine kinase pathway
b. cAMP
c. cGMP
d. IP3-DAG system

Ans. is 'd' IP3-DAG system

88. Which hormone acts through IP3–DAG? *(NEET 2016)*

a. LH
b. FSH
c. ADH
d. Oxytocin

Ans. is 'd' Oxytocin

89. Steroids are transported inside the cell using which mechanism? *(NEET 2016)*

a. Simple diffusion
b. Facilitated diffusion
c. Active transport
d. Osmosis

Ans. is 'a' Simple diffusion

Explanation: Steroid hormones pass easily across a plasma membrane by simple diffusion as they are lipid soluble.

90. Mechanism of action of atrial natriuretic peptide (ANP) is through: *(NEET 2016)*

a. cAMP
b. cGMP
c. JAK-STAT- kinase
d. Tyrosine kinase

Ans. is 'b' cGMP

91. Mechanism of action of steroid hormone: *(NEET 2016)*

a. Activation of G-protein coupled receptors
b. Activation of intrinsic ion channels
c. Regulation of gene expression
d. JAK-STAT kinase receptors

Ans. is 'c' Regulation of gene expression

92. All are true regarding intracellular receptors except: *(NEET 2016)*

a. Act by regulating gene expression
b. Fastest acting receptors
c. Glucocorticoid receptors
d. DNA contains hormone responsive elements

Ans. is 'b' Fastest acting receptors

Explanation: This is slowest acting transduction mechanism because protein synthesis takes some time.

93. Which of the following is not a second messenger? *(NEET 2016)*

a. cAMP
b. NO
c. CO
d. Protein kinase

Ans. is 'd' Protein kinase

Explanation: Some gaseous molecules can diffuse across cell membranes and act as second messenger. These are nitric oxide (NO), carbon monoxide (CO) and hydrogen sulphide (H_2S).

PHOSPHOLIPASE IP3- DAG SYSTEM

- **Activation of phospholipase C (by stimulatory G protein) hydrolyses the membrane phospholipid phosphatidyl inositol 4, 5 bisphosphate (PIP_2) to generate the second messengers inositol 1, 4, 5-triphosphate (IP_3) and diacylglycerol (DAG).**
- IP_3 mobilizes Ca^{2+} from intracellular organelles→ increased cytosolic Ca^{2+}.
- **DAG enhances Protein Kinase C activation by Ca^{2+}.**
- Ca^{2+} acts as third messenger in this type of transduction mechanism.
- **Protein kinase-C phosphorylates various intracellular proteins (threonine, serine or tyrosine residue)**, causing their activation or inactivation. **(ċ-AMP pathway activates Protein kinase-A).**

94. True about protein kinase: *(NEET 2016)*

a. Phosphorylates threonine residue
b. Involved in IP_3–DAG mechanism
c. Activated by Ca^{2+}
d. All of the above

Ans. is 'd' All of the above

95. Which enzyme breaks up compound into IP3 and DAG? *(NEET 2016)*

a. Adenylyl cyclase
b. Guanylyl cyclase
c. Phospholipase C
d. Phospholipase A

Ans. is 'c' Phospholipase C

SOMATOMEDIN

- Growth hormone (GH) is important for linear growth in childhood, bone and protein metabolism.
- GH acts through membrane-bound receptor and activates cytoplasmic tyrosine kinase (JAK 2 enzyme).
- Liver contains many GH receptors and secretes Insulin-like growth factor/Somatomedin that mediates many GH effects
- GH → Liver → IGF-I secreted
- IGF-I (Somatomedin C) acts on bones and protein metabolism. A specific effect of growth hormone (GH) on skeletal growth is to **convert chondrocytes into osteogenic cells**, thus, causing deposition of new bone.
- IGF-II plays an important role in growth of fetus.

96. Insulin-like growth factor is secreted by which organ? *(NEET 2018)*

a. Liver b. Kidney
c. Pancreas d. Brain

Ans. is 'a' Liver

97. Conversion of chondrocyte into osteogenic cells is caused by: *(NEET 2016)*

a. Insulin b. Corticosteroids
c. Growth hormone d. Thyroxine

Ans. is 'c' Growth hormone

CALCITONIN

- Produced by parafollicular C cells of thyroid
- Lowers serum calcium
  - Suppresses reabsorption of bone; inhibits osteoclasts
  - Inhibits renal reabsorption of calcium, phosphorus
  - Increased calcium in urine
- Normally minimal effect on calcium levels
- Used as pharmacologic therapy for hypercalcemia
- Produced by medullary carcinoma–Hypocalcemia
- **Regulation–Calcitonin levels are raised in response to high Ca^{2+} levels (Hypercalcemia)**

98. Calcitonin levels are raised in: *(NEET 2019)*

a. Hyperthyroidism b. Hyperparathyroidism
c. Hypoparathyroidism d. Cushing syndrome

Ans. is 'b' Hyperparathyroidism

Explanation: **Causes of Hypercalcemia**

- Hyperparathyroidism
- Malignancy (Multiple myeloma, squamous cell carcinoma lung)
- Drugs (Thiazides)
- Granulomatous diseases (Sarcoidosis)
- Milk alkali syndrome
- Hypervitaminosis D

INSULIN STRUCTURE

Protein hormone synthesized by beta cells in pancreatic islets:

- Synthesized as preproinsulin in rough endoplasmic reticulum
- Preproinsulin cleaved to proinsulin (Removal of 23-amino acid peptide takes place) and transported to Golgi apparatus
- Packaged into secretory granules
- Proinsulin cleaved into Insulin and C-peptide in granules
- **Insulin is a two chain polypeptide having 51 amino acids**: The α chain has 21 amino acids while β chain has 30 amino acids.

Proinsulin = Alpha chain + Beta chain + C-peptide
Insulin = Alpha chain + Beta chain (bound by disulfide bridges)

C-peptide

- Detached from proinsulin before secretion
- Secreted with insulin in equimolar amounts

- Long half-life
- Indicator of insulin production

99. C-peptide is seen: *(NEET 2019)*

a. As part of insulin structure
b. In proinsulin
c. As combined entity with insulin after secretion
d. As gastrointestinal proactive molecule

Ans. is 'b' In proinsulin

THYROID HORMONE EFFECTS

Calorigenic effects

- ↑ oxygen consumption
- ↑ basal metabolic rate (BMR)
- Raise body temperature
- ↑respiratory rate
- Loss of body weight

Metabolic effects

- ↑glycogenolysis and gluconeogenesis
- ↑lipolysis
- ↓concentrations of cholesterol, triglycerides
- ↑low-density lipoprotein receptors in liver (↓LDL)
- ↑cholesterol secretion in bile

Cardiac effects

- ↑heart rate, cardiac contractility, stroke volume and cardiac output

CNS and bone effects

- Required for normal bone growth/CNS maturation

100. True about thyroxine are all except: *(NEET 2016)*

a. Increase BMR
b. Increase oxygen consumption
c. Decrease rate of respiration
d. Causes lipolysis

Ans. is 'c' Decrease rate of respiration

ADRENOCORTICOTROPIC HORMONE (ACTH)

- Adrenocorticotropic Hormone (ACTH) is derived from precursor molecule pro-opiomelanocortin (POMC)
- Secreted from anterior pituitary
- ACTH stimulates the adrenal cortex to increase the synthesis and release of glucocorticoids. The effect of ACTH on secretion of mineralocorticoid (aldosterone) and androgen is minimal. However, at higher concentration of ACTH, synthesis and release of these hormone can also increase.
- The secretion of ACTH is subjected to **negative feedback (inhibition) by glucocorticoids.**
- ACTH secretion shows diurnal (circadian) rhythm with minimum secretion at evening and maximum secretion at early morning.
- ACTH secretion is increased by stress, exercise, depression, alcohol abuse, severe obesity and ACTH producing tumors.

101. True about ACTH and cortisol (corticosteroid) secretion: *(NEET 2016)*

a. Maximum secretion in the evening
b. ACTH has negative feedback control
c. ACTH has major effect on mineralocorticoid secretion
d. ACTH secretion is increased by glucocorticoids

Ans. is 'b' ACTH has negative feedback control

ADRENAL INSUFFICIENCY

- Secondary adrenal insufficiency occurs as a result of pituitary ACTH deficiency.
- It is characterized by fatigue, weakness, anorexia, nausea, vomiting and occasionally, hypoglycemia.
- In contrast to primary adrenal failure, hypocortisolism associated with pituitary failure is not accompanied by hyperpigmentation or mineralocorticoid deficiency.

Signs and Symptoms of adrenal insufficiency
Signs and symptoms caused by Glucocorticoid deficiency
Fatigue, lack of energy
Weight loss, anorexia
Myalgia, joint pain
Fever
Normochromic anemia, lymphocytosis, eosinophilia
Slightly increased TSH (due to loss of feedback inhibition of TSH release)
Hypoglycemia (more frequent in children)
Low blood pressure, postural hypotension
Hyponatremia (due to loss of feedback inhibition of AVP release)
Signs and symptoms caused by mineralocorticoid deficiency (primary adrenal insufficiency only)
Abdominal pain, nausea, vomiting
Dizziness, postural hypotension
Salt craving
Low bloodpressure, postural hypotension
Increased serum creatinine (due to volume depletion)
Hyperkalemia
Signs and symptoms caused by adrenal androgen deficiency
Lack of energy
Dry and itchy skin (in women)
Loss of libido (in women)
Loss of axillary and pubic hair (in women)
Other Signs and symptoms
Hyperpigmentation (primary adrenal insufficiency only) (due to excess of proopiomelanocortin [POMC]-derived peptides)
Alabaster-colored pale skin (secondary adrenal insufficiency only) (due to deficiency of POMC-derived peptides)

(AVP: arginine vasopressin; TSH: thyroid-stimulating hormone).

102. Clinical features of ACTH deficiency are all *except*: *(NEET 2020)*

a. Anorexia
b. Hyperpigmentation
c. Nausea
d. Fatigue

Ans. is 'b' Hyperpigmentation

Algorithm for management of the patient with suspected cushing's syndrome

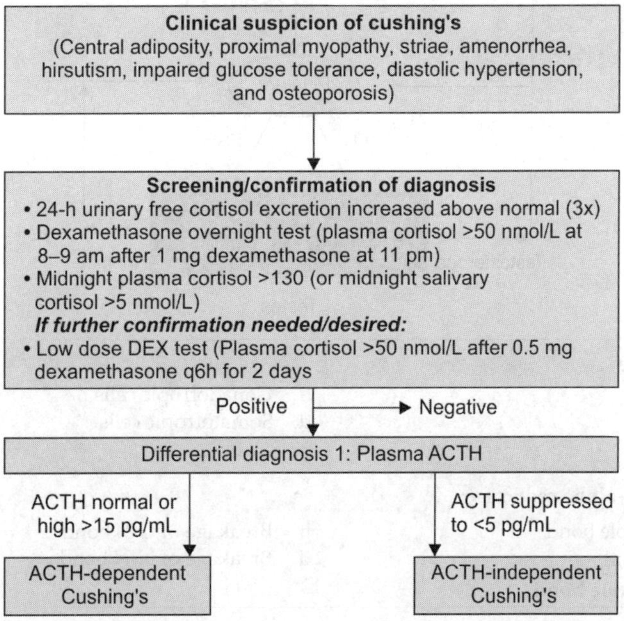

103. Compared to minimal baseline levels of cortisol in evening, rise in both ACTH and cortisol levels are likely to be seen in: *(NEET 2020)*

a. Normal patient in early morning
b. Addison disease
c. Cushing disease
d. Normal patient after taking dexamethasone

Ans. is 'c' Cushing disease

REPRODUCTIVE PHYSIOLOGY

TESTOSTERONE

Secreted by Leydig cells; small contribution to male androgens from adrenal cortex

Leydig cells have **receptors for LH** and secrete androgens, **i.e. testosterone, androstenedione, and dehydroepiandrosterone (DHEA).**

Dihydrotestosterone

- Testosterone converted to dihydrotestosterone (DHT) in peripheral tissues by **enzyme 5-α reductase**
- 5-α reductase causes **reduction (breakage) of C4–C5 double bond** ($\Delta^{4,5}$) with the help of NADH as a cofactor
- Many testosterone effects mediated by DHT
- DHT binds to androgen receptor with ↑potency
- Effects
  - Development of internal genitalia requires testosterone; external genitalia requires DHT
  - Secondary sexual characteristics at puberty
  - Male pattern balding–DHT is key androgen
  - Prostate growth

Sertoli Cells

- **Have receptors for FSH and testosterone**
- Stimulated by FSH
- Supported by testosterone in paracrine fashion
- Need FSH and LH for normal spermatogenesis
- Form blood-testis barrier
- Secrete inhibin B
- Secrete androgen-binding Protein (ABP)–Maintains local testosterone levels
- Produce Mullerian inhibiting hormone during male development

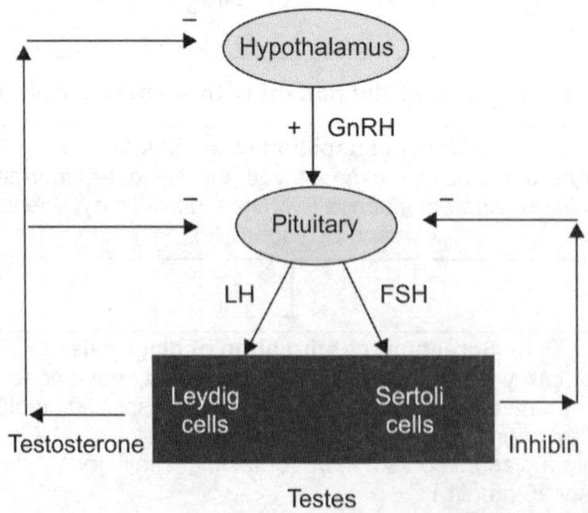

104. Testosterone is secreted by: *(NEET 2019)*

a. Leydig cells
b. Gonadotropic cells
c. Sertoli cells
d. Somatotropic cells

Ans. is 'a' Leydig cells

105. Mechanism of action of 5–alpha reductase: *(NEET 2016)*

a. Breakage of C_4C_5 double bond
b. Breakage of C-N bond
c. Breakage of amide bond
d. Breakage of N-N bond

Ans. is 'a' Breakage of C_4C_5 double bond

Physiology

MENSTRUAL CYCLE

Three Phases

1. **Follicular phase/Proliferative phase (Growth of follicles)**
   - ↑ GnRH pulse frequency
   - ↑ **FSH** → ↑**estradiol** production from ovaries
   - Recruitment of follicles
   - ↑estradiol →↓FSH/LH (Negative feedback)
   - Selection of one dominant/ovulatory follicle
   - 10–14 days (Varies in length)
2. **Ovulation**
   - Mid-cycle surge
   - Switch from negative feedback to positive feedback
   - **Estradiol triggers ↑ frequency GnRH pules → LH surge**
   - Oocyte released from follicle ~36 hours after LH surge
   - Basis for ovulation testing-urine detection of LH
3. **Luteal phase/Secretory phase (Preparation for pregnancy)**
   - Corpus luteum forms
     - Temporary endocrine gland formed from follicle
     - **Produces large amounts of progesterone**
     - Also some estradiol
   - Progesterone/estradiol →↓LH/FSH (Negative feedback)
   - Eventually corpus luteum degrades
   - ↓ progesterone → menstruation - Occurs 14 days after ovulation
   - If fertilization occurs:
     - Embryo makes human chorionic gonadotropin (hCG)
     - Maintains the corpus luteum and progesterone production
     - Progesterone maintains suppression of LH/FSH

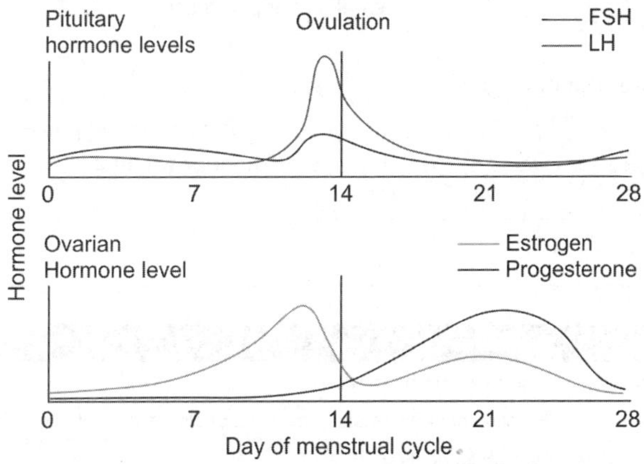

106. Hormone predominantly secreted after day 14 of menstrual cycle is:	*(NEET 2019)*
a. Progesterone	b. Estrogen
c. LH	d. FSH

Ans. is 'a' Progesterone

PROLACTIN PROMOTES LACTATION

❖ Although estrogen and progesterone are essential for the physical development of the breasts during pregnancy, a specific effect of both these hormones is to inhibit the actual secretion of milk. Conversely, the hormone prolactin has exactly the opposite effect and promotes milk secretion.

- Prolactin is secreted by the mother's anterior pituitary gland, and its concentration in her blood rises steadily from the fifth week of pregnancy until birth of the baby, at which time it has risen to 10 to 20 times the normal nonpregnant level. In addition, the placenta secretes large quantities of human chorionic somatomammotropin, which probably has lactogenic properties, thus supporting the prolactin from the mother's pituitary during pregnancy.
- Even so, because of the suppressive effects of estrogen and progesterone, no more than a few milliliters of fluid are secreted each day until after the baby is born. The fluid secreted during the last few days before and the first few days after parturition is called colostrum. Immediately after the baby is born, the sudden loss of both estrogen and progesterone secretion from the placenta allows the lactogenic effect of prolactin from the mother's pituitary gland to assume its natural milk-promoting role, and during the next 1 to 7 days, the breasts begin to secrete copious quantities of milk instead of colostrum.
- After the birth of the baby, the basal level of prolactin secretion returns to the nonpregnant level during the next few weeks. However, each time the mother nurses her baby, nervous signals from the nipples to the hypothalamus cause a 10- to 20-fold surge in prolactin secretion that lasts for about 1 hour. This prolactin acts on the mother's breasts to keep the mammary glands secreting milk into the alveoli for the subsequent nursing periods. If this prolactin surge is absent or blocked as a result of hypothalamic or pituitary damage or if nursing does not continue, the breasts lose their ability to produce milk within 1 week or so. However, milk production can continue for several years if the child continues to suckle, although the rate of milk formation normally decreases considerably after 7 to 9 months.

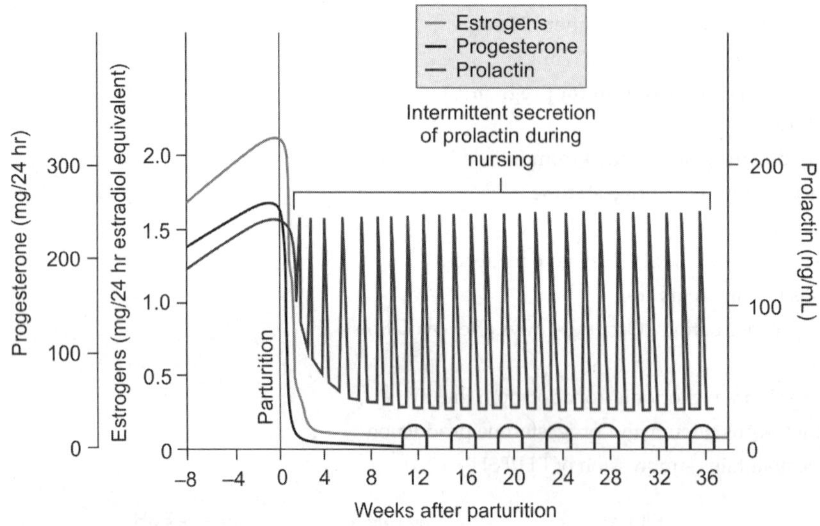

107. Highest levels of prolactin are seen during:	*(NEET 2020)*
a. 24 hrs after delivery	b. During lactational phase
c. REM sleep	d. 1 hr after walking

Ans. is 'a' 24 hrs after delivery

SEXUAL RESPONSE CYCLE

Stage	Response
Excitement phase	Increased BP, heart rate
	Erection of penis (males); swelling of clitoris and labia minora (females)
	Vaginal lubrication
Plateau phase	Further increase in BP and heart rate
Orgasm phase	Reflexive pelvic muscle contraction occurs; **Shortest phase**
	Premature ejaculation occurs
Resolution phase	Body returns to pre-arousal state

108. Premature ejaculation occurs in which phase of sexual cycle?	*(NEET 2016)*
a. Excitement phase	b. Plateau phase
c. Orgasmic phase	d. Resolution

Ans. is 'c' Orgasmic phase

Previously Asked Facts

- Glucose-6-phosphatase is a marker of endoplasmic reticulum.
- Plasmin is a proteolytic enzyme which belongs to serine protease family. Its functions are:
  - **Fibrinolysis** by break down of fibrin → It is the major function.
  - **Activation of collagenase**
  - Break down of matrix proteins (fibrin, fibronectin, thrombospondin, laminin) and **von Willebrand factor**.
- Speed of conduction is fastest in Purkinje fibres.
- Innervation of heart – Parasympathetic supply from Vagus; sympathetic supply from T1–T5
- **Pulmonary arteries and arterioles constrict in response to hypoxia**. This is opposite to the effect observed in systemic vessels, which dilate rather than constrict in response to low oxygen.
- **Mid-expiratory flow rate (MEFR)** for 25–75% of vital capacity is a measure of **small airway resistance**.
- Certain events like coughing, **valsalva maneuver** (Forced expiration against closed glottis), and crying **increase the CSF pressure** by decreasing absorption. Compression of IJV (Internal jugular vein) also raises the CSF pressure.
- In optic pathway, afferents from lateral geniculate body terminate onto the visual cortex, through the **magnocellular pathway (detection of movement depth and flickers)** and **parvocellular pathway (color vision, texture, shape and finer details).**
- Suprachiasmatic nucleus of hypothalamus regulates circadian rhythms.
- **Fatty acids and monoglycerides are absorbed mainly in jejunum**. In side the enterocyte, fatty acids and monoglycerides again form triglycerides. These triglycerides are incorporated into **chylomicrons** and transported to lymphatics.
- Bile ¡s reabsorbed into terminal ileum. The major constituent of bile is bile salts. Thus **excision of ileum will cause increased bile salts in stool.**
- Bile acids are present in the form of bile salts in bile, and not as free bile acids.
- **Iron and calcium are absorbed in duodenum.**
- **Vitamin B_{12} (cyanocobalamine)** is absorbed in the **ileum**. **Intrinsic factor (of castle)** secreted by parietal cells in stomach; is necessary for its absorption. Vitamin B12-IF complex binds with a specific receptor on the surface of the epithelial cells of the ileum. Vitamin B_{12} is transported into the enterocytes leaving behind IF at the brush border.
- **Disaccharidases** (sucrase, lactase) are present in brush border of **small intestinal cells** (duodenum and jejunum).
- **Emulsification** is the process which breaks down ingested fats (mainly triglycerides) into smaller droplets so that they can be digested more efficiently. Thus emulsification mainly **helps in digestion of ingested fats.**
- **Micelles formation** is the process in which digested fats (FFAs and monoglycerides) are incorporated into much smaller droplets (micelles) so that they can be absorbed more efficiently. Thus, micelles formation **helps in absorption of digested fats.**
- Detergent action of **bile salts is necessary for both emulsification and micelles formation.**
- Lactulose is not digested in humans.
- **Gatekeeper in GIT** – Epithelial Calcium channels
- **Melatonin** is a hormone secreted by pineal gland. It is involved in **sleep-wake cycle.**
- Most of the anterior pituitary hormones are under stimulatory control of hypothalamic releasing hormones, **but prolactin is mainly under the inhibitory control**. Therefore, damage to pituitary stalk causes reduction in all the anterior pituitary hormones except prolactin, which is increased.
- Oxytocin is produced in paraventricular nuclei of hypothalamus. It causes milk release in response to suckling by causing contraction of myoepithelial cells in breast. It causes uterine contraction. Increased contractility is limited to uterine body and fundus; **lower segment is not contracted.**
- Maturation of spermatozoa takes place in epididymis.
- Nutrition to sperm is provided mainly by fructose which is present in seminal vesicle secretions.

CHAPTER 3 Biochemistry

AMINO ACIDS

Amino acids	Synthesized biological important compound
Tyrosine (phenylalanine is the precursor of tyrosine)	Catecholamines (epinephrine, norepinephrine), thyroxine, triiodothyronine, **melanin**
Tryptophan	Vitamin niacin, melatonin, serotonin
Glycine, Arginine, Methionine	**Creatine**
Glycine, cysteine	Bile salts
Glycine	Heme
β-alanine	Coenzyme –A
Arginine	**Nitric oxide**
Histidine, arginine, lysine	Keratin
Methionine, lysine	Carnitine
GABA	Glutamine
Glutamate, cysteine, glycine	Glutathione

1. Nitric oxide is produced by: *(NEET 2020)*

a. Lysine
b. Arginine
c. Histidine
d. Citrulline

Ans. is 'b' Arginine

2. Which amino acid is used to synthesize nitric oxide? *(NEET 2019)*

a. Glycine
b. Arginine
c. Tyrosine
d. Threonine

Ans. is 'b' Arginine

3. Creatine is formed from all *except*:

a. Glycine
b. Arginine
c. Methionine
d. Asparagine

Ans. is 'd' Asparagine

4. Melanin is formed from which amino acid?

a. Phenylalanine
b. Tyrosine
c. Tryptophan
d. Histidine

Ans. is 'b' Tyrosine

Urea Cycle

- **Urea cycle is active only in liver for detoxification of ammonia**
- It is partly mitochondrial, partly cytoplasmic.
- CPS I is the rate limiting enzyme of urea cycle

During urea cycle, ornithine should get into mitochondria and citrulline should leave the mitochondria via citrulline transporter present in mitochondrial membrane.

Defect of ornithine citrulline transporter results in HHH syndrome:

- **Hyperammonemia** (as urea cycle is inhibited and accumulates)
- **Hyperornithinemia** (as ornithine is not being utilised for urea cycle)
- **Hyperhomocitrullinemia** (cytoplasmic carbamoyl phosphate reacts with lysine to form homocitrulline)

Property	CPS-I	CPS-II
Pathway	Urea cycle	Pyrimidine synthesis
Location	Mitochondria	Cytoplasm
Amino group	Ammonia	Glutamine
Allosteric regulation	Stimulates by N- acetyl glutamate (NAG)	Inhibited by pyrimidine nucleotides–uridine, cytidine and thymidine

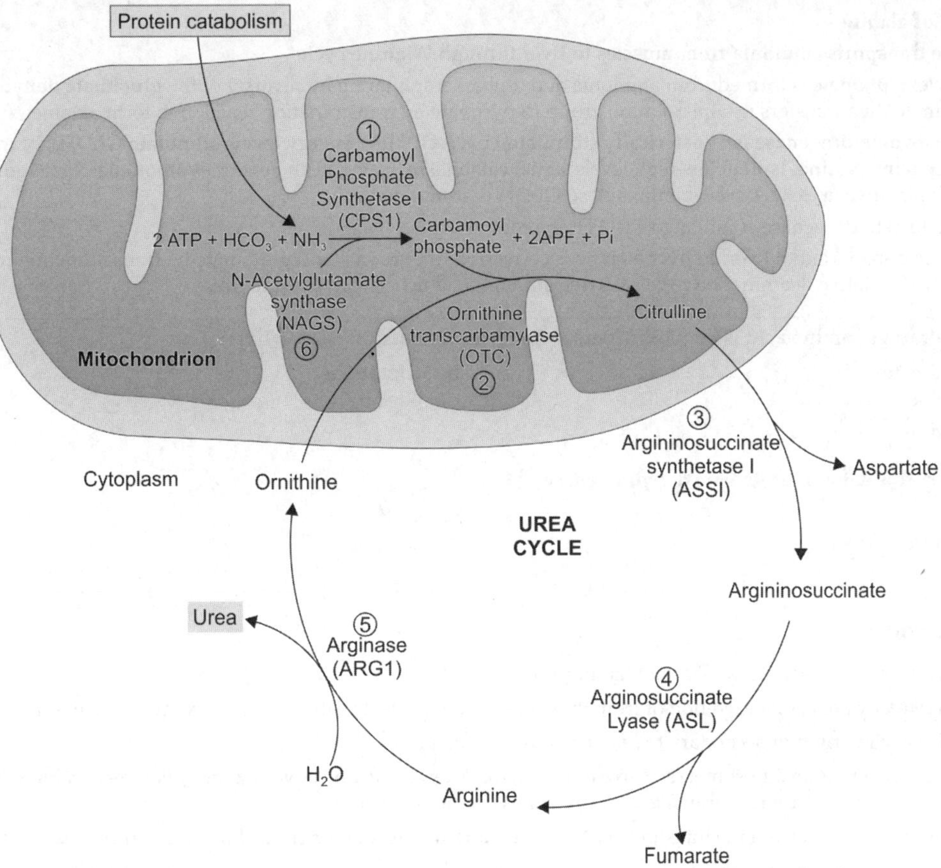

Treatment of urea cycle disorders:

- Phenylbutyrate a pro-drug is used to treat urea cycle disorders, because its metabolites offer an alternative pathway to the urea cycle to allow excretion of excess nitrogen.
- Phenylacetate conjugates with glutamine via acetylation to phenylacetylglutamine, which is eliminated with the urine. It contains the same amount of nitrogen as urea, which makes it an alternative to urea for excreting nitrogen.

5. Urea cycle takes place in:

a. Liver b. Kidney
c. Muscle d. Brain

Ans. is 'a' Liver

6. HHH syndrome is characterized by all *except*:

a. Hyperammonemia b. Hyperornithinemia
c. Hyperhomocitrullinemia d. Hypercitrullinemia

Ans. is 'd' Hypercitrullinemia

7. Carbamoyl Phosphate synthetase I [CPS I) true is:

a. It is present in cytoplasm
b. It is involved in pyrimidine synthesis
c. N-acetyl glutamate is an allosteric stimulator of CPS I
d. Glutamine is the amino group donor for CPS I

Ans. is 'c' N-acetyl glutamate is an allosteric stimulator of CPS I

Transport of Ammonia to Liver

Two mechanisms

1. **In the form of glutamine**
   - In many tissues like liver, kidney and brain, ammonia combines with glutamate to yield glutamine by action of glutamine synthase. The brain predominantly detoxifies ammonia by this route. Glutamine is a nontoxic major transport form of ammonia. The glutamine is transported by blood to liver where glutaminase cleaves glutamine and yields glutamate and free ammonia (ammonium ion). Ammonia is converted by liver to urea.
2. **In the form of alanine**
   - **Alanine transports ammonia from muscles to liver through 'Alanine cycle'.**
   - In muscle, glutamate is formed from ammonia and alpha-ketoglutarate by reversal of the **glutamate dehydrogenase** reaction. L-glutamate then transfers its alpha-amino group to pyruvate by transmination reaction to form alanine.
   - **Glutamate dehydrogenase is allosterically stimulated by: ADP (low energy levels stimulate GLDH), branched chain amino acids (Leucine, Valine, Isoleucine**–high levels signal catabolism. Catabolism generates ammonia. To favour the detoxification of ammonia, urea cycle has to be stimulated, so GLDH is stimulated).
   - Glutamate dehydrogenase is inhibited by–ATP, palmitoyl CoA.
   - Alanine is transported to liver. In liver alanine is converted to pyruvate and glutamate by transamination reaction. Glutamate undergoes oxidative deamination to release free ammonia, which is converted to urea.

8. In which form of amino acid is ammonia transported from skeletal muscle to liver?

a. Glutamate b. Glutamine
c. Alanine d. Glycine

Ans. is 'c' Alanine

9. Allosteric stimulator of glutamate dehydrogenase:

a. ATP b. GTP
c. Palmitoyl CoA d. Leucine

Ans. is 'd' Leucine

Fish Odor Syndrome

- Fish odor syndrome, also known as Trimethylaminuria.
- It is characterized by abnormal excretion of trimethylamine in the urine, breath, sweat and vaginal secretions.
- It may be primary in origin or secondary to liver or kidney damage.
- The primary syndrome is an autosomal recessive inherited disorder due to defective enzyme—flavin-containing mono-oxygenase 3, which normally converts trimethylamine to oxide which is excreted in urine.
- Trimethylamine is derived from the intestinal bacterial **degradation of foods rich in choline, lecithin and carnitine.**
- The biochemical diagnosis is established by measuring the ratio of trimethylamine N-oxide to trimethylamine in the urine. In patients with the condition, the ratio is reduced.
  - Treatment includes counselling and dietary modifications. Dietary adjustments include **avoidance of choline-rich foods such as egg yolk, liver, kidney, peas, soybeans and sea fish.**
  - A short course of low-dose neomycin or metronidazole can be used to suppress production of trimethylamine in the gut.
  - However, restricting dietary choline may result in hepatocellular injury, neurological disease, and even a predisposition to cancer. Notably, pregnant women have an increased choline requirement so restricting intake may be even less desirable in this demographic group.

10. To avoid fish odor syndrome, what to be avoided in the food? *(NEET 2018)*

a. Pantothenic acid b. Choline
c. Biotin d. Pyridoxine

Ans. is 'b' Choline

STRUCTURE OF AMINO ACIDS

Acidic and Basic Amino Acids

Negative charged (acidic side chains)

- Aspartic acid and glutamic acid
  - These amino acids have additional carboxyl groups in the side chain.
- At a pH higher than their pK, carboxylic side chains lose an H^+ ion (proton) and are negative charged. They are therefore acidic.
- At a pH lower than their pK, aspartic acid and glutamic acid side chains are uncharged.

Positive charged (basic side chains)

- **Histidine, arginine and lysine**
  - **These amino acids have additional amino groups in the side chain.**
- At a pH higher than their pK, amine side chains are uncharged.
- At a pH lower than their pK, histidine, arginine and lysine side chains accept an H^+ ion (proton) and are positive charged. They are therefore basic.

Essential and non-essential amino acids

Nutritionally essential	Nutritionally nonessential
Arginine	Alanine
Histidine	Asparagine
Isoleucine	Asparatate
Leucine	Cysteine
Lysine	Glutamate
Methionine	Glutamine
Phenylalamine	Glycine
Threonine	Proline
Tryptophan	Serine
Valine	Tyrosine

Glucogenic and Ketogenic amino acids	Ketogenic amino acids
Isoleucine	***Leucine***
Phenylalanine	Lysine
Threonine	
Tryptophan	
Tyrosine	

Glucogenic amino acids	Component of TCA cycle produced
Histidine, proline, glutamine, arginine, glutamate	**α-ketoglutarate**
Isoleucine, methionine, valine	Succinyl CoA
Tyrosine, phenylalanine	Fumarate
Tryptophan, Alanine	Pyruvate
Hydroxyproline, serine cysteine, threonine, **glycine**	Pyruvate

11. Which of the following has two amino groups in the side chain?

a. Glycine
b. Arginine
c. Lysine
d. Asparagine

Ans. is 'b' Arginine

12. Essential amino acid is:

a. Glycine
b. Alanine
c. Valine
d. Tyrosine

Ans. is 'c' Valine

13. Both glucogenic and ketogenic amino acid is:

a. Leucine
b. Isoleucine
c. Valine
d. Lysine

Ans. is 'b' Isoleucine

14. Which is a purely glucogenic amino acid?

a. Leucine
b. Lysine
c. Phenylalanine
d. Alanine

Ans. is 'd' Alanine

15. All of the following are converted to a-ketoglutarate on catabolism *except*:

a. Glutamate
b. Histidine
c. Proline
d. Glycine

Ans. is 'd' Glycine

ABSORPTION OF UV LIGHT

- Conjugated double bonds in the rings are responsible for UV light absorption.
- Nucleic acids absorb UV light at 260 nm due to nitrogenous base. This absorption is more for purines as compared to pyrimidines.
- Proteins and amino acids absorb UV-light at 280 nm, due to aromatic nature of these amino acids. Maximum absorption occurs by tryptophan as it has 2 rings in its side chain.
- Porphyrins absorb at 400 nm. This absorption band of porphyrins is known as Soret band.

16. Absorption of UV rays can be increased at 280 nm by replacing alanine with: *(NEET 2020)*

a. Tryptophan
b. Lysine
c. Leucine
d. Arginine

Ans. is 'a' Tryptophan

MAPLE SYRUP URINE DISEASE

- Caused by a defect of branched chain keto acid dehydrogenase, in enzyme which is involved in the catabolism of **branched chain amino acids—valine, leucine and isoleucine.**
- The disorder is so called because of the classic sweet odour observed in urine. This classic odour is because of the presence of sotolone (a metabolite of branched chain keto acids) in urine.
- Neurodegenerative features are observed in early onset illness.
- In late onset disease, clinical features appear during metabolic crisis states like starvation or catabolic states. **The patient presents with—Weight loss, Hypoglycemia, Ketoacidosis, Diarrhea, vomiting, dehydration, Neurological manifestations like alternating hypotonia and hypertonia, ataxia, seizures, coma and pancreatitis.**
- Diagnosis can be done using dried blood spot analysed using HPLC and Tandem mass spectrometry. Screening tests includes DNPH test (Dinitrophenylhydrazine test). DNPH reacts with the carbonyl groups of aldehydes and ketone to give a red or yellow complex.
- Treatment involves diet restriction of valine, leucine and isoleucine with formula foods and supplementation of vitamins, minerals and omega 3 fatty acid.

17. Branched chain ketoaciduria is a defect in catabolism of all the following amino acids *except*:

a. Leucine
b. Isoleucine
c. Valine
d. Methionine

Ans. is 'd' Methionine

18. Maple syrup urine disease is characterized by all *except*:

a. Hypotonia
b. Hypertonia
c. Pancreatitis
d. Hypopigmentation

Ans. is 'd' Hypopigmentation

Nitrogen Balance

- Nitrogen balance is the difference between ingested nitrogen and excreted nitrogen.
- Nitrogen balance is an important index of protein and amino acid metabolism.
- In healthy adults, nitrogen balance is zero, i.e. nitrogen intake is equal to nitrogen excretion.
- Negative nitrogen balance (excreted nitrogen exceeds ingested nitrogen): If dietary intake drops below the normal amount of amino acids degraded each day (30–40 grams), a negative nitrogen balance occurs and the body protein is lost. Essential amino acid deficiency has the same effect because relative deficiency of even a single essential amino acid results in corresponding decrease in protein synthesis. Thus, even with normal degradation of protein, there is negative nitrogen balance due to decreased protein synthesis.

Note: Essential amino acids cannot be synthesized in the body whereas nonessential amino acids can be synthesized from other amino acids.

19. Essential amino acid deficiency affect Nitrogen balance by:

a. Increasing protein degradation
b. Decreasing protein degradation
c. Decreasing protein synthesis
d. Increasing protein synthesis

Ans. is 'c' Decreasing protein synthesis

Hartnup's Disease

- Caused by a defect of a neutral amino acid transporter which is specific for tryptophan absorption along intestine and renal tubules.
- Leads to tryptophan deficiency. As tryptophan is necessary for formation of niacin, Hartnup's disease **presents with niacin deficiency or pellagra**—Photosensitive dermatitis, Diarrhoea, Psychiatric manifestations.
- Also presents with amino aciduria. **There is increased excretion of neutral amino acids like: Tryptophan, Phenylalanine, Leucine, Isoleucine, Histidine and Lysine**
- Characteristically in amino aciduria due to Hartnup's disease, levels of proline, hydroxyproline and arginine levels are normal. This differentiates Hartup's disease amino aciduria in Fanconi's syndrome.

20. Pellagra is caused by:

a. Hartnup's disease
b. Cystinuria
c. Cystinosis
d. Type I Tyrosinemia

Ans. is 'a' Hartnup's disease

21. The amino acid excreted in Hartnup's disease is:

a. Arginine
b. Hydroxyproline
c. Tryptophan
d. Proline

Ans. is 'c' Tryptophan

Selenocysteine

- **Selenocysteine is the 21st amino acid** and acts as cofactor for various enzymes that catalyze redox reactions. Examples: thioredoxin reductase, glutathione peroxidase, and deiodinase (that converts thyroxine to triiodothyronine)
- Replacement of selenocysteine by cysteine can significantly decrease catalytic activity.
- Selenium deficiency results in cardiomyopathy (Keshan disease) and impairments in human selenoproteins have been implicated in tumorigenesis and atherosclerosis.
- Carbon skeleton of selenocysteine is provided by serine. Selenophosphate, formed from ATP and selenate, serves as the selenium donor.
- Selenocysteine is coded by UGA which normally acts as a stop codon. The tRNA is designated as tRNASec.

22. 21st amino acid is:

a. β alanine
b. Selenocysteine
c. Pyrrolysine
d. Hydroxyproline

Ans. is 'b' Selenocysteine

Catecholamines

- Include monoamines: Dopamine, norepinephrine, epinephrine
- Specialised products obtained from the two aromatic amino acids—phenylalanine and tyrosine
- **Tyrosine hydroxylase [Tyrosine Dihydroxyphenylalanine (DOPA)] is the rate limiting enzyme of catecholamine synthesis.**
- **Catecholamine breakdown** via two enzymes:
  - Monoamine oxidase (MAO): Amine group COOH
  - Catechol-O-methyltransferase (COMT): Methyl group to oxygen
- **Epinephrine, Norepinephrine → Vanilly mandelic acid (VMA)**
- Dopamine → homovanillic acid (HVA)
- End products - HVA and VMA are excreted in urine.

23. End product of catecholamine metabolism is:

a. Metanephrine
b. Vanillylmandelic acid
c. Normetanephrine
d. Dihydroxyphenyl glycol

Ans. is 'b' Vanillylmandelic acid

24. Rate limiting step in catecholamine synthesis is:

a. Phenylalanine hydroxylase
b. Tyrosine hydroxylase
c. Dopa decarboxylase
d. Dopamine β hydroxylase

Ans. is 'b' Tyrosine hydroxylase

Energy Source for Muscle Contraction

	Immediate energy system	Anaerobic glycolytic system	Oxidative (aerobic) system
Substrates	ATP, creatine phosphate	Glucose or glycogen	Glucose or glycogen, fatty acids
Energy production	Very fast	Fast	Slow
Peak at	0–30 sec	20–180 sec	>3 min
Limiting factor	Depletion of CrP, ATP	↑ Lactic acid	Glycogen depletion
Example	Power lifting and weight lifting, short sprints	Longer sprints	Endurance events Ball games (soccer, field hockey)

25. During muscle contraction, the immediate source of energy is:

a. Glucose
b. Glycogen
c. Fatty acid
d. Creatinine phosphate

Ans. is 'd' Creatinine phosphate

PROTEINS

PROTEIN SYNTHESIS IN LIVER

- The liver serves several metabolic functions within the body including protein synthesis and metabolism.
- The liver plays a crucial role in the production of nearly all plasma proteins (albumin, alpha-1-acid glycoprotein, majority of coagulation cascade, and fibrinolytic pathways).
- Notable exceptions include: Globulins, Factors III, IV, VIII
- Immunoglobulins are synthesized in plasma cells which are end products of the differentiation of cells called B-lymphocytes.
- Other proteins produced by liver: Protein C, Protein S, Protein Z, Plasminogen activator inhibitor, antithrombin III.
- Vitamin K dependent proteins synthesized by the liver include: Factors II, VII, IX, and X, protein S and C.

26. Protein which is not synthesized in liver is: *(NEET 2019)*

a. Phase protein b. Immunoglobulins
c. Albumin d. Plasma hormone

Ans. is 'b' Immunoglobulins

CHAPERONES

- Chaperones are proteins concerned primarily with **protein folding.**
- Major function of chaperones is to prevent both newly synthesized polypeptide chains and assembled subunits from aggregating into non-functional structures.
- Many of these proteins are heat-shock proteins.

27. Chaperones are helpful in: *(NEET 2018)*

a. Folding of proteins b. Denaturation of proteins
c. Promote aggregation of proteins d. Protein degradation

Ans. is 'a' Folding of proteins

COLLAGEN

- Collagen is the most abundant protein in the body.
- Collagen is a triple helix. It is made up of 3 polypeptide chains—each polypeptide chain is made up of repetitive units of (Gly - X - Y), where X and Y are most commonly proline and hydroxyproline. Hence, 33% of amino acid residues of collagen is **glycine—the most abundant amino acid of collagen.**
- **Collagen is synthesized as procollagen by fibroblasts intracellularly**.
- After translation, the polypeptide chains undergo post-translational modifications in the form of hydroxylation and glycosylation.
- Hydroxylation of proline and lysine residues happen at 4th and 5th position by prolyl and lysyl hydroxylase respectively. **Both prolyl and lysyl hydroxylases are dioxygenases and require vitamin C to keep the iron in the enzyme in Fe^{2+} form.**
- Some of the lysyl residues are oxidized by lysyl oxidase to form aldehydes. **Lysyl oxidase is a copper dependent enzyme.**
- **Hydroxylated lysyl residues (not prolyl residues) are next glycosylated** with galactose and glucose by galactosyl and glucose transferases.
- The procollagen molecules are then released out of fibroblasts and extracellular procollagen is cleaved by specific peptidases to form tropocollagen.
- Each of the three polypeptide chains is held in a helical conformation by winding around each other and are held together by hydrogen bonds.
- **Two amino acids help in formation of triple-helix**
  - **Proline: Introduces sharp bends in the polypeptide chains**
  - **Glycine: It plays an indirect role in permitting extremely tight interwinding of the chains due to its small size.**

Distribution of collagen fibres in connective tissue

Type I: Connective tissue of skin, bone, tendon, ligaments, fibrocartilage, dentin, sclera, fascia, and organ capsules.

Type II: Cartilage (hyaline and elastic), notochord, and intervertebral disc

Type III: Loose connective tissue and organs (uterus, liver, spleen, kidney, lung, etc.), blood vessels and fetal skin. It forms reticular fibers.

Type IV: Basal laminae of epithelia and lens capsule. Provides support and filtration barrier

- **Menkes disease**, also known as Menkes syndrome, is an X-linked recessive disorder caused by mutations in genes coding for the copper-transport protein ATP7A, leading to copper deficiency. This decreases the function of Cu-dependent enzymes necessary for the structure and function of bone, skin, hair, blood vessels and the nervous system such as lysyl oxidase.

28. All of the following are true about collagen structure *except*:

a. Collagen is secreted by fibroblasts as procollagen b. Lysyl oxidase is dependent on vitamin C
c. Hydroxylysine undergoes glycosylation d. Glycine is the most abundant amino acid of collagen

Ans. is 'b' Lysyl oxidase is dependent on vitamin C

29. The most abundant amino acid of collagen is:

a. Glycine
b. Proline
c. Lysine
d. Tryptophan

Ans. is 'a' Glycine

30. Folds in collagen are due to:

a. Glycine
b. Proline
c. Hydroxyproline
d. Lysine

Ans. is 'b' Proline

31. Menkes disease is associated with which enzyme deficiency?

a. Lysyl oxidase
b. Methionine synthase
c. Glutamyl aminopeptidase
d. Lysyl hydroxylase

Ans. is 'a' Lysyl oxidase

PROTEIN STRUCTURE

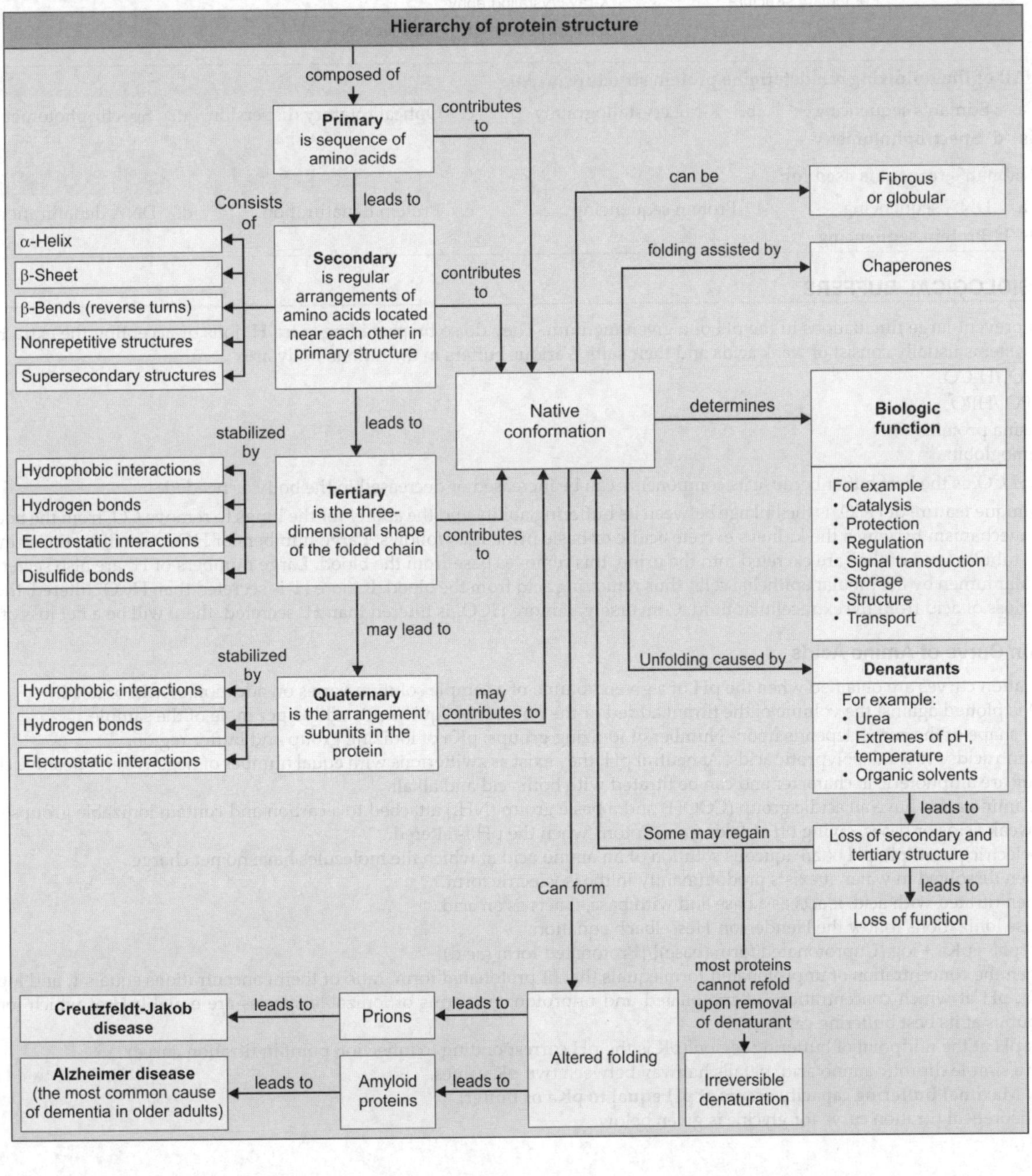

32. Which of the following is true regarding the structural organisation of proteins? *(NEET 2020)*

a. Primary, secondary and tertiary structures are destroyed by denaturation
b. Tertiary structure is stabilized by disulfide bonds
c. Secondary structure is 3 dimensional
d. Structure of secondary and tertiary structure depends on AA sequence

Ans. is 'b' Tertiary structure is stabilized by disulfide bonds

METHODS USED FOR STUDYING PROTEIN STRUCTURE

Structure	Methods
For primary structure	Sanger's sequencing (reagent–1 fluoro 2,4–dinitrobenzene)
	Edman's sequencing (reagent–Phenyl isothiocyanate)
	Reverse sequencing
For secondary structure	Optical rotator dispersion
	Ocular dichroism
For tertiary structure	X-ray crystallography
	UV spectroscopy, NMR spectroscopy

33. All of the following can determine protein structure *except*:

a. Edman's sequencing b. X-ray crystallography c. Optical rotatory dispersion d. Spectrophotometry

Ans. is 'd' Spectrophotometry

34. Edman's reagent is used for:

a. DNA sequencing b. Protein sequencing c. Protein denaturation d. DNA denaturation

Ans. is 'b' Protein sequencing

PHYSIOLOGICAL BUFFERS

Buffers prevent large fluctuations in the pH of a given medium. They do so by providing extra H^+ ions or accepting the extra H^+ ions. Buffer systems usually consist of weak acids and their salts. Various buffers in the human body are:

1. HCO_3^-/H_2CO_3
2. H_2PO_4/HPO_4^-
3. Plasma proteins
4. Hemoglobin

HCO_3^-/H_2CO_3 is the best buffer because its components can be increased or decreased in the body as needed.

A unique feature of HCO_3^- is the linkage between its buffering ability and the ability for the lungs to remove CO_2 from the body. The overall mechanism by which the kidneys excrete acidic or basic urine is as follows: Large numbers of HCO^- are filtered continuously into the tubules, and of they are excreted into the urine, this removes base from the blood. Large numbers of H^+ are also secreted into the tubular lumen by the tubular epithelial cells, thus removing acid from the blood. If more H^+ is secreted than HCO_3^- filtered, there will be a net loss of acid from the extracellular fluid. Conversely, if more HCO_3^- is filtered than H^+ secreted, there will be a net loss of base.

Titration Curve of Amino Acids

- Titration curves are obtained when the pH of a given volume of a sample solution varies on addition of acid or alkali.
- pH is plotted against the volume of the titrant added or the number of equivalents added per mole of the sample.
- The shape of the curve depends upon- Number of ionizing groups, pKa of ionizing group and buffer region.
- Amino acids are weak polyprotic acids. At neutral pH, they exist as zwitterions with equal number of negative and positive charges. They are amphoteric in character and can be titrated with both acid and alkali.
- All amino acids have an acidic group (COOH) and a basic group (NH_2) attached to a carbon and contain ionizable groups that act as weak acids or bases, giving off or taking on protons when the pH is altered.
- Isoelectric point (pl): pH of an aqueous solution of an amino acid at which the molecules have no net charge.
- When dissolved in water, it exists predominantly in the isoelectric form.
- When titrated with acid, it acts as a base and with base, it acts as an acid.
- These ionizations follow the Henderson-Hesselbach equation:
  - pH = pKa + log [Unprotonated form (base)]/[Protonated form (acid)]
- When the concentration of unprotonated form equals that of protonated form, ratio of their concentrations equals 1, and log 1 = 0.
- pKa: pH at which concentrations of protonated and unprotonated forms of ionizable species are equal (pH at which ionizable group is at its best buffering capacity)
- pK: pH at the midpoint of buffering region (pK is the pH corresponding to inflection point in titration curve)
- For a simple diprotic amino acid, pl falls halfway between two pK values.
  - **Maximal buffering capacity occurs at pH equal to pKa of buffer.**
- A theoretical titration curve for glycine is given below:

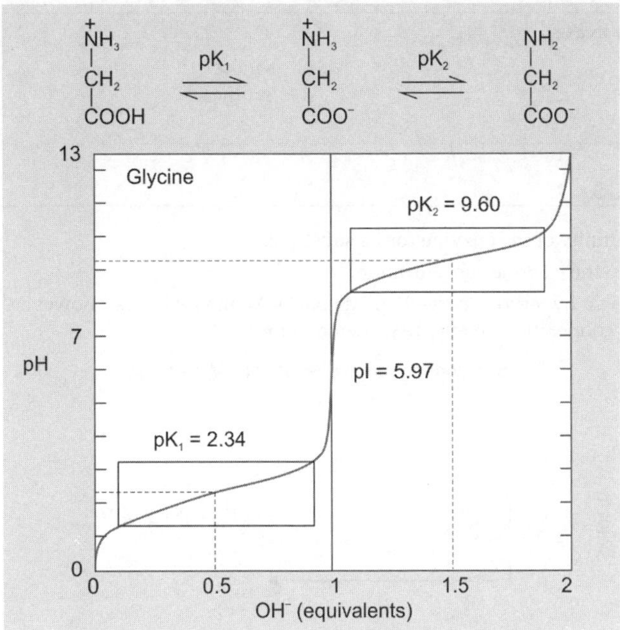

35. Maximum buffering capacity of amino acid is maximum at pH:

a. Less than pKa
b. More than pKa
c. Equal to pKa
d. Has no relation with pKa

Ans. is 'c' Equal to pKa

ENZYMES

TYPES OF ENZYMES

1. Oxidoreductases–Remove hydrogen or add oxygen
   - **Dehydrogenases**–Use NAD/FAD/NADP as acceptor to remove hydrogen
     - NAD-linked dehydrogenases: Pyruvate dehydrogenase, isocitrate dehydrogenase, malate dehydrogenase, a-Icetoglutarate dehydrogenase, glutamate dehydrogenase, glyceraldehyde-3-P dehydrogenase, lactate dehydrogenase, glycerol 3-P dehydrogenase
     - NADP-linked dehydrogenases: Glucose-6-P dehydrogenase, 6-Phosphogluconate dehydrogenase, 3-ketoacyl reductase
     - FAD-linked dehydrogenases: Succinate dehydrogenase, fatty acyl CoA dehydrogenase , glycerol 3P dehydrogenase
   - Oxidases–Use oxygen as acceptor to remove hydrogen
   - Hydroxylases (Mono-oxygenases)–Add oxygen atom; e.g. - Phenylalanine hydroxylase, tyrosine hydroxylase
   - Dioxygenases–Add both oxygen atoms
2. Transferases–Kinase/Phosphotransferase, Transketolase, Transaldolase
3. Hydrolases–Catalyse cleavage of a covalent linkage by addition of water; e.g.–Amidases, Peptidases, Esterases, Phospholipases
4. Lyases–catalyse cleavage of a C-N/C-C linkage without adding water; e.g.–Decarboxylases, Hydratase, Aldolase, Dehydratase
5. Isomerases–catalyse the conversion of one form of a substance to another form of substance without altering the molecular composition; e.g.–Isomerase, Epimerase, Mutase
6. Ligases–catalyse the synthesis of a covalent linkage using ATP as a source of energy; e.g.–Synthetases, Carboxylases.

36. Which of the following is not a source of NADPH? *(NEET 2019)*

a. Isocitrate dehydrogenase
b. ATP citrate lyase
c. Malic enzyme
d. G6PD

Ans. is 'b' ATP citrate lyase

37. Enzyme involved in the transfer of hydrogen:

a. Hydratase
b. Oxidase
c. Peroxidase
d. Dehydrogenase

Ans. is 'd' Dehydrogenase

Biochemistry

38. Which of the following is a Lyase?

a. Hydratase
b. Kinase
c. Oxygenase
d. Syntheses

Ans. is 'a' Hydratase

MICHAELIS-MENTEN KINETICS

- Km is inversely related to the affinity of the enzyme for its substrate.
- Vmax is directly proportional to the enzyme concentration.
- Most enzymatic reactions follow a hyperbolic curve (i.e., Michaelis-Menten kinetics); however, enzymatic reactions that exhibit a sigmoid curve usually indicate cooperative kinetics (e.g., hemoglobin).

[S] = concentration of substrate; V = velocity

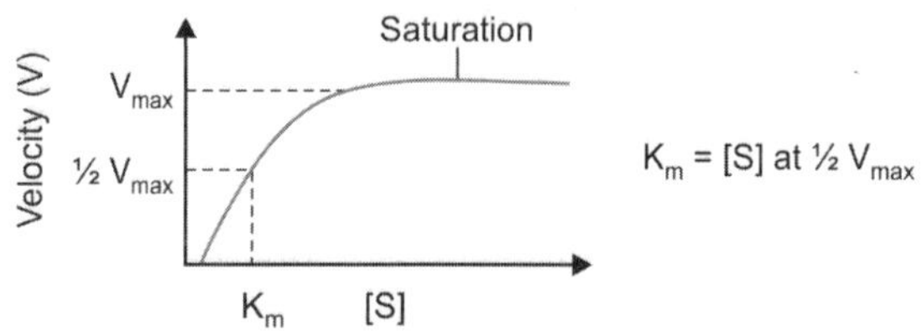

Effects of enzyme inhibition

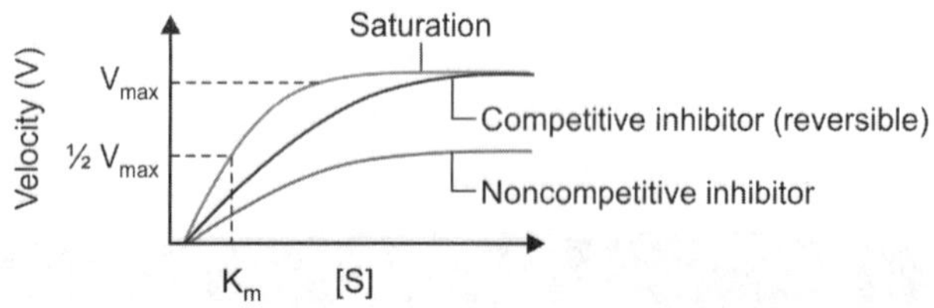

	Competitive inhibitors, reversible	Competitive inhibitors, irreversible	Noncompetitive inhibitors
Resemble substrate	Yes	Yes	No
Overcome by ↑ (S)	Yes	No	No
Bind active site	Yes	Yes	No
Effect on V_{max}	Unchanged	↓	↓
Effect on K_m	↑	Unchanged	Unchanged
Pharmacodynamics	↓ Potency	↓ efficacy	↓ efficacy

39. Which of the following is true regarding non-competitive inhibition? *(NEET 2020)*

a. Km and Vmax increase
b. Km decrease, Vmax increases
c. Km remains same, Vmax decreases
d. Km increases, Vmax remains same

Ans. is 'c' Km remains same, Vmax decreases

RIBOZYMES

- RNA molecules capable of catalyzing specific biochemical reactions.
- Within the ribosome, ribozymes function as part of the large subunit ribosomal RNA to link amino acids during protein synthesis.
- They are also a part of RNA processing reactions–RNA splicing, viral replication and transfer RNA synthesis.
- **Examples of ribozymes include–Ribonuclease P, Peptidyl transferase (transpeptidase), GIR 1 branching ribozyme, self-splicing intron, HDV ribozyme**

40. Which of the following is not a Ribozyme? *(NEET 2019)*

a. Poly A polymerase
b. Ribonuclease
c. Transpeptidase
d. Peptidyl Transferase

Ans. is 'a' Poly A polymerase

GLUTAMATE DEHYDROGENASE (GLDH)

- Catalyzes conversion of glutamate to alpha-ketoglutarate and ammonia (goes into urea cycle)
- **Present in mitochondrial matrix;** considered as a marker enzyme for mitochondria.
- **Unlike AST and ALT levels which get elevated in acute viral hepatitis, GLDH levels rise only following necrotic damage to liver parenchyma.**
- **GLDH is used as a marker to assess drug safety.**
- GLDH is activated by ADP ribosylation in starvation, so that alpha-ketoglutarate is generated to get into citric acid cycle.

41. True about glutamate dehydrogenase:

a. It is present in inner mitochondrial membrane
b. It is elevated in acute viral hepatitis
c. It favours formation of glutamate
d. It is used as a marker to assess drug safety

Ans. is 'd' It is used as a marker to assess drug safety

CONSTITUTIVE ENZYMES

- An enzyme which is constantly present in the same quantity regardless of substrate concentration or physiological or metabolic demands
- They are continuously synthesized because they are indispensable for cell's survival.
- For example–Glycolytic enzymes (like Hexokinase), Cyclo-oxygenase 1 (COX 1)

Regulatory Enzymes

- An enzyme whose concentration is altered depending upon the availability of substrate concentration or physiological or metabolic demands
- Not always required for the survival of a cell or organ
- For example–Cyclo-oxygenase 2 (COX2–expressed only in conditions of inflammation)
- Glucokinase present in liver and pancreatic cells–is expressed more in presence of insulin. So, although Glucokinase is a glycolytic enzyme, it is an inducible enzyme.
- All Lac operon genes β-galactosidase, lactose permease and thiogalactosyl transacetylase, expression happens only in the presence of lactose are regulatory enzymes.

Property	Hexokinase	Glucokinase
Location	All cells	Liver and pancreatic β cells
Affinity	High	Low
Km	**Low**	**High**
Inhibition by glucose 6 phosphate	Yes	No
Induction by insulin	No (constitutive enzyme)	Yes (inducible enzyme)

42. Which of the following is a constitutive enzyme?

a. Hexokinase
b. Glucokinase
c. β galactosidase
d. Cyclo-oxygenase-2

Ans. is 'a' Hexokinase

43. True about glucokinase is:

a. It is present in all cells
b. It is a constitutive enzyme
c. It has a high km
d. It is inhibited by glucose 6 phosphate

Ans. is 'c' It has a high km

ENZYME DEFICIENCY DISEASES

Metabolic disease	Enzyme deficient
Maple syrup urine disease	Branched chain ketoacid dehydrogenase
Methylmalonic aciduria	Methylmalonyl CoA dehydrogenase
Sweaty feet odor in body	Isovaleric acid-CoA dehydrogenase
Tyrosinemia I (tyrosinosis)	**Fumaryl acetoacetate hydroxylase**
Tyrosinemia II	Tyrosine transaminase (tyrosine aminotransferase)
Neonatal tyrosinemia	Hydroxyphenyl pyruvate hydroxylase
Albinism	Tyrosinase
Alkaptonuria	Homogentisate oxidase
Phenylketonuria	**Phenylalanine hydroxylase**
Orotic aciduria	OMP decarboxylase
Homocystinuria	Cystathionine synthase
Leschnyhan syndrome	Hypoxanthine Guanine Phospho RIbosyl Transferase (HGPRT)
Cystinosis	Cystine reductase

ALKAPTONURIA

- Congenital deficiency of homogentisate oxidase in the degradative pathway of tyrosine to fumarate
- Pigment-forming homogentisic acid builds up in tissue.
- Autosomal recessive. Usually benign.
- Findings: bluish-black connective tissue, ear cartilage, and sclerae (ochronosis); urine turns black on prolonged exposure to air. May have debilitating arthralgias (homogentisic acid is toxic to cartilage).

44. A patient suffering from multiple joint pains. His urine turns dark on standing. What is the enzyme deficiency? *(NEET 2020)*

a. FAA hydrolase
b. Homogentisic acid oxidase
c. PHPP oxidase
d. Phenylalanine hydroxylase

Ans. is 'b' Homogentisic acid oxidase

45. The enzyme deficient in Tyrosinemia type-I:

a. Tyrosine transaminase
b. Fumaryl acetoacetate hydroxylase
c. Homogentisate oxidase
d. p-Hydroxyphenylpyruvate hydroxylase

Ans. is Ans. 'b.' Fumaryl acetoacetate hydroxylase

CARBOHYDRATES

REGULATION OF METABOLISM

Activity in						
	Carbohydrate feeding	*Fasting and Diabetes*	*Inducer*	*Repressor*	*Activator*	*Inhibitor*
Glycogen synthase	↑	↓			Insulin, glucose 6- phosphate	Glucagon
Hexokinase						Glucose-6 phosphate
Glucokinase	↑	↓	Insulin	Glucagon		
	Carbohydrate feeding	*Fasting and Diabetes*	*Inducer*	*Repressor*	*Activator*	*Inhibitor*
Phosphofructokinase	↑	↓	Insulin	Glucagon	5' AMP fructose 6- phosphate fructose 2,6 biophosphate, P_i	Citrate ATP, glucagon
Pyruvate kinase	↑	↓	Insulin, fructose	Glucagon	Fructose 1,6 bisphosphate, induline	ATP, alanine, glucagon norepinephrine
Pyruvate dehydrogenase	↑	↓			CoA, NAD^+, insulin ADP, pyruvate	Acetyl CoA NADH ATP (fatty acids, ketone bodies)
Gluconeogenesis						
Pyruvate carboxylase	↓	↑	Glucocorticoids, glucagon, epinephrine	Insulin	Acetyl CoA	ADP
Phosphoenolpyruvate carboxykinase	↓	↑	Glucocorticoids glucagon, epinephrine	Insulin	Glucagon	
Glucose 6 phosphatase	↓	↑	Glucocorticoids glucagon, epinephrine	Insulin		

Hormonal Regulation of Metabolism

Insulin-anabolic and Glucagon-catabolic		
Metabolic Action	*Insulin*	*Glucagon*
Glycogen synthesis	↑	↓
Glycolysis (energy release)	↑	↓
Lipogenesis	↑	↓
Protein synthesis	↑	↓
Glycogenolysis	↓	↑
Gluconeogenesis	↓	↑
Lipolysis	↓	↑
Ketogenesis	↓	↑

The actions of various hormones are depicted in the following diagram:

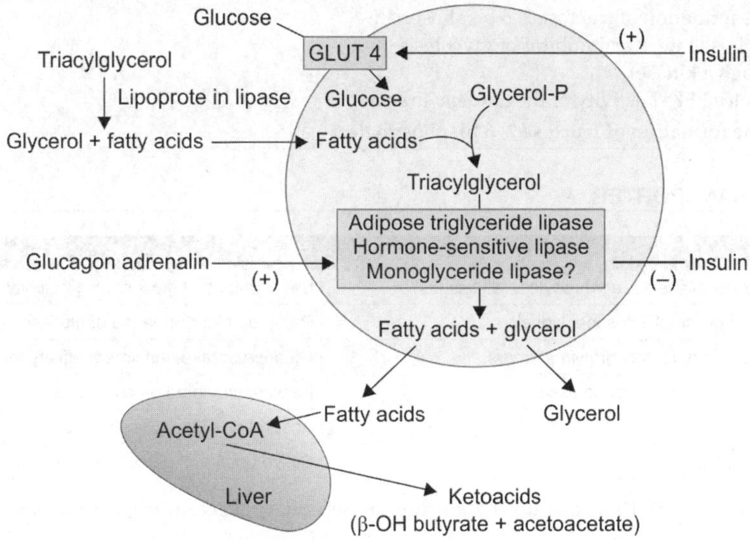

Details of major metabolic pathways have been summarized in the following Table.

Metabolic pathways (cycle or reactions)	Organs/tissues	Cell compartment	Rate limiting enzyme
Cholesterol biosynthesis	All tissues	Cytosol	HMG CoA reductase
Glycolysis	All tissues	Cytosol	Phosphofructokinase 1
HMP shunt	All tissues	Cytosol	Glucose 6 phosphate dehydrogenase
Glycogenesis	Liver, muscle	Cytosol	None
glycogenolysis	Liver, muscle	Cytosol	Glycogen phosphorylase
gluconeogenesis	Liver, kidney	Mitochondria, cytoplasm and ER	Fructose 1,6 bisphosphatase
Fatty acid synthesis	All tissues	Cytosol	Acetyl CoA carboxylase
Beta oxidation of fatty acids	All tissues except brain and RBC	Mitochondria	None
Ketone body synthesis	Liver	Mitochondria	HMG CoA synthase
TCA cycle	All tissues except RBCs	Mitochondria	Isocitrate dehydrogenase
Urea cycle	Liver	Mitochondria and cytoplasm	Carbamoyl phosphate synthase 1
Pyrimidine synthesis	Liver	Cytosol	Carbamoyl phosphate synthase 2
Purine synthesis	Liver	Cytosol	De novo pathway-PRPP glutamyl amidotransferase Salvage pathway-none
Bile acid synthesis	Liver	Cytosol, mitochondria, peroxisome, ER	7 alpha hydroxylase
Oxidation of very long chain fatty acids		Peroxisomes	

46. Enzyme active in low insulin:glucagon ratio is: *(NEET 2020)*

a. PFK-1
b. Hexokinase
c. Glucokinase
d. Glucose 6-phosphatase

Ans. is 'd' Glucose 6-phosphatase

47. Site of glycolysis:

a. Cytoplasm
b. Mitochondria
c. Nucleus
d. Endoplasmic reticulum

Ans. is 'a' Cytoplasm

48. Site of Krebs cycle:

a. Cytoplasm
b. Mitochondria
c. Smooth endoplasmic reticulum
d. Nucleus

Ans. is 'b' Mitochondria

49. Which of the following is true about effect of insulin and glucagon on gluconeogenesis?

a. Insulin favors the formation of fructose 2, 6 bisphosphate
b. Fructose 2, 6 bisphosphate is an inhibitor of glycolysis
c. Insulin acts through a kinase
d. Glucagon stimulates PFK-2 activity of the tandem enzyme

Ans. is 'a' Insulin favors the formation of fructose 2, 6 bisphosphate

TYPES OF GLUCOSE TRANSPORTER

Transporter	Location	Function
GLUT-1	Brain, kidney, colon, placenta, erythrocytes, (all tissues)	Basal uptake of glucose, high affinity
GLUT-2	Liver, pancreatic cell, small intestine, kidney	Rapid uptake or release of glucose
GLUT-3	Brain, kidney, placenta, rapidly growing tumors	Glucose uptake, maximum affinity for glucose
GLUT-4	Heart and skeletal muscle, adipose tissue	Insulin-stimulated glucose uptake
GLUT-5	Small intestine	Absorption of glucose, fructose
SGLT-1	Small intestine and kidney	Active uptake of glucose against a concentration gradient

On the luminal side of enterocytes, SGLT-1 take up the glucose via secondary active transport mediated through a symporter for glucose and sodium.

On the basolateral side, the glucose is transported into the hepatic circulation via the dedicated GLUT-2.

50. Method of transport of glucose in the intestine is:

a. Primary active transport
b. Secondary active transport
c. Simple diffusion
d. Counter transport

Ans. is 'b' Secondary active transport

GLYCOLYSIS

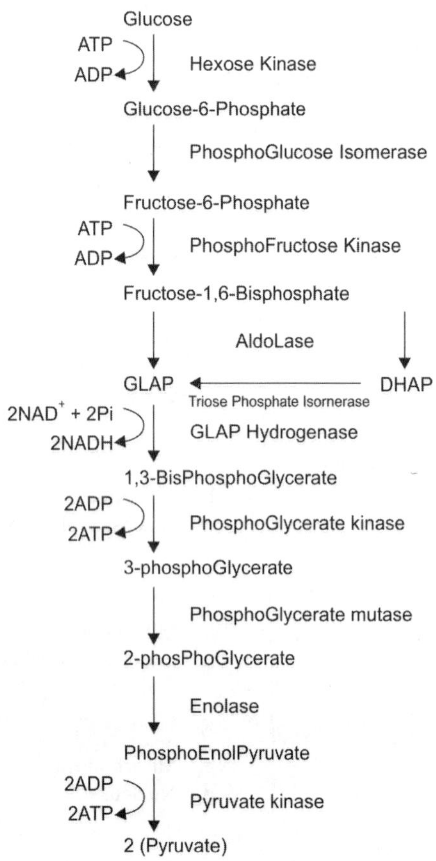

Number of molecules formed in one cycle of glycolysis are given below

- Pyruvate-2
- Net ATP-2
- NADH-2- equivalent to 5 ATP

ATPs production per unit glucose consumed.

- Glycogen = 3 ATPs
- Galactose = 2 ATPs
- Fructose = 2 ATPs

51. Name the enzyme which catalyses substrate phosphorylation in glycolysis:

a. Glyceraldehyde 3 phosphate dehydrogenase
b. Enolase
c. Pyruvate kinase
d. Phosphofructokinase I

Ans. is 'c' Pyruvate kinase

KREBS CYCLE

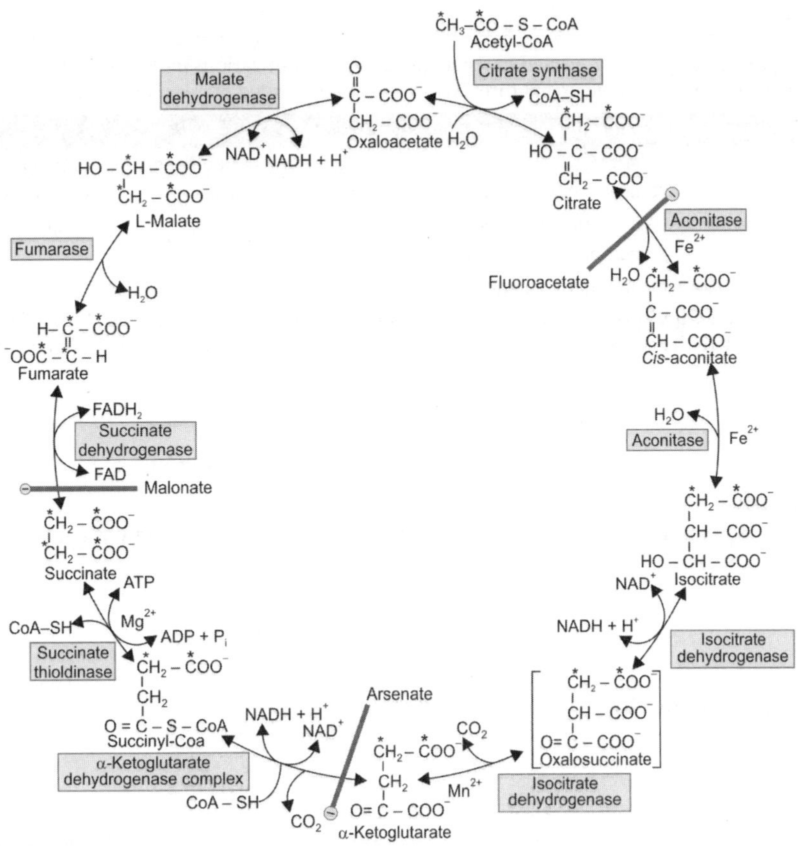

Number of molecules formed in each cycle:

- **GTP** by substrate level phosphorylation - 1
- **NADH**- 3
- **FADH**- 1
- Total ATP formed- 10

Krebs cycle and Urea cycle Link: Fumarate is released during urea cycle, which is an intermediate of Krebs cycle, thus linking the two.

- To detoxify ammonia in hyperammonemia, more glutamate is required (Glutamate + NH_4+ → Glutamine). This glutamate is formed from α-ketoglutarate.
- Thus in hyperammonemia, excessive alpha–ketoglutarate is consumed leading to decrease availability of alpha–ketoglutarate for TCA cycle.

52. In Krebs cycle and Urea cycle the linking amino acid is: *(NEET 2019)*

a. Fumarate
b. Alanine
c. Arginine
d. Aspartate

Ans. is a' Fumarate

53. Hyperammonemia inhibits TCA cycle by depleting: *(NEET 2019)*

a. Succinate
b. α-ketoglutarate
c. Malate
d. Fumarate

Ans. is 'b' α-ketoglutarate

54. Used in citric acid cycle are all *except*:

a. NAD
b. FAD
c. NADP
d. GDP

Ans. is 'c' NADP

55. Substrate level phosphorylation of citric cycle is catalyzed by:

a. Isocitrate dehydrogenase
b. A ketoglutarate dehydrogenase
c. Succinate dehydrogenase
d. Succinyl thiokinase

Ans. is 'd' Succinyl thiokinase

GLUCONEOGENESIS

In gluconeogenesis, the steps of glycolysis are reversed to regenerate glucose from various molecules to supply energy for various tissues of the body. All steps in glycolysis are reversible except three, which are circumvented by reactions undertaken by the following enzymes:

Regulatory and adaptive enzymes associated with gluconeogenesis				
	Inducer	*Repressor*	*Activator*	*Inhibitor*
Pyruvate carboxylase	Glucocorticoids, glucagon, epinephrine	Insulin	Acetyl CoA	ADP
Phosphoenol pyruvate carboxykinase	Glucocorticoids, glucagon, epinephrine	Insulin	Glucagon	
Glucose 6-phosphatase	Glucocorticoids, glucagon, epinephrine	Insulin		

- Liver and kidneys are the major gluconeogenic tissues.
- Allosteric activation by acetyl CoA appears to play the most essential part in gluconeogensis: Acetyl CoA derived from fatty acid oxidation inhibits pyruvate dehydrogenase (PDH) enzyme and stimulates pyruvate carboxylase, shunting pyruvate to gluconeogenesis.

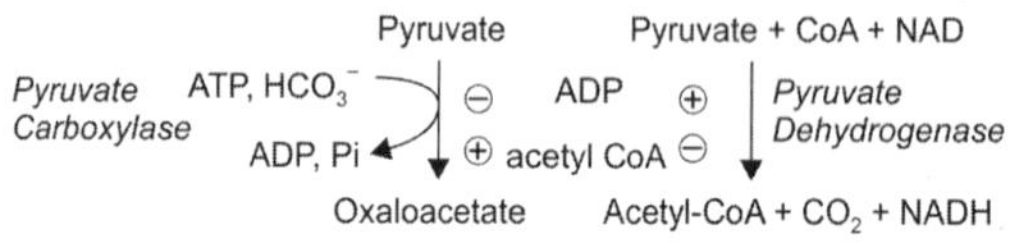

Substrates of gluconeogenesis

- Glucogenic amino acids (all except leucine and lysine which are purely ketogenic); most important is alanine
- Lactate
- Pyruvate
- Propionate
- Glycerol
- Fumarate

56. Pyruvate carboxylase is activated by:

a. Insulin
b. Acetyl CoA
c. ADP
d. NAD

Ans. is 'b' Acetyl CoA

Inhibitors of glycolysis and citric acid cycle		
Process	*Enzyme*	*Inhibitor*
Glycolysis	Glyceraldehyde 3 phosphate dehydrogenase **Enolase** Phosphoglycerate kinase	Iodoacetate **Fluoride** Arsenate
Pyruvate → acetyl CoA	Pyruvate dehydrogenase	Arsenite
Citric acid cycle	Aconitase ά ketoglutarate dehydrogenase Succinate dehydrogenase	Fluoroacetate Arsenite Malonate

Step of Respiratory Chain	Inhibitors
Inhibitors of electron transport chain	
Complex I	Barbiturates, Chlorpromazine, Guanethidine
Complex II	Malanate, Carboxin
Complex III	Dimercaprol, British Anti-Lewisite (BAL)

Contd...

Contd...

Inhibitors of electron transport chain	
Complex IV	Cyanide, Carbon monoxide, Hydrogen Sulphide
Inhibitors of Oxidative Phosphorylation	Oligomycin, Atractiloside
Uncouplers (uncoupling the linkage between ETC and phosphorylation)	2, 4-dinitrophenol (2, 4-DNP), 2, 4-dinitrocresol (2, 4-DNC), and CCCP (chlorocarbonyl cyanide phenylhydrazone)

57. Which enzyme is inhibited by sodium fluoride?

a. Enolase
b. Aconitase
c. Glyceraldehyde 3 phosphate dehydrogenase
d. Pyruvate dehydrogenase

Ans. is 'a' Enolase

58. Which complex of electron transport chain is inhibited by cyanide?

a. Complex I
b. Complex II
c. Complex III
d. Complex IV

Ans. is 'd' Complex IV

GALACTOSEMIA

Galactosemia may be caused by deficiency of any of the enzymes involved in galactose metabolism.

- Classic galactosemia - **galactose 1-phosphate uridylyl transferase (GALT)** deficiency.
- Galactosemia due to deficiency of **galactokinase** results in cataracts
- Deficiency of **uridine diphosphate galactose 4-epimerase**

Pathophysiology

- Since lactose is the most important source of calories in newborns, defect in galactose metabolism leads to accumulation of metabolites, resulting in injury to parenchymal cells of kidney, liver and brain.

Clinical Features

- Infants present with vomiting, diarrhea, hypotonia, jaundice and hepatomegaly.
- They are at an increased risk for *E. coli* neonatal sepsis
- Hyper gonadotropic hypogonadism is seen in 80–90% of women with classic galactosemia

Diagnosis

- Urine of patient shows reducing sugar (galactose), which can be detected by Benedict's reagent.
- Negative glucose oxidase test in spite of presence of a reducing sugar in urine suggests the diagnosis.

Treatment

- Dietary restriction: Elimination of galactose from diet

59. Galactosemia is possible due to deficiency of the following enzyme *except*: *(NEET 2018)*

a. Galactose-1-phosphate uridylyl transferase
b. HGPRT
c. Galactokinase
d. Epimerase

Ans. is 'b' HGPRT

CORI'S CYCLE

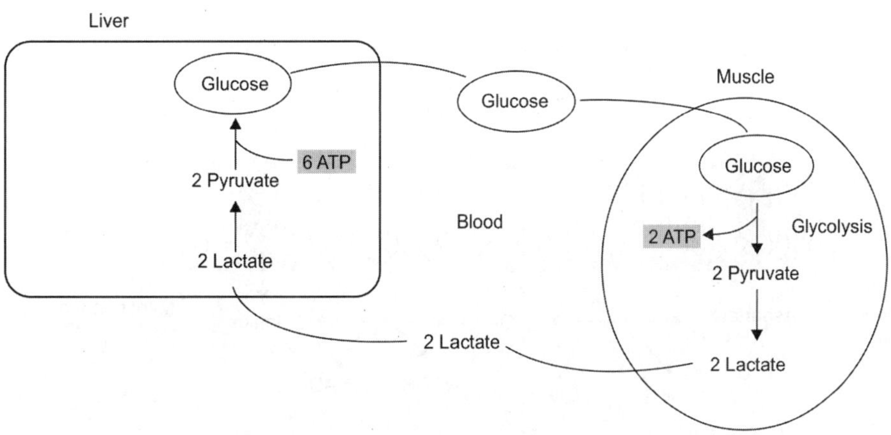

- For 2 ATPs to be produced by muscle, liver generates glucose by spending 6 ATPs. So Cori's cycle shifts the energy burden from muscle to liver.
- It is an energetically unfavourable state as there is a net loss of 4 ATPs. Hence Cori's cycle cannot be sustained for long.
- The glucose that is generated from liver is used in muscle for anaerobic glycolysis if the muscle continues exercising. If the muscle stops exercising, the glucose is used for glycogen synthesis.

60. All of the following are true about lactate utilization in liver *except*:

a. Total net number of ATP formed because of Cori's cycle is 6
b. Cori's cycle shifts the metabolic burden from muscle to liver
c. Cori's cycle cannot be sustained indefinitely because it is energetically unfavourable
d. Cori's cycle is linked to glycogen synthesis in muscle

Ans. is 'a' Total net number of ATP formed because of Cori's cycle is 6

FATES OF PYRUVATE

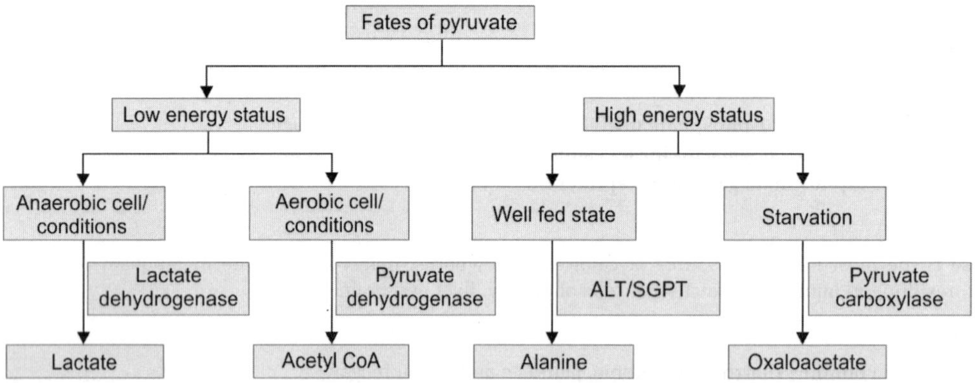

61. Pyruvate can be a substrate of all *except*:

a. Lactate dehydrogenase
b. Pyruvate dehydrogenase
c. Aspartate transaminase
d. Alanine transaminase

Ans. is 'c' Aspartate transaminase

MALATE SHUTTLE

- Malate "shuttles" molecules between cytosol and mitochondria
- Key points:
  - Malate can cross mitochondrial membrane (transporter)
  - NADH and oxaloacetate cannot cross
- Two key uses:
  - Transfer of NADH into mitochondria to get into electron transport chain (Aerobic glycolysis)
  - Transfer of oxaloacetate OUT of mitochondria to get into **gluconeogenesis** by action of Phosphoenolpyruvate Kinase present in cytoplasm

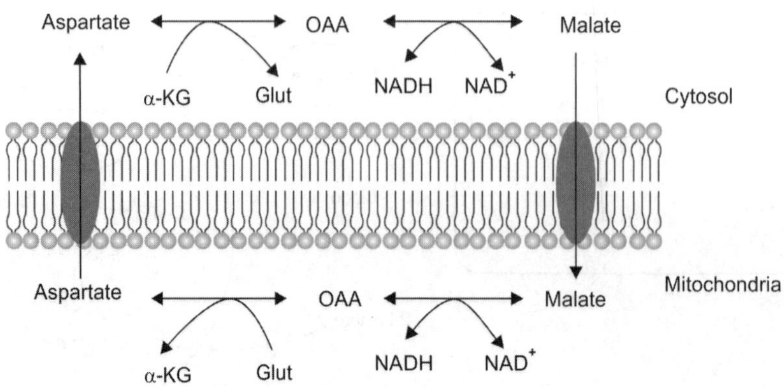

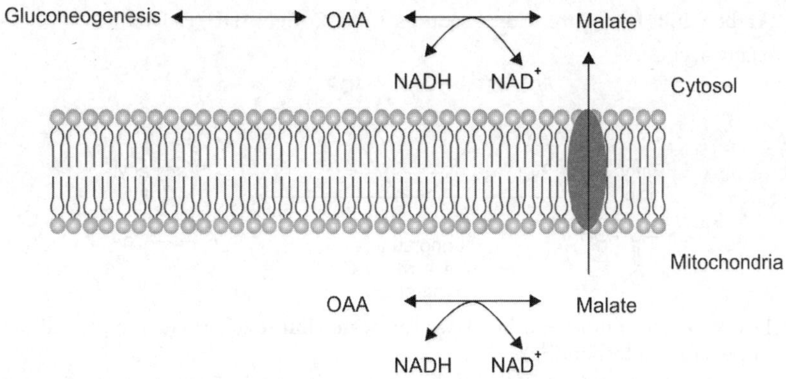

62. Malate shuttle is required for:

a. Gluconeogenesis
b. Anaerobic glycolysis
c. Glycogen synthesis
d. Glycogenolysis

Ans. is 'a' Gluconeogenesis

LIPIDS

HYPERLIPOPROTEINEMIAS

	Type I	Type IIa	Type IIb	Type III	Type IV	Type V
Problem	Decreased lipoprotein lipase or Apo C-II	LDL receptor deficiency	↓LDL receptor increased Apo B-100	**Defect in Apo-E**	Increased VLDL production and decreased elimination (due to apo V deficiency)	Same as in type IV, but more severe
Lipoprotein	**Elevated chylomicrons** (also VLDL same times)	↑ LDL	↑**VLDL** ↑LDL	Increased chylomicron remnants and LDL	↑**VLDL**	↑**VLDL** and chylomicron
Cholesterol	↑↑	↑↑↑	↑↑	↑↑	N	↑↑↑
Triglyceride	↑↑↑↑	N	↑↑	↑↑	↑↑	↑↑↑
Nomenclature	Familial lipoprotein lipase deficiency	Familial hyper cholesterolemia	Familial combined hyperlipidemia	Familial dysbeta-lipoproteinemia	Familial hypertriglyceridemia	Endogenous hypertriglyceridemia

63. Type-I hyperlipoproteinemia is characterized by: *(NEET 2019)*

a. Elevated LDL
b. Elevated HDL
c. Elevated chylomicrons
d. Elevated lipoprotein lipase

Ans. is 'c' Elevated chylomicrons

64. Type III hyperlipoproteinemia is caused by a defect of:

a. ApoCII
b. ApoBlOO
c. ApoAl
d. ApoE

Ans. is 'd' ApoE

FATTY ACID OXIDATION

- Fatty acid oxidation happens in mitochondria and in peroxisomes.
- Very short chain, short chain, medium chain and long chain fatty acids get oxidised in mitochondria. Very long chain fatty acid oxidation cannot happen in mitochondria. It happens in peroxisomes.
- Both mitochondria and peroxisomes oxidise fatty acids by β oxidation, which means β-carbon atom of a fatty acid gets oxidised to form COOH. Hence, alpha-carbon atom and COOH group is released as Acetic acid (CH_3COOH). The active form of acetic acid is acetyl CoA. As acetyl CoA has 2 carbon atoms, whenever *n* number of carbon atom containing fatty acid gets oxidised, we get *n*/2 acetyl CoA in both mitochondria and in peroxisome.
- In mitochondria, removed hydrogen atoms are used for reducing NAD and FAD to form NADH and $FADH_2$ which enter into electron transport chain to form ATP. In peroxisome the hydrogen atom removed from β-carbon atom is used to reduce O_2 forming H_2O_2.

Key enzyme: **Hormone sensitive lipase -** Removes fatty acids from Triacyl glycerol (TAG) in adipocytes; Activated by glucagon and epinephrine

β-oxidation - Removal of 2-carbon units from fatty acids; Produces acetyl-CoA, NADH, FADH2

Step 1: Convert fatty acid to fatty acyl CoA

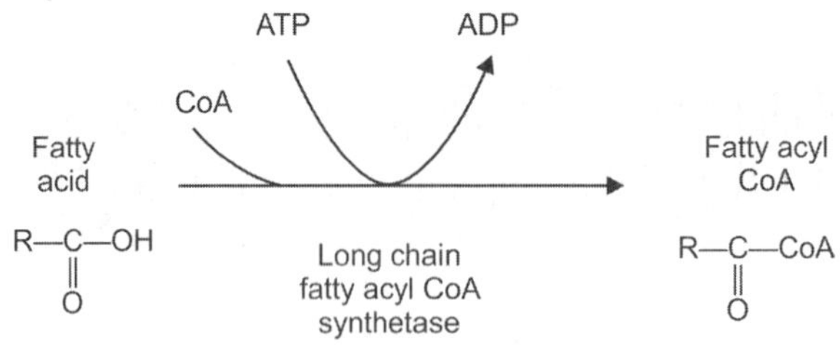

Step 2: Transport fatty acyl CoA to inner mitochondria - **Uses carnitine shuttle** (short chain and medium chain fatty acids are not dependent on carnitine to cross mitochondria)

Step 3: Begin "cycles" of beta oxidation - Removes two carbons, Generates NADH, FADH2, Acetyl CoA. Even chain fatty acids are beta-oxidized to acetyl CoA. Odd chain fatty acids are also beta-oxidized normally but the last step produces a 3-carbon propionyl CoA along with an acetyl CoA (instead of 2 molecules of acetyl CoA that occurs in even chain fatty acids).

ATP yield–Palmitic acid (16C) = 106 ATP; **Stearic acid (18C) = 120 ATP**

Fatty acid oxidation defects present with: Hypoglycemia (more glucose is consumed), Nonketotic hypoglycaemia (Without acetyl CoA ketone bodies are not formed), Hyperammonemia (Amino acid is as a fuel), Dicarboxylic aciduria. Carnitine Palmitoyl Transferase I (CPT-I) defect is an example of fatty acid oxidation defects.

Oxidation of Very Long Chain Fatty Acids

Peroxisomes oxidize very long chain fatty acids. A modified form of β-oxidation is found in peroxisomes and leads to the formation of acetyl-CoA and H_2O_2 (from the flavoprotein- linked dehydrogenase step), which is broken down by catalase. Thus, the dehydrogenation in peroxisomes is not linked directly to phosphorylation and the generation of ATP. The system facilitates the oxidation of very long chain fatty acids (e.g., C20, C22). The enzymes responsible are induced by high-fat diets and in some species by hypolipidemic drugs such as clofibrate. The enzymes in peroxisomes do not attack shorter chain fatty acids; the β-oxidation sequence ends at octanoyl-CoA. Octanoyl and acetyl groups are both further oxidized in mitochondria. Another role of peroxisomal β-oxidation is to shorten the side chain of cholesterol in bile acid formation.

Zellweger (cerebrohepatorenal) syndrome occurs in individuals with inherited absence of peroxisomes in all tissues. They accumulate C26–C38 polyenoic acids in brain tissue and also exhibit a generalized loss of peroxisomal functions. The disease causes severe neurological symptoms, and most patients die in the first year of life.

Refsum Disease

- **Refsum disease is a peroxisomal disorder caused by defective alpha-oxidation of branched chain fatty acids** resulting in build up of phytanic acid and its derivatives in plasma and tissues.
- Refsum's disease presents in adolescence with neurological involvement like cerebellar degeneration and peripheral neuropathy. Other features include ichthyosis, senorineural deafness and retinitis pigmentosa.
- Treatment includes Phytanic acid restriction (Ruminant fats should not be consumed).

65. All are true about beta oxidation of fatty acids *except*:

a. Occurs in mitochondria
b. Occurs in peroxisome
c. Results in hydrogen peroxide generation
d. Fatty- acid oxidation defects present with ketosis

Ans. is 'd' Fatty-acid oxidation defects present with ketosis

66. Carnitine required for which process in fatty acid cycle?

a. Fatty acid synthesis
b. Fatty acid oxidation
c. Fatty acid storage
d. Ketone body synthesis

Ans. is 'b' Fatty acid oxidation

67. Which of the following is true about Beta oxidation of fatty acids?

a. Stearic acid on oxidation provides 106 ATPs
b. Odd chain fatty acid oxidation provides only propionyl CoA
c. Fatty acid oxidation defects cause hypoglycaemia
d. Ketone bodies are formed by incomplete oxidation of fatty acid during starvation to increase energy production

Ans. is 'c' Fatty acid oxidation defects cause hypoglycaemia

68. Refsum's disease is due to defect of:

a. β oxidation of long chain fatty acid
b. α oxidation of long chain fatty acid
c. β oxidation of branched chain fatty acid
d. α oxidation of branched chain fatty acid

Ans. is 'd' α oxidation of branched chain fatty acid

69. Zellweger syndrone is due to absence of: *(NEET 2019)*

a. Lysosomal
b. Mitochondria
c. Peroxisome
d. Nucleus

Ans. is 'c' Peroxisome

KETONE BODIES

- **Ketone body formation (ketogenesis)** occurs when there is a high rate of fatty acid oxidation in liver which provides excessive acetyl CoA - substrate for ketogenesis. Ketone bodies are formed by incomplete oxidation of fatty acids; hence, the **energy obtained is low.**
- Ketone bodies are acetone, acetoacetate and β-hydroxybutyrate. They are **polar** (acids)
- Ketone bodies get **synthesized in liver** during conditions of starvation and uncontrolled diabetes
- Low insulin levels stimulate Hormone sensitive lipase which cleaves adipose tissue triacylglycerol to form glycerol and fatty acids.
  - In liver, glycerol is used as a substrate for gluconeogenesis and fatty acids get oxidized to acetyl CoA.
  - For further utilisation of acetyl CoA through citric acid cycle, oxaloacetate is required. Because in this scenario, there is active gluconeogenesis, oxaloacetate will be used for gluconeogenesis. As Oxaloacetate is not available, acetyl CoA accumulates and undergoes ketogenesis.
- Hence, ketone body is formed in liver because of low availability of oxaloacetate. Though ketone body is formed in liver, **ketone body cannot be utilised in liver**, because liver lacks the enzyme Thiophorase or Succinyl CoA Acetoacetate CoA Transferase.
- In extremes of starvation, **neurons** start utilizing ketone body.
- The preferred fuel for **cardiac muscle fibre** is fatty acid, in starvation cardiac muscle fibre can utilise ketone body.

70. All are true about ketone bodies *except*:

a. Ketone bodies are nonpolar
b. Ketone bodies can be synthesized by liver
c. Ketone bodies cannot be utilised by liver
d. Ketone bodies can be utilised by cardiac muscle

Ans. is 'a' Ketone bodies are nonpolar

71. The fuel used by neurons during starvation is:

a. Glucose
b. Fatty acid
c. Amino acid
d. Ketone body

Ans. is 'd' Ketone body

ACETYL COA CARBOXYLASE

- Acetyl CoA carboxylase (ACC) is the rate limiting step of fatty acid synthesis.
- ACC converts acetyl CoA (the building block of fatty acid) to malonyl CoA in the presence of ATP (source of energy), Biotin (coenzyme) and bicarbonate (source of CO_2).
- **Stimulators–Insulin, Citrate, Other dicarboxylic acids, Glutamate, ATP**
- **Inhibited by Glucagon and Epinephrine, Acyl CoA**

72. Activators of Acetyl CoA carboxylase are all *except*:

a. Acyl CoA
b. Citrate
c. Glutamate
d. Dicarboxylic acid

Ans. is 'a' Acyl CoA

LIPID TRANSPORT

Lipoprotein electrophoresis - **HDL, VLDL, LDL in that order from anode to cathode**

Type of cholesterol	Characteristic feature
Chylomicrons	• Involved in transport of exogenous lipids from the intestine to the liver. • Maximum lipid content overall • Maximum triglyceride • Maximum exogenous (dietary) triglyceride content • Minimum cholesterol content • Minimum phospholipid content • Least density and largest size • Minimum protein content • Least electrophoretic mobility

Contd...

Contd...

Type of cholesterol	Characteristic feature
HDL	• Minimum lipid content overall • Minimum triglyceride content • Maximum phospholipid content • Maximum density and smallest size • Maximum protein content • Maximum electrophoretic mobility
VLDL	Transports endogenous triglycerides from liver to peripheral tissues **Maximum endogenous triglyceride content** • Transport of endogenous triglycerides
LDL	• Maximum cholesterol content; 98% of LDL is formed from VLDL • Cholesterol is transported to peripheral (extrahepatic) tissues by LDL
IDL (VLDL remnants)	• IDL is the immediate precursor for LDL after being acted on by Hepatic Lipase • IDL is removed by liver via LDL-receptor mediated endocytosis.

Reverse Cholesterol Transport

- **Reverse cholesterol transport is the transport of cholesterol ester and phospholipid from extrahepatic tissues to liver.**
- HDL is released by both liver and intestinal cells as discoidal HDL.
- **Apo AI activates lecithin cholesterol acyl transferase (LCAT) and it converts discoidal HDL to Spheroidal HDL (HDL3) (by esterification of cholesterol).**
- HDL3 activates ABC1 (ATP binding casette transporter 1) to collect cholesterol and phospholipids from extra hepatic tissue membranes - HDL3 size increases and density decreases. Hence it forms HDL2.
- This HDL2 reaches liver to empty its contents into liver.
- Cholesterol ester transfer protein (CETP) transfers cholesterol ester from HDL2 to IDL, converting IDL to LDL. Hence **CETP decreases HDL level and increases LDL level.**

73. Which of the following is true about properties of VLDL/LDL?

a. In electrophoresis, VLDL migrates more cathodal than LDL
b. LDL is formed from liver
c. LDL is formed from chylomicron
d. VLDL remnants reach extrahepatic tissues

Ans. is 'b' LDL is formed from liver

74. Maximum content of endogenous triacylglycerol is found in:

a. Chylomicron
b. VLDL
c. IDL
d. LDL

Ans. is 'b' VLDL

75. All are true about Reverse cholesterol transport, *except*:

a. Transport of cholesterol from tissues to liver
b. ATP Binding Cassette Transporter involved in the conversion of HDL3 to HDL2
c. Lecithin Cholesterol Acyl catalyses the conversion of discoidal HDL to Spheroidal HDL
d. Cholesterol ester transfer increases HDL level

Ans. is 'd' Cholesterol ester transfer increases HDL level

APOLIPOPROTEINS

Type	*Found in*	*Function*
Apo-A		
A-I	HDL, Chylomicrons	Major structural protein of HDL, **major activator of LCAT.**
A-II	HDL, chylomicrons	Structural protein of HDL, inhibits lipoprotein lipase (LPL) stimulate hepatic lipase, inhibits LCAT
A-IV	HDL, Chylomicrons VLDL; IDL	Promotes lipoprotein lipase (LPL) mediated triglyceride lipolysis
Apo-B		
B-100	LDL, VLDL, IDL	Structural protein of VLDL, IDL; only apoprotein of LDL; mediate uptake of LDL by LDL receptors of liver

Contd...

Contd...

Type	Found in	Function
Apo-C		
C-I	Chylomicrons,VLDL, Liver HDL	
C-II	Chylomicrons VLDL, HDL	
C-III	Chylomicrons VLDL, HDL liver	
Apo-D	HDL	
Apo-E	Chylomicrons, Chylomicrons Remnants, VLDL, HDL	Mediates uptake of chylomicrons remnants and IDL, by LDL receptors in liver

LCAT Deficiency

- A deficiency of Lecithin cholesterol acyl transferase (LCAT) causes accumulation of unesterified cholesterol in certain body tissues. Cholesterol effluxes from cells as free cholesterol and is transported in HDL as esterified cholesterol.
- LCAT is the enzyme that esterifies the free cholesterol on HDL to cholesterol ester and allows the maturation of HDL.
- LCAT deficiency does not allow for HDL maturation resulting in its rapid catabolism of circulating apoA-1 and apoA-2. The remaining form of HDL resembles nascent HDL.
- **Lipid panel: Severely Low HDL levels, elevated VLDL and triglycerides, high plasma unesterified cholesterol and low plasma cholesterol ester.**

The distribution of apolipoproteins characterizes the lipoprotein.

- The major apolipoproteins of HDL are apo As.
- The main apolipoprotein of LDL is apo B (B-100), which is also found in VLDL.
- Chylomicrons contain a truncated form (48% of apo B-100) of apo-B (B-48) that is synthesized in intestine, while B-100 is synthesized in liver.
- Apo B-100 is one of the longest single polypeptide chains known, having 4536 amino acids and a molecular mass of 550,000 Da.
- To produce Apo B-48, a stop signal is introduced into the mRNA transcript for apo B-100 by an RNA editing enzyme.
- Apo C-I, C-II and C-III are smaller polypeptides freely transferable between several different lipoproteins.
- Apo E found in VLDL, HDL, chylomicrons and chylomicron remnants, is also freely transferable; it accounts for 5–10% of total VLDL apolipoproteins in normal subjects.

76. Genetic basis for the formation of intestine specific Apo B48 is: *(NEET 2020)*

a. RNA editing
b. Alternate splicing
c. DNA translocation
d. Histone modification

Ans. is 'a' RNA editing

77. Activator of LCAT is:

a. Apo CII
b. Apo CIII
c. Apo AI
d. Apo B100

Ans. is 'c' Apo AI

78. LCAT deficiency leads to low levels of : *(NEET 2019)*

a. HDL
b. Triglycerides
c. VLDL
d. Unesterified plasma cholesterol

Ans. is 'a' HDL

ABETALIPOPROTEINEMIA

- Autosomal recessive disorder
- Defect in MTP (Microsomal triglyceride transfer protein)-MTP forms/secretes lipoproteins with apo-B i.e. Chylomicrons from intestine (B48) and VLDL from liver (B100)
- Clinical features
  - Presents in infancy with steatorrhea, failure to thrive
  - Fat-soluble (A, D, E, K) vitamin deficiencies-Vitamin E deficiency is found to have profound effects.
  - Vitamin E deficiency presents as **retinitis pigmentosa** and sabacute combined degeneration
  - Acanthocytes (star shaped RBCs in peripheral smear)
- Treatment involves vitamin E administration.

79. Abetalipoproteinemia affects:

a. Retinal pigment epithelium
b. Optic nerve
c. Occipital cortex
d. Bipolar neurons

Ans. is 'a' Retinal pigment epithelium

Biochemical tests used to detect abnormal constituents of urine	
Abnormal constituent	***Test***
Reducing sugar	Benedict's test
Galactose	Mucic acid test
Ketone body	**Rothera's test (acetoacetate and acetone) Gerhardt's test (acetoacetate)**
Blood	Benzidine test
Protein	Sulphosalicylic acid test
Albumin	Heat coagulation test
Bile salt	Hay's test
Bile pigment	Fouchet's test

80. Rothera's test is used for the detection of:

a. Reducing sugar
b. Blood
c. Ketone body
d. Protein

Ans. is 'c' Ketone body

NUCLEIC ACIDS

NUCLEOTIDE SYNTHESIS

Purine Synthesis

Purine ring atoms	Source
N_1	Aspartate
C_2	N_{10} Formyl THFA
C_8	N_5, N_{10} Methenyl THFA
N_3,N_9	Glutamine
C_4, C_5, N_7	Glycine
C_6	Carbon dioxide

- In purine nucleotide synthesis, first Ribose-5-phosphate is activated by PRPP synthetase to form PRPP (5-Phosphoribosyl-1-Pyrophosphate).
- This PRPP gets attached to N9 (source is glutamine) in the presence of PRPP glutamine amidotransferase. This is the rate limiting enzyme of purine synthesis.
- In purine synthesis, **Inosine inonophosphate (IMP) is first formed**; which is then converted into Adenosine monophosphate (AMP) and Guanosine monophosphate (GMP).

Pyrimidine Synthesis

Pyrimidine ring atoms	Source
N_3	Glutamine
C_2	CO_2
C_4, C_5, C_6, N_1	Aspartate

- First step of pyrimidine synthesis involves carbamoyl phosphate synthetase II (CPS II) which allows Carbon dioxide, Glutamine and 2 molecules of ATP to react together to form Carbamoyl Phosphate.
- When Carbamoyl phosphate is acted upon by Aspartyl transcarbamoylase, it gets diverted to pyrimidine synthesis. Hence, Aspartyl transcarbamoylase is considered as the rate limiting enzyme of pyrimidine synthesis.
- Carbamoyl Aspartate gets converted to Orotic Acid.
- Orotic acid gets attached to PRPP, it forms OMP.
- Uridine monophosphate (UMP) is formed first. Cytosine monophosphate (CMP) and Thymidine monophosphate (TMP) are derived from UMP.

81. Pyrimidine ring is derived from all *except*:

a. Carbon dioxide
b. Glutamine
c. Aspartate
d. Glycine

Ans. is 'd' Glycine

82. All of the following are sources of atoms in purine ring *except*:

a. Carbon dioxide
b. Aspartate
c. Glycine
d. ATP

Ans. is 'd' ATP

83. True about purine synthesis:

a. Glutamine is the source of amino group
b. PRPP synthesis is the rate limiting step in purine synthesis
c. THFA is the source of nitrogen atoms
d. GMP is the first nucleotide to be synthesized

Ans. is 'a' Glutamine is the source of amino group

84. Carbamoyl phosphate is used in:

a. Purine synthesis
b. Pyrimidine synthesis
c. Purine catabolism
d. Pyrimidine catabolism

Ans. is 'b' Pyrimidine synthesis

PYRIMIDINE CATABOLISM

- In pyrimidine catabolism, first cytidine and thymidine are converted to uridine by deamination and demethylation respectively.
- Uridine in the presence of phosphorylase gets converted into uracil.
- Uracil undergoes hydrogenation in the presence of dihydrouracil dehydrogenase to form dihydrouracil.
- Dihydrouracil hydratase opens the ring of dihydrouracil to form a linear structure.
- The linear structure undergoes deamination to form β-alanine or β-amino iso butyrate.
- Hence, pyrimidines on catabolism do not form uracil, they form Carbon dioxide, water and urea (from ammonia generated by deamination).
- B-alanine or β-aminoisobutyrate is an intermediate of pyrimidine catabolism.
- B-alanine gets converted into acetyl CoA and gets into citric acid cycle.
- As β-alanine is a precursor of carnosine and anserine, an increase in the pyrimidine catabolism results in increased generation of carnosine.

85. β-Alanine is a product of metabolism of:

a. Purine
b. Pyrimidine
c. Histidine
d. Glycine

Ans. is 'b' Pyrimidine

86. True about pyrimidine catabolism is:

a. It is a source of uric acid
b. β-aminoisobutyrate is generated
c. Unlike other catabolic pathways, it does not generate intermediates of citric acid cycle
d. Increased pyrimidine catabolism causes decreased synthesis of carnosine

Ans. is 'b' β-aminoisobutyrate is generated

STRUCTURE OF DNA

- The DNA double helix illustrates the contribution of multiple forces to the structure of biomolecules.
- While each individual DNA strand is held together by covalent bonds, the two strands of the helix are held together exclusively by noncovalent interactions such as hydrogen bonds between nucleotide bases (Watson-Crick base pairing) and van der Waals interactions between the stacked purine and pyrimidine bases.
- The double helix presents the charged phosphate groups and polar hydroxyl groups from the ribose sugars of the DNA backbone to water while burying the relatively hydrophobic nucleotide bases inside. The extended backbone maximizes the distance between negatively charged phosphates, minimizing unfavorable electrostatic interactions.

Structure of nucleic acid	Bond
Nucleoside (Pentose sugar + nitrogenous base)	N-glycosidic bond
Nucleotide (Nucleoside + Phosphate group)	Phosphoester linkage
Diphosphate and Polyphosphate nucleotide (Mononucleotide + additional phosphate group)	Acid anhydride linkage
Polynucleotide chain (b/w 3' hydroxyl group of nucleotide with 5' phosphate group of next nucleotide)	**3'5' phosphodiester linkage**

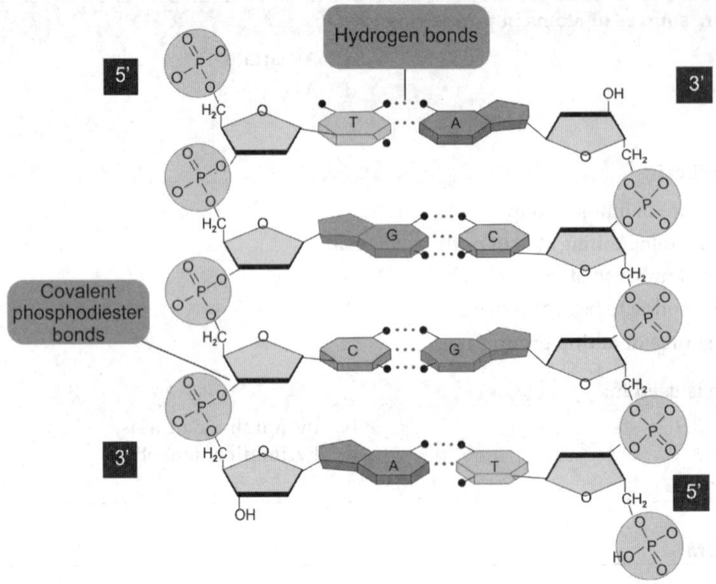

87. The linkage which links individual nucleotides in a polynucleotide chain is:

a. β N- Glycosidic linkage
b. α N−glycosidic linkage
c. 3'5' Phosphodiester linkage
d. 5'3' Phosphodiester linkages

Ans. is 'c' 3'5' Phosphodiester linkage

88. If the thymine content in DNA is 28%, what is the cytosine content? *(NEET 2020)*

a. 28%
b. 56%
c. 22%
d. 44%

Ans. is 'c' 22%

Explanation: By Chargaff's rule, number of purines equal the number of pyrimidines in a double stranded DNA. In DNA, Adenine-Thymine and Guanine-Cytosine pair together. Given that thymine content is 28%, thus adenine content is also 28% as adenine and thymine pair together. Thus, the rest 44% content must be guanine and cytosine–i.e. 22% each.

DNA CONFORMATIONS

	A-DNA	B-DNA	Z-DNA
Direction	Right-handed	Right-handed	**Left-handed**
Major groove	Deep and narrow	Wide	Not real groove
Minor groove	Wide	Narrow	Narrow
Base pairs	Displaced away from the helical axis	Centred over the helical axis	Zig-zag pattern (nearly perpendicular to the helical axis)
Base pairs per turn	11	10	12

89. Left handed helix is seen in:

a. B-DNA
b. A-DNA
c. Z-DNA
d. F-DNA

Ans. is 'c' Z-DNA

NUCLEOSOME

- Chromatin condenses into chromosomes–with help of histones.
- Histones are basic proteins (positively charged) rich in lysine and arginine (basic amino acids)–Binds negatively charged phosphate backbone of DNA
- There are five types of histones–H1, H2A, H2B, H3 and H4.
- **Of these all except H1, the remaining four form dimers to form a histone octamer**. This histone octamer sits in the center and that is surrounded by a segment of dsDNA of length approx 146 bp (in a left handed supercoiling). This string on bead appearance is called as Nucleosome.
- Several such nucleosomes exist, which are connected by a linker fragment. H1 histone is found in the linker fragment.

Biochemistry

90. Nucleosome core proteins include all *except*:

a. H1
b. H2A
c. H2B
d. H4

Ans. is 'a' H1

HUMAN MITOCHONDRIAL DNA

- It is circular, **double-stranded.**
- Contains 16 kbp (nuclear genome- 3.3 billion bp)
- **Encodes 13 protein subunits of the respiratory chain (of a total of about 67 i.e 20%)**
- Encodes large (16S) and small (12S) mt ribosomal RNAs
- Encodes 22 mt tRNA molecules
- Genetic code differs slightly from the standard code
  - UGA (standard stop codon) is read as Trp
  - AGA and AGG (standard codons for Arg) are read as stop codons
- Contains very few untranslated sequences (3% noncoding vs 93% in nuclear DNA)
- **High mutation rate** (5–10 times that of nuclear DNA)
- **Inheritance is strictly maternal.**

91. All are true regarding mitochondrial DNA, *except*? *(NEET 2019)*

a. Double stranded
b. Inherited from mother
c. High mutation rate
d. All respiratory proteins are synthesized within mitochondria itself

Ans. is 'd' All respiratory proteins are synthesized within mitochondria itself

TELOMERASE

- Telomerase is an **RNA-dependent DNA polymerase** that adds DNA to 3′ ends of chromosomes to avoid loss of genetic material with every duplication.
- Often dysregulated in cancer cells, allowing unlimited replication.
- As cells go through cell cycle, during replication, the telomeric end is progressively shortened due to replacement with labile RNA primers.
- After 50 to 70 cell divisions, the telomeric ends reach a critical or minimum length called as Hayflick limit beyond which chromosomes become unstable and cell cycle is stopped. This leads to aging.
- Based on the RNA fragments left back in the terminals as a result of replication, telomerase synthesizes and replaces DNA fragments. Hence, the length of telomeric ends can be maintained and aging is prevented. Hence, telomerase is an anti-aging enzyme.

92. Which enzyme prevents aging?

a. DNA ligase
b. DNA polymerase A
c. Telomerase
d. RNA polymerase H

Ans. is 'c' Telomerase

93. Telomerase is:

a. RNA dependent DNA polymerase
b. DNA dependent DNA polymerase
c. RNA dependent RNA polymerase
d. DNA depenent RNA polymerase

Ans. is 'a' RNA dependent DNA polymerase

94. A young child presented with the signs of premature ageing. Diagnosis of Werner's syndrome was made. What is the genetic basis for this? *(NEET 2020)*

a. Telomere lengthening
b. Lipid peroxidation
c. Telomere shortening due to helicase defect
d. Increased advanced glycation end product

Ans. is 'c' Telomere shortening due to helicase defect

Explanation: Patients with Werner syndrome show premature aging and the defective gene product is a DNA helicase, a protein involved in DNA replication and repair. This leads to rapid telomere shortening that may mimic the cell injury normally accumulated during cellular aging.

DISEASES DUE TO DEFECTS IN DNA REPAIR MECHANISMS

Defective DNA repair mechanism	Disease
Single Strand repair	
Mismatch repair	HNPCC
Base excision repair	MUTYH-associated polyposis
Nucleotide excision repair	Xeroderma pigmentosa Cockayne syndrome Trichothiodystrophy
Double Strand repair	
Homologous repair	Bloom syndrome Werner syndrome BRCA1 and 2 gene mutations
Non-homologous end joining repair (dsDNA break repair)	SCID **Ataxia Telangiectasia**

95. Ataxia telangiectasia is caused by a defect of:

a. Base excision repair
b. Nucleotide excision repair
c. Mismatch repair
d. ds DNA break repair

Ans. is 'd' ds DNA break repair

RECOMBINANT DNA

- Chimeric DNA or recombinant DNA is formed by linking DNA fragments of two unrelated genome.
- Involved in recombinant DNA technology. It is done to introduce a favorable quality into an organism like ability to produce insulin by *E. coli* or insect resistance in crops.
- Requires restriction endonucleases
- Restriction endonucleases are enzymes that cut DNA at specific DNA sequences within the molecule– called the palindromic regions. A palindromic sequence, is a sequence made up of nucleic acids within the double helix of DNA/RNA that is same when read from 5′ to 3′ end on either i.e. complimentary strands.
- Example: 5′- GAATTC- 3′ is the palindromic sequence for Eco R1 and Hpa1

5′ ——— G A A T T C ——→ 3″

3′ ←—— C T T A A G ——— 5″

- Steps involved in recombinant DNA formation are:
  - Cleaving the vector with restriction endonucleases (Sticky end producing restriction endonucleases are favorable than blunt end for formation of recombinant DNA)
  - Introducing the DNA fragment with gene of interest
  - Both the vector and DNA fragment with gene of interest are linked by DNA ligases
  - The recombinant vector or the chimeric DNA is then introduced into the host cell and the host expresses the desired trait.

96. Chimeric DNA are all true *except*:

a. Formed by linking DNA fragments of unrelated genome
b. Sticky end producing restriction endonucleases favor formation of chimeric DNA
c. They don't require DNA ligase
d. The organism harboring a chimeric DNA has features of themselves and the properties of the insert

Ans. is 'c' They don't require DNA ligase

POST-TRANSCRIPTIONAL MODIFICATIONS

Initial transcript is heteronuclear RNA (hnRNA); which undergoes three key modifications before leaving nucleus

1. **5′ capping** - Addition of 7-methylguanosine to 5′ end soon after transcription begins; distinguishes mRNA from other RNA
2. **RNA Splicing**
   - Introns removed from mRNA in nucleus
   - Primary transcript combines with Small nuclear ribonucleoproteins (snRNPs)-Short RNA polymers complexed with proteins containing high content of uridine (U-RNAs). Five different U-RNAs defined: U1, U2, U4, U5, and U6.
   - snRNPs and mRNA forms spliceosome - Loop of mRNA with intron is formed ("lariat")

- Lariat released → removes intron and Exons are joined
- Splicing is never 100%. Not all noncoding intervening sequences are removed (UnTranslated regions)
- Splicing occurs only in eukaryotes.
- Histone genes are of prokaryotic type. Hence they do not have introns. Histone mRNAs do not undergo splicing.

3. **3′-polyadenylation** - Enzyme: Poly-A polymerase (PAP) adds ~200 adenosine nucleotides to 3′ end of mRNA without a template

97. Gene splicing all are true *except*:

a. Complete removal of introns
b. Histone mRNAs do not undergo splicing
c. SnRNAs help in splicing
d. Prokaryotic mRNAs do not undergo splicing

Ans. is 'a' Complete removal of introns

LAC OPERON

The molecular mechanisms responsible for the regulation of the genes involved in the metabolism of lactose are now among the best-understood in any organism. β-Galactosidase hydrolyzes the β-galactoside lactose to galactose and glucose. **The gene encoding β-galactosidase (lacZ) is clustered with the genes encoding galactoside permease (lacY) and thiogalactoside transacetylase (lacA).** The genes encoding these three enzymes, along with the lac promoter and lac operator (a regulatory region), and the lacI gene encoding the LacI repressor are physically linked and constitute the lac operon. This genetic arrangement of the lac operon allows for coordinate expression of the three enzymes concerned with lactose metabolism. Each of the linked operon genes is transcribed into one large polycistronic mRNA molecule that contains multiple independent translation start (AUG) and stop (UAA) codons for each of the three cistrons. Thus, each protein is translated separately, and they are not processed from a single large precursor protein.

a. When no inducer (lactose) is present, the constitutively synthesized lacI gene products form a repressor tetramer that binds to the operator. Repressor-operator binding prevents the binding of RNA polymerase and consequently prevents transcription of the lacZ, lacY, and lacA structural genes.

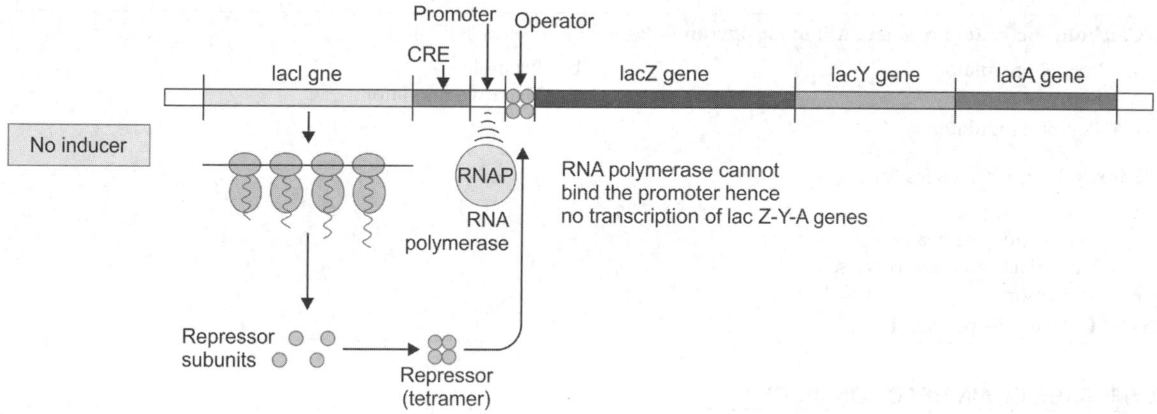

b. When inducer (lactose) is present, but glucose is also present in the culture medium, the tetrameric repressor molecules are conformationally altered by inducer, and cannot efficiently bind to the operator locus (affinity of binding reduced >1000-fold). However, RNA polymerase will not efficiently bind the promoter and initiate transcription because positive protein–protein interactions between CRE-bound CAP protein fail to occur; thus, the lac operon is not efficiently transcribed.

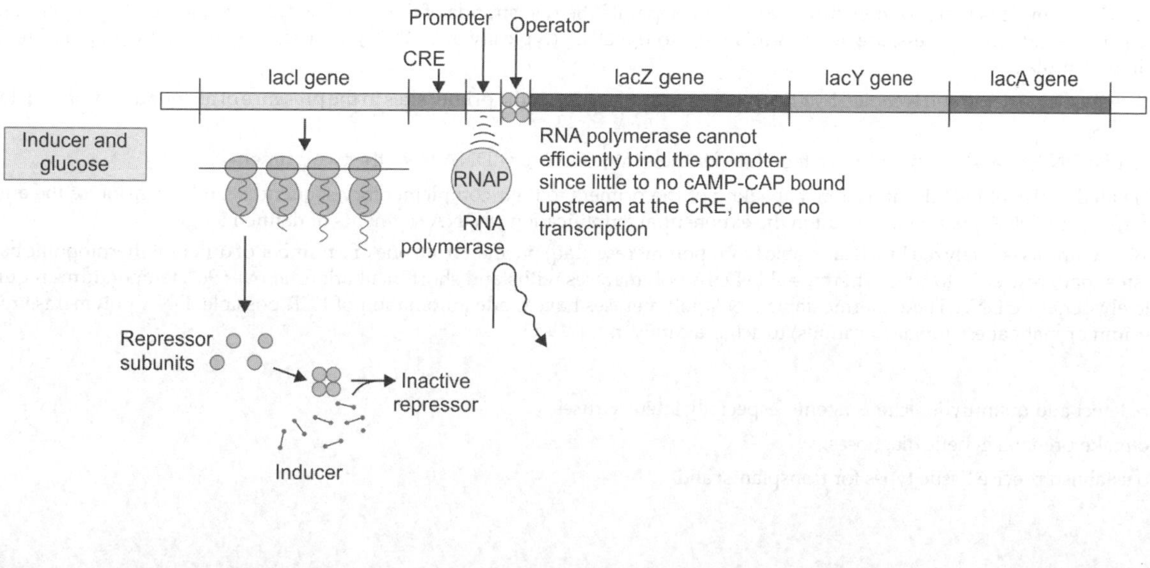

c. However, when inducer is present, and glucose is depleted from the medium, adenylyl cyclase is activated and cAMP is produced. This cAMP binds with high affinity to its binding protein the catabolite activator protein, or CAP. The CAP-cAMP complex binds to its recognition sequence (CRE, the cAMP response element) at lac operon. Direct protein–protein contacts between the CRE-bound CAP and the RNA polymerase increases promoter binding >20-fold; hence RNAP will efficiently transcribe the lac operon and the polycistronic lacZ-lacY-lacA mRNA molecule formed can be translated into the corresponding protein molecules β-galactosidase, permease, and transacetylase as shown.

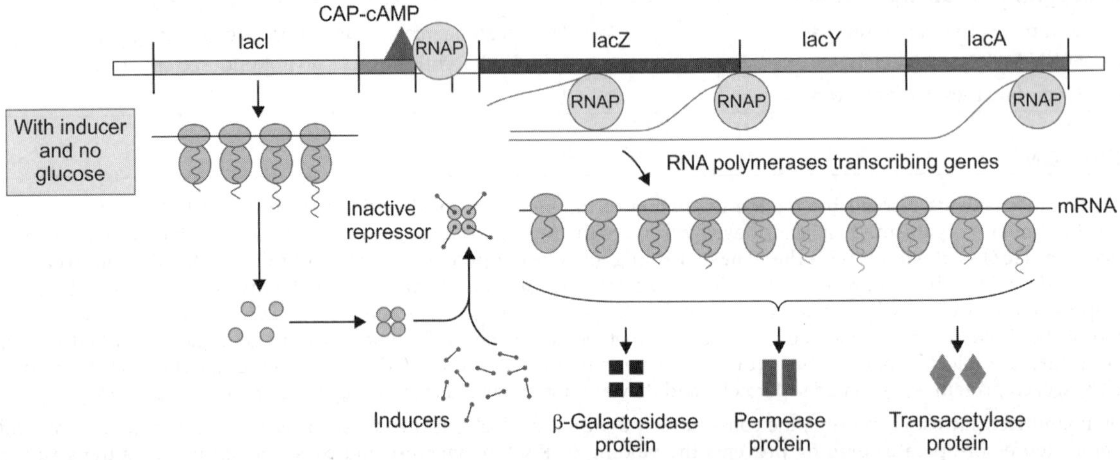

98. Catabolite activator protein (CAP) in lac operon is a:

a. Positive regulator
b. Promoter
c. Repressor
d. Negative regulator

Ans. is 'a' Positive regulator

99. LacY in lac operon codes for:

a. β-Galactosidase
b. Galactoside permease
c. Thiogalactosyl transacetylase
d. Repressor

Ans. is 'b' Galactoside permease

POLYMERASE CHAIN REACTION (PCR)

PCR provides a sensitive, selective, and extremely rapid means of amplifying any desired sequence of DNA. Specificity is based on the use of two oligonucleotide primers that hybridize to complementary sequences on opposite strands of DNA and flank the target sequence.

Steps:

- The DNA sample is first heat denatured (> 90°C) to separate the two strands of the template DNA containing the target sequence; the primers, added in excess, are allowed to anneal to the DNA (typically at 50-75°C) in order to generate the required template-primer complex.
- Subsequently, each strand is copied by a DNA polymerase, starting at the primer sites in the presence of all four deoxyribonucleotides (dNTPs).
- The two DNA strands each serve as a template for the synthesis of new DNA from the two primers.
- Repeated cycles of heat denaturation, annealing of the primers to their complementary sequences, and extension of the annealed primers with DNA polymerase result in the exponential amplification of DNA segments of defined length.

DNA synthesis is catalyzed by a heat-stable DNA polymerase (Taq) purified from one of a number of different thermophilic bacteria, organisms that grow at 70 to 80°C. Thermostable DNA polymerases withstand short incubations at over 90°, temperatures required to completely denature DNA.These thermostable DNA polymerases have made automation of PCR possible. DNA polymerase requires magnesium or manganese (divalent cations) to act as a catalyst.

Uses

1. To detect and quantify infectious agents, especially latent viruses;
2. To make prenatal genetic diagnoses;
3. To establish precise tissue types for transplants; and

4. For quantitative RNA analyses after RNA copying and mRNA quantification by the so-called RT-PCR method (cDNA copies of mRNA generated by a retroviral reverse transcriptase)

100. Not a component of PCR:

a. dNTP
b. Primer
c. Divalent cation
d. Restriction enzyme

Ans. is 'd' Restriction enzyme

FLOW CYTOMETRY

- Laboratory technique to assess size, granularity and protein expression (immunophenotype) of individual cells in a sample.
- Cells are tagged with antibodies specific to surface or intracellular proteins. Antibodies are then tagged with a unique fluorescent dye. Sample is analyzed one cell at a time by focusing a laser on the cell and measuring light scatter and intensity of fluorescence.
- Commonly used in workup of hematologic abnormalities (e.g.–leukemia, PNH) and immunodeficiencies (e.g. CD4 count in HIV)

101. Flow cytometry is used for studying:

a. Cell size
b. Type of cell
c. Surface antigens
d. All of the above

Ans. is 'd' All of the above

FLUORESCENCE IN-SITU HYBRIDIZATION (FISH)

- Fluorescent oligonucleotides or RNA probe binds to specific gene site of interest on chromosomes.
- Used for specific localization of genes and direct visualization of chromosomal anomalies at the molecular level:
  - Microdeletion—no fluorescence on a chromosome compared to fluorescence at the same locus on second copy of that chromosome
  - Translocation—fluorescence signal that corresponds to one chromosome is found in a different chromosome
  - Duplication—extra copy of a chromosome resulting in a trisomy or tetrasomy

102. Regarding FISH all are true *except*:

a. Used to detect copy number variations
b. Used to detect balanced translocations
c. Requires oligonucleotides
d. Requires DNA polymerase

Ans. is 'd' Requires DNA polymerase

IMMUNOCHROMATOGRAPHY

- Also known as lateral flow test or simply strip test which are the devices intended to detect the target analyte in sample without the need for specialized and costly equipment.
- The principle is based on dye labelled antibody specific for target analyte which is present on the lower end of nitrocellulose strip or in the plastic well along with the strip. The antibody which is specific for target antigen is also bound to the strip in a thin test line and antibody antigen specific for labelled antibody bound to control line. So when the sample and buffer are placed on strip or in a well-mixed with labelled antibody to draw across the lines of bound antibody. If the antigen is present, then some of the labelled antibody will be trapped on the test line and the excess labelled antibodies are trapped on the control line.
- Benefits: User-friendly, inexpensive, quick results, long shelf-life
- Examples: Pregnancy test, strep throat, chlamydia, rapid HBsAg test. These are conditions for which a quantitative assay is not necessary.

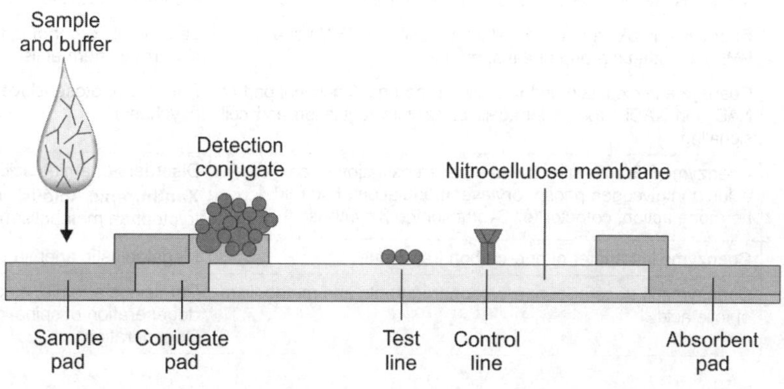

103. What is the principle of the test shown below? *(NEET 2020)*

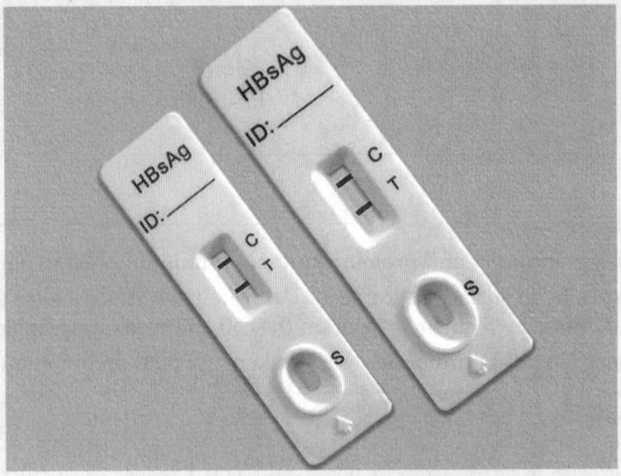

a. Immunochromatography
b. Chemiluminescent assay
c. Immunofluorescence assay
d. Enzyme linked immunosorbent assay

Ans. is 'a' Immunochromatography

VITAMINS

FAT AND WATER SOLUBLE VITAMINS

Fat soluble vitamins include Vitamin A, Vitamin D, Vitamin E and Vitamin K.

- Fat soluble vitamins are stored in adipose tissue and in liver. Hence deficiency manifestations of fat soluble vitamins are relatively rare. There is a risk of toxicity of fat soluble vitamins when the intake is increased.

Water soluble vitamins include Vitamin B1 (thiamine), Vitamin B2 (Riboflavin), Vitamin B3, Vitamin B5 (Pantothenic acid), Vitamin B6 (Pyridoxal), Vitamin B7 (Biotin), Vitamin B9 (Folate), Vitamin (cyanocobalamine), and Vitamin C (ascorbic acid).

- Water soluble vitamins are not stored and they get lost in urine—the only exception is vitamin B12 which is stored in liver. Hence, deficiency manifestations are relatively common. They do not present with toxicity as they are not stored.

104. Water soluble vitamin is:

a. Thiamine
b. Retinoic acid
c. Cholecalciferol
d. Tocopherol

Ans. is 'a' Thiamine

Important Vitamins

Vitamin	Chemical name	Functions	Deficiency disease
A	Retinal, β-carotene	Forms visual pigments in retina; regulation of gene expression and cell differentiation (beta-carotene is an antioxidant)	Night blindness, xerophthalmia; hyperkeratinization of skin
B1	Thiamine	Coenzyme in pyruvate and α-ketoglutarate dehydrogenases and transketolase; regulates Cl channel in nerve conduction	Peripheral nerve damage (beriberi) or central nervous system lesions (Wernicke Korsakoff syndrome)
B2	Riboflavin	Coenzyme in oxidation and reduction reactions (FAD and FMN); prosthetic group of flavoproteins	Lesions of corner of mouth, lips, and tongue, seborrheic dermatitis
Niacin B3	Nicotinic acid, nicotinamide	Coenzyme in oxidation and reduction reactions, functional part of NAD and NADP; role in intracellular calcium regulation and cell signaling	Pellagra-photosensitive dermatitis, depressive psychosis
B6	Pyridoxine, pyridoxal, pyridoxamine	Coenzyme in transamination and decarboxylation of amino acids and glycogen phosphorylase; modulation of steroid hormone action, cofactor for Cystathionine β synthase	Disorders of amino acid metabolism, convulsions **Xanthurenic Aciduria** (alternative pathway for tryptophan metabolism)
B9	Folic acid	Coenzyme in transfer of one-carbon fragments	Megaloblastic anemia
B12	Cobalamin	Coenzyme in transfer of one-carbon fragments and metabolism of folic acid.	Pernicious anemia, megaloblastic anemia with degeneration of spinal cord (Subacute Combined Degeneration)

Contd...

Contd...

Vitamin	Chemical name	Functions	Deficiency disease
B5	Pantothenic acid	Functional part of CoA and acyl carrier protein: fatty acid synthesis and metabolism	Peripheral nerve damage (nutritional melalgia or burning foot syndrome)
C	Ascorbic acid	Coenzyme in hydroxylation of proline and lysine in collagen synthesis, antioxidant; enhances absorption of iron; cofactor for Dopamine β-hydroxylase (Dopamine → Norepinephrine)	Scurvy-impaired wound healing, loss of dental cement, subcutaneous hemorrhage
D	Calciferol	Calcium homeostasis- enhances intestinal absorption and renal reabsorption of Ca^{2+}; regulation of gene expression and cell differentiation	Rickets in children; osteomalacia in adults
E	Tocopherols	Antioxidant, especially in cell membranes; role in cell signaling	Extremely rare—serious neurologic dysfunction, ataxia
K	Phylloquinone: menaquinones	Coenzyme in formation of γ-carboxyglutamate in enzymes of blood clotting (Factors II, VII, IX, X, Protein C and S) and bone matrix	Impaired blood clotting, hemorrhagic disease of newborn
H	Biotin	Coenzyme in carboxylation reactions in gluconeogenesis and fatty acid synthesis; role in regulation of cell cycle	Impaired fat and carbohydrate metabolism, dermatitis

Vitamins synthesized within the human body:

1. Niacin- is produced from amino acid tryptophan.
2. Vitamin D- synthesized from cholesterol

Note: Pantothenic acid, vitamin K and biotin are produced within the human body, but not by human cells. They are produced by colonic bacteria.

Hypervitaminosis A

- Caused by consumption of food rich in vitamin A like fish or liver
- Features include anorexia, irritability, headache, skin peeling, vomiting. Headache, vomiting and papilledema are found due to raised intracranial tension (pseudotumor cerebri). Hypercalcemia and pathological fractures (vitamin A stimulates osteoclasts).
- Teratogenic in large doses

Vitamin B12 is cofactor for:

1. *Methylmalonyl CoA mutase*
    - It converts methylmalonyl CoA to succinyl CoA (odd chain fatty acid metabolism).
    - The activity of this enzyme is greatly reduced in vitamin B12 deficiency, leading to an accumulation of methylmalonyl CoA. Amount of this compound excreted in urine serves as a means of assessing vitamin B12 nutritional status.
2. *Methionine synthase*
    - It catalyses the conversion of homocysteine into methionine using methyl tetrahydrofolate.
    - Impairment of methionine synthase in vitamin B12 deficiency results in the accumulation of methyl tetrahydrofolate that cannot be used for further reactions. This is called the 'folate trap' because it results in functional deficiency of folate
        - Both folate and B12 required to covert homocysteine to methionine - Elevated homocysteine in both deficiencies
3. *Homocysteine methyl transferase:* Transfers methyl groups as methylcobalamin.

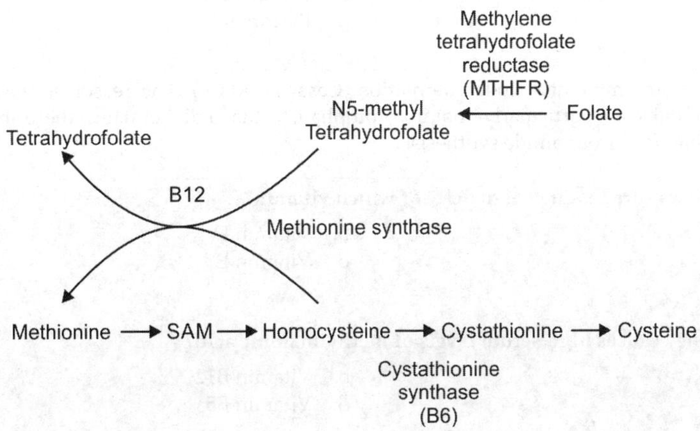

NIACIN (Vitamin B_3)

Functions

- Constituent of NAD+, NADP+ (used in redox reactions).
- Derived from tryptophan. Synthesis requires vitamins B2 and B6.
- Used to treat dyslipidemia; lowers levels of VLDL and raises levels of HDL

Deficiency

- Glossitis.
- Severe deficiency leads to pellagra, which can also be caused by Hartnup disease, malignant carcinoid syndrome (increased tryptophan metabolism), and isoniazid (reduced vitamin B6)
- Symptoms of pellagra: Diarrhea, Dementia (also hallucinations), Dermatitis (C3/C4 dermatome circumferential "broad collar" rash [Casal necklace], hyperpigmentation of sun exposed limbs

Excess

- Facial flushing (induced by prostaglandin, not histamine; can avoid by taking aspirin with niacin)
- Hyperglycemia, hyperuricemia
- Several cases of niacin-induced cystoid macular edema have been reported with different dosages

105. Macular edema and macular cysts is caused by supraphysiological levels of which vitamin? *(NEET 2020)*

a. Niacin
b. Vitamin A
c. Vitamin D
d. Vitamin E

Ans. is 'a' Niacin

106. A child presents with diarrhoea and skin rash. He consumes only maize in the diet. Image is shown below. Which vitamin is deficient in this child? *(NEET 2020)*

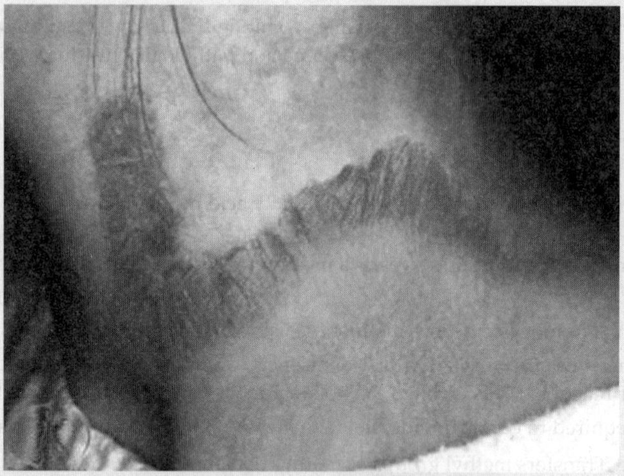

a. Niacin
b. Pantothenate
c. Riboflavin
d. Pyridoxine

Ans. is 'a' Niacin

Explanation: The image shows circumferential collar dermatitis (Casal necklace). The reason a maize-based diet predisposes to pellagra is that the proteins of maize are particularly poor in tryptophan, so that a diet in which there are few other sources of protein provides insufficient tryptophan for nicotinamide synthesis.

107. Headache and papilledema are features of toxicity of which vitamin?

a. Vitamin A
b. Vitamin D
c. Vitamin C
d. Vitamin E

Ans. is 'a' Vitamin A

108. Which vitamin deficiency causes high serum levels of methylmalonic acid?

a. Vitamin B1
b. Vitamin B12
c. Vitamin B6
d. Vitamin B5

Ans. is 'b' Vitamin B12

109. Deficiency of which vitamin leads to Wernicke's encephalopathy?

a. Riboflavin
b. Pyridoxine
c. Thiamine
d. Biotin

Ans. is 'c' Thiamine

110. Vitamin B12 deficiency causes all *except*:

a. Homocysteinuria
b. Methylmalonic aciduria
c. Subacute combined degeneration
d. Epinephrine excess

Ans. is 'd' Epinephrine excess

111. Vitamin B12 is obtained from: *(NEET 2020)*

a. Animal sources
b. Legumes
c. Vegetables
d. Dairy products

Ans. is 'a' Animal sources

112. Biotin is essential for:

a. Decarboxylases
b. Oxidative decarboxylases
c. Transaminases
d. Carboxylases

Ans. is 'd' Carboxylases

113. Which vitamin is required for transfer of 1 carbon unit?

a. Vitamin B3
b. Vitamin B5
c. Vitamin B7
d. Vitamin B9

Ans. is 'd' Vitamin B9

114. Vitamin given in homocysteinuria are all *except*:

a. Vitamin B6
b. Vitamin B12
c. Folate
d. Thiamine

Ans. is 'd' Thiamine

115. Which vitamin in large doses is teratogenic?

a. Vitamin A
b. Vitamin D
c. Vitamin E
d. Vitamin K

Ans. is 'a' Vitamin A

116. Vitamin K dependent dotting factors are *except*:

a. Factor III
b. Factor VII
c. Factor IX
d. Factor X

Ans. is 'a' Factor III

117. Which is an antioxidant vitamin?

a. Vitamin A
b. Vitamin D
c. Vitamin E
d. Vitamin K

Ans. is 'c' Vitamin E

COBALAMIN (VITAMIN B12)

Found in animal products. Synthesized only by microorganisms. Very large reserve pool (several years) stored primarily in the liver. Deficiency caused by malabsorption (e.g., sprue, enteritis, *Diphyllobothrium latum*, achlorhydria, bacterial overgrowth, alcohol excess), lack of intrinsic factor (e.g., pernicious anemia, gastric bypass surgery), absence of terminal ileum (surgical resection, eg, for Crohn disease), certain drugs (e.g., metformin), *or* insufficient intake (e.g., veganism).

Function: Cofactor for methionine synthase (transfers CH_3 groups as methylcobalamin) and methylmalonyl-CoA mutase. Important for DNA synthesis.

Deficiency: Macrocytic, megaloblastic anemia; hypersegmentecl PMNs; paresthesias and subacute combined degeneration (degeneration of dorsal columns, lateral corticospinal tracts and spinocerebellar tracts) due to abnormal myelin. Associated with raised serum homocysteine and methylmalonic acid levels, along with 2° folate deficiency. Prolonged deficiency → irreversible nerve damage. Folate supplementation can mask the hematologic symptoms of B12 deficiency, but not the neurologic symptoms.

Pernicious anemia is a specific form of megaloblastic anemia caused by an autoimmune gastritis that impairs the production of intrinsic factor, which is required for vitamin B_{12} uptake from the gut. The stomach typically shows diffuse chronic gastritis. The most characteristic alteration is fundic gland atrophy, affecting both chief cells and parietal cells, the latter being virtually absent.

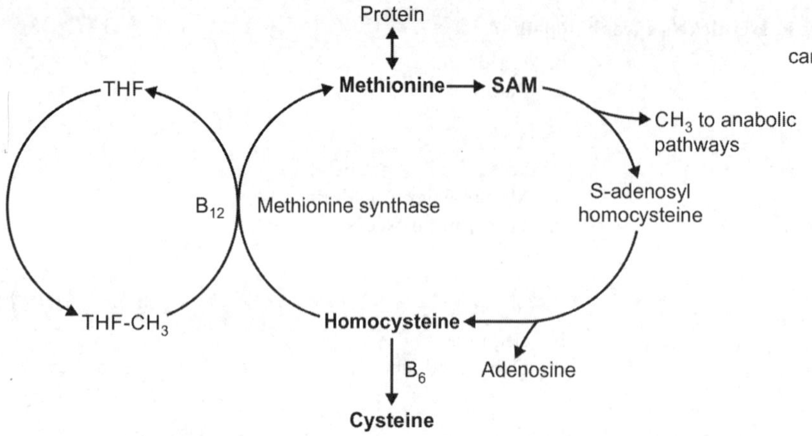

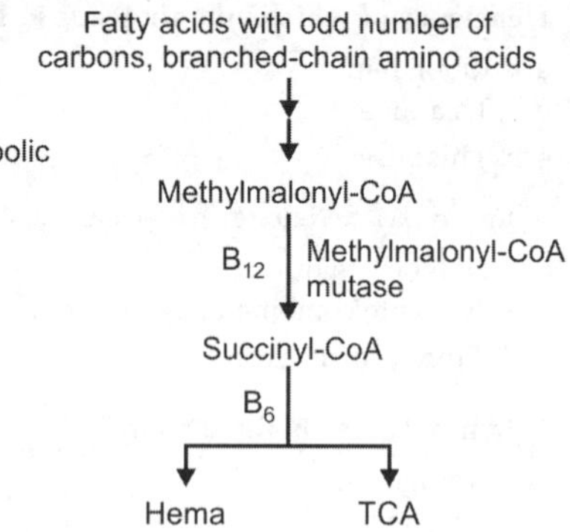

118. A 30-year old female complains of fatigue, dyspnea and weight loss. She has tingling and numbness in lower limbs and decreased vibration sense and ataxia gait. CBC reveals Hb = 7 gm%. She was treated with folate. Her anemia improved but neurological symptoms worsened. What is the likely explanation for this? *(NEET 2020)*

a. Folate not absorbed
b. Abnormal folate reductase in CNS
c. Unmasked pyridoxine deficiency
d. Folate caused rapid depletion of meagre B12 stores in body

Ans. is 'd' Folate caused rapid depletion of meagre B12 stores in body

119. A female presents with anorexia, fatigue and dyspnea. CBC reveals MCV = 101 fl, Hb = 8 gm% and anisopikilocytosis. PBS showed hypersegmented neutrophils and gastric biopsy showed atrophic fundus. What is the likely etiology? *(NEET 2020)*

a. Folate deficiency
b. B12 deficiency
c. Iron deficiency
d. Copper deficiency

Ans. is 'b' B12 deficiency

120. A young male presented with history of fatigue and tiredness. On investigating, he had a hemoglobin of 8 g/dL, MCV of 101fl, hematocrit of 33% with the peripheral smear showing macrocytes and hypersegmented neutrophils. Which of the following is the most likely cause of the findings in this patient? *(NEET 2020)*

a. Lead poisoning
b. Chronic alcohol abuse
c. Chronic renal failure
d. Hemolytic anemia

Ans. is 'b' Chronic alcohol abuse

METALLOENZYMES

Metal	Metalloenzymes
Ca	Lipase, Lecithinase
Cu	Tyrosinase, Superoxide dismutase, Ceruloplasmin, Lysyl oxidase
Fe	Catalase, Peroxidase, Xanthine oxidase
Zn	Carbonic anhydrase, Carboxypeptidase, Glutamate dehydrogenase, Lactate dehydrogenase
Mg	Hexokinase, Phosphofructokinase, Glucose-6-phosphatase, Enolase, Phosphatases, Glutathione synthase
Mn	Arginase, Pyruvate carboxylase, Phosphoglucomutase
Se	Glutathione peroxidase
K	Pyruvate kinase
Ni	Urease
Mo	Xanthine oxidase

121. Which of the following enzymes does not use copper?

a. Prolyl hydroxylase
b. Tyrosinase
c. Ceruloplasmin
d. Superoxide dismutase

Ans. is 'a' Prolyl hydroxylase

HEME

Heme Biosynthesis

- Heme biosynthesis occurs in most mammalian cells except RBCs, which do not contain mitochondria.
- *Sites:* 85% of heme synthesis occurs in erythroid precursor cells in the bone marrow, and the majority of the remainder in hepatocytes.
- The enzymatic process that produces heme is properly called porphyrin synthesis. In humans, this pathway serves almost exclusively to form heme.
- The pathway is initiated by the synthesis of δ-Aminolevulinic acid (δALA) from glycine and succinyl- CoA.
- This step is catalyzed by the rate-limiting enzyme of the pathway, ALA synthase, which is negatively regulated by glucose and heme concentration. Vitamin B6 acts as a co-factor for this step.
- It takes place in both cytoplasm and mitochondria.
- Most important heme containing molecule is hemoglobin, but it also forms part of other biologically important proteins such as myoglobin, cytochrome, catalase and endothelial nitric oxide synthase.

Steps of heme synthesis are depicted in the following diagram:

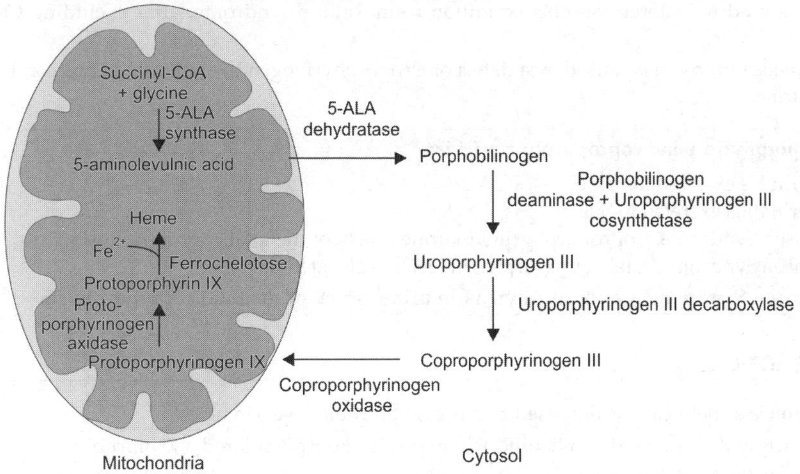

High levels of lead can affect heme metabolism by combining with SH groups in enzymes such as ferrochelatase and ALA (delta-amino levulinic acid) dehydratase. This affects porphyrin metabolism. Elevated levels of protoporphyrin are found in red blood cells, and elevated levels of ALA and of coproporphyrin are found in urine.

122. Ferrochelatase is inhibited by:

a. Arsenic b. Lead
c. Chromium d. Mercury

Ans. is 'b' Lead

123. Heme synthesis requires:

a. Vitamin B6 b. Vitamin B1
c. Vitamin B12 d. THFA

Ans. is 'a' Vitamin B6

124. Name the amino acid that is used in heme synthesis:

a. Glutamine b. Glutamate
c. Glycine d. Histidine

Ans. is 'c' Glycine

Porphyrias

Enzyme defect	Name of the disorder
ALA synthase	X-linked sideroblastic anemia
ALA dehydratase	ALA dehydratase deficient porphyria (ADP)
Hydroxymethylbilane synthase/Porphobilogen deaminase	Àcute intermittent porphyria
Uroporphyrinogen III synthase	Congenital Erythropoietic porphyria
Uroporphyliinogen decarboxylase	Porphyria cutanea tarda
Protoporphyrinogen oxidase	Variegate porphyria
Ferrochelatase	Erythropoietic protoporphyria

125. Enzyme deficient in porphyria cutanea tarda is:

a. Coproporphyrinogen oxidase
b. Protoporphyrinogen oxidase
c. ALA dehydratase
d. Uroporphyrinogen decarboxylase

Ans. is 'd' Uroporphyrinogen decarboxylase

Coproporphyrins

- Intermediates of heme synthesis.
- Normally coproporphyrin I is excreted in bile and is lost in feces. Coproporphyrin III is excreted in urine. Hence in normal urine Coproporphyrin I is 25% of total coproporphyrin levels in urine
- Dubin Johson syndrome, is a form of conjugated hyperbilirubinemia and is caused by a defect of Multi Drug Resistant Protein 2 (MRP-2), which is responsible for secreting bile components (conjugated bile pigments) from hepatocytes into biliary canaliculi. In this disorder, the ratio of Coproporphyrin I:Coproporphyrin III is reversed and coproporphyrin I is more than 80% of the total Coproporphyrin levels. But the total coproporphyrin levels is normal. Hence the increase in the proportion of Coproporphyrin I in urine (Coproporphyrin I >80% of total coproporphyrins). This can be used as a pathognomonic feature of Dubin Johnson syndrome, and can be used to differentiate this condition from Rotor's syndrome, after excluding Congenital Erythropoietic porphyria.
- Congenital Erythropoietic porphyria is caused by a defect of Uroporphyrinogen III synthase. In this condition too, coproporphyrin I level is elevated in urine.

126. True about coproporphyrin I and coproporphyrin III is:

a. Coproporphyrin I is excreted in urine
b. Coproporphyrin III is excreted in bile
c. In Dubin Johnson Syndrome, Coproporphyrin I in urine is 80% of the total coproporphyrin
d. In Dubin Johnson Syndrome, total coproporphyrin levels is elevated

Ans. is 'c' In Dubin Johnson Syndrome, Coproporphyrin I in urine is 80% of the total coproporphyrin

VAN DEN BERGH REACTION

- **Van den Bergh reaction** is a chemical reaction used to measure bilirubin levels in blood
- Principle: bilirubin reacts with diazotised sulphanilic acid to produce purple colored azo bilirubin
- This test helps to identify the type of jaundice.
- The serum of patient is mixed with diazo reagent. If red colour develops immediately it is called direct positive. It happens if conjugated bilirubin is present.
- In indirect positive test, patient's serum is first treated with alcohol and later mixed with diazo reagent. This causes development of red colour. It is seen if unconjugated bilirubin is present.
- If both conjugated and unconjugated bilirubin are present the reaction is termed biphasic reaction.

Differential diagnosis of jaundice

Parameter	*Pre-hepatic*	*Hepatocellular*	*Obstructive*
Basic mechanism of raised bilirubin	Hemolysis leading to excess production	Deficient uptake, conjugation, or excretion by hepatocytes	Deficient excretion due to obstruction of biliary tract
Type of serum bilirubin increased	Mainly unconjugated	Unconjugated + conjugated	Mainly conjugated (>50%)
Urine bilirubin	Absent	Present	Present
Urine urobilinogen	Increased	Variable	Decreased/absent
Prototype	Hemolytic anemia	Viral hepatitis	Common duct stone
Prothrombin time	Normal	Abnormal that is not corrected with Vitamin K	Abnormal that is corrected with Vitamin K
Additional features	Features of hemolysis on blood smear (reticulocytosis, low haptoglobin, low Hb	Marked rise of serum ALT and AST	Marked rise of serum ALP (>3 times normal)

127. A patient presents with dense icterus, clay coloured stools and yellow urine with pruritus. Lab findings reveal highly elevated ALP. What will be the result of van den Berg-test?

a. Normal
b. Direct positive
c. Indirect positive
d. Biphasic

Ans. is 'b' Direct positive

Explanation: Icterus, clay colored stools, yellow urine, pruritus with highly elevated ALP levels is suggestive of Obstructive jaundice.

Dietary fibre:

❖ **Constituents of dietary fibre:**
- Cellulose
- Hemicellulose
- Inulin
- Pectins
- Mucilages
- Gums
- Lignin
- Algal polysaccharides

❖ Dietary fibre consists of unabsorbable cell wall and other constituents of vegetable food like cellulose, lignin, hemicellulose, gums, pectins, glycoproteins and other polysaccharides.

❖ Dietary fibre absorbs water in the intestine, swells, increase bulk of stool by increasing water content of faeces and soften it, decreases transit time by facilitating colonic transit.

❖ The presence of fibre shortens the transit times and increases the stool bulk.

Dietary fibre is of two types:

1. **Soluble fibre/Well fermented:** It absorbs up to 15 times its weight in water as it moves through GIT, producing softer stools. Its good sources are oat, flaxseeds, peas, beans, apple, citrus fruits, carrots, barley and psyllium. Examples–Pectins, Gums, Mucilages
2. **Insoluble fibre/Less fermented:** It promotes movement of material through digestive system and increases stool bulk. Its good sources are wheat flour, wheat bran, nuts and vegetables. Examples–Cellulose, Hemicellulose, Lignin.

Classification of dietary fibre components based on water solubility/fermentability

Characteristic	*Fibre component*	*Description*	*Main food sources*
Water insoluble/ Less fermented	Cellulose	Main structural component of plant cell wall. Insoluble in concentracted alkali, soluble in concentrated acid.	Plants (vegetables, sugar beet, various brans)
	Hemicellulose	Cell wall polysaccharides, which contain backbone of β-1, 4 glucosidic linkages. Soluble in dilute alkali.	Cereal grains
	Lignin	Non-carbohydrate cell wall component. Complex cross-linked phenyl propane polymer. Resists bacterial degradation.	Woody plants
Water soluble/ Well fermented	Pectin	Components of primary cell wall with D-galacturonic acid as principal components. Generally water soluble and gel forming	Fruits, vegetables, legumes, sugar beet, potato
	Gums	Secreted at site of plant injury by specialized secretary cells. Food and pharmaceutical use.	Leguminous seed plants (guar, locust bean), seaweed extracts (carrageenan, alginates), microbial gums (xanthan, gellan)
	Mucilages	Synthesized by plant, prevent desiccation of seed endosperm. Food industry use, hydrophilic, stabilizer.	Plant extracts (gun acacia, gum karaya, gum tragacanth)

128. Which dietary fibres have least water solubility? *(NEET 2020)*

a. Hemicellulose b. Gums
c. Mucilage d. Pectin

Ans. is 'a' Hemicellulose

Previously Asked Facts

❖ Molecular mimicry is often found in the presence of cysteine (forms disulphide bridges), arginine or lysine (form hydrogen bonds) in the binding site of antigens.

❖ Formation and secretion of ammonia by renal tubular cells helps in maintaining acid base balance. Ammonia is formed from glutamine by glutaminase. Excretion of ammonia increases in metabolic acidosis and decreases in metabolic alkalosis.

❖ Methionine is an essential amino acid that is required for synthesis of cysteine. Thus, adequate dietary cysteine can spare the requirement of methionine in diet.

❖ Transaminase enzyme transfers amino group from an amino acid to a keto acid, converting the amino acid to a keto acid. The keto acid which accepts the amino group becomes an amino acid.

❖ FIGLU test or formiminoglutamate test is done to detect the deficiency of folate. FIGLU level is high in urine in folate deficiency.

❖ Glutamate is the most abundant free amino acid found in brain.

❖ Cysteine with a sulfhydryl group can get oxidised and forms a dimer (2 molecules) called as cystine.

❖ Melanin is formed from Tyrosine by the action of enzyme Tyrosinase.

❖ Biologically important tripeptidase include glutathione and thyrotropin releasing hormone (TRH).

- Antioxidant role of glutathione is operative mainly in RBCs. Cysteine acts as the reducing agent in glutathione by donating hydrogen atom from sulfhydryl group.
- Examples of serine proteases (have serine in active site and form covalent bonds) include trypsin, chymotrypsin, thrombin and elastase. Examples of Aspartyl proteases (have aspartic acid in active site and mediate acid based catalysis) include pepsin, cathepsin and HIV protease.
- Histones (proteins in nucleosomes) are made up of positively charged or basic amino acids—Histidine and Arginine.
- The term denaturation refers to disruption of higher order (secondary, tertiary and quaternary) structure of protein. Primary structure is not affected by denaturation.
- Extracellular proteins and intracellular long lived proteins get degraded in lysosomes with the help of cathepsin. Intracellular short lived proteins undergo degradation with ubiquitin-proteasome pathway in an ATP dependent manner once their life span gets over.
- Selenium acts as a co-factor for enzymes–Glutathione peroxidase, Thioredoxine reductase and Deiodinase.
- Serum Glutamate Oxaloacetate Transaminase (SGOT) catalyses the transamination between Aspartate and alpha –Ketoglutarate to form oxaloacetate and glutamate.
- Enzymes act by decreasing activation energy of a biochemical reaction.
- Enzymes active in acidic pH–Pepsinogen (gastric chief cells), lysosomal enzymes, acid phosphatase. Enzymes active in alkaline pH–Pancreatic enzymes (Trypsinogen, chymotrypsinogen, carboxypeptidases).
- Out of the five LDH isoenzymes, LDH1 isoenzyme is specific for heart. In blood generally LDH2 isoenzyme concentration is higher. In myocardial infarction, LDH1 concentration as increased–flipped pattern of LDH suggestive of myocordial infarction.
- Guthrie's test is done to detect Phenylketonuria. It is based on the fact that organism Bacillus subtilis needs phenyl ketone for its growth.
- Disaccharide not digested in intestine is Sucralose.
- Alpha-ketoglutarate is the precursor for Proline in TCA cycle.
- Glucose is virtually the sole fuel for the brain, except in prolonged starving when ketone bodies are the major source. Fatty acids do not serve as fuel for the brain, because they are bound to albumin in plasma; hence cannot cross blood-brain barrier.
- Storage form of energy in liver is Glycogen.
- Glycemic index defined as the ratio of incremental area under the blood glucose response curve (AUC) following ingestion of a food and the AUC of the standard (glucose) and multiplied by 100. Glycemic index is used to assess the rate of absorption of a particular food's carbohydrate. Carbohydrates with a low GI value (55 or less) are more slowly digested, absorbed and metabolised and cause a lower and slower rise in blood glucose.
- Inhibition of glycolysis by excess of oxygen is Pasteur effect. Preferable utilization of anaerobic metabolism over aerobic metabolism is Warburg effect, seen in malignant cells.
- Reducing and non-reducing sugars

Reducing sugars	Non-reducing sugars
• All monosaccharides (glucose, fructose, galactose) • Disaccharide: lactose, maltose, cellobiose, melibiose	• Disaccharide: sucrose, trehalose

- APOE4 allele is associated with increased risk for AD, whereas APOE2 is associated with decreased risk.
- Granulosa cells use follicular fluid HDL as a source of cholesterol for the synthesis of progesterone.
- The products of HMG CoA (3-Hydroxy 3-methyl glutaryl CoA) are cholesterol, Bile acids, Ubiquinone, Dolichol, Heme A, Prenylated protein and ketone bodies (acetoacetate).
- MDA (Malondialdehyde) is one of the most known secondary products of lipid peroxidation, and it can be used as a marker of cell membrane injury.
- High density lipoprotein is involved in reverse cholesterol transport and is found to be protective against atherosclerosis.
- Nutritionally essential fatty acids are linoleic acid and alpha-linolenic acid. Arachidonic acid is considered as conditionally essential because it has to be supplied in the diet if linoleic acid is not supplemented.
- Lipoprotein- X is an abnormal discoidal lipoprotein that is present either in obstructive jaundice or in LCAT deficiency.
- There are two types of fatty acids: Saturated and Unsaturated. Cis-trans isomerism is seen in unsaturated fatty acids. Stearic acid is a saturated fatty acid (No cis-trans isomerism). Important unsaturated trans-fatty acid is Elaidic acid (trans-9-octadecenoic). Oleic acid and Arachidonic acid are cis-fatty acids.
- Genotype is the genetic expression of a trait. Phenotype is the physical expression of a trait.
- Small RNAs are less than 200 nucleotides in length, coded by intronic sequences of DNA. They post-transcriptionally regulate gene expression (Gene Silencing) by targeting 3′ untranslated region of specific mRNAs for degradation or translational repression.
- Transposons or Jumping Genes are moderately repetitive sequences in DNA that can change its position within a genome. These transposable elements form a large fraction of genome of eukaryotic DNA.
- tRNAs are known for their modified bases including—Pseudouridine of T ψc arm, Dihydrouridine of D arm, inosine of anticodon arm, methylated bases and alkylated bases.

- In tRNA, T ψc arm is for attachment to ribosome. D arm is for attachment to aminoacyl tRNA synthetase attachment.
- Since thymidine is present in RNA, it can include 3 of the 4 nucleotides—A, U, G, C (never thymidine).
- Out of 64 codons, 3 are stop codons. The three stop codons are UGA, UAG, UAA. Exception–In mitochondrial DNA, UGA is not a stop codon. It codes for Tryptophan. Instead AGA and AGG act as stop codons in mitochondrial DNA.
- Agarose gel or Polyacrylamide gel electrophoresis is used to separate DNA fragments cut using restriction endonucleases.
- Enzymes in DNA replication:

Function in DNA replication	Enzyme
Leading stand synthesis	DNA polymerase δ
Okazaki fragment synthesis	**RNA primase + DNA polymerase α + DNA polymerase δ**
Removal of RNA printer and gap filling	DNA polymerase δ + Flap endonuclease I
Proof reading and repair	DNA polymerase ε and β
Mitochondrial DNA synthesis	DNA polymerase γ

- In DNA replication, leading strand replication is continuous. Lagging strand replication is discontinuous–with help of RNA primers and Okazaki fragments by DNA polymerase delta. After RNA primer removal, Okazaki fragments are joined by DNA Ligase.
- Plamid pBR322 is the most widely used vector for DNA cloning. It has two resistance genes Ampicillin resistance gene and Tetracycline resistance gene.

Procedure	Sample analyzed	Gel electrophoresis	Probe
Southern blot	DNA	Yes	Radio-labelled DNA
Northern blot	RNA	Yes	DNA probe
Western blot	Protein	Yes	Labelled antibody
Southwestern blot	DNA-binding proteins	No	Double-stranded DNA probes

- Heme is Type III porphyrin (Type III series). It is series IX porphyrin (Fischer series).
- Fetal hemoglobin (HbF) is resistant to alkali denaturation unlike adult hemoglobin.
- Hemopexin is a glycoprotein which exhibits the highest affinity for free heme and protects the cell and tissues from oxidative damage caused by heme. Haptoglobin binds hemoglobin (which is released following intravascular hemolysis) not to free heme.

CHAPTER 4 Pathology

CELL INJURY AND ADAPTATION

GRANULOMATOUS INFLAMMATION

Granulomatous inflammation is a distinctive pattern of chronic inflammation that is encountered in a limited number of infectious and some noninfectious conditions. Briefly, a granuloma is a cellular attempt to contain an offending agent that is difficult to eradicate. In this attempt there is often strong activation of T lymphocytes leading to macrophage activation, which can cause injury to normal tissues. Tuberculosis is the prototype of the granulomatous diseases, but sarcoidosis, cat-scratch disease, Q fever, lymphogranuloma inguinale, lymphoma, leprosy, brucellosis, syphilis, some mycotic infections, berylliosis, reactions of irritant lipids, and some autoimmune diseases are also included. Recognition of the granulomatous pattern in a biopsy specimen is important because of the limited number of possible conditions that cause it and the significance of the diagnoses associated with the lesions.

Disease	Cause	Tissue reaction
Tuberculosis	*Mycobacterium tuberculosis*	Caseating granuloma (tubercle): focus of activated macrophages (epithelioid cells), rimmed by fibroblasts, lymphocytes, histiocytes, occasional Langhans giant cells; central necrosis with amorphous granular debris; acid-fast bacilli
Leprosy	*Mycobacterium leprae*	Acid-fast bacilli in macrophages; noncaseating granulomas
Syphilis	*Treponema pallidum*	Gumma: microscopic to grossly visible lesion, enclosing wall of histiocytes; plasma cell infiltrate; central cells necrotic without loss of cellular outline
Cat-scratch disease	Gram-negative bacillus	Rounded or stellate granuloma containing central granular debris and recognizable neutrophils; giant cell uncommon
Sarcoidosis	Unknown etiology	Noncaseating granulomas with abundant activated macrophages
Crohn disease (inflammatory bowel disease)	Immune reaction against intestinal bacteria, self-antigens	Occasional noncaseating granulomas in the wall of the intestine, with dense chronic inflammatory infiltrate

- Very often, giant cells are seen in granulomas. However, they can also be seen in wide variety of conditions as described below.
- A giant-cell is formed by the union of several distinct cells. Most of the times these giant cells are produced by fusion of the macrophages:

Foreign body giant cells

- These cells contain multiple nuclei (10–100). Nuclei are scattered throughout the cytoplasm haphazardly. They can arise directly by fusion of macrophages or from Langhans type of giant cells. These cells are seen in infective granulomatous conditions, e.g. TB, Leprosy, syphilis, Brucellosis.

Langhans type giant cells

- These cells contain 3–5 nuclei. Nuclei are arranged around periphery in the form of horseshoe. These cells may also act as precursors of foreign body giant cells. These cells are seen in TB and sarcoidosis.

Touton giant cells

- These cells are seen in Xanthomas.

Aschoff cells in rheumatic nodule: Osteoclasts

Reed-Sternberg cells in Hodgkin's disease

Warthin Finkeldey giant cells: measles

Giant Cells

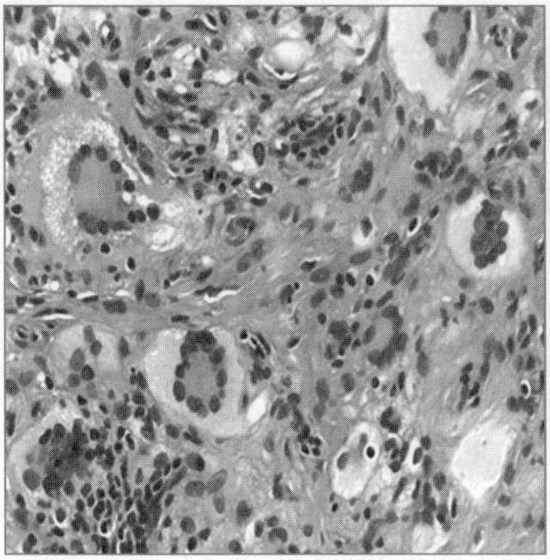

Touton type giant cell

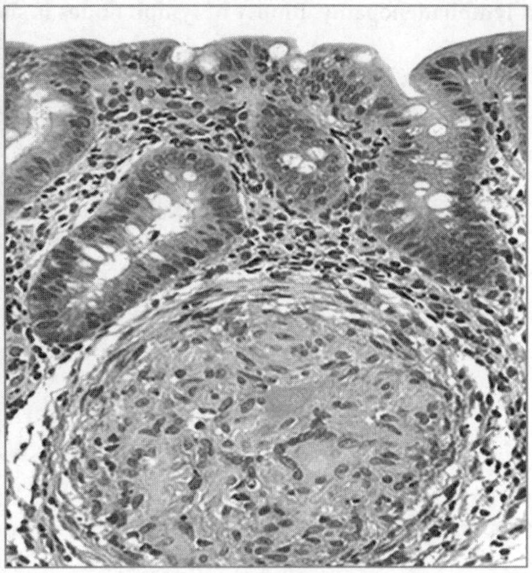

Epithelioid giant cell

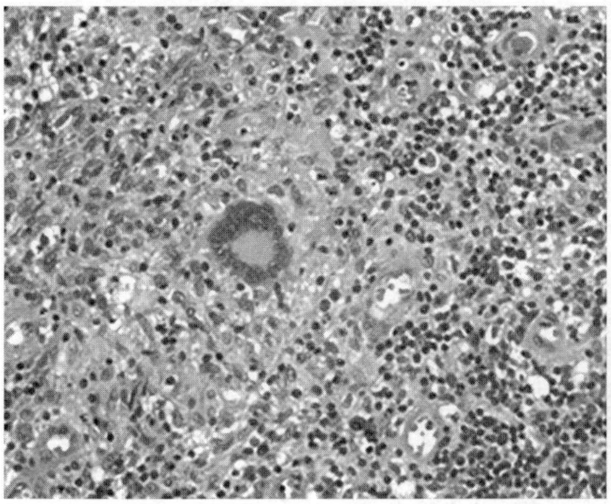

Langhans giant cell

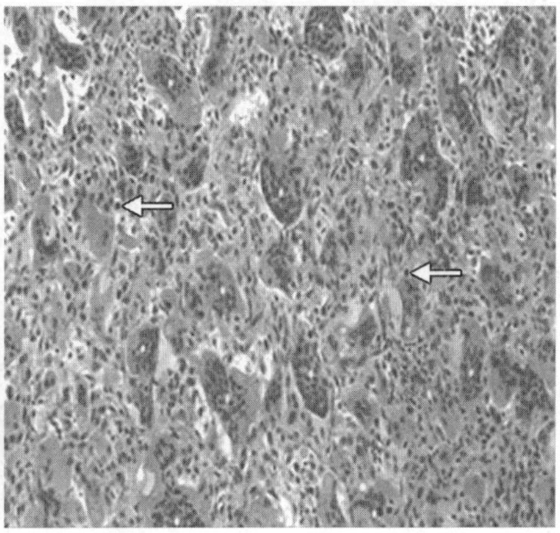

Osteoclastic giant cells

1. Nuclei are arranged at cell periphery in which type of cell? *(NEET 2016)*

a. Langhans giant cell
b. Merkel's cells
c. NK cells
d. Neutrophills

Ans. is 'a' Langhans giant cell

2. Stellate granuloma with necrotic debris with neurtrophils is seen in: *(NEET 2018)*

a. Crohn's disease
b. Syphilis
c. Sarcoidosis
d. Cat-scratch disease

Ans. is 'd' Cat-scratch disease

3. Granuloma formation is not seen in: *(NEET 2018)*

a. Asthma
b. Hodgkin's disease
c. Sarcoidosis
d. Q-Fever

Ans. is 'a' Asthma

4. Warthin Finkeldey bodies are found in: *(NEET 2016)*

a. Tuberculosis
b. Sarcoidosis
c. Herpes
d. Measles

Ans. is 'd' Measles

5. An 11-year-old boy presents with history of cough, weight loss and low grade fever for 15 days. On examination he had cervical lymphadenopathy. Biopsy of lymph nodes is shown below. What is the diagnosis? *(NEET 2020)*

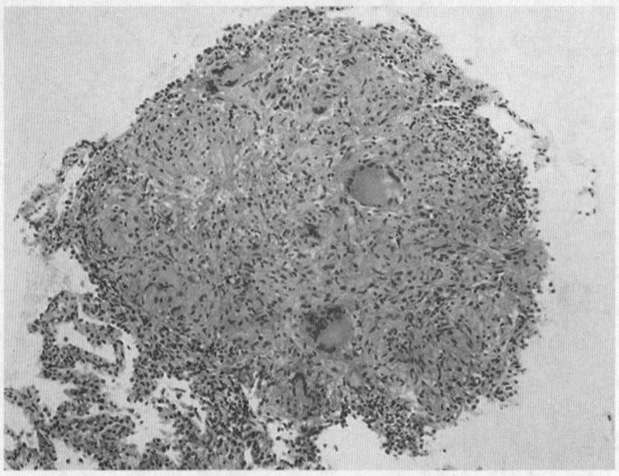

a. Syphilis
b. Sarcoidosis
c. TB
d. Leprosy

Ans. is 'c' TB

LIPOFUSCIN

Lipofuscin is an insoluble pigment, also known as lipochrome or wear-and-tear pigment. Lipofuscin is composed of polymers of lipids and phospholipids in complex with protein, suggesting that it is derived through lipid peroxidation of polyunsaturated lipids of subcellular membranes. Lipofuscin is not injurious to the cell or its functions. Its importance lies in its being a telltale sign of free radical injury and lipid peroxidation. The term is derived from the Latin (fuscus, brown), referring to brown lipid. In tissue sections it appears as a yellow-brown, finely granular cytoplasmic, often perinuclear, pigment. It is seen in cells undergoing slow, regressive changes and is particularly prominent in the liver and heart of aging patients or patients with severe malnutrition and cancer cachexia.

The following figures show lipofuscin granules in a cardiac myocyte shown by (A) light microscopy and (B) electron microscopy (note the perinuclear, intralysosomal location).

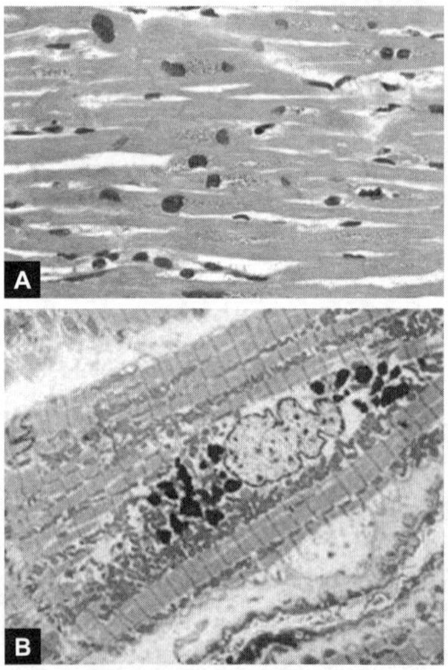

6. Lipofuscin containing macrophages are a feature of: *(NEET 2016)*

a. Wear and tear
b. Fat deposit
c. Iron deficiency
d. Calcification

Ans. is 'a' Wear and tear

7. Cell debris with golden yellow appearance is : *(NEET 2016)*

a. Melanin
b. Hemosiderin
c. Hematin
d. Lipofuscin

Ans. is 'd' Lipofuscin

CELL DEATH

Reversible Injury

Reversible injury is characterized by generalized swelling of the cell and its organelles; blebbing of the plasma membrane; detachment of ribosomes from the ER; and clumping of nuclear chromatin. Mitochondria are the first organelles to get affected in case of cell injury. These morphologic changes are associated with decreased generation of ATP, loss of cell membrane integrity, defects in protein synthesis, cytoskeletal damage, and DNA damage. Within limits, the cell can repair these derangements and, if the injurious stimulus abates, will return to normalcy. Persistent or excessive injury, however, causes cells to pass the rather nebulous "point of no return" into irreversible injury and cell death. Cellular swelling (hydropic change) due to intracellular accumulation of water is the earliest change in cell injury.

Irreversible Injury

Feature	Necrosis	Apoptosis
Cell size	Enlarged (swelling)	Reduced (shrinkage)
Nucleus	Pyknosis → karyorrhexis → karyolysis	Fragmentation into nucleosome-size fragments
Plasma membrane	Disrupted	Intact; altered structure, especially orientation of lipids
Cellular contents	Enzymatic digestion; may leak out of cell	Intact; may be released in apoptotic bodies
Adjacent inflammation	Frequent	No
Physiologic or pathologic role	Invariably pathologic (culmination of irreversible cell injury)	Often physiologic, means of eliminating unwanted cells; may be pathologic after some forms of cell injury, especially DNA damage
Agarose gel electrophoresis of DNA	Diffuse smearing of DNA	Ladder pattern of DNA fragments

Fibrinoid necrosis is a special form of necrosis usually seen in immune reactions involving blood vessels. This pattern of necrosis typically occurs when complexes of antigens and antibodies are deposited in the walls of arteries. Deposits of these "immune complexes", together with fibrin that has leaked out of vessels, result in a bright pink and amorphous appearance in HandE stains, called "fibrinoid" (fibrin-like) by pathologists.

Mechanisms of Apoptosis

❖ The process of apoptosis may be divided into
- **Initiation phase**—caspases become catalytically active
- **Execution phase**—caspases trigger the degradation of critical cellular components
- Initiation phase—intrinsic or mitochondrial pathway
- Extrinsic, or death receptor—initiated pathway.

In both pathways, cysteine aspartyl-specific proteases (caspases) are activated that cleave cellular substrates.

The Intrinsic (Mitochondrial) Pathway

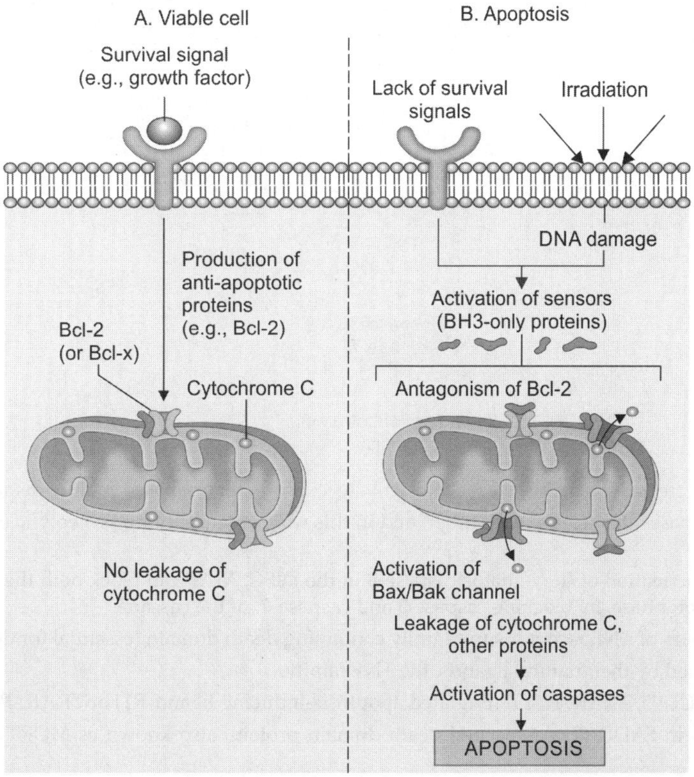

The Extrinsic (Death Receptor- Initiated) Pathway

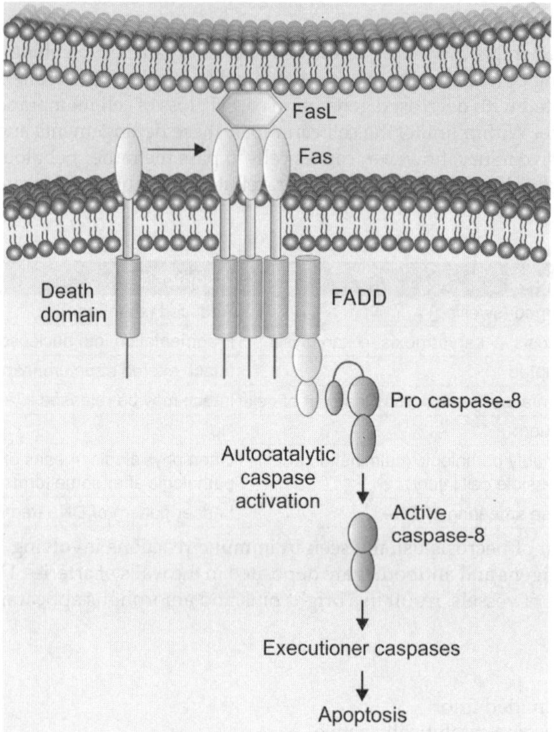

Execution of Apoptosis

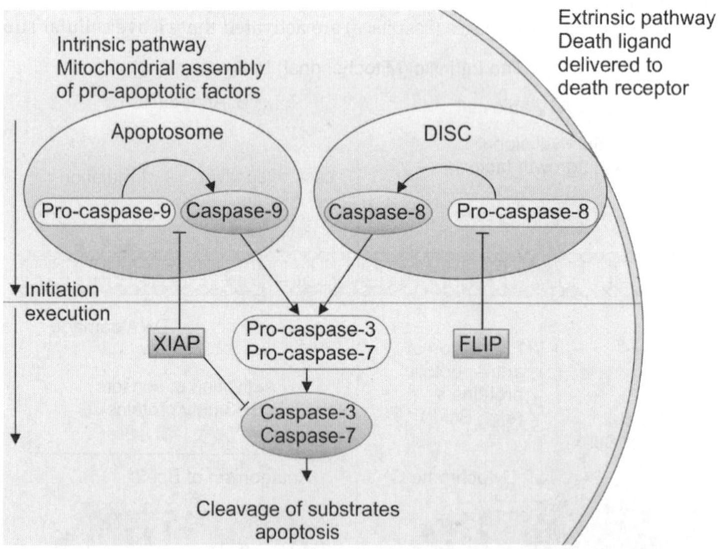

- Once the initiator caspases are activated, they cleave and activate 'executioner' caspases, mainly caspase-3, caspase-6 and caspase-7.
- The active executioner caspases then cleave each other, and in this way, an amplifying proteolytic cascade of caspase activation is started.

  Whereas FLIP blocks the activation of the initiator caspase-8 in the DISC, XIAP can block both the initiation phase, by inhibiting caspase-9, and the execution phase, by blocking caspase-3 and caspase-7, of the cascade.
- Death receptors are members of TNF receptor superfamily containing death domain (essential for delivering apoptotic signal).
- Death receptors are activated by their natural ligands, the TNF family.
- Death receptors—such as CD95, TRAIL-R1 (TNF-related apoptosis-inducing ligand-R1) or TRAIL-R2 —binds to FASL.
- Intracellular adaptor protein FADD (Fas-associated death domain protein, also known as MORT1 is activated), which, in turn, recruits the procaspases.

Bcl-2 Family Members

A very large family with 30 members identified and belongs to both

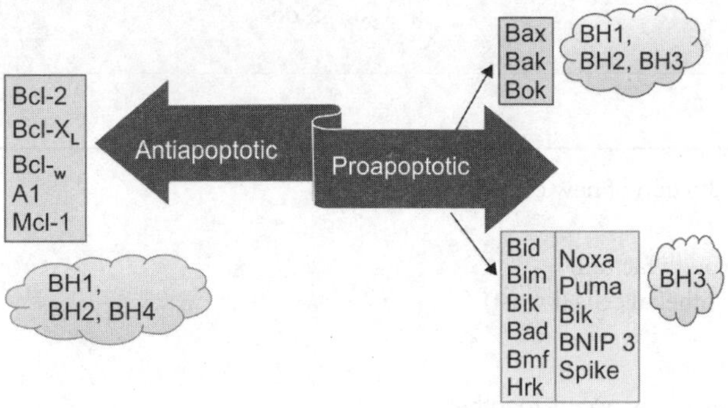

Genes Related to Apoptosis (Apoptotic Genes)

- *Proapoptotic*: Apaf-l, cytochrome C, BaK, Bar, Bim, AIF, P53, Caspases, TNFRI, FAS (CD95), FADD, BH3 (Bim, Bid, Bad), Snac/ DIABLO.
- *Antiapoptotic*: BCL-2, BCL-X, Mci-l, TAPs, FLIP.

8. Hydropic change is due to: *(NEET 2016)*

a. Accumulation of water intracellularly
b. Fat accumulation intracellularly
c. Lysozyme degeneration
d. Glycogen accumulation intracellularly

Ans. is 'a' Accumulation of water intracellularly

9. In reversible cell injury, microscopic change seen is: *(NEET 2016)*

a. Leakage of enzymes
b. Mitochondrial densities
c. Cytoplasmic vacuole
d. Pyknosis

Ans. is 'c' Cytoplasmic vacuole

10. What is the first sign of injury? *(NEET 2016)*

a. Mitochondrial dysfunction
b. Membrane damage
c. Diminished ATP
d. Release of lysosomal enzymes

Ans. is 'a' Mitochondrial dysfunction

11. Not true about apoptosis is: *(NEET 2016)*

a. Cellular swelling
b. Nuclear compaction
c. Intact cell membrane
d. Cytoplasmic eosinophilia

Ans. is 'a' Cellular swelling

12. Antiapoptotic gene is: *(NEET 2016)*

a. FLIP
b. P53
c. BAX
d. BIM

Ans. is 'a' FLIP

13. Gene associated with apoptosis is: *(NEET 2016)*

a. FAS
b. RET
c. Rb
d. ICAM

Ans. is 'a' FAS

14. Pro-apoptotic gene is: *(NEET 2018)*

a. Bax
b. Bcl2
c. Bclx
d. Mcl

Ans. is 'b' Bcl2

15. Blebs are found in which type of injury? *(NEET 2016)*

a. Reversible
b. Irreversible
c. Both
d. None

Ans. is 'a' Reversible

16. Type of necrosis seen in blood vessels due to immune reactions? *(NEET 2018)*

a. Coagulation
b. Liquefaction
c. Fibrinoid
d. None

Ans. is 'c' Fibrinoid

HYPERPLASIA

- Increase in number of cells (production of new cells from stem cells)
- Mostly occurs in dividing cells
- Physiological (hormones and growth factors)
  - Proliferation of glandular epithelial cells (breast)
  - Liver regeneration
  - Bone marrow.

  In general hyperplasia and hypertrophy occurs together
- **Physiological hyperplasia**
  - It occurs due to increased physiological demand, e.g.
    - *Hormonal*: Hyperplasia of endometrium during pregnancy, hyperplasia of breast during puberty.
    - *Compensatory*: Increase in tissue mass after damage or partial resection (regeneration of liver or kidney after partial hepatectomy or nephrectomy, respectively).
- **Pathological hyperplasia**
  - It occurs due to persistent stimulus under pathological conditions, e.g. endometrial hyperplasia due to estrogen producing tumors.

17. Which of the following is an example of physiological hyperplasia? *(NEET 2016)*

a. Endometrium during pregnancy
b. Liver regeneration after rejection
c. Breast during pregnancy
d. All of the above

Ans. is 'd' All of the above

18. Definition of hypertrophy is: *(NEET 2016)*

a. Increased protein content of the cells
b. Increased in size of cells
c. Increase in number of cells
d. None of the above

Ans. is 'b' Increased in size of cells

ATROPHY

- Reduction in size of organ or tissue
- Decrease in size and number
- Physiological (notochord and thyroglossal duct, decrease in size of uterus).

Pathological Atrophy (Causes)

- Decreased workload-skeletal muscle atrophy
- Loss of innervation
- Diminished blood supply-senile atrophy
- Inadequate nutrition-cachexia
- Loss of endocrine stimulation
- Pressure.

Mechanism

- Decreased protein synthesis (reduced metabolic activity) and increased protein degradation
- Ubiquitin –proteasome pathway
- Autophagy
- Apoptosis.

19. Example of physiological atrophy is: *(NEET 2016)*

a. Decrease in uterus size after delivery
b. Disuse atrophy
c. Atrophy of a muscle after nerve damage
d. Senile atrophy

Ans. is 'a' Decrease in uterus size after delivery

REGENERATIVE CAPACITY OF CELLS

Cells can be divided based on their proliferative capacity:

Labile cells (continuously dividing cells) or inter mitotic cells

These cells have capacity to proliferate and regenerate throughout the life. They always remain in cell cycle and have very short G0-phase (quiescent phase). Examples are:

- Surface epithelium (stratified squamous) of skin, oral cavity, vagina and cervix.
- Lining mucosa of all excretory ducts of glands (Salivary gland, pancreas, biliary duct).
- Columnar epithelium of GIT (Intestinal mucosa) and uterus.
- Transitional epithelium of the urinary tract.
- Bone marrow cells and hematopoietic cells.
- Basal cells of epithelia.

Stable or quiescent or reversible post mitotic cells

They have limited capacity to proliferate and regenerate. They remain in G0 phase of cell cycle but can enter in G1 phase when stimulated, i.e. they usually remain quiescent, but proliferate in response to stimulate. Examples are:

- Parenchymal cells of liver, kidney and pancreas.
- Mesenchymal cells, e.g. fibroblast and smooth muscles.
- Vascular endothelium
- Osteoblast, chondroblast
- Resting lymphocytes and other leukocytes.

Permanent or nondividing or irreversible postmitotic cells

They cannot divide and regenerate. These cells are nondividing and have left the cell cycle, i.e. they do not belong to any phase of cell cycle. Examples are:

- Neurons
- Cardiac muscle
- Skeletal muscle.

  Smooth muscle cells are stable cells whereas cardiac muscle and skeletal muscle cells are permanent cells.

20. Which of the following is a permanent cell? *(NEET 2016)*

a. Bone marrow
b. Intestinal mucosa
c. Epithelium of skin
d. Cardiac muscle

Ans. is 'd' Cardiac muscle

EDEMA

Edema, is an abnormal accumulation of fluid in the interstitium, located beneath the skin and in the cavities of the body, which can cause severe pain. Clinically, edema manifests as swelling. The amount of interstitial fluid is determined by the balance of fluid homeostasis and the increased secretion of fluid into the interstitium. Net outflow of fluid from venules surpasses the capacity of lymphatics to remove fluid; hence, there is swelling of tissue. It can be either an exudate or a transudate. When total plasma protein is below 5 g/dL (normal 6–8 g/dL) or albumin is below 2.5 g/dL (normal 3.5–5 g/dL) edema takes place. Severe generalized edema is called anasarca.

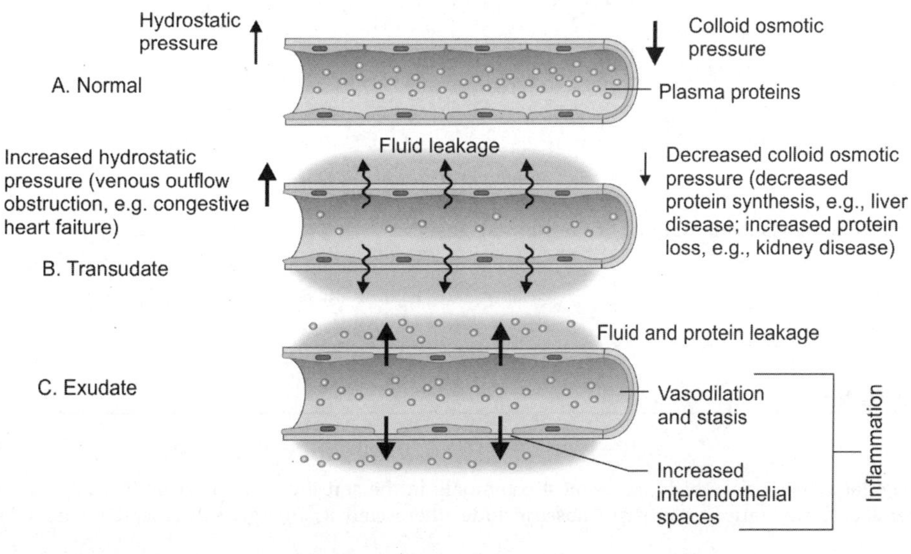

Transudate	Exudate
• Result of hydrostatic or osmotic imbalance • Ultrafiltrate of plasma • Low protein content • Specific gravity < 1.015	• Result of inflammation • Altered vascular permeability (cell debris) • High protein content • Specific gravity > 1.020

21. Edema occurs when plasma protein level is below: *(NEET 2016)*

a. 20 mg/dL b. 15 mg/dL
c. 10 mg/dL d. 5 mg/dL

Ans. is 'd' 5 mg/dL

22. Generalized body edema is associated with deficiency of: *(NEET 2016)*

a. Vitamin B12 b. Sodium
c. Albumin d. EFAs

Ans. is 'c' Albumin

23. Characteristic of exudative fluid is: *(NEET 2016)*

a. Low proteincontent b. Specific gravity <1.012
c. Normal vascularpermeability d. Cellular debris

Ans. is 'd' Cellular debris

FIBRINOID NECROSIS

Fibrinoid necrosis is special form of necrosis typically occurs when complexes of antigen and antibodies are deposited in the walls of arteries. Deposits of these "immune complexes", together with fibrin that has leaked out of vessels, result in a bright pink and amorphous appearance in H and E stains, called "fibrinoid" (fibrin like) by pathologists.

Diseases causing fibrinoid necrosis are malignant hypertension (most common), PAN, SLE, SABE, acute rheumatic fever (Aschoffs nodule), RA, HSP, HBV, near peptic ulcer and malignancy. Nain: In fibrinoid necrosis, there is no deposition of fibrin. It is fibrin like matter, which is deposited.

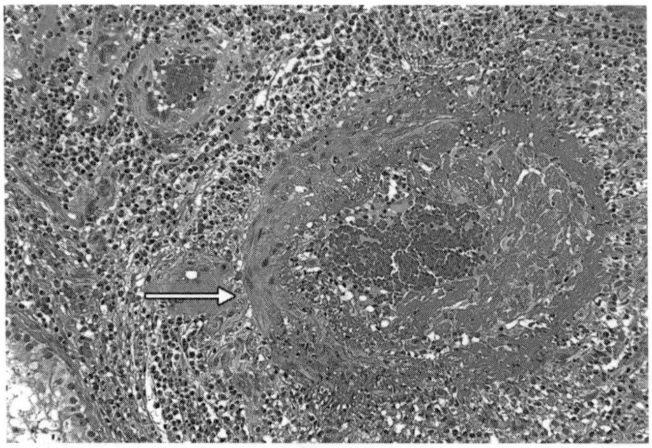

Fibrinoid necrosis

24. Which of the following is not an example of fibrinoid necrosis? *(NEET 2016)*

a. PAN b. Rheumatoid arthritis
c. Pancreatitis d. Rheumatic fever

Ans. is 'c' Pancreatitis

TYPES OF GANGRENE

Dry Gangrene

It is a variant of coagulative necrosis, which occurs most commonly in the soft tissue of lower limbs (Leg; foot, toes) as a result of ischemia due to arterial occlusion (arteriosclerosis). Causes include atherosclerosis, Buerger's disease, Raynaud's disease, trauma.

Wet Gangrene

- When bacterial infection is superimposed there is more liquefactive necrosis because of the actions of degradative enzymes in the bacteria and the attracted leukocytes (giving rise to so-called wet gangrene). More commonly due to venous occlusion then arterial occlusion.
- Occurs in diabetic foot and bedsores. There are two distinct subtypes of wet gangrene:
  - **Gas gangrene**
    - It is caused by Clostridium, most commonly alpha toxin producing Clostridium perfringens, or various non-clostridial species, and is characterized by production of gas within the tissues. It is a medical emergency.
  - **Fournier gangrene**
    - It is a type of necrotizing fasciitis involving the scrotum and perineal region. It is more likely to occur in those with diabetes, alcoholics, or those who are immune compromised.

25. All are associated with diabetic gangrene *except*: *(NEET 2016)*

a. Wet gangrene b. Dry gangrene
c. Gas gangrene d. Fournier's gangrene

Ans. is 'c' Gas gangrene

COAGULATIVE NECROSIS

Coagulative necrosis is a form of necrosis in which the architecture of dead tissues is preserved for a span of at least some days. The affected tissues exhibit a firm texture. Presumably, the injury denatures not only structural proteins but also enzymes and so blocks the proteolysis of the dead cells; as a result, eosinophilic, anucleate cells may persist for days or weeks. Ultimately the necrotic cells are removed by phagocytosis of the cellular debris by infiltrating leukocytes and by digestion of the dead cells by the action of lysosomal enzymes of the leukocytes. Ischemia caused by obstruction in a vessel may lead to coagulative necrosis of the supplied tissue in all organs except the brain. A localized area of coagulative necrosis is called an infarct.

The causes of coagulative necrosis are:

- Ischemia in solid organs such as heart (MI), Kidney, Liver, adrenal gland, spleen. One exception is the brain, where ischemia leads to liquefactive necrosis and not coagulative necrosis.
- Toxic products of bacteria, such as diphtheria.
- Poisons. e.g. mercuric chloride.
- Thermal injury- heat, electricity; or X-rays.

26. Type of necrosis seen in MI is: *(NEET 2016)*

a. Coagulative necrosis b. Liquefactive necrosis
c. Caseous necrosis d. Fat necrosis

Ans. is 'a' Coagulative necrosis

27. Example of coagulative necrosis is: *(NEET 2016)*

a. Acute tubular necrosis b. Stroke
c. Malignant hypertension d. Acute pancreatitis

Ans. is 'a' Acute tubular necrosis

MEMBRANE TRANSPORT

Various modes of membrane transport are summarized below:

- *Channels* are used when concentration gradients can drive the solute movement.
- *Carriers* are required when solute is moved *against* a concentration gradient. Receptor-mediated and fluid-phase uptake of material involves membrane bound vacuoles.
- *Caveolae* endocytose extracellular fluid, membrane proteins, and some receptor bound molecules (e.g. folate) in a process driven by caveolin proteins concentrated within lipid rafts (*potocytosis*).
- *Pinocytosis* of extracellular fluid and most surface receptor-ligand pairs involves *clathrin-coated pits and vesicles*. After internalization, the clathrin dissociates and can be re-used, while the resulting vesicle progressively matures and acidifies. In the early and/or late endosome, ligand can be released from its receptor (e.g. iron released from transferrin bound to the transferrin receptor) with receptor recycling to the cell surface for another round. Alternatively, receptor and ligand within endosomes can be targeted to fuse with lysosomes (e.g. epidermal growth factor bound to its receptor); after complete degradation, the late endosome-lysosome fusion vesicle can regenerate lysosomes.
- *Phagocytosis* involves the non-clathrin-mediated membrane invagination of large particles—typically by specialized phagocytes (e.g. macrophages or neutrophils). The resulting phagosomes eventually fuse with lysosomes to facilitate the degradation of the internalized material.
- *Transcytosis* involves the transcellular endocytotic transport of solute and/or bound ligand from one face of a cell to another.

- *Exocytosis* is the process by which membrane-bound vesicles fuse with the plasma membrane and discharge their contents to the extracellular space.

28. Clathrin mediated ingestion in cells are for: *(NEET 2016)*

a. Pinocytosis
b. Phagocytosis
c. Endocytosis
d. Exocytosis

Ans. is 'c' Endocytosis

AMYLOIDOSIS

Approximately 95% of the amyloid material consists of fibril proteins, the remaining 5% being the P component and other glycoproteins. Three most common types are: (1) AL (amyloid light chain) is derived from Ig light chains produced in plasma cells; (2) AA (amyloid-associated) is derived from a unique non-Ig protein synthesized by the liver; and (3) Aβ amyloid is produced from β amyloid precursor protein and is found in the cerebral lesions of Alzheimer disease.

- The AL protein is made up of complete immunoglobulin light chains, the amino-terminal fragments of light chains, or both. Most of the AL proteins analyzed are composed of λ light chains or their fragments, but in some cases κ chains have been identified. The amyloid fibril protein of the AL type is produced from free Ig light chains secreted by a monoclonal population of plasma cells, and its deposition is associated with certain forms of plasma cell tumors.
- The second major class of amyloid fibril protein (AA) does not have structural homology to immunoglobulins. AA fibrils are derived by proteolysis from a larger precursor in the serum called SAA (serum amyloid–associated) protein that is synthesized in the liver and circulates in association with high density lipoproteins. The production of SAA protein is increased in inflammatory states as part of the "acute phase response"; therefore, this form of amyloidosis is associated with chronic inflammation, and is often called secondary amyloidosis.
- β-amyloid protein (Aβ) constitutes the core of cerebral plaques found in Alzheimer disease as well as the amyloid deposited in walls of cerebral blood vessels in individuals with this disease. The Aβ protein is derived by proteolysis from a much larger transmembrane glycoprotein, called amyloid precursor protein.
- Transthyretin (TTR) is a normal serum protein that binds and transports thyroxine and retinol. A mutant form of TTR (and its fragments) is deposited in a group of genetically determined disorders referred to as familial amyloid polyneuropathies. TTR is also deposited in the heart of aged individuals (senile systemic amyloidosis), but in such cases the amino acid sequence of the TTR molecule is normal.
- β2-microglobulin, a component of MHC class I molecules and a normal serum protein, has been identified as the amyloid fibril subunit (Aβ2m) in amyloidosis that complicates the course of patients on long-term hemodialysis.

29. Substance deposited in senile cardiac amyloidosis is: *(NEET 2016)*

a. AA
b. AL
c. Beta-2 microglobulin
d. ATTR

Ans. is 'd' ATTR

30. Secondary amyloidosis is associated with: *(NEET 2016)*

a. Multiple myeloma
b. Plasmacytosis
c. Ankylosing spondylitis
d. All of them

Ans. is 'c' Ankylosing spondylitis

31. Secondary amyloidosis is a complication of: *(NEET 2016)*

a. RA
b. Plasmacytosis
c. Multiple myeloma
d. None

Ans. is 'a' RA

32. Amyloidosis associated with transthyretin deposition is: *(NEET 2016)*

a. Multiple myeloma
b. Hemodialysis
c. Familial Mediterranean fever
d. Senile systemic amyloidosis

Ans. is 'd' Senile systemic amyloidosis

DYSTROPHIC CALCIFICATION

Dystrophic calcification is encountered in areas of necrosis, whether they are of coagulative, caseous, or liquefactive type, and in foci of enzymatic necrosis of fat. Calcification is almost always present in the atheromas of advanced atherosclerosis. It also commonly develops in aging or damaged heart valves, further hampering their function. Whatever the site of deposition, the calcium salts appear macroscopically as fine, white granules or clumps, often felt as gritty deposits. Sometimes a tuberculous lymph node is virtually converted to stone.

METASTATIC CALCIFICATION

Metastatic calcification may occur in normal tissues whenever there is hypercalcemia. Hypercalcemia also accentuates dystrophic calcification. There are four principal causes of hypercalcemia: (1) increased secretion of parathyroid hormone (PTH) with subsequent bone resorption, as in hyperparathyroidism due to parathyroid tumors, and ectopic secretion of PTH-related protein by malignant tumors; (2) destruction of bone tissue, secondary to primary tumors of bone marrow (e.g., multiple myeloma, leukemia) or diffuse skeletal metastasis (e.g., breast cancer), accelerated bone turnover (e.g., Paget's disease), or immobilization; (3) vitamin D–related disorders, including vitamin D intoxication, sarcoidosis (in which macrophages activate a vitamin D precursor), and idiopathic hypercalcemia of infancy (Williams syndrome), characterized by abnormal sensitivity to vitamin D; and (4) renal failure, which causes retention of phosphate, leading to secondary hyperparathyroidism. Less common causes include aluminum intoxication, which occurs in patients on chronic renal dialysis, and milk-alkali syndrome, which is due to excessive ingestion of calcium and absorbable antacids such as milk or calcium carbonate.

33. Dystrophic calcification is found in: *(NEET 2016)*

a. Pulmonary veins
b. Old scars
c. Renal failure
d. Vitamin A intoxication

Ans. is 'b' Old scars

34. Metastatic calcification is seen in: *(NEET 2016)*

a. TB lymph nodes
b. Fungal granuloma
c. Renal failure
d. Atheromatous plaque

Ans. is 'c' Renal failure

INFLAMMATION AND REPAIR

TOLL-LIKE RECEPTORS

The Toll-like receptors are membrane proteins that recognize a variety of microbe-derived molecules and stimulate innate immune responses against the microbes. The Toll-like receptors are expressed on many different cell types that participate in innate immune responses including macrophages, dendritic cells, neutrophils, NK cells, mucosal epithelial cells and endothelial cells.

Signaling by Toll like receptors results in the activation of transcription factors, notably NF-Kß and AP- genes that are expressed in response to TLR signaling encode proteins important in many different components of innate immune response. These include inflammatory cytokines (TNF, IL-l); endothelial adhesion molecules (E-selectin); and proteins involved in microbial killing mechanism.

Different TLRs recognize different molecules of microbes: TLR-2 - LPS (endotoxin) of leptospira, peptidoglycan of gram positive bacteria, Zymosan of fungi, lipoarabinomannan of mycobacteria.

TLR-3: Double-stranded DNA of virus.

TLR-4: LPS (endotoxin) of all gram negative bacteria ***except*** leptospira.

TLR-5: Flagellin of bacteria.

35. All are true about Toll-like receptors *except*: *(NEET 2016)*

a. Recognize microbial molecules
b. Activation of immune system
c. Regulation of calcium channel
d. Activation of transcription factors

Ans. is 'c' Regulation of calcium channel

36. Toll-like receptors are: *(NEET 2016)*

a. Membrane proteins
b. Cytoplasmic proteins
c. Nuclear proteins
d. Mitochondrial proteins

Ans. is 'a' Membrane proteins

INFLAMMATORY MEDIATORS AND THEIR EFFECTS

- *Increased vascular permeability*: Histamine, serotonin (5-hydroxytryptamine), anaphylotoxins (C3a, C4a,C5a), PAF, leukotrienes (LTC4, D4, E4), bradykinin. PAF is the most potent one to increase permeability.
- *Chemo attractant*: C5a (most potent), IL-8, LTB4, PAF, bacterial products, Lymphokine, Kallikrejn. C5a is the most potent chemo attractant.
- *Vasodilatation*: Histamine, prostaglandins (PG D2, PGE2), prostacyclins (PGI2), serotonin, Nitric oxide, bradykinin.
- *Vasoconstriction*: Leukotrienes (LTC4, D4, E4), Thromboxane A2.

- *Bronchoconstriction*: Leukotrienes (LTC4, D4, E4), PFA, histamine, bradykinin. Leokotrienes (LTC4, D4, E4) are most potent bronchoconstrictors.
- *Pain*: Prostaglandins, bradykinin.
- *Fever (pyrogens)*: IL-1, TNF-a, IL-6, prostaglandins, interferon.

TGF-Beta

The most important fibrogenic mediator (causing fibrosis) is transforming growth factor-beta. It induces proliferation of fibroblasts, endothelial cells and specialized fibrogenic cells. It is chemotactic for fibroblasts, neutrophils, macrophages, lymphocytes and smooth muscle cells. It is not an activator of macrophages, instead it is secreted by alternatively activated macrophages.

Vascular Endothelial Growth Factor (VEGF)

- Inducer of extracellular proteinase expression, increased expression of specific integrins for migration, and initiation of cell proliferation and migration.
- Binds to endo-specific receptors Fit-l and Flic-1 (of the tyrosine kinase family).
- Expression of VEGF potentiated by hypoxia and inactivation of p53.

IL-1 – Formerly known as Lymphocyte Activating Factor

- Augments the activity of many cell types, especially T-cells is an endogenous pyrogen (EP).
- Induces an increase in acute phase reactants.

Caspase-1/Interleukin-1 converting enzyme (ICE) is an evolutionarily conserved enzyme that proteolytically cleaves other proteins, such as the precursors of the inflammatory cytokines interleukin 1β and interleukin 18 as well as the pyroptosis inducer Gasdermin D, into active mature peptides. It plays a central role in cell immunity as an inflammatory response initiator.

Prostaglandin Analogues

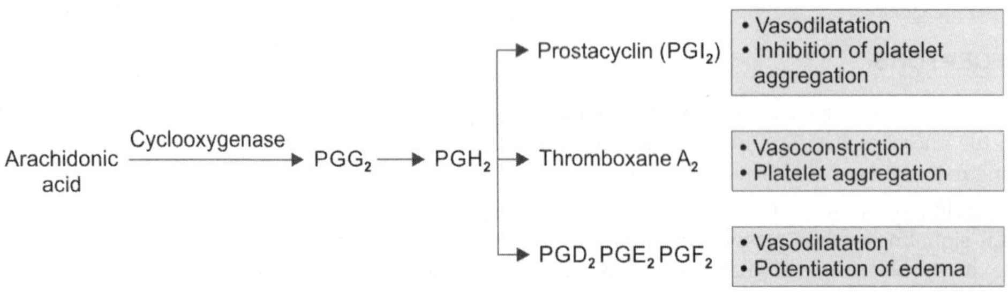

37. Fibroblast proliferation is stimulated by: *(NEET 2016)*

a. TGF-β
b. IFN-γ
c. TNF-α
d. IL-10

Ans. is 'a' TGF-β

38. True about TGF-β is: *(NEET 2016)*

a. Activates macrophages
b. Involved in fibrogenesis
c. Proinflammatory
d. All of the above

Ans. is 'b' Involved in fibrogenesis

39. Not true about VEGF is: *(NEET 2016)*

a. Highly specific for endothelium
b. Hypoxia potentiates its expression
c. Inhibits angiogenesis
d. Helps in tumor metastasis

Ans. is 'c' Inhibits angiogenesis

40. VEGF action is: *(NEET 2016)*

a. Vasodilatation
b. Angiogenesis
c. Fibrogenesis
d. Chemotaxis

Ans. is 'b' Angiogenesis

41. True about thromboxane -A2 is: *(NEET 2016)*

a. Vasodilatation
b. Platelet aggregation
c. Potentiation of edema
d. Formed in endothelium

Ans. is 'b' Platelet aggregation

42. Vasodilatation following endothelial damage is due to: *(NEET 2016)*

a. Histamine
b. IL-2
c. TGF-β
d. FGF

Ans. is 'a' Histamine

43. Which among the following is a vasoconstrictor? *(NEET 2016)*

a. Histamine
b. PGI2
c. Bradykinin
d. TXA2

Ans. is 'd' TXA2

44. What is the function of IL-1? *(NEET 2018)*

a. Enhances hematopoiesis
b. Stimulates mast cells
c. Has antiviral properties
d. Endognous pyrogen

Ans. is 'd' Endognous pyrogen

45. IL-1 is activated by:

a. Caspase 1
b. Caspase 3
c. Caspase 8
d. Caspase 5

Ans. is 'a' Caspase 1

HEALING OF AN INJURY

Skin wounds can heal by primary intention or secondary intention.

Healing by Primary Intention:

❖ It occurs in wounds with opposed edegs, e.g. surgical incision. It is characteristic of clean uncontaminated (non-infected) wound. It follows a series of sequential steps:

Immediately after incision: Incision is filled with blood clot containing fibrin and blood cells (including platelets), dehydration of surface clot forms scab on surface.

- *Within 24 hours*: Nentrophils appear at the margin of wound, which is filled with blood clot.
- *24–48 hours*: Epithelial cells move from wound edges and fuse in the midline beneath the surface scab, producing a continuous but thin epithelium layer that closes the wound.
- *Day 3*: Neutrophils are replaced by macrophages, granulation tissue appears, collagen fibers are present in the argin but do not bridge the incision.
- *Day 5*: Abundant granulation tissue, maximum neovascularization, abundant collagen which bridges the incision, the epidermis recovers its normal thickness.
- *2" week*: Disappearance of leukocytes and edema, presence of fibroblasts (derived from local mesenchyme) and maximum collagen.
- *End of 1 month*: There is scar which is made up of cellular connective tissue devoid of inflammatory infiltrate covered now by intact epidermis. There is replacement of collagen type III with collagen type I.

Healing by Secondary Intention:

❖ It occurs in wounds with separated edges in which there is more extensive loss of cells and tissue. Much larger amounts of granulation tissue are formed. Wound contraction occurs—Feature that most clearly differentiate secondary from primary healing.

❖ Permanent wound contraction requires the action of myofibroblasts—Fibroblasts that have the ultrastructural characteristic of smooth muscle cells.

❖ In presence of infection there is secondary healing.

46. Which type of healing occurs in an incisional wound with infections: *(NEET 2016)*

a. Primary
b. Delayed primary
c. Secondary
d. Tertiary

Ans. is 'c' Secondary

47. Normal time taken for scar formation after injury: *(NEET 2016)*

a. 2 weeks
b. 3 weeks
c. 4 weeks
d. 5 weeks

Ans. is 'c' 4 weeks

48. Scar tissue replaces infarcted myocardium in how much time? *(NEET 2016)*

a. 3 weeks
b. 5 weeks
c. 6 weeks
d. 12 weeks

Ans. is 'd' 12 weeks

FREE RADICALS

Properties	$O_2^{\bullet-}$	H_2O_2	•OH	$ONOO^-$
Mechanisms of production	Incomplete reduction of O_2 during oxidative phosphorylation; by phagocyte oxidase in leukocytes	Generated by SOD from O_2^- and by oxidases in peroxisomes	Generated from H_2O by hydrolysis, e.g., by radiation; from H_2O_2 by Fenton reaction; from $O_2^{\bullet-}$	Produced by interaction of $O_2^{\bullet-}$ and NO generated by NO synthase in many cell types (endothelial cells, leukocytes, neurons, others)
Mechanisms of inactivation	Conversion to H_2O_2 and $O_2^{\bullet-}$ by superoxide dismutase (SOD)	Conversion to H_2O and $O_2^{\bullet-}$ by catalase (peroxisomes), glutathione peroxidase (cytosol, mitochondria)	Conversion to H_2O by glutathione peroxidase	Conversion to HNO_2 by peroxiredoxins (cytosol, mitochondria)
Pathologic effects	Stimulates production of degradative enzymes in leukocytes and other cells; may directly damage lipids, proteins, DNA; acts close to site of production	Can be converted to **•OH** and OCl^-, which destroy microbes and cells; can act distant from site of production	Most reactive oxygen-derived free radical; principal ROS responsible for damaging lipids, proteins, and DNA	Damages lipids, proteins, DNA

Vitamins A, C and E act as antioxidant agents. Vitamin C and other water soluble compounds, such as uric acid, thiols including glutathione and dihydrolipoic acid and possibly other substances such as metallothionein, serve to defend against hydroxyl radicals. Vitamin E, in contrast, is less effective in eliminating hydroxyl radicals.

49. Peroxidase enzyme found in neutrofils is used for: *(NEET 2016)*

a. Macrophage activation
b. Chemotactic agent
c. Microbial killing
d. Vasodilatation

Ans. is 'c' Microbial killing

50. Which among the following is not a free radical: *(NEET 2016)*

a. Superoxide dismutase
b. Hydrogen peroxide
c. Superoxide anion
d. Nitric oxide

Ans. is 'a' Superoxide dismutase

51. Hydroxyl ions are destroyed in the body by: *(NEET 2016)*

a. Vitamin C
b. Vitamin A
c. Vitamin K
d. Vitamin D

Ans. is 'a' Vitamin C

CHEMOKINES

- Chemokines are a family of small proteins that act primary as chemo attractants for specific types of leukocytes.
- They are classified into four major groups according to the arrangement of the conserved cysteine (C) residues in mature proteins. *C-x-c chemokines*: They primarily act on neutrophils, e.g. li-8, IL-1 and TNF.
- *c—C chemokines*: Attract all leukocytes ***except*** neutrophils. Examples are Eotaxin (specific for eosinophils), MCP-1 (monocyte chemo attractant protein), RANTES (regulated and normal T-cell expressed and secreted), and MIP-la (macrophage inflammatory proteinla).
- *C—chemokines*: They are specific for lymphocytes, e.g. lymphotactin.
- *cxc chemokines*: They promotes strong adhesion between monocytes and t cells, e.g. fractalkine.

52. Limphotactin is which type of chemokine? *(NEET 2016)*

a. C
b. C-C
c. C-X-C
d. C-X3-C

Ans. is 'a' C

CONTENTS OF NEUTROPHIL GRANULES

Primary (Azeurophilic granules)	Secondary (Specific granules)	Tertiary (C-particle) granules (from internet)
1. Myeloperoxidase 2. Lysozyme 3. Acid hydrolases 4. Elastases 5. Nonspecific collagenase 6. Bacterial permeability protein 7. Defensin (BPI)	1. Lactoferrin 2. Lysozyme 3. Alkaline phosphatase 4. Type IV Collagenase 5. Phospholipase A2 6. Lenkocyte adhesion molecules 7. Plasminogen activator	Contains gelatinase and acid hydrolases

Contd...

Contd...

Primary (Azeurophilic granules)	Secondary (Specific granules)	Tertiary (C-particle) granules (from internet)
8. Cathepsin G 9. PliospholipaseA2	8. Vit B12 binding protein 9. Gelatinase 10. Histaminase 11. β2-microglobulin 12. Cytochrome B	

53. Primary granules contain which enzyme? *(NEET 2016)*

a. Myeloperoxidase   b. Hydrolases
c. Lactoferrin   d. Phospholipase A2

Ans. is 'a' Myeloperoxidase

54. Active compound secreted by neutrophills against pathogen is known as: *(NEET 2016)*

a. Major basic protein   b. Myeloperoxidase
c. Hydrolase   d. Proteoglycans

Ans. is 'b' Myeloperoxidase

ACUTE INFLAMMATION

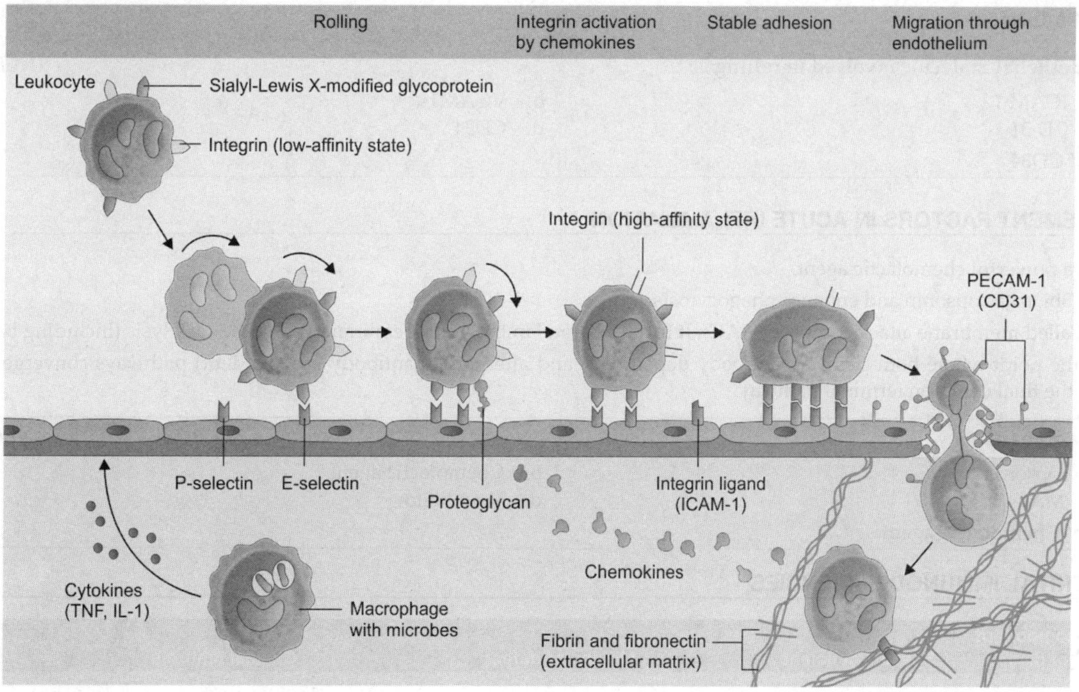

- ❖ Neutrophils are the major cells in early phase of acute inflammation.
- ❖ Macrophages are the major cells in late phase of acute inflammation and in chronic inflammation.
- ❖ ICAM (intracellular adhesion molecule-1) and VCAM (Vascular cell adhesion molecule-1) act as adhesion molecules in the process of diapedesis.
- ❖ Platelet endothelial cell adhesion molecule (PECAM or CD-31) is present on both endothelium and leukocytes. It is the major adhesive molecule for diapedesis.

Endothelial–leukocyte adhesion molecules		
Endothelial molecule	***Leucocyte molecule***	***Major role***
P-selectin	Sialyl-Lewis X-modified proteins	Rolling
E-selectin	Sialy-Lewi X-modified proteins	Rolling and adhesion
GlyCam-1, CD34	L-selectin	Rolling
ICAM-1 (immunoglobulin family)	(LFA-1, Mac-1)	Adhesion, arrest, transmigration
VCAM-1 (immunoglobulin family)	VLA-4	Adhesion
PECAM-I (CD-31)	PECAM-1 (CD -31)	Diapedesis (transmigration)

Post capillary venules are an important point of interchange between the lumen of the vessels and the surrounding tissue. Moreover both vascular leakage and leucocyte exudation occur preferentially in venules in many types of inflammation.

55. What types of cells are predominant in early phase of inflammations? *(NEET 2016)*

a. Macrophages
b. Basophill
c. Mast cells
d. Neutrophils

Ans. is 'd' Neutrophils

56. Leukocyte migration occurs mainly in: *(NEET 2016)*

a. Arterioles
b. Venules
c. Arteries
d. Capillaries

Ans. is 'b' Venules

57. Endothelial ligands VCAM and ICAM are involved in: *(NEET 2016)*

a. Phagocytosis
b. Adhesion
c. Chemotaxis
d. Leukocyte activation

Ans. is 'b' Adhesion

58. Main function of cell adhesion molecule PECAM1 is: *(NEET 2016)*

a. Rolling arrest
b. Arrest
c. Adhesion
d. Diapedesis

Ans. is 'c' Adhesion

59. Endothelial molecule involved in rolling is: *(NEET 2016)*

a. ICAM 1
b. VCAM1
c. CD 31
d. CD34

Ans. is 'd' CD34

COMPLEMENT FACTORS IN ACUTE INFLAMMATION

- C5a is a powerful chemotactic agent.
- C3b, C3bi act as opsonin and enhance phagocytosis.
- C5-9 Called membrane attack complex (MAC). It forms channel in the lipid membrane and causes cell lysis (including bacteria).
- C5 is the point where both classical (antibody dependent) and alternative (antibody independent) pathways converge. Thus C5 forms the final common terminal pathway.

60. C5a act as a/an: *(NEET 2016)*

a. Opsonin
b Chemotactic agent
c. MAC
d. Vasodilator

Ans. is 'b' Chemotactic agent

CONGENITAL IMMUNODEFICIENCIES

Deficient component and name of disease	Specific deficiency	Molecular defect	Clinical features
B cell			
X-linked (Bruton's)	Absence of B cells; very low immunoglobulin (Ig) levels, which results in defective opsonization	Mutant tyrosine kinase	Recurrent bacterial infections, especially of respiratory tract, caused by pyogenic bacteria such as pneumococci
Selective IgA	Very low IgA levels	Failure of heavy-chain gene switching	Recurrent infections, especially of the sinuses and lung, caused by pyogenic bacteria
T cell			
Thymic aplasia (DiGeorge's)	Absence of T cells	Defective development of pharyngeal pouches; not a genetic disease	Viral, fungal, and protozoal infections; tetany
Chronic mucocutaneous candidiasis	Deficient T-cell response to Candida	Unknown	Skin and mucous membrane infections with Candida
Combined B and T cell			
Severe combined immunodeficiency (SCID)	Deficiency of both B-cell and T-cell function	Either defective IL-2 receptor, defective recombinases, defective kinases, absence of class II MHC proteins, or ADA or PNP deficiency	Bacterial, viral, fungal, and protozoal infections

Contd...

Contd...

Deficient component and name of disease	Specific deficiency	Molecular defect	Clinical features
Complement			
Hereditary angioedema	Deficiency of C1 protease inhibitor	Too much C3a, C4a, and C5a -generated	Edema, especially laryngeal edema
C3b	Insufficient C3	Unknown	Pyogenic infections, especially with Staphylococcus aureus
C6,7,8	Insufficient C6,7,8	Unknown	Neisseria infections
Phagocytes			
Chronic granulomatous disease	Defective bactericidal activity because no oxidative burst	Deficient NADPH oxidase activity	Pyogenic infections, especially with S. aureus and Aspergillus
Chédiak-Higashi Syndrome	Defective lysosomal killing of microbes	Failure of the lysosomes of neutrophils to fuse with phagosomes	Recurrent pyogenic infections, caused primarily by staphylococci and streptococci

Chronic Granulomatous Disorder

CGD is characterized by defective NADPH oxidase. Leukocytes do not undergo degranulation during phagocytosis. The diminished production of H_2O_2 appears to be the major reason for defective bactericidal activity.

There is recurrent infections by catalase positive bacteria (staphylococci, coliform), but catalase negative pathogens (streptococci and pneumococci) are handled normally.

Screening test for CGD is Nitroblue tetrazolium (NBT) test which is negative in CGD. Other tests used are Dihydrorhodamine (DHR) oxidation test, cytochrome C reduction assay and immunoblot for NADPH oxidase component.

Most common mode of inheritance of CGD is X-linked followed by autosomal recessive.

Autosomal Dominant Hyper-IgE Syndrome (Job Syndrome)

- Deficiency of Th 17 cells due to STAT3 mutation – impaired recruitment of neutrophils to sites of infection.
- Cold (noninflamed) staphylococcal abscesses, retained Baby teeth, Coarse facies, Dermatologic problems (eczema), raised IgE, bone Fractures from minor trauma.
- Raised IgE and eosinophils

Wiskott-Aldrich Syndrome

- Mutation in WAS gene; leukocytes and platelets unable to reorganize actin cytoskeleton → defective antigen presentation; X-linked recessive
- Thrombocytopenia, Eczema, Recurrent (pyogenic) infections
- Increased risk of autoimmune disease and malignancy
- Reduced to normal IgG, IgM. Raised IgE and IgA. Fewer and smaller platelets.

61. A child presents with recurrent infections, eczema and thrombocytopenia. What is the diagnosis? *(NEET 2020)*

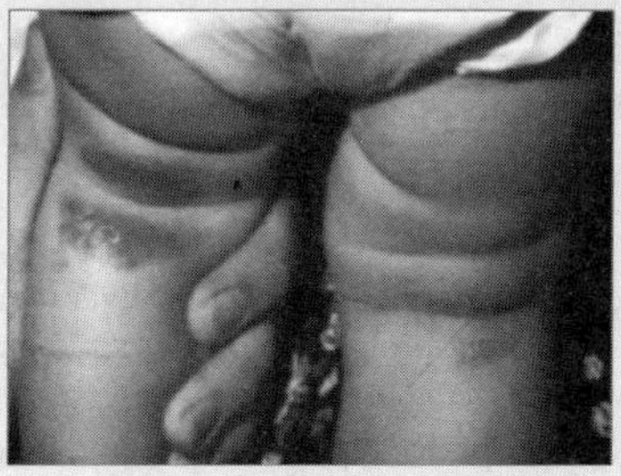

a. Job syndrome
b. Wiskott-Aldrich syndrome
c. HSP
d. CGD

Ans. is 'b' Wiskott-Aldrich syndrome

62. Which one of the following statements is not correct regarding chronic granulomatous disease? *(NEET 2016)*

a. It is an autosomal recessive disease
b. It is characterized by abnormal bacterial phagocytosis
c. Function of macrophages is defective
d. Nitro blue tetrazolium test is useful for screening.

Ans. is 'c' Function of macrophages is defective

63. All of the following organisms can cause serious infection in chronic granulomatous disease *except*: *(NEET 2016)*

a. Streptococcus pneumoniae
b. Staphylococcus aureus
c. Pseudomonas
d. H.influenza

Ans. is 'a' Streptococcus pneumoniae

Pathology

64. Nitro blue tetrazolium test is used to detect defect in: *(NEET 2016)*

a. Cellular immunity
b. Humoral immunity
c. Phagocytosis
d. Complement pathway

Ans. is 'c' Phagocytosis

65. Defect in Chediak-Higashi syndrome is: *(NEET 2016)*

a. Fusion of lysosome
b. T-cell
c. B-cell
d. Complement

Ans. is 'a' Fusion of lysosome

66. Phagolysosome fusion defect is seen in: *(NEET 2016)*

a. Chronic granulomatous disease
b. Chediak-Higashi disease
c. LAM 1
d. LAM 2

Ans. is 'b' Chediak-Higashi disease

Miscellaneous

67. Destruction of Heinz bodies in spleen is performed by: *(NEET 2016)*

a. Macrophages
b. Lymphocytes
c. Neutrophils
d. Fibroblasts

Ans. is 'a' Macrophages

68. Foam cells are formed by: *(NEET 2016)*

a. Neutrophils
b. Fibroblasts
c. Macrophages
d. All of them

Ans. is 'c' Macrophages

Foam cells are lipid-laden cells that derive predominantly from macrophages (M2 type), but smooth muscle cells can also imbibe lipid to become foam cells. They are seen in atherosclerosis.

69. Delayed umbilical cord detachment leukocytosis is seen in: *(NEET 2016)*

a. Leukocyte adhesion deficiency
b. Chronic granulomatous disease
c. Severe combined immunodeficiency
d. None of the above

Ans. is 'a' Leukocyte adhesion deficiency

HEMODYNAMIC DISORDERS

PASSIVE VENOUS CONGESTION OF LIVER

Hepatic manifestations of systemic circulatory compromise-passive congestion and centrilobular necrosis can be seen in both left and right-sided heart failure.

Pathology

- Right-sided cardiac decompensation leads to passive congestion of the liver. The liver is slightly enlarged, tense, and cyanotic, with rounded edges. Microscopically there is congestion of centrilobular sinusoids. With time, centrilobular hepatocytes become atrophic, resulting in markedly attenuated liver cell plates.
- Left-sided cardiac failure or shock may lead to hepatic hypoperfusion and hypoxia, causing ischemic coagulative necrosis of hepatocytes in the central region of the lobule (centrilobular necrosis).
- Combination of hypoperfusion and retrograde congestion acts synergistically to cause centrilobular hemorrhagic necrosis. The liver takes on a variegated mottled appearance, reflecting hemorrhage and necrosis in the centrilobular regions. This finding is known as nutmeg liver due to its resemblance to the cut surface of a nutmeg.

70. Nutmeg liver is seen in: *(NEET 2016)*

a. Right sided heart failure
b. Left sided heart failure
c. Increased pulmonary pressure
d. Decreased pulmonary pressure

Ans. is 'a' Right sided heart failure

71. The zonal necrosis most commonly affected in chronic passive hepatic congestion is: *(NEET 2016)*

a. Central
b. Peripheral
c. Mid zonal
d. None

Ans. is 'a' Central

Causes of Edema

Increased hydrostatic pressure of capillaries: It causes increase in outward driving force. It may be due to impaired venous return, e.g. in CHF or DVT.

Decreased plasma osmotic pressure of capillaries: It causes decreases in inward driving force. It results from Hypoproteinemia. When total plasma protein is below 5 g/dL (normal 6–8 g/dL) or albumin is below 2.5 g/dL (normal 3.5–5 g/dL) edema takes place. Conditions causing hypoproteinemia are nephrotic syndrome, liver cirrhosis, protein losing enteropathy, and PEM.

Defective removal of interstitial fluid by lymphatics: It is due to lymphatic obstruction, which may be inflammatory, neoplastic, post-surgical and post-irradiation.

Increased vascular permeability: It occurs in acute and chronic inflammation, and during angiogenesis (new vessels are leaky).

Sodium (salt) and water retention: It causes expansion of plasma volume (hydrostatic pressure) and dilution of plasma proteins (1- osmotic pressure).

72. Decrease in plasma osmotic pressure is cause of edema in: *(NEET 2016)*

a. CHF
b. DVT
c. Nephrotic syndrome
d. None

Ans. is 'c' Nephrotic syndrome

DISTRIBUTIVE SHOCK

It is characterized by abnormal distribution of blood flow in the smallest blood vessels results in inadequate supply of blood to the body's tissues and organ. It results from excessive vasodilatation due to decreased systemic vasomotor tone, usually qualified as a decreased systemic vascular resistance (SVR). There is venous pooling of blood with decreased preload. With fluid resuscitation, effective circulating volume increases and often creates a hyperdynamic pattern and increased cardiac output associated with a low-to-normal blood pressure.

Septic shock is the most common form of distributive shock.

Other causes of distributive shock include systemic inflammatory response syndrome (SIRS) due to noninfectious inflammatory conditions such as burns and pancreatitis; toxic shock syndrome (TSS); anaphylaxis; reactions to drugs or toxins, including insect bites, transfusion reaction, and heavy metal poisoning; Addisonian crisis; hepatic insufficiency; and neurogenic shock due to brain or spinal cord injury.

Summary of Pathophysiologic Findings in Hypovolemic, Cardiogenic, and Septic Shock

Type of Shock	CO	PVR	LVEDP	MVO_2
Hypovolemic	↓	↑	↓	↓
Cardiogenic	↓	↑	↑	↓
Endotoxic (septic)	↑	↓	↓	↑

(CO: Cardiac output; LVEDP: Left ventricular end-diastolic pressure; MVO_2: Mixed venous oxygen content; PVR: Peripheral vascular resistance).

73. Feature characteristic of distributive shock is: *(NEET 2016)*

a. Normal or high cardiac output
b. Vasoconstriction
c. Most common cause in neurogenic
d. Increased preload

Ans. is 'a' Normal or high cardiac output

GENETICS AND GENETIC DISORDERS

Denver System for classification of human chromosomes:

Group	Chromosome number	Characteristics
A	1	Longest with median kinetochore
	2	Second longest, kinetochore slightly off center
	3	Third longest with median kinetochore
B	4–5	Four long chromosomes with kinetochore close to one end
C	6–12	Fourteen medium tenth chromosomes with slightly sub-median kinetochore.
D	13–15	Six chromosomes slightly smaller than the C group with the kinetochores in a near terminal position.
E	16–18	Six chromosomes; short with median kinetochores in 16 and sub-median in 17 and 18.
F	19–20	Four chromosomes, shorter than E group with median kinetochores.
G	21–20	Four shortest chromosomes with sub-median kinetochores. It is difficult to see any short aims.
X	23	Similar to C group but often the largest in this group.
Y		Similar to G group but the chromatids tend to remain dose together.

74. Group-D chromosome is: *(NEET 2016)*

a. Chromosome 3
b. Chromosome 6
c. Chromosome 12
d. Chromosome 15

Ans. is 'd' Chromosome 15

MODES OF INHERITANCE

Autosomal dominant

- Often due to defects in structural genes. Many generations, both males and females are affected.
- Often pleiotropic (multiple apparently unrelated effects) and variably expressive (different between individuals). Family history crucial to diagnosis. With one affected (heterozygous) parent, on average, half of children affected.

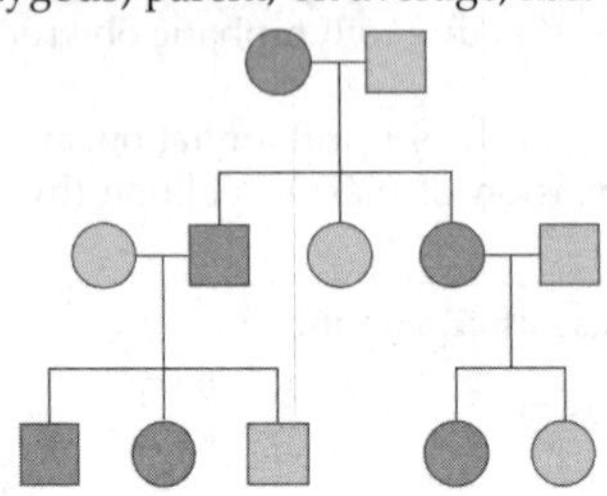

Autosomal recessive

- With 2 carrier (heterozygous) parents, on average: 1/4 of children will be affected (homozygous), 1/2 of children will be carriers, and 1/4 of children will be neither affected nor carriers.
- Often due to enzyme deficiencies. Usually seen in only 1 generation. Commonly more severe than dominant disorders; patients often present in childhood. Increased risk in consanguineous families. Unaffected individual with affected sibling has 2/3 probability of being a carrier.

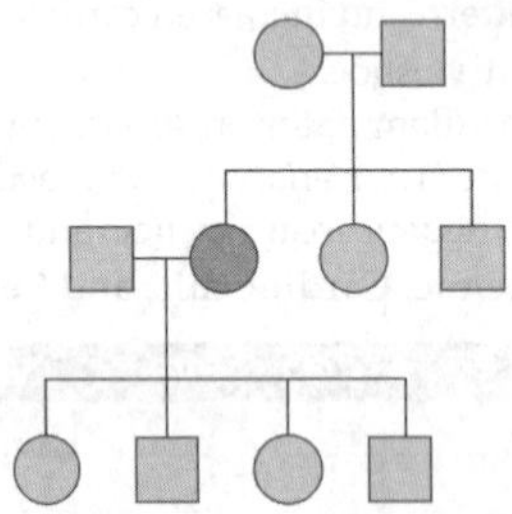

X-linked recessive

- Sons of heterozygous mothers have a 50% chance of being affected. No male-to-male transmission. Skips generations.
- Commonly more severe in males. Females usually must be homozygous to be affected.

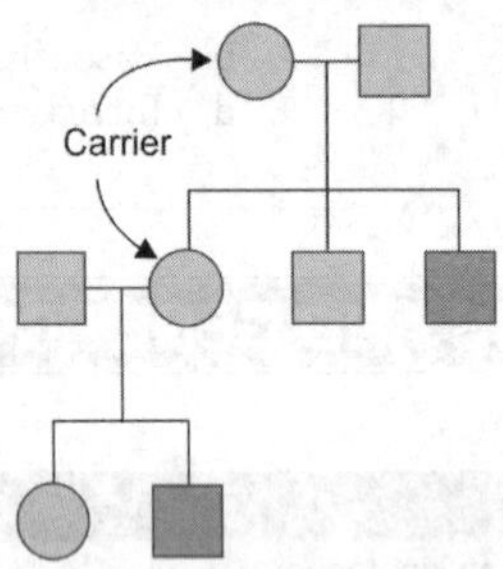

X-linked dominant

- Transmitted through both parents. Mothers transmit to 50% of daughters and sons; fathers transmit to all daughters but no sons.

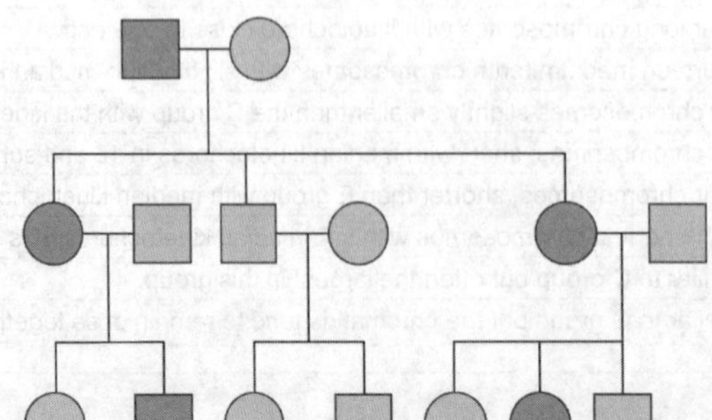

Mitochondrial inheritance

- Transmitted only through the mother. All offspring of affected females may show signs of disease.

❖ Variable expression in a population or even within a family due to heteroplasmy.

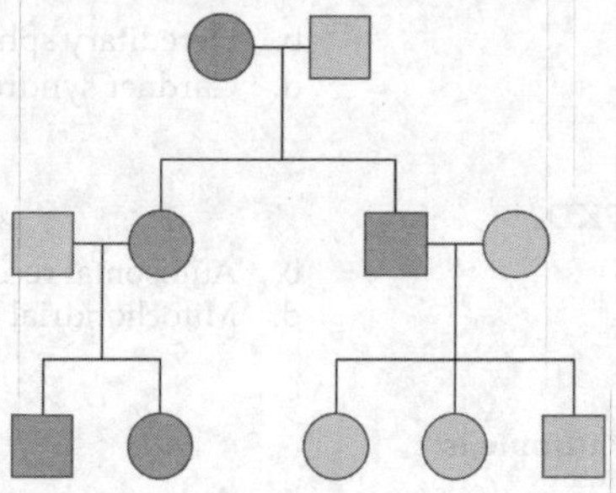

75. A young male, very tall and thin with long fingers and audible murmur on CVS examination. Pedigree chart shown below. What is the likely inheritance? *(NEET 2020)*

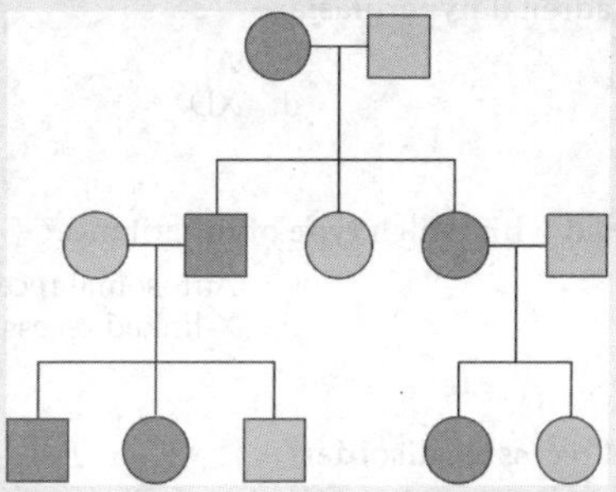

a. Autosomal dominant
b. Autosomal recessive
c. X linked dominant
d. X linked recessive

Ans. is 'a' Autosomal dominant

Explanation: History of arachnodactyly with cardiac murmur (likely secondary to aortic regurgitation) is suggestive of Marfan syndrome.

Autosomal dominant disorders					
Nervous	***Urinary***	***GIT***	***Hematological***	***Skeletal***	***Metabolic***
• Huntington disease • Neurofibromatosis • Myotonic dystrophy • Tuberous sclerosis • Retinoblastoma	• ADPKD	• Familial polyposis coli • Gardner's syndrome • Turcot's syndrome • Lynch syndrome • Peutz Jagher's syndrome • Juvenile polyposis	• Hereditary spherocytosis • Von Willibrand disease	• Marfan syndrome • EDS (soine variant) • Osteogenesis imperfècta • Achondroplasia • Tuberous scleosis • Crouzon syndrome • Hereditary multiple exostoses	• Familial hypercholestero-lesterlemia • Acute intermittent porphyria

X-linked recessive disorders				
Musculoskeletal	***Hematological***	***Immune***	***Metabolic***	***Nervous***
Duchene muscular Chronic granulomatous disease	Hemophilla A and B G-6-PD deficiency	Agammaglobulinemia Wiskott Aldrich syndrome	Diabetes insipidus Lesch Nyhan syndrome	Fragile X syndrome Color blindness

X-linked dominant disorders
Vitamin D resistant (X-linked hypophosphatemic) Rickets
Familial hypophosphatemia
Fragile X-syndrome
Incontinentia pigmenti
Rett syndrome

76. All of the following are X-linked recessive disorders *except*: *(NEET 2016)*

a. G-6PD deficiency
b. Duchene muscular dystrophy
c. Wiskott- Aldrich syndrome
d. Hypophosphatemic rickets

Ans. is 'd' Hypophosphatemic rickets

77. Which of the following is not an X-linked recessive disorder? *(NEET 2016)*

a. G-6PD deficiency
b. Diabetes insipidus
c. Hemophilia
d. Incontinentia pigmenti

Ans. is 'd' Incontinentia pigmenti

78. Not an autosomal dominant disorder: *(NEET 2016)*

a. Alkaptonurea
b. Hereditary spheocytosis
c. Osteogenesis imperfecta
d. Gardner syndrome

Ans. is 'a' Alkaptonurea

79. What is the mode of inheritance of ADPKD? *(NEET 2016)*

a. Autosomal dominant
b. Autosomal recessive
c. X-linked recessive
d. Mitochondrial inheritance

Ans. is 'a' Autosomal dominant

80. Inheritance associated with fragile X-syndrome is: *(NEET 2016)*

a. Autosomal dominant
b. Autosomal recessive
c. X-linked dominant
d. X-linked recessive

Ans. is 'c' X-linked dominant

81. Inheritance associated with congenital adrenal hyperplasia: *(NEET 2016)*

a. AR
b. AD
c. XR
d. XD

Ans. is 'a' AR

82. Acute intermittent porphyria is associated with which type of inheritance? *(NEET 2016)*

a. Autosomal dominant
b. Autosomal recessive
c. X-linked dominant
d. X-linked recessive

Ans. is 'a' Autosomal dominant

83. Which of the following is an autosomal recessive disorder? *(NEET 2019)*

a. Albinism
b. Huntington's syndrome
c. Marfan's syndrome
d. Neurofibromatosis-1

Ans. is 'a' Albinism

CONSANGUINITY

- Increases risk of—autosomal recessive disease
- No change in risk of—autosomal dominant, X-linked recessive (if neither parent affected)
- Not Proven—complex late onset diseases like diabetes, schizophrenia, cardiovascular diseases

84. Most common type of inheritance associated with consanguinity: *(NEET 2016)*

a. Autosomal dominant
b. Autosomal recessive
c. X-linked dominant
d. X-linked recessive

Ans. is 'b' Autosomal recessive

TREATMENT OF MITOCHONDRIAL DISORDERS

- "Mito Cocktail" is the name given to a variety of vitamins and supplements which are commonly used by adults and children who have been diagnosed with mitochondrial disease. It includes:
  - Coenzyme Q-10
  - L-Carnitine
  - B-Vitamins—Thiamine (Bi), Riboflavin (B2), B3, B6, B12 and folic acid (B9)
  - Antioxidants—Vitamin C (ascorbic acid) and Vitamin E (tocopherol).

85. Treatment for mitochondrial disorder is: *(NEET 2016)*

a. Ascorbic acid
b. Folic acid
c. Coenzyme Q-10
d. All of the above

Ans. is 'd' All of the above

X-LINKED ADRENOLEUKODYSTROPHY

- X-linked adrenoleukodystrophy (ALD/X-ALD) is a disease caused by mutations in ABCDI, a gene located on the X chromosome, that codes for ALD, a peroxisomal membrane transporter protein.
- ALD is the most common peroxisomal inborn error of metabolism. It is a disorder of peroxisomal fatty acid beta oxidation which results in the accumulation of very long chain fatty acids in tissues throughout the body. The most severely affected tissues are the myelin in the central nervous system, the adrenal cortex and the Leydig cells in the testes.
- As an X-linked disorder, ALD presents most commonly in males.

86. X-linked adrenoleukodystrophy is:	(NEET 2016)
a. Fatty acid disorder	b. Lysosomal storage disorder
c. Mucoplysacchardoses	d. Glycogen storage disorder

Ans. is 'a' Fatty acid disorder

Diseases associated with trinucleotide repeat mutation are:

- Huntington's disease (CAG repeat)
- Spinocerebellar ataxia (CAG repeat)
- Friedreich ataxia (GAA repeat)
- Fragile-X-syndrome (GGG or GCC repeat)
- Dystrophia myotonica (CTG/CUG repeat)
- X-linked spinobulbar muscular atrophy (GAG repeat)
- Dentatorubral pallidoluysian atrophy (GAG repeat).

87. Trinucleotide sequence associated with spinocerebellar ataxia is:	(NEET 2016)
a. CTG	b. CUG
c. GGG	d. CAG

Ans. is 'd' CAG

HUNTINGTON DISEASE

- Autosomal dominant trinucleotide (CAG) repeat expansion in the Huntington (HTT) gene on chromosome 4.
- Symptoms manifest between ages 20 and 50: chorea, athetosis, aggression, depression, dementia (sometimes initially mistaken for substance abuse).
- Anticipation results from expansion of CAG repeats.
- Caudate shows reduced levels of ACh and GABA
- Atrophy of caudate and putamen with ex vacuo venticulomegaly
- Neuronal death via NMDA-R binding and glutamate excitotoxicity.

88. Which of the following is correct regarding Huntington chorea?	(NEET 2020)
a. It is a trinucleotide repeat related mutational disorder	b. Loss of function type of mutation
c. Abnormal CUG repeats	d. Locus of mutation is on chromosome 6

Ans. is 'a' It is a trinucleotide repeat related mutational disorder

GENOTYPE AND PHENOTYPE

- The genotype (The genetic makeup of an individual) of an organism is the inherited map it carries within its genetic code.
- The genotype is the part (DNA sequence) of the genetic makeup of a cell. Genotype is one of three factors that determine phenotype, the other two being inherited epigenetic factors, and non-inherited environmental factors.
- A phenotype is the detectable expression of the genotype. An expressed and observable trait, e.g. hair color.
- By definition a phenotype is the composite of an organism's observable characteristics or traits, such as its morphology, development, biochemical or physiological properties, behavior, and products of behavior. A phenotype results from the expression of an organism's genetic code, its genotype, as well as the influence of environmental factors and the interactions between the two.

89. Expression of a gene is known as:	(NEET 2016)
a. Genotype	b. Phenotype
c. Genome	d. Morphology

Ans. is 'b' Phenotype

KRABBE DISEASE

Krabbe disease, also known as globoid cell leukodystrophy or galactosyl ceramide lipidosis, is an autosomal-recessive sphingolipidosis caused by deficient activity of the lysosomal hydrolase galactosylceramide beta-galactosidase (GALC). GALC degrades galactosyl ceramide, a major component of myelin, and other terminal beta-galactose–containing sphingolipids, including psychosine (galactosyl sphingosine). Increased psychosine levels are believed to lead to widespread destruction of oligodendroglia in the CNS and to subsequent demyelination.

90. Krabbe's disease is:	
a. Deficiency of Beta-galactosylceramidase	b. Deficiency of arylsulphatase
c. Alpha galactosidase	d. Acid lipase

Ans. is 'a' Deficiency of Beta-galactosylceramidase

DUCHENNE MUSCULAR DYSTROPHY

- X-linked disorder typically due to frameshift deletions or nonsense mutations → truncated or absent dystrophin protein → progressive myofiber damage
- Dystrophin gene (DMD) is the largest protein-coding human gene → high chance of spontaneous mutation. Dystrophin helps anchor muscle fibers, primarily in skeletal and cardiac muscle. It connects the intracellular cytoskeleton (actin) to the transmembrane proteins α- and β- dystroglycan, which are connected to the extracellular matrix (ECM)
- Weakness begins in pelvic girdle muscles and progresses superiorly
- Pseudohypertrophy of calf muscles due to fibrofatty replacement of muscle
- Waddling gait
- Onset before 5 years of age
- Raised creatine kinase and aldolase; genetic testing confirms diagnosis
- Dilated cardiomyopathy is common cause of death
- *Gowers sign*: Patient uses upper extremities to help stand up. Classically seen in Duchenne muscular dystrophy, but also seen in other muscular dystrophies and inflammatory myopathies (e.g., polymyositis)

91. Absence of dystrophin protein is seen in: *(NEET 2020)*

a. Duchenne muscular dystrophy
b. Beckers dystrophy
c. Myotonic dystrophy
d. Spinomuscular dystrophy

Ans. is 'a' Duchenne muscular dystrophy

NEOPLASIA

HAMARTOMA

- It is a focal developmental malformation. It represents a mass of disorganized but mature specialized cells indigenous to the particular site. For example, hamartoma of lung contains bronchial structures like cartilage, blood vessels, etc.

CHORISTOMA

- Choristoma is the ectopic rest of normal tissue, i.e. the normal tissue is present at a different anatomical site of the body. For example, presence of pancreatic tissue in mucosa of small intestine.
- Normally differentiated tissue at abnormal (ectopic) site Choristoma.
- Abnormally ciliated tissue at normal site Hamartoma.

92. All are pre-malignant conditions *except*: *(NEET 2016)*

a. Anaplasia
b. Metaplasia
c. Hamartoma
d. Dysplasia

Ans. is 'c' Hamartoma

93. Choristoma is defined as: *(NEET 2016)*

a. Normal tissue in abnormal site
b. Normal tissue in excess at normal site
c. Abnormal tissue at any site
d. None of the above

Ans. is 'a' Normal tissue in abnormal site

Cellular adaptations	
Hypertrophy	↑ structural proteins and organelles → ↑ in size of cells
Hyperplasia	Controlled proliferation of cells → ↑ in number of cells Physiological—Endometrium during pregnancy, breast during puberty, liver regeneration after partial resection Pathological—Endometrial hyperplasia due to estrogen producing tumors → can progress to dysplasia/cancer
Atrophy	↓ in tissue mass due to ↓ in size (cytoskeletal degradation via ubiquitin-proteasome pathway) and/or number (apoptosis) of cells. Physiological—During embryogenesis, senile atrophy of uterus Pathological—Disuse, denervation, loss of blood supply, loss of hormonal stimulation, poor nutrition
Metaplasia	Reprogramming of stem cells → replacement of one cell type by another that can adapt to a new stress. Usually due to exposure to an irritant, such as gastric acid (Barrett esophagus) or cigarette smoke. May progress to dysplasia→ malignant transformation with persistent insult (Barrett esophagus →esophageal adenocarcinoma). Metaplasia of connective tissue can also occur (myositis ossificans)
Dysplasia	Disordered, precancerous epithelial cell growth; not considered a true adaptive response. Characterized by loss of uniformity of cell size and shape (pleomorphism); loss of tissue orientation; nuclear changes (↑ nuclear:cytoplasmic ratio and clumped chromatin).

94. A chronic smoker presents with cough. Biopsy shows which of the following adaptive changes? *(NEET 2020)*

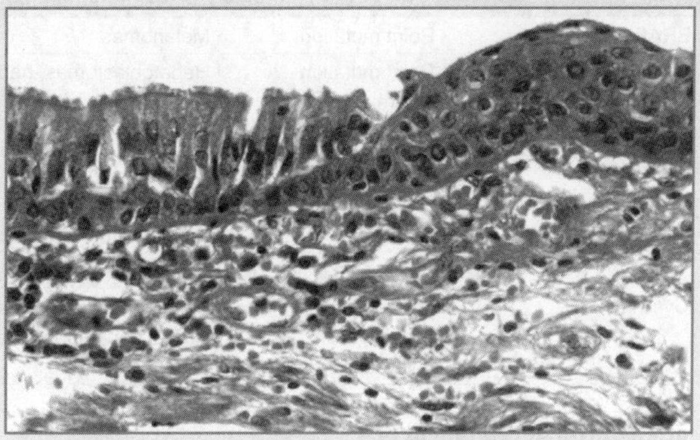

a. Atrophy
b. Metaplasia
c. Hypertrophy
d. Dysplasia

Ans. is 'b' Metaplasia

Explanation: Slide shows metaplasia of columnar epithelium (left) to squamous epithelium (right) in a bronchus.

ANAPLASIA

Differentiation refers to the extent to which neoplastic parenchymal cells resemble the corresponding normal parenchymal cells, both morphologically and functionally; lack of differentiation is called anaplasia. In general, benign tumors are well differentiated. The neoplastic cell in a benign adipocyte tumor—a lipoma—so closely resembles the normal cell that it may be impossible to recognize it as a tumor by microscopic examination of individual cells. Only the growth of these cells into a discrete mass discloses the neoplastic nature of the lesion. One may get so close to the tree that one loses sight of the forest. In well differentiated benign tumors, mitoses are extremely scant in number and are of normal configuration.

95. Anaplasia is: *(NEET 2018)*

a. Changing one type of epithelium to another
b. Nuclear chromatin changes
c. Lack of differentiation
d. Morphological changes

Ans. is 'c' Lack of differentiation

PROTO-ONCOGENES

Proto-oncogenes have multiple roles, participating in cellular functions related to growth and proliferation. Proteins encoded by proto-oncogenes may function as growth factors or their receptors, signal transducers, transcription factors, or cell cycle components. Oncoproteins encoded by oncogenes generally serve functions similar to their normal counterparts. However, mutations convert proto-oncogenes into constitutively active cellular oncogenes that are involved in tumor development because the oncoproteins they encode endow the cell with self-sufficiency in growth.

Oncogenes involved in various cancers are given below:

Category	Proto-oncogene	Mode of activation	Associated human tumor
Growth factors			
HGF	HGF	Overexpression	Thyroid cancer
Growth factor receptors			
EGF-receptor family	ERBB1 (EGFR), ERBB2	Overexpression	Squamous cell carcinoma of lung, gliomas
Receptor for neurotrophic factors	RET	Point mutation Point mutation	Leukemia Multiple endocrine neoplasia 2A and B, familial medullary thyroid carcinomas
Receptor for stem cell (steel) factor	KIT	Point mutation	Gastrointestinal stromal tumors, seminomas, leukemias
Proteins involved in signal transduction			
GTP-binding	KRAS HRAS NRAS	Point mutation Point mutation Point mutation	Colon, lung, and pancreatic tumors Bladder and kidney tumors Melanomas, hematologic malignancies
Nonreceptor tyrosine kinase	ABL	Translocation	Chronic myeloid leukemia Acute lymphoblastic leukemia

Contd...

Pathology

Contd...

Category	Proto-oncogene	Mode of activation	Associated human tumor
RAS signal transduction	BRAF	Point mutation	Melanomas
WNT signal transduction	β-catenin	Point mutation Overexpression	Hepatoblastomas, hepatocellular carcinoma
Nuclear-regulatory proteins			
Transcriptional activators	C-MYC N-MYC L-MYC	Translocation Amplification Amplification	Burkitt lymphoma Neuroblastoma, small-cell carcinoma of lung Small-cell carcinoma of lung
Cell cycle regulators			
Cyclins	Cyclin D Cyclin E	Translocation Amplification Overexpression	Mantle cell lymphoma Breast and esophageal cancers Breast cancer

96. RET proto-oncogene is associated with development of: *(NEET 2018)*

a. Medullary carcinoma thyroid
b. Astrocytoma
c. Paraganglioma
d. Hurthle cell tumor

Ans. is 'a' Medullary carcinoma thyroid

TUMOR MARKERS

Tumor markers	Cancer
Hormones • Human chorionic gonadotropin • Calcitonin • Gastrin	• Gestational trophoblastic disease, gonadal germ cell tumor • Medullary cancer of the thyroid • Gastrinoma (Pancreatic neurocrine tumor)
Oncofetal antigens • Alphafetoprotein • Carcinoembryonic antigen	• Hepatocellular carcinoma gonadal germ cell tumor • Adenocarcinomas of the colon, pancreas, lung, breast, ovary
Enzymes • Prostatic acid phosphatase • Neuron–specific enolase and chromogranin A • Lactate dehydrogenase	• Prostate cancer • Small cell cancer of the lung, neuroblastoma • Lymphoma, Ewing's Sarcoma
Tumor associated protein • Prostatic-specific antigen • Monoclonal immunoglobulin • CA-125 • CA19-9 • CA-15-3 • β2 -Microglobulin • S-100, HMB-45,TA-90 • NMP-22 • CD-99 • BRCA-1 and BRCA-2	• Prostate cancer • Myeloma • Ovarian cancer • Colon, pancreatic, breast cancer • Breast cancer • Multiple myeloma • Malignant melanoma • Urinary bladder Ca • Ewing's sarcoma • Carcinomas of ovary and breast

97. Following is tumor marker for lung: *(NEET 2016)*

a. S-100
b. CEA
c. CD-99
d. Beta 2 microglobulin

Ans. is 'b' CEA

98. CA-125 is: *(NEET 2016)*

a. Mucin glycoprotein
b. Carcinoma transmigration antigen
c. Mucopolysaccharide
d. Lipid

Ans. is 'a' Mucin glycoprotein

99. Both BRAC-1 and BRAC-2 is associated with: *(NEET 2016)*

a. Endometrial carcinoma
b. Colon carcinoma
c. Ovarian carcinoma
d. Testicular carcinoma

Ans. is 'c' Ovarian carcinoma

100. All of the following are associated increased CA- 125 *except*: *(NEET 2016)*

a. Fibroid
b. PID
c. Prostate enlargement
d. Endomteriosis

Ans. is 'c' Prostate enlargement

GENETIC ABNORMALITIES IN SOFT-TISSUE SARCOMAS

Tumor	Cytogenetic abnormality	Genetic abnormality
Ewing sarcoma/primitive neuroectodermal tumor	t (11;22)(q24;q12)	FLI1-EWS fusion gene
	t(21;22) (q22;q12)	ERG-EWS fusion gene
	t(7;22)(q22;q12)	ETV1-EWS fusion gene
Liposarcoma—myxoid and round-cell type	t(12;16)(q 13;p11)	CHOP/TLS fusion gene
Synovial sarcoma	t(x;18) (p 11;q11)	SYT-SSX fusion gene
Rhabdomyosarcoma—alveolar type	t(2;13)(q35;q14)	PAX3-FKHR fusion gene
	t(1;13)((p36;q14)	PAX7-FKHR fusion gene
Extraskeletal myxoid chondrosarcoma	t(9;22)(q22;q12)	CHN-EWS fusion gene
Desmoplastic small round-cell tumor	t(11;22)(q13;q12)	EWS-WT1 fusion gene
Clear-cell sarcoma	t(12;22)(q13;q12)	EWS-ATF1 fusion gene
Dermatofibrosarcoma protuberans	t(17;22)(q22;q15)	COLA1-PDGFB fusion gene
Alveolar soft-part sarcoma	t(X;17)(p11;q25)	TFE3-ASPL fusion gene
Congenital fibrosarcoma	t(12;15)(q13;q23)	ETV6-NTRK3 fusion gene

101. Most common genetic mutation in PNET/Ewing's sarcoma is: *(NEET 2016)*

a. t[2:;3][q13;p25]
b. t[11;22][q24;q12]
c. t[11;14][q13;q32]
d. t[8;14][q24;q32]

Ans. is 'b' t[11;22][q24;q12]

TUMOR SUPPRESSOR GENES AND ASSOCIATED CANCERS

Subcellular locations	Gene	Function	Tumors associated with somatic mutations	Tumors associated with inherited mutations
Cell surface	TGF-β receptor	Growth inhibition	Carcinomas of colon	Unknown
	E-cadherin	Cell adhesion	Carcinoma of stomach	Familial gastric cancer
Inner aspect of plasma membrane	NF1	Inhibition of RAS signal transduction and of p21 cell cycle inhibitor	Neuroblastomas	Neurofibromatosis type 1 and sarcomas
Cytoskeleton	NF2	Cytoskeletal stability	Schwannomas meningiomas	Neurofibromatosis type 2, acoustic schwannomas, and meningiomas
Cytosol	APC/β-catenin	Inhibition of signal transduction	Carcinomas of stomach, colon, pancreas; melanoma	Familial adenomatous polyposis coli/colon cancer
	PTEN	P13 kinase signal transduction	Endometrial and prostate cancers	Cowden syndrome
	SMAD2 and SMAD4	TGF-β signal transduction	Colon, pancreas tumors	Unknown
Nucleus	RB1	Regulations of cell cycle	Retinoblastoma, osteosarcoma carcinomas of breast, colon, lung	Retinoblastomas, osteosarcoma
	P53	Cell cycle arrest and apoptosis in response to DNA damage	Most human cancers	Li-Fraumeni syndrome; multiple carcinomas and sarcomas
	WT1	Nuclear transcription	Wilms' tumor	Wilms' tumor
	P16/INK4a	Regulation of cell cycle by inhibition of cyclin-dependent kinases	Pancreatic, breast, and esophageal cancers	Malignant melanoma
	BRCA1 and BRCA2	DNA repair	Unknown	Carcinomas of female breast of ovary; carcinomas of male breast

102. APC gene is involved in: *(NEET 2016)*

a. Colorectal carcinoma
b. Gastric carcinoma
c. Gastric lymphoma
d. Esophageal adenocarcinoma

Ans. is 'a' Colorectal carcinoma

103. Gene affected in endometrial cancer is: *(NEET 2016)*

a. p16
b. RET
c. PTEN
d. APC

Ans. is 'c' PTEN

104. Gene affected in breast cancer: *(NEET 2016)*

a. WT1
b. p53
c. RAS
d. p83

Ans. is 'b' p53

105. Which of the following is a tumor suppressor gene? *(NEET 2016)*

a. k-RAS gene
b. Rb gene
c. FOS gene
d. MYC gene

Ans. is 'b' Rb gene

106. Most common tumor suppressor gene involved in cancer genesis is: *(NEET 2016)*

a. Rb
b. p53
c. p16
d. p73

Ans. is 'b' p53

IMMUNOHISTOCHEMISTRY FOR CANCERS

- Intermediate filaments of cytoskeleton are the major antigens used in immunohistochemistry. There are five major types of intermediate filaments.
  - Cytokeratin—Carcinoma
  - Vimentin—Sarcoma
  - Desmin—Leiomyoma/Leiomyosarcoma, Rhabdomyoma/Rhabdomyosarcoma
  - Glial fibrillary acid protein (GFAP)—Astrocytoma, Ependymoma
  - Neurofilament—Pheochromocytoma, Neuroblastoma

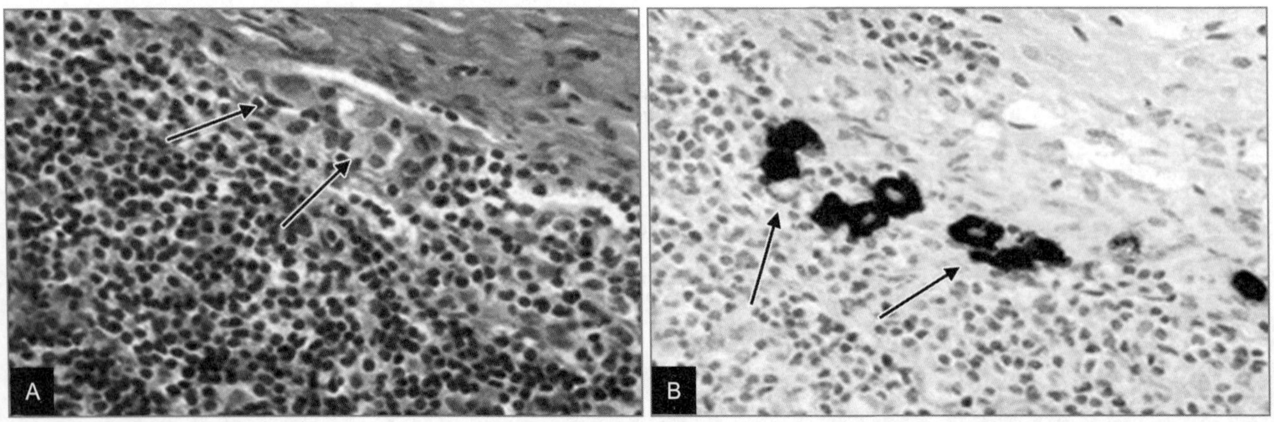

Cytokeratin staining in sentinel lymph node, individual tumor cells (ITCs). (A) Arrows show few atypical cells in subcapsular sinus of sentinel lymph node. (B) Cytokeratin AE1/AE3 stain confirms the epithelial nature of subcapsular cells.

- Neuroendocrine markers:
  - CD-56
  - Chromogranin-A
  - Synaptophysin.

107. Marker for neuroblastoma among the following is: *(NEET 2016)*

a. NMP22
b. Chromogranin A
c. LDH
d. β 2 microglobulin

Ans. is 'b' Chromogranin A

108. Immunohistochemical marker for sentinel node biopsy for breast carcinoma is: *(NEET 2016)*

a. Cytokeratin
b. Vimentin
c. Calretinin
d. CD45

Ans. is 'a' Cytokeratin

HARMFUL EFFECTS OF RADIATION

The effects of biological changes caused by radiation can be categorized into:

Stochastic Effects

A stochastic effect is one where the probability of the effect occurring is governed by the law of chance. The greater the radiation dose received, the greater the probability of the effect occurring.

There is no safe dose limit: All doses of radiation carry some risk and there is no threshold.

- Severity of the effect is unrelated to the radiation dose received, since the probability of the effect occurring is chance related.
- Stochastic effects cannot be definitely associated with radiation exposure and occur in both general population as well as in irradiated people.
- Two important stochastic effects due to exposure to ionizing radiation are : Radiation induced cancers and Genetic effects.
- Susceptibility of various phases of cell cycle to effects of radiation is as given below:

G2M > G2 ≥ M >G1 >early S >Late S

Deterministic Effects

- A deterministic effect of radiation is one : Whose severity increases with radiation dose
- For which there is usually a threshold below which the effect will not occur.
- These effects are definitely associated with radiation exposure and occur only in irradiated people.
- Examples of deterministic effects include erythema, cataract, hair loss, impairment of fertility, Myelosuppression.

109. Radiation most commonly affects which phase of cell cycle? *(NEET 2016)*

a. G1
b. G2
c. S
d. M

Ans. is 'b' G2

110. Mechanism of radiation induced carcinogenesis: *(NEET 2016)*

a. Direct effect
b. Indirect effect
c. Stochastic effect
d. Deterministic effect

Ans. is 'c' Stochastic effect

CELL-CYCLE CHECKPOINTS

G1/S Checkpoint

- It is the most important checkpoint during cell division, in which the cell checks for DNA damage before replication in 'S' phase.
- In case of DNA damage, the cell cycle is arrested and DNA repair mechanisms are activated.
- If repair fails, the cell undergoes apoptosis.
- Defects at G1/S checkpoint results in carcinogenesis.

G2/M Checkpoint

- DNA damage occurring during replication, is repaired at this checkpoint.
- DNA replication is monitored.
- Checks whether cell can safely initiate mitosis and separate sister chromatids.
- Defects in this checkpoint give rise to chromosomal abnormalities.

111. At which cell cycle checkpoint is the cell cycle halted if the cell's DNA is damaged? *(NEET 2016)*

a. G1-S
b. S-G2
c. G2-M
d. G0-G1

Ans. is 'a' G1-S

FAMILIAL CANCER SYNDROMES

Syndrome	Gene	Chromosome
Familial adenomatous polyposis	APC	5q21
Familial Wilm's tumor	SWT 1	11p13
Hereditary breast/ovarian cancer	BRCA 1	17q21
Hereditary retinoblastoma	mCa 2	13q12.3
Multiple endocrine neoplasia type 1	MEN1	13q142
Multiple endocrine neoplasia type 2a	KET	11q13
Neurofibromatosis type 1	NF	17qIL2
Neurofibromatosis type 2	NP	22q122
Li-Fraumenl syndrome	p53	17
Melanoma	p16 INK4a	

112. Gene involved in Cowden syndrome is: *(NEET 2018)*

a. PTEN b. Rb
c. P 53 d. Ras

Ans. is 'a' PTEN

113. Gene associated with familial adenomatous polyposis is: *(NEET 2018)*

a. p 53 b. Rb
c. APC d. RET

Ans. is 'c' APC

114. Familial polyposis coli is associated with following genetic defect: *(NEET 2018)*

a. MLH1 b. MSH2
c. APC d. RET

Ans. is 'c' APC

115. Li-Fraumeni syndrome occurs due to mutation in gene: *(NEET 2018)*

a. p53 b. p16
c. p14 d. p12

Ans. is 'a' p53

PARANEOPLASTIC SYNDROMES

Clinical syndromes	Major forms of underlying cancer	Causal mechanism
Endocrinopathies		
Cushing syndrome	Small-cell carcinoma of lung Pancreatic carcinoma Neural tumors	ACTH or ACTH-like substance
Syndrome of inappropriate antidiuretic hormone secretion	Small-cell carcinoma of lung; intracranial neoplasms	Antidiuretic hormone or atrial natriuretic hormones
Hypercalcemia	Squamous cell carcinoma of lung Breast carcinoma Renal carcinoma Adult t-cell leukemia/lymphoma	Parathyroid hormone–related protein (PTHRP), TGF-A, TNF, IL-1
Hypoglycemia	Ovarian carcinoma Fibrosarcoma Other mesenchymal sarcomas	Insulin or insulin-like substance
Carcinoid syndrome	Hepatocellular carcinoma Bronchial adenoma (carcinoid) Pancreatic carcinoma	Serotonin, bradykinin
Polycythemia	Gastric carcinoma Renal carcinoma Cerebellar hemangioma Hepatocellular carcinoma	Erythropoietin

Contd...

Pathology

Contd...

Clinical syndromes	Major forms of underlying cancer	Causal mechanism
Nerve and muscle syndromes		
Myasthenia	Bronchogenic carcinoma	Immunological
Disorders of the central and peripheral nervous system	Breast carcinoma	
Dermatologic disorders		
Acanthosis nigricans	Gastric carcinoma Lung carcinoma Uterine carcinoma	Immunological; secretion of epidermal growth factor
Dermatomyositis	Bronchogenic, breast carcinoma	Immunological
Osseous, articular, and soft-tissue changes		
Hypertrophic osteoarthropathy and clubbing of the fingers	Bronchogenic carcinoma	Unknown
Vascular and hematologic changes		
Venous thrombosis (Trousseau phenomenon)	Pancreatic carcinoma Bronchogenic carcinoma Other cancers	Tumor products (mucins that activate clotting)
Nonbacterial thrombotic endocarditis	Advanced cancers	Hypercoagulability
Red cell aplasia	Thymic neoplasms	Unknown
Others		
Nephrotic syndrome	Various cancers	Tumor antigens, immune complexes

116. Which type of paraneoplastic syndrome is most commonly associated with lung carcinoma? *(NEET 2016)*

a. SIADH
b. Gynecomastia
c. Acanthosis nigricans
d. Hypocalcemia

Ans. is 'a' SIADH

117. Malignancy associated hypercalcemia is due to: *(NEET 2016)*

a. Tumor lysis syndrome
b. Parathyroid related peptide
c. IL-7
d. IGF-β

Ans. is 'b' Parathyroid related peptide

TYPES OF STEM CELLS

Potency refers to ability of stem cells to differentiate into specialized (mature) cell type:

- *Totipotent stem cells*: These cells are produced from fertilization of sperm and ovum and cells that are produced by first few division after fertilization are also totipotent. These cells can differentiate into all the tissues of embryonic or extraembryonic cell types.
- *Pluripotent stem cells*: These are descendants of totipotent stem cells and can differentiate into cells derived from any of the three germ layers.
- *Multipotent stem cells*: These cells can differentiate only into cells of a closely related family, e.g. hematopoietic stem cells differentiate into RBC, WBC, platelets but not into other types.
- *Unipotent stem cells*: Can differentiate only into one cell type (e.g. muscle stem cell), but have property of self-renewal which distinguishes them from non-stem cells.

118. Totipotency of embryonic stem cell is due to that they: *(NEET 2016)*

a. Can differentiate into all the tissues of embryonic or extraembryonic cell types
b. Can differentiate into cells derived from any of the three germ layers
c. Can differentiate only into cells of a closely related family
d. Can differentiate only into one cell type

Ans. is 'a' Can differentiate into all the tissues of embryonic or extraembryonic cell types

BARR BODY (SEX-CHROMATIN)

- It is a densely staining inactivated condensed 'X' chromosome that is present in each somatic cells of female. It is found in the nucleus. It is used as a test of genetic femaleness → it is possible to determine the genetic sex of an individual according as to whether there is a chromatin mass present on the inner surface of the nuclear membrane of cells with resting or intermittent nuclei.
- Chroma Ud body (Barr body or sex chromatin) is derived from one of the two X-chromosomes which becomes inactivated. The number of Barr bodies is thus one less than the number of X-chromosomes.
- It is particularly visible when the cell is in interphase, meaning it is not currently undergoing cell division.

119. Barr body is found in following phase of cell cycle: *(NEET 2016)*

a. Interphase
b. Metaphase
c. G1phase
d. Telophase

Ans. is 'a' Interphase

Miscellaneous

120. Most common site for carcinoid tumor is: *(NEET 2016)*

a. Pituitary
b. Pancreas
c. Small intestine
d. Lungs

Ans. is 'c' Small intestine

Carcinoid tumors arise from the neuroendocrine cells (Argentaffin cells of Kulchitsky cells). The majority are found in GI tract, and more than 40% in small intestine (jejunum and ileum). The tracheobronchial tree and lungs are the next common sites involved.

IMMUNITY AND IMMUNE DISORDERS

TYPES OF GRAFT REJECTION

Hyperacute rejection: Graft rejection occurring within minutes to hours, usually due to ABO incompatibility or pre-formed anti-HLA antibodies.

- Antibodies activate complement pathway, resulting in their deposition in the vessel wall, inducing thrombosis.
- Hyperacute rejection of kidneys result in kidney becoming cyanotic, mottled and flaccid.

Acute rejection: It occurs within 6 months of the transplant and is further divided into 2 types:

- Acute cellular (T cell-mediated) rejection
    - It is characterized by mononuclear cell infiltration and is usually reversible
    - It may present as tubulitis associated with presence of both CD4+ and CD8+ T lymphocytes or endotheliitis.
- Acute antibody-mediated rejection
    - Lesions consist of inflammation of glomeruli and peritubular capillaries, with deposition of complement breakdown product C4d
- *Chronic Rejection*: It is most type of graft rejection and it occurs 6 months after the transplant.
    - It is characterized by myointimal proliferation in graft arteries leading to ischemia and fibrosis.
    - In kidneys, it presents with glomerulopathy with duplication of basement membrane and peritubular capillaritis with multilayering of peritubular capillary basement membranes.
    - Interstitial fibrosis and tubular atrophy with loss of renal parenchyma also occurs.

121. Hyperacute graft rejection is seen within: *(NEET 2018)*

a. 24 hours
b. 2 weeks
c. 1 year
d. In minutes

Ans. is 'd' In minutes

122. Nude mice can accept xenograft because it lacks which immunal cells? *(NEET 2018)*

a. T-cells
b. B-cells
c. Dendritic cells
d. Memory cells

Ans. is 'a' T-cells

OPSONIZATION

Opsonization involves the binding of an opsonin, e.g. antibody, to an epitope on an antigen. After opsonin binds to the membrane, phagocytes are attracted to the pathogen.

The Fab portion of the antibody binds to the antigen, whereas the Fc portion of the antibody binds to an Fc receptor on the phagocyte, facilitating phagocytosis.

The core receptor + opsonin complex also creates byproducts like C3b and C4b which are important components for the efficient function of the complement system. These components are deposited on the cell surface of the pathogen and aid in its destruction.

The cell can also be destroyed by a process called antiphagocytic cell-mediated cytotoxicity in which the pathogen does not need to be phagocytosed to be destroyed. During this process, the pathogen is opsonized and bound with the antibody IgG via its Fab domain. This allows the antibody binding of an immune effector cell via its Fc domain.

Antibody-dependent cell-mediated inherent mediation then triggers a release of lysis products from the bound immune effect or cell (monocytes, neutrophils, eosinophils and NK cells). Lack of mediation can cause inflammation of surrounding tissues and damage to healthy cells.

123. Opsonization is done by: *(NEET 2018)*

a. C_{3a}
b. C_{3b}
c. C_{5a}
d. C_{5d}

Ans. is 'b' C_{3b}

HYPERSENSITIVITY REACTIONS

Type	Mechanism	Clinical manifestation or Disease
I (Immediate, anaphylactic)	Antigen (allergen) induces IgE antibody whose Fc region binds to mast cells and basophils. When exposed to the allergen again, the allergen cross-links the bound IgE on those cells. This causes degranulation and release of mediators (e.g., histamine).	Systemic anaphylaxis, urticaria (hives), asthma, hay fever, allergic rhinitis, allergic conjunctivitis, food allergies (e.g., nuts, shellfish, eggs), drug allergies especially penicillin, eczema (atopic dermatitis), bee venom, latex gloves, angioedema
II (Cytotoxic)	Antigens on a cell surface combine with IgG antibody. This leads to complement-mediated lysis of the cells.	Hemolytic anemia, neutropenia, thrombocytopenia, ABO transfusion reactions, Rh incompatibility (erythroblastosis fetalis, hemolytic disease of the newborn), rheumatic fever, Goodpasture's syndrome
III (Immune complex)	Antigen–antibody immune complexes are deposited in tissues, complement is activated, and polymorphonuclear cells are attracted to the site. They release lysosomal enzymes, causing tissue damage.	Systemic lupus erythematosus, rheumatoid arthritis, poststreptococcal glomerulonephritis, IgA nephropathy, serum sickness, hypersensitivity pneumonitis (e.g., farmer's lung), Arthus reaction
IV (Delayed)	T lymphocytes activated/sensitized by an antigen release lymphokines upon second contact with the same antigen. The lymphokines induce inflammation and activate macrophages, which, in turn, release various inflammatory mediators.	Contact dermatitis, poison oak/ivy, tuberculin skin test reaction, drug rash, Stevens-Johnson syndrome, toxic epidermal necrolysis, erythema multiforme, Takayasu arteritis

124. Type 1 hypersensitivity reaction differs from type 2 hypersensitivity reaction being: *(NEET 2016)*

a. Type 1 reaction is IgE mediated
b. Type 1 reaction is compliment mediated
c. Type 1 reaction is involves opsonization
d. All of the above

Ans. is 'a' Type 1 reaction is IgE mediated

125. Which part of the IgE antibody is responsible for binding to mast cells and basophils? *(NEET 2016)*

a. Light chain
b. Immunoglobulin fold
c. Fc region
d. Complement binding site

Ans. is 'c' Fc region

126. Cell most important in causation of asthma are: *(NEET 2016)*

a. Macrophages
b. Mast cells
c. Neutrophils
d. Lymphocytes

Ans. is 'b' Mast cells

127. Non IgE mediated anaphylactic reaction includes: *(NEET 2016)*

a. IgG
b. IgM
c. Complement factors
d. All of the above

Ans. is 'd' All of the above

128. Complement mediated hypersensitivity reaction is: *(NEET 2016)*

a. Type -1 hypersensitivity
b. Type -2 hypersensitivity
c. Type -4 hypersensitivity
d. None

Ans. is 'b' Type -2 hypersensitivity

129. T-cell mediated disease is: *(NEET 2016)*

a. Asthma
b. Myasthenia gravis
c. SLE
d. Sarcoidosis

Ans. is 'd' Sarcoidosis

130. Type 4 hypersensitivity reaction to TB antigen is similar to which of the following? *(NEET 2016)*

a. Serum sickness
b. Asthma
c. Myasthenia gravis
d. Temporal arteritis

Ans. is 'd' Temporal arteritis

HEAVY CHAIN DISEASE

- Heavy chain diseases are plasma cell disorders that are typically malignant. They are a form of paraproteinemias in which incomplete monoclonal immunoglobulins (true paraproteins) are produced. They consist of only heavy chain components (either alpha [a], gamma [y], mu [t], or delta [s]) without light chains.
- The clinical picture is more like lymphoma than multiple myeloma
- There are four forms:
  - Alpha chain disease (Seligmann's disease)—most common type
  - Gamma chain disease (Franklin's disease)
  - Mu chain disease
  - Delta chain disease

131. Most common type of heavy chain disease is: *(NEET 2016)*

a. Alpha chain disease
b. Gama chain disease
c. Mu chain disease
d. Delta chain disease

Ans. is 'a' Alpha chain disease

ANTIGEN PRESENTING CELLS

Professional APCs: Express MHC class II molecules

- *Dendritic cells*: most efficient
- Langerhans cells
- Macrophages
- B-cells

Nonprofessional APCs: Do not express MHC class II for interaction with naïve T cells.

- Fibroblasts
- Thymic epithelial cells
- Thyroid epithelial cells
- Glial cells
- Pancreatic beta cells
- Endothelial cells

132. Most potent antigen presenting cell is: *(NEET 2016)*

a. B-cells
b. Dendritic cells
c. T-cells
d. NK cells

Ans. is 'b' Dendritic cells

133. Cell which do not participate in cell mediated immunity are: *(NEET 2016)*

a. T- cells
b. B-cells
c. Macrophages
d. Plasma cells

Ans. is 'd' Plasma cells

T-LYMPHOCYTES

T-cells constitutes 60–70% of the circulating peripheral lymphocytes. Based on their surface markers, target cells and functions the following T-cell category have been identified.

A. Helper T-cells (Inducer T-cells)

- These cells constitute 60% of total T-cells. These have CD4 surface marker and bind to MHC class II (MHC class II restricted). There are following types of CD4 cells (Helper T-cells): Effector cells (Effector CD4 helper T-cells)
- There are divided into: TH-1 cells: These are activated by IFN-y and themselves produce IL-2, IFN-y and IL-12. These are the primary cells involved in delayed hypersensitivity, cell mediated immunity, macrophage activation and killing of intracellular microbes (*M. tuberculosis, M. leprae*).
- These cells also induce destruction of target cells by activating T-cells to become cytotoxic T-cells and by activating NK cells: Tif-2 cells

- These are activated by IL-4 and themselves produce IL-4, IL-5, IL-6 and IL-13. These cells induce synthesis of IgE more efficiently and cause activation of mast cells and eosinophils. Therefore these cells provide defence against Helminthic parasites: TH-17 cells
- These cells are powerful recruiters of neutrophils and monocytes to play a role in severe inflammatory diseases. These cells produce IL-17, IL-22 and chemokines which recruit neutrophils and monocytes. TH-17 cells produce IL-21, which amplifies the TH-17 (self) response. Memory cells (Memory CD4 helper T-cells). Provide memory, i.e. retain the antigenic affinity of the originally activated T-cells and are used to act as later effector cells during a second immune response.

b. Cytotoxic T-cells (Cytolytic T-cells)

- These cells constitute 30% of total T-cells. These cells have CDS surface marker and are MHC class I restricted
- They kill and lyse target cells including tumor cells, virus infected cells and allograft; and participate in type II Hypersensitivity.

c. Suppressor T-cells

- These cells have CD8 surface marker and are MHC class I restricted. These cells down regulate immune response.

CD4:CD8 Ratio

The CD4+/CD8+ ratio in the peripheral blood of healthy adults is about 2:1, and an altered ratio can indicate diseases relating to immunodeficiency or autoimmunity. An inverted CD4+/CD8+ ratio (less than 1) indicates an impaired immune system.

A declining CD4+/CD8+ ratio is associated with ageing, and is an indicator of immunosenescence. HIV infection leads to low levels of CD4+ T cells (lowering the CD4+/CD8+ ratio) through a number of mechanisms, including killing of infected CD4+ T cells by CD8 cytotoxic lymphocytes that productively infected cells. When CD4+ T cell numbers decline below a critical level, cell-mediated immunity is lost, and the body becomes progressively more susceptible to opportunistic infections.

T-cell growth factors: (TCGF(s)) are signaling molecules collectively called growth factors which stimulate the production and development of T-cells. A number of them have been discovered, among them many members of the interleukin family (IL-2, IL-4, IL-7, IL-9, IL-15 and IL-21). The thymus is one organ which releases TCGFs

134. Which interleukin is T-cell growth factor? *(NEET 2016)*

a. IL-3
b. IL-7
c. IL-11
d. IL-5

Ans. is 'b' IL-7

135. IL-2 is a growth factor for: *(NEET 2016)*

a. RBCs
b. T-cells
c. Fibroblasts
d. All of the above

Ans. is 'b' T-cells

136. CD8 is a marker for which of the following cell? *(NEET 2016)*

a. T- cell
b. B-cell
c. NK-cells
d. Macrophages

Ans. is 'a' T-cell

137. Memory cells are best provided by: *(NEET 2016)*

a. Helper cells
b. Cytotoxic cells
c. Macrophages
d. NK cells

Ans. is 'a' Helper cells

138. What is the function of Helper T-cell? *(NEET 2016)*

a. Immunogenic memory
b. Produce immunoglobulins
c. Killing tumor cells
d. All of the above

Ans. is 'a' Immunogenic memory

139. TH1 helper cells act via: *(NEET 2016)*

a. Cell mediated immunity
b. Activating macrophages
c. Activating cytotoxic T-cells
d. All of the above

Ans. is 'd' All of the above

140. CD4 is associated with HLA: *(NEET 2016)*

a. HLA1
b. HLA2
c. HLA3
d. All of them

Ans. is 'b' HLA2

141. Most important factor associated with progression of HIV positive to AIDS is: *(NEET 2016)*

a. Nutrition
b. Viral load
c. Age
d. CD4 count

Ans. is 'd' CD4 count

142. Normal value of CD4:CD8 ratio is: *(NEET 2016)*

a. 0.5
b. 1
c 1.5
d. 2

Ans. is 'd' 2

T-cell subsets			
	Th1 cell	*Th2 cell*	*Th17 cell*
Secretes	IFN-γ, IL-2	IL-4, IL-5, IL-6, IL-10, IL-13	IL-17, IL-21, IL-22
Function	Activates macrophages and cytotoxic T cells to kill phagocytosed microbes	Activates eosinophils and promotes production of IgE for parasite defense	Immunity against extracellular microbes, through induction of neutrophilic inflammation
Induced by	IFN-γ, IL-12	IL-2, IL-4	TGF-β, IL-1, IL-6
Inhibited by	IL-4, IL-10 (from Th2 cell)	IFN-γ (from Th1 cell)	IFN-γ, IL-4
Immunodeficiency	Mendelian susceptibility to mycobacterial disease		Hyper-IgE syndrome

143. A 33-year-old man presents with a 5-week history of calf pain and swelling and low-grade fever. Serum levels of creatine kinase are elevated. A muscle biopsy reveals numerous eosinophils. Also he had peripheral blood eosinophilia. Which of the following interleukins is primarily responsible for the increase in eosinophils in this patient? *(NEET 2020)*

a. IL-2
b. IL-4
c. IL-1
d. IL-17

Ans. is 'b' IL-4

ANTI NUCLEAR ANTIBODIES

Pattern	Disease	Remarks
Homogenous (diffuse)	SLE, mixed connective tissue disease, and drug-induced lupus	Antibodies to chromatin, histones and, occasionally, double-stranded DNA
Rim/Peripheral	SLE	Antibodies to double-stranded DNA
Speckled	SLE, Sjogren syndrome, scleroderma, polymyositis, rheumatoid arthritis, and mixed connective tissue disease	Antibodies to non-DNA nuclear constituents: Sm antigen, ribonucleoprotein, and SS-A and SS-B reactive antigens
Nucleolar	Scleroderma and polymoysitis	Antibodies to nucleolar RNA
Centromere Pattern (peripheral)	Limited scleroderma and CREST	

For SLE, anti ds DNA antibody is the most specific antibody.
Anti-Ro and anti-La antibodies are associated with congenital heart block in babies born to patients with SLE.

Peripheral (rim)	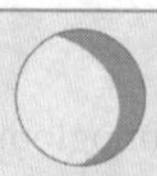	Anti-DNA (not seen on HEp-2)	SLE
Homogeneous (diffuse)	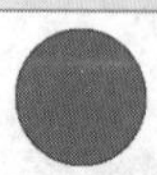	Anti-DNA Anti-histone Anti-DNA	RA and SLE Misc. disorders (anti-ssDNA)
Speckled	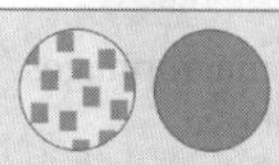	Anti-5 m and RNP Anti-Ro and La Anti-Ja-1 and MI-2	SLE and SS PM/DM PSS (Systemic)
Centromere	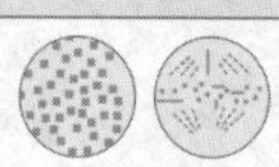	Anti-centromere	PSS (CRESS)
Nucleolar	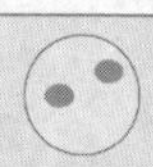	Anti-nucleolar	SLE and PSS

144. Best marker for SLE is: *(NEET 2016)*

a. Anti Sm antibodies
b. Anti-ds DNA antibodies
c. Anti-Histone antibodies
d. Anti Ro (ss-A) antibodies

Ans. is 'b' Anti-ds DNA antibodies

145. Anti- Jo-1 antibodies are a features associated with: *(NEET 2016)*

a. SLE
b. Systemic sclerosis
c. Polymyositis
d. Rheumatoid arthritis

Ans. is 'c' Polymyositis

146. CREST syndrome is associated with: *(NEET 2016)*

a. Anti-Scl-70 antibodies
b. Anti-dsDNA antibodies
c. Anti-centromere antibodies
d. Anti-histone antibodies

Ans. is 'c' Anti-centromere antibodies

147. Anti-Ro antibody is found in: *(NEET 2016)*

a. SLE
b. Scleroderma
c. MCTD
d. Neonatal lupus

Ans. is 'd' Neonatal lupus

148. Anti-histone antibodies are diagnostic of: *(NEET 2016)*

a. Drug induced LE
b. Systemic sclerosis
c. Mixed connective tissue disorder
d. Sicca syndrome

Ans. is 'a' Drug induced LE

MAJOR HISTOCOMPATIBILITY COMPLEX

Class I MHC molecules are expressed on all nucleated cells and platelets. They are encoded by three closely linked loci, designated HLA-A, HLA-B, and HLA-C. Each class I MHC molecule is a heterodimer consisting of a polymorphic α, or heavy, chain (44-kD) linked noncovalently to a smaller (12-kD) nonpolymorphic peptide called β2-microglobulin, which is not encoded within the MHC. The extracellular region of the α chain is divided into three domains: α1, α2, and α3. Crystal structure of class I molecules has revealed that the α1 and α2 domains form a cleft, or groove, where peptides bind. The polymorphic residues line the sides and the base of the peptide-binding groove; the variation in this region explains why different class I alleles bind different peptides. MHC class I is responsible for graft rejection and cell mediated cytolysis of viral infected or tumor cells.

Class II MHC molecules are encoded in a region called HLA-D, which has three subregions: HLA-DP, HLA-DQ, and HLA-DR. Each class II molecule is a heterodimer consisting of a noncovalently associated α chain and β chain, both of which are polymorphic. The extracellular portions of the α and β chains have two domains each: α1, α2 and β1, β2. Crystal structure of class II molecules has revealed that, similar to class I molecules, they have peptide-binding clefts facing outward. This cleft is formed by an interaction of the α1 and β1 domains, and it is in this portion that most class II alleles differ. Thus, as with class I molecules, polymorphism of class II molecules is associated with differential binding of antigenic peptides.

149. MHC-I is involved in: *(NEET 2016)*

a. Tumor lysis
b. Mixed leukocyte reaction
c. Autoimmune disease susceptibility
d. All of the above

Ans. is 'a' Tumor lysis

150. The following is true about MHC 2 molecules: *(NEET 2016)*

a. Not involved in innate immunity
b. Cytotoxic T- cell involved
c. Present in all nucleated cells
d. Contains 'D' loci

Ans. is 'd' Contains 'D' loci

151. Cell type which lacks HLA {MHC} antigen is: *(NEET 2016)*

a. Monocyte
b. Thrombocytes
c. Neutrophil
d. Red blood cell

Ans. is 'd' Red blood cell

152. Cell mediated lysis of tumor cells is mediated by: *(NEET 2016)*

a. HLA1
b. HLA2
c. HLA3
d. All of the above

Ans. is 'a' HLA1

ACUTE GVHD

Acute GVHD occurs within 100 days (usually 10–50 days) of bone marrow transplantation. The manifestations of acute GVHI are:

1. **Skin**
   - It is the most commonly affected tissue in acute GVHD. There is generalized rash (maculopapular). Histological findings are—Perivascular mononuclear infiltrates.
   - Vacuolar degradation of dermo-epidermal junction
   - Dyskeratotic cells or eosinophilic bodies in the epidermis.
   - Epidermolysis and bullae.
   - Denudation of epidermis (separation of epidermis from dermis).
2. **Gut**
   - The primary clinical manifestation of gut GVHD is diarrhea and abdominal pain. There is lymphocytic infiltrates at the crypts with accompanied necrosis and dropout of crypt cells.
3. **Liver**
   - Lymphocytic infiltrates in the interlobular and marginal bile ducts are characteristic histopathologic findings. This results in hepatitis with necrosis of hepatocytes and bile duct epithelial cells. There is inflammation of the parenchyma and portal tracts. These findings lead to clinically identifiable cholestatic picture.

153. Most common organ to be involved in acute phase of GVHD is: *(NEET 2016)*

a. Bone marrow b. Skin
c. Liver d. Gut

Ans. is 'b' Skin

TYPES OF GRAFTS

- *Autograft (autogenic graft)*: Graft from self.
- *Isograft (syngraft)*: Graft from genetically identical person, e.g. identical twin.
- *Allograft (homograft or allogeneic graft)*: Graft from genetically unrelated member of same species.
- *Xenograft (heterograft)*: Graft from different species.

154. Autologous transplant means: *(NEET 2016)*

a. Graft from individuals of same genetic constitution b. Graft from self
c. Graft from twins d. Graft from members of different species

Ans. is 'b' Graft from self

155. Graft obtained from identical twin is known as: *(NEET 2020)*

a. Allograft b. Isograft
c. Xenograft d. Autograft

Ans. is 'b' Isograft

ANTI-LKM ANTIBODIES

Type	Antigen	Disease
Anti LKM 1	Cytochrome P450 2D6	Autoimmune hepatitis type II and chronic hepatitis C
Anti LKM 2	Cytochrome P450 2C9	Drug induced hepatitis
Anti LKM 3	Cytochrome P450 1A2	Chronic hepatitis D, chronic active hepatitis in associated with autoimmune polyendocrine syndrome type 1

156. Anti LKM antibodies are found in: *(NEET 2016)*

a. Inflammatory myopathies b. SLE
c. Autoimmune hepatitis d. CREST syndrome

Ans. is 'c' Autoimmune hepatitis

Miscellaneous

157. RA factor is: *(NEET 2016)*

a. IgG b. IgM
c. IgD d. IgA

Ans. is 'b' IgM

Rheumatoid factor is an autoantibody, usually IgM, directed against the Fc region of IgG.

158. HLA marker associated with diabetes mellitus type 1 is: *(NEET 2016)*

a. B7
b. DR4
c. DQ 3
d. DQ4

Ans. is 'b' DR4

HLA associated with DM-1 are DR3, DR4, DR8, DQ8.

RED BLOOD CELL DISORDERS

PAROXYSMAL NOCTURNAL HEMOGLOBINURIA

Paroxysmal nocturnal hemoglobinuria (PNH) is a rare acquired clonal hematopoietic stem cell disorder that results in abnormal sensitivity of the red blood cell membrane to lysis by complement and therefore hemolysis. The underlying cause is an acquired defect in the gene for phosphatidyl inositol class A (PIG-A), which results in a deficiency of the glycosyl phosphatidyl inositol (GPI) anchor for cellular membrane proteins. In particular, the complement-regulating proteins CD55 and CD59 are deficient, which permits unregulated formation of the complement membrane attack complex on red cell membranes and intravascular hemolysis. Free hemoglobin is released into the blood that scavenges nitric oxide and promotes esophageal spasms, male erectile dysfunction, kidney damage, and thrombosis. Patients with significant PNH live about 10–15 years following diagnosis; thrombosis is the primary cause of death.

Clinical Findings

Symptoms and Signs

Classically, patients report episodic hemoglobinuria resulting in reddish-brown urine. Hemoglobinuria is most often noticed in the first morning urine due to the drop in blood pH while sleeping (hypoventilation) that facilitates this hemolysis. Besides anemia, these patients are prone to thrombosis, especially within mesenteric and hepatic veins, central nervous system veins (sagittal vein), and skin vessels (with formation of painful nodules). As this is a hematopoietic stem cell disorder, PNH may appear de novo or arise in the setting of aplastic anemia or myelodysplasia with possible progression to acute myeloid leukemia (AML). It is common that patients with idiopathic aplastic anemia have a small PNH clone (less than 2%) on blood or bone marrow analysis; this should not be considered PNH per se, especially in the absence of a reticulocytosis or thrombosis.

Laboratory Findings

Anemia is of variable severity and frequency, so reticulocytosis may or may not be present at any given time. Abnormalities on the blood smear are nondiagnostic but may include macro-ovalocytes and polychromasia. Since the episodic hemolysis is mainly intravascular, urine hemosiderin is a useful test. Serum LD is characteristically elevated. Iron deficiency is commonly present, related to chronic iron loss from hemoglobinuria.

The white blood cell count and platelet count may be decreased and are always decreased in the setting of aplastic anemia. The best screening test is flow cytometry of blood erythrocytes, granulocytes, or monocytes to demonstrate deficiency of CD55 and CD59. The proportion of erythrocytes deficient in these proteins might be low due to the ongoing destruction of affected erythrocytes. The FLAER assay (fluorescein-labeled proaerolysin) by flow cytometry is more sensitive. Bone marrow morphology is variable and may show either generalized hypoplasia or erythroid hyperplasia or both. The bone marrow karyotype may be either normal or demonstrate a clonal abnormality.

159. What is the cause of intracorpuscular defects in hemolysis? *(NEET 2018)*

a. Uremic syndrome
b. PCH
c. PNH
d. Portal hypertension

Ans. is 'c' PNH

160. CD59 deficiency leads to: *(NEET 2018)*

a. Chediak-Higashi syndrome
b. Lysosomal disorders
c. Chronic granulomatous disease
d. Paroxysmal nocturnal hemoglobinuria

Ans. is 'd' Paroxysmal nocturnal hemoglobinuria

Sickle Cell Anemia Symptoms

- Vaso-occlusion symptoms—Strokes, acute chest syndrome (associated with fever, hypoxia and pulmonary infarcts, most common cause of death in adults with sickle cell anemia), hand and feet swelling (ischemic dactylitis), aseptic necrosis of femoral or humeral head, splenic infarcts as well as autosplenectomy leads to increased susceptibility to encapsulated bacteria (most common cause of death from bacterial infections in children with sickle cell).
- Sequestration symptoms—Acute pooling of RBCs in spleen, usually post-infection; presents with acute spenomegaly and septic shock-like state
- Hemolytic symptoms—Pallor from chronic hemolytic anemia, mostly intravascular hemolysis. Massive erythroid hyperplasia due to expansion of hematopoiesis into skull (crewcut), facial bone (chipmunk face) and extramedullary hematopoiesis.
- Aplastic symptoms— ↑ risk of Parvovirus B19 infection

161. A 10-year-old boy develops sudden onset of abdominal pain. He complains of chronic fatigue and painful swelling of digits in past. USG reveals a shrunken spleen. What is the likely diagnosis? *(NEET 2020)*

a. Acute pancreatitis
b. Sickle cell anemia
c. Thalassemia
d. Iron deficiency anemia

Ans. is 'b' Sickle cell anemia

Important causes of megaloblastic anemia

Vitamin B12 deficiency

- Decrease intake in adequate diet, vegetarianism.
- *Impaired absorption*: Intrinsic factor deficiency (pernicious anemia, gastrectomy), intestinal diseases (Crohn' disease, ileitis, ileal resection, lymphoma, systemic sclerosis), Fish tapeworm infestation (D latum), blind loop syndrome (bacterial overgrowth), diverticuli of bowel, chronic pancreatitis.
- *Increased requirement*: Pregnancy, hyperthyroidism, disseminated cancer.

Folate deficiency

- *Decrease intake*: Inadequate diet, alcoholism, infancy
- *Impaired absorption*: Malabsorption state, intestinal diseases
- *Increased requirement*: Pregnancy infancy disseminated cancer
- *Others*: Hemodialysis antifolate drugs (methotrexate, phenobarbitone, phenytoin, trimethoprim primidone triametrene, azathioprine

162. Megaloblastic anemia is due to: *(NEET 2016)*

a. Folic acid deficiency
b. Vitamin B6 deficiency
c. Defect in RNA synthesis
d. Defect in protein synthesis

Ans. is 'a' Folic acid deficiency

PLUMMER-VINSON SYNDROME

- Plummer-Vinson syndrome (PVS), also called Paterson-Brown-Kelly syndrome or sideropenic dysphagia, is a rare disease characterized by: Dysphagia (difficulty in swallowing)
- Odynophagia (painful swallowing)
- Pain, Weakness
- Atrophic glossitis
- Angular stomatitis
- Cheilosis
- Esophageal webs (on serial contrasted gastrointestinal radiography)
- Blood tests show a hypochromic microcytic anemia that is consistent with an iron-deficiency anemia

163. All are true about Patterson Kelly syndrome *except*: *(NEET 2016)*

a. Iron deficiency anemia
b. Cheilosis
c. Esophageal webs
d. Gastric polyps

Ans. is 'd' Gastric polyps

164. False about Patterson-Kelly-Brown syndrome is: *(NEET 2016)*

a. Anemia
b. Esophageal webs
c. Glossitis
d. Risk factor for adenocarcinoma

Ans. is 'd' Risk factor for adenocarcinoma

MULTIPLE MYELOMA

The proliferation and survival of myeloma cells are dependent on several cytokines, most notably IL-6. A variety of cytokines prod by the tumor cells, particularly MIP1a and the receptor activator NF-KB ligand (RANKL), serve as osteoclast-activating factors.

- The most frequent karyotypic abnormalities are deletions of 13q translocations involving the 1g heavy chain locus on 14q32.
- Microscopic examination of the marrow reveals an increased number of plasma cells, which usually constitute more than 30% marrow cellularity. Like their benign counterparts, neoplastic plasma cells must have a perinuclear clearing (due to a prominent Golgi apparatus and an eccentrically placed nucleus).
- Other cytologic variants stem from the dysregulated synthesis and secretion of immunoglobulin, which sometimes leads intracellular accumulation of intact or partially degraded Ig.
- Such variants include flame cells, with fiery red cytoplasm, Mott cells having multiple blue grape-like cytoplasmic Russell bodies (cytoplasmic) or Dutcher bodies (nuclear).

- Commonly, the high levels of serum M proteins causes red cells smears of peripheral blood to stick to one another in linear arrays, a finding referred to as Rouleaux formation.
- Bence Jones proteins are excreted in the kidney and contribute to a form of renal disease called myeloma kidney
- Amyloidosis of the AL (amyloid light chain) type occurs in some patients owing to secretion of amyloidogenic 1g light chains

165. Dutcher bodies are seen in: *(NEET 2016)*

a. Brain b. Liver
c. Spleen d. Bone marrow

Ans. is 'd' Bone marrow

GLUCOSE-6-PHOSPHATE DEHYDROGENASE DEFICIENCY

- G6PD deficiency is an X-linked recessive disorder, characterized by hemolytic anemia on exposure to oxidative stress.
- Normally RBCs are protected from oxidant injury by reduced glutathione. Reduced glutathione is generated from oxidized glutathione and the reducing equivalent for this reaction is provided by NADPH. This NADPH is generated in HMP shunt by enzyme Glucose-6-phosphate dehydrogenase, while oxidizing glucose-6-phosphate.
- If G6PD is deficient, NADPH production will be reduced that results in increased susceptibility of RBC to oxidative damage because of unavailability of reduced glutathione. So, whenever there is oxidant stress, e.g. by drugs, infection or foods, hemolysis occurs. G6PD deficiency causes episodic intravascular and extravascular hemolysis.
- There are three types of G6PD deficiency:
  - Type-1 (mildest form)
  - Type-2 (moderately sever)
  - Type-3 (most severe form).
- Important peripheral smear findings are Heinz bodies (precipitate of denatured globin in RBC), bite cells and spherocytes.

166. Not a feature of G6PD deficiency: *(NEET 2016)*

a. Intravascular hemolysis b. Oxidative stress
c. Membrane defect d. Bite cells

Ans. is 'c' Membrane defect

167. Which is the cause of hemolysis in G6PD deficiency? *(NEET 2016)*

a. Hemoglobin defect b. Oxidative stress
c. Membrane defect d. Vitamin B12 deficiency

Ans. is 'b' Oxidative stress

THALASSEMIA

Thalassemia is an autosomal recessive disorder characterized by defective synthesis of hemoglobin chains.

Morphological features in Thalassemia: Blood smears show severe red cell abnormalities, including marked variation in size (anisocytosis) and shape (poikilocytosis), microcytosis, and hypochromia. Target cells (so called because hemoglobin collects in the center of the cell), basophilic stippling, and fragmented red cells are also common. Inclusions of aggregated α chains are efficiently removed by the spleen and not easily seen. The reticulocyte count is elevated, but it is lower than expected for the severity of anemia because of the ineffective erythropoiesis. Variable numbers of poorly hemoglobinized nucleated red cell precursors (normoblasts) are seen in the peripheral blood as a result of "stress" erythropoiesis and abnormal release from sites of extramedullary hematopoiesis.

Other major alterations involve the bone marrow and spleen. In the untransfused patient there is a striking expansion of hematopoietically active marrow. In the bones of the face and skull the burgeoning marrow erodes existing cortical bone and induces new bone formation, giving rise to a "crew-cut" appearance on X-ray. Both phagocyte hyperplasia and extramedullary hematopoiesis contribute to enlargement of the spleen, which can weigh as much as 1500 gm. The liver and the lymph nodes can also be enlarged by extramedullary hematopoiesis.

Hemosiderosis and secondary hemochromatosis, the two manifestations of iron overload, occur in almost all patients. The deposited iron often damages organs, most notably the heart, liver, and pancreas.

In thalassemia major, The major red cell hemoglobin is HbF, which is markedly elevated. HbA2 levels are sometimes high but more often are normal or low.

168. Thalassemia is inherited as an: *(NEET 2016)*

a. AR b. AD
c. XR d. XD

Ans. is 'a' AR

169. Diagnosis of beta Thalassemia is established by: *(NEET 2016)*

a. Elevated HbA2
b. Decreased HbF
c. Fragility test
d. Coomb's test

Ans. is 'a' Elevated HbA2

GAMNA-GANDY BODIES

- ❖ Gandy-Gamna bodies are foci of fibrosis containing iron and calcium salts deposits on connective tissue and elastic fibres.
- ❖ Gandy-Gamna bodies are seen in congestive splenomegaly e.g. in sickle cell anemia, CML and liver cirrhosis.

170. Gamna Gandy bodies are not seen in: *(NEET 2016)*

a. Cirrhosis with portal hypertension
b. Chronic myeloid leukemia
c. Sickle cell anemia
d. Thalassemia

Ans. is 'd' Thalassemia

Miscellaneous

171. Gallstones in sickle cell anemia are made up of: *(NEET 2016)*

a. Cholesterol
b. Calcium carbonate
c. Bilirubin
d. None

Ans. is 'c' Bilirubin

In sickle cell disease, chronic hemolysis with its accelerated bilirubin turnover leads to a high incidence of pigment gallstones. They are composed primarily of bilirubin and calcium (calcium phosphate) salts that are found in bile.

DISORDERS OF WHITE BLOOD CELLS, LYMPH NODE, SPLEEN AND THYMUS

LEUKOCYTOSIS

Neutrophilic leukocytosis	Acute bacterial infections (pyogenic)
Eosinophilic leukocytosis (eosinophilia)	Allergic disorders such as asthma, hay fever, allergic skin diseases parasitic infestations, drug reactions, certain malignancies (e.g. Hodgkin disease and some non-Hodgkin lymphomas);
Basophilic leukocytosis (Basophilia)	Rare, indicative of CML
Monocytosis	Chronic infections (TB, SLE) inflammatory bowel diseases (ulcerative colitis)
Lymphocytosis	Accompanies monocytosis in many disorders viral infections (e.g. hepatitis A, cytomegalovirus, Epstein-Barr virus); Bordetella pertussis infection

172. Basophilic leukocytosis is associated with: *(NEET 2016)*

a. Acute myeloid leukemia
b. Acute lymphoblastic leukemia
c. Chronic myelogenous leukemia
d. Burkett's lymphoma

Ans. is 'c' Chronic myelogenous leukemia

ARNETH COUNT

- ❖ The Arneth count or Arneth index describes the percentage distribution of different type of neutrophills on the basis of their nuclear lobes.
- ❖ Neutrophills typically have two or three lobes. The Arneth count determines the percentage of neutrophills with one, two, three, four, and five or more lobes and the normal count is: Nl — 2–10%
- ❖ N2 — 20–30%
- ❖ N3 — 40–50%
- ❖ N4—10–15% y
- ❖ N5—2–5%

Hyperactive bone marrow

- ❖ Individuals who have a larger percentage of neutrophills with fewer lobes (mainly Nl and N2) have a left shift which can be indicative of disease processes such as infections (pyogenic and TB), malignant tumors, hemolytic crises, myocardial infarction, acidosis, irradiation etc.

Shift to right (Inadequate hematopoiesis)

- Individuals with a larger percentage of neutrophills with more lobes have a right shift and most commonly have diseases such as vitamin B12 or folate deficiency, aplastic anemia, septicemia, chronic uremia, liver disease, etc.

173. Left side shift in Arneth's count is seen in: *(NEET 2016)*

a. Megaloblastic anemia
b. Septicemia
c. TB
d. Liver disease

Ans. is 'c' TB

MEDIASTINAL TUMOURS

- Thymoma is the most common mediastinal mass
- Neurogenic tumors are most common in the posterior mediastinum in children

Superior mediastinum	Anterior mediastinum	Posterior mediastinum	Middle mediastinum
• Lymphoma • Thymoma • Thyroid lesions • Metastatic carcinoma • Parathyroid tumors	• Thymoma (MC) • Teratoma • Lymphoma • Thyroid lesions • Parathyroid tumors	• Neurogenic tumors (MC) (schwannoma, neurofibroma) • Lymphoma • Gastroenteric hernia	• Bronchogenic cyst • Pericardial cyst • Lymphoma

174. Not commonly seen in anterior mediastinal space is: *(NEET 2018)*

a. Thymoma
b. Neural tumors
c. NHL
d. Thyroid carcinoma

Ans. is 'b' Neural tumors

HODGKIN'S LYMPHOMA

Subtype	Clinical features	Immuno-phenotype	Association with EBV	Morphology
Nodular sclerosis	Most common subtype; usually stage I or II disease; frequent mediastinal involvement Mostly seen in young females.	CD15+, CD30+	Usually EBV	Frequent lacunar cells (clear space around nucleus) and occasional diagnostic RS cells Background infiltrate composed of T lymphocytes, eosinophils, macrophages and plasma cells and fibrous bands
Mixed cellularity	Most common subtype in India; >50% present as stage III or IV disease; M > F; Biphasic incidence, peaking in young adults and again in >55 years Good prognosis	CD15+, CD30+	70% EBV+	Frequent mononuclear and diagnostic RS cells
Lymphocyte rich	Uncommon; M > F; seen in older adults Good prognosis	CD15+, CD30+	40% EBV+	Frequent mononuclear and diagnostic RS cell
Lymphocyte depletion	Uncommon; more common in older males, HIV-infected individuals and in developing countries; often presents with advanced disease Worst prognosis	CD15+, CD30+	Most EBV+	Reticular variant: Frequent diagnostic RS cells
Lymphocyte predominance	Uncommon; young males with cervical or axillary lymphadenopathy Best prognosis	CD20+, CD15–, C30–	EBV–	Lymphocytic and Histiocytic (popcorn cell)

Reed-Sternberg Cells

- Although seen in Hodgkin's lymphoma, Reed-Sternberg cells alone are not diagnostic, since they are also seen in infectious mononucleosis, immunoblastic NHL, carcinoma and sarcoma.
- Histological diagnosis is established by presence of Reed-Sternberg cells along with background of mixed inflammation consisting of neutrophils, plasma cells, eosinophils and histiocytes.
- Reed–Sternberg cells are large and are either multinucleated or have a bilobed nucleus (thus resembling an "owl's eye" appearance) with prominent eosinophilic inclusion-like nucleoli.
- Reed–Sternberg cells are CD30 and CD15 positive, usually negative for CD20 and CD45.
- The presence of these cells is necessary in the diagnosis of Hodgkin's lymphoma – the absence of Reed–Sternberg cells has very high negative predictive value.

175. H and L variety of Reed-Sternberg cells are seen in: *(NEET 2018)*

a. Lymphocytic predominance
b. Nodular sclerosis
c. Lymphocyte-depleted
d. Mixed cellularity

Ans. is 'a' Lymphocytic predominance

176. Hodgkin's lymphoma with lacunar cells is: *(NEET 2018)*

a. Mixed cellularity type
b. Nodular sclerotic type
c. Lymphocyte predominant type
d. Lymphocytic depletion type

Ans. is 'b' Nodular sclerotic type

177. RS cells are seen in: *(NEET 2018)*

a. Hodgkins disease
b. Sickle cell anaemia
c. Thalassemia
d. CML

Ans. is 'a' Hodgkins disease

Langerhans Cell Histiocytosis (Histiocytosis-X)

- Histiocytosis X is characterized by proliferation of Langerhans histiocytes (tissue macrophages). It is subdivided into three categories:
  - Letterer-Siwe syndrome
  - Hand-Schuller-Christian disease
  - Eosinophilic granuloma

Tumor cells in each are derived from dendritic cells and express S-100, CD1a and HLA-DR. The presence of Birbeck granules in the cytoplasm is characteristic. Under the electron microscope, Birbeck granules have a pentalaminar, rod-like, tubular appearance and sometimes a dilated terminal end (tennis - racket appearance).

178. Birbeck's granule is seen in: *(NEET 2016)*

a. Granulomatous vasculitis
b. Histiocytic necrotizing lymphadenitis
c. Langerhans cells histiocytosis
d. Multiple myeloma

Ans. is 'c' Langerhans cells histiocytosis

Burkitt's Lymphoma

- Burkitt's lymphoma is a B-cell lymphoma arising from germinal center B-cells. As this a tumor of mature B-cells it expresses IgM, CD19, CD2O, CD10 and BCL 6 a phenotype consistent with a B-cell origin.
- **Microscopy:** Diffuse pattern of growth.
- Starry sky appearance is characteristic but not pathognomonic.
- Monotonous infiltrate of medium sized cells, having multiple nucleoli.
- Atypical variant—greater variation in size and shape of nuclei.
- However, unlike other tumors of germinal center origin, Burkitt lymphoma almost always fails to express the anti-apoptotic protein BCL-2.
- **Genetics:** Ig genes are rearranged, somatic mutations seen.
- t(8;14)(q24;q32) most common translocation.
- Less commonly seen t(2;8)(p12;q24), t(8;22)(q24;q11).
- C-myc oncogene is translocated to the Ig heavy or light chain on chr.2, 4, 22.
- Burkitt's lymphoma presents with peripheral lymphadenopathy or an intra-abdominal mass. The disease is typically rapidly progressive and has a propensity to metastasize to CNS.
- Chemotherapy is the treatment of choice in Burkitt's Lymphoma. Burkitt's Lymphoma was one of the first cancers shown to be curable by chemotherapy.

179. True about Burkitt's lymphoma is: *(NEET 2016)*

a. Radiotherapy is the best treatment
b. Commonly express the anti-apoptotic protein BCL-2
c. CD34 + ve and surface Ig-ve
d. C-myc gene is involved

Ans. is 'd' C-myc gene is involved

180. Protooncogene associated with Burkitt's lymphoma is: *(NEET 2016)*

a. C-MYC
b. N-MYC
c. L-MYC
d. RET

Ans. is 'a' C-MYC

RICHTER'S SYNDROME

Richter's syndrome (RS), also known as Richter's transformation, is a transformation which occurs in about 5–10% of B-cell chronic lymphocytic leukemia (CLL) and hairy cell leukemia into a fast-growing diffuse large B-cell lymphoma, a variety of non-Hodgkin lymphoma which is refractory to treatment and carries a bad prognosis.

181. Ritcher's transformation is associated with: *(NEET 2016)*

a. CML
b. CLL
c. AML
d. ALL

Ans. is 'b' CLL

ACUTE MYELOID LEUKEMIA

Class	Blast cells	Remarks
M0 minimally differentiated AML	• Myeloperoxidase negative • Auer rods negative • Express myeloid linease antigen	
M1 AML without differentiated	• ≥3% blasts myeloperoxidase positive • Auer rods positive • Sudan black positive	
M2 AML with maturation (most common)	• Full range of myeloid maturation • Myeloperoxidase positive • Auer rods positive • Sudan black positive	t(8:21)
M3 acute promyelocytic leukemia	• Maximum Auer rods • Myeloperoxidase positive • Sudan black positive	t(15:17) 'Faggot cells'
M4 acute myelomonocytic leukemia (naegeli type)	• Both myeocytic and monocytic differentiation • Myeloperoxidase (+) ve • Auer rods (+) ve [Myeloblastic] • Nonspecific esterase (+) ve → monoblastic • Sudan black positive	Inv (16)
M5 acute monocytic leukemia (schilling type)	• Nonspecific esterase (+) ve • Myeloperoxidase and auer rods (-1) ve • Sudan black positive	
M6 acute erythroleukemia (diguglielmo disease)	• Dysplastic erythroid precursors • Myeloblasts seen in advanced age	
M7 acute megakaryocytic (least common)	• Blasts of megakaryocytic lineage • GP IIb /IIIa or VwF (+) ve	

182. AML is associated with which of the following translocation? *(NEET 2016)*

a. T[18,21]
b. T[15,17]
c. T[15,21]
d. T[9,11]

Ans. is 'b' T[15,17]

ALL-TRANS RETINOIC ACID

- Acute Promyelocytic Leukemia (APML) is virtually always associated with a reciprocal translocation between chromosomes 15 and 17 that produces a PML-RARA fusion gene.
- The fusion gene encodes a chimeric protein consisting of part of a protein called PML and part of the retinoic acid receptor-α (RARα). Normal RARα binds to DNA and activates transcription in the presence of retinoids. Among the RARα responsive genes are a number that are needed for the differentiation of myeloid progenitors into neutrophils.
- The PML-RARα oncoprotein has diminished affinity for retinoids, such that at physiologic levels retinoids do not bind to PML-RARα to any significant degree. In this "unliganded" state, it retains the capacity to bind DNA, but instead of activating transcription, it inhibits transcription through recruitment of transcriptional repressors. This interferes with the expression of genes that are needed for differentiation, leading to a "pile-up" of proliferating myeloid progenitors that replace normal bone marrow elements.
- When given in pharmacologic doses, all-trans retinoic acid binds to PML-RARα and causes a conformational change that results in the displacement of repressor complexes and the recruitment of different complexes that activate transcription. This exchange overcomes the block in gene expression, causing the neoplastic myeloid progenitors to differentiate into neutrophils and die, clearing the marrow over several days and allowing for recovery of normal hematopoiesis.

- This highly effective therapy is the first example of differentiation therapy, in which immortal tumor cells are induced to differentiate into their mature progeny, which have limited life spans.

183. All trans retinoic acid is used in treatment of tumour associated with: *(NEET 2020)*

a. BCR-ABL
b. PML-RARA
c. C-myc
d. CEBPA

Ans. is 'b' PML-RARA

GENETIC ALTERATIONS IN MYELODYSPLASTIC SYNDROME

Very good (4%)	Y, del (11q)
Good (72%)	Normal, del (5q), del (12p), del (20q), double including del (5q)
Intermediate (13%)	del (7q), + 8, +19, i(17q), any other single or double independent clones
Poor (4%)	-7, inv(3)/t(3q)/del(3q), double including -7/del(7q), complex: 3 abnormalities
Very poor (7%)	Complex:> 3 abnormalities

184. Acute myelodyspalstic syndrome is associated with following cytogenetic abnormality? *(NEET 2016)*

a. Trisomy 8
b. 20q
c. 5q-
d. Monosmy 7

Ans. is 'd' Monosmy 7

GRADING OF NHL

Low grade	Intermediate grade	High grade
• Small lymphocytic • Follicular small cleaved cells • Follicular mixed	• Follicular large cell • Diffuse small cleaved cell • Diffuse large cell • Diffuse mixed	• Large cell immunoblastic • Lymphoblastic • Small non-cleaved cells.

185. Most malignant form of Non Hodgkin's lymphoma is: *(NEET 2016)*

a. Small cell lymphocytic lymphoma
b. Follicular cleavage
c. Large cell follicular
d. Small non-cleaved cell

Ans. is 'd' Small non-cleaved cell

EXTRANODAL LYMPHOMA

- Although extra-nodal lymphomas can arise in virtually any tissue, they do so most commonly in the GI tract and stomach is the most common site for extranodal lymphoma.
- Nearly all gastric lymphomas are B-cell ymphomas of mucosa-associated lymphoid tissue (MALT lymphoma).
- Majority of cases (80%) are associated with chronic gastritis and H. Pylori infection.
- Cag A (cytotoxin-associated gene A) is a virulence factor for Helicobacter pylori, encoded on the cag pathogenicity island (PAT).

186. Cag A gene is associated with: *(NEET 2016)*

a. Hepatocellular carcinoma
b. Esophageal carcinoma
c. MALT lymphoma
d. Lung carcinoma

Ans. is 'c' MALT lymphoma

187. What is most frequent site of extranodal lymphoma? *(NEET 2016)*

a. Lung
b. Stomach
c. Liver
d. Kidney

Ans. is 'b' Stomach

MANTLE CELL LYMPHOMA

- The immunophenotype of the cells resembles the lymphocytes in the mantle zone of normal germinal follicles, and is characterized by co-expression of B-cell antigens (CD 19+, CD20+, CD22+, CD43+, CD79+, surface immunoglobulin sIgM+, sIgD+) and the T-cell associated marker CD5+.

- ❖ MCL cells stain strongly for the antiapoptotic protein BCL-2, but are negative for germinal center markers like CD10 and BCL-6.
- ❖ MCL has pathognomonic chromosomal translocation t(11;14), leading to constitutive cyclin D1 overexpression. Cyclin D1 (CCND1) overexpression has been detected in 90% of MCL patients.
- ❖ SOX11 has been found to be specifically expressed **in more than 90% of MCL cases**.
- ❖ SOX11 can serve as a biomarker for diagnosis and prognosis **(bad prognosis)** of a subset of MCL.

188. Tumor marker for mantle cell lymphoma is: *(NEET 2016)*

a. CD 23 b. CD 20
c. CD 8 d. CD 4

Ans. is 'b' CD 20

Causes of thymic hyperplasia	
True thymic hyperplasia	***Lymphoid hyperplasia***
• Rebound hyperplasia to chemotherapy/steroids	• Myasthenia gravis
• Radiation therapy	• Systemic lupus erythematosus rheumatoid arthritis
• Burns	• Scleroderma
• Other severe systemic stresses	• Graves disease

189. Thymic follicular hyperplasia is seen in: *(NEET 2016)*

a. DiGorge syndrome b. Myasthenia gravis
c. Multiple myeloma d. B-cell lymphoma

Ans. is 'b' Myasthenia gravis

Miscellaneous

190. TEL-AML 1 fusion is associated with: *(NEET 2016)*

a. CLL b. CML
c. ALL d. AML

Ans. is 'c' ALL

- ❖ TEL-AML 1 gene fusion is the most common genetic alteration in childhood acute lymphoblastic leukemia. It is created by balanced translocation t(12:21).
- ❖ Cytogenetic abnormalities associated with ALL are gain of function mutation in NOTCH-i gene in T-cell ALL. Whereas, B-cell ALL is associated with loss of function mutation in PAX-5 (B-cell transcription factor), E2A and EBF; or balanced translocation t (12: 21) (TEL-AML. fusion).

191. Follicular lymphomas associated with: *(NEET 2019)*

a. Bcl-1 b. Bcl-6
c. Bcl-2 d. None of the above

Ans. is 'c' Bcl-2

A translocation between chromosome 14 and 18 results in the over-expression of the bcl-2 gene. As the bcl-2 protein is normally involved in preventing apoptosis, cells with an overexpression of this protein are basically immortal. The bcl-2 gene is normally found on chromosome 18, and the translocation moves the gene near to the site of the immunoglobulin heavy chain enhancer element on chromosome 14.

BLEEDING AND COAGULATION DISORDERS

COAGULATION CASCADE

Initial primary hemostasis is caused by vasoconstriction. Further clotting involves aggregation of platelets followed by formation of fibrin. Fibrin is derived from fibrinogen with the help of thrombin. Thrombin is formed by activation of prothrombin by factor X and V. Factor X can be activated by either of two systems, known as intrinsic and extrinsic. The initial reaction in the intrinsic system is conversion of inactive factor XII to active factor XII (XIIa). This activation, which is catalyzed by high-molecular-weight kininogen and kallikrein, can be brought about *in vitro* by exposing the blood to glass, or *in vivo* by collagen fibers underlying the endothelium. Active factor XII then activates factor XI, and active factor XI activates factor IX. Activated factor IX forms a complex with active factor VIII, which is activated when it is separated from von Willebrand factor. The complex of IXa and VIIIa activate factor X. Phospholipids from aggregated platelets (PL) and Ca^{2+} are necessary for full activation of factor X. The extrinsic system is triggered by the release of tissue thromboplastin (TPL), a protein–phospholipid mixture that activates factor VII. Tissue thromboplastin and factor VII activate factors IX and X. In the presence of PL, Ca^{2+}, and factor V, activated factor X catalyzes the conversion of prothrombin to thrombin.

Pathology

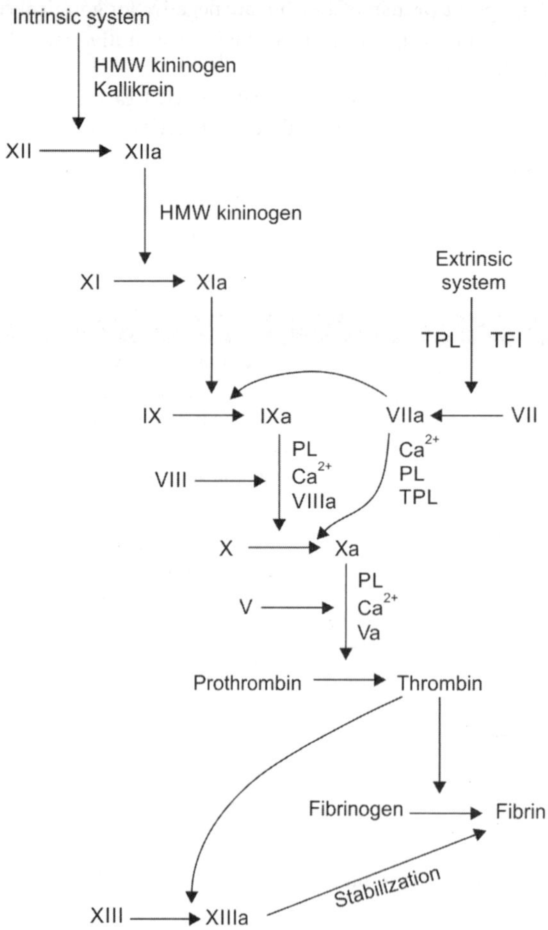

Platelet Plug Formation (Primary Hemostasis)

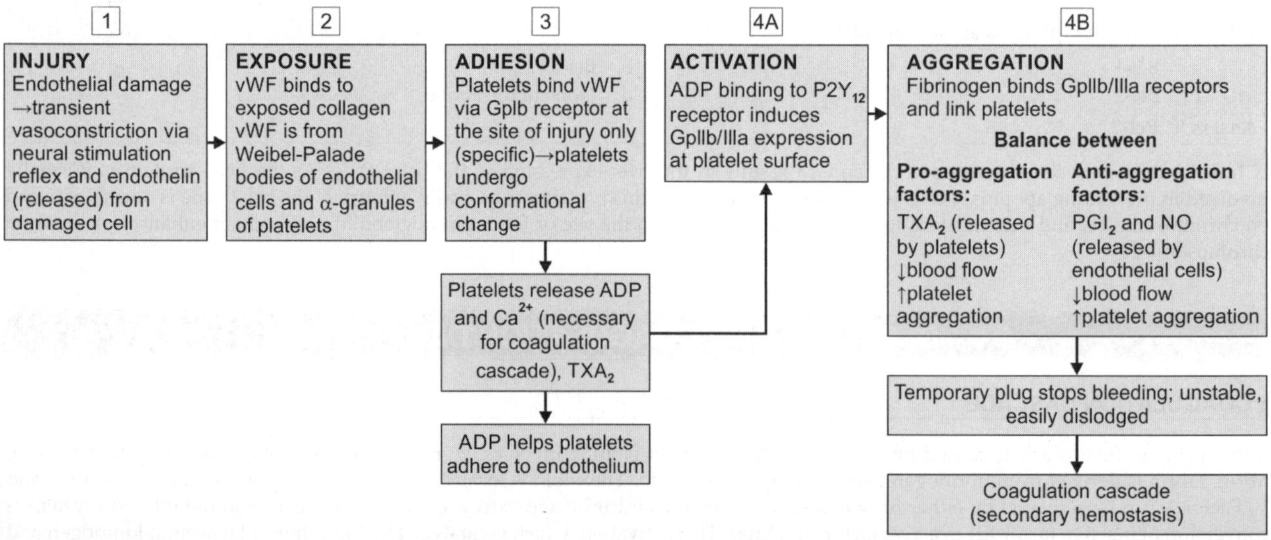

192. Which of the following initiates hemostatic cascade? *(NEET 2020)*

a. Vasoconstriction
b. Activation of tissue thromboplastin
c. Platelet activation
d. Endothelial injury

Ans. is 'd' Endothelial injury

193. First step in initiation of primary hemostasis for clot formation is: *(NEET 2016)*

a. Fibrin deposition b. Vasoconstriction
c. Platelet adhesion d. Thrombosis

Ans. is 'b' Vasoconstriction

194. Which of the following is a pro-coagulant? *(NEET 2016)*

a. Thrombomodulin b. Protein C
c. Protein S d. Thrombin

Ans. is 'd' Thrombin

TYPES OF HEMATOMAS

- Hematomas can be subdivided by size. By definition, ecchymoses are 1 centimeter in size or larger, and are therefore larger than petechiae (less than 2 millimeters in diameter) or purpura (2 millimeters to 1 centimeter in diameter).
- Ecchymoses also have a more diffuse border than other purpura.

195. Size of ecchymosis is: *(NEET 2016)*

a. 2 mm b. 2–5 mm
c. 5 mm–1 cm d. 1 cm or more

Ans. is 'd' 1 cm or more

COMMONLY USED TESTS FOR COAGULATION DISORDERS

- *Partial thromboplastin time (PTT)*: It tests the intrinsic and common coagulation pathways. So, a prolonged PTT can results from deficiency of factor V, VIII (Von Willebrand factor), IX, X, XI, XII, prothrombin or fibrinogen.
- *Prothrombin time (PT)*: It tests the extrinsic and common coagulation pathways. So, a prolonged PT can results from deficiency of factor V, VII, X, prothrombin or fibrinogen.
- Thus in common coagulation pathway defect both PT and PTT are elevated.
- *Activated clotting time (clotting time)*: It also tests the intrinsic and common coagulation system. So it is prolonged in deficiency of same factors as for prolonged PTT
- *Thrombin time*: It tests the conversion of fibrinogen to fibrin and is elevated in fibrinogen deficiency.
- *Ristocetin agglutination test*: It is used the ability of ristocetin to promote the interaction between vWF and platelet membrane glycoprotein lb-IX. Defective ristocetin agglutination test is seen in Von-Willebrand disease.
- *Fibrin degradation products (FDPs)*: They are used to assess the fibrinolytic activity and are increased in DIC.

196. Which test is used for both intrinsic and common clotting pathways? *(NEET 2016)*

a. Thrombin time b. Partial thromboplastin time
c. Ristocetin agglutination test d. FDPs

Ans. is 'b' Partial thromboplastin time

Features of Various Bleeding Disorders

	Platelet count	BT	PT	aPTT	Clotting time	Fibrogen	Fibrin degradation	Confirmatory test
Thrombocytopenia	↓	↑	N	N	N or ↑	N	Negative	
DIC	↓	↑	↑	↑	↑	↓	Positive	
vWD	N	↑	N	↑	↑	N	Negative	↓ vWF on assay
Factor VIIIc deficiency (Hemophilia A)	N	N	N	↑	↑	N	Negative	↓ VIIIc on assay
Factor IX deficiency (hemophilia B) Factor XI deficiency (hemophilia C) factor XII deficiency	N	N	N	↑	↑	N	Negative	Specific factor assay
Factor VII deficiency	N	N	↑	N	N	N	Negative	Specific factor assay
Factor X deficiency Prothrombin deficiency Factor V deficiency (parahemophilia)	N	N	↑	↑	↑	N	Negative	Specific factor assay
Platelet function defect	N	↑	N	N	N	N	Negative	
Liver disease	N	N	↑	↑	↑	↓	Negative	Liver function tests
Warfarin poisoning vitamin k deficiency	N		↑	↑	↑	N	Negative	↓ bleeding on Vitamin k administration

197. BT is increased in deficiency of: *(NEET 2018)*

a. vWF
b. Hemophilia A
c. Hemophilia B
d. HSP

Ans. is 'a' vWF

198. Von Willebrand disease is associate with: *(NEET 2018)*

a. Increased aPTT, increased PT
b. Decreased PT, increased aPTT
c. Normal PT, Normal aPTT
d. Normal PT, increased aPTT

Ans. is 'd' Normal PT, increased aPTT

VITAMIN K-DEPENDENT COAGULATION COMPONENTS

- Vitamin K deficiency: reduced synthesis of factors II, VII, IX, X, protein C, protein S
- Warfarin inhibits vitamin K epoxide reductase. Vitamin K administration can potentially reverse inhibitory effect of warfarin on clotting factor synthesis (delayed). Fresh Frozen Plasma (FFP) or Prothrombin Complex Concentrate (PCC) administration reverses action of warfarin immediately and can be given with vitamin K in cases of severe bleeding.
- Neonates lack enteric bacteria, which produce vitamin K. Early administration of vitamin K overcomes neonatal deficiency/ coagulopathy.
- Factor VII (Seven): Shortest half life. Factor II (Two) - Longest half life

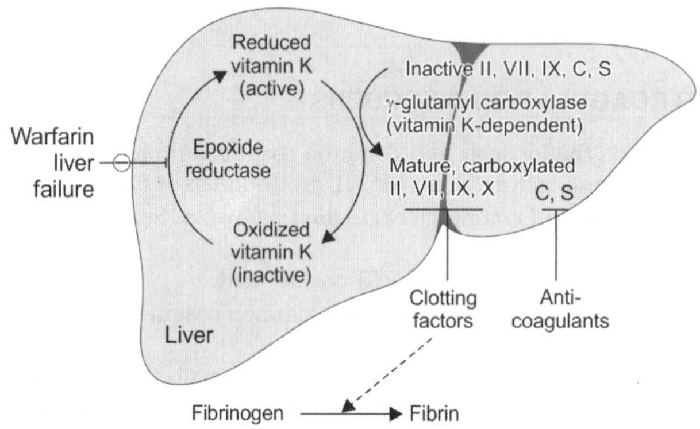

199. A patient admitted in ICU is on warfarin treatment. Which clotting factor would have decreased gamma carboxyglutamate residues? *(NEET 2020)*

a. Factor II
b. Factor V
c. Factor XI
d. Factor XII

Ans. is 'a' Factor II

DISORDERS OF PLATELET FUNCTION

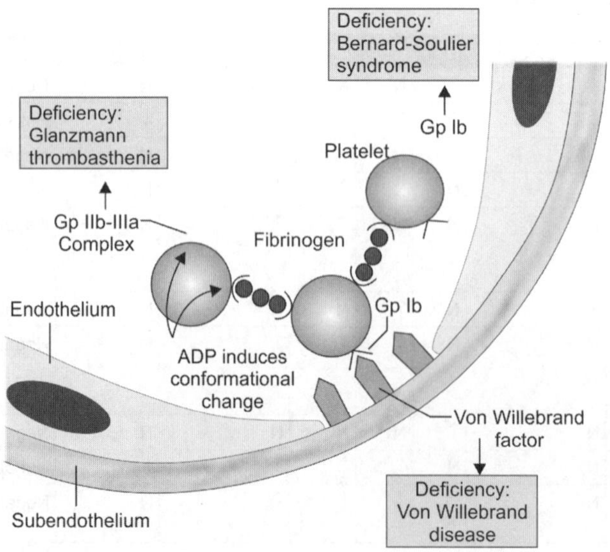

200. Bernard-Soulier syndrome is due to deficiency of: *(NEET 2018)*

a. GpIIb/IIIa
b. Gp1b
c. vWF
d. TNF

Ans. is 'b' Gp1b

201. Glanzmann thrombasthenia is due to defect in: *(NEET 2016, 2019)*

a. GpIIB/IIIA
b. GpIB/IX
c. GpIB/IIIA
d. GpIIB/IX

Ans. is 'a' GpIIB/IIIA

THROMBOTIC THROMBOCYTOPENIC PURPURA

Patients with TTP are deficient in an enzyme called ADAMTSB.13 also known as vWF metalloprotease leading to platelet macroaggregate formation throughout the microcirculation.

Clinical Features

- TTP is characterized by a pentad of:
  - Microangiopathic henzolytic anemia
  - Thrombocytopenia
  - Neurological symptoms (platelet thrombin in cerebral vessels)
  - Renal dysfunction
  - Fever
- There is intravascular hemolysis.
- BT is raised with normal PT and aPTT.
- Hemolytic syndrome is classically included in the spectrum of thrombotic microangiopathies. Hemolytic uremic syndrome is characterized by the triad of: Anemia (microangiopathic hemolytic anemia).
- Renal failure (microangiopathy of kidney involving glomerular capillaries and arterioles).
- Thrombocytopenia (due to platelet consumption).

202. Following is specific for hemolytic uremic syndrome: *(NEET 2016)*

a. Thrombotic microangiopathy
b. Coomb's positive hemolytic anemia
c. Neural manifestations
d. None of the above

Ans. is 'a' Thrombotic microangiopathy

203. Thrombotic thrombocytopenic purpura involves all *except*: *(NEET 2016)*

a. Microangiopathy
b. Neural dysfunction
c. High complement level
d. Intravascular hemolysis

Ans. is 'c' High complement level

Idiopathic Thrombocytopenic Purpura

Idiopathic thrombocytopenic purpura (ITP) is an acquired autoimmune disorder characterized by impaired platelet production and antibody-mediated platelet destruction. Platelet function is always normal. Patients are likely to present to the emergency department with nonblanching petechiae in dependent areas, purpura, epistaxis, or gingival bleeding. Severe hemorrhage (intracranial, gastrointestinal, and genitourinary) is uncommon (<10%), and up to one-third of patients may be asymptomatic at presentation.

Clinical Findings

ITP is a diagnosis of exclusion and the work-up involves ruling out other causes of thrombocytopenia. History taking should investigate recent infections, medications, changes in diet, history of collagen vascular disease, thyroid disease, and liver disease. The physical examination should look for stigmata of liver disease, splenomegaly, and evidence of lymphadenopathy that may indicate a secondary cause. Laboratory testing should include a peripheral blood smear, HIV testing, and hepatitis C virus (HCV) testing. A bone marrow biopsy was previously considered routine in adults older than 60 to exclude the possibility of myelodysplastic syndrome, but this is no longer recommended.

Treatment

The treatment of ITP depends primarily on platelet count, risk factors, and presence of active bleeding. Emergency department treatment generally falls into one of four categories. (1) No emergency treatment is indicated in a healthy, nonbleeding patient with a platelet count more than 30,000 platelets/μL because the risks generally outweigh the benefits. (2) High-risk patients (prior bleeding, predisposing conditions, surgery, or anticoagulation) may be treated at platelet counts more than 30,000 platelets/μL. (3) Patients with active bleeding or severe thrombocytopenia fewer than 30,000 platelets/μL should receive high-dose dexamethasone 1–2 mg/kg/d for 4 weeks and/or a one-time dose of intravenous immune globulin (IVIg) at 1 g/kg for 1–2 days. In patients with functioning spleens, anti-D immune globulin given at 50–75 μg/kg in a single dose is an alternative. IVIg and anti-D globulin are immediately effective, but the effects are transient. Glucocorticoids are slower but can provide a more sustained response. (4) Patients with severe bleeding, including intracranial hemorrhage, should receive immediate platelet transfusion combined with dexamethasone and IVIg. The best treatment remains splenectomy

204. What is the treatment of choice for Idiopathic Thrombocytopenic Purpura (ITP)? *(NEET 2019)*

a. Blood transfusion
b. Spontaneous recovery
c. IV infusion
d. Splenectomy

Ans. is 'd' Splenectomy

LEIDEN MUTATION

- Of the inherited causes of hypercoagulability, mutation in factor V gene is the most common.
- Factor V mutations (called the Leiden mutation) causes substitution of arginine residue (at position 506) by glutamine.
- This mutation makes factor V resistant to cleavage by protein 'C' (normally protein 'C' is one of the factor that regulates coagulation by inactivating factor V and VIII).
- This results in unchecked coagulation.

205. Most common type of inherited disease of hypercoagulability is: *(NEET 2016)*

a. Protein C deficiency
b. Leiden mutation
c. DIC
d. Antithrombin III deficiency

Ans. is 'b' Leiden mutation

Miscellaneous

206. Which of the following is absent in cryoprecipitate? *(NEET 2016)*

a. vWf
b. Factor XIII
c. Factor VIIIc
d. Protein C

Ans. is 'd' Protein C

- Cryoprecipitate contains fibrinogen, factor VIIIc and vWF, and factor XIII. It is most commonly used in hypofibrinogenemia (e.g. in DIC).
- It can also be used in hemophilia A and von-Willebrand disease (but recombinant factor and desmopressin are preferred in these conditions).

BLOOD VESSELS

HYPERCOAGULABLE STATES

Primary (Genetic)

Common

- Factor V mutation (G1691A mutation; factor V Leiden)
- Prothrombin mutation (G20210A variant)
- 5,10-Methylenetetrahydrofolate reductase (homozygous C677T mutation)
- Increased levels of factors VIII, IX, XI, or fibrinogen

Rare

- Antithrombin III deficiency
- Protein C deficiency
- Protein S deficiency

Very Rare

- Fibrinolysis defects
- Homozygous homocystinuria (deficiency of cystathione β synthetase)

Secondary (Acquired)

High Risk for Thrombosis

- Prolonged bedrest or immobilization
- Myocardial infarction
- Atrial fibrillation

- ❖ Tissue injury (surgery, fracture, burn)
- ❖ Cancer
- ❖ Prosthetic cardiac valves
- ❖ Disseminated intravascular coagulation
- ❖ Heparin-induced thrombocytopenia

207. DVT is a manifestation of: *(NEET 2018)*

a. Hemophilia
b. Leiden mutation
c. Vitamin K deficiency
d. Chronic liver failure

Ans. is 'b' Leiden mutation

HEMANGIOMAS

Hemangiomas are the most common tumors of infancy. Both cavernous and capillary hemangiomas may be encountered, although the latter often are more cellular than in adults and thus may be deceptively worrisome-appearing. In children, most hemangiomas are located in the skin, particularly on the face and scalp where they produce flat to elevated, irregular, red-blue masses; the flat, larger lesions are referred to as port wine stains. They may enlarge as the child gets older, but in many instances they spontaneously regress.

The vast majority of superficial hemangiomas have no more than a cosmetic significance; rarely, they may be the manifestation of a hereditary disorder associated with disease within internal organs, such as the von Hippel-Lindau and Sturge-Weber syndromes.

A subset of CNS cavernous hemangiomas can occur in the familial setting; affected families harbor mutations in one of three cerebral cavernous malformation (CCM) genes.

208. In 20-year-old girl reddish brown soft to firm nodule seen on the chest not increasing in size, histopathology image is given, what is the diagnosis? *(NEET 2018)*

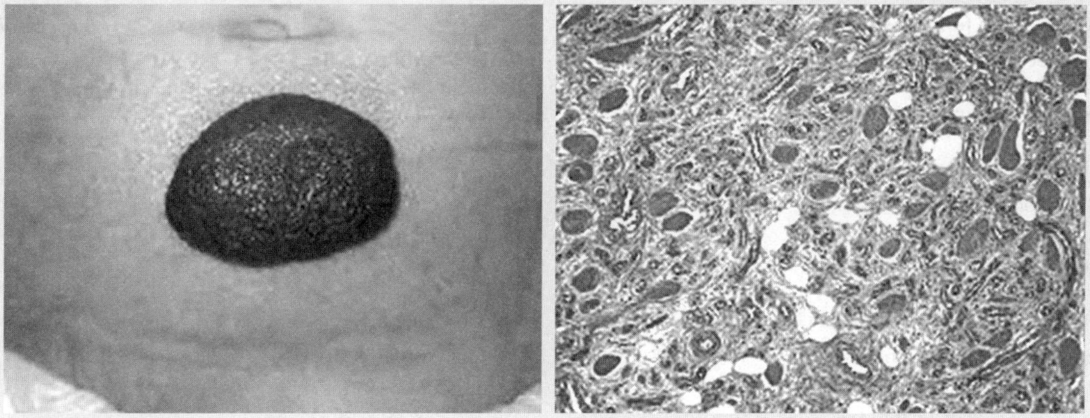

a. Hemangioma
b. Nevus
c. Lipoma
d. Paget's disease

Ans. is 'a' Hemangioma

OXIDIZED LDL

- ❖ Oxidized LDL are particularly important relation to atherosclerosis.
- ❖ Macrophages and endothelial cells generate oxygen free radicals that induce chemical change in LDL to yield oxidized (modified) LDL. Oxidized LDL has following effects: Ingested by macrophages through the scavenger receptor, distinct from LDL receptors, thus forming foam cells.
- ❖ Increases monocyte accumulation in lesions.
- ❖ Stimulates release of growth factors and cytokines.
- ❖ Is cytotoxic to smooth muscle cells and endothelial cells.

209. Scavenger receptors are for: *(NEET 2016)*

a. Oxidized LDL
b. Reduced LDL
c. HDL
d. VLDL

Ans. is 'a' Oxidized LDL

VASCULITIS

Wegener's Granulomatosis

- Wegener's granulomatosis is a necrotizing and granulomatous vasculitis characterized by triad of: Acute necrotizing granulomas of upper and lower respiratory tract
- Necrotizing granulomatous vasculitis affecting mainly lung, but other site as well.
- Renal disease focal proliferative crescentic glomerulonephritis (focal necrotizing glomerulonephritis).
- Wegener's granulomatosis is associated with c-ANCA.
  Note: Vasculitis causing strawberry tongue → Kawasaki disease.

Takayasu Arteritis

- Takayasu arteritis is granulomatous vasculitis of large and medium arteries. It is characterized principally by ocular disturbance and marked weakening of pulses in the upper extremities → Pulseless disease. It is also characterized by a strong predilection for aortic arch and its branches—Aortic arch syndrome.
- It is more common in adolescent girls and young women. Morphological changes in vessel wall are same as in giant-cell arteritis.
- Subclavian artery is involved most commonly, causing arm claudication, lower BP and weaker pulse in upper limb than lower limb. Other vessels involved are common carotid, abdominal aorta, coeliac, superior mesenteric, renal, vertebral, iliac, pulmonary, and coronary arteries.

Polyarteritis Nodosa

- *Presentation*: Medium-vessel vasculitis in middle-aged men. Hepatitis B seropositivity in 30% of patients. Fever, weight loss, malaise, headache. GI: abdominal pain, melena. Hypertension, neurologic dysfunction, cutaneous eruptions, renal damage.
- *Pathology*: Typically involves renal and visceral vessels, not pulmonary arteries. Transmural inflammation of the arterial wall with fibrinoid necrosis. Different stages of inflammation may coexist in different vessels. Innumerable renal microaneurysms and spasms on arteriogram.
- Treat with corticosteroids, cyclophosphamide.

210. Which of the following is true about PAN? *(NEET 2020)*

a. Necrotizing vasculitis of large arteries
b. ANCA positive in 90% cases
c. 30% are HBsAg positive
d. Patient has hypogammaglobulinemia

Ans. is 'c' 30% are HBsAg positive

211. Strawberry gums are seen in: *(NEET 2016)*

a. Goodpasture's syndrome
b. Classic polyarteritis nodosa
c. Wegener's granulomatosis
d. Kawasaki syndrome

Ans. is 'c' Wegener's granulomatosis

212. True about Takayasu arteritis is: *(NEET 2016)*

a. More common in males
b. Small vessel disease
c. Involves primarily upper extremities
d. Common carotid is the most common artery involved

Ans. is 'c' Involves primarily upper extremities

CEAP CLASSIFICATION OF CHRONIC VENOUS INSUFFICIENCY

CEAP classification of chronic venous disease	Clinical classification
C0	No visible or palpable signs of venous disease
C1	Telangiectasias or reticular veins
C2	Varicose veins
C3	Edema
C4a	Pigmentation or eczema
C4b	Lipodermatosclerosis or atrophie blanche
C5	Healed venous ulcer
C6	Active venous ulcer

213. CEAP score is used for: *(NEET 2019)*

a. Arterial disorders
b. Venous disorder
c. Neurological disorder
d. Trauma disorder

Ans. is 'b' Venous disorder

THE HEART

CHRONIC CONSTRICTIVE PERICARDITIS

- Characterized by dense fibrous or fibrocalcific thickening of the pericardium resulting in mechanical interference with the function of the heart and reduced cardiac output.
- Important causes of constrictive pericarditis: TB (most common cause), purulent pericarditis, hemopericardium, SLE, RA, sarcoidosis, radiation, Dressler syndrome, uremia, drugs (hydralazine, procainamide), infections (bacterial, histoplasmosis, toxoplasma), and neoplasms.

214. Not a cause of constrictive pericarditis: *(NEET 2016)*

a. TB
b. Sarcoidosis
c. SLE
d. Trauma

Ans. is 'd' Trauma

RHEUMATIC CARDITIS

Rheumatic carditis is seen in 40–60% of patients and develops within 3 weeks. It can be divided into:

1. **Acute rheumatic carditis**
   - Characteristically, all three layers of heart are involved, i.e. Pancarditis.
   - Pericardial involvement causes fibrinous or serofibrinous pericarditis also called 'bread and butter' pericarditis.
   - Myocardium involvement results in myocarditis with Aschoff bodies. Endocardium involvement leads to formation of small warty projections (verrucae) along the line of closure of valvular leaflets, mostly on mitral valve.
   - The characteristic histological finding of rheumatic carditis is Aschoff bodies/or Aschoff nodules, which can be found in all three layers of heart, but mostly seen in myocardium (myocarditis).
   - Aschoff bodies (Aschoff nodules) are characteristic inflammatory lesions of acute rheumatic fever found any of the three layers of heart. They consist of foci of collagen surrounded by following cells: Lymphocytes (especially T-cells), plasma cells, Aschoff giant cells, anitschkow Cells, histiocytes and fibroblasts. Neutrophils (polymorphonuclear cells) are characteristically absent.
2. **Chronic rheumatic carditis**
   - There is organization of acute inflammation with subsequent fibrosis. There is fish mouth' or Buttonhole stenosis of mitral valve (most commonly involved valve). Aortic (2'° most common) and tricuspid valves may also be involved. The pulmonary valve is least frequently involved.
   - Irregular thickening of posterior wall of left atrium produces MacCallum plaque/patch due to subendothelial collection of Aschoff nodules.
   - Most commonly involved valve in rheumatic carditis in mitral valve. Most common lesion in acute rheumatic carditis is mitral regurgitation acid in chronic rheumatic carditis is mitral stenosis. Overall most common lesion is mitral regurgitation. Pulmonary valve is least frequently involved.

215. Fish mouth appearance of valve in RHD is due to: *(NEET 2019)*

a. Rupture of valve
b. Calcification and fibrosis
c. Hypertrophy of ventricular wall
d. None

Ans. is 'b' Calcification and fibrosis

216. Characteristic histopathological feature of rheumatic heart failure is: *(NEET 2016)*

a. Aschoff's nodule
b. MacCallum patch
c. Bread and butter pericarditis
d. Shaggy vegetation

Ans. is 'a' Aschoff's nodule

VEGETATIVE ENDOCARDITIS

- Small, warty vegetations along the lines of closure of valve leaflets.
- Friable, bulky masses on the valve cusps that can extend onto the chordae
- Small sterile vegetations, usually attached at the line of closure; seen in debilitated patients (e.g. cancer, sepsis)
- Small to medium-sized vegetations on either or both sides of the valve leaflets; seen with systemic lupus erythematosus (SLE)

217. Bulky friable vegetations on surface of cardiac valves is seen in: *(NEET 2020)*

a. Rheumatic carditis
b. Infective endocarditis
c. Nonbacterial thrombotic endocarditis
d. Libman Sach carditis

Ans. is 'b' Infective endocarditis

COMPLICATIONS OF PROSTHETIC HEART VALVES

- Thromboembolic events
- Bleeding
- Prosthetic heart valve obstruction or stenosis
- Prosthetic heart valve regurgitation (valvular and paravalvular)
- Infective endocarditis
- Hemolytic anemia
- Patient-prosthesis mismatch.

218. Prosthetic valves are predisposed to: *(NEET 2016)*

a. Thromboembolism b. Infection
c. Hemolysis d. All of the above

Ans. is 'd' All of the above

CARCINOID SYNDROME OF HEART

Carcinoid heart disease is the cardiac manifestation of the systemic syndrome caused by carcinoid tumors. It generally involves the endocardium and valve of the right side of heart.

Cardiovascular lesions consist of firm plaque like endocardial fibrous thickenings on the inside surfaces of the cardiac chambers and the tricuspid and pulmonary valves.

219. Carcinoid tumor of heart most commonly involves: *(NEET 2016)*

a. Epicardium b. Pericardium
c. Endocardium d. Valves of the left side of heart

Ans. is 'c' Endocardium

Important complications of MI are:

- **Acute effects of myocardial infarction**
  - Contractile dysfunction
  - Arrhythmias ventricular premature contractions are the most common arrhythmia.
  - Most common cause of death is ventricular fibrillation. Frequently associated with cardiogenic shock
  - Heart block occurs in 5% of inferior AMIs
  - Occurs in 3% of anterior AMIs
- **Cardiac rupture**
  - Most commonly occurs between days 3 and 7 (range is 1–10 days)
  - Anterior wall rupture produces cardiac tamponade
  - Associated with thrombosis of the LAD coronary artery
  - Posteromedial papillary muscle rupture or dysfunction—Most often associated with inferior AMIs due to thrombosis of the RCA
  - Presents with an acute onset of MV regurgitation and LHF
  - Interventricular septum (IVS) rupture—Most often associated with a thrombosis in the LAD coronary artery
  - Produces a left-to-right shunt, causing RHF
- **Fibrinous pericarditis with or without effusion**
  - Most often occurs between day 1 to 7 of a STEMI. Presents with substernal chest pain that is relieved by leaning forward and aggravated by leaning backward
  - Precordial friction rub is present on auscultation
  - Due to increased vessel permeability in the pericardium (exudate of acute inflammation)
- **Autoimmune pericarditis (Dressler syndrome)**
  - Usually occurs 1 to 8 weeks after a STEMI infarction.
  - Autoantibodies are directed against the damaged pericardial antigens (type II hypersensitivity reaction)
  - Fever and a precordial friction rub are present.
- **Ventricular aneurysm**
  - Clinically recognized within 4 to 8 weeks after a STEMI.
    - Begins to develop in the first 48 hours
  - Precordial bulge occurs during systole
    - Blood enters the aneurysm, causing anterior chest wall movement.
  - Complications
    - SHF occurs because of the lack of contractile tissue.
    - Clot material may embolize.
    - Rupture is uncommon.
    - Scar tissue has good tensile strength.
- **Myocardial rupture Ventricular free wall**
- **Septal**
- **Papillary muscle**

220. Most frequent time period between myocardial infarction and subsequent myocardial rupture is: *(NEET 2016)*

a. 3–4 days
b. 4–8 days
c. 1–3 days
d. 3–6 days

Ans. is 'a' 3–4 days

221. Which type of MI is most commonly associated with formation of aneurysms? *(NEET 2016)*

a. Posterior
b. Inferior
c. Subendocardial
d. Anterior

Ans. is 'd' Anterior

POST-MI REPERFUSION

- Reperfusion is the restoration of blood flow to ischemic myocardium threatened by infarction; the goal is to salvage cardiac muscle at risk and limit infarct size.
- Reperfused infarcts are usually hemorrhagic because the vasculature is injured during ischemia and there is bleeding after flow is restored.
- Microscopic examination reveals that irreversibly injured myocytes exhibit contraction bands, intensely eosinophilic intracellular stripes composed of closely packed sarcomeres
- Reperfusion not only salvages reversibly injured cells but also alters the morphology of lethally injured cells.
- Reperfusion can trigger deleterious complications, including arrhythmias as well as damage superimposed on original ischemia, so-called reperfusion injury.

222. Which of the following would be seen on cardiac biopsy of a patient with post-MI reperfusion injury? *(NEET 2020)*

a. Waviness of fibres
b. Neutrophilic infiltration in muscle
c. Eosinophilic contraction bands
d. Swelling of cells

Ans. is 'c' Eosinophilic contraction bands

CARDIAC TUMOURS

- The most common cardiac tumor is metastasis (secondaries).
- The most common primary cardiac tumor (overall) is cardiac myxoma.
- Most common primary cardiac tumor in adults is cardiac myxoma. The most common primary cardiac tumor in infant and children is rhabdomyoma.

223. Most common primary cardiac tumor is: *(NEET 2016)*

a. Myxoma
b. Rhabdomyosarcoma
c. Fibroma
d. Lipoma

Ans. is 'a' Myxoma

CARDIOMYOPATHIES

Restrictive Cardiomyopathy

- Restrictive cardiomyopathy is characterized by a primary decrease in ventricular compliance, i.e. ventricles become stiff. Resulting in impaired ventricular filling during diastole because heart cannot relax normally during diastole → Diastolic dysfunction. Ventricles are normal in size (or slightly enlarged) without any dilatation of cavity. Atrial cavities are dilated. There is interstitial fibrosis.
- Important causes of restrictive cardiomyopathy are: Three most common causes → Amyloidosis, Radiation, myocardial fibrosis after open heart surgery.
- Others → Sarcoidosis, hemochromatosis, carcinoid syndrome, Fabry's disease, Loeffler's syndrome, scleroderma, glycogen deposition, neoplasm.
- RCM-associated mutations have been reported in four genes that encode key sarcomeric proteins/myofilaments MYH7 gene–β-Myosin heavy chain
- TNNI3 gene—Cardiac troponin I type 3
- TNNT2 gene—Cardiac troponin T type 2
- ACTC gene—a-actin

Mutations in the TNNI3 gene and MYH7 gene are the major causes of this condition.

Hypertrophic Cardiomyopathy

- Hypertrophic cardiomyopathy is caused by a mutation in one of nine genes that encode sarcomere proteins.
- Mutations in thick filament proteins called cardiac b-myosin heavy chain or cardiac myosin binding protein-C appear to account for approximately 82% of hypertrophic cardiomyopathy.
- Mutations in thin filament proteins cardiac troponin T and a tropomyosin account for about 13% of hypertrophic cardiomyopathy.
- Mutations in two other sarcomere proteins, the myosin regulatory and essential light chains are quite rare and contribute less than 5% to hypertrophic cardiomyopathy.
- A tenth gene has been identified that is a non-sarcomere protein (a subunit of protein kinase A) is associated with individuals who have both hypertrophic cardiomyopathy and Wolf-Parkinson-White syndrome.

224. Restrictive cardiomyopathy is not associated with: *(NEET 2016)*

a. Alcohol
b. Hemochromatosis
c. Amyloidosis
d. Sarcoidosis

Ans. is 'a' Alcohol

225. Mutation in protein associated with restrictive cardiomyopathy? *(NEET 2016)*

a. Myosin regulatory proteins
b. Myosin binding protein-C
c. Troponin I
d. Tropomyosin

Ans. is 'c' Troponin I

226. Mutation in which of the following is a cause of hypertrophic cardiomyopathy? *(NEET 2016)*

a. Myosin regulatory proteins
b. Myosin binding protein-C
c. Troponin I
d. Troponin T

Ans. is 'b' Myosin binding protein-C

Miscellaneous

227. Deposition of which substance leads to tigroid appearance of heart? *(NEET 2016)*

a. Calcium
b. Fat
c. Protein
d. Fibrous tissue

Ans. is 'b' Fat

Tigroid effect is grossly apparent bands of yellowed myocardium (containing fat) alternating with bands of darker, red-brown, uninvolved heart.

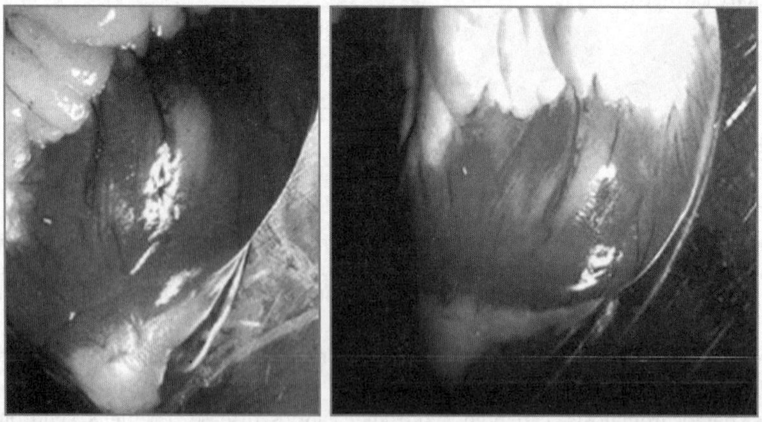

THE LUNG

TUBERCULOSIS

It is the classic granulomatous infection. The disease is divided into primary and secondary (or reactivation) tuberculosis.

- *Primary tuberculosis*: The disease is acquired from the initial exposure to *M. tuberculosis*, most commonly as a result of inhaling infected aerosols generated when a person with cavitary tuberculosis coughs.

Pathology

- The Ghon complex is the first lesion of primary tuberculosis and consists of a peripheral parenchymal granuloma, often in the upper lobes.
- When it is associated with an enlarged mediastinal lymph node a Ranke complex is formed.
- Microscopically, a granuloma with central caseous necrosis shows varying degrees of fibrosis. Apical scarring with the appearance of a fibronodular patch or ill-defined reticular shadow in the upper lung fields on chest X-ray is known as 'Simon's focus'.
- *Puhl's lesion*: Lesion at the apex of lung in chronic cases.
- *Assmann's focus*: Typically apical (site of highest oxygen tension)
- *TB Simon's focus*: Early hematogenous seedling in apex of lungs.
- *Ghon's complex*: Parenchymal subpleural lesion + draining lymphatics + enlarged caseous lymph nodes in primary tuberculosis
- *Ranke complex*: Healed lesions in lung parenchyma and hilar lymph nodes undergoing calcification due to TB
- *Rich focus*: Tuberculous caseous foci in brain, meninges and spinal cord.

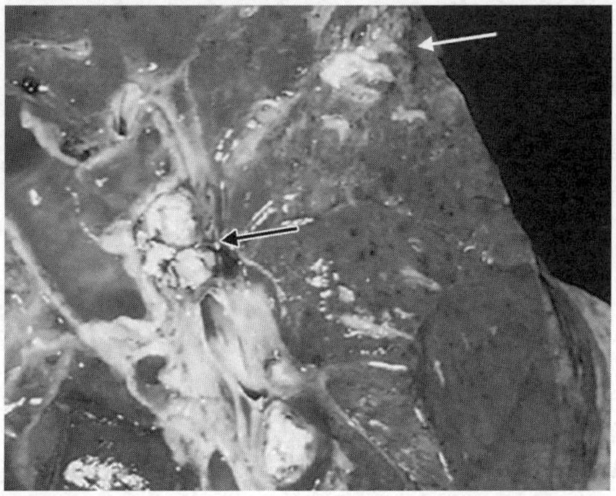

- ***Primary pulmonary tuberculosis (Ghon complex)*: The gray-white parenchymal focus is under the pleura in the lower part of the upper lobe *(White arrow). Hilar lymph nodes with caseation are seen on the left.*** Combination of parenchymal lung lesion and nodal involvement is referred to as the Ghon complex.
- *Secondary tuberculosis*: This stage represents either reactivation of primary pulmonary tuberculosis or a new infection in a host previously sensitized by primary tuberculosis.
- **Secondary tuberculosis is associated with a number of complications:**
  - Miliary tuberculosis refers to the presence of multiple, small (size of millet seeds), tuberculous granulomas in many organs. 'Miliary pattern' of granulomas are a multitude of small tan granulomas about 2 to 4 mm in size, scat tered throughout the lung parenchyma. The miliary pattern gets its name from the resemblance of the granulomas to millet seeds.
  - Miliary TB can occur when TB lung lesions erode pulmonary veins or when extra-pulmonary TB lesions erode systemic veins.
  - This results in hematogenous dissemination of tubercle bacilli producing myriads of 1–2 mm lesions throughout the body insusceptible hosts.
  - Miliary spread limited to the lungs can occur following erosion of pulmonary arteries by TB lung lesions.
  - Hemoptysis
  - Broncho pleural fistula occurs when a subpleural cavity ruptures into the pleural space. In turn, tuberculous empyema and pneumothorax result.
  - Tuberculous laryngitis
  - Intestinal tuberculosis.
  - Most common site of extrapulmonary tuberculosis is lymph nodes.
  - Other extrapulmonary sites of involvement are pleura, pericardium, meninges, brain, genitourinary system, GIT and skeletal system.

IGRA: Assay Principles

IGRAs are in vitro blood tests of cell-mediated immune response; they measure T-cell release of IFN-γ following stimulation by antigens specific to the *M. tuberculosis* complex (with the exception of BCG substrains), i.e. early secreted antigenic target 6 (ESAT-6) and culture filtrate protein 10 (CFP10). These antigens are encoded by genes located within the region of difference 1(RD 1) locus of the *M. tuberculosis* genome. They are more specific than PPD for *M. tuberculosis* because they are not encoded in the genomes of any BCG vaccine strains or most species of NTM, other than *M. marinum, M. kansasii, M. szulgai, and M. flavescens.* However, not all NTMs have been studied for cross-reactivity. There is some evidence of cross-reactivity between ESAT-6 and CFP-10 of *M. tuberculosis* and *M. leprae,* but the clinical significance of this in settings where leprosy and TB are endemic (e.g. India and Brazil) is poorly characterized.

228. What does the given specimen of lung show? *(NEET 2018)*

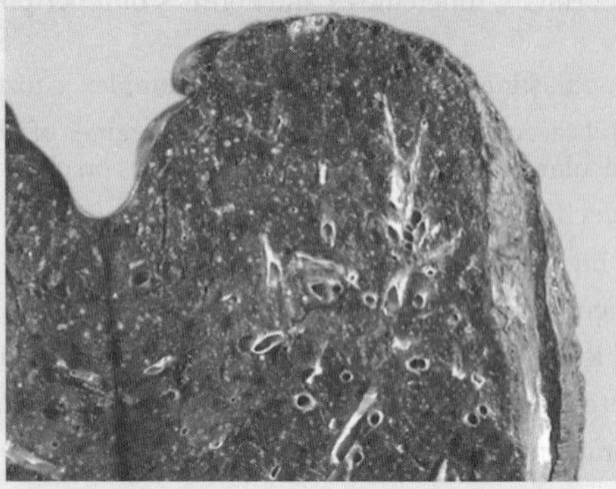

a. Miliary TB
b. Pneumoconiosis
c. Bronchiectasis
d. Pneumonia

Ans. is 'a' Miliary TB

229. Whole blood is used in diagnosis of TB in: *(NEET 2018)*

a. Gamma interferon assay
b. GeneXpert
c. Bactec test
d. Blood culture

Ans. is 'a' Gamma interferon assay

230. What is the most common site for extrapulmonary tuberculosis is: *(NEET 2016)*

a. Lymph nodes
b. Pleura
c. GIT
d. Brain

Ans. is 'a' Lymph nodes

Granulomatous lung disease refers a broad group of infection and well as non-infections conditions characterized by formation of granulomas

The spectrum includes:

❖ **Infectious**
- **Mycobacterial** pulmonary tuberculosis
- Pulmonary non-tuberculous mycobacterial infection
- **Fungal** pulmonary coccidioidomycosis
- Pulmonary cryptococcosis
- Pulmonary histoplasmosis
- Pulmonary blastomycosis
- Pulmonary aspergillus infections
- **Parasitic** pulmonary dirofilaria infection

❖ **Non-infectious**
- Sarcoidosis
- Wegener granulomatosis
- Churg-Strauss syndrome
- Chronic granulomatous disease
- Hypersensitivity pneumonitis
- Bronchocentric granulomatosis
- Pulmonary manifestations of rheumatoid arthritis
- Granulomatosis secondary to substances—Pulmonary talc granulomatosis, Berylliosis
- Changes secondary to chronic aspiration pneumonitis
- Lymphoproliferative—Lymphocytic interstitial pneumonitis
- Pulmonary Langerhans cell histiocytosis
- Erdheim-Chester disease
- Granulomatous lung disease associated with common variable immunodeficiency.

231. Granulomatous lung disease is caused by: *(NEET 2016)*

a. Hypersensitivity pneumonitis
b. Sarcoma
c. Bronchogenic carcinoma
d. Bronchogenic cyst

Ans. is 'a' Hypersensitivity pneumonitis

Pneumoconiosis

The term *pneumoconiosis* was originally coined to describe the non-neoplastic lung reaction to inhalation of mineral dusts encountered in the workplace. Now it also includes diseases induced by organic as well as inorganic particulates and chemical fumes and vapors.

Agent	Disease	Exposure
Mineral dusts		
Coal dust	Anthracosis Macules Progressive massive fibrosis Caplan syndrome	Coal mining (particularly hard coal)
Silica	Silicosis Caplan syndrome	Foundry work, sandblasting, hard rock mining, stone cutting, others
Asbestos	Asbestosis Pleural plaques Caplan syndrome Mesothelioma Carcinoma of the lung, larynx, stomach, colon	Mining, milling, fabrication, and installation and removal of insulation
Beryllium	Acute berylliosis Beryllium granulomatosis Lung carcinoma(?)	Mining, fabrication
Iron oxide	Siderosis	Welding
Barium sulfate	Barilosis	Mining
Tin oxide	Stannosis	Mining

Caplan syndrome is coexistence of rheumatoid arthritis with coal worker pneumoconiosis

Asbestosis

Histology

- Asbestosis is marked by diffuse pulmonary interstitial fibrosis.
- Asbestos bodies are present, which appear as golden brown, fusiform or beaded rods with a translucent center and consist of asbestos fibers coated with an iron-containing proteinaceous material. They arise when macrophages attempt to phagocytose asbestos fibers; the iron is presumably derived from phagocyte ferritin.
- Other inorganic particulates may become coated with similar iron-protein complexes and are called ferruginous bodies.
- Asbestosis begins as fibrosis around respiratory bronchioles and alveolar ducts and extends to involve adjacent alveolar sacs and alveoli. The fibrous tissue distorts the architecture, creating enlarged airspaces enclosed within thick fibrous walls; eventually the affected regions become honeycombed.
- The pattern of fibrosis is similar to that seen in UIP.
- Asbestosis begins in the lower lobes and subpleurally.
- Pleural plaques, the most common manifestation of asbestos exposure, are well-circumscribed plaques of dense collagen, often containing calcium. They develop most frequently on the anterior and posterolateral aspects of the parietal pleura and over the domes of the diaphragm.
- Both lung carcinomas and mesotheliomas (pleural and peritoneal) develop in workers exposed to asbestos. Concomitant cigarette smoking greatly increases the risk of lung carcinoma but not that of mesothelioma.

Silicosis

- Silicosis is a slowly progressive lung disease caused by inhalation of crystalline silicon dioxide (silica). Currently, it is the most prevalent occupational disease in the world.
- Silica occurs in both crystalline and amorphous forms but crystalline forms are much more fibrogenic. The crystalline form are quartz, and cristobalite.
- Silicosis is characterized in its early stages by nodules in the upper zones of the lung. As the disease progresses these nodules may coalesce into hard collagenous scars. Fibrotic lesions occur in the hilar lymph node and pleura. Sometimes thin sheets of calcification occur in the lymph nodes and are seen radiographically as egg shell calcification i.e. (calcium surrounding a zone lacking calcification. If the disease continues to progress, expansion and coalescence of lesions produce progressive massive fibrosis.
- Silicosis is associated with an increased susceptibility to TB. It is postulated that silicosis results in depression of cell mediated immunity and the crystalline silica may inhibit the ability of pulmonary macrophages to kill phagocytosed mycobacteria. Nodules of silicotuberculosis often display a central zone of caseation.

- Histologically the lesions of silicosis consist of concentric layers of hyalinized collagen surrounded by a dense capsule of more condensed collagen. Examination of the nodules by polarized microscopy reveals the birefringent silica particles

Anthracosis (Coal Worker Pneumoconiosis/Black Lung)

Caused by long exposure to coal dust. Coal worker's pneumoconiosis has following spectrum:

- *Asymptomatic anthracosis*: Inhaled carbon pigment is engulfed by alveolar or interstitial macrophages, which then accumulate in the connective tissue along the lymphatics. Patient is completely asymptomatic.
- *Simple coal worker's pneumoconiosis*: Characterized by coal macules (composed of carbon laden macrophages) and coal nodules (carbon laden macrophages + collagen). The upper lobes and upper zones of the lower lobes are involved. They are located primarily adjacent to respiratory bronchioles, the site of initial dust accumulation, centriacinar emphysema may develop. Dust cells are alveolar macrophages with anthracoid pigment (carbon).
- *Complicated coal worker's pneumoconiosis*: Requires many years to develop. Characterized by intensely blackened multiple scar larger than 2 cm. This is also known as Progressive massive fibrosis.

232. Finding associated with anthracosis is: *(NEET 2016)*

a. Ferruginous bodies
b. Egg shell calcification
c. Increased susceptibility to TB
d. Centriacinar emphysema

Ans. is 'd' Centriacinar emphysema

233. Most common type of pneumoconiosis, associated with TB is: *(NEET 2016)*

a. Silicosis
b. Byssinosis
c. Asbestosis
d. Bagassosis

Ans. is 'a' Silicosis

234. On polarising microscopy, refractile body in the centre of granuloma is seen in: *(NEET 2016)*

a. Sarcoidosis
b. Silicosis
c. Tuberculosis
d. Asbestosis

Ans. is 'b' Silicosis

235. True about silicosis is: *(NEET 2016)*

a. Starts in upper zone of lungs
b. Crystalline form of silica is more fibrogenic
c. Associate with pleural thickening
d. All of the above

Ans. is 'd' All of the above

236. Most common cancer found in coal mine workers: *(NEET 2016)*

a. Anal canal
b. Testicular
c. Lung
d. Liver

Ans. is 'c' Lung

237. Ferruginous bodies are seen in: *(NEET 2016)*

a. Silicosis
b. Byssinosis
c. Asbestosis
d. Bagassosis

Ans. is 'c' Asbestosis

238. Association of coal worker pneumoconiosis and rheumatoid arthritis is known as: *(NEET 2016)*

a. Kartagener's syndrome
b. Good pasture syndrome
c. Caplan syndrome
d. Hamman-Rich syndrome

Ans. is 'c' Caplan syndrome

KARTAGENER'S SYNDROME

Kartagener's syndrome (KS) is a subset of a larger group of ciliary motility disorders called primary ciliary dyskinesias (PCDs). It is a genetic condition with an autosomal recessive inheritance, comprising a triad of situs inversus, bronchiectasis and sinusitis. Although Siewart first described this condition in 1904, it was Kartagener who recognized the etiological correlation between the elements of the triad and reported four cases in 1933. The estimated prevalence of PCD is about 1 in 30,000, though it may range from 1 in 12,500 to 1 in 50,000. In KS, the ultrastructural genetic defect leads to impaired ciliary motility which causes recurrent chest, ear/nose/throat (ENT), and sinus infections, and infertility. A high index of suspicion is needed to make an early diagnosis so that timely treatment options may be offered for infertility in these young patients, wherever feasible. Also, although unproven, it seems likely that early diagnosis is important for the preservation of pulmonary function, quality of life, and life expectancy in this disease.

239. Kartagener's syndrome is characterized by: *(NEET 2016)*

a. Pancreatic insufficiency
b. Bronchiectasis
c. Glomerulonephritis
d. All of the above

Ans. is 'b' Bronchiectasis

STAGES OF PNEUMONIA

In **lobar pneumonia**, four stages of the inflammatory response have classically been described: congestion, red hepatization, gray hepatization, and resolution. Current effective antibiotic therapy frequently slows or halts the progression. In the first stage of **congestion** the lung is heavy, boggy, and red. It is characterized by vascular engorgement, intra-alveolar fluid with few neutrophils, and often the presence of numerous bacteria. The stage of **red hepatization** that follows is characterized by massive confluent exudation with neutrophils, red cells, and fibrin filling the alveolar spaces. On gross examination, the lobe now appears distinctly red, firm, and airless, with a liver-like consistency, hence the term **hepatization**. The stage of **gray hepatization** follows with progressive disintegration ofred cells and the persistence of a fibrinosuppurative exudate, giving the gross appearance of a grayish brown, dry surface. In the final stage of **resolution** the consolidated exudate within the alveolar spaces undergoes progressive enzymatic digestion to produce granular, semifluid debris that is resorbed, ingested by macrophages, expectorated, or organized by fibroblasts growing into it. The patients develops expectoration at this stage. Pleural fibrinous reaction to the underlying inflammation, often present in the early stages if the consolidation extends to the surface **(pleuritis)**, may similarly resolve. More often it undergoes organization, leaving fibrous thickening or permanent adhesions.

240. A patient of pneumonia develops sputum expectoration. What is the stage of pneumonia? *(NEET 2016)*

a. Congestion
b. Red hepatization
c. Grey hepatization
d. Resolution

Ans. is 'd' Resolution

OBSTRUCTIVE LUNG DISEASES

	Pre-dominant bronchitis	Predominant emphysema
Age (yr)	40–45	50–75
Dyspnea	Mid; late	Severe; early
Cough	Early; copious sputum	Late; scanty sputum
Infections	Common	Occasional
Respiratory insufficiency	Repeated	Terminal
Cor pulmonale	Common	Rare; terminal
Airway resistance	Increased	Normal or slightly increased
Elastic recoil	Normal	Low
Chest radiograph	Prominent vessels; large heart	Hyperinflation; small heart
Appearance	*Blue bloater*	*Pink puffer*

- Chronic bronchitis is defined as persistent cough with sputum production for at least 3 months in at least 2 consecutive years, in the absence of any other identifiable cause. It is strongly associated with smoking.
- The earliest feature of chronic bronchitis is hypersecretion of mucus in the larger airways, associated with hypertrophy of submucosal gland of trachea and bronchi.
- Although the numbers of glands increase slightly, the major increase is in the size of mucous glands. This increase can be assessed by Reid index which is the ratio of between thickness of the submucosal glands to that of the bronchial wall. The Reid index (normal 0.4) is increased in chronic bronchitis.
- Later, small airways (small bronchi and bronchioles) are also involved and show goblet cell hyperplasia, and intraluminal and peribronchial fibrosis.
- In most severe cases, there may be obliteration of lumen due to fibrosis → Bronchiolitis obliterans.
- The bronchial epithelium may undergo squamous metaplasia and dysplasia.

Bronchiectasis

- Bronchiectasis refers to abnormal permanent dilatation of bronchi and bronchioles resulting from chronic necrotizing infection.
- Two major factors in pathogenesis of bronchiectasis are obstruction and infection. Bronchial obstruction impairs normal clearing mechanism and results in pooling of mucus. This predisposes to infection and infection of the bronchi lead to inflammation, often with necrosis, fibrosis, and eventually dilatation of airways.
- Bronchiectasis commonly affects lower lobe bronchi, the left side being involved more frequently than right. The airways are dilated, sometimes up to four times normal size.
- Important complications of bronchiectasis are massive hemoptysis, purulent pericarditis, lung abscess, empyema, amyloidosis, metastatic abscess (in brain, bones etc.) , and cor pulmonale. It is not a premalignant condition.

EMPHYSEMA

- *Findings*: Barrel-shaped chest, exhalation through pursed lips (increases airway pressure and prevents airway collapse).
- *Centriacinar*: Associated with smoking. Frequently in upper lobes.
- *Panacinar*: Associated with 1-antitrypsin deficiency. Frequently in lower lobes.
- Enlargement of air spaces → increased compliance, reduced D from destruction of alveolar walls. Imbalance of proteases and antiproteases → increased elastase activity → loss of elastic fi bers → increased lung compliance

241. A 35-year-old male, non smoker, non alcoholic suffered from long history of cough, sputum and dyspnea and died following a bout of lobar pneumonia. Lung autopsy is shown below. What is the likely pathology shown here? *(NEET 2020)*

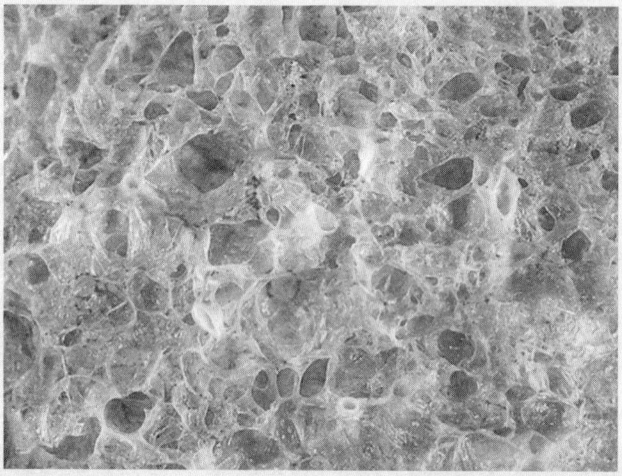

a. Mutation in dynein arms of cilia
b. Cystic fibrosis
c. Alpha1 antitrypsin deficiency
d. Antibodies against type 4 collagen

Ans. is 'c' Alpha1 antitrypsin deficiency

Explanation: Autopsy specimen shows marked emphysematous damage involving the entire pulmonary lobule – Panacinar emphysema.

242. Condition not associated with bronchiectasis is: *(NEET 2016)*

a. Pericarditis
b. Lung cancer
c. Amyloidosis
d. Hemoptysis

Ans. is 'b' Lung cancer

243. Chronic bronchitis is associated with: *(NEET 2016)*

a. Increase in number of glands without any change in size
b. Bronchiolitis obliterans
c. Decrease in Reid index
d. Only large airways are involved

Ans. is 'b' Bronchiolitis obliterans

244. Which lobe in the lungs is most commonly involved in bronchiectasis: *(NEET 2016)*

a. Right upper lobe
b. Right middle lobe
c. Left upper lobe
d. Left lower lobe

Ans. is 'd' Left lower lobe

245. Pink puffers are associated with: *(NEET 2016)*

a. Emphysema
b Chronic bronchitis
c. Pneumonia
d. Bronchiectasis

Ans. is 'a' Emphysema

Lung Carcinoma

Different Genes Involved in Lung Carcinoma

- c-MYC and RB: Small cell cancer
- RAS and p16: Non-small cell cancer

Pathology

- p53: Both small and non-small cell, but highest in squamous cell carcinoma
- K-RAS: Adenocarcinoma
- Adenocarcinoma is the overall most common type of lung carcinoma.
- Adenocarcinoma is the most common type of lung carcinoma in non-smokers and females.
- Squamous cell (epidermoid) carcinoma is the most common type of lung carcinoma in India.
- Squamous cell carcinoma is the most common type of lung carcinoma in smokers and males.
- MC variety in young Patients → Adenocarcinoma
- Histological variety that cavitates → Squamous cell Ca
- MC Histological variety to metastasize → Small cell Ca
- Ca which metastasize to opposite lung → Adenocarcinoma
- Clubbing least common in which Ca → Small cell Ca
- Gynecomastia is seen in which type of Ca → Large cell Ca
- Thrombophlebitis is seen with which Ca→ Adenocarcinoma
- Most common site for metastasis from ca lung → Brain
- Lung Ca with worst prognosis → Small cell Ca
- Variety most responsive to chemotherapy → Small cell Ca
- Variety most responsive to radiotherapy → Small cell Ca
- MC Endocrine gland to be involved by metastasis → Adrenal
- Variety with best prognosis → Squamous cell Ca
- In relative order of frequency, metastatic tumor to lung originate from carcinoma in the breast, colon, stomach, pancreas, kidney, prostate, liver, thyroid, adrenal, male genital tract and female genital tract. Sarcomas from bone, soft tissues and visceral sites are prone to disseminate via blood stream and frequently metastasize to lung

246. Deficiency of p53 mutation is maximum in which lung carcinoma? *(NEET 2016)*

a. Small cell carcinoma
b. Squamous cell carcinoma
c. Adenocarcinoma
d. Lymphoma

Ans. is 'b' Squamous cell carcinoma

247. Tumor suppressor gene responsible for lung squamous cell carcinoma is: *(NEET 2016)*

a. p53
b. Rb
c. PTEN
d. p63

Ans. is 'a' p53

248. Most common variety of lung carcinoma in women and children is: *(NEET 2016)*

a. Small cell carcinoma
b. Adenocarcinoma
c. Squamous cell carcinoma
d. Large cell carcinoma

Ans. is 'b' Adenocarcinoma

249. Lung cancer most commonly associated with smoking: *(NEET 2016)*

a. Small cell carcinoma
b. Adenocarcinoma
c. Squamous cell carcinoma
d. Large cell carcinoma

Ans. is 'c' Squamous cell carcinoma

250. Metastasis to lungs come most commonly from: *(NEET 2016)*

a. Breast carcinoma
b. Brain carcinoma
c. Bone carcinoma
d. Melanoma

Ans. is 'a' Breast carcinoma

Sarcoidosis

- Sarcoidosis is an immune system disorder characterized by the presence of non-caseating granulomas (aggregate of tightly clustered epithelioid cells, often with langhans or foreign body type giant cells. Central necrosis is unusual).
- Granulomas most often appear in the lung or the lymph nodes —Bilateral hilar lymphadenopathy or lung involvement is visible on chest radiograph in 90% of cases.

Histology

- Noncaseating epithelioid granulomas with tightly packed epithelioid cells, Langhans giant cells and lymphocytes (T cells), usually in interstitium adjacent to bronchioles and around and within vessel walls, pleura and connective tissue septa
- May also be hyalinization, diffuse interstitial fibrosis, fibrinoid necrosis, fibrosis within granulomas, intra- and extracellular inclusions
- Pleural involvement in 10%
- *Schaumann bodies*: Laminated concretions of calcium and protein

- *Asteroid bodies*: Stellate inclusions within giant cells, in 60% of granulomas
- Neither is specific for sarcoid (also seen in Berylliosis)
- *Necrotizing sarcoid granulomatosis*: Extensive, vascular, noncaseating sarcoid-like granulomas invading pulmonary arteries and veins with diffuse necrosis of lung parenchyma.

Clinical Features

Lung and Lymph Nodes (95%)

- Respiratory complaints including cough and dyspnea are the most common presenting symptoms. Usually the infiltrate in sarcoidosis are predominantly an upper lobe process. There is bilateral hilar lymphadenopathy.
- 'Potato nodes' are seen in sarcoidosis.

Skin (24–43%)

- Skin lesions include erythma nodosum, maculopapular lesion, subcutaneous nodules, hypo or hyperpigmentation, keloid formation and lupus pernio.
- Lupus pernio is involvement of bridge of nose, area beneath the eyes and cheek. It is diagnostic for a chronic form of sarcoidosis.

Eye (12–29%)

- Eye lesions include uveitis, retinitis, pars planitis and dry eye due to lacrimal gland involvement.
- Uveoparotid fever (Heerfordt-Waldenstrom syndrome) include classical triad of Uveitis, parotitis and 7th nerve palsy.

Other Organs Involved

These are salivary glands particularly parotid (causing dry mouth), spleen (splenomegaly), liver, heart and brain (neurosarcoidosis). Granuloma in sarcoidosis can secrete 1-25 (OH)2 vitamin-D which causes hypercalcemia. Heerfordt syndrome or uveoparotid fever, is an uncommon acute presentation of sarcoidosis manifesting as fever, parotid and lacrimal gland enlargement, uveitis, bilateral hilar adenopathy and often cranial neuropathy.

251. Uveo-parotitis is seen in: *(NEET 2016)*

a. SLE
b. Sjogren's syndrome
c. Rheumatoid arthritis
d. Sarcoidosis

Ans. is 'd' Sarcoidosis

252. True about sarcoidosis is: *(NEET 2016)*

a. Skin is the most common organ involved
b. Premalignant condition
c. Non-caseating granuloma
d. May be associated with hypocalcemia

Ans. is 'c' Non-caseating granuloma

Miscellaneous

253. Vitamin deficiency associated with cystic fibrosis is: *(NEET 2016)*

a. K
b. B6
c. C
d. B12

Ans. is 'a' K

Patients with cystic fibrosis (CF) are at risk of developing deficiencies of fat-soluble vitamins (A, D, E, and K) because of pancreatic insufficiency, hepatobiliary disease, or both.

254. In allergic bronchopulmonary aspergillosis, the location of lesion is: *(NEET 2016)*

a. Pleura
b. Bronchi and bronchioles
c. Alveoli
d. All of the above

Ans. is 'b' Bronchi and bronchioles

Allergic bronchopulmonary, aspergillosis (ABPA) is a condition characterised by a hypersensitivity response to the Aspergillus (most commonly Aspergillus fumigatus). It occurs most often in patients with asthma or cystic fibrosis. ABPA causes airway inflammation, leading to bronchiectasis._a condition marked by abnormal dilation of the bronchi and bronchioles.

255. Heart failure cells are seen in: *(NEET 2016)*

a. Pulmonary infarction
b. Pulmonary edema
c. Pneumonia
d. Pulmonary embolism

Ans. is 'b' Pulmonary edema

- Heart failure cells are hemosiderin laden alveolar macrophages.
- Heart failure cells are a manifestation of pulmonary congestion and edema (as seen in heart failure).

256. Alpha-1 antitrypsin works by:

a. Inhibition of trypsin
b. Inhibition of trypsinogen
c. Inhibition of elastase
d. Inhibition of chymotrypsin

Ans. is 'c' Inhibition of elastase

Alpha-1 antitrypsin (A1AT) is produced in the liver, and one of its functions is to protect the lungs from neutrophil elastase, an enzyme that can disrupt connective tissue.

GASTROINTESTINAL TRACT

WHO HISTOLOGICAL CLASSIFICATION OF GASTRIC TUMORS

Intraepithelial neoplasia	Non- epithelial tumors
• Adenoma • Carcinoma – Adenocarcinoma – Intestinal type – Diffuse type	• Leiomyoma • Schwannoma • Granular cell tumor • Glomus tumor • Leiomyosarcoma
– Papillary adenocarcinoma – Tubular adenocarcinoma – Mucinous adenocarcinoma potential – Signet-ring cell carcinoma – Adenosquamous carcinoma – Squamous cell carcinoma – Small cell carcinoma – Undifferentiated carcinoma – Others • Carcinoid (well differentiated endocrine neoplasm)	• GI stromal tumor – Benign – Uncertain malignant – Malignant • Kaposi sarcoma • Others • Malignant lymphoma

RISK FACTORS FOR GASTRIC CARCINOMA

Genetic factors	Environmental factors	Other factors
Sex	*Helicobacter pylori*	Gastric adenomas
Familial adenomatous polyposis	Epstein-Barr virus	Barrett's esophagus
Hereditary nonpolyposis colorectal cancer (Lynch II)	Nitrites	Hamartomas
Genetic diffuse gastric cancer (E-cadherin-CDH1 mutation)	Excess alcohol ingestion	Menetier's disease
Genetic polymorphisms for pro- and anti-inflammatory cytokines	High intake of salted, pickled, or smoked foods	Chronic atrophic gastritis
Polymorphisms for cell receptors of innate immune response	Low intake of fiber, fruits and vegetables	Gastric metaplasia
Peutz-Jeghers syndrome	Antioxidant consumption (especially ascorbic acid, carotenoids, folates and tocopherols)	Pernicious anemia
Blood group A	Tobacco smoking (adenocarcinoma of cardia)	Benign gastric ulcers
		Fundic gland polyps
		Hyperplastic polyps
		Gastric biopsy revealing high-grade dysplasia
		History of subtotal gastrectomy (> 20 year)

257. Which of the following is an epithelial tumor of stomach? *(NEET 2018)*

a. Leiomyosarcoma
b. Lymphoma
c. GIST
d. Gastric adenocarcinoma

Ans. is 'd' Gastric adenocarcinoma

258. Most common type of gastric carcinoma is: *(NEET 2016)*

a. Squamous cell carcinoma
b. Adenocarcinoma
c. Lymphoma
d. Leiomyosarcoma

Ans. is 'b' Adenocarcinoma

259. Blood group most commonly associated with gastric carcinoma is: *(NEET 2016)*

a. Blood Group O
b. Blood Group A
c. Blood Group AB
d. Blood Group B

Ans. is 'b' Blood Group A

WHIPPLE'S DISEASE

Microscopic (Histologic) Appearance

Noncaseating Granulomas

- Numerous foamy macrophages in lamina propria containing PAS+ (diastase resistant) granules and rod shaped bacilli by EM
- Dilated lymphatics or fat vacuoles
- Often multinucleated giant cells; rarely epithelioid granulomas in minority
- In mesentery or retroperitoneal nodes, resembles lipogranulomatous inflammation with round empty spaces.

260. Biopsy of small intestine with foamy macrophages are seen. What is the diagnosis? *(NEET 2018)*

a. Whipple's disease
b. Abetalipoproteinemia
c. Lysosomal disorder
d. Giardiasis

Ans. is 'a' Whipple's disease

SQUAMOUS CELL CARCINOMA OF ESOPHAGUS

Squamous cell carcinoma is the most common type of esophageal carcinoma worldwide and in India. It usually occurs in middle 1/3" (not common) and upper 1/3'" of esophagus. Some may also arise in lower 1/3".

- *Distribution*: 20%—upper third
- 50%—middle third
- 30%—lower third
- Morphologic patterns
- Polypoid exophytic
- Flat
- Ulcerative
- Most are moderately/well differentiated

261. Carcinoma associated most commonly with upper one third of esophagus is: *(NEET 2016)*

a. Adenocarcinoma
b. Squamous cell carcinoma
c. Adenosquamous carcinoma
d. Leiomyosarcoma

Ans. is 'b' Squamous cell carcinoma

GIST

- GISTs are the most common mesenchymal neoplasm of gastrointestinal tract. GIST represents a distinct group of gastrointestinal tumors that originate from the interstitial cells of cajal which control gastrointestinal peristalsis.
- GISTs can occur anywhere in the gastrointestinal tract; the most common site being the stomach followed by small intestine.
- The most useful marker of GIST is c-kit (CD-1 17). Other markers are CD 34, smooth muscle actin and vimentin.
- Although CD 117 (c- kit) is considered the most specific marker for GIST. It is not pathognomonic of GIST as other tumors may also express CD 117. These tumors include mast cell tumor, germ cell tumors (seminomas), leukemias, malignant melanoma, angiolipomas, and some sarcomas.

262. Most common organ involved in GIST: *(NEET 2016)*

a. Ileum
b. Duodenum
c. Colon
d. Stomach

Ans. is 'd' Stomach

263. GIST associated marker is: *(NEET 2016)*

a. CD 117
b. CD34
c. CD 23
d. S-100

Ans. is 'a' CD 117

BARRETT'S ESOPHAGUS

- Barrett's esophagus is a metaplasia in which normal squamous epithelium of lower part of esophagus is replaced by columnar epithelium due to prolonged esophageal reflux.
- Most common type of metaplasia in Barrett's esophagus is intestinal metaplasia which is characterized by presence of intestinal goblet cells in the metaplastic columnar epithelium.
- The squamocolumnar junction normally may occur anywhere within the distal 2–3 cm esophagus. Proximal extension of the squamocolumnar junction beyond the distal 2–3 cm of esophagus is abnormal and is suggestive of Barrett's esophagus.

Types

- Long segment Barrett's esophagus (LSBE)
- Short segment Barrett's esophagus (SSBE)

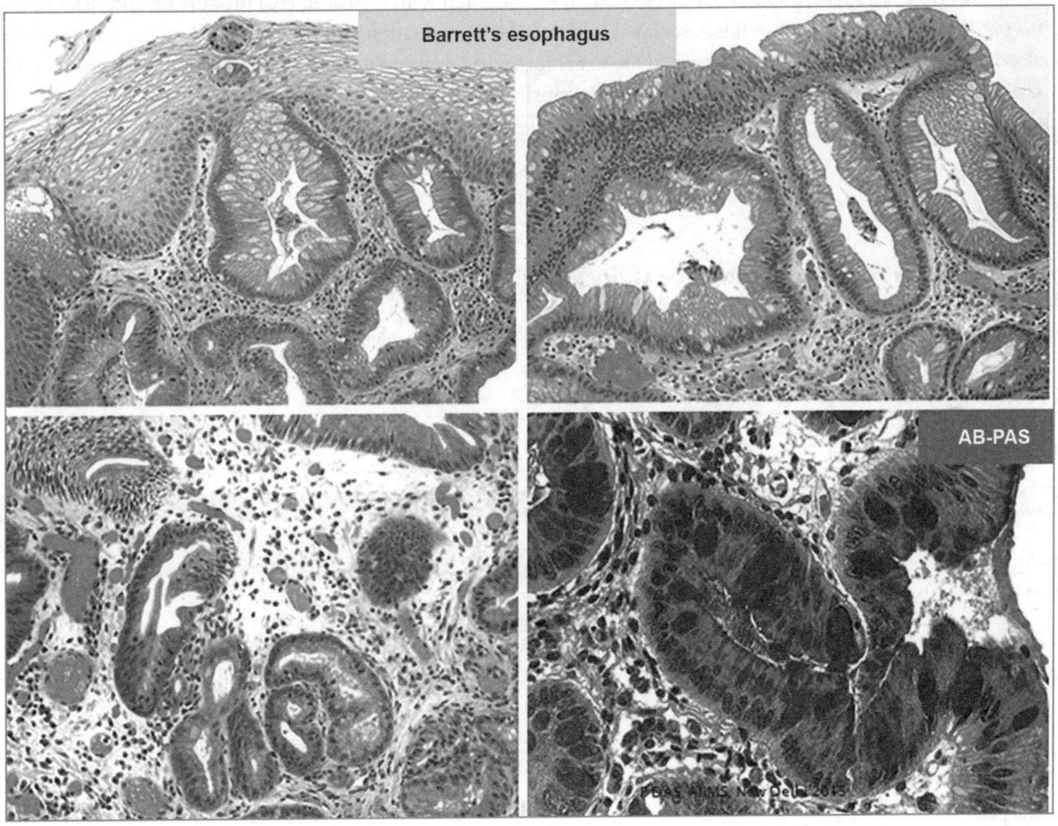

- **True esophageal adenocarcinomas** are unusual
- The majority arise from the Barrett's mucosa
- The life time risk for cancer development from Barrett esophagus is approximately 10%
- Usually arise from the distal third and most of them are mucin producing
- Poor prognosis than other forms esophageal cancer
- M/I risk factor for adenocarcinoma of the distal esophagus is Barrett's, irrespective of the length of the segment with intestinal metaplasia

264. Normally squamocolumnar junction is usually located at: *(NEET 2016)*

a. Distal 2–3 cm of esophagus
b. Proximal 2–3 cm of stomach
c. In esophagus more than 3 cm proximal to GEJ
d. None of the above

Ans. is 'a' Distal 2–3 cm of esophagus

265. True about Barrett's esophagus is: *(NEET 2016)*

a. More incidence of adenocarcinoma
b. Squamous metaplasia
c. Most commonly in upper one third of esophagus
d. All are true

Ans. is 'a' More incidence of adenocarcinoma

GASTRITIS

Type 'A' Gastritis (Autoimmune Gastritis)

- The two important autoantibodies causing damage are anti-parietal cell antibodies (most common) and antibodies against intrinsic factor; anti-IF (most specific). Anti-parietal cell antibodies are directed against proton pump ($H^+ K^+$ ATPase). The effect of these antibodies are: - *Achlorhydria*: Due to loss of parietal cells.
- *Vitamin B-12 deficiency and pernicious anemia*: Due to deficiency of IF cells (secreted by parietal cells) as well as damage of IF by anti-IF antibodies.
- *Antral endocrine cell hyperplasia (G-call hyperplasia)*: Due achlorhydria (normally gastric acid has inhibitory effect on G-cells).
- *Reduced serum pepsinogen I*: Only pepsinogen I is reduced (pepsinogen II is normal).

Type 'B' Gastritis (H. Pylori associated Gastritis)

- *Antral predominant gastritis (Type B chronic atrophic gastritis)*: It is associated with increased HCl production and risk of duodenal ulcer.
- *Pangastritis (multifocal atrophic gastritis)*: It is associated with low HCl production and higher risk of gastric adenocarcinoma.
- *Antral endocrine cell hyperplasia (G-cell hyperplasia)*: Due to achlorhydria (normally gastric acid has inhibitory effect on G-cells).
- *Reduced serum pepsinogen I*: Only pepsinogen I is reduced (pepsinogen II is normal)

266. Autoimmune gastritis is associate with deficiency of vitamin: *(NEET 2016)*

a. A
b. B12
c. C
d. D

Ans. is 'b' B12

267. Which of the following is most likely to be associated with type A gastritis resulting from autoimmune destruction of parietal cells? *(NEET 2016)*

a. Pernicious anemia
b. Atrophic gastritis
c. Pangastritis
d. All of the above

Ans. is 'a' Pernicious anemia

SMALL BOWEL BIOPSY

Lesion seen on a small bowel biopsy		
Specific		*Non specific (Biopsy is not diagnostic)*
Diffuse specific	*Patchy specific*	*Diffuse nonspecific*
Whipples disease	• Intestinal lymphoma • Intestinal lymphangiectasia • Eosinophilic gastroenteritis • Amyloidosis • Crohn's disease • Infection by one or more microorganisms • Mastocytosis	• Celiac sprue • Tropical sprue • Bacterial overgrowth • Folate deficiency • Vitamin B12 deficiency • Radiation enteritis • Zollinger-Ellison syndrome • Protein-calorie malnutrition • Drug-induced enteritis
Agammaglobulinemia		
Abetalipoproteinemia		

268. Which of the following diseases is diagnosed by jejunal biopsy? *(NEET 2016)*

a Celiac disease
b. Intestinal lymphoma
c. Argentaffinoma of intestine
d. Tropical sprue

Ans. is 'b' Intestinal lymphoma

HIRSCHSPRUNG DISEASE

- Hirschsprung disease (Congenital aganglionic megacolon) is caused by defective migration of neural crest into the mesodermal layer of gut. There is aganglionosis (absence of ganglions) in a portion of intestinal tract. Intestinal segment lacks both Meissner submucosal and Auerbach myenteric plexuses.
- Total colonic aganglionosis (Zuelzer-Wilson syndrome) is particular variant of Hirschsprung's disease (5–8% cases) in which aganglionic portion extends to entire length of colon. In rare cases aganglionosis may extent from duodenum to rectum.

269. What is the embryological basis of Hirschsprung disease? *(NEET 2020)*

a. Failure of migration of neural crest cells in intestine
b. Failure of canalization of gut tube
c. Atresia of distal colon
d. Failure of neuroendocrine relaxation

Ans. is 'a' Failure of migration of neural crest cells in intestine

270. Total colonic aganglionosis is a variant of: *(NEET 2016)*

a. Crohn's disease
b. Ulcerative colitis
c. Hirschsprung's disease
d. Tropical sprue

Ans. is 'c' Hirschsprung's disease

PATHOGENESIS OF ACHALASIA CARDIA

- Achalasia cardia is a disorder of esophageal smooth muscles. The most common type of achalasia is primary achalasia with unknown etiology. Secondary achalasia may occur in Chaga's disease (Trypanosoma Cruzi), Allgrove syndrome (Triple A syndrome), multiple endocrine neoplasia, and cancer invading LES (Pseudoachalasia).
- It is due to dysfunction of inhibitory neurons containing nitric oxide and vasoactive intestinal polypeptide in the distal esophagus, The cholinergic innervation of the LES is intact or affected only in the advanced stage.
- The degenerative changes are either intrinsic (degeneration of ganglion cells of Auerbach's myenteric plexus) or extrinsic (extra esophageal vagus nerve or the dorsal motor nucleus of vagus).
- As a result of the abnormality; LES fails to relax and there is progressive dilatation of esophagus above the level of LES.
- Both sexes are equally affected. There is progressive dysphagia for both solids and liquids (in initial stages, dysphagia is more for the liquids than for solids). Other features may include regurgitation and pulmonary aspiration, and esophagitis with ulceration.
- It is due to dysfunction of inhibitory neurons containing nitric oxide and vasoactive intestinal polypeptide in the distal intestine. The cholinergic innervation of the LES is intact or affected only in the advanced stage. There is neurogenic degeneration either idiopathic or due to infection. As a result of the abnormality, LES fails to relax and there is progressive dilatation of esophagus above the level of LES
- The degenerative changes are either intrinsic (degeneration of ganglion cells of Auerbach's myenteric plexus) or extrinsic (extra esophageal vagus nerve or the dorsal motor nucleus of vagus).

271. Achalasia cardia true statement is: *(NEET 2020)*

a. Decreased esophageal peristalsis
b. Decreased resting LES tone
c. Decreased release of NO and VIP at lower end of esophagus
d. Premature esophageal contractions

Ans. is 'c' Decreased release of NO and VIP at lower end of esophagus

272. True about esophageal motility disorder is: *(NEET 2016)*

a. Dysphagia to solid food only
b. Cholinergic nerve endings are affected first
c. More common in males
d. Primary achalasia is more common than secondary

Ans. is 'd' Primary achalasia is more common than secondary

273. Pathology in achalasia cardia is: *(NEET 2016)*

a. Degeneration of nerves
b. Muscular atrophy
c. Hypertrophy of nerves
d. Hypertrophy of muscles

Ans. is 'a' Degeneration of nerves

PREMALIGNANT LESIONS FOR ORAL CANCER

- Leukoplakia is the most common premalignant lesions.
- The risk of malignant transformation of erythroplakia is much higher than that seen with leukoplakia.
- The most common predisposing factor for both these conditions is smoking.

274. True about erythroplakia is: *(NEET 2016)*

a. Most common malignant premalignant lesion of oral mucosa
b. More malignant capacity than leukoplakia
c. Most common risk factor is alcohol consumption
d. Most common site in oral cavity is the floor of the mouth

Ans. is 'b' More malignant capacity than leukoplakia

RISK FACTORS ASSOCIATED WITH ORAL CANDIDIASIS

Wearing Dentures

- A course of antibiotic medicine
- Excessive use of antibacterial mouthwash
- Taking steroid tablets or inhalers

- Dry mouth
- Diabetes
- Severe anemia (Iron, folate or vitamin B12 deficiency)
- Immunosuppression
- General poor health
- Smoking.

275. Which of the following is not associated with oral candidiasis? (NEET 2016)

a. Smoking
b. Severe anemia
c. Alcoholism
d. Antibiotic treatment

Ans. is 'c' Alcoholism

INFLAMMATORY BOWEL DISEASE

Feature	Crohn disease	Ulcerative colitis
Macroscopic		
Bowel region	Ileum ± colon	Colon only
Distribution	Skip lesions	Diffuse
Stricture	Yes	Rare
Wall appearance	Thick	Thin
Microscopic		
Inflammation	Transmural	Limited to mucosa
Pseudopolyps	Moderate	Marked
Ulcers	Deep, knife-like	Superficial, broad-based
Lymphoid reaction	Marked	Moderate
Fibrosis	Marked	Mild to none
Serositis	Marked	Mild to none
Granulomas	Yes (~ 35%)	No
Fistulae/sinuses	Yes	No
Clinical		
Perianal fistula	Yes (in colonic disease)	No
Fat/Vitamin malabsorption	Yes	No
Malignant potential	With colonic involvement	Yes
Recurrence after surgery	Common	No
Toxic megacolon	No	Yes

276. In ulcerative colitis and Crohn's disease, what is the histological difference between them? (NEET 2019)

a. Diffuse distribution of pseudopolyps
b. Mucosal edema
c. Crypt abscess
d. Lymphoid aggregates in mucosa

Ans. is 'c' Crypt abscess

277. Characteristic feature of Crohn's disease is: (NEET 2016)

a. Skip lesions
b. Toxic megacolon
c. Fibrosisis rare
d. Involvement is superficial

Ans. is 'a' Skip lesions

278. Best differentiating feature between ulcerative colitis and Crohn's disease is: (NEET 2016)

a. Distributions of pseudopolyps
b. Mucosal edema
c. Crypt abscesses
d. Lymphoid aggregate in the mucosa

Ans. is 'a' Distributions of pseudopolyps

279. Collar button ulcer is found in: (NEET 2016)

a. Ulcerative colitis
b. Crohn's disease
c. Shigella
d. All of the above

Ans. is 'd' All of the above

DIAGNOSIS OF CELIAC DISEASE

- The definitive diagnosis is based on histopathological findings which show: *Villous atrophy and Crypt hyperplasia with decrease in villus*: crypt ratio.
- Loss of microvilli brush border.
- *Inflammatory cells are present in lamina propria*: plasma cells, macrophages, lymphocytes, eosinophils and mast cells.
- One of the characteristic features is that overall mucosal thickness remains same (as villous atrophy is compensated by crypt hyperplasia).
- Mainly proximal intestine is involved.
- Other characteristic diagnostic finding is symptom resolution on gluten free diet.
- The most sensitive non-invasive serological tests are the presence of IgA antibodies to tissue transglutaminase or IgA/IgG antibodies to deamidated gliadin. Anti-endomysial antibodies are highly specific but less sensitive.

280. An 8-month-old infant who was recently weaned from breast milk presented with malabsorptive diarrhea and failure to thrive. Biopsy from duodenum revealed villous atrophy, crypt hyperplasia and CD8+ cell infiltrates in lamina propria. What is the likely diagnosis? *(NEET 2020)*

a. Environmental enteropathy
b. Celiac disease
c. Tropical sprue
d. Whipples disease

Ans. is 'b' Celiac disease

281. Histopathological finding of gluten hypersensitivity is: *(NEET 2016)*

a. Crypt hyperplasia
b. Increase in thickness of the mucosa
c. Distal intestine involvement
d. Villous hypertrophy

Ans. is 'a' Crypt hyperplasia

282. Antigliadin antibodies are seen in: *(NEET 2016)*

a. Tropical sprue
b. Whipple's disease
c. Celiac disease
d. Intestinal lymphoma

Ans. is 'c' Celiac disease

Phlegmonous Gastritis

- Life threatening condition
- Characterized by suppurative bacterial infection of gastric wall
- Predisposing factors: Immunosuppression
- Disability
- Gastritis
- Chronic alcoholism

Causative Organisms

- *Streptococci* (mainly)
- *Staphylococci*
- *Hemophilus influenzae*
- *E. coli*
- *Proteus sp.*

283. Phlegmonous gastritis occurs due to: *(NEET 2016)*

a. *H. Pylori*
b. *E. Coli*
c. *C. Jejuni*
d. *Cl. Tetani*

Ans. is 'b' *E. Coli*

Miscellaneous

284. Newly erupted tooth is covered by: *(NEET 2018)*

a. Perikymata
b. Nasmyth's membrane
c. Fibrous tissue
d. All of the above

Ans. is 'b' Nasmyth's membrane

Primary enamel cuticle also called Nasmyth's membrane is thin membrane of tissue also known as reduced enamel epithelium (REE) produced by the ameloblast that covers the tooth once it has erupted.

285. Most common benign tumor of esophagus is: *(NEET 2016)*

a. Lipoma
b. Fibroma
c. Leiomyoma
d. Lymphangioma

Ans. is 'c' Leiomyoma

Tumors of smooth muscle origin, leiomyomas are most common; fibromas, lipomas, hemangiomas, neurofibromas bromas and lymphangiomas also occur.

286. In a patient with lipoprotein lipase deficiency, which of these is increased following a fatty meal?

a. Chylomicron
b. LDL
c. HDL
d. Apo-A

Ans. is 'a' Chylomicron

Lipoprotein lipase deficiency (Type I hyperlipoproteinemia): is a rare, autosomal recessive disorder caused by a deficiency of lipoprotein lipase. Resulting in fasting chylomicronemia and hypertriglycerolemia. There is slow clearance of chylomicrons and VLDL. Low levels of LDL and HDL. There is no increased risk of coronary disease.

GASTROINTESTINAL POLYPOSIS SYNDROMES

- *Familial adenomatous polyposis:* Autosomal dominant mutation of APC tumor suppressor gene on chromosome 5q22. 2-hit hypothesis. Thousands of polyps arise starting after puberty; pancolonic; always involves rectum. Prophylactic colectomy or else 100% progress to CRC.
- *Gardner syndrome:* FAP + osseous and soft tissue tumors (e.g., osteomas of skull or mandible), congenital hypertrophy of retinal pigment epithelium, impacted/supernumerary teeth.
- *Turcot syndrome*: FAP or Lynch syndrome + malignant CNS tumor (e.g., medulloblastoma, glioma)
- *Peutz-Jeghers syndrome*: Autosomal dominant syndrome featuring numerous hamartomas throughout GI tract, along with hyperpigmented macules on mouth, lips, hands, genitalia. Associated with increased risk of breast and GI cancers (e.g., colorectal, stomach, small bowel, pancreatic).
- *Juvenile polyposis syndrome*: Autosomal dominant syndrome in children (typically < 5 years old) featuring numerous hamartomatous polyps in the colon, stomach, small bowel. Associated with increased risk of CRC.
- *Lynch syndrome:* Previously known as hereditary nonpolyposis colorectal cancer (HNPCC). Autosomal dominant mutation of DNA mismatch repair genes with subsequent microsatellite instability. ~ 80% progress to CRC. Proximal colon is always involved. Associated with endometrial, ovarian, and skin cancers.

287. A 5-year-old child presented with rectal bleeding. He has a polypoidal mass located in the rectum. The biopsy is shown in the image below. What is the likely diagnosis for this patient? *(NEET 2020)*

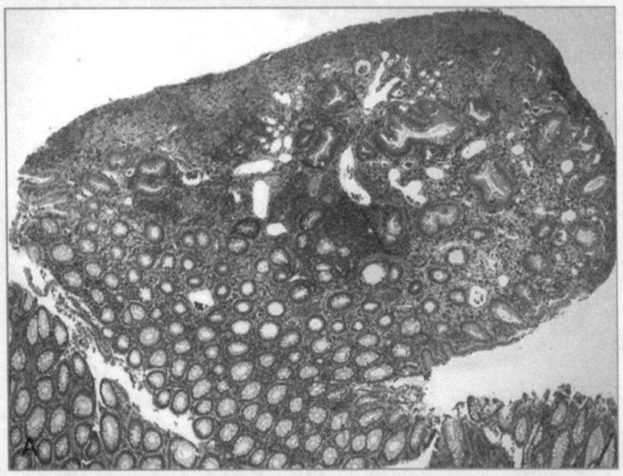

a. Serrated adenoma
b. Villous adenoma
c. Angiodysplasia
d. Juvenile polyp

Ans. is 'd' Juvenile polyp

Explanation: Biopsy shows multiple cystically dilated glands filled with mucin and inflammatory debris; suggestive of juvenile polyp.

LIVER, GALLBLADDER AND THE PANCREAS

HEPATIC STELLATE CELLS

HSCs (hepatic stellate cells) (also called vitamin A-storing cells, lipocytes, interstitial cells, fat-storing cells or Ito cells) exist in the space between parenchymal cells and liver sinusoidal endothelial cells of the hepatic lobule and store 50–80% of vitamin A in the whole body as retinyl palmitate in lipid droplets in the cytoplasm.

288. Vitamin A is stored in:

a. Cells of Ito
b. Hepatocyte
c. Endothelial cell
d. Kupffer cell

Ans. is 'a' Cells of Ito

HSCs (hepatic stellate cells) (also called vitamin A-storing cells, lipocytes, interstitial cells, fat-storing cells or Ito cells) exist in the space between parenchymal cells and liver sinusoidal endothelial cells of the hepatic lobule and store 50-80% of vitamin A in the whole body as retinyl palmitate in lipid droplets in the cytoplasm.

Amebic Liver Disease

- Amebic liver abscess is the most common extraintestinal manifestation of amebiasis (primary site of infection is intestine).
- Most common in postero-superior surface of the right lobe. Usually there is one large solitary abscess.
- The necrotic contents of liver abscess are classically described as anchovy-sauce pus.
- Although colon is the primary site of infection, diarrhea is not common.
- Common clinical features are right upper quadrant pain, fever, weight loose and hepatomegaly.
- Pleuropulmonary involvement is the most frequent complication of amebic liver abscess.
- Erythrophagocytosis is seen in amebiasis.
- Metronidazole is the drug of choice. Response is dramatic.

289. Amebic liver disease is characterized by: *(NEET 2016)*

a. Most common in right lobe of the liver
b. Diarrhea is the most common presentation
c. Resistant to metronidazole
d. Liver is the most common primary site of infection

Ans. is 'a' Most common in right lobe of the liver

Mitogenic factors involved in hepatic regeneration:

Hepatocyte growth factor (HGF/ scatter factor) levels rise to high levels soon after partial hepatectomy. This is the only factor tested that acts by itself as a potent mitogen for isolated hepatocytes cultured in vitro. This factor is also of critical importance in development of the liver, as target deletions of its gene lead to fetal death due to hepatic insufficiency.

- TNF-alpha, which stimulates proliferation of hepatic endothelial cells.
- Interleukin-6, which acts as a biliary epithelial mitogen.
- Epidermal growth factor and transforming growth factor-α (TGF-α)
- Norepinephrine potentiates the mitogenic activity of EGF and HGF.

290. What is responsible for regeneration of liver cells: *(NEET 2016)*

a. HGF
b. VEGF
c. TGF-β
d. IFN-γ

Ans. is 'a' HGF

HEPATOCELLULAR CARCINOMA

Clinical Features

- *Symptoms*: Abdominal pain, ascites, hepatomegaly and obstructive jaundice; also systemic manifestations
- *Laboratory*: Elevated serum AFP (70% sensitive); AFP sensitivity reduced in alcohol related cirrhosis (65% sensitive), tumors arising in noncirrhotic liver (33% sensitive), tumors 2 cm or less (25% sensitive)
- *Screening*: Recommended to use ultrasound and serum AFP in patients with chronic liver disease; leads to diagnosis of tumors 2 cm or less, may not reduce deaths; des-gamma-carboxy prothrombin (DCP/protein induced by vitamin K absence or antagonist II/ PIVKAII): more specific than serum AFP and marker of poor prognosis; abnormal prothrombin produced by HCC, associated with early portal vein invasion, intrahepatic metastasis and capsular infiltration
- *Other causes of elevated serum AFP*: Chronic hepatitis, cirrhosis, fetal death, fetal neural tube defect, fetal distress, hepatoblastoma, hepatoid adenocarcinoma, massive liver necrosis, normal pregnancy, yolk sac tumors of gonads
- *Metastases*: Initially within liver, distant metastases late to adrenal gland, bone, lung, porta hepatis lymph nodes
- *Classification*: Either **small** (< 2 cm) or advanced (2 cm or more).

Microscopic (Histologic) Description

- Patterns are trabecular (most common) with 4+ cells surrounded by layer of flattened endothelial cells; also clear cell, giant cell, pelioid (vascular lakes), pseudoglandular (acinar with proteinaceous material or bile in lumina, may resemble thyroid follicles), sarcomatoid, solid (compact).
- **Fibrolamellar carcinoma (fibrolamellar variant of HCC).** It is a distinctive variant of hepatocellular carcinoma. It is seen in young adults (20–40 yrs of age). It has equal sex incidence. It has better prognosis. It has no association with HBV or cirrhosis. It is grossly encapsulated mass. APP elevation is not seen in Fibrolamellar Ca.
- Presence of sinusoidal vessels surrounding tumor cells is an important diagnostic feature.

291. HCC marker is: *(NEET 2016)*

a. CEA
b. AFP
c. CA-125
d. HMB99

Ans. is 'b' AFP

292. Immature variant of HCC is: *(NEET 2016)*

a. Pseudoglandular
b. Fibrolamellar
c. Pleomorphic
d. Giant cell

Ans. is 'b' Fibrolamellar

CHRONIC HEPATITIS

Chronic hepatitis is divided into following types:

- *Chronic active hepatitis*: There is active continuing necrosis of liver cells. There is disruption of limiting plate of hepatocytes, causing inflammation of both parenchyma and portal tracts.
- Characteristic features are:
  - Portal fibrosis (fibrosis of porta hepatis)
  - Bridging necrosis
  - Piecemeal necrosis
  - Interface hepatitis.
- *Chronic persistent hepatitis*: Inflammation is mild and restricted to portal tracts with no disruption of limiting plates. Lobular architecture is maintained with minimal or no necrosis and fibrosis.

293. Bridging necrosis is seen in: *(NEET 2016)*

a. Alcoholic liver disease
b. Chronic persistent hepatitis
c. Non- alcoholic fatty liver disease
d. Chronic active hepatitis

Ans. is 'd' Chronic active hepatitis

Mallory Bodies

- Mallory bodies are eosinophilic intracytoplasmic inclusion bodies which are composed predominantly of keratin intermediate filaments. They are also known as alcoholic hyaline.
- These inclusions are characteristic but not specific feature of alcoholic liver disease, as they are also seen in other conditions such as:
  - Alcoholic liver disease
  - Primary biliary cirrhosis
  - Indian childhood cirrhosis
  - Wilson's disease
  - Hepatocellular carcinoma
  - Focal nodular hyperplasia
  - Chronic cholestatic syndrome
  - α1 - antitrypsin deficiency.

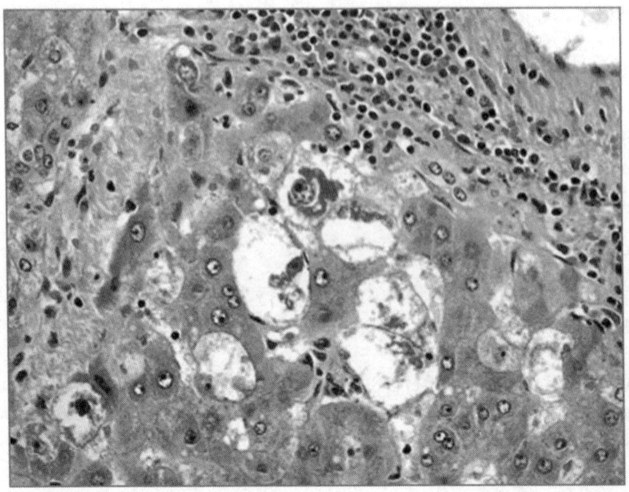

294. Mallory bodies are seen in:	*(NEET 2016)*
a. Hepatitis B infection	b. Hydatid cyst
c. α1-antitrypsin deficiency	d. Autoimmune hepatitis

Ans. is 'c' α1-antitrypsin deficiency

Cholesterosis

- In Cholesterosis, there are deposits of cholesterol in the epithelial cells and in the submucosal macrophages. This gives appearance of multiple small yellow spots on a red hyperplastic muscosa, the strawberry gallbladder.

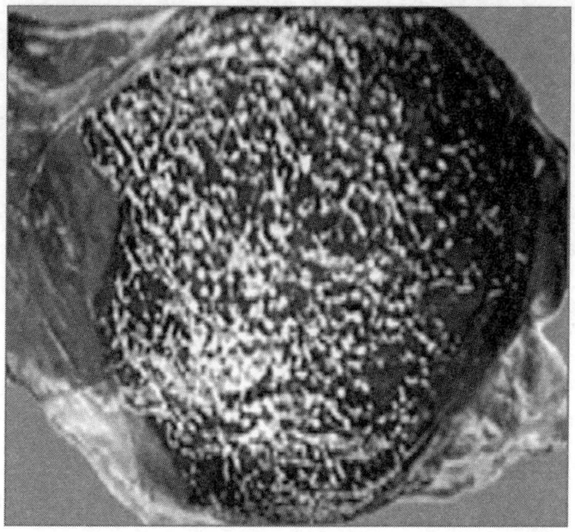

Yellow, flat deposits on mucosal surface, focal or diffuse. May have speckled appearance ("strawberry gallbladder"), 20% are associated with cholesterol polyps.

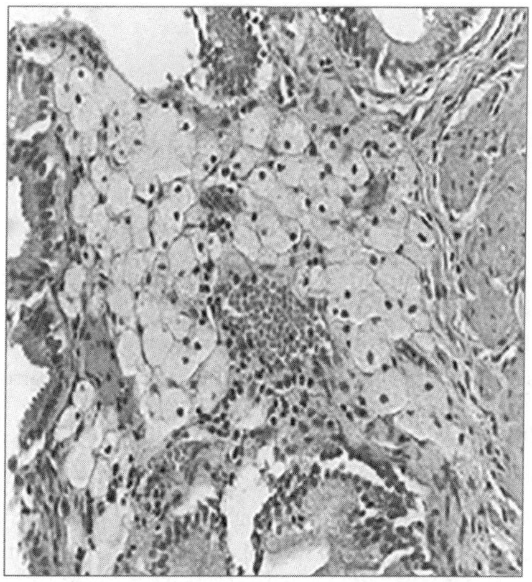

Lipid laden histiocytes in lamina propria

295. Strawberry gallbladder is seen in:	*(NEET 2016)*
a Cholesterosis	b. Primary sclerosing cholangitis
c. Cholestasis	d. Primary biliary cirrhosis

Ans. is 'a' Cholesterosis

Miscellaneous

296. Condition associated with ground glass hepatocytes is:	*(NEET 2016)*
a. HAV	b. HBV
c. HCV	d. HDV

Ans. is 'b' HBV

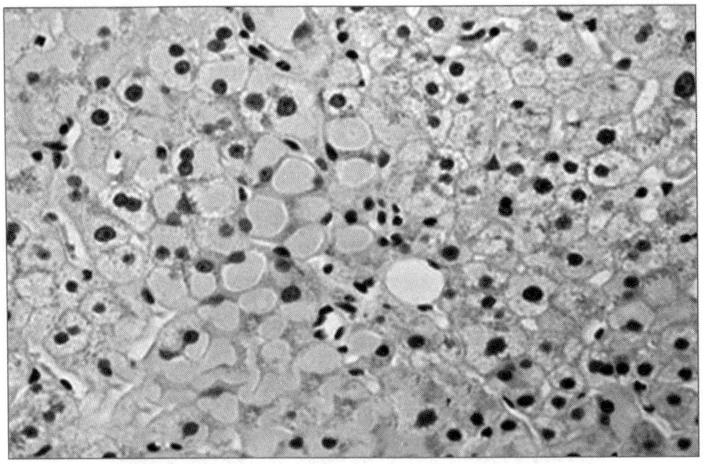

Chronic hepatitis due to HBV shows ground-glass hepatocytes —* HBs Ag in cytoplasm of hepatocytes produce finely granular appearance.

PANCREATIC NEUROENDOCRINE TUMORS

Insulinoma

- Most common of pancreatic neuroendocrine neoplasms
- Tumor of pancreatic β cells → overproduction of insulin → hypoglycemia.
- *Whipple triad*: Low blood glucose, symptoms of hypoglycemia (e.g., lethargy, syncope, diplopia), and resolution of symptoms after normalization of glucose levels.
- Symptomatic patients have low blood glucose and high C-peptide levels (vs exogenous insulin use).
- 10% of cases associated with MEN I syndrome.
- *Treatment*: Surgical resection

Glucagonoma

- Tumor of pancreatic α cells → overproduction of glucagon.
- Presents with 5D's: Dermatitis (necrolytic migratory erythema), Diabetes (hyperglycemia), DVT, Declining weight, Depression
- *Treatment*: Octreotide, surgery

Somatostatinoma

- Tumor of pancreatic δ cells → overproduction of somatostatin—decreased secretion of secretin, cholecystokinin, glucagon, insulin, gastrin, gastric inhibitory peptide (GIP).
- May present with diabetes/glucose intolerance, steatorrhea, gallstones, achlorhydria.
- *Treatment*: Surgical resection; somatostatin analogs (e.g., octreotide) for symptom control

Zollinger-Ellison Syndrome (Gastrinoma)

- Gastrin-secreting tumor (gastrinoma) of pancreas or duodenum.
- Acid hypersecretion causes recurrent ulcers in duodenum and jejunum.
- Presents with abdominal pain (peptic ulcer disease, distal ulcers), diarrhea (malabsorption)
- *Positive secretin stimulation test*: Gastrin levels remain elevated after administration of secretin, which normally inhibits gastrin release.
- May be associated with MEN I.
- Over 90% of gastrinomas are found within an anatomic triangle referred to as the gastrinoma triangle. Sporadic gastrinomas are usually single and are most commonly located in the pancreas. By contrast, gastrinomas found in patients with MEN1 are usually multiple and are most often located in the duodenal wall.

VIPoma

- Rare neuroendocrine tumor that secretes vasoactive intestinal peptide (VIP).
- Most commonly arises in pancreas.
- Associated with MEN I.
- Primary symptom is secretory diarrhea.
- Associated with WDHA (Watery Diarrhea, Hypokalemia, Achlorhydria) syndrome.

MULTIPLE NEUROENDOCRINE NEOPLASIAS

Subtype	Characteristics
MEN 1	Pituitary tumors (prolactin or GH) Pancreatic endocrine tumors—Zollinger-Ellison syndrome, insulinomas, VIPomas, glucagonomas (rare) Parathyroid adenomas Associated with mutation of *MEN1* (menin, a tumor suppressor, chromosome II), angiofibromas, collagenomas, meningiomas
MEN 2A	Parathyroid hyperplasia Medullary thyroid carcinoma—neoplasm of parafollicular C cells; secretes calcitonin; prophylactic thyroidectomy required Pheochromocytoma (secretes catecholamines) Associated with mutation in *RET* (codes for receptor tyrosine kinase)
MEN 2B	Medullary thyroid carcinoma Pheochromocytoma Mucosal neuromas (oral/intestinal ganglioneuromatosis) Associated with marfanoid habitus; mutation in *RET* gene

297. Most common pancreatic neuroendocrine tumor is: *(NEET 2020)*

a. Insulinoma
b. Gastrinoma
c. VIPoma
d. Glucagonoma

Ans. is 'a' Insulinoma

298. Most common site for gastrinoma in MEN-1 syndrome is: *(NEET 2020)*

a. Distal ileum
b. Duodenum
c. Head of pancreas
d. Stomach

Ans. is 'b' Duodenum

KIDNEY AND THE LOWER URINARY TRACT

Summary of major primary glomerulonephritides

				Glomerular pathology	
Disease	***Most frequent clinical presentation***	***Pathogenesis***	***Light microscopy***	***Fluorescence microscopy***	***Electron microscopy***
Post infectious glomerulonephritis	Nephritic syndrome	Immune complex mediated; circulating or planted antigen	Diffuse endocapillary proliferation; leukocytic infiltration	Granular IgG and C3 in GBM and mesangium; Granular IgA in some cases	Primarily subepithelial humps; subendothelial deposits in early disease stages.
Goodpasture syndrome	Rapidly progressive glomerulonephritis	Anti-GBM COL4-A3 antigen	Extracapillary proliferation with crescents; necrosis	Linear IgG and C3; fibrin in crescents	No deposits; GBM disruptions; fibrin
Chronic glomerulonephritis	Chronic renal failure	Variable	Hyalinized glomeruli	Granular or negative	
Membranous nephropathy	Nephrotic syndrome	In situ immune complex formation; PLA Rantigen in most cases of primary disease mostly unknown	Diffuse capillary wall thickening	Granular IGG and C3; diffuse	Subepithelial deposits
Minimal change disease	Nephrotic syndrome	Unknown; loss of glomerular polyanion; podocyte injury	Normal; lipid in tubules	Negative	Loss of foot processes; no deposits
Focal segmental glomerulosclerosis	Nephrotic syndrome; nonnephrotic proteinuria	Unknown Ablation nephrophathy Plasma factor (?); podocyte injury	Focal and segmental sclerosis and hyalinosis	Focal; IgM + C3 in many cases	Loss of foot processes; epithelial denudation
Membranoproliferative glomerulonephritis (NPGN) type I	Nephrotic/nephrotic syndrome	Immune complex	Mesangial proliferative or membranoproliferative patterns of proliferation; GBM thickening; splitting	IgG ++ C3; C1q++ C4	Subendothelial deposits
Dense-deposit disease (MPGN type II)	Hematuria chronic renal failure	Autoantibody; alternative complement pathway	Mesangial proliferative or membranoproliferative patterns of proliferation; GBM thickening; splitting	C3; no C1q or C4	Dense deposits
IgA nephropathy	Recurrent hematuria or proteinuria	Unknown	Focal mesangial proliferative glomerulonephritis; mesangial widening	IgA ± IgA, IgM, and C3 in mesangium	Mesangial and paramesangial dense deposits

299. Loss of foot process of podocytes is classically seen in: *(NEET 2020)*

a. MPGN
b. IgA nephropathy
c. Minimal change disease
d. Diabetic nephropathy

Ans. is 'c' Minimal change disease

300. An elderly normotensive patient presents with hematuria and pedal edema. Creatinine was elevated and glycosuria was absent. Immunofluorescene image is shown below. What investigation should be done to identify the etiology of disease? *(NEET 2020)*

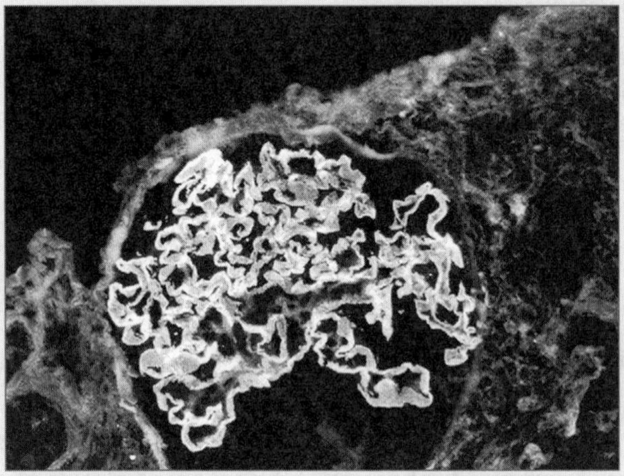

a. ANA levels
b. Anti-GBM antibodies
c. HIV RNA
d. Urine immunoelectrophoresis

Ans. is 'b' Anti-GBM antibodies

Explanation: Immunofluorescence image shows linear pattern of deposition characteristic of anti-GBM disease.

301. True about RCC is: *(NEET 2016)*

a. Most common site is lower lobe of kidney
b. Most common variety is papillary type
c. Invasion of renal vein is more common than renal artery
d. Most common site of metastasis is lymph nodes

Ans. is 'c' Invasion of renal vein is more common than renal artery

302. Choroid metastasis is associated most commonly with: *(NEET 2016)*

a. Gastric carcinoma
b. Renal carcinoma
c. Brain tumor
d. Bone tumor

Ans. is 'b' Renal carcinoma

303. Hebnail appearance is seen in: *(NEET 2016)*

a. Clear cell carcinoma
b. Endodermal sinus tumor
c. HCC
d. Choriocarcinoma

Ans. is 'a' Clear cell carcinoma

304. Most common type of renal adenocarcinoma is: *(NEET 2016)*

a. Clear cell type
b. Chromophobe type
c. Papillary type
d. Tubular type

Ans. is 'a' Clear cell type

COLLAPSING GLOMERULOPATHY

- Most common (80%) kidney lesion in AIDS is FSGS (especially collapsing variant). Mesangioproliferative GN is 2nd most common kidney lesion (10–15%).
- Other kidney lesions in AIDS are acute diffuse proliferative GN, MPGN, IgA nephropathy, membranous GN and minimal change disease.

Characterized by collapse and sclerosis of the entire glomerular tuft in addition to the usual FSGS lesions. A characteristic feature is proliferation and hypertrophy of glomerular visceral epithelial cells (podocytes). There is prominent tubular injury with formation of microcysts. It is the most characteristic lesion of HIV nephropathy.

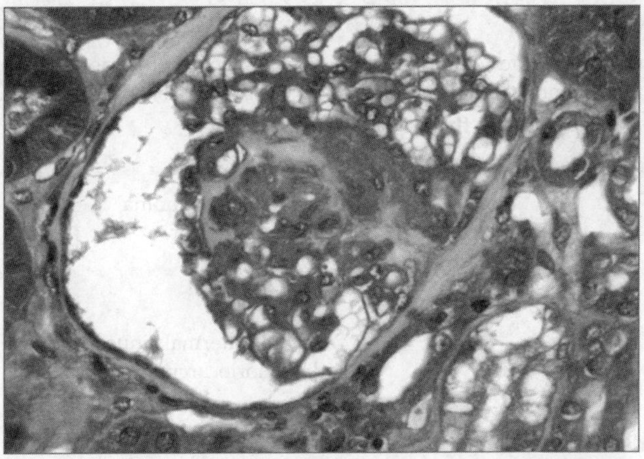

305. Collapsing glomerulopathy is seen in: *(NEET 2016)*

a. Poststreptococcal GN
b. HIV
c. IgA nephropathy
d. Tuberculosis

Ans. is 'b' HIV

306. Most common type of nephropathy found in HIV patient is: *(NEET 2016)*

a. Membranous glomerulonephritis
b. Fibrillary glomerulopathy
c. Collapsing glomerulonephritis
d. RPGN

Ans. is 'c' Collapsing glomerulonephritis

RENAL CELL CARCINOMA

Important risk factors for RCC are smoking (most significant), obesity, hypertension, asbestos exposure, estrogen therapy, CRF, tuberous sclerosis and familial conditions (Von Hippel-Landau syndrome).

RCC is an adenocarcinoma and most commonly arises from upper pole.

Clear cell carcinoma is the most common type of renal cancer accounting for about 70% to 80% of the renal cell cancer. Papillary carcinoma, Chromophobic (oncocytic) carcinoma, collecting duct (Bellini duct) carcinoma are the other three varities.

The three classical diagnostic features (classical triad) of renal cell carcinoma are costovertebral pain, palpable mass and hematuria. The most reliable of three is hematuria.

The one of the striking characteristics of RCC is to invade renal vein and is associated with poor prognosis.

Metastasis usually occur by hematogenous route to lung (most commonly), bone, lymph nodes, liver, adrenal and brain.

Types of Renal Cell Carcinoma

Important histological types of renal-cell carcinoma are:

- *Clear cell carcinoma*: It is the most common type of renal cancer accounting for about 70% to 80% of the renal cell cancer. They are so named because they are made up to cells with clear or granular cytoplasm and are nonpapillary.
  - They occur as solitary unilateral lesions. It arises from proximal tubular epithelium.
  - Hobnail cell is a cell with a characteristic appearance, including a bulbous nucleus and nuclear projections into the cytoplasm. Hobnail cells are found in clear cell ovarian adenocarcinoma, collecting duct carcinoma, and in end-stage cirrhosis.
- *Papillary carcinoma*: It accounts for 10% to 15% of renal cancers. It is characterized by papillary growth pattern. It arises from distal convoluted tubule. It can be multifocal and bilateral. These are most common type of renal cancer in patients who develop dialysis associated cystic disease. Papillary carcinoma also occurs in two forms hereditary and sporadic.
- *Chromophobe (oncocytic) renal cell carcinoma*: These tumors arise from intercalated cells of 'cortical' collecting ducts. The cells have pale eosinophilic cytoplasm with perinuclear halo with a plant cell appearance. Electron microscopic finding consisting of numerous 150–300 nm microvesicles is the single most distinctive and defining fracture of chromophobe cell carcinoma.
- *Collecting duct (Bellini duct) carcinoma*: It is the least common type of RCC. It arises from 'medullary' collecting duct. Cells have prominent fibrotic stroma.

307. Large cells with plant like appearance with Perinuclear halo is seen in which type of renal cell carcinoma? *(NEET 2016)*

a. Granular cell carcinoma
b. Angiosarcoma
c. Chromophobic
d. Clear cell carcinoma

Ans. is 'd' Clear cell carcinoma

308. True about RCC is: *(NEET 2016)*

a. Most common site is lower lobe of kidney
b. Most common variety is papillary type
c. Invasion of renal vein is more common than renal artery
d. Most common site of metastasis is lymph nodes

Ans. is 'c' Invasion of renal vein is more common than renal artery

309. Choroid metastasis is associated most commonly with: *(NEET 2016)*

a. Gastric carcinoma
b. Renal carcinoma
c. Brain tumor
d. Bone tumor

Ans. is 'b' Renal carcinoma

310. Hebnail appearance is seen in: *(NEET 2016)*

a. Clear cell carcinoma
b. Endodermal sinus tumor
c. HCC
d. Choriocarcinoma

Ans. is 'a' Clear cell carcinoma

311. Most common type of renal adenocarcinoma is: *(NEET 2016)*

a. Clear cell type
b. Chromophobe type
c. Papillary type
d. Tubular type

Ans. is 'a' Clear cell type

Miscellaneous

312. What is the incidence of renal ectopia? *(NEET 2016)*

a. 1 in 500
b. 1 in 1000
c. 1 in 1500
d. 1 in 2000

Ans. is 'b' 1 in 1000

- The average occurrence is 1 in 900
- The renal ectopia occurs in approximately 1 in 1000 people with equal sex distribution.

ACID-BASE DISORDERS

Acidosis and Alkalosis

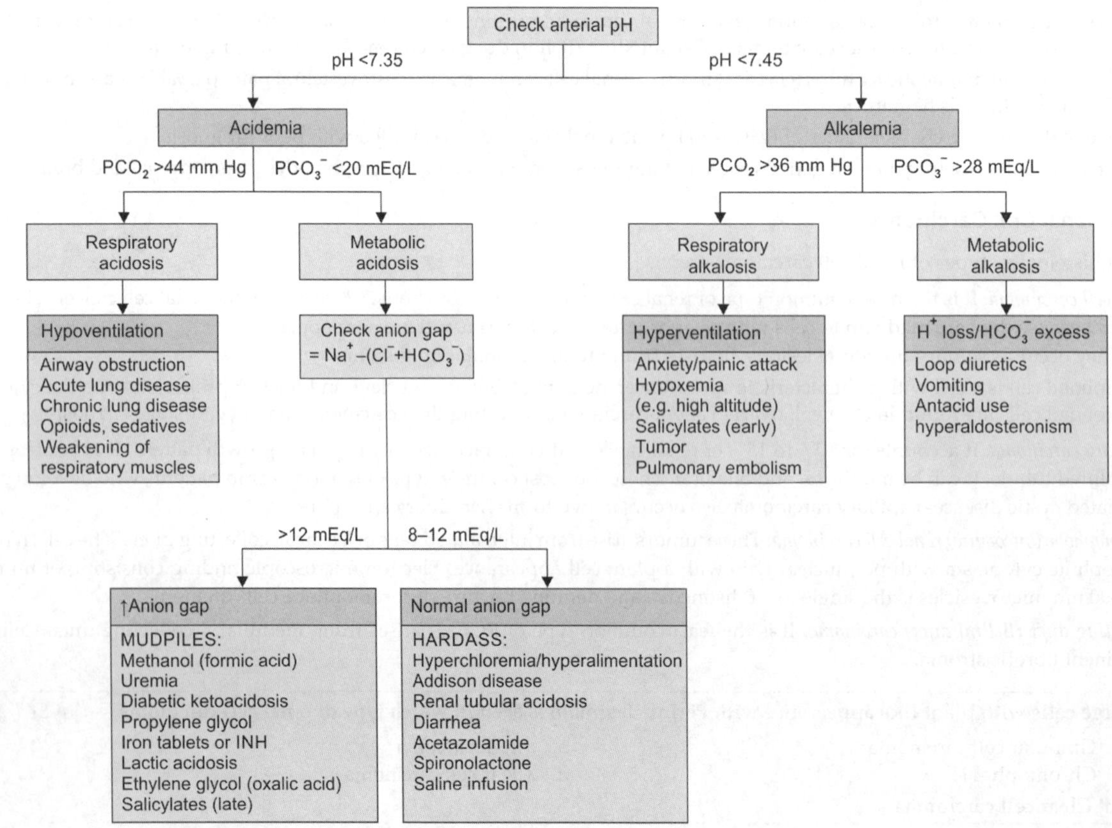

Prediction of compensatory responses to simple acid-base disturbances and pattern on changes				
			Range of values	
Disorder	*Prediction of compensation*	*pH*	*HCO_3^-*	*$PaCO_2$*
Metabolic acidosis	$PaCO_2 = (1.5 \times HCO_3) + 8 \pm 2$ Or $PaCO_2$ will ↓ 1.25 mmHg per mmol/L ↓ in $[HCO_3^-]$ Or $PaCO_2 = [HCO_3^-] + 15$	Low	Low	Low
Metabolic alkalosis	$PaCO_2$ will ↑ 0.75 mmHg per mmol/L ↑ in (HCO_3^-) Or $PaCO_2$ will ↑ 6 mmHg per 10 mmol/L ↑ in $[HCO_3^-]$ Or $PaCO_2 = [HCO_3^-] + 15$	High	High	High
Respiratory alkalosis		High	Low	Low
Acute	$[HCO_3^-]$ will ↓ 0.2 mmol/L per mmHg ↓ in $PaCO_2$			
Chronic	$[HCO_3^-]$ will ↓ 0.4 mmol/L per mmHg ↓ in $PaCO_2$			
Respiratory acidosis		Low	High	High
Acute	$[HCO_3^-]$ will ↑ 0.1 mmol/L per mmHg ↑ in $PaCO_2$			
Chronic	$[HCO_3^-]$ will ↑ 0.4 mmol/L per mmHg ↑ in $PaCO_2$			

DIABETIC KETOACIDOSIS

- One of the most feared complications of diabetes. Usually due to insulin noncompliance or raised insulin requirements from stress (e.g., infection). Excess fat breakdown and increased ketogenesis from raised free fatty acids, which are then made into ketone bodies (β-hydroxybutyrate > acetoacetate).
- Usually occurs in type I diabetes, as endogenous insulin in type 2 diabetes usually prevents lipolysis and ketogenesis.
- *DKA is Deadly*: Delirium/psychosis, Kussmaul respirations (rapid, deep breathing}, Abdominal pain/nausea/vomiting, Dehydration. Fruity breath odor (due to exhaled acetone)
- *Labs*: Hyperglycemia, metabolic acidosis, reduced HCO_3^- (raised anion gap metabolic acidosis}, raised urine and blood ketone levels, leukocytosis. hyperkalemia, but depleted intracellular K^+ due to transcellular shift from raised insulin and acidosis. Osmotic diuresis → increased K^+ loss in urine → total body K^+ depletion
- *Complication*: Life-threatening mucormycosis (usually caused by Rhizopus infection), cerebral edema, cardiac arrhythmias, heart failure
- *Treatment*: IV fluids, IV insulin, and K^+ (to replete intracellular stores); glucose if necessary to prevent hypoglycemia

313. A patient presented with vomitting and abdominal pain. Blood sugar levels were 350 mg/dL and pH was 7.2. What is the diagnosis? *(NEET 2020)*

a. Metabolic acidosis
b. Metabolic alkalosis
c. Respiratory acidosis
d. Respiratory alkalosis

Ans. is 'a' Metabolic acidosis

Explanation: History and high glucose levels are suggestive of Diabetic ketoacidosis.

314. Comment on the diagnosis based on the given ABG analysis: pH 7.2, bicarbonates = 10 mmol/L, pCO_2 = 30 mmHg. *(NEET 2020)*

a. Uncompensated metabolic acidosis
b. Uncompensated metabolic alkalosis
c. Uncompensated respiratory acidosis
d. Uncompensated respiratory alkalosis

Ans. is 'a' Uncompensated metabolic acidosis

Explanation: Low pH with reduced bicarbonate suggests metabolic acidosis. Predicted CO = 1.5 × 10 + 8 ± 2 = 23 ± 2 mmHg. Since the prevailing pCO_2 is above predicted value, it is suggestive of uncompensated metabolic acidosis.

315. A patient of chronic renal failure with ABG values as shown: pH = 7.24, HCO_3^- = 10 mmol/L, pCO_2 = 25 mmHg. What is the basis of this acidosis? *(NEET 2020)*

a. Renal bicarbonate loss
b. Tubular H^+ secretion
c. CO_2 expired by lungs
d. Exogenous HCO_3^- loads

Ans. is 'a' Renal bicarbonate loss

Explanation: Low pH with reduced bicarbonate suggests metabolic acidosis.

MALE AND FEMALE GENITAL SYSTEM

SEMINOMA

- Most common type of testicular tumor
- Germ cell origin arising in the seminiferous epithelium
- Peak incidence: 30–50 years

- *Histological subtypes*: Classical-lymphocytic stromal infiltrate; spermatocytic; anaplastic; with syncytiotrophoblast giant cells-contain human chorionic gonadotropin (hCG); combined with other types of tumor
- Five histological subtypes of seminoma are recognized: Classical
- Spermatocytic
- Anaplastic
- With syncytiotrophoblast giant cells
- Combined with other types of germ cell tumor.

Morphology

- The histologic appearances of germ cell tumors may be pure (i.e. composed of a single histologic type) or mixed (seen in 40% of cases).
- Seminomas are soft, well-demarcated, gray-white tumors that bulge from the cut surface of the affected testis.
- Large tumors may contain foci of coagulation necrosis usually without hemorrhage.
- Microscopically, seminomas are composed of large, uniform cells with distinct cell borders, clear, glycogen-rich cytoplasm, and round nuclei with conspicuous nucleoli. The cells often are arrayed in small lobules with intervening fibrous septa. A lymphocytic infiltrate usually is present and may, on occasion, overshadow the neoplastic cells.
- Seminomas may also be accompanied by an ill- defined granulomatous reaction. In approximately 15% of cases, syncytiotrophoblasts are present that are the source of the minimally elevated serum hCG concentrations encountered in some males with pure seminoma. Their presence has no bearing on prognosis.

Tumor markers for various testicular tumors

Testicular tumor	Tumor markers
Seminoma	• Placental alkaline phosphatase, keratin • Classical seminomas are negative for hCG, but 7–15% may be positive for IICO
Embryonal carcinoma	• hCG, AFP
Yolk sac tumor	AFP, α-1 antitrypsin
Choriocarcinoma	hCG

AFP is a glycoprotein synthesized normally early in fetal life by yolk sac, fetal liver and fetal GIT. It is structurally and genetically related to albumin.

AFP is raised in liver cancer (hepatocellular carcinoma), lung carcinoma, pancreatic carcinoma, colon carcinoma, and non-seminoma germ cell tumor of testis/ovary (yolk sac tumor/endodermal sinus tumor, embryonal carcinoma, teratoma).

316. After surgery in scrotum, tumor specimen obtained is shown below. What is the diagnosis? *(NEET 2018)*

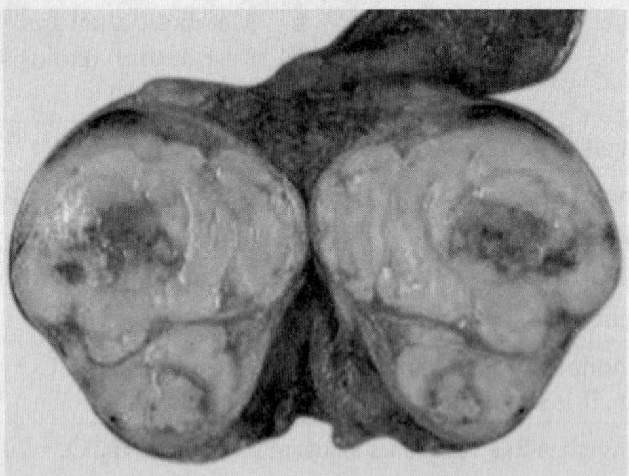

a. Seminoma
b. Teratoma
c. Dysgerminoma
d. Yolk sac tumor

Ans. is 'a' Seminoma

317. Most common type of germinal cell tumor in testis is: *(NEET 2016)*

a. Teratoma
b. Embryonal carcinoma
c. Seminoma
d. Endodermal sinus tumor

Ans. is 'c' Seminoma

318. Which tumor is associated with raised AFP and β-hCG? *(NEET 2016)*

a. Seminoma
b. Embryonal cell carcinoma
c. Yolk sac tumor
d. Choriocarcinoma

Ans. is 'b' Embryonal cell carcinoma

319. What is the marker for endodermal sinus tumor: *(NEET 2016)*

a. CA-125
b. hCG
c. Alpha-1 antytrypsin
d. Inhibin

Ans. is 'c' Alpha-1 antytrypsin

320. Seminoma testis marker is: *(NEET 2016)*

a. Alfa fetoprotein
b. Carcinoembryonic antigen
c. Acid phosphatase
d. Alkaline phosphatase

Ans. is 'd' Alkaline phosphatase

321. AFP is produced by: *(NEET 2016)*

a. Fetal yolk sac
b. Fetal liver
c. Fetal GIT
d. All of the above

Ans. is 'd' All of the above

322. Testicular tumor associated with high hCG level is: *(NEET 2016)*

a. Choriocarcinoma
b. Seminoma
c. Endodermal sinus tumor
d. All of the above

Ans. is 'a' Choriocarcinoma

323. Tumor marker for dysgerminoma is: *(NEET 2016)*

a. AFP
b LDH
c. hCG
d. CA-125

Ans. is 'b' LDH

Penile Carcinoma

- ❖ Most of the penile cancers are squamous cell carcinoma and arise on glans or inner surface of prepuce.
- ❖ Two most common growth patterns are papillary and flat. A third uncommon variant is verrucous carcinoma (Giant condyloma or Buschke- Lowenstein tumor) which is well-differentiated with low malignant potential.

324. Penile carcinoma is usually: *(NEET 2016)*

a. Squamous cell carcinoma
b. Basal cell carcinoma
c. Adenocarcinoma
d. Small cell carcinoma

Ans. is 'a' Squamous cell carcinoma

Specific Histologic Types of Breast Carcinoma

ER-positive tumors

- ❖ *Lobular carcinoma:* Most commonly forms hard irregular masses similar to other breast cancers, but may also have a diffuse infiltrative pattern with minimal desmoplasia. This is the most common type of breast carcinoma to present as an occult primary. The histologic hallmark is the presence of discohesive infiltrating tumor cells, often including signet-ring cells containing intracytoplasmic mucin droplets.
- ❖ *Mucinous (colloid) carcinoma:* is soft or rubbery and has the consistency and appearance of pale gray-blue gelatin. The borders are pushing or circumscribed. The tumor cells are arranged in clusters and small islands of cells within large lakes of mucin
- ❖ *Tubular carcinoma* consists exclusively of well-formed tubules and is sometimes mistaken for a benign sclerosing lesion. Apocrine snouts are typical, and calcifications may be present within the lumens. Tubular carcinomas are frequently associated with flat epithelial atypia, atypical lobular hyperplasia, LCIS, or low-grade DCIS.
- ❖ *Papillary carcinoma,* as the name implies, produces true papillae, fronds of fibrovascular tissue lined by tumor cells.

ER-negative, HER2-negative tumors

- ❖ Chief among these is *medullary carcinoma* is softer than other carcinomas due to minimal desmoplasia, and often presents as a well-circumscribed mass. It is characterized by (1) solid, syncytium-like sheets of large cells with pleomorphic nuclei, and prominent nucleoli, which compose more than 75% of the tumor mass; (2) frequent mitotic figures; (3) a moderate to marked lymphoplasmacytic infiltrate surrounding and within the tumor; and (4) a pushing (non-infiltrative) border.

325. A 40-year-female presents with palpable lump in upper outer quadrant of right breast. Biopsy revealed densely packed cells with bland nuclei and mucin pools in stroma. What is the likely diagnosis? *(NEET 2020)*

a. Colloid carcinoma
b. Tubular carcinoma
c. Papillary carcinoma
d. Medullary carcinoma

Ans. is 'a' Colloid carcinoma

CENTRAL NERVOUS SYSTEM

DEFECTS OF PROTEIN FOLDING

- Defective protein folding disorders (DPFDs) are a group of diverse neurological and systemic diseases in which the hallmark pathological event is the misfolding, aggregation and accumulation of a protein in different organs, inducing cellular apoptosis, tissue damage and organ dysfunction.
- This group includes Alzheimer's disease, transmissible spongiform encephalopathies, serpin-deficiency disorders, sickle cell anemia, Huntington's disease, diabetes type II, amyotrophic lateral sclerosis, Parkinson's disease, dialysis-related amyloidosis, spinocerebellar ataxias, secondary or reactive amyloidosis, cystic fibrosis and prion diseases.

326. Folding defect is associated with which disease? *(NEET 2016)*

a. Parkinson's disease
b. Marfan syndrome
c. Acute intermittent porphyria
d. Wermer syndrome

Ans. is 'a' Parkinson's disease

Alzheimer's Disease

Morphology

Grossly, the brain shows a variable degree of cortical atrophy marked by widening of the cerebral sulci that is most pronounced in the frontal, temporal, and parietal lobes. With significant atrophy, there is compensatory ventricular enlargement (hydrocephalus ex vacuo) secondary to loss of parenchyma and reduced brain volume. Structures of the medial temporal lobe, including hippocampus, entorhinal cortex and amygdala, are involved early in the course and are usually severely atrophied in the later stages. The major microscopic abnormalities of AD, which form the basis of the histologic diagnosis, are neuritic (senile) plaques and neurofibrillary tangles. There is progressive and eventually severe neuronal loss and reactive gliosis in the same regions that bear the burden of plaques and tangles.

Neuritic plaques are focal, spherical collections of dilated, tortuous, neuritic processes (dystrophic neurites) often around a central amyloid core, which may be surrounded by clear halo. Neuritic plaques range in size from 20 to 200 μm in diameter; microglial cells and reactive astrocytes are present at their periphery. Plaques are found in the hippocampus, amygdala, and neocortex, although there is usually relative sparing of primary motor and sensory cortices (this also applies to neurofibrillary tangles). The amyloid core, which can be stained by Congo Red, contains several abnormal proteins. The dominant component of the amyloid plaque core is Aβ, a peptide derived through specific processing events from a larger molecule, amyloid precursor protein (APP). The two dominant species of Aβ, called Aβ40 and Aβ42, share an N-terminus and differ in length by two amino acids at the C-terminus.

Neurofibrillary tangles are bundles of filaments in the cytoplasm of the neurons that displace or encircle the nucleus. In pyramidal neurons, they often have an elongated "flame" shape; in rounder cells, the basket weave of fibers around the nucleus takes on a rounded contour ("globose" tangles). Neurofibrillary tangles are visible as basophilic fibrillary structures with HandE staining but are dramatically demonstrated by silver (Bielschowsky) staining. They are commonly found in cortical neurons, especially in the entorhinal cortex, as well as in other sites such as pyramidal cells of the hippocampus, the amygdala, the basal forebrain, and the raphe nuclei. Neurofibrillary tangles are insoluble and apparently resistant to clearance in vivo, thus remaining visible in tissue sections as "ghost" or "tombstone" tangles long after the death of the parent neuron. Ultrastructurally, neurofibrillary tangles are composed predominantly of paired helical filaments along with some straight filaments that appear to have a comparable composition. A major component of paired helical filaments is abnormally hyperphosphorylated forms of the protein tau, an axonal microtubule-associated protein that enhances microtubule assembly.

327. Which of the following is not a feature of Alzheimer's disease? *(NEET 2016)*

a. Intracellular neurofibrillary tangles
b. Intracellular neuritic plaques
c. Loss of cholinergic neurons in nucleus basalis of Meynert
d. Loss of recent memory

Ans. is 'd' Loss of recent memory

328. Alzheimer's disease is due to: *(NEET 2016)*

a. Increase in cerebral acetyl cholinelevel
b. Abnormal phosphorylation of tau proteins
c. Ventricular atrophy
d. All of the above

Ans. is 'b' Abnormal phosphorylation of tau proteins

Brain Tumors

- Metastasis to brain is the most common brain tumor. Most common primary malignancy metastatizing to brain is lung carcinoma, followed by (in decreasing order of frequency) breast, skin (melanoma), kidney (genitourinary) and GIT cancers.
- Prostate carcinoma, ovarian carcinoma and Hodgkin's disease are very unlikely to metastatize to brain.
- Most common primary neoplasms of CNS are gliomas.
- Most common primary brain tumor in adults is Astrocytoma (glioma) of cerebral hemisphere (lateral hemisphere).
- Most common type of astrocytoma is glioblastoma multiforme.

Locations of common brain tumours

- Location of craniopharyngiomas can be: Sellar-suprasellar (most cases)—most commonly arising on the pituitary stalk and projecting into the hypothalamus.
- Infrasellar or intrasellar.
- Prechiasmic.
- Retrochiasmic.
- Rare locations include extradural and extracranial nasophageal posterior fossa or extending down the cervical spine.
- Ependymal can both supra and infratentorial.
- Medulloblastoma is an infratentorial tumor.

329. Cystic supratentorial tumor is: *(NEET 2016)*

a. Craniopharyngioma
b. Ependymoma
c. Medulloblastoma
d. None of the above

Ans. is 'a' Craniopharyngioma

330. Most common site of occurrence of craniopharyngioma is: *(NEET 2016)*

a. Infrasellar
b. Suprasellar
c. Posterior fossa
d. Nasopharynx

Ans. is 'b' Suprasellar

331. Most common type of primary brain tumor is: *(NEET 2016)*

a. Meningioma
b. Ependymoma
c. Medulloblastoma
d. Astrocytoma

Ans. is 'd' Astrocytoma

332. Most common cause of brain metastasis is: *(NEET 2016)*

a. Carcinoma lung
b. Prostate cancer
c. HCC
d. Seminoma

Ans. is 'a' Carcinoma lung

Froin's Syndrome

- Caused by meningeal irritation (e.g. During spinal meningitis) and CSF flow blockage by tumor mass or abscess.
- Characterized by coexistence of xanthochromia, high protein level and marked coagulation of CSF.

333. Froin syndrome is associated with: *(NEET 2016)*

a. Spinal meningitis
b. Coagulation of CSF
c. High protein level
d. All of the above

Ans. is 'd' All of the above

Neurofibromatosis

NF-1 is diagnosed if two of following sevens are present:

1. Six or more cafe-au-lait macules: > 5 mm in prepubertal age and > 15 mm in postpubertal age.
2. Axillary or inguinal freckling.
3. Two or more Lisch nodules (hamartomas on fris).
4. Two or more neurofibroma or one plexiform neurofibroma.
5. A distinctive osseous lesion: Sphenoid dysplasia or cortical thinning of long bones.
6. Optic glioma.
7. A first degree relative with NF–1.
    - Other findings are pseudarthrosis of tibia, scoliosis (most common orthopedic problem), short stature, mental retardation, hypertension, epilepsy, meningiomas, ependymomas, astrocytomas, pheochromocytomas and leukemia (most common juvenile myelomonocytic leukemia.

334. Sphenoid dysplasia is seen in: *(NEET 2016)*

a. NF-1
b. Tuberous sclerosis
c. Sturge-Weber syndrome
d. Creutzfeldt- Jakob disease

Ans. is 'a' NF-1

335. Most common CNS tumor associated with NF-1 is: *(NEET 2016)*

a. Optic nerve glioma
b. Meningioma
c. Medulloblastoma
d. Ependymoma

Ans. is 'a' Optic nerve glioma

SCHWANNOMA

- It is a benign tumour of schwann cells. It is associated with NF2.
- Most of them arise from the vestibular branch of eighth nerve at the cerebellopontine angle. Tinnitus and sensorineural hearing loss are the common symptoms.
- On gross examination, it appears as a well-circumscribed, encapsulated mass attached to the nerve but can be separated from it
- On microscopic examination, it shows two different growth patterns
  - Antoni A areas show moderate to high cellularity and scant stromal matrix containing elongated cells with cytoplasmic processes arranged in fascicles. Verocay bodies are seen, which are the zones free of nuclei, lying in between the regions of palisading nuclei.
  - Antoni B areas have less cellularity, with a loose meshwork of cells, microcysts and myxoid stroma.
- The lesions are positive for S-100.

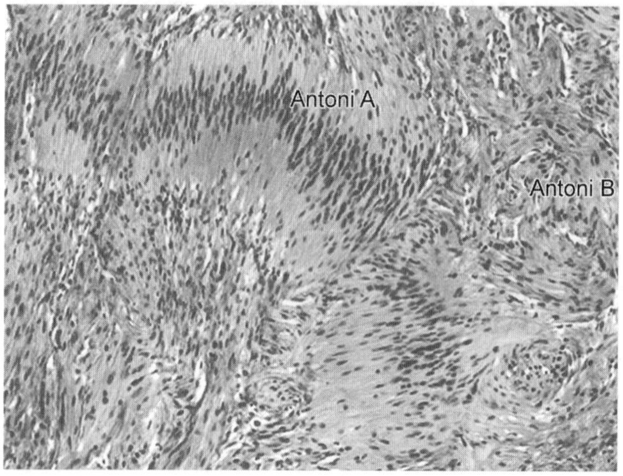

336. A young female presented with a firm nontender swelling near the wrist joint since 2 years. Biopsy revealed spindle cells and areas of hypocellularity and verrocay bodies. What is the diagnosis? *(NEET 2020)*

a. Neurofibroma
b. Schwannoma
c. Lipoma
d. Dermoid cyst

Ans. is 'b' Schwannoma

BONES, JOINTS AND SOFT TISSUE TUMORS

Extra-articular Manifestations of Rheumatoid Arthritis

Dermatologic	• Rheumatoid nodules with and without ulceration • Periungual vasculitic infarcts • Vasculitic leg ulcers • Pyoderma gangrenosum (rare)
Mucosal	• Sicca symptoms – Ocular, oral, vaginal mucosa • Sjögren syndrome
Ocular	• Keratoconjunctivitis sicca • Episcleritis • Scleritis • Scleromalacia perforans • Peripheral ulcerative keratitis
Pulmonary	• Nonspecific interstitial pneumonitis – Usual interstitial pneumonitis • Cryptogenic organizing pneumonitis • Bronchiectasis • Bronchiolitis obliterans • Pleuritis and pleural effusion • Rheumatoid nodulosis in the lungs • Caplan syndrome

Contd...

Pathology

Contd...

Cardiac	• Pericarditis and pericardial effusion • Constrictive pericarditis • Valvular thickening and nodulosis • Conduction abnormalities • Coronary vasculitis • Myocarditis
Hematologic and Lymphatic System	• Anemia of chronic disease • Felty syndrome • Large granular lymphocyte leukemia • Extremity lymphedema—unilateral or bilateral • Neutropenia • Lymphocytosis
Neurologic	• Compression neuropathies • Atlantoaxial subluxation • Peripheral neuropathy • Mononeuritis multiplex • Rheumatoid pachymeningitis
Renal	• AA amyloidosis • Necrotizing crescentic glomerulonephritis (rare)

337. Rheumatoid arthritis is associated with all *except*: *(NEET 2018)*

a. Decreased neutrophils
b. Increased macrophages
c. Increased lymphocytes
d. Increased neutrophils

Ans. is 'd' Increased neutrophils

Types of Collagen

Type of collagen	Distribution
Type I	Skin, tendon bone, cornea
Type II	Articular, cartilage, intervertebral disc, vitreous humor
Type III	Fetal skin, cardiovascular system, lung, reticular fiber
Type IV	Basement membrane
Type V	Placenta, skin

338. Collagen found in intervertebral disc is: *(NEET 2016)*

a. Type I
b. Type II
c. Type III
d. Type IV

Ans. is 'b' Type II

Ollier's Disease

- Ollier's disease is a form of bone dysplasia where there are multiple enchondromas of the metaphysis and diaphysis of bones.
- Enchondroma is a benign cartilage tumor.
- Most commonly the tumor arises from the short tubular bones of hand (phalanges and metatarsals). However, other bones may also be affected, like femur, humerus and ribs.
- Multiple enchondromas with multiple hemangiomas—Maffucci's syndrome.

339. True about Ollier's disease is: *(NEET 2016)*

a. Malignant disease
b. Cartilage involvement
c. Most common site is legs
d. Always associated with hemangioma

Ans. is 'b' Cartilage involvement

LIPOSARCOMA

- One of the most common sarcoma in adulthood
- Occurs in 5th to 6th decade in deep soft tissues of proximal extremities and in retroperitoneum
- Amplification of 12q13-q15 and t(12;16) are characteristic of well-differentiated and myxoid liposarcomas, respectively.
- Liposarcomas are histologically divided into three morphologic subtypes:
  - Well-differentiated liposarcoma contains adipocytes with scattered atypical spindle cells

- Myxoid liposarcoma contains abundant basophilic extracellular matrix, arborizing capillaries and primitive cells at various stages of adipocyte differentiation reminiscent of fetal fat
- Pleomorphic liposarcoma consists of sheets of anaplastic cells, bizarre nuclei and variable amounts of immature adipocytes (lipoblasts)

340. A 40-year-old patient presented with 10 × 8 cm retroperitoneal mass. Molecular analysis revealed t(12;16). Biopsy is shown below. What is the diagnosis? *(NEET 2020)*

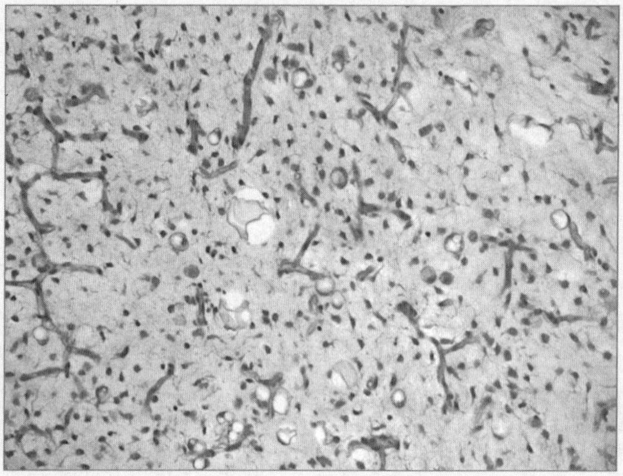

a. Myxoid liposarcoma b. Lipoma
c. Pleomorphic liposarcoma d. Spindle cell lipoma

Ans. is 'a' Myxoid liposarcoma

Explanation: Biopsy slide shows myxoid liposarcoma with abundant ground substance and a rich capillary network in which are scattered immature adipocytes.

Miscellaneous

341. Painless burn in hand is a characteristic feature of: *(NEET 2016)*

a. Thalamic syndrome b. Syringomyelia
c. Cord compression d. SLE

Ans. is 'b' Syringomyelia

In Syringomyelia, there sensory deficit in upper extrimities in the form of loss of pain and temperature sensations with touch and vibration being intact.

SKIN AND ENDOCRINE SYSTEM

CHRONIC LYMPHOCYTIC (HASHIMOTO) THYROIDITIS

Hashimoto's thyroiditis is the most common cause of hypothyroidism in areas of the world where iodine levels are sufficient.

It is characterized by the gradual thyroid failure secondary to autoimmune destruction of the thyroid gland.

It is most prevalent between the ages of 45 and 65 years and is more common in women than in men, with female predominance in a ratio of 10:1 to 20:1.

Although it is primarily a disease of older women, it can occur in children and is a major cause of nonendemic goiter in children.

Morphology

The thyroid usually is diffusely and symmetrically enlarged, although more localized enlargement may be seen in some cases.

The cut surface is pale and gray-tan in appearance, and the tissue is firm and somewhat friable. Microscopic examination reveals widespread infiltration of the parenchyma by a mononuclear inflammatory infiltrate containing small lymphocytes, plasma cells, and well-developed germinal centers.

The thyroid follicles are atrophic and are lined in many areas by epithelial cells distinguished by the presence of abundant eosinophilic, granular cytoplasm, termed Hurthle or oxyphil cells. This is a metaplastic response of the normally low cuboidal follicular epithelium to ongoing injury; on ultra-structural examination, the Hurthle cells are characterized by the numerous prominent mitochondria. Interstitial connective tissue is increased and may be abundant.

Less commonly, the thyroid is small and atrophic as a result of more extensive fibrosis (fibrosing variant). Unlike in Reidel thyroiditis, the fibrosis does not extend beyond the capsule of the gland.

342. A 30-year-old female presents with thyroid swelling. TSH levels were elevated. Biopsy revealed lymphocytic infilterates and Hurthle cells. What is the diagnosis? *(NEET 2020)*

a. Graves disease
b. Hashimoto's thyroiditis
c. Medullary carcinoma
d. Follicular carcinoma

Ans. is 'b' Hashimoto's thyroiditis

343. A 38-year-old female with neck swelling shown is gross and histology of the tissue, what is the diagnosis? *(NEET 2018)*

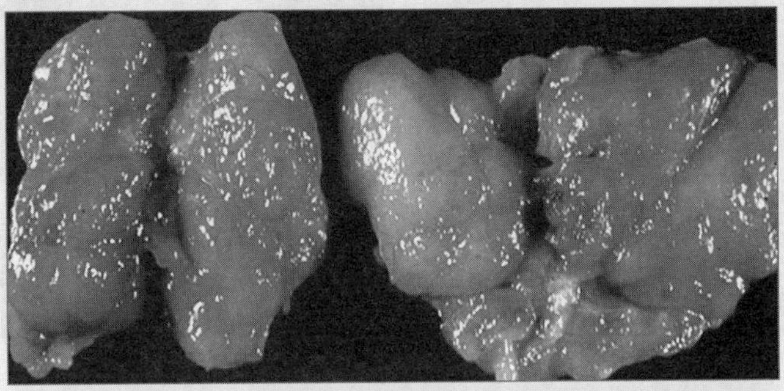

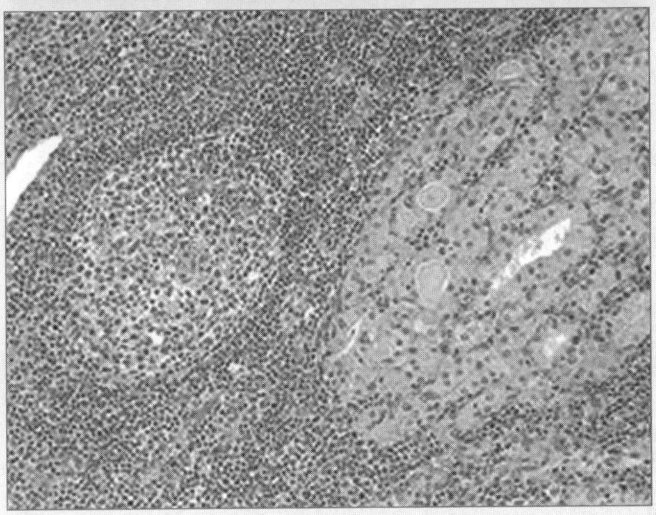

a. NHL
b. MCT
c. Melanoma
d. Hashimoto's thyroiditis

Ans. is 'd' Hashimoto's thyroiditis

Basal Cell Carcinoma: Types

Nodular: Cystic, pigmented, keratotic; the most common type of BCC; usually presents as a round, pearly, flesh-colored papule with telangiectasias.

Infiltrative: Tumor infiltrates the dermis in thin strands between collagen fibers, making tumor margins less clinically apparent.

Micronodular: Not prone to ulceration; may appear yellow-white when stretched, is firm to the touch, and may have a seemingly well-defined border.

Morpheaform: Appears as a white or yellow, waxy; sclerotic plaque that rarely ulcerates; is flat or slightly depressed, fibrotic, and firm.

Superficial: Seen mostly on the upper trunk or shoulders; appears clinically as an erythematous, well-circumscribed patch or plaque, often with a whitish scale.

344. Most common variety of basal cell carcinoma is: *(NEET 2016)*

a. Morpheaform
b. Micronodular
c. Nodular
d. Superficial

Ans. is 'c' Nodular

Turban Tumor

In dermatologic pathology, a dermal cylindroma, also dermal eccrine cylindroma and (less specifically) cylindroma, is a benign adnexal tumor, which occurs on the scalp and forehead.

Multiple cylindromas may grow together in a "hat-like" configuration, sometimes referred to as a turban tumor.

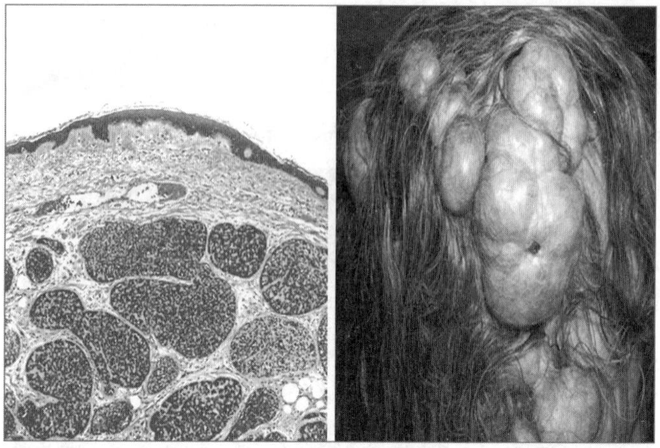

345. Turban tumor is: *(NEET 2016)*

a. Basal cell carcinoma
b. Squamous cell carcinoma
c. Cutaneous cylindroma
d. Dermatofibroma

Ans. is 'c' Cutaneous cylindroma

Malignant Melanoma—Markers

- S-100: 90% of tumors are positive
- HMB-45: More specific but less sensitive than s-100
- TA-90 : Melan-A
- Tyrosinase.

346. Which condition is associated with s-100 marker? *(NEET 2016)*

a. Multiple myeloma
b. Malignant melanoma
c. Prostate carcinoma
d. Medullary carcinoma thyroid

Ans. is 'b' Malignant melanoma

Multiple Endocrine Neoplasia

Syndrome	Gene	Chromosome
• Multiple endocrine neoplasia type 1 • Multiple endocrine neoplasia type 2a	• MEN 1 • RET	• 11q13 • 10q11.2

347. Chromosome for MEN2 gene is: *(NEET 2016)*

a. 11q13
b. 13q11
c. 10q11.2
d. 11q10.2

Ans. is 'c' 10q11.2

Miscellaneous

348. Most common cancer to occur in organ transplant patient is: *(NEET 2016)*

a. Squamous cell carcinoma
b. Melanoma
c. Lung cancer
d. Colorectal cancer

Ans. is 'a' Squamous cell carcinoma

Skin cancer is the most common cancer to develop in organ transplant patients who are on immune suppressive therapy. Interestingly, organ transplant recipients have an inverse ratio of BCC to SCC.

Squamous cell carcinoma is the most type of skin cancer in transplant patients.

Infections in Transplant Recipients

Common infections after hematopoietic stem cell transplant		
Early (<1 month)	***Middle (1-4 months)***	***Late (> 6 months)***
Bacterial pneumonia	CMV (diarrhea, pneumonia, bone marrow)	Encapsulated bacterial infections (*Streptococcus, Haemophilus, Neisseria*)
HSV (mucous membrane)	CNS toxoplasmosis	*Pneumocystis pneumonia*
Pulmonary Aspergillosis	Pneumocystis pneumonia	CNS toxoplasmosis
Costridium difficile (diarrhea)	EBV (disseminated)	CMV infection
	BK virus (kidney)	

Common infections after solid organ transplant		
Early (<1 month)	***Middle (1-4 months)***	***Late (> 6 months)***
Bacterial infections (disseminated, pneumonia)	CMV (diarrhea, pneumonia, bone marrow)	Encapsulated bacterial infections (*Streptococcus, Haemophilus, Neisseria*)
Graft infections	CNS toxoplasmosis	*Pneumocystis pneumonia*
	Pneumocystis pneumonia	CNS toxoplasmosis
	BK virus (kidney)	CMV infection
		EBV infection

349. Which of the following infections is common within 1–4 months post-transplant? *(NEET 2020)*

a. CMV
b. Herpes zoster
c. Varicella
d. EBV

Ans. is 'a' CMV

IMPORTANT STAINS

TYPES OF STAINS

1. *Gordon and Sweet's stain for reticulin*: Connective tissue stain, stains reticular fibers in lives, spleen and lymph nodes via argyrophil metallic impregnation
   - Shows nuclei as Red, cytoplasm as light Red, reticular fibers as black.
   - Used to diagnose Hemangiopericytoma, endothelial cells tumors, myelofibrosis and liver fibrosis.

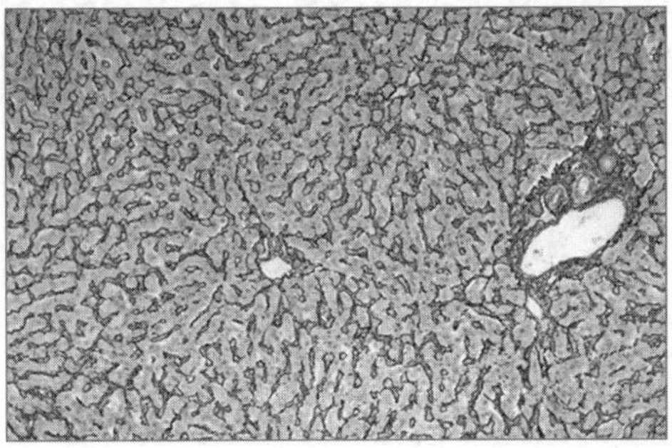

2. *Masson's trichrome stain*: The stain imparts a blue color to collagen against a red background of hepatocytes and other structures.
   - It stains type 1 collagen, normally present in the portal tracts and vessel walls.
   - It is used for staging of chronic liver diseases, and helps to delineate perisinusoidal fibrosis associated with steatohepatitis and periductal fibrosis in primary sclerosing cholangitis.

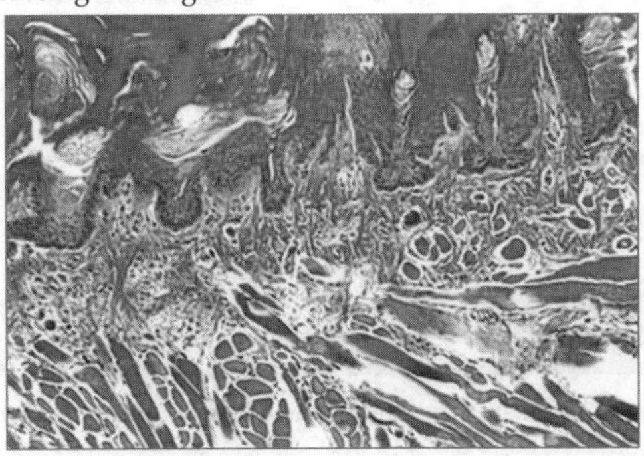

3. *Perl's iron stain (Prussian blue reaction)*: Iron is stored within hepatocytes in 2 forms (a) soluble form as ferritin: not seen on H and E stain (b) Insoluble form as hemosiderin: seen as coarsely granular, brown refractile granules in cytoplasm.
   - Pearl's stain highlights hemosiderin as coarse blue granules, while ferritin is seen as a faint blue cytoplasmic blush.
   - In hemochromatosis, iron accumulates primarily in the cytoplasm and initially in the periportal hepatocytes. In secondary iron overload, the accumulation is mainly in the Kupffer cells.

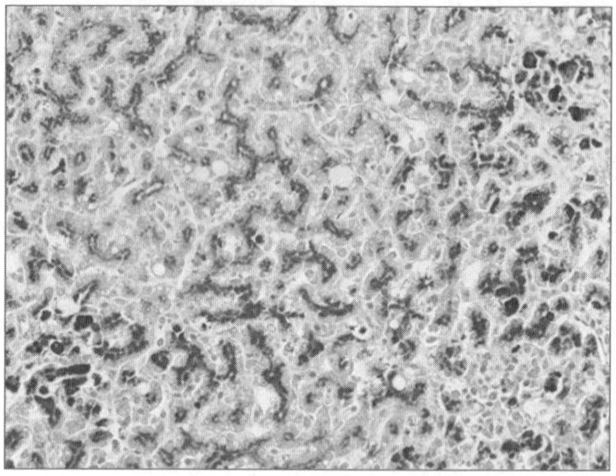

4. *Periodic acid-Schiff stain*: Stains glycogen is helpful in diagnosis of alpha-1-antitrypsin globules, basement membrane, debris within macrophages, and fungal organisms, e.g. various glycogen storage diseases. In patients with alpha-1-antitrypsin deficiency, accumulation is seen as bright magenta globules, typically in periportal hepatocytes.

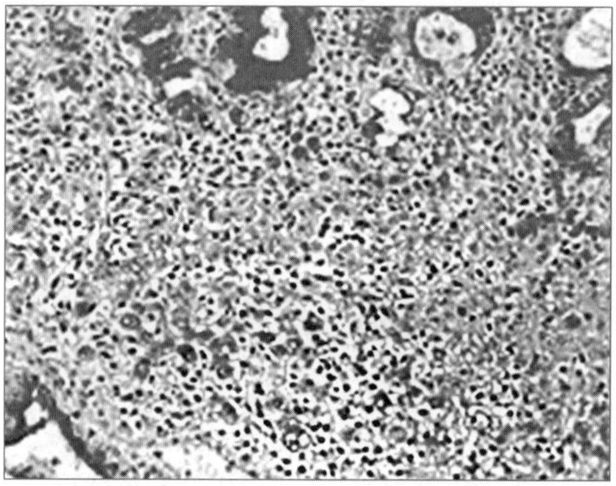

5. *Rhodamine stain* is used to detect copper-binding protein and is thus useful for (1) Evaluation of Wilson disease (2) For differential diagnosis of biliary vs non-biliary disease.

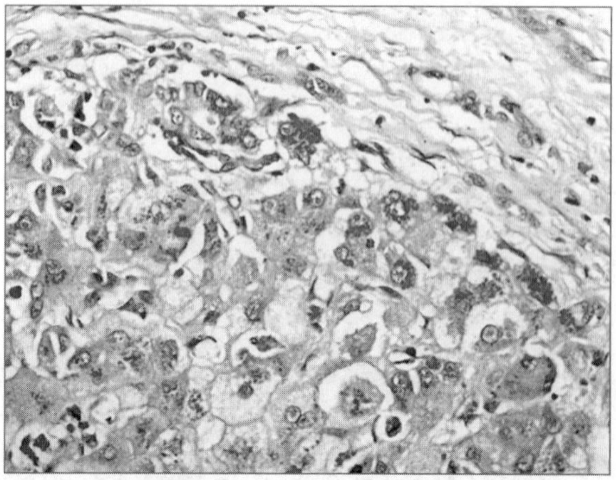

6. *Toluidine blue stains the Mast cells*: Their cytoplasm contains metachromatic granules composed of heparin and histamine. It stains the mast cells violet with blue background.

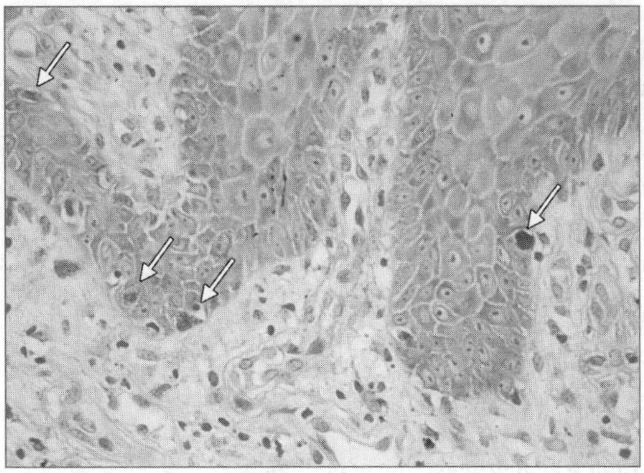

7. *Sudan IV or Oil Red-O* are used for lipids both of which impart an orange color to the contained lipids.
8. *Spirochrome* recently released unique fluorescent stains for monitoring both major components of the cytoskeleton easily in living cells. These fluorescent stains (SiR-Actin and SiR-Tubulin) are cell permeable compounds which stain F-actin (and microtubules, respectively).

350. Stain used for tissue fats is: *(NEET 2016)*

a. PAS
b. Prussian blue
c. Sudan IV
d. Alcian blue

Ans. is 'c' Sudan IV

351. Stain used for tubulin is: *(NEET 2016)*

a. Luna stain
b. Cajal stain
c. SiR stain
d. Masson's trichrome

Ans. is 'c' SiR stain

352. Stain used for staining the nucleus is: *(NEET 2016)*

a. Safranin
b. Fast green
c. Hematoxylin
d. Erythrosine

Ans. is 'c' Hematoxylin

353. Pearl's stain is used to detect: *(NEET 2016)*

a. Glycogen
b. Iron
c. Fungal cell wall
d. Basement membrane of bacteria

Ans. is 'b' Iron

HEAD AND NECK

THYROID CARCINOMA

• Most common thyroid carcinoma	• Papillary carcinoma
• Least common thyroid carcinoma	• Follicular carcinoma
• Radiation induced thyroid carcinoma	• Anaplastic carcinoma
• Thyroid carcinoma arising in long standing goiter	• Papillary carcinoma
• Thyroid carcinoma arising in thyroglossal cyst	• Follicular
• Thyroid carcinoma associated with MEN syndrome	• Papillary carcinoma
• Most common primary cancer with metastasis to thyroid	• Kidney

Genes involved in thyroid cancers:

Papillary	• Tyrosine kinase receptors RET or NTRK1 • RAS mutation • BRAF oncogene
Follicular	• RAS oncogene NRAS • HRAS and KRAS • PAX8- PPARr1 translocation
Medullary	• RET proto-oncogene

- Hurthle cells are large epithelial cells with abundant pink cytoplasm.
- They are found in follicular adenoma, follicular carcinoma and Hashimoto's thyroiditis.
- Amyloid deposition is seen in medullary thyroid cancers.

354. Hurthle cells are seen in: *(NEET 2016)*

a. Medullary carcinoma thyroid
b. Papillary carcinoma thyroid
c. Hashimoto's thyroiditis
d. Pituitary adenoma

Ans. is 'c' Hashimoto's thyroiditis

355. Amyloidosis is associated with which thyroid carcinoma? *(NEET 2016)*

a. Papillary
b. Follicular
c. Anaplastic
d. Medullary

Ans. is 'd' Medullary

356. Metastasis to thyroid comes from which primary site of malignancy? *(NEET 2016)*

a. Liver
b. Testis
c. Prostate
d. Kidney

Ans. is 'd' Kidney

357. Translocation associated with follicular thyroid carcinoma is: *(NEET 2016)*

a. PAX8-PPARr1
b. RET-PTC
c. ALK-NMP1
d. JAK-TEL

Ans. is 'a' PAX8-PPARr1

THYROID CANCER

Typically diagnosed with fine need le aspiration; treated with thyroidectomy. Complications of surgery include hypocalcemia (due to removal of parathyroid glands), transection of recurrent laryngeal nerve during ligation of inferior thyroid artery (leads to dysphagia and dysphonia), and injury to the external branch of the superior laryngeal nerve during ligation of superior thyroid vascular pedicle (may lead to loss of tenor usually noticeable in professional voice users).

Papillary Carcinoma: Most common, excellent prognosis. Empty-appearing nuclei with central clearing ("Orphan Annie" eyes), psammoma bodies, nuclear grooves. Increased risk with *RET/PTC* rearrangements and *BRAF* mutations, childhood irradiation.

Follicular Carcinoma: Good prognosis. Invades thyroid capsule and vasculature (unlike follicular denoma), uniform follicles; hematogenous spread is common. Associated with *RAS* mutation and PAX8-PPAR-γ translocations.

Medullary Carcinoma: From parafollicular C cells; produces calcitonin, sheets of cells in an amyloid stroma (stains with Congo red). Associated with MEN 2A and 2B (RET mutations).

Undifferentiated/Anaplastic Carcinoma: Older patients; presents with rapidly enlarging neck mass→ compressive symptoms (e.g., dyspnea, dysphagia); very poor prognosis. Associated with *TP53* mutation.

358. A 20-year-old female was diagnosed with thyroid mass. Histology revealed orphan annie eyed nuclei as shown in figure. What is the diagnosis? *(NEET 2020)*

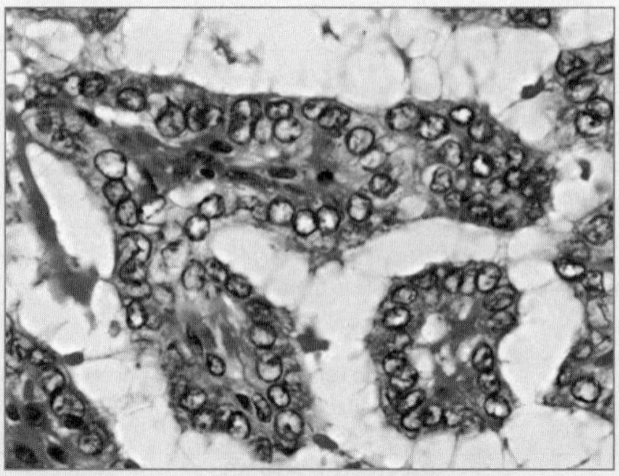

a. Papillary carcinoma
b. Follicular carcinoma
c. Anaplastic carcinoma
d. Medullary carcinoma

Ans. is 'a' Papillary carcinoma

Pathology

Pheochromocytoma

Pheochromocytoma is composed of polygonal to spindle shaped chromaffin cells or chief cells, clustered with sustentacular cells into small nests or alveoli (zellballen) by a rich vascular network. The nuclei are usually round to ovoid, with a stippled "salt and pepper" chromatin that is characteristic of most neuroendocrine tumors.

Zellballen pattern is also seen in paraganglioma.

Urinary VMA, along with other catecholamine metabolites, including homovanillic acid (HVA), metanephrine, and normetanephrine are elevated in patients with tumors that secrete catecholamines (e.g. neuroblastoma, pheochromocytoma, or other neural crest tumors).

These tests are used to diagnose neuroblastomas, and to monitor treatment of these conditions.

Elevated values of homovanillic acid (HVA), vanillylmandelic acid (VMA), and other catecholamine metabolites (e.g., dopamine) may be suggestive of the presence of a catecholamine-secreting tumor.

359. Zellballen pattern is seen in: *(NEET 2016)*

a. Pheochromocytoma
b. Schwannoma
c. Acoustic neuroma
d. Transitional renal cell carcinoma

Ans. is 'a' Pheochromocytoma

360. Which of the following condition is associated with increased VMA? *(NEET 2016)*

a. Rhabdomyosarcoma
b. Pheochromocytoma
c. Nephroblastoma
d. RCC

Ans. is 'b' Pheochromocytoma

Prognostic Factors for Neuroblastoma

Prognostic factors in neuroblastomas

Variable	*Favorable*	*Unfavorable*
Stage	Stage 1, 2A, 2B, 4S	Stage 3, 4
Age	≤1 year	>1 year
Histology • Evidence of schwannian stroma and gangliocytic differentiation • Mitotic rate • Mitosis- karhorrhexis index • Intratumoral calcification	 Present Low ≤200/500 cells Present	 Absent High >200/500 cells Absent
DNA ploidy	Hyperdiploid or near-triploid	Diploid, near-diploid or near tetraploid
N-myc	Not amplified	Amplified
a Chromosome 17q gain	Absent	Present
Chromosome 1p loss	Absent	Present
Chromosome 11q loss	Absent	Present
TrK-B expression	Absent	Present
TrK –A expression	Present	Absent
Telomerase expression	Low or Absent	Highly expressed
MRP expression	Absent	Present
CD-44 expression	Present	Absent
Serum biochemical markers • Ferritin • Lactate dehydrogenase	 Normal ≤1500 U/mL	 Elevated >1500 U/mL

361. What is the most important good prognostic factor for neuroblastoma: *(NEET 2016)*

a. Telomerase expression
b. MRP expression
c. Loss of 11q
d. CD44 expression

Ans. is 'd' CD44 expression

Accessory Salivary Gland

An accessory salivary gland is ectopic salivary gland tissue with a salivary gland duct system. The most common location of accessory salivary gland tissue is an extra major salivary gland in front of the parotid gland.

Salivary gland heterotopia is where salivary gland acini cells are present in an abnormal location without any duct system. The most common location is the cervical lymph nodes.

Most common ectopic salivary gland tissue is Stafne bone cyst.

It presents as asymptomatic, clearly demarcated radiolucency of the angle of mouth, characteristically, below inferior dental neurovascular bundle.

362. Most common site of ectopic salivary gland is: *(NEET 2016)*

a. Cheek b. Palate
c. Angle of mandible d. Tongue

Ans. is 'c' Angle of mandible

Salivary Scintigraphy

- Technetium pertechnetate scans (Salivary scintigraphy) tests the size, shape and function of the salivary glands. It is useful. To help determine the cause of salivary gland swelling (e.g. bacteria or veins).
- To detect a blockage of the salivary ducts.
- To detect a growth in the salivary glands (e.g. Warthin's Tumor).
- To help diagnose abnormal mouth dryness as Sjogren's Syndrome.

363. Salivary schintigraphy is useful in: *(NEET 2016)*

a. Monomorphic adenoma b. Pleomorphic adenoma
c. Sialadenitis d. Sjogren syndrome

Ans. is 'd' Sjogren syndrome

Pleomorphic Adenoma

Pleomorphic adenoma or mixed cell tumor is the most common benign salivary gland neoplasm characterized by neoplastic proliferation of parenchymatous glandular cells along with myoepithelial components, having a malignant potentiality. It is the most common type of salivary gland tumor and the most common tumor of the parotid gland. It arises most commonly from the parotid. It derives its name from the architectural Pleomorphism (variable appearance) seen by light microscopy. It is also known as "Mixed tumor, salivary gland type", which refers to its dual origin from epithelial and myoepithelial elements as opposed to its pleomorphic appearance.

364. Parotid mass with mixed consistency: *(NEET 2019)*

a. Pleomorphic adenoma b. Sebaceous cyst
c. Dermoid cyst d. All

Ans. is 'a' Pleomorphic adenoma

365. Most common variety of benign salivary gland tumor is: *(NEET 2016)*

a. Mucoepidermoid tumor b. Mixed cell tumor
c. Warthin's tumor d. Oncocytoma

Ans. is 'b' Mixed cell tumor

366. Most common site of salivary gland tumor is: *(NEET 2016)*

a. Parotid salivary gland b. Submandibular salivary gland
c. Sublingual gland d. Submaxillary gland

Ans. is 'a' Parotid salivary gland

Warthin Tumor

- Warthin tumor has very characteristic appearance resulting front two main components—epithelial oncocytes arranged in cystic papillary structures and lymphoid stroma.
- They are well encapsulated.
- The epithelium forms cysts with papillary processes extending into them, cystic spaces are lined by bilayered epithelium with oncocytic change—abundant eosinophilic granular cytoplasm (filled with abnormal mitochondria) with centrally placed pyknotic nuclei.
- The stoma contains a variable amount of lymphoid tissue with well-differentiated germinal centers of follicles.
- Very few of Warthin tumors (8%) show squamous metaplasia and regressive changes.

367. Not true about histopathology of Warthin tumor: *(NEET 2016)*

a. Encapsulation b. Pyknotic nuclei
c. Eosinophilic cytoplasm d. Columnar metaplasia

Ans. is 'd' Columnar metaplasia

Miscellaneous

368. Soft wood exposure leads to: *(NEET 2016)*

a. Nasal adenocarcinoma
b. Skin cancer
c. Liver cancer
d. Bladder cancer

Ans. is 'a' Nasal adenocarcinoma

369. Trilateral retinoblastoma is: *(NEET 2016)*

a. Bilateral retinoblastoma plus medulloblastoma
b. Bilateral retinoblastoma plus pineoblastoma
c. Bilateral retinoblastoma plus neuroblastoma
d. Bilateral retinoblastoma plus ependymoma

Ans. is 'b' Bilateral retinoblastoma plus pineoblastoma

370. Most common type of hypopharyngeal carcinoma is: *(NEET 2016)*

a. Adenocarcinoma
b. Lymphoma
c. SCC
d. Neuro-endocrine tumor

Ans. is 'c' SCC

Squamous cell carcinoma is by far the most malignant tumor of the larynx and hypopharynx.

BLOOD TRANSFUSION

BLOOD PRODUCTS

Blood product	Volume in one unit	Storage	Content	Clinical response
Whole blood	350 mL	2–6°C for 42 days	Contains RBCs, WBCs, plasma and platelets	It is not used routinely. Used for massive bleeding if packed RBCs are not available
Packed RBCs	350 mL	2–6°C for 42 days	RBCs with variable leukocyte content and small amount of plasma	Increase Hb 1 g/dL hematocrit 3%
Platelets Random donor Single donor	 40–50 mL 200–240 mL	22–24°C for 5 days	 0.5×10^{10} 3×10^{10}	Increase platelet count 5000–10,000/μL 60,000/μL
FFP	200–250 mL	–18°C for 1 year	Plasma proteins: Coagulation factors, proteins C and S, antithrombin	Increases coagulation factors about 2%
Cryoprecipitate	10–15 mL	–18°C for 1 year	Cold-insoluble plasma proteins, fibrinogen, factor VIII, vWF	Topical fibrin glue, also 80 IU factor VIII

371. Platelets are usually stored at? *(NEET 2016)*

a. 1–6°C
b. 22°C
c. –25°C
d. 40°C

Ans. is 'b' 22°C

Transfusion-related Acute Lung Injury (TRALI)

- TRALI is the most common cause of death after blood transfusion.
- It is frequently associated with multiparous female donors.
- Features predisposing to TRALI
  - Smoking
  - Chronic alcohol use
  - Shock
  - Liver surgery (transplantation)
  - Mechanical ventilation
  - Positive fluid balance

Pathogenesis

- Presence of high-titer of anti-HLA class II antibodies in donor plasma that bind recipient leukocytes.
- Leukocytes aggregate in pulmonary vessels, releasing inflammatory mediators.

Clinical Features

- Hypoxia (PaO_2/FIO_2 <300 mm Hg) with signs of non-cardiogenic pulmonary edema, including bilateral interstitial infiltrates on chest X-ray, within 6 hours of transfusion.

Treatment

- Treatment is supportive with proper oxygenation.
- No definitive treatment is available for TRALI.
  Most cases resolve within 3 days.

372. TRALI usually is due to: *(NEET 2016)*

a. High titer anti-HLA antibodies in recipient plasma
b. Low titer anti-HLA antibodies in donor plasma
c. High titer anti-HLA antibodies in donor plasma
d. HPA-1a on the platelet glycoprotein IIIa receptor

Ans. is 'c' High titer anti-HLA antibodies in donor plasma

Miscellaneous

373. Chromosome for ABO gene is: *(NEET 2016)*

a. 9q
b. 10p
c. 11q
d. 12p

Ans. is 'a' 9q

The ABO gene (Histo-blood group ABO system transferase enzyme) resides on chromosome 9 at the band 9q34.2.

Anticoagulants used for Blood Storage

Acid Citrate Dextrose (ACD)	Citrate Phosphate Dextrose (CPD)
Citric acid, sodium citrate, dextrose	Citric acid, sodium citrate, monobasic sodium phosphate, dextrose
Shelf life of 21 days	Shelf life of 35 days
Acid pH does not help in maintaining 2,3-DPG levels	Alkaline pH and phosphate help in maintaining 2,3-DPG levels
Used in plasmapheresis, tissue typing	Commonly used

374. Why is CPD stored blood better than ACD stored blood for transfusion in a hypoxia patient? *(NEET 2020)*

a. Because it is less acidic
b. Fall in 2,3-DPG is less
c. Hypertonicity of blood
d. More citrate ions

Ans. is 'b' Fall in 2,3-DPG is less

CHAPTER 5 Pharmacology

GENERAL PHARMACOLOGY

THERAPEUTIC INDEX

The therapeutic index (TI) of a drug is the ratio the dose that produces toxicity to the dose that produces a clinically desired or effective response in a population of individuals:

$$TI = TD50/ED50$$

Where TD50 = the drug dose that produces a toxic effect in 50% the population and ED50 = the drug dose that produces a therapeutic or desired response in 50% of the population.

More the TD50, safer is the drug. More the ED50, lower is the potency.

TI is a measure of a drugs' safety, because a larger value indicates a wide margin between doses that are effective and doses that are toxic.

Drugs with Narrow Therapeutic Index: Lithium, TCAs, Aminoglycosides, Amphotericin B, Phenytoin, Valproate, Theophylline, Warfarin

1. ED50 of a drug is a measure of its:

a. Safety
b. Potency
c. Efficacy
d. Marketability

Ans. is 'b' Potency

BIOAVAILABILITY

- Bioavailability describes the fractional extent to which an administered dose of drug reaches its site of action or a biological fluid (usually the systemic circulation) from which the drug has access to its site of action.
- A drug given orally must be absorbed first from the GI tract, but net absorption may be limited by the characteristics of the dosage form, by the drug's physicochemical properties, by metabolic attack in the intestine, and by transport across the intestinal epithelium and into the portal circulation.
- The absorbed drug then passes through the liver, where metabolism and biliary excretion may occur before the drug enters the systemic circulation. Accordingly, less than all of the administered dose may reach the systemic circulation and be distributed to the drug's sites of action.
- If the metabolic or excretory capacity of the liver and the intestine for the drug is large, bioavailability will be reduced substantially (first-pass effect).
- This decrease in availability is a function of the anatomical site from which absorption takes place; for instance, intravenous administration generally permits all of the drug to enter the systemic circulation.
- Bioavailability F is defined as:

$$F = \frac{\text{Quantity of drug reaching systemic circulation}}{\text{Quantity of drug administered}}$$

2. What explains correctly about the fraction of drug given via nonintravenous route reaching the systemic circulations?

a. Efficacy
b. Potency
c. Bioavailability
d. Maintenance dose

Ans. is 'c' Bioavailability

BIOTRANSFORMATION

- Biotransformation means chemical alteration of the drug in the body.
- It is needed to render nonpolar (lipid soluble) compounds to polar (lipid insoluble or water soluble) so that they are not reabsorbed in the renal tubules and are excreted.
- Biotransformation reactions (metabolism) of drugs can be classified:

Non-synthetic/Phase I/Functionalization Reactions

- The enzymes involved in Phase I reactions are primarily located in the endoplasmic reticulum of the liver they are called microsomal enzymes (CYP-450 enzymes – superfamily of mono-oxygenases).
- Metabolism brings about a change in the drug molecule by: Oxidation, Reduction, Hydrolysis, Cyclization, Decyclization.

Synthetic/Phase II/Conjugation Reactions

- Metabolism involves union of the drug with one of several polar (water-soluble) endogenous molecules that are products of intermediary metabolism, to form a water-soluble conjugate which is readily eliminated by kidney or bile. Metabolite is mostly inactive.
- Reactions involved are: Acetylation, Glucuronide conjugation, Glycine conjugation, Glutathione conjugation, Sulfate conjugation, Methylation, Nucleotide synthesis.

Drugs Metabolized by Acetylation

- Compounds having amino or hydralazine residues are conjugated with the help of Acetyl CoA.
- *Examples*: Clonazepam, Hydralazine, INH, PAS, Procainamide, Sulfonamides including dapsone.

CYP Enzyme Inducers and Inhibitors

Enzyme inducers	Enzyme inhibitors
All antiepileptics except valproate	Propoxyphene
All antitubercular drugs except isoniazid	Erythromycin
DDT	Amiodarone, verapamil, diltiazem
Phenytoin, phenobarbital	Ciprofloxacin
Griseofulvin	Omeprazole Cimetidine, clopidogrel
Smoking Ethanol	Ketoconazole/itraconazole Ritonavir Grape fruit juice

3. Drug not causing enzyme inhibition is:

a. Phenobarbitone
b. Omeprazole
c. Disulfiram
d. Diltiazem

Ans. is 'a' Phenobarbitone

4. All of the following are Phase II reactions *except*:

a. Acetylation
b. Methylation
c. Cyclization
d. Glycine conjugation

Ans. is 'c' Cyclization

5. Which of the following drug is not metabolized by acetylation?

a. PAS
b. Dapsone
c. Hydrocortisone
d. Hydralazine

Ans. is 'c' Hydrocortisone

6. Which of the following antimicrobials should not be given to a chronic asthmatic patient managed on theophylline therapy? *(NEET 2020)*

a. Erythromycin
b. Cefotaxime
c. Cotrimoxazole
d. Amoxicillin

Ans. is 'a' Erythromycin

Explanation: Drugs which inhibit theophylline metabolism and increase its plasma level are—erythromycin, ciprofloxacin, cimetidine, oral contraceptives, allopurinol, etc.

SYNERGISM

When the action of one drug is facilitated or increased by the other, they are said to be synergistic. In a synergistic pair, both the drugs can have action in the same direction or given alone one may be inactive but still enhance the action of the other when given together.

Synergism can be:

- *Additive:* The effect of the two drugs is in the same direction and simply adds up: effect of drugs A + B = effect of drug A + effect of drug B
- ***Supra-additive (potentiation):*** The effect of combination is greater than the individual effects of the components: effect of drug A + B > effect of drug A + effect of drug B. This is always the case when one component is inactive as such.

Pharmacology

Additive drug combination	
Aspirin + paracetamol	As analgesic/antipyretic
Nitrous oxide + halothane	As general anesthetic
Amlodipine + atenolol	As antihypertensive
Glibenclamide + metformin	As hypoglycemic
Ephedrine + theophylline	As bronchodilator

Supra-additive drug combination	
Drug pair	***Basis of potentiation***
Acetylcholine + physostigmine	Inhibition of break down
Levodopa + carbidopa/benseramine	Inhibition of peripheral metabolism
Adrenaline + cocaine/desipramine	Inhibition of neuronal uptake
Sulfamethoxazole + trimethoprim	Sequential blockade
Antihypertensives (enalapril + hydrochlorothiazide)	Tackling two contributory factors
Tyramine + MAO inhibitors	Increasing release of CA store

7. Synergistic action is shown by the following drug combinations *except*:

a. Glibenclamide and metformin
b. Enalapril and hydrochlorothiazide
c. Levodopa and carbidopa
d. Hydrochlorothiazide and triamterene

Ans. is 'd' Hydrochlorothiazide and triamterene

P-GLYCOPROTEIN

- P-glycoprotein (P-gp) is a product of multidrug resistance 1 gene.
- P-glycoprotein plays an important role in pharmacokinetics of drugs.
- P-glycoprotein is an ATP-binding cassette (ABC) transporter and is an important factor to limit membrane permeability, in several tissues and/or elimination pathways into urine (renal tubules) and bile (liver).
- P-glycoprotein has following effects on drugs
  - Decreasing the absorption of drugs and toxins in intestine by efflux transport from enterocytes
  - Decreasing the distribution of drug in brain by efflux transport at BBB
  - Excretion of drug by kidney (renal tubular secretion) and liver (secretion into bile)
  - Multiple drug resistance of a cancer by export (explusion) of anticancer drugs from the cells.

Inhibitors of P-glycoprotein
Verapamil Quinidine Erythromycin
Inducers of P-glycoprotein
Phenobarbitone Rifampicin

8. Which of the following drugs is not an inhibitor of P-glycoprotein?

a. Quinidine
b. Erythromycin
c. Verapamil
d. Phenobarbitone

Ans. is 'd' Phenobarbitone

PHASES OF CLINICAL TRIAL

Phase	Name	Blinding and control	Subject population	Purpose
I	Human pharmacology and safety	No blinding or control	Healthy volunteers (20–100)	To know maximum tolerable dose Safety and tolerability
II	Therapeutic exploratory	Single blinded with control	100–150 patients in a single centre	To establish therapeutic efficacy Dose ranging and celling efficacy
III	Therapeutic confirmatory	Double blinded trial with standard drug being given to the control population.	A large number of patients from several centers	To confirm therapeutic efficacy To establish the value of drug in relation to existing therapy

Contd...

Contd...

Phase	Name	Blinding and control	Subject population	Purpose
IV	Post marketing surveillance	–	Patients being treated by the doctors	To ascertain long-term adverse effects and effect of the drug on special groups like children, pregnant ladies, elderly
0	Microdosing studies	No blinding or control	Small number of healthy volunteers	The drug is administered in very low doses- 1/100th of human dose, to ascertain the pharmacokinetics

9. Phase II in a clinical drug trial is:

a. Human pharmacology and safety
b. Therapeutic exploration and dose ranging
c. Therapeutic comparison
d. Post-marketing surveillance

Ans. is 'b' Therapeutic exploration and dose ranging

DOSE RESPONSE CURVE

- It is a graphical representation of response plotted against the log of dose given. It can be used to evaluate and compare the potencies and efficacies of various drugs.
- Potency refers to the amount of drug needed to produce a certain response. The drug which requires a lower dose to produce the same response is said to be more potent.
- ED50, which is the dose required to produce half the maximum response is used to compare the potencies of two drugs.
- Efficacy refers to the maximum response produced by the drug. It is by far more clinically relevant than potency in most cases.

Dose responce curve (DRC) can also be used to study various types of antagonisms:

Competitive Antagonism

- It has affinity but no intrinsic activity. It is structurally similar to the agonist and competes with it for the receptor binding site.
- DRC of the agonist is shifted to the Right, but the maximum response remains the same.

Non-competitive Antagonism

- It binds to an allosteric site different from the agonist binding site, altering the receptor in such a way that it is unable to combine with agonist.
- Maximum response of the agonist is reduced.
- The antagonism is irreversible regardless of the agonist concentration.

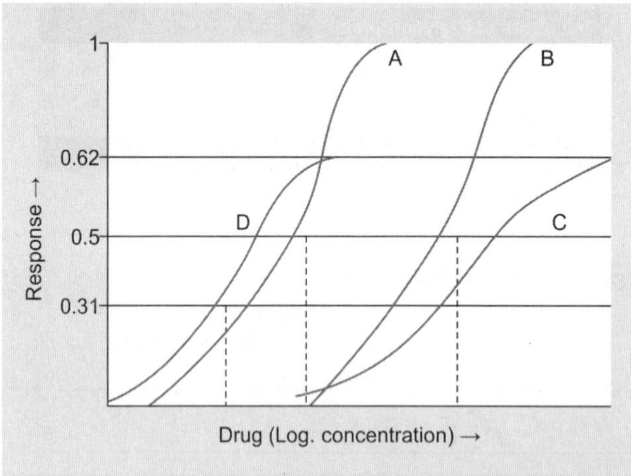

In the given DRC:

- Drug B is less potent but equally efficacious as drug A
- Drug C is less potent and less efficacious than drug A
- Drug D is more potent than drugs A, B & C but less efficacious than drugs A & B, and equally efficacious as drug C.

10. Variation in sensitivity of response to different doses of a drug in different individuals is obtained from? *(NEET 2019)*

a. Dose response curve
b. Therapeutic index
c. Bioavailability
d. Phase 1 clinical trials

Ans. is 'a' Dose response curve

Pharmacology

11. Which of the drugs shown in the graph below has highest potency? *(NEET 2020)*

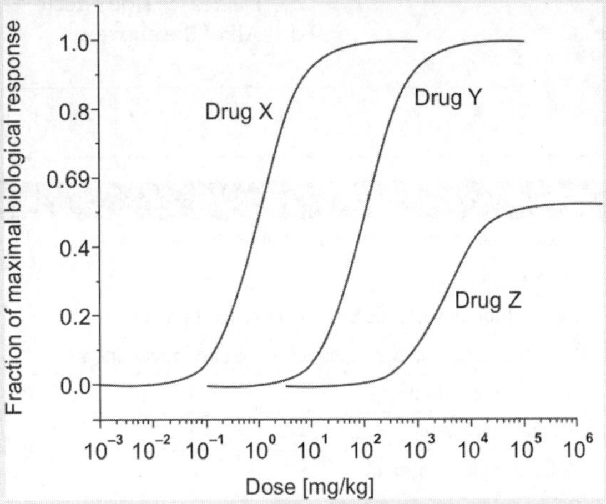

a. Drug X
b. Drug Y
c. Drug Z
d. Equal for drug X and Y

Ans. is 'a' Drug X

PLASMA PROTEIN BINDING

- Most drugs get reversibly bound to plasma proteins.
- Acidic drugs generally bind to plasma albumin and basic drugs bind to α_1-acid glycoprotein.

Clinical Implications

- Highly plasma protein bound drugs are largely restricted to vascular compartment. They have smaller volume of distribution.
- The bound fraction is not available for action. However, it is in equilibrium with free drug concentration in plasma. Plasma protein binding thus tantamount to temporary storage of drug.
- High protein binding makes the drug long-lasting, because bound fraction is not available for metabolism or glomerular filtration. Active tubular secretion however, is not affected by protein binding. Highly protein bound drugs are not removed by hemodialysis and need special techniques for treatment for poisoning.
- One drug can bind to many sites on the albumin molecule. Conversely, more than one drug can bind to the same site. This can give rise to displacement interactions among drugs.
- In hypoalbuminemia, high concentrations of free drug may be attained (e.g. phenytoin, furosemide).

12. A drug with high plasma protein binding has which of these properties? *(NEET 2019)*

a. Less GFR
b. Less drug interaction
c. Higher volume of distribution
d. Less tubular secretion

Ans. is 'a' Less GFR

FIXED DOSE COMBINATIONS (FDCs) OF DRUGS

Advantages

- Convenience and better compliance
- Synergistic combinations; e.g. sulfamethoxazole + trimethoprim
- If the components act by different mechanisms, the therapeutic effect of two components may add up while side effects may not; e.g. amlodipine + atenolol
- The side effect of one component may be counteracted by the other; e.g. thiazide + potassium sparing diuretic
- Combined formulation ensures that a single drug will not be administered; important in TB, HIV and falciparum malaria.

Disadvantages

- Patient may not actually need all component drugs
- Dose of most drugs needs to be individualized
- Time course of action of the components may be different
- Adverse effect cannot be easily ascribed to the particular drug causing it
- Contraindication to one component contraindicates the whole product.

13. What is the advantage of fixed dose combination of drugs? *(NEET 2019)*

a. Increases efficacy of drugs
b. Decreases side effects
c. Patient compliance improved
d. All of the above

Ans. is 'd' All of the above

TERATOGENS

Teratogen	Effects on Fetus
ACE inhibitors	Oligohydramnios, renal failure, hypocalvaria
Aminoglycosides	Ototoxicity
Antiepileptic drugs	Neural tube defects, cardiac defects, cleft palate
Diethylstilbestrol (DES)	Mullerian anomalies, Vaginal clear cell adenocarcinoma
Folate antagonists	Neural tube defects
Lithium	Ebstein anomaly
Methimazole	Aplasia cutis congenita
Tetracyclines	Discolored teeth, inhibited bone growth
Thalidomide	Limb defects (phocomelia, micromelia – 'flipper' limbs)
Warfarin	Bone deformities, fetal hemorrhage
Maternal diabetes	Caudal regression syndrome (anal atresia to sirenomelia – fused legs), congenital heart defects (e.g. VSD, TGA), neural tube defects, macrosomia, neonatal hypoglycemia, polycythemia
Vitamin A excess	Extremely high risk for spontaneous abortions and birth defects (cleft palate, cardiac)

14. A female gave birth to a child as shown below. What is the likely cause of this malformation? *(NEET 2020)*

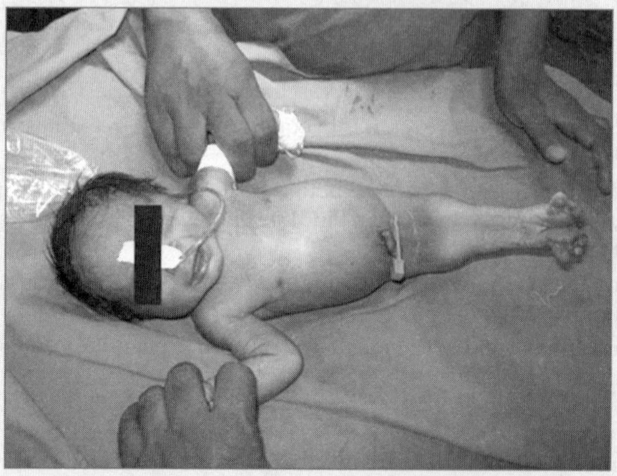

a. Diabetes
b. Lithium
c. Valproate
d. ACEI

Ans. is 'a' Diabetes

AUTONOMIC NERVOUS SYSTEM

CHOLINERGIC RECEPTORS

Receptor	Cellular and tissue location	Cellular response	Functional response	Disease relevance
M_1	CNS; most abundant in cerebral cortex, hippocampus, striatum, and thalamus Autonomic ganglia Glands (gastric and salivary) Enteric nerves	Couples by $G_{q/11}$ to activate PLC-IP_3-Ca^{2+}-PKC pathway Depolarization and excitation (↑ sEPSP) Activation of PLD_2, PLA_2; ↑AA	Increased cognitive function (learning and memory) Increased seizure activity Decrease in dopamine release and locomotion Increase in depolarization of autonomic ganglia Increase in secretions	Alzheimer disease Cognitive dysfunction Schizophrenia

Contd...

Pharmacology

Contd...

Receptor	Cellular and tissue location	Cellular response	Functional response	Disease relevance
M_2	Widely expressed in CNS, hindbrain, thalamus, cerebral cortex, hippocampus, striatum, heart, smooth muscle, autonomic nerve terminals	Couples by G_i/G_o (PTX sensitive) Inhibition of AC, ↓ cAMP Activation of inwardly rectifying K^+ channels Inhibition of voltage-gated Ca^{2+}channels Hyperpolarization and inhibition	***Heart:*** SA node: slowed spontaneous depolarization; hyperpolarization, ↓ HR AV node: decrease in conduction velocity Atrium: ↓ refractory period, ↓ contraction Ventricle: slight ↓ contraction ***Smooth muscle:*** ↑ Contraction ***Peripheral nerves:*** Neural inhibition via autoreceptors and heteroreceptor ↓ Ganglionic transmission. ***CNS:*** Neural inhibition ↑ Tremors; hypothermia; analgesia	Alzheimer disease Cognitive dysfunction Pain
M_3	Widely expressed in CNS (< other mAChRs), cerebral cortex, hippocampus Abundant in smooth muscle and glands Heart	Couples by $G_{q/11}$ to activate PLC-IP_3/DAG-Ca^{2+}-PKC pathway Depolarization and excitation (↑ sEPSP) Activation of PLD_2, PLA_2; ↑AA	***Smooth muscle:*** ↑ Contraction (predominant in some, e.g., bladder) ***Glands:*** ↑ Secretion (predominant in salivary gland) Increases food intake, body weight, fat deposits Inhibition of DA release Synthesis of NO	Chronic obstructive pulmonary disease (COPD) Urinary incontinence Irritable bowel disease
M_4	Preferentially expressed in CNS, particularly forebrain, also striatum, cerebral cortex, hippocampus	Couples by G_i/G_0 (PTX sensitive) Inhibition of AC, ↓ cAMP Activation of inwardly rectifying K^+ channels Inhibition of voltage-gated Ca^{2+}channels Hyperpolarization and inhibition	Autoreceptor- and heteroreceptor-mediated inhibition of transmitter release in CNS and periphery Analgesia; cataleptic activity Facilitation of DA release	Parkinson disease Schizophrenia Neuropathic pain
M_5	Substantia nigra Expressed in low levels in CNS and periphery Predominant mAChR in neurons in VTA and substantia nigra	Couples by $G_{q/11}$ to activate PLC-IP_3–Ca^{2+}–PKC pathway Depolarization and excitation (↑ sEPSP) Activation of PLD_2, PLA_2; ↑AA	Mediator of dilation in cerebral arteries and arterioles (?) Facilitates DA release Augmentation of drug-seeking behavior and reward (e.g., opiates, cocaine)	Drug dependence Parkinson disease Schizophrenia

Receptor (primary receptor subtype)	Main synaptic location	Membrane response	Molecular mechanism	Agonists	Antagonists
Skeletal muscle (Nm)	Skeletal neuromuscular junction (postjunctional)	Excitatory; end-plate depolarization; skeletal muscle contraction	Increased cation permeability (Na^+; K^+)	ACh Nicotine Succinylcholine	Atracurium Vecuronium d-Tubocurarine Pancuronium α-Conotoxin α-Bungarotoxin
Peripheral neuronal (Nn)	Autonomic ganglia; adrenal medulla	Excitatory; depolarization; firing of postganglion neuron; depolarization and secretion of catecholamines	Increased cation permeability (Na^+; K^+)	ACh Nicotine Epibatidine Dimethylphenyl- piperazinium	Trimethaphan Mecamylamine
CNS neuronal α-BTX-insensitive	CNS; pre- and postjunctional	Pre- and postsynaptic excitation; prejunctional control of transmitter release	Increased cation permeability (Na^+; K^+)	Cytosine, epibatidine Anatoxin A	Mecamylamine DHbE Erysodine Lophotoxin
α-BTX-sensitive	CNS; pre- and postsynaptic	Pre- and postsynaptic excitation; prejunctional control of transmitter release	Increased permeability (Ca^{2+})	Anatoxin A	Methyllycaconitine α-Bungarotoxin α-Conotoxin Iml

15. Mechanism of action of curare like drugs: *(NEET 2019)*

a. Blocks ACh synthesis
b. Blocks ACh receptors
c. Persistent depolarization
d. Agonistic with ACh receptors

Ans. is 'b' Blocks ACh receptors

Pharmacology

USES OF ANTIMUSCARINIC AGENTS

- CNS effects
  - Motion sickness: Scopolamine (transdermal patch)
  - Drug-induced parkinsonism: Trihexiphenidyl, benztropine
  - Atropine is CNS stimulant whereas scopolamine is CNS depressant
- Mydriatic and cycloplegic agents: Atropine. Homatropine, cyclopentolate, tropicamide
  - Tropicamide is the shortest acting mydriatic, Atropine is longest acting mydriatic
  - Anticholinergic agents are contraindicated in glaucoma
- Arrhythmias like AV block: Atropine
- COPD and Bronchial asthma: Ipratropium, tiotropium
- Preanesthetic medication to reduce secretions: Glycopyrrolate
  - Glycopyrrolate is a quarternary synthetic compound, which is potent and rapidly acting antimuscarinic lacking CNS penetration and central effects. It is almost exclusively used in preanesthetic medication.
- GIT
  - Anti-spasmodics: Hyoscine, dicyclomine, propantheline
  - Irritable bowel syndrome: Darifenacin, solefenacin (selective M3 blockers)
- Genitourinary tract
  - Urinary incontinence (detrusor instability): Oxybutynin, dicyclomine
- Atropine is contraindicated in children due to the risk of hyperthermia (due to decreased sweating).

16. A patient was recently started on Fluphenazine. Few weeks later, he developed tremors, rigidity, bradykinesia and excessive salivation. First line of management for this patient is: *(NEET 2020)*

a. Selegiline
b. Trihexiphenidyl
c. Pramipexole
d. Amantadine

Ans. is 'b' Trihexiphenidyl

Explanation: Trihexyphenidyl is anticholinergic and it is the most commonly used drug for drug-induced parkinsonism. Selegiline, Pramipexole, Amantadine are used in Parkinson disease but not in drug-induced parkinsonism.

17. Oxybutynin acts by:

a. Adrenergic receptor antagonist
b. Muscarinic receptor antagonist
c. Histaminic antagonist
d. Serotonergic antagonist

Ans. is 'b' Muscarinic receptor antagonist

Cholinomimetic Agents

Direct Agonists

- Bethanechol: Urinary retention (activates bladder smooth muscle; no nicotinic activity)
- Carbachol: Constricts pupil and relieves intraocular pressure in open-angle glaucoma
- Methacholine: Challenge test for diagnosis of asthma
- Pilocarpine: Potent stimulator of sweat, tears and saliva. Contracts ciliary muscle of eye (open-angle glaucoma), pupillary sphincter (closed-angle glaucoma). Used in xerostomia (Sjogren syndrome)

Indirect Agonists (Anti-cholinesterases)

- Donepezil, rivastigmine, galantamine: First line for Alzeihmer's disease
- Edrophonium: Historically used to diagnose myasthenia gravis; replaced by anti-AChR Ab (anti-acetylcholine receptor antibody) test
- Neostigmine: Postoperative and neurogenic ileus and urinary retention, myasthenia gravis, reversal of postoperative neuromuscular junction blockade. No CNS penetration.
- Physostigmine: Antidote for anticholinergic toxicity
- Pyridostigmine: Myasthenia gravis (long acting)

18. A patient with diabetes and COPD developed postoperative urinary retention. Which of the following drugs can be used for short-term treatment to relieve the symptoms of this person? *(NEET 2020)*

a. Bethanechol
b. Tamsolusin
c. Terazosin
d. Methacholine

Ans. is 'a' Bethanechol

19. Perioperative patient was given a skeletal muscle relaxant that acts by competitive inhibition of nicotinic ACh receptors. What agent can be used for the reversal of its effects? *(NEET 2020)*

a. Physostigmine
b. Neostigmine
c. Succinylcholine
d. Carbachol

Ans. is 'b' Neostigmine

ORGANOPHOSPHATE POISONING

The anticholinesterase action of organophosphates causes increased cholinergic activity in both muscarinic and nicotinic receptors.

Various anticholinesterases are:

- Organophosphates: malathion, dyflos, echothiophate, diazinon (TIK-20)
- Carbamates: Carbaryl (Sevin), Propoxur (Baygon).

Clinical Manifestations

Action at neuromuscular junction results in fatigability & generalized weakness, fasciculations & eventually paralysis.

Involvement of respiratory muscles leads to respiratory failure.

Miosis and ciliary spasm results in diminished vision

- *Respiratory effects*: Chest tightness and dyspnea
- Nausea, vomiting, and diarrhea
- Excessive salivation, lacrimation, bradycardia, hypotension

Red Tears or Chromo-lacryorrhea—Occurs rarely due to accumulation of porphyrin pigments in lacrimal glands.

Treatment

- Avoiding further exposure to the toxin.
- Maintain patent airway, provide adequate ventilation and maintain fluid balance.
- *Gastric lavage*: Effective only when given within the initial 2 hrs.
- Activated charcoal without cathartic: It can bind the unabsorbed toxin and prevent further worsening of symptoms.
- *Specific antidotes*: Atropine, being an anticholinergic agent, can reverse the symptoms.
- *Pralidoxime*: Reactivates cholinesterase enzyme, by preventing the formation of phosphorylated enzyme & directly detoxify organophosphates. It can thus decrease the amount of atropine required & potentiates the action of atropine.

Oximes are ineffective in carbamate poisoning. In fact, pralidoxime is contraindicated in carbamate poisoning, because not only it does not reactivate carbamylated enzyme, it has weak anti-ChE activity of its own.

20. Drug given in organophosphate poisoning is:

a. Hyoscine
b. Atropine
c. Propantheline
d. Physostigmine

Ans. is 'b' Atropine

BETA-BLOCKERS

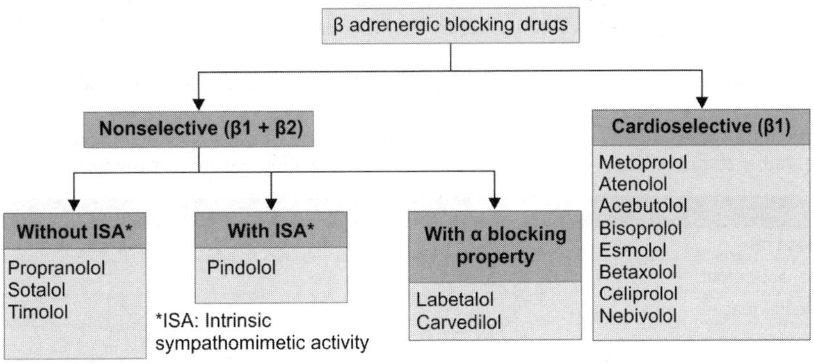

Generation-wise classification

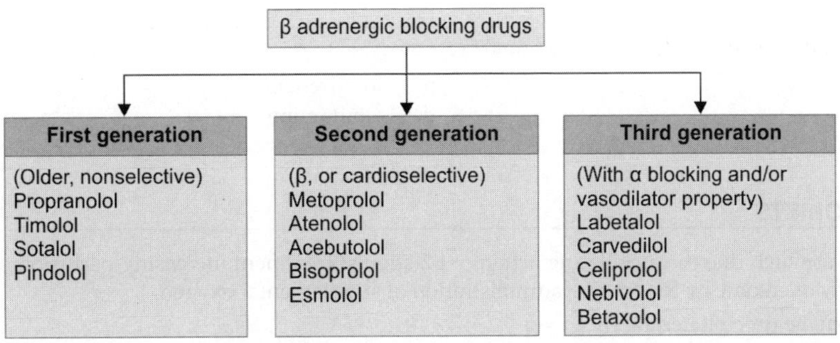

Beta-blockers with Membrane Stabilizing Activity

- These drugs possess Na^+ channel blocking (local anesthetic) activity. It can contribute to anti-arrhythmic action.
- These drugs should be avoided in glaucoma due to the risk of corneal anesthesia.
- *Examples:* Propranolol (maximum), Metoprolol, Labetalol, Acebutolol, Pindolol, Carvedilol.

21. β-blocker/s which should be avoided in glaucoma is/are:

a. Pindolol
b. Carvedilol
c. Labetalol
d. All the above

Ans. is 'd' All the above

ADRENERGIC DRUGS

Nonselective adrenergic drugs
Adrenaline: α1 + α2 + β1 + β2 + β3 (β2 > β1)
Noradrenaline: α1 + α2 + β1 + β3 (but no β2)
Isoprenaline: β1 + β2 + β3 (but no α action)
Selective adrenergic drugs
α1 agonists—Phenylephrine, methoxamine, naphazoline, oxymetazoline, xylometazoline
α2 agonists—Clonidine, methyldopa, brimonidine, apraclonidine
β1 agonists—Dobutamine
β2 agonists—Salbutamol, terbutaline, salmeterol, ritodrine

Properties of Adrenaline

Adrenaline acts on-α1, α2, β1, β2 and β3 receptors
α1- present in blood vessels–causes vasoconstriction—increases blood pressure
β2 – present in blood vessels—causes vasodilation–decreases blood pressure

At lower concentration of adrenaline, β2–receptors are more sensitive

At higher concentration, adrenaline acts on all receptors.

When we give adrenaline intravenously, initially the concentration of adrenaline is high.

So it will act on α1, β2. But action of α1 (vasoconstriction), will predominate over actions of β2.(vasodilatation). So there will be rise in blood pressure within few seconds.

Level of adrenaline will decrease due to its rapid metabolism and neuronal reuptake

At lower concentration only action of β2 will predominate, so only fall in blood pressure is seen

So at this level you can observe initial rise in blood pressure and then fall in blood pressure. This is called biphasic response (it is not vasomotor reversal of dale)

After biphasic response if we administer non-selective alpha blocker, it blocks the alpha receptors, hence α1 mediated vasoconstriction gets blocked.

Now, if you give adrenaline again, only β2 mediated action occurs (because α1 receptors are blocked by alpha blocker). So only fall in blood pressure is seen, rather than biphasic response. The phenomenon is called vasomotor reversal of Dale.

	Adrenaline	Noradrenaline	Isoprenaline
Heart rate	↑	↓	↑↑
Cardiac output	↑↑	-	↑↑
Blood Pressure			
Systolic	↑↑	↑↑	↓↑
Diastolic	↓↑	↑↑	↑↑
Mean	↑	↑↑	↓

22. Which of the following acts on α1, α2, β1 but not on β2 receptors?

a. Adrenaline
b. Noradrenaline
c. Isoprenaline
d. Dobutamine

Ans. is 'b' Noradrenaline

TOXICITIES OF β2-AGONISTS

- Ventilation-perfusion mismatch due to vasodilating action of β2-agonist treatment increasing perfusion of poorly ventilated lung units. This effect is easily overcome by the routine administration of supplemental oxygen.
- Cardiac arrhythmias may be precipitated rarely.

Pharmacology

- *Tachyphylaxis*: A reduction in the bronchodilator response to low-dose β-agonist treatment can be shown after several days of regular β-agonist use, but maximal bronchodilation is still achieved well within the range of doses usually given.
- Tremors occur β2-agonists directly stimulate β-2 receptors present in the skeletal muscles.
- Hypokalemia due to intracellular shift of potassium.
- The commonest adverse effects are muscle tremors and palpitations which are more common in elderly patients.

23. Commonest side effect of short β2-agonist used in asthma is:

a. Muscle tremors　　b. Hypokalemia
c. Hypoglycemic attacks　　d. Sedation

Ans. is 'a' Muscle tremors

DRUGS USED FOR GLAUCOMA

Action of Autonomic System on Intraocular Muscles

	Parasympathetic nervous system	Sympathetic nervous system
Radial muscles of iris	—	Mydriasis via alpha1 receptors
Circular muscles of iris	Miosis	—
Ciliary muscles	Contraction for near vision	—

Drugs used for glaucoma (Open angle)

Group	*Drugs*	*Mechanism of action*	*Adverse-effects*
Miotics: Direct acting AChE inhibitor	Pilocarpine Physostigmine	↑ Trabecular outflow	• Blurred vision (induced myopia) • Headache, brow pain • Cataract formation • Retinal detachment • Iris cysts & corneal hypoesthesia
Beta-blockers: Non-selective (beta-1 & beta-2) Selective (beta-1)	Timolol Levobunolol Carteolol Betaxolol	↓ Aqueous formation	• Allergic blepharoconjunctivitis • Transient stinging • Acquired nasolacrimal duct obstruction
Carbonic anhydrase inhibitors	Dorzolamide Brinzolamide	↓ Aqueous formation	• Ocular allergy, bitter taste • Corneal edema
Alpha-2 agonists	Apraclonidine Brimonidine	↓ Aqueous formation	• Lid retraction • Allergic follicular conjunctivitis • Blepharitis & anterior uveitis • Dry mouth, drowsiness & apnea in children <6 years with apraclonidine
Alpha-1 agonists	Dipivefrine adrenaline	↑ Trabecular & uveoscleral outflow	• Maculopathy, black adrenochrome deposits with adrenaline • Ocular allergy • Conjunctival hyperemia
Prostaglandin 2- alpha	Latanoprost Bimatoprost Travoprost Unoprostone Tafluprost	↑ Uveoscleral outflow	• Iris pigmentation (Hyperchromia) • Darkening of periocular skin • Conjunctival congestion (Least with latanoprost) • Growth of eyelashes • Macular edema • Mild iridocyclitis

Management of Acute Congestive (Angle Closure) Glaucoma

It is an emergency condition with marked congestion of eyes and severe headache.

- Hypertonic mannitol or glycerol – given IV; decongest the eye by osmotic action
- Acetazolamide – started concurrently
- Miotic – When IOP is very high, iris muscle fails to respond to miotics; tension should be reduced by other measures before miotics can act
- Topical beta-blocker
- Apraclonidine / Latanoprost may be added.

24. IV mannitol is used for treatment of: *(NEET 2019)*

a. Acute congestive glaucoma　　b. Pulmonary edema
c. Acute renal failure　　d. CHF

Ans. is 'a' Acute congestive glaucoma

25. Which of the following is alpha-2-agonist? *(NEET 2019)*

a. Apraclonidine
b. Timolol
c. Prostaglandin analogues
d. Verapamil

Ans. is 'a' Apraclonidine

26. Anti-glaucoma drug that acts by increasing uveoscleral outlfow is: *(NEET 2020)*

a. Latanoprost
b. Timolol
c. Dorzolamide
d. Pilocarpine

Ans. is 'a' Latanoprost

Explanation: Mode of action of ocular hypotensive drugs

Drug/class	Aqueous secretion	Trabecular outflow	Uveoscleral outflow
1. β-blockers (Timolol)	↓	–	–
2. Adrenaline/Dipivefrine	↓	↑	↑
3. Brimonidine/apraclonidine	↓	–	↑
4. Prostaglandins (Latanoprost)	–	↑	↑
5. Miotics (Pilocarpine)	–	↑	–
6. Carbonic anhydrase inhibitors	↓	–	–

AUTACOIDS

TREATMENT AND PROPHYLAXIS OF MIGRAINE

- For aborting an acute attack of migraine, sumatriptan (or any other triptan) is the drug of choice. Other drugs used for treatment are NSAIDs, ergotamine and dihydroergotamine, and intranasal butorphanol.
- For Prophylaxis, Beta-blocker (propranolol) is the drug of choice. Other drugs used for prophylaxis are tricyclic antidepressants (amitriptyline), calcium channel blockers (cinnarizine, verapamil), serotonin antagonists (methysergide, cyproheptadine), MAO inhibitors, and anticonvulsants (valproate, topiramate, gabapentin), papaverine and phenelzine.

Triptans

- These are 5-HT ID/IB receptor agonists.
- Sumatriptan is the 1st triptan to be developed. It is the drug of choice for aborting an acute attack of migraine.
- Other triptans include almotriptan, eletriptan, frovatriptan, rizatriptan, naratriptan, and zolmitriptan.
- All triptans can cause coronary vasospasm and are contraindicated in IHD. Other contraindications are hypertension, epilepsy, hepatic or renal impairment and during pregnancy.

27. Drug of choice for aborting the acute attack of migraine is:

a. NSAIDs like indomethacin
b. Opioids like morphine
c. Triptans like sumatriptan
d. Glucocorticoids

Ans. is 'c' Triptans like sumatriptan

H_1 ANTIHISTAMINICS

First generation H1 antihistaminics			Second generation H1 antihistaminics
Highly sedative	*Moderately sedative*	*Mild sedative*	
• Diphenhydramine • Dimenhydrinate • Promethazine • Hydroxyzine	• Pheniramine • Cyproheptadine • Meclizine • Cinnarizine	• Chlorpheniramine • Dexchlorpheniramine • Triprolidine • Clemastine	• Fexofenadine • Loratadine • Desloratadine • Cetirizine • Levocetizine • Azelastine • Mizolastine • Ebastine • Rupatadine • Acrivastine
Some authors describe the term 3rd generation antihistaminics for the active enantiomer (like levocetirizine) or active metabolites of second generation antihistaminics (desloratadine and fexofenadine).			

Pharmacology

Second Generation H1-antihistaminics

- Absence of CNS depressant property
- Higher H1 selectivity; no anticholinergic activity
- Additional anti-allergic mechanisms apart from histamine blockade.

Cetirizine

- Cetirizine is a 2nd generation antihistaminic
- It is a metabolite of hydroxyzine with marked affinity for the peripheral H1 receptors
- It penetrates CNS poorly and has mild sedating effect
- It inhibits release of histamine from mast cells and therefore has been used for urticarial and atopic dermatitis.

First-generation H1-antihistaminics	Second-generation H1-antihistaminics
Cross Blood-brain barrier, cause sedation	Do not cross Blood-brain barrier, no sedation
Anti-cholinergic side-effects occur	No anti-cholinergic activity
Useful in • Motion sickness • Drug-induced Parkinsonism • Muscular dystonias • Allergy	Useful only for allergy

28. A patient of motion sickness wants to undertake a road trip. What drug can be helpful for him? *(NEET 2020)*

a. Fexofenadine
b. Cetirizine
c. Loratadine
d. Promethazine

Ans. is 'd' Promethazine

29. Which of the following antihistaminics has minimal or no CNS depressant activity?

a. Promethazine
b. Meclizine
c. Cinnarizine
d. Ebastine

Ans. is 'd' Ebastine

Explanation: From the given options, Ebastine is the only second generation antihistaminic.

30. About cetirizine all are true *except*:

a. It is a 2nd generation antihistaminic
b. It is metabolite of hydroxyzine
c. Good CNS penetration
d. Inhibits release of histamine

Ans. is 'c' Good CNS penetration

SEROTONIN (5-HYDROXYTRYPTAMINE) RECEPTORS

5HT1

- $5HT_{1A}$: Presynaptic autoreceptors; partial agonists (Buspirone, gepirone) used as anti-anxiety drugs
- $5HT_{1B/1D}$: Causes constriction of cranial vessels; Agonists (triptans) used in treatment of migraine attacks.

$5HT_{2A/2C}$

- Responsible for most direct actions of serotonin
- Antagonists (Ketanserin and ritanserin) used as anti-hypertensive agents
- Clozapine, risperidone are atypical antipsychotics that through antagonistic activity.

$5HT_3$

- Inotropic receptor (all other 5-HT receptors are G-protein coupled receptors)
- Mediates most of the reflex and indirect actions of serotonin
- Antagonists (Ondansetron, granisetron) used as drug of choice for chemotherapy-induced vomiting

$5HT_4$

- Present in GIT, responsible for increase in peristalsis
- Agonists (Cisapride, mosapride, renzapride, tegaserod) are useful in treatment of gastroesophageal reflux disease.

Non-selective Drugs

- *Cyproheptadine*: It blocks $5HT_{2A}$, H1 and muscarinic receptors. It increases appetite and can be used in children to promote weight gain.
- *Methysergide*: It is a $5HT_{2A/2C}$ antagonist and $5HT_1$ agonist. It is indicated for prophylaxis of migraine attacks. Prolonged use can result in pulmonary, endocardial and retroperitoneal fibrosis.

31. Which of the following actions of drugs on serotoninergic system is not correctly matched?

a. Buspirone partial agonist 5-HT1A
b. Cyproheptadine blocks 5-HT2A receptor
c. Tropisetron 5-HT3 antagonist
d. Tegaserod 5-HT1D receptor agonist

Ans. is 'd' Tegaserod 5-HT1D receptor agonist

32. Drug action on 5HT4 receptor is:

a. Loxiglumide
b. Renzapride
c. Atractyloside
d. Metoclopramide

Ans. is 'b' Renzapride

33. Adverse effect of methysergide is:

a. Metabolic syndrome
b. Endocardial fibrosis
c. Peyronie's syndrome
d. Dry mouth

Ans. is 'b' Endocardial fibrosis

34. Mechanism of action of buspirone? *(NEET 2019)*

a. 5HT1A partial agonism
b. 5HT1B partial agonism
c. 5HT1B antagonism
d. 5HT1C antagonism

Ans. is 'a' 5HT1A partial agonism

DISEASE-MODIFYING ANTIRHEUMATOID DRUGS (DMARD)

Drug	Class or action
Small molecules	
Methotrexate	Antifolate
Leflunomide	Pyrimidine synthase inhibitor (Inhibits dihydro-orotate dehydrogenase)
Hydroxychloroquine	Antimalarial
Minocycline	5-Lipoxygenase inhibitor, tetracycline antibiotic
Sulfasalazine	Salicylate
Azathioprine	Purine synthase inhibitor
Cyclosporine	Calcineurin inhibitor
Cyclophosphamide	Alkylating agent
Penicillamine	Chelating agent
Auranofin	Gold compound
Biologicals	
Adalimumab	Ab, TNF-α antagonist
Golimumab Etanercept	Ab, TNF-α antagonist Ab, TNF-α antagonist
Infliximab	IgG-TNF receptor fusion protein (anti-TNF)
Certolizumab	Fab fragment toward TNF-α
Abatacept	T-cell costimulation inhibitor (binds B7 protein on antigen-presenting cell)
Rituximab	Ab toward CD20 (cytotoxic toward B cells)
Anakinra	IL-1 receptor antagonist
Tocilizumab	IL-6 receptor antagonist
Tofacitinib	Janus kinase inhibitor

Therapy

- NSAIDs are used to provide symptomatic relief, they have no effect on the progression of the disease.
- Current recommendation is to start DMARDs as soon as the diagnosis of RA is confirmed.
- Methotrexate is the DMARD of first choice for initial treatment of moderate to severe RA. Failure to achieve adequate improvement with methotrexate therapy calls for a transition to effective **combination therapy**.
- Effective combinations include – Methotrexate, sulfasalazine & hydroxychloroquine (Oral triple therapy); methotrexate and leflunomide; and methotrexate plus a biological.

35. A patient of Rheumatoid arthritis is taking methotrexate, steroids and NSAIDs since 4 months, but activity of disease progression is same. What should be next probable step? *(NEET 2019)*

a. Start monotherapy with Anti-TNF alpha drugs
b. Continue methotrexate and steroids
c. Start parenteral methotrexate
d. Add sulfasalazine

Ans. is 'd' Add sulfasalazine

36. Anakinra is:

a. TNFα antagonist
b. IL-1 antagonist
c. IL-2 antagonist
d. IL-6 antagonist

Ans. is 'b' IL-1 antagonist

37. Tocilizumab acts as an antagonist at which receptor?

a. IL-1
b. IL-2
c. IL-6
d. TNF

Ans. is 'c' IL-6

TREATMENT OF GOUT

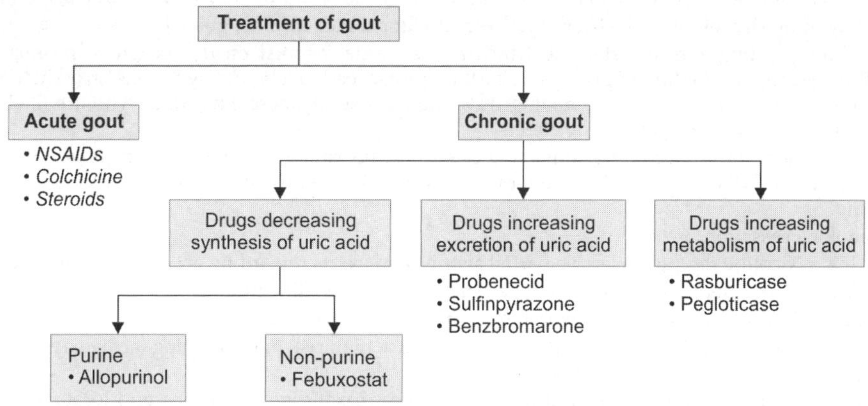

Acute Gout

- NSAIDs like indomethacin are drug of choice due to better tolerability. Aspirin is not used as it may cause hyperuricemia.
- Colchicine is more effective and faster acting than NSAIDs but is used rarely due to high toxicity. It acts by inhibiting granulocyte migration into the inflamed joint. It causes metaphase arrest (other drugs causing metaphase arrest are vinca alkaloids and taxanes). Most common and dose-limiting toxicity is diarrhea. It can also cause kidney damage, myopathy and bone marrow depression.
- Two indications for daily colchicines are:
  - To prevent further attacks
  - Along with urate-lowering therapy to suppress attacks precipitated by abrupt changes in serum uric acid.
- Intra-articular corticosteroids can be used in refractory cases.

Drugs Increasing Metabolism of Uric Acid

- Urate oxidase metabolizes insoluble uric acid to soluble allantoin.
- Recombinant urate oxidase is now available as Rasburicase. Pegloticase is another similar drug that is pegylated to increase duration of action.

38. Pegloticase is used for: *(NEET 2020)*

a. Resistant RA
b. Tophaceous gout
c. CPPD
d. Ankylosing spondylitis

Ans. is 'b' Tophaceous gout

39. True about Colchicine: *(NEET 2019)*

a. Acts by inhibiting neutrophil recruitment
b. Causes metaphase arrest
c. Causes bone marrow depression
d. All of the above

Ans. is 'd' All of the above

40. Rasburicase is an analogue of:

a. Xanthine oxidase
b. IMP dehydrogenase
c. Adenosine deaminase
d. Urate oxidase

Ans. is 'd' Urate oxidase

Previously Asked Facts

- pKa is the pH at which 50% of the drug is ionized and 50% is non-ionized.
- The clearance of a drug is the theoretical volume of plasma from which the drug is completely removed in unit time. Clearance (CL) = Rate of elimination/Plasma concentration.
- First dose effect (postural hypotension) is now uncommon and occurs mainly with drugs having a vasodilatory action on veins (α-adrenoreceptor blockers like prazosin, ACE inhibitors) when baroreceptors reflex is impaired, e.g. old age.
- Tizanidine is a centrally acting muscle relaxant with alpha-2 adrenergic activity.
- Physostigmine (anti-ChE) is rapidly absorbed from GIT and parenteral sites, penetrates cornea freely and crosses BBB (blood brain barrier).
- DOC for anaphylactic shock is – Adrenaline.
- Atenolol, sotalol and nadolol are primarily excreted by kidney-> should not be given in renal failure.
- The specific antidote in beta-blocker toxicity is glucagon. Glucagon acts to stimulate the formation of cyclic adenosine monophosphate which in turn has positive ionotropic and chronotropic effects on the heart.
- Specific adverse effect of Thalidomide is phocomelia (teratogenic effect).
- Drugs associated with priapism – Hydralazine, Prazosin, Risperidone, Papaverine, Phenothiazines, Trazodone
- Botulinum toxin (inhibits ACh release) is used in treatment of blepharospasm, spastic cerebral palsy, strabismus, spasmodic torticollis, nystagmus, hemifacial spasm, axillary hyperhidrosis, spastic cerebral palsy which is due to cholinergic excess.
- Central sympatholytic anti-hypertensives – Clonidine, α-methyldopa, moxonidine, guanabenz.
- Clonidine is a centrally acting anti-hypertensive which acts a partial agonist on α_{2A} receptors in brainstem and decreases sympathetic outflow. Abrupt discontinuation of clonidine therapy can lead to rebound hypertension (treated with phentolamine); therefore this drug is not suitable for people having traveling job like business executives who are likely to miss the doses. Constipation and impotency can be seen as side effects.
- Aprepitant is an antiemetic substance that belongs to a class of drugs called substance P antagonists. It mediates its effect by blocking the neurokinin 1 (NK1) receptor. Aprepitant is used for chemotherapy induced nausea & vomiting and postoperative nausea & vomiting.
- Drugs used in smoking cessation
    - Varenicline: It is a Nicotine receptor selective partial agonist and exerts rewarding action of nicotine through a4β2 receptors
    - Bupropion: Atypical anti-depressant; inhibits dopamine and noradrenaline uptake.
    - Mecamylamine: It is nicotine ganglion blocker, blocks the reward effect of nicotine.
- FDA has issued a black box warning for metoclopramide because of high risk of developing tardive dyskinesia if its use extends beyond 12 weeks.
- H2-receptor antagonists include cimetidine, ranitidine, famotidine, roxatidine, nizatidine and loratadine. These drugs inhibit gastric secretion by blocking H2 receptors on parietal cells. Cimetidine is the least potent H2 blocker. Famotidine is the most potent H2 blocker.
- Cimetidine (but not other H2 blockers) has antiandrogenic action (displaces dihydrotestosterone from its cytoplasmic receptor), increases plasma prolactin and inhibits degradation of estradiol by liver. High doses given for long periods have produced gynecomastia, loss of libido, impotence and temporary decrease in sperm count.
- Tianeptine is an atypical anti-depressant; acts by increasing 5-HT uptake.
- PGF2α analogues are smooth muscle constrictor which bring about contraction of smooth muscles. Carboprost is used for postpartum hemorrhage. Latanoprost has been used for glaucoma and is a first line drug for open angle glaucoma. It is contraindicated in bronchial asthma as it causes bronchial muscle contraction.
- Tachyphylaxis is rapidly diminishing response to repeated administration of a drug. It occurs in asthmatics who use α2-agonists excessively (due to downregulation of receptors) or with indirectly acting drugs like amphetamine, tyrosine, ephedrine (due to depletion of neuro-transmitters).

CARDIOVASCULAR SYSTEM

Drugs that prolong Q-T interval (Have potential to precipitate Torsades de pointes)	
Antiarrhythmics	Quinidine, Procainamide, Disopyramide, Propafenone, Amiodarone
Antimalarials	Quinine, Mefloquine, Artemisinin, Halofantrine
Antibacterials	Sparfloxacin, Moxifloxacin
Antihistaminics	Terfenadine, Astemizole, Ebastine
Antidepressants	Amitriptyline and other tricyclics
Antipsychotics	Thioridazine, Pimozide, Aripiprazole, Ziprasidone
Prokinetic	Cisapride

41. Which of the following can prolong Q-T interval?

a. Quinidine
b. Lignocaine
c. Ciprofloxacin
d. Propranolo

Ans. is 'a' Quinidine

ANTIARRHYTHMIC DRUGS

Subclass, drug	Mechanism of action	Effects	Clinical applications	Pharmacokinetics, toxicities, interactions
CLASS				
• Procainamide	I_{Na} (primary) and I_{Kr} (secondary) blockade	• Slows conduction velocity and pacemaker rate • Prolongs action potential duration and dissociates from I_{Na} channel with intermediate kinetics • Direct depressant effects on sinoatrial (SA) and atrioventricular (AV) nodes	• Most atrial and ventricular arrhythmias • Drug of second choice for most sustained ventricular arrhythmias associated with acute myocardial infarction	• Oral, IV, IM • Eliminated by hepatic metabolism to N-acetylprocainamide (NAPA; see text) and renal elimination • NAPA implicated in torsades de pointes in patients with renal failure • Toxicity: Hypotension • Long-term therapy produces reversible lupus-related symptoms
• Quinidine: Similar to procainamide but more toxic (cinchonism, torsades); rarely used in arrhythmias; • Disopyramide: Similar to procainamide but significant antimuscarinic effects; may precipitate heart failure; not commonly used				
CLASS				
• Lidocaine	Sodium channel (INa) blockade	• Blocks activated and inactivated channels with fast kinetics • Does not prolong and may shorten action potential	Terminates ventricular tachycardias and prevents ventricular fibrillation after cardioversion	• IV • First-pass hepatic metabolism • Reduce dose in patients with heart failure or liver disease • *Toxicity*: Neurologic symptoms
• *Mexiletine*: Orally active congener of lidocaine; used in ventricular arrhythmias, chronic pain syndromes				
CLASS				
• Flecainide	Sodium channel (INa) blockade	• Dissociates from channel with slow kinetics • No change in action potential duration	• Supraventricular arrhythmias in patients with normal heart • Do not use in ischemic conditions (post-myocardial infarction)	• Oral • Hepatic and kidney metabolism • Half life ~20 h • *Toxicity:* Proarrhythmic
• *Propafenone*: Orally active, weak β-blocking activity; supraventricular arrhythmias; hepatic metabolism				
CLASS				
• Propranolol	β-Adrenoceptor blockade	Direct membrane effects (sodium channel block) and prolongation of action potential duration Slows SA node automaticity and AV nodal conduction velocity	Atrial arrhythmias and prevention of recurrent infarction and sudden death	• Oral, parenteral • Duration 4–6 h • *Toxicity:* Asthma, AV blockade, acute heart failure • *Interactions:* With other cardiac depressants and hypotensive drugs
• *Esmolol:* Short-acting, IV only; used for intraoperative and other acute arrhythmias				
CLASS				
• Amiodarone	Blocks I_{Kr}, I_{Na}, $I_{Ca\text{-}L}$ channels, β adrenoceptors	• Prolongs action potential duration and QT interval • Slows heart rate and AV node conduction • Low incidence of torsades de pointes	Serious ventricular arrhythmias and supraventricular arrhythmias	• Oral, IV • Variable absorption and tissue accumulation • Hepatic metabolism, elimination complex and slow • *Toxicity*: Bradycardia and heart block in diseased heart, peripheral vasodilation, pulmonary and hepatic toxicity • Hyper- or hypothyroidism • *Interactions:* Many, based on CYP metabolism
• Dofetilide	I_{Kr} block	Prolongs action potential, effective refractory period	Maintenance or restoration of sinus rhythm in atrial fibrillation	• Oral • Renal excretion • *Toxicity*: Torsades de pointes (initiate in hospital with monitoring) • *Interactions*: Additive with other QT-prolonging drugs
• *Sotalol:* β-Adrenergic and I_{Kr} blocker, direct action potential prolongation properties, use for ventricular arrhythmias, atrial fibrillation • *Ibutilide*: Potassium channel blocker, may activate inward current; IV use for conversion in atrial flutter and fibrillation • *Dronedarone*: Amiodarone derivative; multichannel actions, reduces mortality in patients with atrial fibrillation • *Vernakalant*: Investigational in the USA, multichannel actions in atria, prolongs atrial refractoriness, effective in atrial fibrillation				

Contd…

Contd...

Subclass, drug	Mechanism of action	Effects	Clinical applications	Pharmacokinetics, toxicities, interactions
CLASS				
• Verapamil	Calcium channel ($I_{Ca\text{-}L}$ type) blockade	• Slows SA node automaticity and AV nodal conduction velocity • Decreases cardiac contractility • Reduces blood pressure	Supraventricular tachycardias, hypertension, angina	• Oral, IV • Hepatic metabolism • Caution in patients with hepatic dysfunction • AV block occurs if given with beta blockers
• *Diltiazem*: Equivalent to verapamil				
Miscellaneous				
• Adenosine	• Activates inward rectifier I_K • Blocks I_{Ca}	Very brief due to uptake into RBCs and endothelial cells, usually complete AV blockade	Paroxysmal supraventricular tachycardias	• IV only • Duration 10–15 s • *Toxicity*: Flushing, chest tightness, dizziness • *Interactions*: Minimal
• Magnesium	• Poorly understood • Interacts with Na^+/K^+ ATPase, K^+, and Ca^{2+} channels	Normalizes or increases plasma Mg^{2+}	• Torsades de pointes • Digitalis-induced arrhythmias	• IV • Duration dependent on dosage • *Toxicity*: Muscle weakness in overdose
• Potassium	Increases K^+ permeability, K^+ currents	• Slows ectopic pacemakers • Slows conduction velocity in heart	• Digitalis-induced arrhythmias • Arrhythmias associated with hypokalemia	• Oral, IV • *Toxicity*: Reentrant arrhythmias, fibrillation or arrest in overdose

Amiodarone

- Amiodarone is a broad spectrum anti-arrhythmic drug which belongs to class III of the anti-arrhythmic drugs.
- Following are the adverse effects:
  - Fall in BP, bradycardia and myocardial depression occurs on IV injection.
  - Photosensitization and skin pigmentation occurs in about 10% of patients.
  - Corneal microdeposits may cause headlight dazzle, but is reversible on discontinuation.
  - Pulmonary fibrosis and alveolitis is most serious side effect seen on prolonged use.
  - Peripheral neuropathy generally manifests as the pelvic and shoulder muscle weakness.
  - Amiodarone interferes with thyroid function and prevents peripheral conversion of T4 to T3 and causes hypothyroidism

42. Which of the following is NOT a side effect of amiodarone?

a. Pulmonary fibrosis
b. Corneal microdeposits
c. Photosensitivity
d. Tachycardia

Ans. is 'd' Tachycardia

43. Why adenosine has a short half life?

a. Spontaneous hydrolysis
b. Uptake in subcutaneous tissue
c. Uptake in RBC and endothelial cells
d. Renal excretion

Ans. is 'c' Uptake in RBC and endothelial cells

44. Which of the following antiarrhythmic drug is contraindicated in a patient with interstitial lung disease? *(NEET 2020)*

a. Amiodarone
b. Sotalol
c. Quinidine
d. Lignocaine

Ans. is 'a' Amiodarone

Explanation: Pulmonary alveolitis and fibrosis is the most serious toxicity of prolonged use of Amiodarone.

Arrhythmias and their Drugs of Choice

Supraventricular Tachycardias

- Atrial fibrillation (AF)/Atrial flutter (AFL) without heart failure (to control ventricular rate)—β-blockers (Propranolol, esmolol)
- AF/AFL with heart failure (to control ventricular rate)—Digoxin
- AF (to maintain sinus rhythm)—Propafenone or Flecainide or Ibutilide
- PSVT—Adenosine (DOC), β-blockers or CCBs
- WPW Syndrome
  - *PSVT*: Adenosine (DOC), CCBs (2nd choice)
  - *AF*: Procainamide (DOC), Lidocaine

Ventricular Tachycardia

- Ventricular premature beat (ventricular extrasystole)—β-blockers
- Ventricular tachycardia or VF—Lidocaine, Amiodarone, Procainamide
- Digitalis induced ventricular arrythmia—Lidocaine (DOC), Phenytoin
- Congenital QT prolongation - β-blockers

Bradyarrhythmias

- AV Block—Atropine, Isoprenaline
- Sinus bradycardia—Atropine, Isoprenaline

Management of PSVT

Immediate Treatment

- Vagal stimulation (Valsalva maneuver or carotid sinus massage) can slow conduction in AV node sufficiently to terminate PSVT
- If physical maneuvers do not terminate tachyarrhythmia, 1st-line treatment: Adenosine
- 2nd-line treatment: IV beta blockade or calcium channel therapy
- In hemodynamically unstable patients, R-wave synchronous DC cardioversion using 100–200 J can terminate the tachyarrhythmia

Catheter Ablation:

- Catheter ablation of slow AV nodal pathway is recommended for recurrent or severe episodes or when drug therapy is ineffective, not tolerated, or not desired by the patient
- Catheter ablation is curative in over 95% of patients
- **Major risk**: Heart block requiring permanent pacemaker implantation

45. An elderly male presented with tachycardia, palpitations and dyspnea. He is a hypertensive on treatment and underwent CABG for MI 4 years back. His ECG on presentation showed supraventricular tachycardia. Soon after, he collapsed with feeble pulses and unrecordable BP. ECG rhythm of SVT was maintained. What is the best step in management? *(NEET 2020)*

a. IV flecainide
b. IV amiodarone
c. IV ibutilide
d. Cardioversion

Ans. is 'd' Cardioversion

ISCHEMIC HEART DISEASE

Drug	Therapeutic uses	Major toxicity and clinical pearls
Organic Nitrates		
Glyceryl trinitrate (GTN, nitroglycerin) Isosorbide dinitrate (ISDN) Isosorbide mononitrate (ISMN)	• Angina (sublingual) • Acute pulmonary edema (IV) • Acute hypertension (IV)	• NO-mediated vasodilation of large (venous, arterial) > small (resistance) vessels → preferential preload reduction without steal effect • Short-acting formulations of GTN or ISDN are standby drugs for all patients with CAD • First choice for vasospastic angina, along with Ca^{2+} channel blockers • Second choice for the prevention of exertional angina (longer-acting formulations) • Adverse effects: headache, dizziness, postural hypotension, syncope • Tolerance after >16 h (leave nitrate-free interval of >8 h) • Do not use concurrently with PDE5 inhibitor
Molsidomine	• Angina	• Direct NO donor • Second choice for the prevention of angina • Adverse effects same as above • No documented advantage over GTN/ISDN/ISMN
Inhaled NO	• Pulmonary hypertension in neonates	• Relatively selective effect on pulmonary vascular bed
Ca^{2+} Channel Blockers		
Dihydropyridines Amlodipine Felodipine Lercanidipine Nifedipine Nitrendipine ***Others*** Diltiazem Verapamil	• Angina • Hypertension • Rate control in atrial fibrillation (verapamil, diltiazem)	• Preferential arterial vasodilation → afterload reduction • First choice for vasospastic angina (dihydropyridines) • Second choice for preventing exertional angina • Immediate-release nifedipine and short-acting dihydropyridines can cause tachycardia and hypotension and trigger angina • Diltiazem and verapamil can ↓ heart rate and AV conduction; should not be used with β blockers • CYP3A4-mediated drug interactions with verapamil and diltiazem • Other unwanted effects: peripheral edema (dihydropyridines), obstipation (verapamil)

Contd...

Contd…

Drug	Therapeutic uses	Major toxicity and clinical pearls
β Blockers		
Atenolol Bisoprolol Carvedilol Metoprolol Nadolol Nebivolol Many others	• Angina • Heart failure • Hypertension • Widely used for other indications (prevention of arrhythmias, rate control in atrial fibrillation, migraine, etc.)	• First choice for prevention of exertional angina • Only antianginal drug class with proven prognostic benefits in CAD • Adverse effects: bradycardia, AV block, bronchospasm, peripheral vasoconstriction, worsening of acute heart failure, depression, worsening of psoriasis • Polymorphic CYP2D6 metabolism (metoprolol) • Additional vasodilation (carvedilol, nebivolol)
Ranolazine		
	• Angina	• Inhibits late Na^+ and other cardiac ion currents • Has weak β blocking and metabolic effects • Second choice in the prevention of exertional angina • CYP3A4-dependent metabolism
Ivabradine		
	• Angina • Heart failure	• Selectively ↓ heart rate by inhibiting HCN currents in SA node • Second choice in the prevention of exertional angina; approved in patients not tolerating β blockers or having heart rate > 75 under β blockers • Unwanted effects: bradycardia, QT prolongation, atrial fibrillation, phosphenes • Contraindication: combination with diltiazem or verapamil
Nicorandil		
	• Angina	• Dual nitrate-like and I_{KATP}-stimulatory action (K^+ channel opener) • Hemodynamic profile between nitrates and dihydropyridines; ↓ afterload more than nitrates • Second choice in the prevention of exertional angina • Adverse effects: hypotension, headache, buccal and GI ulcers • Do not combine with PDE5 inhibitor
Trimetazidine		
	• Angina	• Metabolic shift from fatty acid to glycolytic metabolism in the heart • Second choice in the prevention of exertional angina • May increase the incidence of Parkinson disease
Antiplatelet, Anti-integrin, and Antithrombotic Drugs		
Aspirin $P2Y_{12}$ receptor antagonists (clopidogrel, prasugrel, ticagrelor cangrelor [IV])	• Prevention of thrombotic events (MI, stroke) • Acute coronary syndromes • Prevention of stent thrombosis	• ↓ Platelet aggregation by inhibiting COX-1–mediated TxA_2 production (aspirin) or ADP receptors ($P2Y_{12}$ receptor antagonists) • Oral use only: clopidogrel, prasugrel, ticagrelor • Irreversible action: aspirin, clopidogrel, prasugrel • Prodrugs: clopidogrel, prasugrel • Variable, CYP2C9-dependent metabolism (clopidogrel) • Withdraw 5–7 days before surgery • First choice in NSTEMI and STEMI • Dual platelet inhibition after stenting
Abciximab Eptifibatide Tirofiban	• Percutaneous coronary interventions	• Antibody (abciximab) or small molecule antagonists at platelet GpIIb/IIIa receptor • Parenteral use only • Highly efficient platelet inhibition • Therapeutic value in the era of highly effective dual platelet inhibition unclear
Heparin Low-molecular-weight heparins (e.g., enoxaparin)	• Acute coronary syndromes • Percutaneous coronary interventions	• Endogenous polysaccharide, inhibits thrombin (factor IIa) and factor Xa in an antithrombin III–dependent manner • Parenteral use only • Heparin: short $t_{1/2}$, complex pharmacokinetics, low bioavailability after subcutaneous. injection • Low-molecular-weight heparin: longer half-life, renal excretion; accumulation in renal insufficiency • Heparin-induced thrombocytopenia
Fondaparinux	• Acute coronary syndromes • Percutaneous coronary interventions	• Synthetic pentasaccharide, antithrombin III-dependent, factor Xa inhibitor • Most favorable efficacy-safety ratio
Bivalirudin Lepirudin	• Percutaneous coronary interventions (bivalirudin) • Heparin-induced thrombocytopenia (HIT II) recombinant lepirudin	• Direct thrombin (factor IIa) inhibitors • Parenteral use only • Advantage of bivalirudin over heparin unclear

Pharmacology

46. Which of the following drugs acts on K^+ channels? *(NEET 2019)*

a. Spironolactone
b. Amiloride
c. Nicorandil
d. Methyldopa

Ans. is 'c' Nicorandil

47. Which of the following drugs block late inward sodium ion channels? *(NEET 2020)*

a. Ranolazine
b. Trimetazidine
c. Ivabradine
d. Fasudil

Ans. is 'a' Ranolazine

Explanation: Fasudil is a potent Rho-kinase inhibitor and vasodilator. Since it was discovered, it has been used for the treatment of cerebral vasospasm, which is often due to subarachnoid hemorrhage, as well as to improve the cognitive decline seen in stroke patients.

Thiazide Diuretics

Hydrochlorothiazide, chlorthalidone, metolazone

Mechanism: Inhibit NaCl reabsorption in early DCT → reduced diluting capacity of nephron. Also reduces Ca^{2+} excretion

Clinical uses: Hypertension, heart failure, idiopathic hypercalciuria, nephrogenic diabetes insipidus, osteoporosis

Adverse Effects

- Hypokalemic metabolic alkalosis
- Hyponatremia
- Hyperglycemia
- Hyperlipidemia
- Hyperuricemia
- Hypercalcemia
- Sulfa allergy

48. Which of the following antihypertensive drug is avoided in patients with high serum uric acid levels? *(NEET 2020)*

a. Hydrochlorothiazide
b. Atenolol
c. Prazosin
d. Enalapril

Ans. is 'a' Hydrochlorothiazide

ENDOCRINOLOGY

DRUGS USED FOR BENIGN PROSTATIC HYPERPLASIA

Tamsulosin: Alpha1a-antagonist. Decreases smooth muscle tone of prostate and bladder neck which leads to improved urine flow, but it will not lead to reduction in size of prostate.

Finasteride: 5-alpha reductase (type II) inhibitor. Prevents conversion of testosterone to dihydrotestosterone. DHT is the main androgen in the prostate which is produced from testosterone by 5 alpha reductase and causes growth and differentiation in the prostate. Type 2 isoform of this enzyme is expressed by stromal cells in the prostate. Reduction in levels of DHT prevents further growth and sometimes reduces the size of prostate as well.

Flutamide: Oral nonsteroidal antiandrogen which inhibits androgen binding to its receptor. No studies yet to show decrease in size of prostate and decrease in symptoms of BPH. It is used in the treatment of metastatic prostatic cancer.

Treatment with PDE-5 inhibitors can be considered **in patients who have erectile dysfunction** and mild or moderate symptoms of BPH. **Tadalafil** is approved by the FDA for use in BPH. PDE-5 inhibitors can potentiate the hypotensive effects of alpha-1-adrenergic antagonists. **But it does not cause decrease in size.**

49. Mechanism of action of finasteride is:

a. Androgen receptor antagonist
b. 5-α reductase inhibitor
c. 17-α hydroxylase inhibitor
d. Aromatase inhibitor

Ans. is 'b' 5-α reductase inhibitor

DRUGS USED FOR OSTEOPOROSIS

Inhibit Bone Resorption

- Bisphosphonates
- Calcium receptor agonist: Cinacalcet
- Calcitonin

- *SERMs*: Tamoxifen, raloxifene
- Gallium nitrate
- *RANKL inhibitors*: Denosumab.

Stimulate Bone Formation

- Teriparatide
- Calcium
- Calcitriol
- Fluoride.

Both actions: Inhibits resorption and stimulates bone formation—Strontium ranelate.

Bisphosphonates

- They are pyrophosphate analogs.
- Examples of commonly available bisphosphonates include etidronate, pamidronate, alendronate, risedronate, tiludronate, ibandronate, and zoledronate.

Mechanism of Action

They bind hydroxyapatite in bone, inhibiting osteoclast activity.

Some of the newer bisphosphonates appear to increase bone mineral density well beyond the 2-year period predicted for a drug whose effects are limited to slowing bone resorption. This may be due to their other cellular effects, which include inhibition of 1,25(OH)2D production, inhibition of intestinal calcium transport, metabolic changes in bone cells such as inhibition of glycolysis, inhibition of cell growth, and changes in acid and alkaline phosphatase activity.

Clinical Uses

Osteoporosis, hypercalcemia associated with malignancy, Paget disease of bone.

Side Effects

- Corrosive esophagitis, osteonecrosis of jaw.
- Esophageal irritation can be minimized by taking the drug with a full glass of water and remaining upright for 30 minutes or by using the intravenous forms of these compounds.

Teriparatide

- This is recombinant preparation of 1–34 molecules of amino terminal of human PTH.
- It duplicates all the actions of long (1–84) PTH.
- Injected SC once daily, it has been found to increase bone mineral density in osteoporotic women.

50. Mechanism of action of Teriparatide is:

a. Recombinant PTH [rPTH]
b. Recombinant calcitonin
c. Recombinant insulin
d. Recombinant prolactin

Ans. is 'a' Recombinant PTH [rPTH]

ANTI-THYROID DRUGS

Side Effects

- Most serious—agranulocytosis. Propylthiouracil has got maximum chance of causing agranulocytosis. It is mostly reversible.
- Most common—purpuric rash.
- Pain & stiffness in joints, paresthesias. headache, skin pigmentation & loss of hair.
- ANCAs in 50% of patients receiving propylthiouracil.
- Cholestatic jaundice is common with methimazole.
- Propylthiouracil causes hepatic dysfunction, especially in children & pregnant women.
- Methimazole is rarely associated with aplasia Cutis & choanal atresia.
- Carbimazole rarely associated with congenital gut abnormalities.

Propylthiouracil should not be used in children except in the case of methimazole allergy.

Therapeutic Uses

- Used in treatment of hyperthyroidism
- Methimazole is the preferred drug for Grave's disease
- Thyrotoxicosis in pregnancy: Carbimazole is the preferred drug
- Propylthiouracil is preferred in thyroid storm since it inhibits peripheral conversion of T4→ T3.

51. Which of the following antithyroid medications has the maximum chances of causing agranulocytosis?

a. Carbimazole
b. Clotrimazole
c. Propylthiouracil
d. Methimazole

Ans. is 'c' Propylthiouracil

DIABETES MELLITUS

Oral antidiabetic agents for type 2 diabetes mellitus treatment

Agent	*Mechanism of action*	*Side effects*
Insulin secretagogues Sulfonylureas Meglitinides	Increases insulin secretion by inhibiting β-cell K+ ATP channels	Hypoglycemia Weight gain
Biguanides Metformin	Stimulates AMP Kinase, decreasing glucose production and insulin resistance	Lactic acidosis
Thiazolidinediones Pioglitazone Rosiglitazone	Activates transcription regulator PPAR-g, decreasing insulin resistance	Risk of bladder cancer Fluid retention/heart failure Weight gain
GLP-1 (Glucagon-Like Peptide) agonists Exenatide Liraglutide	Increases glucose-dependent insulin secretion, decreases glucagon secretion, delays gastric emptying	Pancreatitis
DPP4 (Dipeptidyl Peptidase) Inhibitors Sitagliptin Saxagliptin	Increases endogenous GLP-1 and GIP levels	Pancreatitis Nasopharyngitis
α-glucosidase inhibitors Acarbose Miglitol	Reduces intestinal disaccharide absorption	Diarrhea Flatulence
SGLT2 (Sodium-Glucose Transport Protein) inhibitors Canagliflozin Dapagliflozin	Increases renal glucose excretion	Urinary tract infections Hypotension Polyuria (osmotic diuresis) Weight loss

Side Effects of Metformin

- Abdominal pain, anorexia, nausea, metallic taste, mild diarrhea and tiredness are the frequent side effects.
- Lactic acidosis: Small increase in blood lactate level occurs with metformin, but lactic acidosis is rare (<1% per 10,000 patient years). Alcohol ingestion can precipitate severe lactic acidosis.
- Vitamin B12 deficiency due to interference with its absorption.
- In addition to general restrictions for use of oral hypoglycemic, metformin is contraindicated in hypotension severe respiratory, renal and hepatic failure, heart failure and alcoholics as it may aggravate lactic acidosis.

Parenteral Anti-hyperglycemics

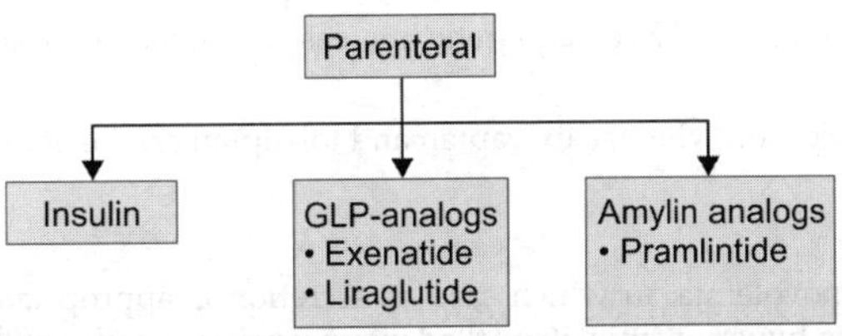

Insulin Preparations

Insulin preparations	Onset of action	Peak action	Effective duration
Insulins lispro, aspart, glulisine	5–15 min	1–1.5 h	3–4 h
Human regular	30–60 min	2 h	6–8 h
Technosphere inhaled insulin	5–15 min	1 h	3 h
Human NPH/ Lente insulin (30% Amorphous + 70% Crystalline insulin)	2–4 h	6–7 h	10–20 h
Insulin glargine	0.5–1 h	Flat	~24 h
Insulin detemir	0.5–1 h	Flat	17 h
Insulin degludec	0.5–1.5 h	Flat	>42 h

52. All of the following are contraindications for the use of metformin *except*:

a. Hypotensive state
b. Alcoholics
c. Renal failure
d. Hypokalemia

Ans. is 'd' Hypokalemia

53. Which of the following is a side effect of dapagliflozin?

a. Increased weight loss
b. Polyuria
c. Increased incidence of urinary tract infections
d. All of the above

Ans. is 'd' All of the above

54. Mechanism action of sulfonylureas is:

a. Na ATP channel blocker
b. K ATP channel blocker
c. Cl ATP channel blocker
d. Ca ATP channel blocker

Ans. is 'b' K ATP channel blocker

55. Mechanism of action of Voglibose is:

a. β galactosidase inhibitor
b. β lactase inhibitor
c. α glucosidase inhibitor
d. β glucosidase inhibitor

Ans. is 'c' α glucosidase inhibitor

56. Which of the following pairs is correct?

a. Glibenclamide—Na^{+}ATP blocker
b. Biguanides—AMP kinase activation
c. Vildagliptin—SGLT2 inhibitor
d. Voglibose—DPP4 inhibitor

Ans. is 'b' Biguanides—AMP kinase activation

57. Mechanism of action of exenatide is:

a. Bile acid sequestrant
b. LPL activator
c. CETP inhibitor
d. GLP-1 analogue

Ans. is 'd' GLP-1 analogue

58. Longest acting insulin is:

a. Neutral protamine Hagedorn
b. Insulin glulisine
c. Insulin glargine
d. Lente insulin

Ans. is 'c' Insulin glargine

VASOPRESSIN RECEPTOR ANTAGONISTS

- V1 receptor antagonists may be useful when total peripheral resistance is increased (e.g. CHF and hypertension) whereas V2 antagonists may be useful for the treatment of SIADH.
- Relcovaptan is selective V1 antagonist whereas Lixivaptan, Mozavaptan and Tolvaptan are selective V2 antagonists.
- Conivaptan is V1a/V2 receptor antagonist used as an aquaretic (increase water excretion without affecting electrolytes like sodium) in CHF.
- Conivaptan is administered by IV. injection whereas lixivaptan and tolvaptan can be given orally.

SIADH

- ADH is secreted in response to hypovolemia, in which case its secretion is appropriate. However, if ADH is secreted in high quantities in presence of euvolemia or hypervolemia, it is called inappropriate secretion (SIADH). The resultant water retention can result in hyponatremia. Thus, SIADH is characterized by normovolemic or hypervolemic hyponatremia.
- Fluid restriction is treatment of choice for SIADH.
- Hypertonic saline (3% NaCl) + loop diuretics (depending upon volume status) is treatment of choice for severe symptomatic hyponatremia.
- Among drugs, tolvaptan (oral), conivaptan (IV) are preferred for long-term use.

59. Which of the following drug is used in SIADH? *(NEET 2019)*

a. Tolvaptan
b. Desmopressin
c. vWb factor
d. Terlipressin

Ans. is 'a' Tolvaptan

Previously Asked Facts

- Nitrates act by activating Guanylyl cyclase and increasing cGMP levels.
- Drug of choice for Digitalis-induced ventricular arrhythmias – Lignocaine.
- Rubidomycin and doxorubicin are the anthracycline anti-tumor antibiotics. They have cardiotoxicity as an adverse effect. This can manifest either acutely with ECG changes, arrhythmias and hypotension, which are reversible, or be delayed like CHF. To prevent the chances of anthracycline-induced cardiomyopathy, antioxidants like dexrazoxane can be used.
- Drugs causing pulmonay fibrosis: Amiodarone, Bleomycin, Busulphan, Cyclophosphamide, Nitrofurantoin, Methysergide, Penicillamine, Methotrexate, Vinblastine.
- Drugs causing gynecomastia: Spironolactone, Digitalis, Phenytoin, Cimetidine, Griseofulvin, Ketoconazole, Flutamide, Goserelin, Cyproterone acetate.
- Mechanism of action of aspirin is Nonselective irreversible inhibition of cyclo-oxygenase. Anti-inflammatory action is exerted at high doses of 3–6 g/day or 100 mg/day. Analgesic effect is maximal at 1000 mg/day.

Drugs causing AV block	
Beta blockers	Adenosine
Calcium channel blockers	Antiarrhythmics (class I and III)
Digitalis	Lithium

- The Na^+K^+ATPase and inhibits the enzyme causing rise in the intracellular levels of Na^+. The raised Na^+ in turn inhibits the Na^+–Ca^{2+} exchanger and causes rise in intracellular Ca^{2+}. This raised intracellular Ca^{2+} is responsible for the positive ionotropic effect. Thus, digitalis increases the cardiac contractability and force of contraction.

Drugs acting on RAS
ACE inhibitors: captopril, enalapril, lisinopril, ramipril
Renin inhibitors: aliskiren, remikiren, enakiren
AT1 blockers: losartan, candesartan, irbesartan, valsartan, telmisartan

- Digitalis increases the force of contraction by a direct action independent of the innervation. It binds to the extracellular face of
- ACE inhibitors are contraindicated in renal artery stenosis (either unilateral or bilateral).
- Diuretic which causes maximum amount of the kaliuresis for the same amount of natriuresis is Acetazolamide.
- Diuretic that causes impaired glucose tolerance – Thiazides.
- Physiological dose of hydrocortisone is 15 mg/kg/day.
- Most potent topical steroids are: Halobetasol propionate, Betamethasone dipropionate, Clobetasol propionate.
- Metyrapone inhibits 11-beta hydroxylase in adrenal cortex and decreases synthesis of hydrocortisone. It is used to test responsiveness of pituitary and its ACTH producing capacity.
- BW755 is a drug that inhibits both cyclo-oxygenase and lipoxygenase.
- Selective estrogen receptor modulators (SERMs): These drugs act as estrogen receptor agonist at some sites and antagonists in other tissues. Agonistic action is beneficial at bone and (resorption of bone) and lipid profile, whereas deleterious in uterus (cause endometrial proliferation and endometrial carcinoma) and in coagulation profile causing increased risk of thromboembolism. Antagonistic action is beneficial in breast (can be used in breast cancer). Drugs in this group are clomiphene, tamoxifen, doloxifene, toremifene, fulvestrant, raloxifene and ormeloxifene.
- Fulvestrant is a pure estrogen receptor antagonist. It has been used in postmenopausal females suffering from Ca Breast which has stopped responding to tamoxifen.
- Sildenafil (Viagra) acts to increase cGMP by inhibiting its breakdown by phosphodiesterase-5 (PDE5). It is an orally active drug which is used for treatment of erectile dysfunction. It is recommended that at least 6 hours pass between use of a nitrate and the ingestion of sildenafil. Sildenafil also has effects on color vision, causing difficulty in blue-green discrimination. Two similar PDE-5 inhibitors, tadalafil and vardenafil, are available. Other uses – Pulmonary artery hypertension.
- Antiandrogens include – Danazol, Cyproterone acetate, Flutamide, Finasteride, Dutasteride. Other drugs with anti-androgenic effect – Spironolactone, Ketoconazole, Cimetidine.
- Danazol–The most prominent action is suppression of gonadotropin (FSH/LH) from pituitary. The most important use is endometriosis. Other uses are fibrocystic breast disease, infertility, hereditary angioneurotic edema, menorrhagia, ITP, and hemophilia.
- Mifepristone is a partial agonist and competitive antagonist at both A and B forms of progesterone receptor (PR). Its uses include – Termination of pregnancy, cervical ripening, contraception.
- Pegvisomant is polyethylene glycol complexed mutant GH. It acts as a CH receptor antagonist. Approved for treatment of acromegaly due to small pituitary adenomas.
- Tibolone is a 19-norsteroid developed specifically to be used for hormone replacement therapy, which combines estrogenic and progestational properties with weak androgenic activity.
- Metyrosine is a competitive inhibitor of Tyrosine Hydroxylase, which is limiting enzyme of catecholamine synthesis. It is hence used in the treatment of pheochromocytoma.

- Estramustine is a complex of estradiol and nitrogen mustard (normustine) which has weak estrogenic but no alkylating property. It binds to beta tubulin and interferes with its organization of microtubules exerting anti-mitotic action. It gets concentrated in the prostatic tissues and therefore, only indication is: Advanced or metastatic Ca Prostate.
- Among sulfonylureas, chlorpropamide has the longest half-life.
- Drug of choice for Tyrosinemia is Nitisinone, which inhibits tyrosine degradation by 4-HPPD.
- Octreotide is somatostatin analogue. It is used in acromegaly, bleeding esophageal varices, insulinoma and secretory diarrhea associated with carcinoid.
- GnRH analogues are buserelin, goserelin, leuprolide, nafarelin, deslorelin and triptorelin.
  - Pulsatile administration of GnRH analogues stimulate gonadotropins release; used in hypogandotropic hypogonadism, delayed puberty and anovulatoy infertility.
  - Continuous administration of GnRH analogues suppresses gonadotropins secretion; used in pharmacological orchiectomy, precocious puberty, prostatic carcinoma, endometriosis, premenopausal breast cancer and PCOD.
  - GnRH analogues are used by SC route, however nafarelin and buserelin can be used as intranasal spray.
- Aromatase inhibitors are of two types - Type I (steroidal) aromatase inhibitor: They cause irreversible inhibition of aromatase, e.g. Exemestane, formestane. Type II (non-steroidal) aromatase inhibitor: They cause reversible inhibition of aromatase, e.g. Anastrozole. Letrozole.

CENTRAL NERVOUS SYSTEM (CNS)

PARKINSON'S DISEASE

Drugs for parkinsonism	
Increasing brain dopaminergic activity • Dopamine Precursor →Levodopa • Peripheral decarboxylase inhibitors → Carbidopa, Benserazide • Dopaminergic agonists →Bromocriptine, Ropinirole, Pramipexole, Rotigotine • MAO-B inhibitor – Selegiline, Rasagiline • COMT inhibitor - Entacapone, Tolcapone • Dopamine facilitator (NMDA receptor agonist)→Amantadine	*Decreasing brain cholinergic activity* • Central anticholinergic → trihexyphenidyl, procyclidine, biperiden • Antihistaminic → Orphenadrine, Promethazine

Management of Parkinsonism

- The most disabling symptoms in parkinsonism are motor symptoms especially bradykinesia. So, the main treatment is directed to decrease motor symptoms.
- Levodopa and dopamine agonists resolve motor symptoms. Dopamine agonist (Ropinirole, pramipexole, rotigotine) monotherapy is the initial treatment of choice. (But levodopa remains the most effective drug for Parkinsonism).
- If motor symptoms are not adequately controlled, levodopa (along with carbidopa) is added.
- If there is inadequate control or wearing-off symptoms (on-off effect), add COMT inhibitor or MAO-B inhibitor.
- If maximal therapy fails, surgical options should be considered.

Levodopa

- Levodopa is inactive by itself, but is the immediate precursor of the neurotransmitter dopamine.
- 95% of the oral dose is decarboxylated in the peripheral tissues.
- About 1–2% of the administered levodopa crosses the blood-brain barrier to reach the brain, which is taken up by the surviving dopaminergic neurons and converted to dopamine.

RESTLESS LEG SYNDROME

- Peculiar sensory-motor disorder affecting the legs especially during sleep
- Patient feels an irrestible urge to constantly move the legs, usually associated with tingling, itching, discomfort, aching or cramps. The symptoms abate by walking.
- The disorder may be primary (idiopathic) or secondary to iron-deficiency anemia, folate or other vitamin deficiencies.
- *Management*: Nonergot dopaminergic agonists are the most effective drugs. Relatively low doses of Ropinirole or Pramipexole taken 2–3 hours before bedtime each day afford dramatic relief. Other drugs used are—benzodiazepines, gabapentin or pregabalin, but these are mostly reserved for nonresponsive cases.

60. A young patient presents to OPD with complains of crawling sensation under his skin on legs. This feeling is relieved as soon as he starts moving his legs. What is the appropriate treatment for him? *(NEET 2020)*

a. Pramipexole
b. Gabapentin
c. Iron supplementation
d. Vit B12

Ans. is 'a' Pramipexole

61. All of the following pairs are correct *except*:

a. Peripheral decarboxylase inhibitor—Benserazide
b. MAO- B inhibitor—Clorgyline
c. COMT inhibitor—Entacapone
d. Dopamine facilitation—Amantadine

Ans. is 'b' MAO- B inhibitor—Clorgyline

62. True about anti-Parkinson drug levodopa is:

a. Levodopa an active metabolite of dopamine
b. About 50% of administered levodopa is peripherally converted to carbidopa
c. About 2% of the administered levodopa crosses blood-brain barrier
d. Levodopa has no role in hepatic coma

Ans. is 'c' About 2% of the administered levodopa crosses blood-brain barrier

63. Which of the following is used for the patient on antiparkinsonian medication levodopa + carbidopa, but patient showing marked on-off effect?

a. Bromocriptine
b. Amatidine
c. Selegiline
d. Rimonabant

Ans. is 'c' Selegiline

MECHANISM OF ACTION OF BENZODIAZEPINES

- BZDs act on GABA-A receptors.
- GABA binding site is on β subunit, while BZD binding site is on α/γ subunit.
- BZDs increase the conductance of Cl channel. BZDs do not themselves increase Cl conductance, i.e. they have only GABA facilitatory but no GABA mimetic action. (Barbiturates have both GABA facilitatory and GABA mimetic actions).
- In contrast to barbiturates, BZDs are not general depressant, but exert relatively selective anxiolytic, hypnotic, muscle relaxant and anticonvulsant effects.
- Stage 2 sleep is increased, while REM, Stage 3 & 4 sleep are decreased.
- Muscle relaxation is produced by action on medulla. Ataxia is due to action on cerebellum.

MECHANISM OF ACTION OF BARBITURATES

- Barbiturates act at the GABA-BZD receptor-Cl channel complex and potentiate GABAergic inhibition by increasing the lifetime of Cl channel opening caused by GABA (Vs benzodiazepines which enhance frequency of Cl channel opening) - GABA excitatory action.
- At high concentrations, barbiturates directly increase Cl conductance—GABA mimetic action.
- At very high concentrations, barbiturates depress voltage sensitive Na and K channels as well.
- Barbiturates depress all areas of CNS, but the reticular activating system is most sensitive.
- Sleep architecture is disturbed (REM, stage 3 and 4 sleep are decreased).
- They have no analgesic action, may even cause hyperalgesia (Diazepam has analgesic action).

Long acting barbiturates: Phenobarbitone, Mephobarbitone.
Short acting barbiturates: Butobarbitone, Secobarbital, Pentobarbital.
Ultrashort acting barbiturates: Thiopentone, Methohexitone.

64. Which of the following is not true about benzodiazepines?

a. Can produce ataxia
b. Has GABA facilitatory but not GABA mimetic action
c. REM, and stage 3 and 4 sleep is increased
d. Produces muscle relaxation by action on medulla

Ans. is 'c' REM, and stage 3 and 4 sleep is increased

65. Which of the following is not true about the mechanism of action of benzodiazepines?

a. Acts on midbrain, ascending reticular formation andlimbic system
b. It exerts effects through the GABA A receptors
c. It increases conductance of Cl–channels
d. It has GABA mimetic action

Ans. is 'd' It has GABA mimetic action

66. Which of the following is not true about barbiturate?

a. Shows GABA mimetic action
b. Shows GABA facilitatory action
c. It can depress voltage gated Na^+ and K^+ channels at high concentrations
d. Limbic system is most sensitive to the depressive action of barbiturates to CNS

Ans. is 'd' Limbic system is most sensitive to the depressive action of barbiturates to CNS

ANTIDEPRESSANTS

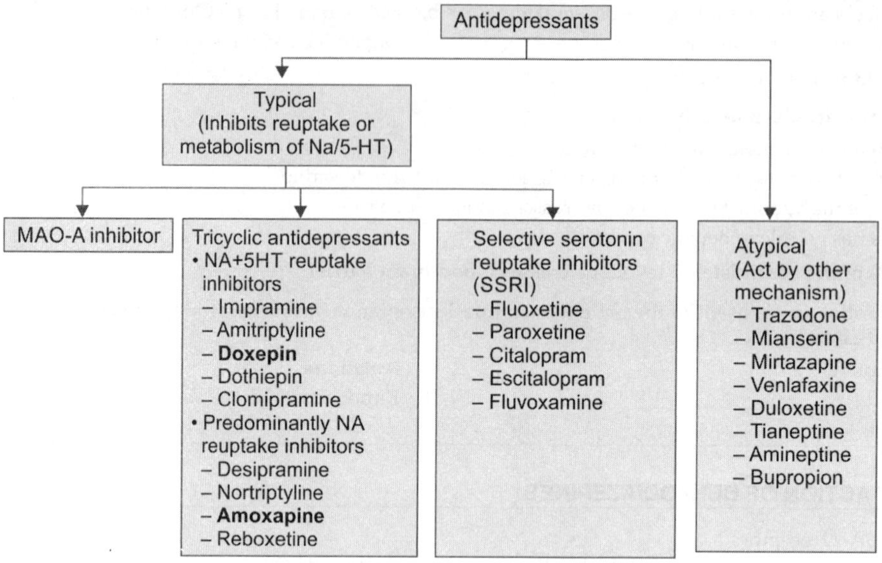

MAO-A inhibitors include—Moclobemide, Clorgylline

67. Mechanism of action of amoxapine is:

a. SNRI
b. SSRI
c. NA+ 5HT reuptake inhibitor
d. Predominantly NA reuptake inhibitor

Ans. is 'd' Predominantly NA reuptake inhibitor

LITHIUM

Mechanism: Not established; possibly related to inhibition of phosphoinositol cascade.
Clinical use: Mood stabilizer for bipolar disorder; treats acute manic episodes and prevents relapse.
Pharmacokinetics: Almost exclusively excreted by kidneys; most is reabsorbed at PCT via Na+ channels.

Adverse Effects

- Tremor (MC side effect), thyroid abnormalities (e.g. hypothyroidism), polyuria (causes nephrogenic diabetes insipidus), teratogenesis.
- Causes Ebstein anomaly in newborn if taken by pregnant mother.
- Narrow therapeutic window—requires close monitoring of serum levels.

Interactions: Diuretics (thiazide, furosemide) by causing Na+ loss promote proximal tubular reabsorption of Na+ as well as Li+ → plasma levels of lithium rise. Potassium sparing diuretics cause milder Li+ retention. Tetracyclines, NSAIDs and ACE inhibitors can also cause lithium retention.

Plasma concentration norms

- Acute mania: 0.8 – 1.2 mEq/L
- Prophylaxis: 0.5 – 0.8 mEq/L
- Toxic: > 2 mEq/L

68. A patient of bipolar disorder was treated with lithium. Hydrochlorothiazide was prescribed for his hypertension. He developed nausea, vomiting, coarse tremors and brisk reflexes 2 weeks after taking drugs. What is the likely reason for this presentation? *(NEET 2020)*

a. Side effects of hydrochlorothiazide
b. Decreased metabolism of HCTZ by lithium
c. Increased renal tubular reabsorption of lithium
d. Thiazide act as addon drug to lithium

Ans. is 'c' Increased renal tubular reabsorption of lithium

69. A female patient was on lithium therapy for bipolar disorder for 6 months. She kept the fast for few days due to religious reasons and presented with seizures, coarse tremors, confusion and weakness of limbs. Which of the following should be done to diagnose her condition? *(NEET 2020)*

a. Serum electrolytes
b. Serum lithium levels
c. ECG
d. MRI

Ans. is 'b' Serum lithium levels

SIDE EFFECTS OF ANTIPSYCHOTICS

Extrapyramidal side effects				
Effect	***Feature***	***Time of risk***	***Mechanism?***	***Treatment***
Acute dystonia	Spasm of muscles of tongue, face, neck, back	1 to 5 days	Unknown	Antimuscarinic agents
Akathisia	Motor restlessness, Anxiety	5 to 60 days	Unknown	Reduce dose, propranolol
Parkinsonism	Bradykinesia, rigidity, tremor	5 to 30 days	DA antagonism	Quetiapine or clozapine
Neuroleptic malignant syndrome	Catatonia, stupor fever, can be fatal	Weeks, can persist for days	DA antagonism	Stop neuroleptic immediately
Tardive dyskinesia	Stereotyped or choreic involuntary movements of face, tongue, trunk	After months of years of treatment, seen when withdraw drug	Excess function of DA due to hypersensitivity of dopamine receptors	Prevention crucial, switch to clozapine or quetiapine

Tardive Dyskinesia

- Typically composed of choreiform movements involving the mouth, lips, and tongue.
- Atypical antipsychotics (e.g. Clozapine, Risperidone, Olanzapine, Quetiapine, Ziprasidone and Aripiprazole) are associated with a significantly lower risk of TD in comparison to traditional antipsychotics.
- If the patient is receiving a traditional antipsychotic and withdrawal is not possible, replacement with an atypical antipsychotic should be tried.
- Abrupt cessation of a neuroleptic should be avoided as acute withdrawal can induce worsening.
- In refractory cases, catecholamine depleters such as tetrabenazine may be helpful. Other approaches include baclofen, clonazepam, or valproic acid.

70. Which of the following can be used in the management of tardive dyskinesia?

a. Cessation of antipsychotic medication
b. Baclofen
c. Tetrabenazine
d. All of the above

Ans. is 'd' All of the above

Drug of choice for various types of seizures	
Type of seizure seizures	***Drug of choice***
• Absence seizures • GTCS (Grand mal) • Tonic seizures • Clonic seizures • Myoclonic seizures • Atonic (Akinetic) seizures	• Valproate
• Partial seizures	• Carbamazepine
• Infantile spasm	• ACTH
• Infantile spasm with tuberous sclerosis	• Vigabatrin
• Febrile seizures	• Diazepam (per rectal)
• Status epilepticus	• Lorazepam (IV)
• Seizures in eclampsia	• Magnesium sulphate

Phenytoin Side Effects

Adverse effects of phenytoin	
At therapeutic level	***At high plasma level (dose related)***
• Hypertrophy of gum—commonest (20% incidence) • Hirsutism • Hypocalcemia • Hypersensitivity reactions, these include: – Rashes – DLE – Lymphadenopathy – Neutropenia • Hyperglycemia—it inhibits release of insulin • Hydantoin syndrome (fetal) • Megaloblastic anemia	• Cerebellar and vestibular manifestations • Ataxia • Vertigo • Diplopia • Nystagmus • Epigastric pain, vomiting, nausea • IV Injection causes local vascular injury • Fall in BP and cardiac arrhythmias • Drowsiness & mental confusion

Fosphenytoin

- This is water soluble prodrug of phenytoin that has been introduced to overcome the difficulties in IV administration of phenytoin.
- On IV injection it is less damaging to the intima; few vascular complications are produced; it can be injected at a faster rate.
- While phenytoin cannot be injected in a drip of glucose solution, fosphenytoin can be injected with both saline and glucose.

Valproic Acid

Mechanism of Action

- It prolongs the recovery of voltage-activated Na channels from inactivation, thus reducing the excitability of neurons.
- It increases the activity of glutamic acid decarboxylase & inhibit enzymes involved in degradation of GABA, thereby increasing its concentration.

Uses

GTCS, partial seizures, absence, myoclonic, and atonic seizures.

Side Effects

- Anorexia, nausea & vomiting
- Sedation, ataxia & tremor
- Rash, alopecia, curling of hair
- Stimulation of appetite & weight gain
- Elevation of hepatic transaminases, microvesicular steatosis
- Acute pancreatitis, increased incidence of PCOS
- Neural tube defects.

Interactions

- Valproate is metabolized by CYP450 enzymes into a minor metabolite, which is hepatotoxic.
- Enzyme inducers like carbamazepine phenytoin and Phenobarbital can induce the microsomal enzyme and increase production of this metabolite. This increases the risk of hepatotoxicity.

Vigabatrin

- Irreversible inhibitor of GABA-transaminase, causing increased concentrations of GABA in the brain.
- Used in Infantile spasms or with complex partial seizures refractory to other treatments.
- Long-term therapy with vigabatrin has been associated with peripheral visual field defects. These are caused by retinal lesions and are irreversible

Gabapentin

- Gabapentin enhances GABA release but itself does not act as an agonist at the GABA-A receptor.
- Uses
  - GTCS and partial seizures
  - Pain due to diabetic neuropathy–DOC
  - Postherpetic neuralgia–DOC
  - Prophylaxis of migraine.

71. All are adverse effects of phenytoin *except*:

a. Hypertrophy of gums
b. Hirsutism
c. Hypertension
d. Hypersensitivity

Ans. is 'c' Hypertension

72. Drug of choice for status epilepticus is:

a. Diazepam
b. Lorazepam
c. Phenytoin
d. Sodium valproate

Ans. is 'b' Lorazepam

73. Neural tube defects are associated with which drugs?

a. Ethosuximide
b. Valproic acid
c. Lamotrigine
d. Topiramate

Ans. is 'b' Valproic acid

74. Fosphenytoin is different from phenytoin as:

a. It is less damaging to intima on intravenous administration
b. It can be injected in a drip of glucose solution
c. It is a prodrug of phenytoin
d. All of the above

Ans. is 'd' All of the above

75. Vigabatrin acts through:

a. Decreasing GABA uptake at synaptic cleft
b. Increasing GABA uptake at synaptic cleft
c. GABA transaminase inhibitor
d. GABA transacetylase inhibitor

Ans. is 'c' GABA transaminase inhibitor

ALCOHOL WITHDRAWAL

Drugs used in Acute Ethanol Withdrawal

Benzodiazepines (chlordiazepoxide, diazepam, lorazepam): They facilitate GABA-mediated activation of GABA receptors.

Thiamine (vitamin B1): Alcoholic patients are deficient in thiamine. Hence, it must be administered to patients suspected of having alcoholism (those exhibiting acute alcohol in toxication or alcohol withdrawal syndrome) to prevent Wernicke-Korsakoff syndrome

Drugs used in Chronic Alcoholism

Naltrexone: Competitive antagonist of opioid receptors. It reduces craving in alcoholics.

Acamprosate: NMDA receptor antagonist & GABAA agonist effects. It also reduces craving.

Disulfiram: It is an inhibitor of aldehyde dehydrogenase and therefore causes accumulation of aldehyde if alcohol is ingested. This results in troublesome symptoms. It is used as a deterrent agent to reduce the consumption of alcohol in motivated individuals.

76. Drug to prevent heavy drinking relapse is:

a. Methadone
b. Naltrexone
c. Naloxone
d. Nalmefene

Ans. is 'b' Naltrexone

77. Acamprosate is used for:

a. Alcohol abstinence
b. Nicotine abstinence
c. Opioid abstinence
d. Cocaine abstinence

Ans. is 'a' Alcohol abstinence

OPIOIDS

Subclass, drug	Mechanism of action	Effects	Clinical applications	Pharmacokinetics, toxicities
Opioid agonists				
• Morphine • Methadone • Fentanyl	• Strong μ-receptor agonists • Variable affinity for δ and κ receptors	• Analgesia • Relief of anxiety • Sedation • Slowed gastrointestinal transit	• Severe pain • Adjunct in anesthesia (fentanyl, morphine) • Pulmonary edema (morphine only) • Maintenance in rehabilitation programs (methadone only)	• First-pass effect • Duration 1–4 h except methadone, 4–6 h • *Toxicity:* Respiratory depression • Severe constipation • Addiction liability • Convulsions • Causes spasm of sphincter of Oddi- increasing biliary colic
• Hydromorphone, oxymorphone: Like morphine in efficacy, but higher potency • Meperidine: Strong agonist with anticholinergic effects • Oxycodone: Dose-dependent analgesia • Sufentanil, alfentanil, remifentanil: Like fentanyl but shorter durations of action				
• Codeine • Hydrocodone	• Less efficacious than morphine • Can antagonize strong agonists	• Like strong agonists • Weaker effects	• Mild-moderate pain • Cough (codeine)	• Like strong agonists, toxicity dependent on genetic variation of metabolism
Mixed opioid agonist-antagonists				
• • Buprenorphine	• Partial μ agonist • Κ antagonist	• Like strong agonists but can antagonize their effects • Also reduces craving for alcohol	• Moderate pain • Some maintenance rehabilitation programs	• Long duration of action 4–8 h • May precipitate abstinence syndrome

Contd...

Contd...

Subclass, drug	Mechanism of action	Effects	Clinical applications	Pharmacokinetics, toxicities
Opioid antagonists				
• Naloxone • Naltrexone • Nalmefene	• Antagonist at μ, δ, and κ receptors	• Rapidly antagonizes all opioid effects	• Opioid overdose	• Duration 1–2 h (may have to be repeated when treating overdose) • *Toxicity:* Precipitates abstinence syndrome in dependent users

- Morphine is contraindicated in Head injury, Bronchial asthma, elderly males (risk of urinary retention).

Opioid dependence: Treated in two stages:

- **Detoxification**: It includes treatment of withdrawal symptoms. Methadone is the drug of choice. Other drugs used are buprenorphine, LAAM (L-alpha-acetylmethadol), clonidine, benzodiazepine (lorazepam or oxazepam), dextropropoxyphene and diphenoxylate.
- **Maintenance therapy**: Methadone is the treatment of choice. Other drugs used are buprenorphine and LAAM.

78. Mechanism of action of methadone is:

a. Opioid receptor agonist
b. Opioid receptor partial agonist
c. Opioid receptor antagonist
d. Opioid receptor inverse agonist

Ans. is 'a' Opioid receptor agonist

79. Which of the following acts as partial/weak μ agonist + κ antagonist on opioid receptor?

a. Nalorphine
b. Naltrexone
c. Buprenorphine
d. Nalmefene

Ans. is 'c' Buprenorphine

80. Drug for opioid dependence is:

a. Naloxone
b. Naltrexone
c. Methadone
d. Nalmefene

Ans. is 'c' Methadone

81. A patient of biliary colic presented to hospital. Intern gave an injection and the pain worsened. Which is the most likely injection given? *(NEET 2020)*

a. Morphine
b. Diclofenac
c. Nefopam
d. Etoricoxib

Ans. is 'a' Morphine

Explanation: Morphine can aggravate certain condition, e.g., biliary colic, pancreatitis, diverticulitis. Diclofenac, Nefopam and Etoricoxib does not cause biliary colic.

Preferred Drugs for Psychiatric Conditions

Psychiatric condition	Preferred drugs
ADHD	Stimulants (methylphenidate, amphetamines)
Alcohol withdrawal	Benodiazepines (e.g. chlordiazepoxide, lorazepam, diazepam)
Bipolar disorder	Lithium, valproic acid, carbamazepine, lamotrigine, atypical antipsychotics
Bulimia nervosa	SSRIs
Depression	SSRIs
Generalized anxiety disorder	SSRIs, SNRIs
Obsessive-compulsive disorder	SSRIs, venlafaxine, clomipramine
Panic disorder	SSRIs, venlafaxine, benzodiazepines
PTSD	SSRIs, venlafaxine
Schizophrenia	Atypical antipsychotics
Social anxiety disorder	SSRIs, venlafaxine Performance only: β-blockers, benzodiazepines
Tourette syndrome	Antipsychotics (e.g. fluphenazine, risperidone), tetrabenazine

82. A patient presented with symptoms of depression and was started with imipramine. Post-treatment, he develops symptoms of excessive energy, elated mood and lack of sleep, excessive cheerfulness and talkativeness. What should be the modification in the treatment? *(NEET 2020)*

a. Stop imipramine and start valproate
b. Add BZD to imipramine
c. Add antipsychotic to imipramine
d. Start SSRI

Ans. is 'a' Stop imipramine and start valproate

Explanation: Since, the patient has both depressive and manic episodes—the diagnosis is bipolar disorder.

HEMATOLOGY

HYPOLIPIDEMIC DRUGS

Drug	Indication
HMG-CoA reductase inhibitors (statins)	Elevated LDL-cholesterol; increased CV risk
Cholesterol absorption inhibitor Ezetimibe	Elevated LDL-cholesterol
Bile acid sequestrants cholestyramine	Elevated LDL-cholesterol
MTP inhibitor lomitapide	Familial hypercholesterolemia
ApoB inhibitor mipomersen	Familial hypercholesterolemia
Nicotinic acid	Elevated LDL-Cholesterol, elevated TG
Fibric acid derivatives Gemfibrozil, Fenofibrate	Elevated TG
Omega-3 fatty acids	Elevated TG

HMG-CoA Reductase Inhibitors (Statins)

Inhibit HMG-CoA reductase, a key enzyme in cholesterol biosynthesis. By inhibiting cholesterol biosynthesis, statins lead to increased hepatic LDL receptor activity and accelerated clearance of circulating LDL, resulting in a dose-dependent reduction in plasma levels of LDL-Cholesterol.

Statins also reduce plasma TGs in a dose-dependent fashion, which is roughly proportional to their LDL-Cholesterol lowering effects (if the TGs are <400 mg/dL).

Statins have a modest HDL-raising effect (5–10%) that is not generally dose-dependent.

Potential side effects include dyspepsia, headaches, fatigue, and muscle or joint pains.

The risk of statin-associated myopathy is increased by renal insufficiency, and coadministration of fibric acid derivatives (particularly gemfibrozil).

Nicotinic Acid

- ❖ Niacin increases lipolysis and triglyceride breakdown by activating lipoprotein lipase and also increases blood HDL levels.
- ❖ Side effects are:
  - Dyspepsia is very common, dryness and hyperpigmentation can be troublesome.
  - Hepatic failure and jaundice.
  - Hyperglycemia and may precipitate DM.
  - Hyperuricemia and gout.

CETP Inhibitors

- ❖ CETP, i.e. Cholesteryl ester transfer proteins inhibitors are class of cholesterol lowering agents.
- ❖ CETP facilitates exchange of cholesterol esters with triglycerides between HDL and chylomicrons, VLDL and LDL which plays an important role in the disposal of HDL associated cholesterol.
- ❖ Examples of CETP inhibitors: Torcetrapib, Anacetrapib.

83. Statins inhibit which of the following enzyme?

a. HMG CoA reductase
b. HMG CoA synthetase
c. HMG CoA oxidase
d. Acetyl CoA synthetase

Ans. is 'a' HMG CoA reductase

84. Mechanism of action of Torcetrapib is:

a. Bile acid sequestrant
b. Sterol absorption inhibitor
c. Lipoprotein lipase activator
d. CETP inhibitor

Ans. is 'd' CETP inhibitor

85. Which anti-lipidemic drug causes hyperuricemia?

a. Gemfibrozil
b. Nicotinic acid
c. Torcetrapib
d. Ezetimibe

Ans. is 'b' Nicotinic acid

ANTIPLATELET DRUGS

Aspirin

Mechanisms of Action

- ❖ Aspirin is an irreversible inhibitor of cyclooxygenase enzyme. Aspirin gets deactivated once it reaches the liver. Therefore, it acts on the platelets within the portal circulation.
- ❖ Aspirin acetylates a serine residue near active site of platelet cyclooxygenase-1 (COX-1) that thromboxane, which is involved in platelet aggregation.
- ❖ Since platelets cannot synthesize new proteins, the action of aspirin lasts for as long as the lifespan of the platelets (7–10 days).

Uses

- It is used as an antiplatelet agent in cerebrovascular accidents, unstable angina, myocardial infarction. It is useful in secondary prevention as well in these cases.
- Long-term use of aspirin is associated with a lower incidence of colon cancer.

Adverse Effects

- Peptic ulcer disease due to inhibition of gastric COX.
- Hepatotoxicity, asthma, rashes, GI bleeding & renal toxicity.

Thienopyridines

Includes clopidogrel, ticlopidine, prasugrel, cangrelor and ticagrelor

- They block ADP receptors (P2Y12 receptors), thus suppressing platelet adhesion
- Uses- Secondary prevention of MI, stroke or PVD
- Decreases thrombus risk in coronary stenting.

Side effects: Increased risk of hemorrhage & GI bleeding, neutropenia with ticlopidine

Prasugrel is about 10-fold more potent than clopidogrel and has a more rapid onset of action because of better absorption. Prasugrel should generally be avoided in older patients, and the drug is contraindicated in those with a history of cerebrovascular disease (due to risk of fatal bleeding).

Clopidogrel is safer than ticlopidine as it is associated with a lower frequency of neutropenia, thrombocytopenia and other bone marrow toxicity.

GP IIb/IIIa inhibitors

- Includes abciximab, eptifibatide, tirofiban
- They Inhibit platelet aggregation by binding to platelet GP IIb/ IIIa receptors
- They are used to reduce the risk of thrombus in unstable angina or following PTCA.

Dipyridamole

- Inhibit activity of adenosine deaminase & phosphodiesterase receptors, thus inhibiting adenosine reuptake.
- Dipyridamole is a powerful coronary dilator; increases total coronary flow by preventing uptake and degradation of adenosine.
- It dilates resistance vessels in nonischemic zone as well → Diverts the already reduced blood flow away from ischemic zone- Coronary steal phenomenon.

Used in combination with aspirin in patients with recent stroke or with warfarin following artificial heart valve replacement.

86. Which of the following statements about prasugrel is true as compared to clopidogrel?

a. It is slower acting than clopidogrel
b. It is contraindicated in stroke
c. It is a reversible antagonist of ADP receptors
d. Decrease the risk of bleeding

Ans. is 'b' It is contraindicated in stroke

87. All are ADP inhibitors *except*:

a. Ticlopidine
b. Tirofiban
c. Clopidogrel
d. Prasugrel

Ans. is 'b' Tirofiban

ANTICOAGULANTS

Heparin

- It acts in conjunction with antithrombin Ill, to inhibit thrombin & factor Xa
- Uses: Immediate anticoagulation for Ml, DVT PE, stroke; Postoperative prophylaxis for DVT & PE
- It is safe in pregnancy.

Side effects are: Thrombocytopenia, hemorrhage, osteoporosis, hypersensitivity

Antidote of heparin is Protamine sulphate. It is a strongly basic, low molecular weight protein obtained from the sperm of certain fish. Given IV, it neutralizes heparin weight for weight.

Low Molecular Weight Heparin (LMWH) (Enoxaparin)

- It differs from unfractionated heparin because it inhibits only factor Xa
- It is more commonly used instead of UFH.

Direct Thrombin Inhibitors

Parenteral: Lepirudin, Argatroban, Bivalirudin
Oral: Dabigatran
They selectively inhibit thrombin to suppress activity of factors V, IX & XIII & platelet aggregation.
They are the preferred drugs in case of heparin induced thrombocytopenia.

Indirect factor Xa inhibitors

- Fondaparinux—inhibits factor Xa using antithrombin as a cofactor, but has no activity against thrombin.
- It does not inhibit factor Xa bound to prothrombinase complex.
- It is used for DVT prophylaxis and acute DVT or PE
- Adverse effects include hemorrhage, fever & anemia, edema & rash.
- It does not require laboratory monitoring.

Oral Direct Factor Xa inhibitors

- It includes rivaroxaban, apixaban.
- They directly engage the active center of factor Xa molecule & inhibit both free factor Xa in plasma & factor Xa attached to prothrombinase complex.
- Used for prevention & treatment of venous thromboembolism & stroke prevention in atrial fibrillation.

Warfarin

It inhibits the synthesis & carboxylation of vitamin K-dependent factors II, VII, IX & X and protein C & protein S.

- Used for long-term anticoagulation, post-thrombotic event or in cases of increased thrombus risk (post-surgery, atrial fibrillation, artificial valves)
- Metabolized by cytochrome P-450 pathway, long half-life.

Adverse effects include hemorrhage, teratogenicity (Conrad's syndrome), calciphylaxis.

Interactions

- Inducers of CYP2C9 like carbamazepine, Phenobarbital and rifampicin increase metabolism of warfarin and hence decrease plasma concentration this can cause thrombosis.
- Inhibitors of CYP2C9 like isoniazid, amiodarone, cimetidine and cotrimoxazole can inhibit metabolism of warfarin and hence increase plasma concentration; this can cause bleeding.

88. Which of the following is orally active direct Xa inhibitor? *(NEET 2019)*

a. Rivaroxaban
b. Agrataban
c. Dabigatran
d. Bivalirudin

Ans. is 'a' Rivaroxaban

Previously Asked Facts

- Venlafaxine is serotonin and noradrenaline reuptake inhibitor (SNRI). It is FDA approved for use in major depression, generalized anxiety disorder, and panic disorder.
- FDA approved drug for refractory schizophrenia – Clozapine.
- A depot injection, usually subcutaneous or intramuscular releases its active compound in a consistent way over a long period of time. Antipsychotic drugs with depot preparations are risperidone, paliperidone, haloperidol, fluphenazine, flupenthixol, zuclopenthixol, olanzapine, clozapine and quetiapine.
- Temazepam is an intermediate acting benzodiazepine. Its metabolism is independent of liver and hence, can be safely given in patients with hepatic failure. Temazepam does not have an active metabolite like diazepam [Note: Diazepam is converted to an active metabolite 'desmethyl diazepam' (oxazepam)].
- Carbamazepine, vigabatrin, and tiagabine are contraindicated in the treatment of absence seizures, irrespective of cause and severity.
- Flumazenil is antagonist of BZDs at GABA receptor. It is not GABA antagonist.
- Phenobarbital is the drug of choice for management of seizures for patients allergic to phenytoin.
- Drugs causing hypothyroidism – Lithium, sulfonamide, phenobarbitone, phenytoin, amiodarone, carbamazepine, ethionamide.
- Aripiprazole is the only antipsychotic with D2 agonistic activity (all others are D2 antagonists).
- Most potent opioid is Sufentanil.
- Atracurium: Unique feature is its inactivation in plasma by spontaneous nonenzymatic degradation called as Hoffman elimination. Following degradation it produces a metabolite—laudanosine. Laudanosine may induce seizures in some patients.

- Cis-atracurium: Undergoes Hoffman elimination, does not provoke histamine release (hence, preferred over atracurium), produces less laudanosine (hence, less risk for seizures).
- Paclitaxel acts by inhibiting microtubulin polymerization and inhibits division of metastatic cells.
- Abraxane is a novel albumin bound paclitaxel which has got lesser propensity to cause hypersensitivity reactions than paclitaxel. Abraxane is used in the treatment of the advanced metastatic breast carcinoma patients.
- GM CSF used in neutropenia is Molgramostim.
- Half-life of alteplase (recombinant-tissue plasminogen activator) is 4–8 minutes.
- Vagiprost is a novel thromboxane receptor antagonist. It is usually used along with r-tPA like alteplase.
- Dazoxiben is an orally active thromboxane synthase inhibitor. It has shown a significant clinical improvement in patients with Raynaud's syndrome. Daltroban and sultroban are TXA2 receptor antagonists.
- The most significant advance in the therapy of sickle cell anemia has been the introduction of hydroxyurea as a mainstay of therapy. Hydroxyurea increases fetal hemoglobin concentration.
- Treatment of clopidogrel toxicity can be done with recombinant factor VIIa infusion.
- Monitoring of unfractionated heparin → aPTT; Monitoring of oral anticoagulants → PT/INR; Monitoring of LMW heparins → No monitoring required.

RESPIRATORY SYSTEM

Drugs used in asthma				
Bronchodilators	***Drugs reducing inflammation***			
	Leukotriene antagonists	***Mast cell stabilizers***	***Corticosteroids***	***Anti-IgE antibody***
β2 Sympathomimetics	• Montelukast	• Sodium cromoglycate	*Systemic*	• Omalizumab
• Salbutamol	• Zafirlukast	• Ketotifen	• Hydrocortisone	
Bronchodilators	***Drugs reducing inflammation***			
	Leukotriene antagonists	***Mast cell stabilizers***	***Corticosteroids***	***Anti-IgE antibody***
• Terbutaline			• Prednisolone	
• Bambuterol			*Inhalation*	
• Salmeterol			• Beclomethasone	
• Formoterol			• Budesonide	
• Ephedrine			• Fluticasone	
Methylxanthines			• Flunisolide	
• Theophylline			• Ciclesonide	
• Aminophylline				
• Doxophylline				
Anticholinergics				
• Ipratropium				
• Tiotropium				
• Selective PGE4 inhibitors are under clinical trial as antiasthma drugs, these are cilomilast and roflumilast.				

THEOPHYLLINE

Mechanisms of Action

1. Inhibition of phosphodiesterase → Increases cAMP levels by inhibiting hydrolysis – PDE3 is responsible for methylxanthine-induced bronchodilation; PDE4 responsible for inhibition of inflammatory cells. Causes bronchodilatation, cardiac stimulation and vasodilation
2. Blockade of adenosine receptors → Adenosine A1 receptor antagonism considered responsible for cardiac arrythmias and seizures occurring in theophylline toxicity. Blockade of A1 receptors can induce diuresis and natriuresis by inhibition of proximal tubular reabsorption. Methylxanthines are weak renal vasodilators and they act as competitive antagonists against adenosine-induced preglomerular vasoconstriction. Since enhanced intrarenal adenosine levels lead to reduced glomerular filtration rate in several pathological conditions, theophylline has been tested for its therapeutic potential in the renal impairment following administration of nephrotoxic substances such as radiocontrast media, cisplatin, calcineurin inhibitors or following ischemia-reperfusion injury.

89. Which mechanism of action of theophylline is responsible for diuresis? *(NEET 2020)*

a. PDE-3 inhibition
b. PDE-4 inhibition
c. A1 antagonism
d. Beta-2 agonism

Ans. is 'c' A1 antagonism

90. Which of the following is not an inhalational steroids?

a. Beclomethasone
b. Betamethasone
c. Budesonide
d. Fluticasone acetonide

Ans. is 'b' Betamethasone

91. Montelukast is a:

a. Leukotriene antagonist
b. Mast cell stabilizer
c. Anti-IgE antibody
d. Lipoxygenase inhibitor

Ans. is 'a' Leukotriene antagonist

GASTROINTESTINAL TRACT (GIT)

ANTI-EMETICS

Types of antiemetics

Type	*Mechanism*	*Examples*	*Clinical indications*
Antiemetic agents	H1 antihistaminics	Promethazine, cyclizine diphenhydramine, dimenhydrinate, cinnarizine	Motion, sickness, inner ear disease
	Anticholinergic	Hyoscine, dicyclomine	Motion sickness, inner ear disease
	Antidopaminergic	Prochlorperazine, thiethylperazine	Medication, toxin or metabolic-induced emesis
	5-HT3 antagonist	Ondansetron, granisetron	DOC for Chemotherapy & radiation-induced emesis, postoperative emesis
	Neurokinin (NK-1) antagonist	Aprepitant, fosaprepitant	Chemotherapy-induced nausea & vomiting
	Tricyclic antidepressant	Amitriptyline, nortriptyline	Chronic idiopathic nausea, functional vomiting, cyclic vomiting syndrome
Prokinetic agents	5-HT4 Agonism improves motility & D2 antagonist action reduce emesis	Metoclopramide	Gastroparesis
	Motilin agonist	Erythromycin	Gastroparesis, intestinal pseudo-obstruction
	Peripheral antidopaminergic	Domperidone	Gastroparesis
	5-HT4 agonist	Tegaserod	Constipation predominant irritable bowel syndrome, gastroparesis
	5-HT4 agonist with weak 5-HT3 antagonism	Cisapride	GERD
	Somatostatin analogue	Octreotide	Intestinal pseudo-obstruction
Adjuvant antiemetics	Benzodiazepines	Lorazepam	Anticipatory nausea & vomiting with chemotherapy
	Glucocorticoids	Methylprednisolone, dexamethasone	Chemotherapy-induced emesis
	Cannabinoids	Tetrahydrocannabinol	Chemotherapy-induced emesis

92. Which of the following is not a prokinetic drug? *(NEET 2020)*

a. 5HT4-agonist
b. D2 blocker
c. Macrolides
d. Diphenoxymethane

Ans. is 'd' Diphenoxymethane

93. DOC for chemotherapy-induced vomiting? *(NEET 2019)*

a. Granisetron
b. Prazosin
c. Clonidine
d. Dimenhydrinate

Ans. is 'a' Granisetron

GLP-2 ANALOG

- Glucagon-like peptide-2 (GLP-2): Important intestinotrophic growth factor & mediator of intestinal adaptation.
- Teduglutide is a GLP-2 analog that is used in short bowel syndrome. It works by promoting mucosal growth and possibly restoring gastric emptying and secretion.

94. What is the mechanism of action of teduglutide in short bowel syndrome? *(NEET 2019)*

a. GLP-2 analog
b. HT-1 inhibitor
c. GLP-1 analogs
d. C-peptide analogs

Ans. is 'a' GLP-2 analog

Irritable Bowel Syndrome

- No structural abnormalities.
- Most common in middle-aged women.
- Chronic symptoms may be diarrhea—predominant, constipation—predominant, or mixed.
- First-line treatment is lifestyle modification and dietary changes.

Rome IV diagnostic criteria for irritable bowel syndrome[a]
Recurrent abdominal pain, on average, at least 1 day per week in the last 3 months, associated with ≥ 2 of the following criteria:
1. Related to defecation
2. Associated with a change in frequency of stool
3. Associated with a change in form (appearance) of stool

[a] Criteria fulfilled for the last 3 months with symptom on set at least 6 months prior to diagnosis.

95. A patient of polycystic kidney disease has hematuria and chronic hypertension. He is also taking tolvaptan. He develops complains of alternating diarrhoea, vomiting, abdominal cramps and bloating. What can be the likely etiology? *(NEET 2020)*

a. Tolvaptan side effects
b. Irritable bowel syndrome
c. Colonic diverticulosis
d. Ischemic bowel disease

Ans. is 'b' Irritable bowel syndrome

Previously Asked Facts

- Salmeterol and Formoterol are long acting β_2-agonists. In comparison to salmeterol, formoterol has faster onset of action and is used on a regular morning-evening schedule for round the clock bronchodilatation.
- Pirenzepine (Gastrozepin), an M1 selective antagonist, is used in the treatment of peptic ulcers, as it reduces gastric acid secretion and reduces muscle spasm.
- Senna is an FDA-approved over-the-counter laxative. Chronic use may cause colonic atony and mucosal pigmentation (melanosis coli).
- Erythromycin stimulates motilin (an upper gastrointestinal peptide hormone) receptors in the GIT which induces gastric contractions, hastens gastric emptying and promotes intestinal motility without significant effect on colonic motility. It has been used to afford short-term symptomatic relief in diabetic gastroparesis.
- In cases of unconjugated hyperbilirubinemia, phenobarbitone induces liver microsomal enzymes, which convert it into conjugated bilirubin and is excreted in urine. Thus, it is used in cases of neonatal jaundice.
- Penicillamine is the drug of choice for treatment of Wilson's disease. Trientine is ind icated especially in patients who are intolerant to penicillamine. Trientine is a less potent cupriuretic agent than penicillamine. Trientine may cause iron deficiency.
- Racecadotril is rapidly converted to thiorphan, an enkephalinase inhibitor which prevents the degradation of encephalin (ENK) which are mainly δ opioid receptor agonists. It decreases intestinal hypersecretion without affecting motility and used for short-term treatment of acute secretory diarrhea.
- The two molecules of Aminosalicylate coupled via azo bond form Olsalazine.
- Lubiprostone is a bicyclic fatty acid that stimulates chloride channels in the apical membrane of intestinal epithelial cells. Chloride secretion induces passive movement of sodium and water into the bowel lumen and improve bowel function. Lubiprostone is used for treatment of chronic constipation with or without Irritable Bowel Syndrome (IBS).
- Proton Pump Inhibitors (PPI) are the DOC for peptic ulcer (gastric or duodenal), prevention of aspiratory pneumonia and NSAID-induced gastric/duodenal ulcers.

ANTI-MICROBIAL AGENTS

MECHANISM OF ACTION OF ANTIBIOTICS

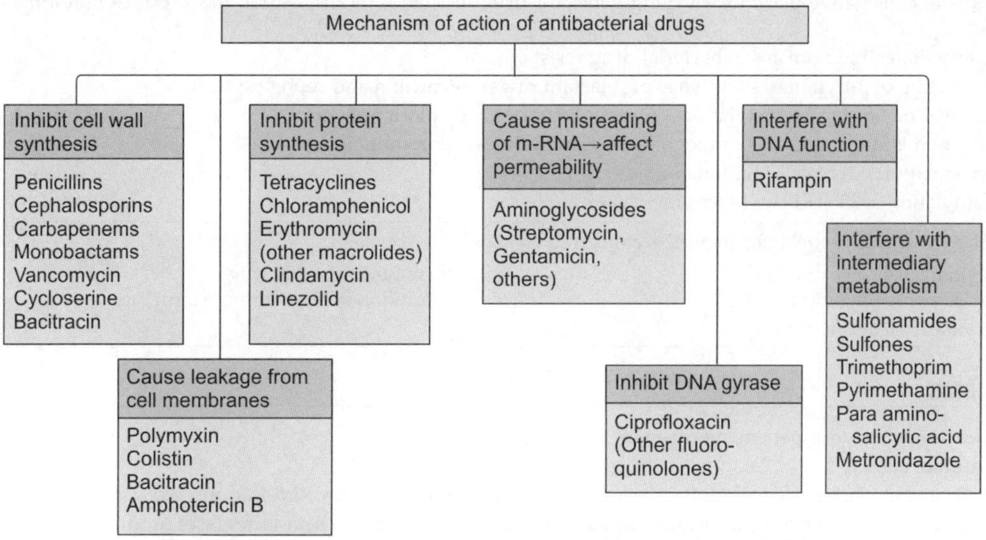

Primarily Bacteriostatic	Primarily Bactericidal
Sulfonamides Tetracyclines Erythromycin Chloramphenicol Clindamycin Linezolid Ethambutol	Penicillins Aminoglycosides Cephalosporins Vancomycin Polypeptides Fluoroquinolones Rifampicin Metronidazole Isoniazid Cotrimoxazole Pyrazinamide

96. Which of the following acts by inhibiting the transcription of DNA to RNA? *(NEET 2020)*

a. Rifampicin
b. Ciprofloxacin
c. Novobiocin
d. Nitrofurantoin

Ans. is 'a' Rifampicin

Explanation: Rifampin interrupts RNA synthesis by binding to β subunit of mycobacterial DNA- dependent RNA polymerase (encoded by rpo β gene) and blocking its polymerizing function. Ciprofloxacin inhibits bacterial DNA gyrase. Novobiocin binds to DNA gyrase, and blocks adenosine triphosphatase (ATPase) activity. Nitrofurantoin, after reduction by bacterial enzymes causes DNA damage.

97. All of the following drugs are bacteriostatic *except*:

a. Vancomycin
b. Clindamycin
c. Tetracycline
d. Linezolid

Ans. is 'a' Vancomycin

Antibiotic Resistance

Three general types of antibiotic resistance: intrinsic, chromosome-mediated and plasmid-mediated.

1. *Intrinsic drug resistance*
   - Bacteria lack target molecule for the drug or their normal anatomy and physiology makes them refractory to drug's action.
   - For example, Mycoplasma are intrinsically resistant to penicillins as they lack peptidoglycan wall. Bacteria that lack mycolic acids are resistant to isoniazid.
2. *Chromosome-mediated resistance*
   - Most commonly, these genes alter target for a drug so that the drug can no longer bind
   - Usually causes low-level drug resistance
     - Alteration of penicillin-binding proteins—Methicillin-resistant Staphylococcus aureus (MRSA)
     - Mutation of catalase-peroxidase gene needed to activate the drug—Isoniazid

- Mutation of arabinosyl transferase gene—Ethambutol
- Ribosomal binding-site mutations—Aminoglycosides

3. *Plasmid-mediated resistance*
   - Often, these genes code for enzymes that modify the drug
   - R factors are conjugative plasmids carrying genes for drug resistance. Transposition has produced multiple drug-resistance plasmids.
   - Plasmid-mediated mechanisms of bacterial drug resistance
     - Production of β-lactamases (cleavage of β-lactam rings) – Penicillin and cephalosporins
     - Inactivation of drug by acetylation – Aminoglycosides and chloramphenicol
     - Increased efflux out of cell (efflux pump) – Tetracyclines, fluoroquinolones
     - Active export out of cell – Sulfonamides
     - Methylation of 23S rRNA - Macrolides

98. Antibiotic resistance by beta lactamases is conferred by: *(NEET 2020)*

a. Enzymatic cleavage of drug
b. Increased efflux of drug
c. Altered penicillin binding site
d. Alteration in 50s ribosome structure

Ans. is 'a' Enzymatic cleavage of drug

CARBAPENEMS

- These include imipenem, doripenem, meropenem and ertapenem
- Wide spectrum of activity
- Carbapenems are beta-lactamase resistant and are drug of choice for *Enterobacter, Klebsiella* and *acinetobacter* species
- Only beta-lactams that are reliably efficacious against ESBL (extended spectrum beta-lactamase) producing organisms
- Imipenem is rapidly inactivated by renal dehydropeptidase I, so it is combined with cilastatin, an inhibitor of this enzyme. Cilastatin increases the half-life of imipenem and also inhibits the formation of nephrotoxic metabolite.
- Main adverse effects of imipenem-cilastatin combination include seizures and gastrointestinal distress.
- Meropenem, doripenem and ertapenem are not metabolized by renal dehydropeptidase and are less likely to cause seizures.

99. Antibiotic used for ESBL [Extended spectrum β lactamase] producing Klebsiella infection is:

a. Spectinomycin
b. Carbapenem
c. Aztreonam
d. Streptomycin

Ans. is 'b' Carbapenem

100. Carbapenem which has tendency to cause maximum seizures: *(NEET 2019)*

a. Imipenem
b. Ertapenem
c. Doripenem
d. Meropenem

Ans. is 'a' Imipenem

101. Imipenem, a new antibiotic with a broad antibacterial spectrum, is co-administered with cilastatin. What is the reason for the same? *(NEET 2019)*

a. Combination is synergistic against Pseudomonas species
b. Cilastatin aids gastrointestinal absorption of active moiety
c. Cilastatin inhibits beta-lactamase enzyme
d. Cilastatin inhibits an enzyme in kidney that destroys imipenem

Ans. is 'd' Cilastatin inhibits an enzyme in kidney that destroys imipenem

FLUOROQUINOLONES

Examples: Ciprofloxacin, norfloxacin, ofloxacin, pefloxacin; respiratory fluoroquinolones – Gemifloxacin, levofloxacin, moxifloxacin

Mechanism: Inhibit prokaryotic enzymes topoisomerase II (DNA gyrase) and topoisomerase IV. FQs are Bactericidal.

Mechanism of resistance: Chromosome-encoded mutation in DNA gyrase

Clinical uses: Gram negative rods of urinary and GI tracts (including Pseudomonas), some gram positive organisms, otitis externa.

Adverse effects

- GI upset, superinfections, skin rashes, headache, dizziness. Less commonly, can cause leg cramps and myalgias.
- Contraindicated in pregnant women, nursing mothers, and children < 18 years old due to possible damage to cartilage.
- May cause tendonitis or tendon rupture in people > 60 years old and in patients taking prednisone.
- Ciprofloxacin inhibits cytochrome P-450.
- Sparfloxacin and moxifloxacin can cause prolonged Q-T interval.
- All FQs are contraindicated in renal failure except Pefloxacin, moxifloxacin and trovafloxacin. Dose of pefloxacin needs to be reduced in liver disease, but not in renal insufficiency.

102. Fluoroquinolone contraindicated in liver disease is: *(NEET 2020)*

a. **Levofloxacin**
b. **Pefloxacin**
c. **Moxifloxacin**
d. **Lomefloxacin**

Ans. is 'b' Pefloxacin

ANTITUBERCULAR DRUGS

Anti TB drugs (First line durgs)	Isoniazid	Rifampicin	Ethambutol	Pyrizinamide	Streptomycin
Mechanism	Inhibits Mycolic acid	Inhibits DNA dependent RNA polymerase	Inhibits Mycolic acid-Arabinosyl transferase	Inhibits Mycolic acid	Inhibits-30s ribosome (Initiation complex)
Route	Oral	Oral	Oral	Oral	Intramuscular
Site	Intra and Extracellular	Intra and Extracellular	Intra and Extracellular	Intracellular only	Extracellular only
Cidal or static	Bactericidal	Bactericidal	Bactericidal	Bactericidal	Bactericidal
Metabolism	Liver-Acetylation	Liver-CYP inducer	Unchanged urine	Liver	Unchanged urine
S/E	• Hepatotoxicity (Fast acetylators) • Peripheral neuropathy (Slow Acetylators)	• Hepatotoxicity • Reddish orange discoloration (urine, sweat, saliva)	• Retrobulbar neuritis (red-green color blindness) • Hyperuricemia (Gout)	• Hepatotoxicity • Hyperuricemia (Gout)	• Ototoxicity • Vestibulotoxicity • Cochleotoxicity • Nephrotoxicy • Neuromuscular blockage

Isoniazid-Induced Neurotoxicity

Isoniazid interferes with the utilization of pyridoxine and increases its urinary excretion, causing pyridoxine deficiency, which manifests as peripheral neuritis and a variety of neurologic manifestations (paresthesias, numbness, mental disturbances), accounting for the most important dose dependent toxic effects of INH.

Management of **INH** toxicity: 0.5 g of IV pyridoxine (Vitamin B6) given over 5 to 10 mins is sufficient to counteract the neurotoxic effects of Isoniazid.

Isoniazid-induced peripheral neuritis is more common in slow acetylators. Hepatotoxic metabolite is produced by CYP2E1 from acetylhydrazine.

103. Which anti-TB drug cause ocular problem?

a. Rifampin
b. Ethambutol
c. Streptomycin
d. Pyrazinamide

Ans. is 'b' Ethambutol

104. Peripheral neuritis induced by isoniazid is prevented by giving which vitamin along with it?

a. Vitamin B1
b. Vitamin B6
c. Vitamin B3
d. Vitamin B12

Ans. is 'b' Vitamin B6

Diphtheria Contacts

- They should be throat swabbed and their immunity status determined.
- Where primary immunization or booster dose was received within the previous 2 years, no further action would be needed
- Where primary course or booster dose of diphtheria toxoid was received more than 2 years before, only a booster dose of diphtheria toxoid need be given
- Non-immunized close contact should receive prophylactic penicillin or erythromycin. They should be given 1000–2000 units of diphtheria antitoxin and actively immunized against diphtheria

105. A 3-year-old child diagnosed with Diphtheria. The child has a 6 years old sibling at home, who is fully immunized as per the Immunization schedule. What is the best measure to prevent disease in the sibling of the child? *(NEET 2020)*

a. Full course of DPT vaccine given
b. Booster dose of DPT
c. Nothing is required to be done
d. Prophylactic erythromycin to be given

Ans. is 'c' Nothing is required to be done

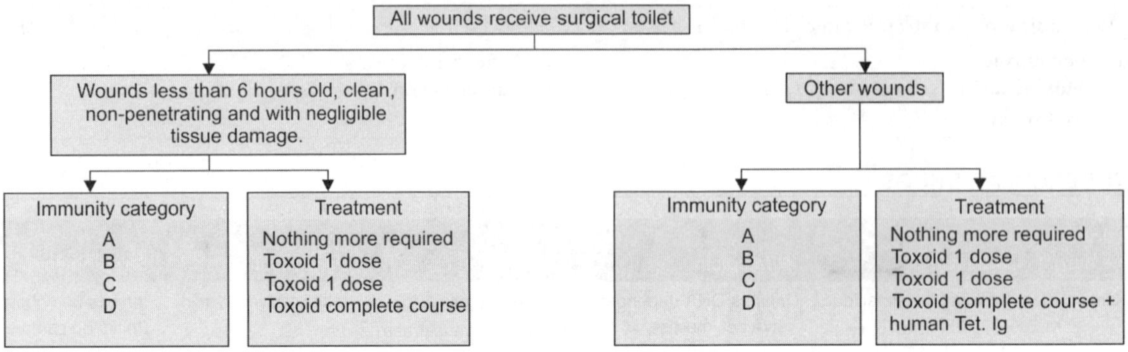

A = Has had a complete course of toxoid or a booster dose within the past 5 years.
B = Has had a complete course of toxoid or a booster dose more than 5 years ago and less than 10 years ago
C = Has had a complete course of toxoid or a booster dose more than 10 years ago
D = Has not had a complete course of toxoid or immunity status is unknown.

Fig. Recommendations of prevention of Tetanus in the wounded

106. A patient came with history of clean cut which was not lacerated. He was fully vaccinated 10 years ago. What to do next? *(NEET 2020)*

a. Give immunoglobulin
b. Give tetanus toxoid single dose
c. Repeat full course of vaccination
d. Tetanus toxoid + Immunoglobulin

Ans. is 'b' Give tetanus toxoid single dose

Vaccination in Disaster Management

- The WHO does not recommend typhoid and cholera vaccines in routine use in endemic areas. The newer typhoid and cholera vaccines have increased efficacy, but because they are multidose vaccines, compliance is likely to be poor. Supervision of sterilization and injection techniques may be impossible, resulting in more harm than good. However, these vaccinations are recommended for health workers. Supplying safe drinking water and proper disposal of excreta continue to be the most practical and effective strategy.
- Significant increase in tetanus incidence have not occurred after natural disasters. Mass vaccination of population against tetanus is usually unnecessary. The best protection is maintenance of a high level of immunity in the general population by routine vaccination before the disaster occurs, and adequate wound cleaning and treatment.
- Natural disasters may negatively affect the maintenance of on-going national or regional eradication programmes against polio and measles. Disruption of these programmes should be monitored closely.

107. Which of the following is true regarding mass vaccination after disaster? *(NEET 2020)*

a. Mass vaccination with cholera
b. Mass vaccination with tetanus
c. Mass vaccination with typhoid
d. Cholera and typhoid vaccination of health workers

Ans. is 'd' Cholera and typhoid vaccination of health workers

MATERNAL IMMUNIZATION

- **Tetanus, Diphtheria and Pertussis (Tdap)**: Health-care personnel should administer a dose of Tdap during each pregnancy irrespective of the patient's prior history of receiving Tdap. To maximize the maternal antibody response and passive antibody transfer to the infant, optimal timing for Tdap administration is between 27 and 36 weeks of gestation although Tdap may be given at any time during pregnancy.
- **Polio (IPV)**: Although no adverse effects of IPV have been documented among pregnant women or their fetuses, vaccination of pregnant women should be avoided on theoretical grounds. However, if a pregnant woman is at increased risk for infection and requires immediate protection against polio, IPV can be administered in accordance with the recommended schedules for adults.

Vaccines in Pregnancy

	General recommendation for use in pregnant women
Hapatitis A	Base decision on risk vs. benefit
Hapatitis B	Recommended in some circumstances
Human papillomavirus (HPV)	Not recommended
Influenza (Inactivated)	Recommended
Influenza (LAW)	Contraindicated

Contd...

Contd…

	General recommendation for use in pregnant women
MMR	Contraindicated
Meningococcal (ACWY)	May be used if otherwise indicated
Meningococcal (B)	Base decision on risk vs. benefit
PCV13	No recommendation
PPSV23	Inadequate data for specific recommendation
Polio	May be used if needed
Td	Should be used if otherwise indicated (Tdap preferred)
Tdap	Recommended
Varicella	Contraindicated
Zoster	Contraindicated

108. Maternal immunization does not provide protective immunity to neonate in: *(NEET 2020)*

a. Diphtheria
b. Pertussis
c. Tetanus
d. Polio

Ans. is 'd' Polio

ANTIMALARIAL DRUGS

Drug indication	Potential adverse effects	Comments
Artemether-lumefantrine *P. falciparum* from chloroquine-resistant or unknown areas	Adults; headache anorexia, dizziness, asthenia, arthralgia myalgia Children: fever, cough, vomiting, loss of appetite, headache	Take with food or whole milk. If patient vomits within 30 min, repeat dose. Contraindicated in pregnancy.
Atovaquone-proguanil *P. falciparum* from chloroquine-resistant areas *P. vivax*	Abdominal pain, nausea, vomiting, diarrhea, headache, rash, mild reversible elevations in liver aminotransferase levels	Not indicated for use in pregnant women due to limited data. Contraindicated if hypersensitivity to atovaquone or proguanil; severe renal impairment (creatinine clearance < 30 mL/min). Should be taken with food to increase absorption of atovaquone.
Chloroquine phosphate *P. falciparum* from chloroquine-sensitive areas *P. vivax* from chloroquine-sensitive areas All *P. ovale* All *P malariae* All *P. knowlesi*	Nausea, vomiting, rash, headache, dizziness, urticaria, abdominal pain, pruritus, retinal pigmentation	Safe in children and pregnant women. Give for chemoprophylaxis (500 mg salt orally every week) in pregnant women with chloroquine-sensitive *P. vivax*. Contraindicated if retinal or visual field change; hypersensitivity to 4-aminoquinolines. Use with caution in those with impaired liver function since the drug is concentrated in the liver.
Clindamycin *(oral or IV)* *P. falciparum* from chloroquine-resistant areas *P. vivax* from chloroquine-resistant areas	Diarrhea, nausea, rash	Always use in combination with quinine-quinidine. Safe in children and pregnant women.
Doxycycline (oral or IV) *P. falciparum* and *P. vivax* from chloroquine-resistant areas	Nausea, vomiting, diarrhea, abdominal pain, dizziness, photosensitivity, headache, esophagitis, odynophagia. Rarely hepatotoxicity, pancreatitis, and benign intracranial hypertension seen with tetracycline class of drugs.	Always use in combination with quinine or quinidine. Contraindicated in children < 8 y, pregnant women, and persons with known hypersensitivity to tetracyclines. Food, milk, and Ca^{2+} antacids decrease absorption and decrease GI disturbances. To prevent esophagitis, take tetracyclines with large amounts of fluids (patients should not lie down for 1 h after taking the drugs).
Hydroxychloroquine (oral) Secondary alternative for treatment of *P. falciparum* and *P. vivax* from chloroquine-sensitive areas All *P. ovale* All *P. malariae*	Nausea, vomiting, rash, headache, dizziness, urticaria, abdominal pain, pruritus	Safe in children and pregnant women. Contraindicated if retinal or visual field change; hypersensitivity to 4-aminoquinolines. Use with caution in those with impaired liver function.
Mefloquine *P. falciparum* from chloroquine-resistant areas, except Thailand-Burmese and Thailand-Cambodian border regions *P. vivax* from chloroquine-resistant areas	Nausea, vomiting, diarrhea, abdominal pain; dizziness, headache, somnolence, sleep disorders; myalgia, mild skin rash, and fatigue; moderate-to-severe neuropsychiatric reactions; ECG changes (sinus arrhythmia, sinus bradycardia, 1° AV block, QTc prolongation, and abnormal T waves.	Contraindicated if hypersensitive to the drug or to related compounds; cardiac conduction abnormalities; psychiatric disorders; and seizure disorders. Do not administer if patient has received related drugs (chloroquine, quinine, quinidine) less than 12 h ago

Contd…

Contd...

Drug indication	Potential adverse effects	Comments
Primaquine phosphate Radical cure of *P. vivax* and *P. ovale* (to eliminate hypnozoites) Gametocidal for all species	GI disturbances, methemoglobinemia (self-limited), hemolysis in persons with G6PD deficiency	Must screen for G6PD deficiency prior to use. Contraindicated in persons with G6PD deficiency; pregnant women. Should be taken with food to minimize GI adverse effects.
Quinine sulfate (oral) *P. falciparum* from chloroquine-resistant areas *P. vivax* from chloroquine-resistant areas	Local irritant (nausea, vomiting), Cinchonism, sinus arrhythmia, junctional rhythms, atrioventricular block, cardiodepressant, hypotension, prolonged QT interval, ventricular tachycardia, ventricular fibrillation (these are rare and more commonly seen with quinidine), hypoglycemia	Combine with tetracycline, doxycycline, or clindamycin, except for *P. Vivax* infections in children < 8 y or pregnant women. Contraindicated in hypersensitivity, including history of blackwater fever, thrombocytopenic purpura, or thrombocytopenia associated with quinine or quinidine use; many cardiac conduction defects and arrhythmias; myasthenia gravis; optic neuritis.

Antimalarial drugs		
Purpose	Acting on	Examples
Causal prophylaxis	Pre-erythrocytic schizogony	For falciparum: proguanil,tetracycline For all species: primaquine
Clinical cure	Erythrocytic schizogony	Fast acting → Artemisinin (fastest acting), chloroquine, amadioquine, quinine, mefloquine, halofantrine, lumefantrine, atovaquone Slow acting→pyrimethamine, proguanil, sulfonamides, tetraclines
Gametocidal	Gametocytes	For all species: primaquine, artimisinins For *P. vivax*: chloroquine, quinine
Radical care	Exoerythrocytic schizogony	Primaquine

109. Primaquine acts on which stage of life cycle of all human malarial parasites for causal prophylaxis?

a. Pre-erythrocyte
b. Erythrocyte
c. Exo-erythrocyte
d. Hypnozoite

Ans. is 'a' Pre-erythrocyte

110. Not true about quinine:

a. Causes hypotension
b. Acts as local irritant
c. Causes hyperglycemia
d. Decreases myocardial contractility

Ans. is 'c' Causes hyperglycemia

111. Which of the following causes retinal pigmentations?

a. Quinine
b. Chloroquine
c. Mefloquine
d. Atovaquone

Ans. is 'b' Chloroquine

112. A patient diagnosed with Rheumatoid arthritis was on medications. After 2 years, he developed blurring of vision and was found to have corneal opacity. Which drug is most likely to cause this? *(NEET 2020)*

a. Sulfasalazine
b. Chloroquine
c. Methotrexate
d. Leflunomide

Ans. is 'b' Chloroquine

Explanation: Prolonged use of high doses of chloroquine (as needed for rheumatoid arthritis, DLE, etc.) may cause loss of vision due to retinal damage. Corneal deposits may also occur and affect vision, but are reversible on discontinuation.

ANTI-INFLUENZA DRUGS

Amantadine and Rimantadine

- Prevent uncoating of influenza A virus (not Influenza B)
- They prevent release of viral nucleic acid into the host cell by interfering with transmembrane domain of viral M2 protein
- Decrease the duration of symptoms of influenza if used prophylactically.
- Rimantadine is longer acting than amantadine.
- Most common adverse effects – GI complaints, minor CNS effects.

Oseltamivir and Zanamivir

- Neuraminidase inhibitors—prevent the virion release.
- Effective against both Influenza A and Influenza B.
- Oseltamivir is an oral prodrug; Zanamivir is administered by inhalational route.

- ❖ Neuropsychiatric disorders are associated with these drugs.
- ❖ Oseltamivir is the drug of choice for bird flu.
- ❖ Peramivir is a newer drug in this category that can be administered intravenously.
- ❖ Laninamivir is a long-acting inhaled neuraminidase inhibitor effective against oseltamivir-resistant virus.

113. Mechanism of action of Oseltamivir: *(NEET 2019)*

a. Protein synthesis inhibitor
b. Thymidylate synthesis inhibitor
c. Neuraminidase inhibitor
d. Pyrimidine analog

Ans. is 'c' Neuraminidase inhibitor

ANTIFUNGALS

Classification

Antibiotics Polyenes: Amphotericin B (AMB), Nystatin, Hamycin, Natamycin (Pimaricin)

Heterocyclic benzofuran: Griseofulvin

Antimetabolite: Flucytosine (5-FC)

Imidazoles: Topical—Clotrimazole, Econazole, Miconazol Oxiconazole. Systemic—Ketoconazole

Triazoles (systemic): Fluconazole, Itraconazole, Voriconazole

Allylamine: Terbinafine

Echinocandins: Anidulafungin, Caspofungin, Micafungin

Other topical agents: Tolnaftate, Undecylenic acid, Benzoic acid, Quiniodochlor, Ciclopirox olamine, Butenafine, Sodium Thiosulfate.

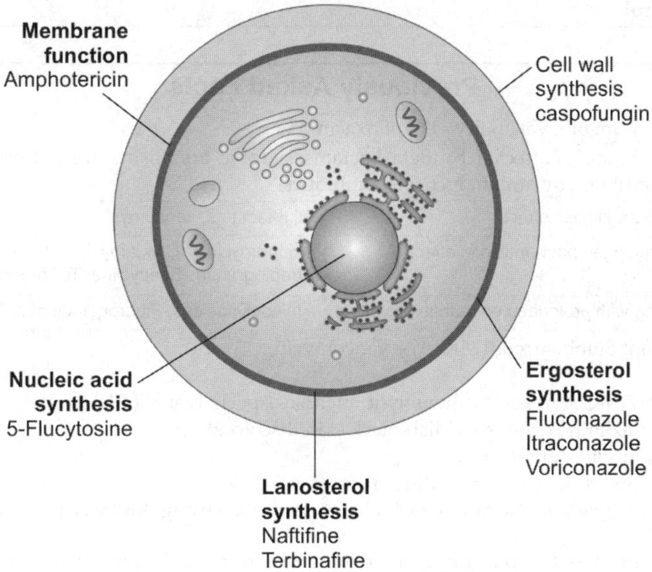

Amphotericin-B: DOC for all serious, life threatening fungal infections (including mucormycosis), except invasive aspergillosis: Voriconazole. Nephrotoxicity is the most important side effect of Amphotericin B which occurs uniformly and dose related and often manifests as azotemia, reduced GFR, acidosis, hypokalemia.

Coccidioidal meningitis: Fluconazole.

Itraconazole: DOC for all non-serious infections including Blastomycosis, Histoplasmosis, Sporotrichosis, Tinea, etc. except Tinea unguium/capitis: Terbinafine.

Fluconazole: DOC for all Candida infections, coccidioidomycosis and localized cryptococcosis.

DOC for cryptococcal meningitis: Amphotericin B + 5-Flucytosine

Caspofungin has been approved for Invasive aspergillosis (in patients who are failing on Amphotericih-B or voriconazole) and Esophageal candidiasis.

Febrile neutropenia prophylaxis: Fluconazole; First drug: Caspofungin; DOC: Voriconazole.

- ❖ Topical antifungal of choice for aspergillus infection of eye is Clotrimazole
- ❖ Fluconazole and itraconazole have largely replaced ketoconazole as therapy for systemic mycosis because of greater efficacy, Longer t1/2, fewer side effects and drug interactions.

Pharmacology

114. Which of the following drugs is used as nail lacquer for fungal infections? *(NEET 2020)*

a. Fluconazole
b. Nystatin
c. Itraconazole
d. Terbinafine

Ans. is 'd' Terbinafine

Explanation: Terbinafine is DOC for dermatophytosis (tinea infections). Nystatin is used topically for local candida infection and orally for gastrointestinal infection.

115. Drug of choice for invasive pulmonary aspergillosis is: *(NEET 2020)*

a. Amphotericin B
b. Voriconazole
c. Caspofungin
d. Posaconazole

Ans. is 'b' Voriconazole

Explanation: Voriconazole is the drug of choice for invasive aspergillosis. Posaconazole is the only azole active against mucormycosis. Caspofungin is approved for invasive aspergillosis not responding to amphotericin-B or voriconazole.

116. Most important side effect of Amphotericin B is:

a. Fever and chills
b. Nephrotoxicity
c. Hyperkalemia
d. Anemia

Ans. is 'b' Nephrotoxicity

117. Which statement best describes mechanism of action of azoles? *(NEET 2019)*

a. Synthesis of ergosterol
b. Thymidylate synthase
c. Targeting Beta 1,3-glucan
d. Disruption of cell wall

Ans. is 'a' Synthesis of ergosterol

Previously Asked Facts

- Fluoroquinolone with maximum bioavailability– Levofloxacin
- Mycoplasma and Chlamydia are unaffected by Beta Lactams; aerobic organisms are not affected by metronidazole; while anaerobic bacteria are not inhibited by aminoglycoside antibiotics.

Time dependent killing, No post-antibiotic effect	All β-lactams, vancomycin
Time dependent killing with prolonged post-antibiotic effect	Azithromycin, Clindamycin, Linezolid, Macrolides, Tetracyclines, Streptogramin, Tigecycline, Telithromycin
Concentration dependent killing with prolonged post-antibiotic effect	Aminoglycosides, Fluoroquinolones, Daptomycin, Metronidazole.

- DOC for Methicillin-Resistant Staph aureus (MRSA) – Vancomycin
- Antileprotic drugs
  - *Sulfones*: Dapsone (DDS) (MC side effect is hemolytic anemia; especially in G6PD)
  - *Phenazine derivative*: Clofazimine (causes reddish-black skin discoloration)
  - *Antitubercular drugs*: Rifampin, Ethionamide
  - *Other antibiotics*: Ofloxacin, Minocycline, Clarithromycin (Macrolide)
- Ivermectin: It is the DOC for single dose treatment of onchocerciasis and strongyloidosis. It is the only oral drug effective against scabies and pediculosis.
- Niclosamide acts by inhibiting oxidative phosphorylation in mitochondria and by interfering with anaerobic generation of ATP. It is mainly active against cestodes—T. solium, T. saginata, Diphyllobothrium latum and H. nana.
- Levamisole is an anti-helminthic agent that is also an immunomodulator.
- Strains of M. tuberculosis resistant to individual drugs arise by spontaneous point mutations in the mycobacterial genome that occur at low but predictable rates.
- All first line drugs are tuberculocidal except ethambutol which is tuberculostatic.
- 1st line anti-tuberculosis drug contraindicated in pregnancy is Streptomycin.
- Most hepatotoxic ATT drug is Pyrazinamide.
- Drug of choice for treatment of B. fragilis infection is Cefoxitin.
- Drug of choice for anaerobic infections is Metronidazole.
- Linezolid acts by inhibiting bacterial protein synthesis by binding to 23s fraction of 50s ribosome.
- Most nephrotoxic cephalosporin is Cephaloridine
- Important drugs with liposomal delivery systems:
  - Anticancer drugs → Doxorubicin, Daunorubicin, vincristine, camptothecin, methotrexate, cisplatin, mitoxantrone
  - Antifungals → Amphotericin B, Nystatin
  - Antibiotics → Amikacin, Ampicillin, ciprofloxacin, Ribavirin, Ganciclovir, chloroquine
  - Others → IL-2, cyclosporine
- Drug of choice for treatment of uncomplicated Chlamydia trachomatis genital infection is Azithromycin.
- Drug of choice for for Neisseria gonorrhoea infection is Ceftriaxone.

ANTI-NEOPLASTIC DRUGS

CLASSIFICATION

1. Cell cycle nonspecific

- These kill cells whether resting or actively cycling. Examples are:
  - Alkylating agents
  - Mitomycin
  - Camptothecins
  - Anthracyclines (doxorubicin)
  - Platinum compounds
  - Dactinomycin

2. Cell cycle specific

- They kill actively cycling cell and their site of action is confined to one phase of the cell cycle
- Drugs causing cell cycle specific inhibition are given below:
  - G1 phase - Vinblastine
  - S phase - MTX, cytarabine, 6-MP, Hydroxyurea, mitomycin
  - G2 phase - Bleomycin, etoposide, daunorubicin, topotecan
  - M phase - Vincristine, vinblastine, paclitaxel, docetaxel, ixabepilone, estramustine

Purine Antagonists

- 6-mercaptopurine (6-MP), 6-thioguanine, fludarabine and cladribine are purine analogues that are used in cancer chemotherapy.
- Azathioprine is also a purine analogue, but it is used primarily as an immunosuppressant.
- These drugs are activated by hypoxanthine guanine phosphoribosyl transferase (HGPRTase), and the resulting nucleotides inhibit enzymes in purine biosynthesis and metabolism.
- 6-MP & azathioprine are metabolized by xanthine oxidase, dose has to be reduced when allopurinol (a xanthine oxidase inhibitor) is given concurrently.
- Cladribine is the DOC for Hairy cell leukemia as it is resistant to degradation by adenosine deaminase.
- Fludarabine is the DOC for CLL.
- Use of pentostatin with fludarabine may result in severe pulmonary fibrosis.

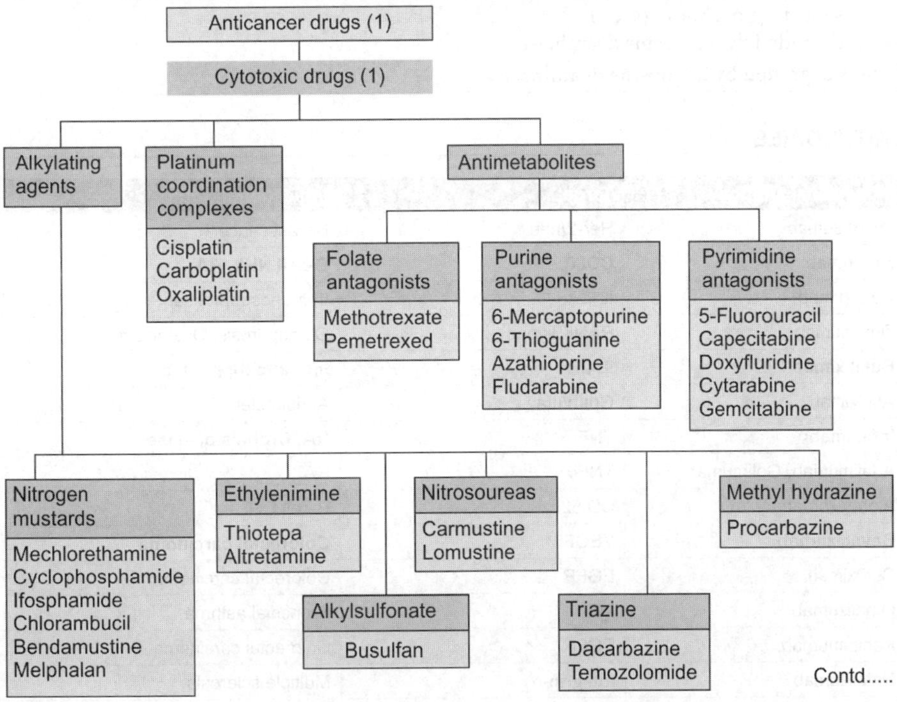

Contd.....

Contd...

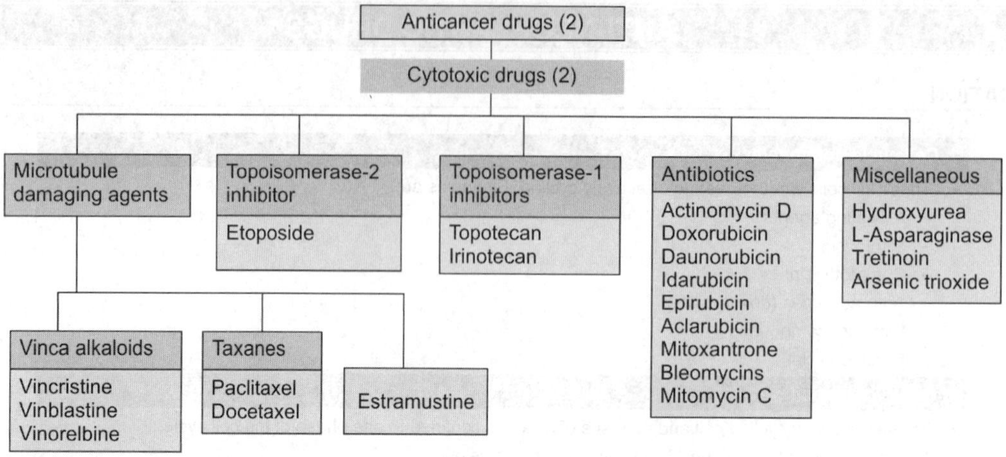

118. Which of the following is an inhibitor of DNA replication? *(NEET 2020)*

a. Actinomycin D
b. Asparaginase
c. Mitomycin
d. 6-mercaptopurine

Ans. is 'd' 6-mercaptopurine

Explanation: 6-Mercaptopurine is purine antimetabolite therefore it prevents DNA replication. Mitomycin is an antitumor antibiotic that inhibits DNA synthesis by producing DNA cross-links which halt cell replication and eventually cause cell death. Actinomycin D acts by inhibiting DNA dependent RNA synthesis. Asparaginase is an enzyme that catalyzes the hydrolysis of L-asparagine to L-aspartic acid and ammonia. They inhibit protein synthesis in tumor cells by depriving them of the amino acid asparagine.

119. Drug acting on 'S' phase of cycle:

a. Chlorambucil
b. Methotrexate
c. Vincristine
d. Paclitaxel

Ans. is 'b' Methotrexate

120. Which of the following is not true about purine antagonists?

a. Azathioprine is used as immunosuppressant
b. Drugs are activated by hypoxanthine guanine phosphoribosyl transferase (HGPRTase)
c. Fludarabine is the drug of choice for CLL
d. Cladribine is degraded by adenosine deaminase

Ans. is 'd' Cladribine is degraded by adenosine deaminase

MONOCLONAL ANTIBODIES

Monoclonal antibody	Target	Indication
Trastuzumab	Her-2/neu	Breast cancer
Rituximab	**CD20**	**B-cell NHL, RA**
Daclizumab	IL-2R	Immunosuppressant
Denosumab	RANK ligand	Osteoporosis, Osteoclastoma
Basiliximab	**IL-2R**	**Immunosuppressant**
Abciximab	GpIIb/IIIa	Antiplatelet
Infliximab	**TNFα**	**RA, Crohn's disease**
Adalimumab, Golimumab	TNFα	RA
Alemtuzumab	CD 52	B-cell CLL
Bevacizumab	**VEGF**	**Colorectal carcinoma**
Cetuximab	EGFR	Colorectal carcinoma
Omalizumab	IgE	Bronchial asthma
Panitumumab	EGFR	Colorectal carcinoma
Natalizumab	Integrin-α_4	Multiple sclerosis

Contd...

Contd...

Monoclonal antibody	Target	Indication
Denosumab	RANK ligand	Osteoporosis
Tocilizumab	**IL-6R**	**SLE**
Ranibizumab	VEGF	Neovascular macular degeneration
Eculizumab	C5 complement	Paroxysmal Nocturnal Hemoglobinuria
Muromonab (OKT3)	**CD3**	**Post-transplant**

121. Basiliximab acts on: *(NEET 2018)*

a. IL-2R
b. IL-6R
c. CD-20
d. VEGF

Ans. is 'b' IL-6R

122. Cetuximab is used to treat:

a. Adamantinoma
b. Basal cell Ca
c. Colorectal Ca
d. Crohn's disease

Ans. is 'c' Colorectal Ca

Previously Asked Facts

• Folinic acid	For preventing methotrexate toxicity
• Allopurinol	To prevent hyperuricemia caused by rapid destruction of cells during cancer chemotherapy
• Lithium carbonate	It has stimulant effect on bone marrow, so used during myelosuppressive drug therapy
• Ondansetron	For controlling cytotoxic drug induced vomiting
• Mesna	For prevention of cyclophosphamide/formamide induced hemorrhagic cystitis

❖ Bendamustine is an alkylating agent used in the treatment of chronic lymphocytic leukemia (CLL), multiple myeloma, and non-Hodgkin's lymphoma.

❖ Amifostine is mainly used for prophylaxis of cisplatin induced neuro/nephrotoxicity and radiotherapy related stomatitis.

❖ Anti-mitotic drugs of natural origin – Vincristine, Vindesine, Paclitaxel, Vinblastine, Vinorelbine, Docetaxel.

❖ Toxicity of Cyclophosphamide - Bone marrow suppression (relative platelet sparing), Pulmonary toxicity, Cardiac toxicity (at higher doses), Hemorrhagic cystitis, Infertility.

❖ Imatinib is a tyrosine kinase inhibitor, which inhibits PDGF (Platelet derived growth factor) receptor as well. Uses: Š CML, DOC for c-kit +ve GIST (Gastrointestinal Stromal Tumor). Adverse effects include - Abdominal pain, vomiting, fluid retention, pleural effusion, periorbital edema, myalgia, liver damage and CHF.

❖ Tacrolimus and cyclosporine are both calcineurin inhibitors which are nephrotoxic. Cyclosporine is the most effective drug for the prevention and treatment of graft rejection reaction. It depresses renal function and should be carefully used along with nephrotoxic drugs.

❖ Pemetrexed is a newer congener of methotrexate which primarily targets the enzyme thymidylate synthase. In combination with cisplatin, pemetrexed is approved for treatment of mesothelioma and non-small cell lung carcinoma.

CHAPTER 6 Microbiology

GENERAL MICROBIOLOGY

- **Louis Pasteur** is known as the Father of Modern Microbiology.

Scientist	Contributions
Louis Pasteur	Father of medical microbiology, developed pasteurization, rabies vaccine, Germ theory of disease
Robert Koch	Discovered *M. tuberculosis* and *V. cholerae*, suggested Koch's postulates
Joseph Lister	Father of Aseptic surgery, proved that sepsis could be prevented by hand hygiene
Antonie Van Leeuwenhoek	Invented microscope (Father of compound microscope), Father of Bacteriology
Edward Jenner	Father of Immunology
Peyton Rous	Isolated virus causing sarcoma (role of viruses in transmission of certain cancer)

CAPSULE

- Many bacteria secrete a viscid material around the cell surface. When this is organized into a sharply defined structure, it is known as capsule.
- Capsules are protective walls that surround the cell membranes of gram-positive and gram-negative bacteria.
- They are usually composed of simple sugar (**polysaccharide**) except in *Bacillus anthracis,* it is made up of **polypeptide** (protein).
- Capsules are protective and protect the bacteria from phagocytosis and from lytic enzymes.
- Important **capsulated** organisms are:
    - *Pneumococcus*
    - *Bacillus anthracis*
    - *Bordetella*
    - *Meningococcus*
    - *Klebsiella*
    - *H. influenzae*
    - *Cl. perfringens, Cl. butyricum*
    - *Yersinia*
    - *V. parahaemolyticus*
    - *Bacteroides*
    - **Fresh strains** of *Staphylococcus, Streptococcus, E. coli.*
    - *Cryptococcus* (a **fungus**).

1. Polysaccharide capsule is seen in which bacteria?

a. *Bacillus anthracis*
b. *Cryptococcus*
c. *Pneumococcus*
d. *Proteus*

Ans. is 'c' *Pneumococcus*

SPORE GERMINATION

- Heating for 20 minutes at 80°C destroys vegetative cells and activates the spores for germination.
- Microorganisms can be grouped into broad categories, according to their temperature ranges for growth.
- Psychrophiles (cold-loving) can grow at 0°C, and some even as low as –10°C; their upper limit is often about 10°C.
- Mesophiles grow in the moderate temperature range, from about 20°C (or lower) to 45°C.
- Thermophiles are heat-loving, with an optimum growth temperature of 50°C or more, a maximum of up to 70°C or more, and a minimum of about 200°C.
- Hyperthermophiles have an optimum above 75°C and thus can grow at the highest temperatuers tolerated by any organism. An extreme example is the genus Pyrodictium, found on geothermally heated areas of the sea bed. It has optimal growth temperature range of 82°C to 105°C.

> **2. Nutrient agar heated at 80°C used for:**
> a. Spore germination
> b. To grow mesophilic bacteria
> c. To grow thermophilic bacteria
> d. For *Clostridium* isolation
>
> **Ans. is 'a' Spore germination**

ACID FAST STAINING

- *Ziehl-Neelsen stain (Hot method):* In first step, smear is poured with hot carbol fuchsin (aniline dye) for 5 minutes.
- After staining with aniline dye, acid fast organisms resist decolorization with acids (20% H_2SO_4) or acid-alcohol (3%).
- In this, 'concentrated' carbol fuchsin is used as primary stain and 20% sulphuric acid is used as decolorizing agent. Methylene blue is used for counter staining:

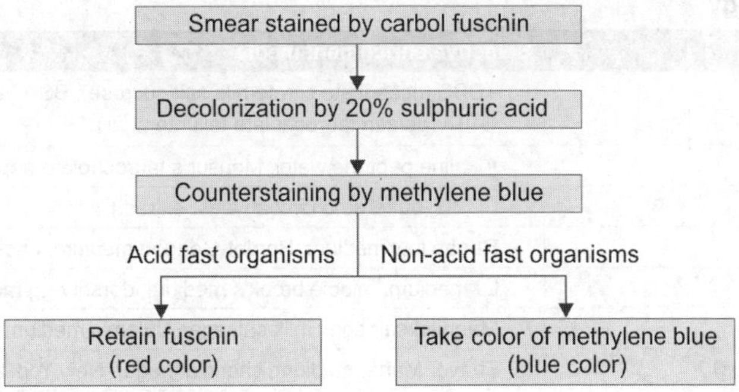

- Partially acid-fast means, organism which shows less affinity for primary stain, thus less concentrated H_2SO_4 (instead of 20% H_2SO_4) is used for decolorization of primary stain (Carbol fuchsin).

Modified Ziehl-Neelsen Stain

- There are some modifications in any of the reagent. These may be:
  - *Use of alcohol as secondary decolorizer*: After primary decolorization, 95% alcohol is used to further decolorize the smear. *M. tuberculosis* resist decolorization with both (i.e. acid fast as well as alcohol fast), while saprophytic mycobacteria are decolorized by alcohol (i.e. they are only acid fast).
  - *Use of acid-alcohol as decolorizer*: Instead of 20% sulfuric acid, 3% HCl in 95% alcohol is used as decolorizer. This also differentiates tubercle bacilli from saprophytic mycobacteria.
  - *Kinyoun's modifications of ZN staining (Cold method)*: In this modification, concentration of primary stain has been increased, so hot Carbol fuchsin is not required, cold carbol fuchsin is used here. Concentration of decolorizer has also been decreased.
- ***Modification** in percentage of sulfuric acid* for different organisms:
  - 5% H_2SO_4 (instead of 20%) – *Mycobacterium leprae*
  - 1% H_2SO_4 – *Nocardia, Actinomycetes*
  - 0.5–1% H_2SO_4 –Oocysts of *Cryptosporidium, Cyclospora* and *Cystoisospora;* Microsporidia, eggs of *Schistosoma mansoni,* eggs of *Taenia saginata,* hooklets of hydatid cysts, Sperm head, *Legionella micdadei*
  - 0.25–0.5% H_2SO_4 –Bacterial spores.

> **3. Partially acid fast organism is:**
> a. *M. tuberculosis*
> b. *M. bovis*
> c. *Nocardia*
> d. None
>
> **Ans. is 'c' *Nocardia***

CULTURE MEDIA

Type of medium	Name of medium	Laboratory use
Liquid media		
• Basal (simple)	• Peptone water • Nutrient broth	• Routine culture, basal medium for sugar fermentation test • Routine culture
• Special (complex) – Enriched – Enrichment	• Glucose broth • Robertson's cooked meat medium • Tetrathionate broth medium • Selenite F broth • Thioglycolate broth • Alkaline peptone water	• Blood culture • Culture of anaerobic bacteria • Enrichment culture for *Salmonella* • Enrichment culture for *Salmonella* and *Shigella* • Culture of anaerobic bacteria • Enrichment culture for *Vibrio*

Contd...

Contd...

Type of medium	Name of medium	Laboratory use
Solid media • Simple • Special – Enriched	Nutrient agar (2–3% agar) • Blood agar (also indicator media) • Chocolate agar • Loeffler's serum • Dorsett's egg	Routine culture • General culture, *Streptococcus;* Most widely used medium • Culture of *H. influenzae, N. gonorrhoeae* • Culture of *C. diphtheriae* • Culture of *Mycobacterium*
Selective (contains inhibitory substance)	• MacConkey agar (also indicator and differential medium • Deoxycholate citrate agar (DCA) • Lowenstein Jensen (LJ)	• Enterobacteriaceae (Lactose fermenter produce pink colonies) • Selective medium for *Salmonella* and *Shigella* • Culture of *M. tuberculosis*

Important Media in Microbiology

Organism	Selective/enrichment media
Plating media for *V. cholerae*	• TCBS (thiosulfate citrate bile salt sucrose), BSA (alkaline bile salt agar) • GTTA (gelatin taurocholate tellurite agar)
Enrichment media for *V. cholerae*	• Alkaline peptone water, Monsur's taurocholate peptone water
Legionella	• BCYE (buffered charcoal yeast extract)
Bordetella	• Regan low medium, Bordet-Gengou medium, Lacey's DFP medium
M. tuberculosis	• LJ medium, middle brook's medium, dorset egg medium
S. aureus	• Mannitol salt agar, milk salt agar, Udlam's medium
Neisseria (gonococcus/meningococcus)	• Thayer Martin medium, chocolate agar, New York agar
Corynebacterium diphtheriae	• Loeffler's serum slope, potassium tellurite agar
Bacillus cereus	• MYPA (mannitol egg yolk phenol red polymyxin agar)
Bacillus anthracis	• PLET (polymyxin lithium EDTA thallous acetate)
Leptospira	• EMJH medium, Fletcher medium, Korthof medium, Stuart's medium
Campylobacter	• Skirrow's medium, campy BAP medium, Butzler's medium
Reiter's treponema	• Smith-Noguchi medium
Salmonella	• Tetrathionate broth, selenite F broth
Pseudomonas	• Cetrimide agar
Anaerobes	• Robertson cooked meat broth, thioglycollate, Smith-Noguchi
Lactose fementing enteric pathogens (*E. coli* and others)	• MacConkey agar, Eosine-methylene blue (EMB), Deoxycholate agar
Haemophilus	• Blood agar with *Staph.* streak (Satellitism), Levinthal's medium, Fildes agar, chocolate agar
Listeria	• PALCAM agar
Burkholderia	• Ashdown's medium
Salmonella, Shigella	• Deoxycholate medium, Hektoen enteric agar (salmonella-shigella agar)
Streptococcus agalactiae	• Todd-Hewitt broth antibiotics
Mycoplasma pneumoniae	• PPLO medium
For culturing urine sample	• CLED (cysteine lactose electrolyte deficient) medium
Clostridium difficile	• CCFA (cefoxitin cycloserine fructose agar) • CCEY (cefoxitin cycloserine egg-yolk agar)
Yersinia	• CIN (cefsulodin-Irgasan-Novobiocin) medium, Ghee broth
Enterococcus	• Bile esculin agar
Actinomyces	• Thioglycollate medium, brain heart infusion agar

Organism	Transport media
Streptococcus pyogenes	Pike's medium
Neisseria	Stuart's medium, amies medium
For stool specimen	Buffered glycerol saline, Cary-Blair, Stuart medium
Salmonella, shigella	Sach's buffered glycerol saline
V. cholerae	VR medium, Cary-Blair medium, autoclaved sea water
Bordetella	Modified Stuart's medium, Mischulow's charcoal agar

Contd...

Organism	Transport media
E. histolytica	• Boeck and Drbohlav's medium • Philip's medium • Shaffer and Frye's medium • Jones medium • Balamuth's medium • Diamond's medium
Lepra bacillus	• Armadillo (**Nine banded armadillo**) is highly susceptible and provides sufficient bacilli for a number of studies and for production of skin test reagent, Lepromin A • **Foot pad of mice** has been used for testing of sensitivity of anti-leprotic drug (replication in foot pad of mice is limited and less numerous than armadillo)

Important Media used for V. cholerae

V. cholerae		
Transport or holding media	*Enrichment media*	*Plating (selective) media*
• Venkatraman-Ramakrishnan (VR) medium • Cary-Blair medium • Autoclaved sea water	• Alkaline peptone water • Monsur's taurocholate peptone water	• Alkaline bile salt agar (BSA) • Monsur's gelatin taurocholate trypticase tellurite agar (GTTA) • TCBS medium (thiuosulfate, citrate, bile salts, sucrose)

New York City (NYC) Medium

- New York City (NYC) medium is primarily designed for isolation of pathogenic *Neisseria*.
- It is superior to other media generally employed for isolation of *Neisseria* species.
- It also supports the growth of genital mycoplasma (*Mycoplasma hominis* and *Ureaplasma urealyticum*).
- It consists of primarily a peptone-corn starch agar-base buffered with phosphates and supplemented with horse plasma, horse hemoglobin, dextrose, yeast autolysate and antibiotics.

4. Loeffler's serum is an example of:

a. Enriched medium
b. Selective medium
c. Enrichment medium
d. Simple medium

Ans. is 'a' Enriched medium

5. TCBS Agar is used for isolation of:

a. *Leptospira*
b. *V. cholerae*
c. *Salmonella*
d. *Pseudomonas*

Ans. is 'b' *V. cholerae*

6. Culture media used for isolation of *Bordetella pertussis*:

a. L-J medium
b. Chocolate media
c. Wilson Blair medium
d. Bordet-Gengou medium

Ans. is 'd' Bordet-Gengou medium

7. Selective media for *Salmonella* and *Shigella*:

a. MacConkey agar
b. Mannitol salt agar
c. BCYE medium
d. XLD agar

Ans. is 'd' XLD agar

8. Modified Thayer-Martin medium is used for:

a. Gonococcus
b. *Legionella*
c. *Helicobacter*
d. *Campylobacter*

Ans. is 'a' Gonococcus

9. Culture medium used for *Entamoeba histolytica:*

a. Blood agar
b. Philip's medium
c. CLED mediu
d. Trypticase serum

Ans. is 'b' Philip's medium

10. Culture of Lepra bacillus is done on:

a. L J medium
b. Robertson's cooked meat medium
c. Foot pad of mice
d. Sabouraud's agar

Ans. is 'c' Foot pad of mice

11. Transport medium for cholera:

a. LJ medium
b. Cary-Blair medium
c. MYPA medium
d. Stewart medium

Ans. is 'b' Cary-Blair medium

12. New York agar is used for:

a. *Salmonella*
b. *Clostridia*
c. *Neisseria*
d. *Bacillus anthracis*

Ans. is 'c' *Neisseria*

Buffered Charcoal Yeast Extract (BCYE) Medium

- It is selective media for *Legionella pneumophila.*
- *Legionella* is nutritionally fastidious, non-spore forming, aerobic, pleomorphic Gram-negative short bacilli.
- There are two types of pulmonary infections caused by *Legionella*:
  - *Pontiac fever*: It is self-limiting flu-like illness with incubation period of 24–48 hours. There is no pneumonia.
  - *Legionnaire's disease*: It is an atypical pneumonia with incubation period of 2–10 days. It is characterized by cough, chest pain, hemoptysis, high grade fever, diarrhea, confusion, 'relative' bradycardia and hyponatremia. If onset of symptoms occur within 10 days of discharge from the hospital, nosocomial legionnaire's disease should be suspected. Case fatality rate is 15–20%.
- Media containing cysteine, yeast extract, α-ketoglutarate, and iron (BCYE) are required for isolation of *Legionella.*
- Selective BCYE (medium containing antibiotics), is recommended for specimens likely to be contaminated with other bacteria.
- *McConkey agar*: It is an indicator, a selective and differential culture medium for bacteria designed to selectively isolate Gram-negative and enteric (normally found in the intestinal tract) bacilli and differentiate them based on lactose fermentation.
- *Baird- Parker agar*: It is a selective medium for the detection and enumeration of coagulase-positive staphylococci from food samples
- *Sabouraud's agar*: It is a selective medium primarily used for the isolation of fungi.

13. What type of culture medium is used for Legionella? *(NEET 2019)*

a. BCYE agar medium
b. McConkey agar
c. Baird- Parker agar
d. Sabouraud's agar

Ans. is 'a' BCYE agar medium

14. True about Pontiac fever:

a. Typical pneumonia
b. Atypical pneumonia
c. Flu-like illness
d. Relative bradycardia

Ans. is 'c' Flu-like illness

ANAEROBIOSIS

- Obligate aerobes *Micrococcus* and *Pseudomonas* are used to create anaerobic condition (anaerobiosis).
- The micrococcus and the anaerobic organism to be cultivated are both inoculated into the same liquid medium.
- During incubation the Micrococcus gradually utilizes the free oxygen creating conditions favorable for the growth of anaerobes.
- After anaerobiosis is achieved, the micrococcus dies (due to lack of oxygen) leaving the anaerobe in pure culture.

15. To create anaerobiosis which organism is used?

a. *Micrococcus*
b. *Clostridium*
c. *B. anthracis*
d. *Corynebacterium*

Ans. is 'a' *Micrococcus*

IMPORTANT BODIES IN MICROBIOLOGY

Name of body	*Disease/infection*
Bollinger bodies	Fowl pox
Brassy body	Dark shrunken blood corpuscle found in malaria
Chromatid bodies	Entamoeba histolytica precyst
Citron bodies	Cl. septicum
Cigar bodies	Sporotrichosis
Councilman bodies	Yellow fever/viral hepatitis
Coccoid X bodies	Psittacosis
Donovan bodies	Granuloma inguinale (LGV)
Guarneri bodies	Inclusion bodies of Vaccínia

Contd...

Contd...

Name of body	*Disease/infection*
• Henderson Patterson bodies	• Molluscum contagiosum
• Levinthal Coles like bodies	• Psittacosis
• Mooser bodies	• Endemic typhus
• Negri bodies	• Rabies
• Paschen bodies	• Vaccinia/Variola
• Ross's bodies	• Syphilis
• Sclerotic bodies	• Chromoblastomycosis
• Asteroid bodies	• Sporotrichosis
• Halber Staedter Prowazek body	• Chlamydia trachomatis
• Cowdry type A	• Herpes, chickenpox, CMV, yellow fever
• Cowdry type B	• Poliovirus, Adenovirus

16. Citron bodies are seen in:

a. Psittacosis
b. Molluscum contagiosum
c. *Clostridium septicum*
d. *Clostridium perfringens*

Ans. is 'c' *Clostridium septicum*

IMPORTANT TYPES OF MOTILITY

Types of motility	
Motility	***Organisms***
Darting	• *V. cholerae* • *Campylobacter* • *Gardnerella vaginalis*
Stately	*Clostridia*
Tumbling	*Listeria*
Lashing	*Borrelia*
Corkscrew motility	*T. pallidum*
Gliding	*Mycoplasma*
Swarming	*Proteus mirabilis and vulgaris, B. cereus, Cl. tetani*

17. A child is presenting with watery stools, Gram staining is showing comma shaped bacilli. The isolated organism will show which type of motility:

a. Tumbling
b. Darting
c. Gliding
d. Stately

Ans. is 'b' Darting

UREASE POSITIVE BACTERIA

- *Proteus*
- *Staph. aureus*
- *Morganella*
- *Klebsiella*
- *Nocardia*
- *H. pylori*
- *Y. pseudotuberculosis*
- *Y. enterocolitica*
- *Cryptococcus* (fungus)
- Diphtheroids
- Mycobacteria except MAC.

18. Urease positive organism:

a. *Proteus*
b. *Streptococcus*
c. *Vibrio cholerae*
d. *Pseudomonas*

Ans. is 'a' *Proteus*

Bacterial structures		
Structure	***Chemical composition***	***Function***
Appendages		
Flagellum	Proteins	Motility
Pilus/fimbria	Glycoprotein	Mediate adherence of bacteria to cell surface; sex pilus forms during conjugation
Specializedstructures		
Spore	Keratin-like coat; dipicolinic acid; peptidoglycan, DNA	Garm ⊕ only Survival: Resist dehydration, heat, chemicals.
Cell envelope		
Capsule	Organized, discrete polysaccharide layer (except poly-D-glutamate on B *anthracis*)	Protests against phagocytosis
Slime (S) layer	Loose network of polysaccharides	Mediates adherence to surfaces, especially foreign surfaces (e.g. indwelling catheters)
Outer membrane	Outer leaflet: contains endotoxin (LPS/LOS) Embedded proteins: Porins and other outer membrane proteins (OMPs) Inner leaflet: phospholipids	Gram ⊖ only Endotoxin: Lipid A induces TNF and IL-I; antigenic O polysaccharide component Most OMPs are antigenic Proins: Transport across outer membrane
Periplasm	Space between cytoplasmic membrane and outer membrane in gram ⊖ bacteria (Peptidoglycan in middle)	Accumulates components exiting gram ⊖ cells, including hydrolytic enzymes (e.g., β-lactamases)
Cell wall	Peptidoglycan is a sugar backbone with peptide side chains cross-linked by transpeptidase	Net-like structure gives rigid support, protects; against osmotic pressure damage
Cytoplasmic membrane	Phospholipid bilayer sac with embedded proteins (e.g. penicillin-binding proteins [PBPs]) and other enzymes Lipoteichoic acids (gram positive) only extend from membrane to exterior	Site of oxidative and transport enzymes; PBP; involved in cell wall synthesis Lipoteichoice acids induce TNF-α and IL-1

19. Which bacterial structure is responsible for adherence? *(NEET 2020)*

a. Mesosomes
b. Cytoplasmic membrane
c. Fimbriae
d. Flagella

Ans. is 'c' Fimbriae

BACTERIAL GENETICS AND ANTIMICROBIAL RESISTANCE

GENE TRANSFER IN BACTERIA

- Transformation: Transfer of genetic material through the agency of free DNA.
- Transduction: Transfer of a portion of DNA by bacteriophage (a virus).
- Conjugation: Transfer of genetic material by physical contact.
- Lysogenic conversion: Incorporation of phage DNA into host DNA.

Transformation

- Ability to take up naked DNA (i.e. from cell lysis) from environment.
- *E.g.: S. pneumoniae, Hib, Neisseria.*

Transduction

Example: Shiga **A** toxin, **B**otulinum toxin, **C**holera toxin, **D**iphtheria toxin, **E**rythrogenic toxin (*Strep. pyogenes*)

Conjugation

- F+ plasmid contains genes required for sex pilus and conjugation. Bacteria without plasmid is F–
- Sex pilus on F+ bacteria contacts F– bacteria → A single stranded plasmid DNA is transferred [No transfer of chromosomal DNA]
- F+ plasmid can become incorporated into bacterial chromosomal DNA, termed high-frequency recombination [Hfr] cell.

Transposition

- Segment of DNA can jump from one location to another
- Plasmid ←→chromosome
- *E.g.*: Van A gene from vancomycin resistant *Enterococcus* to *S. aureus*.

There are two processes of gene transfer:

Microbiology

1. Horizontal gene transfer (HGT) or lateral gene transfer:
   - Horizontal gene transfer is the process by which genetic material is passed between two different organisms, i.e. organism of different species.
   - The recipient is not the offspring of donor.
   - The **most important** example is gene transfer between the bacteria.
   - The processes of horizontal gene transfer in bacteria are:
     - Transduction
     - Transformation
     - Conjugation
2. Vertical gene transfer:
   - Vertical gene transfer is the process of transferring genetic material to organism of same species, i.e. donor receives genetic material from its ancestor, e.g. its parent or a species from which it evolved.
   - Therefore, the donor will have the same general makeup as the parents.
   - Vertical gene transfer is "a mix of two parents", i.e. when two organisms meet, their genes are vertically transferred to their spawn.
   - This process is not important in bacteria.

20. Transduction is mediated by: *(NEET 2018)*

a. Bacteriophage
b. Plasmid
c. Metaphage
d. Cosmids

Ans. is 'a' Bacteriophage

21. Most important method of gene transfer in bacteria: *(NEET 2018)*

a. Lateral gene transfer
b. Vertical gene transfer
c. Medial gene transfer
d. Conjugation

Ans. is 'a' Lateral gene transfer

22. Phage mediated transfer of DNA is seen in: *(NEET 2018)*

a. *Streptococcus*
b. *Corynebacterium diphtheriae*
c. *E. coli*
d. *Vibrio parahemolyticus*

Ans. is 'b' ***Corynebacterium diphtheriae***

23. Method of gene transfer between bacteria in physical contact:

a. Transduction
b. Lysogenic conversion
c. Conjugation
d. Transformation

Ans. is 'c' Conjugation

24. Transfer of genetic material by bacteriophage is: *(NEET 2018)*

a. Transduction
b. Transformation
c. Transcription
d. Integration

Ans. is 'a' Transduction

25. Bacterial R factor is transmitted by which method? *(NEET 2018)*

a. Transduction
b. Transformation
c. Conjugation
d. Fusion

Ans. is 'c' Conjugation

ANTIBIOTIC SENSITIVITY TESTING

- Antibiotic sensitivity testing is carried out to determine appropriate antibiotic to be used for a particular strain isolated from clinical specimens.
- *Antibiotic testing can be carried out mainly by two methods*:
  - Disc diffusion tests
  - Dilution tests.

Disc Diffusion Tests

- Most commonly used methods to determine antibiotic susceptibility.
- Discs impregnated with known concentration of antibiotics are placed on the culture medium that has been inoculated with a culture of bacterium to be tested.
- Antibiotic sensitivity is determined by zone of inhibition of bacterial growth around the disc.

Selection of media

- Medium that supports both test and control strains is selected for carrying out antibiotic susceptibility testing.
- *For example*:
  - Muller-Hinton agar is used for gram-negative bacilli and *Staphylococcus* spp.
  - Blood agar is used for *Streptococcus* spp and *Enterococcus* spp.
  - Chocolate agar is used for *Haemophilus influenzae.*
  - Wellcotest medium uses antibiotics sulfonamide and cotrimoxazole.
- Mueller-Hinton agar is most commonly used medium for antibiotic sensitivity testing.

Type of Disc Diffusion Test

- *Disc diffusion tests are following types*:
  - **Kirby-Bauer disc diffusion method**—most commonly used.
  - Stoke disc diffusion method
  - Primary disc diffusion test.

Dilution Tests

- These tests are used to determine minimum inhibitory concentration (MIC) of antibiotics.
- *Following methods are used to determine MIC*:
  - Broth dilution method
  - Agar dilution method
  - Epsilometer test (E-test).

26. Disc diffusion method is also known as: *(NEET 2019)*

a. Kirby Bauer
b. VDRL
c. Dark field microscopy
d. None of these

Ans. is 'a' Kirby Bauer

27. All culture media are used for antibiotic susceptibility *except*:

a. Tetrathionate F
b. Blood agar
c. Chocolate agar
d. Muller-Hinton agar

Ans. is 'a' Tetrathionate F

METHICILLIN-RESISTANT STAPHYLOCOCCUS AUREUS (MRSA)

- *Staphylococcus aureus* has developed resistance to most of the penicillins.
- Penicillin resistance is of three types:
  1. Production of Beta-lactamase (penicillinase)
     - Beta-lactamase production is controlled by plasmid. Plasmid is transmitted and acquired mainly by transduction and less commonly by conjugation.
     - Staphylococci produce four types of penicillinases. A to D. Hospital strains usually form type 'A' penicillinase.

     Plasmid which is responsible for penicillinase production in *Staphylococcus* is transferred by transduction
     Drug resistance in *Staphylococcus* is mainly transferred by transduction.

  2. Alteration in surface receptors (penicillin binding proteins: PBPs)
     - Penicillin (and other beta lactams) acts on cell wall by binding to penicillin binding proteins, which have high affinity for penicillins and other beta-lactams.
     - Sometimes there is production of altered PBP called PBP2a, which has low affinity for beta lactams. PBP2a production is chromosomally mediated.
     - It is the major mechanism of methicillin resistance → Methicillin resistance *Staphylococcus aureus*.
     - The resistance gene is **mecA gene** which is a part of large mobile genetic element-staphylococcal cassette chromosome (SCCmec).
  3. Development of tolerance to penicillin
     - Bacterium is only inhibited not killed by penicillins.

28. True about resistance in MRSA:

a. MecA gene involved
b. Due to β-lactamase production
c. Plasmid mediated
d. All are correct

Ans. is 'a' MecA gene involved

Microbiology

IMMUNITY

ANTIBODY (IMMUNOGLOBULINS)

- Immunoglobulins are molecules that are produced by plasma cells in response to an immunogen.
- Immunoglobulins are glycoproteins.
- Each immunoglobulin is composed of two light chains (L) and two heavy chains (H).
- The L chain has a molecular weight of 25000, and the H chain of 50000.
- The L chain is attached to H chain by disulphide bond.
- The two H chains are joined together by disulphide bonds.
- Immunoglobulin isotype (i.e. G, M, A, D, E) is determined by the type of Ig heavy chain present.
- Hinge point is the point at which heavy and light chains join. This point can be digested by papain digestion, to produce one Fc fragment and two Fab fragments.
- The infinite range of the antibody specificity of immunoglobulins depends on the variability of the amino acid sequences at the variable units of H and L chains.
- Variable region is present on Fab region.

> - Isotype variation of class of antibody is due to variation in the amino acid sequence in the Constant region of the heavy chain. Because there are five potential variation in the amino acid sequence in the constant region there are five classes of antibody, i.e. IgG, IgM, IgA, IgD, IgE.
> - These H chain differences are called isotypes and are designated by the greek letters gamma, alpha, mu, epsilon and delta respectively.

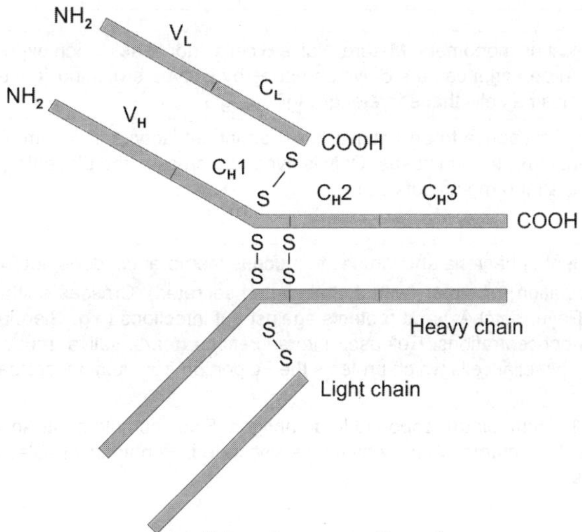

Basic structure of immunoglobulin molecule

- Amino acid sequences of the variable regions are not uniformly variable along their length, but consist of relatively invariable and some highly variable zones. The highly variable zones are involved with the formation of antigen binding sites. The sites on the **hypervariable regions** that make actual contact with the epitopes are called **"complementarity determining regions (CDRs)"**.
- "The idiotype is defined as the specific region of the fab portion of the Ig molecule to which antigen binds".
- The infinite range of the antibody specificity of immunoglobulin depends on the variability of the amino acid sequences at the variable regions of the H and L chains which form the antigen combining sites.
- Antibody specificity is due to variability of the amino acid sequences at the variable unit (at amino terminal) of both H and L chains (not only H or L chains).
- *IgM is more effective than IgG for*:
  - Immunohemolysis
  - Complement fixation by classical pathway
  - Opsonization
  - Bacterial agglutination
- *IgG is more effective than IgM for*:
  - Neutralization of toxins and viruses
  - Precipitation reactions.

29. Specificity of antibody is dependent on:

a. Fc portion
b. Fab region
c. Carboxy terminal
d. All of the above

Ans. is 'b' Fab region

30. Antibody diversity is due to:

a. Hinge region
b. Constant region
c. Variable region
d. Hypervariable region

Ans. is 'd' Hypervariable region

31. Antibody specificity is due to:

a. Amino acid sequence at H chain
b. Amino acid sequence at L chain
c. Amino acid at carboxy terminal
d. Amino acid sequence at amino terminal

Ans. is 'd' Amino acid sequence at amino terminal

32. Most effective antibody for precipitation:

a. IgM
b. IgG
c. IgA
d. IgD

Ans. is 'b' IgG

ANTIBODY ISOTYPES

Immunoglobulin isotypes	All isotypes can exist as monomers. Mature, Naive B cells prior to activation express IgM and IgD on their surfaces. They may differentiate in germinal centers of lymph nodes by isotype switching (gene rearrangement; induced by cytokines and CD40L) into plasma cells that secrete IgA, IgE, or IgG
IgG 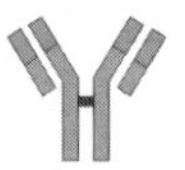	Main antibody in 2° response to an antigen. Most abundant isotype in serum. Fixes complement, opsonizes bacteria, neutralizes bacterial toxins and viruses. Only isotype that crosses the placenta (provides infants with passive immunity that starts to wane after 6 months of age)
IgA 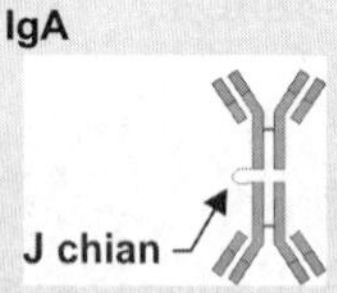	Prevents attachment of bacteria and viruses to mucous membranes; does not fix complement Monomer (in circulation) or dimer (with J chain when secreted). Crosses epithelial cells by transcytosis. Produced in GI tract (e.g. by Peyer patches) and protects against gut infections (e.g. Giardia). Most produced antibody overall, but has lower serum concentrations. Released into secretions (tears, saliva, mucus) and breast milk. Picks up secretory component from epithelial cells which protects the Fc portion from luminal proteases
IgM 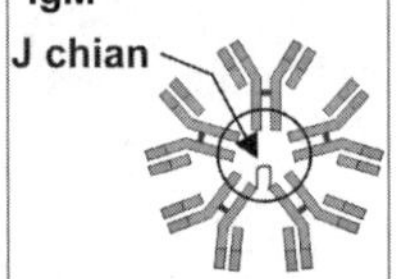	Produced in the 1° (immediate) response to an antigen. Fixes complement. Antigen receptor on the surface of B cells. Monomer on B cell, pentamer with J chain when secreted. Pentamer enables avid binding to antigen while humoral response evolves.
IgD 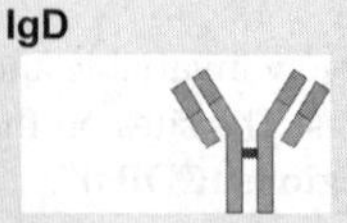	Unclear function. Found on surface of many B cells and in serum.
IgE 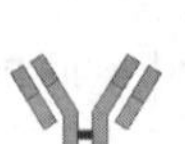	Binds mast cells and basophils; cross-links when exposed to allergen, mediating immediate (type I) hypersensitivity through release of inflammatory mediators such as histamine. Contributes to immunity to parasites by activating eosinophils. Lowest concentration in serum.

33. Identify the shown antibody isotype: *(NEET 2020)*

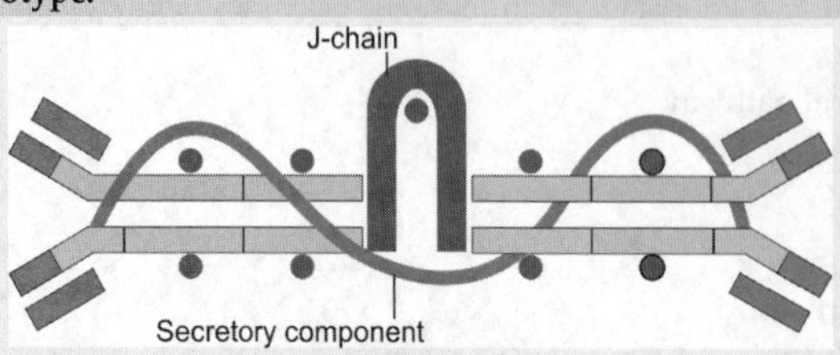

a. IgM
b. IgA
c. IgE
d. IgG

Ans. is 'b' IgA

IGG SUBCLASS DEFICIENCY

- It is defined as the decrease of one or more subclasses of IgG antibodies with normal or near normal levels of other immunoglobulin classes.
- There are four IgG subclasses, IgG1, IgG2, IgG3, and IgG4, and their concentrations change with age. IgG2 subclass deficiency is most common in children, whereas the IgG3 subclass deficiency has the highest prevalence in adults.
- Children with IgG subclass deficiency present most commonly with recurrent ear infections, sometimes as early as the second year of life.
- Symptomatic patients experience recurrent sinopulmonary infections, particularly with *Streptococcus pneumoniae* and *Haemophilus influenzae*, which present as repeated ear infections, bronchitis, pneumonia, sinusitis and diarrhea.
- IgG2 antibodies are predominantly against the **polysaccharide coating (capsule)** of certain disease-producing bacteria (such as, *Streptococcus pneumoniae* and *Haemophilus influenzae*).
- Patients may also present with meningitis, bronchiectasis and severe, recurrent otitis media, which may lead to hearing loss.
- It has also been associated with ataxia telangiectasia and systemic lupus erythematosus (SLE). Children with SLE and IgG2 and IgG4 deficiency may present with cardiac tamponade, instead of the more common nephropathy and arthritis.

34. A child is suffering from recurrent chronic infections with encapsulated bacteria. Deficiency of which Ig subclass is suspected? *(NEET 2019)*

a. IgG1
b. IgG2
c. IgG3
d. IgG4

Ans. is 'b' IgG2

ANTIGEN-ANTIBODY REACTIONS

Precipitation

- When a soluble antigen combines with its antibody in the presence of electrolytes (NaCl) at a suitable temperature and pH, the antigen-antibody complex forms an insoluble precipitate.
- When instead of sedimenting, the precipitate remains suspended as floccules, the reaction is known as flocculation.
- It is very sensitive in detection of antigens and as little as 1 μg of protein can be detected by precipitation tests.

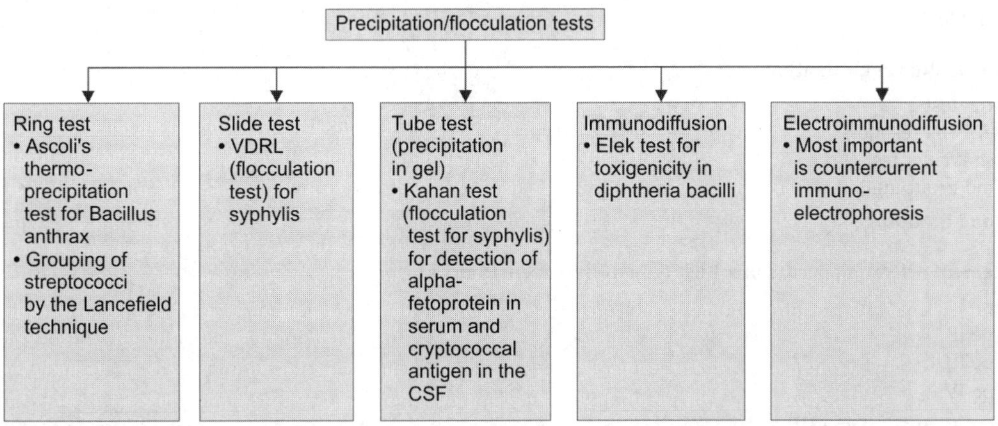

Agglutination

- When a particulate antigen is mixed with its antibody in the presence of electrolytes at a suitable temperature and pH, the particles are clumped or agglutinated.

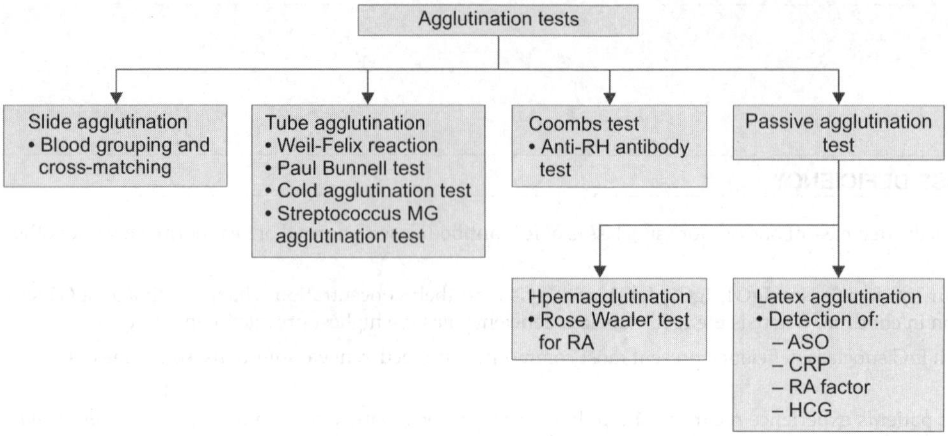

❖ Agglutination is more sensitive than precipitation for the detection of antibodies.

Complement Fixation Test

❖ The avidity of antigen antibody complexes to 'fix' complement is made use of in the complement fixation test.

❖ The source of complement is guinea pig serum.

❖ **Positive complement fixation test is indicated by hemolysis.**

❖ Principle of the complement fixation test is that when antigen and antibodies of the IgM or the IgG classes are mixed, complement is "fixed" to the antigen antibody complex. If this occurs on the surface of RBCs, the complement cascade will be activated and hemolysis will occur.

❖ Examples
- Wassermann CFT for syphilis
- *Treponema pallidum* immobilization test.

❖ Complement activation occurs in Type II and Type III both types of hypersensitivity.
- Type II reactions (Antibody mediated) → Involve immunoglobulin G or Immunoglobulin M bound to cell surface antigen, with subsequent **complement fixation**.
- Type III reactions (Immune complex mediated)→ involve circulating antigen-antibody complexes that deposit in postcapillary venules, with subsequent **complement fixation**.

35. Which of the following is an example of agglutination test:

a. Wassermann test
b. VDRL test
c. Widal test
d. Kahn test

Ans. is 'c' Widal test

36. Example of slide agglutination test:

a. Widal test
b. Weil-Felix reaction
c. Rose Waaler test
d. Blood grouping

Ans. is 'd' Blood grouping

37. Complement activation occurs in which type of hypersensitivity?

a. Type I
b. Type II
c. Type III
d. Type IV

Ans. is 'b' Type II and 'c' Type III

COMPLEMENT DEFICIENCY AND NEISSERIAL INFECTIONS

❖ The complement system is an essential component of the innate immune defence against infection by *Neisseria* (*N. meningitidis* and *N. gonorrhoeae*).

- Terminal complement component (C5 through C9) deficiencies and deficiencies of the alternative pathway (Properdin, C3, Factor D) have a strong effect on susceptibility to, as well as severity of, Neisserial infections.
  - *Deficiency of terminal complement (C5–C9) component*: Deficiency of one of the terminal components that compose membrane attack complex (MAC) predisposes patients to infection with *Neisseria meningitidis* or *Neisseria gonorrhoeae*. However, *N. meningitidis* infection is more common.
  - *Deficiencies of terminal pathway*: Deficiencies in components of alternative pathway, namely properdin, C3 and factor D, have been associated with increased susceptibility, almost exclusively, to meningococcal infection (amongst *Neisseria*).

38. Meningococcal (*Neisseria meningitidis*) infection is predisposed by deficiency of:

a. Late complement
b. Early complement
c. C1 esterase
d. All of the above

Ans. is 'a' Late complement

JOB'S SYNDROME (HYPER-IGE SYNDROME)

- Job's syndrome, also called Hyper-IgE syndrome, is an autosomal dominant disorder due to mutations in Signal Transducer and Activator of Transcription-3 (STAT-3).
- There is defect in phagocytosis. IgE levels are elevated. Other immunoglobulins are normal.
- Clinical manifestations include staphylococcal cold abscess, otitis media, recurrent pulmonary and skin infections, and cavitary pneumonia with pneumatoceles.
- Beside infections, other findings are characteristic facies with broad nose, osteoporosis, kyphoscoliosis, cerebral demyelinating plaques and coronary artery aneurysm.
- Despite very high IgE levels, these patients do not have elevated levels of allergy.
- IL-17 producing cells are which are considered responsible for protection against extracellular and mucosal injections are reduced in Job's syndrome.

39. A patient is presenting with recurrent staphylococcal infection, kyphoscoliosis and typical facies. The patient is suffering from:

a. IgA deficiency
b. Hyper-IgE syndrome
c. Common variable immunodeficiency
d. Bruton's agammaglobulinemia

Ans. is 'b' Hyper-IgE syndrome

SUPERANTIGENS

- **Mechanism:** Cross- links β region of TCR to MHC class II on APCs outside of the antigen binding site $\rightarrow$ overwhelming release of IL-1, IL-2, IFN-γ, and TNF-α $\rightarrow$ shock
- *Staphylococcus aureus*: Toxic shock syndrome toxin (TSST-I). Causes Toxic shock syndrome: fever, vomiting, rash, desquamation, shock, end-organ failure. Associated with prolonged use of vaginal tampons or nasal packing.
- *Streptococcus pyogenes*: Erythrogenic exotoxin A. Causes Toxin shock-like syndrome: fever, rash, shock. Associated with painful skin infection

40. Toxin of which of the following bacteria acts as superantigen? *(NEET 2020)*

a. *V.cholerae*
b. *S.pyogenes*
c. *S.epidermidis*
d. *C.perfringes*

Ans. is 'b' *S.pyogenes*

BACTERIOLOGY

EFFECTS OF pH ON BACTERIAL GROWTH

- **Lactobacillus** is a genus of gram-positive, facultative anaerobic or microaerophilic, rod-shaped, nonspore-forming bacteria. They are a major part of the lactic acid bacteria group (i.e. they convert sugars to lactic acid). They are normally a major part of the vaginal microbiota.
- *Acidophiles*: Organisms that grow best at low pH are called acidophiles. The cytoplasm of these organisms is acidic in nature. Some acidophiles are also thermophiles in nature. Many fungi grow optimum pH 5 or below and few grow well at pH values as level as 2. However, a few bacteria prefer to grow at more extreme pH values, e.g. thiobacillus, thioxydents has an optimum pH of 2–3.5.
- *Neutrophiles*: Most microorganism whose optimum pH for grow this between pH 6 and 8 are refer to as neutrophiles. Most bacteria grow best at the neutral pH 7 with a normal range between 6 and 8, e.g. *E. coil, Kiebsiella, Salmonella*, etc.

- *Alkaliphiles*: Some organisms which have very optimum pH for growth. Sometimes as high as pH 10–12 are called alkaliphiles. Alkaliphilic microorganisms are usually found in highly basic habited such as soda lakes and high carbonate soil. Some alkaliphiles have been found to be industrial importance because they produce hydrolytic enzymes such as proteases and lipases which function well at alkaline and are used as supplements for household detergents, e.g. bacillus alkaliphile, *Vibrio*.

41. Which can grow in acidic medium? *(NEET 2018)*

a. *Lactobacillus* b. *Peptostreptococcus*
c. *Staphylococcus* d. *Streptococcus*

Ans. is 'a' *Lactobacillus*

STREPTOCOCCI: CLASSIFICATION

- On the bases of Oxygen requirement streptococci are divided into two groups:
  - Aerobes and facultative anaerobes (streptococci).
  - Obligate anaerobes (peptostreptococci).
- On the bases of hemolysis, aerobes and facultative anaerobes (streptococci) are further divided into:
  - Alpha hemolytic – Viridans group
  - Beta hemolytic – Hemolytic Streptococci
  - Gamma – *Enterococcus* group
- Hemolytic streptococci were classified by Lancefield serological classification into groups based on nature of 'C' carbohydrate antigen on the cell wall. Called as Lancefield groups, 22 of which have been identified so far and named A to V (without I and J).
- Majority of human infections are caused by group 'A' streptococci, i.e. *Streptococcus pyogenes*.
- Group 'A' streptococci are further subdivided into types based on the protein (M, T and R) antigens present on the cell surface (**Griffith typing**). About 80 types of *Str. pyogenes* have been recognized.

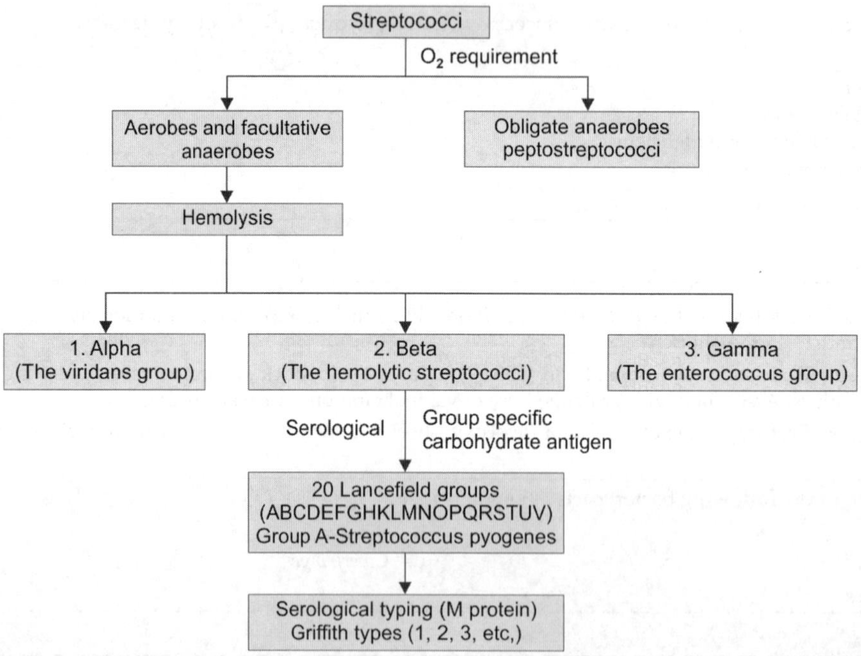

42. Griffith classification is based on:

a. 'C'-carbohydrate
b. M, T, R antigens
c. Type of hemolysis
d. O_2 requirement

Ans. is 'b' M, T, R antigens

CATALASE AND COAGULASE TEST

- Catalase test is used to differentiate staphylococci from streptococci.
- Coagulase test is used to differentiate the different species of Staphylococci (*Staph. aureus, Staph. epidermidis*).

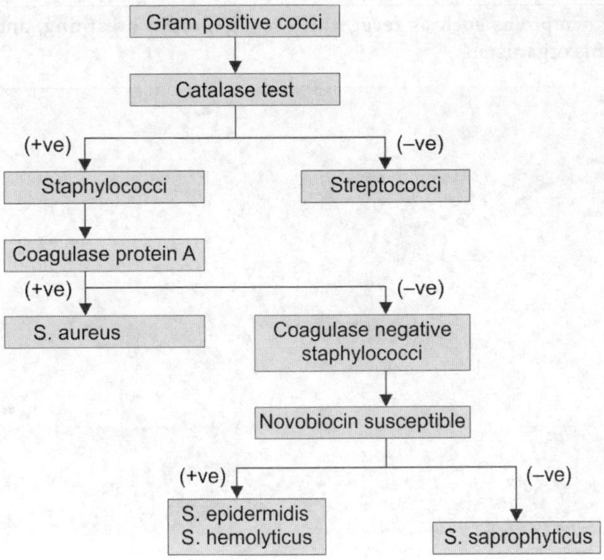

- Medically important staphylococci that causing human disease are divided into two groups:
  1. *Coagulase positive*: *Staphylococcus aureus.*
  2. *Coagulase negative*: *Staphylococcus epidermidis, Staphylococcus haemolyticus, Staphylococcus saprophyticus.*

43. *Staphylococcus* differs from *Streptococcus* by:

a. Coagulase test
b. Catalase test
c. Phosphatase test
d. Gram negative

Ans. is 'b' Catalase test

44. Classification of *Staphylococcus* is based on:

a. Catalase test
b. Coagulase test
c. Mannitol fermentation
d. Optochin sensitivity

Ans. is 'b' Coagulase test

STREPTOCOCCUS PNEUMONIAE (PNEUMOCOCCUS)

- A Gram-positive diplococcus (lanceolate shaped), is the most common cause of community-acquired pneumonia. It also a common cause of acute otitis media in children.
- *S. pneumoniae* is alpha-hemolytic on 5% sheep blood agar, it can break down red blood cells through the production of hydrogen peroxide (H_2O_2). The production of H_2O_2 by the bacterial infection can also cause damage to DNA, and kill cells within the lungs.
- Colonies on blood agar appears as concentric rings when viewed from above (Draughtsman shaped or carom coin shaped appearance) due to autolysin enzymes.
- Pneumococci are catalase negative, soluble in bile (bile solubility) and sensitive to optochin.
- It gives Quellung reaction due to presence of polysaccharide capsule.
- Pneumococcal (lobar) pneumonia causes fever and chills, coughs, difficulty breathing, and chest pain. If the infection spreads to the brain and spinal cord, it can cause pneumococcal meningitis.
- *Streptococcus pneumoniae* is the most common cause of meningitis in adults older than 20 years of age.
- Pneumonia is the most common predisposing condition for the risk of pneumococcal meningitis.
- Additional risk factors include alcoholism, acute and chronic otitis media, diabetes, splenectomy, hypogammaglobulinemia and head trauma with basilar skull fracture and CSF leak.
- ***Treatment:*** Penicillin remains drug of choice for treatment. Cephalosporins and Vancomycin can be given for meningitis. Quinolones may be considered for non-meningeal infections. Oral Amoxicillin recommended for otitis media in children.
- **Pneumococcal vaccines: PPSV23** and **PCV13.**
  - 23-valent pneumococcal polysaccharide vaccine (PPSV23) contains 23 serotypes of *S. pneumoniae* recommended for adult persons.
  - Pneumococcal conjugate vaccine (PCV13) contains 13 serotypes of *S. pneumoniae* recommended for children <2 years of age and also to adult persons.

45. A 6-year-old boy is having symptoms such as fever, chills, cough, rapid breathing, and chest pain. Gram stain from a sample is shown. Identify this organism: *(NEET 2019)*

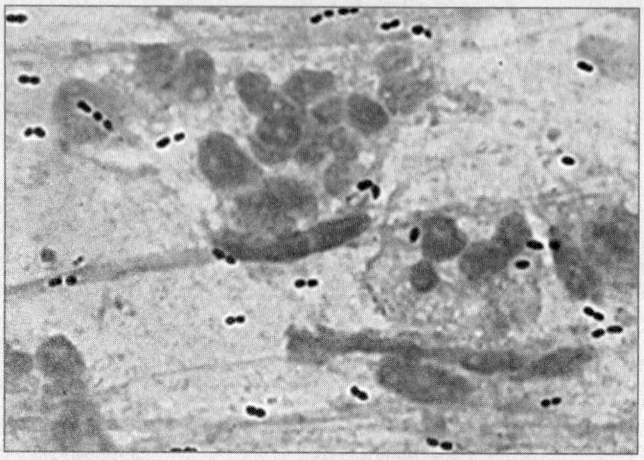

a. *Streptococcus pneumoniae*
b. *Staphylococcus*
c. *Propionibacterium*
d. *Mycobacterium*

Ans. is 'a' *Streptococcus pneumoniae*

46. A 30-year-old patient with CSF leak is presenting with neck rigidity, fever and seizures. What could be the probable infective agent:

a. *Streptococcus pneumoniae*
b. *N. meningitidis*
c. *Listeria monocytogenes*
d. *E. coli*

Ans. is 'a' *Streptococcus pneumoniae*

STAPHYLOCOCCUS EPIDERMIDIS

- Most common coagulase negative *Staphylococci* causing human infections.
- It is present on normal human skin (where it is the most abundant bacterial species) as well as in the oropharynx and vagina.
- It is a common cause of stitch abscesses, can cause cystitis and endocarditis.
- It has a predilection for growth on the implanted foreign bodies such as artificial heart valves, shunts, intravascular catheters and prosthetic appliances leading to bacteremia.
- *S. epidermidis* is uniquely adopted to colonize these devices by its capacity to elaborate the extracellular polysaccharide (slime) that facilitates formation of a protective biofilm (slime layer) on the device surface. This biofilm acts as a barrier protecting bacteria from host defence mechanisms as well as from antibiotics.
- The surface-associated staphylococcal enzyme autolysin **(AmiE)** may play a role in attachment to prosthetic surfaces, which are often coated with host serum or tissue constituents such as fibrinogen or fibronectin.
- *Staphylococcus epidermidis* is the most common cause of prosthetic valve endocarditis (early onset, up to 12 months).

47. Organism which has specific affinity for growing around prosthesis:

a. *Staphylococcus aureus*
b. *Staphylococcus epidermidis*
c. *Streptococcus pyogenes*
d. *Enterococcus faecalis*

Ans. is 'b' *Staphylococcus epidermidis*

ENTEROCOCCI

- Most common enterococci are *E. faecalis* and *E. faecium*. Less frequently isolated species are *E. gallinarum, E. durans, E. hirae* and *E. avium*.
- Previously they were classified as group D streptococci, along with non-enterococcal group.
- Enterococci are normal inhabitants of the large bowel of human adults, although they usually make up < 1% of the culturable intestinal microflora.
- They are catalase negative (as all Streptococci).
- *Their characteristic feature is that they can grow in presence of:*

Microbiology

- 40% bile
- 6.5% Sodium chloride
- At pH 9.6
- At 45 °C (relative heat resistant surving 60°C for 30 minutes)
- In 0.1% methylene blue milk

❖ They hydrolyze esculin. They grow in presence of 40% bile and hydrolyze esculin—Bile esculin positive.

❖ They are PYR (Pyrrolidonyl Arylamidase) positive.

❖ They are usually non-hemolytic (gamma-hemolytic), but sometimes may show alpha or beta hemolysis.

48. Bile esculin test is used to differentiate:

a. *Streptococcus agalactiae* b. *Enterococcus faecalis*
c. *Streptococcus bovis* d. *Streptococcus pneumoniae*

Ans. is 'b' *Enterococcus faecalis*

LISTERIA MONOCYTOGENES

❖ It is a **gram positive** 'coccobacillus' with tendency to occur in chains.

❖ Shows tumbling motility when grown at 25°C but nonmotile at 37°C.

❖ It grows on ordinary media within a temperature range of 1° to 45°C.

❖ Culture media used for isolation are blood agar, chocolate agar and PALCAM agar.

❖ *Listeria monocytogenes* shows 'subtle' beta hemolysis on blood agar.

49. True about Listeria are all *except*:

a. Shows beta hemolysis b. Shows tumbling motility
c. Gram negative d. PALCAM agar selective media

Ans. is 'c' Gram negative

CULTURE CHARACTERISTICS OF B. ANTHRACIS

❖ When grown on blood agar plates, the organisms produce nonhemolytic gray to white colonies with a rough texture and a ground-glass appearance. Comma-shaped outgrowths (**Medusa head**) may project from the colony.

❖ Gram stain shows large gram-positive rods (bamboo stick appearance).

❖ In semisolid medium, anthrax bacilli are always nonmotile, whereas related non-pathogenic organisms (e.g. *B. cereus*) exhibit motility by "swarming".

❖ In gelatin stab culture, a characteristic **inverted fir tree appearance** is seen, with slow liquefaction commencing from the top.

❖ A selective 'PLET' medium consisting of polymyxin, lysozyme, EDTA, and Thallous acetate added to heart infusion agar may be used for isolation.

❖ When grown on the surface of a solid medium containing penicillin, the cells become large, spherical and occur in chains on the surface of agar—**"string of pearls"** appearance.

McFadyean's Reaction

❖ When blood films containing anthrax bacilli are stained with polychrome **methylene blue** for a few seconds and examined under microscope, an amorphous purplish material is noticed around bacilli. This represents the capsular material and is characteristic of the anthrax bacillus.

50. Medusa head colonies on nutrient agar is seen in:

a. Pneumococcus b. *Legionella*
c. *Brucella* d. *Anthrax*

Ans. is 'd' *Anthrax*

51. McFadyean reaction seen with which organism?

a. *Clostridium perfringens*
b. *Clostridium botulinum*
c. *Bacillus cereus*
d. *Bacillus anthracis*

Ans. is 'd' *Bacillus anthracis*

Microbiology

ESCHERICHIA COLI IS CLASSIFIED ACCORDING TO VIRULENCE FACTOR

Specific diseases caused by different types of *E. coli*

- Enteropathogenic *E. coli* (EPEC): Watery diarrhea in infants and children
- Enterotoxigenic *E.coli* (ETEC):Traveler's diarrhea and most common cause of diarrhea in children of developing countries
- Entero invasive *E. coli* (EIEC): Diarrhea and dysentery similar to shigellosis
- Enterohemorrhagic *E. coli* (EHEC): Hemolytic uremic syndrome, Hemorrhagic colitis
- Enteroaggregative *E. coli*: Persistent diarrhea
- Extraintestinal pathogenic strains: UTI, Abdominal and-pelvic infections, meningitis, septicemia

❖ *O157*:H7 is the most prominent serotype of EHEC.

Culture of O157: H7 *E. coli*

❖ *E. coli O157*: H7 is not identified on routine stool cultures.

❖ *E. coli O157*: H7 can be specifically detected by the use of modified MacConkey media which contains sorbitol in place of lactose (SMAC).

❖ O157:H7 strain does not ferment sorbitol.

❖ Nonfermenting colonies on a Sorbitol MacConkey plate (SMAC) therefore suggest the diagnosis of *E. coli* O157:H7.

❖ Sorbitol MacConkey media is the screening method of choice for *E. coli* O157:H7.

Asymptomatic Bacteriuria

❖ Bacteria are typically introduced into the urinary tract during intercourse or when wiping after a bowel movement. ***E. coli*** is responsible for at least 75% to 80% of asymptomatic bacteriuria. *Kiebsiella pneumoniae, Proteus* species, staphylococcal species, enterococci, and group B streptococci can also establish colonization.

❖ Diagnosis can be considered only when the patient does not have local or systemic symptoms referable to the urinary tract. The clinical presentation is usually that of a patient who undergoes a screening urine culture for a reason unrelated to the genitourinary tract and is incidentally found to have bacteriuria.

52. *E. coli* subtypes are divided on the basis of:

a. Lactose fermentation
b. Virulence properties
c. Somatic O antigen
d. Maltose fermentation

Ans. is 'b' Virulence properties

53. Hemorrhagic colitis is caused by which strain of *E. coli*?

a. Enteropathogenic
b. Enterotoxigenic
c. Enteroinvasive
d. Enterohemorrhagic

Ans. is 'd' Enterohemorrhagic

54. ELISA test for virulence antigen is used for which type of *E. coli*?

a. ETEC
b. EIEC
c. EHEC
d. EAEC

Ans. is 'b' EIEC

55. Sorbitol MacConkey agar is used for which strain of EHEC?

a. O157:H7
b. O159:H7
c. O107:H7
d. O55:H7

Ans. is 'a' O157:H7

56. *E. coli* O157: H7 can cause:

a. Guillain-Barre syndrome
b. Hemolytic uremic syndrome
c. Traveler diarrhea
d. All of the above

Ans. is 'b' Hemolytic uremic syndrome

57. Most common organism grown in urine culture of pregnant woman with asymptomatic bacteriuria:

a. Proteus
b. *E. coli*
c. *Staph. aureus*
d. *Pseudomonas*

Ans. is 'b' *E. coli*

58. Which culture media is used for identification of *E.coli* O157:H7?

a. Macconkey agar
b. Sorbitol MacConkey agar
c. TCBS
d. DCA agar

Ans. is 'b' Sorbitol MacConkey agar

SHIGELLA

- It is a highly communicable. The infective dose for Shigella is less (10–100 bacilli). It can be as low as 10–100 bacilli because they survive gastric acidity better than other *Enterobacteriaceae*.
- Shigellae produce following clinical features:
  - *Intestinal*: These are:
    - *Dysentery*: Most common cause is *S. dysenteriae* type 1.
    - *Diarrhea*: Usually by *S. sonnei*.
  - *Extraintestinal*: These are hemolytic uremic syndrome (caused by *S. dysenteriae*-1), arthritis (*S. flexneri*), seizures (*S. flexneri*), pneumonia and Reiter's syndrome (in HLA B27 association).

59. Species of *Shigella* causing arthritis:

a. *S. dysenteriae*-1
b. *S. sonnei*
c. *S. flexneri*
d. *S. boydii*

Ans. is 'c' *S. flexneri*

PROTEUS

- Gram negative, uncapsulated, pleomorphic, motile bacilli.
- Proteus bacilli are divided into three genera.
  - *Proteus* → *Proteus vulgaris, Proteus mirabilis*
  - *Morganella* → *Morganella morganii*
  - *Providencia* → *Prov. alcalifaciens, Prov. stuartii, Prov. rettgeri*
- Most of them except *Providencia* strains, produce powerful Urease.
- A characteristic feature of proteus bacilli is "PPA reaction". It is due to presence of enzyme phenylalanine deaminase which converts phenylalanine to phenyl pyruvic acid.
- Culture of Proteus bacilli have a characteristic putrefactive odor described as **"fishy or seminal".**
- They produce swarming growth over the surface of agar, except for *Morganella morganii* which does not swarm.
- **Dienes phenomenon** is used to detect swarming growth (Note: **Diene's method** is used to study *Mycoplasma* colony).
- Some nonmotile Proteus strains (OX-2, OX-19 and OX-K) are used in Weil-Felix agglutination reaction for the diagnosis of rickettsia infections.
- *Proteus mirabilis* is an important cause of urinary and septic infections, often nosocomial.
- *Proteus* bacilli are resistant to many of common antibiotics. An exception is *P. mirabilis* which is sensitive to ampicillin and cephalosporins.
- Their ability to generate histamine form contaminated fish has implicated in the pathogenesis of **Scombroid poisoning**.
- *Proteus* produces phosphate stones in kidney as it produces ammonia and contributes to alkalinity which leads to necrosis of renal tubular epithelium with precipitation of phosphate stones.

60. Fishy odor is found on growth of which organism?

a. *Proteus*
b. *Pseudomonas*
c. *Yersinia pseudotuberculosis*
d. *Yersinia pestis*

Ans. is 'a' *Proteus*

61. Dienes phenomenon is seen in:

a. *Proteus*
b. *Mycoplasma*
c. *Rickettsia*
d. *Chlamydia*

Ans. is 'a' *Proteus*

62. Scombroid fish poisoning is due to which of the following Gram-negative bacteria? *(NEET 2018)*

a. *E. coli*
b. *Salmonella*
c. *Proteus*
d. *Shigella*

Ans. is 'c' *Proteus*

VIBRIO PARAHEMOLYTICUS

- It is a halophilic capsulated *Vibrio*, shows bipolar staining.
- Inhabits the coastal sea, where it is found in fishes, arthropods such as shrimps and crabs and molluscs such as oyster.
  It resembles the *Vibrio cholerae* except that:
- Produces peritrichous flagella when grown on solid medium (*V. cholerae* has polar flagella), in liquid medium polar flagella are formed.
- It grows, only in media containing NaCl, optimum concentration is 2–4%
- Its enteropathogenicity is closely linked to its ability to cause hemolysis on Wagatsuma agar (a high salt blood agar) → the **Kanagawa phenomenon**.
- *V. parahaemolyticus* causes common source outbreaks of diarrhea after consumption of undercooked or improperly handled seafood or of other food contaminated by seawater.
- It can result in two distinct gastrointestinal presentation:
  - *Watery diarrhea*: It is more common and occurs in North America.
  - *Dysentery*: It is less common and occurs in India and Bangladesh.

63. Kanagawa's phenomenon is seen in:

a. *Pseudomonas aeruginosa* b. *Vibrio parahaemolyticus*
c. *Shigella sonnei* d. *Proteus mirabilis*

Ans. is 'b' *Vibrio parahaemolyticus*

NEISSERIA GONORRHOEAE

- Gram-negative, non-encapsulated kidney shaped diplococci
- It oxidizes only glucose and not maltose.

Clinical Features

- *Men*: May be asymptomatic; urethritis with burning urination and urethral strictures
- Watercan perineum—spread of infection into periurethral tissues forming abscesses and draining sinuses
- *Women*: Cervicitis, urethritis; may progress to pelvic inflammatory disease
- PID may in turn result in infertility
- *Fitz-Hugh-Curtis syndrome*: Perihepatic adhesions due to peritonitis
- Gonococcal ophthalmia neonatorum is seen in neonates due to acquisition during passage through an infected birth canal.
- Gonococcal urethritis:
  - The pili of gonococcus have affinity for the columnar epithelium of urethra.
  - Virulent gonococci have affinity to adhere to urethral epithelial cells even in the presence of the violent flushing of urine.

The important infections caused by gonococci are:

- Males
  - Acute urethritis is the most common manifestation. Prostate, seminal vesical and epididymis may also be involved.
  - Testis is usually spared.
- Females
  - Cervicitis is the most common manifestation, which primarily infects cervical os. Infection may spread to cause salpingitis, urethritis, endometritis, peritonitis and perihepatitis (Fitz-Hugh-Curtis syndrome).

  > The vaginal mucosa of healthy women is lined by stratified squamous epithelium and is usually not infected by *N. gonorrhoeae* however, gonococcal vaginitis can occur in anestrogenic women (e.g. prepubertal girls and postmenopausal women) in whom the vaginal stratified epithelial layers are often thinned down to basilar layer, which can be infected by *N. gonorrhoeae.*

  - *Other infections:* These are anorectal gonorrhea (proctitis), pharyngeal gonorrhea, ocular gonorrhea and in children vulvovaginitis.
- Gonorrhea in neonates:
  - The most common form of gonorrhea in neonates is ophthalmia neonatorum which results from exposure to infected cervical secretions during parturition.
  - Septic arthritis is the most common manifestation of systemic infection.
- Disseminated gonococcal infection (DGI) or Gonococcal arthritis
  - *It has two stages:*
    1. *Stage I (Bacteremic stage)*: There is bacteremia with polyarthralgia and skin lesions (papule, pustules).
    2. *Stage II (Suppurative arthritis)*: There is pyogenic arthritis which may cause complications (endocarditis, meningitis).

Laboratory Diagnosis

Samples - swabs from urethra or cervix is taken for culture and smear.

- *Transport media*: Charcoal impregnated swabs/medium (Stuart/Amies media)
- *Smears:* Gram Stained smears show intracellular diplococci
- *Culture*: Selective media—Chocolate agar, New York City (NYC) medium
- *Selective media useful in chronic cases*: Thayer-Martin medium
- *Nucleic acid Amplification Tests*: High sensitivity and specificity
- *Serology*: Immunoblotting, radioimmunoassay and ELISA.

NEISSERIA MENINGITIDIS INFECTION

- Rash can be seen, which may be erythematous initially, progressing into petechiae.
- Fulminant meningococcemia, most rapid lethal form of septic shock, with prominent hemorrhagic skin lesions.
- *Waterhouse-Friedrichsen syndrome*: is characterized by purpuric rash (purpura fulminans), shock, DIC, bilateral adrenal hemorrhage and multi-organ failure.

Laboratory Diagnosis of Meningococci

- Specimens used are CSF (for cases), nasopharyngeal swab (for carrier), blood (in meningococcemia and early meningitis), and petechial lesions (in meningococcemia).

> - Best specimen for case — CSF (by lumbar puncture).
> - Best specimen for carrier – Nasopharyngeal swab.

- Gram stained smear of CSF shows gram negative diplococci within pus cells.
- Transport medium for meningococci - Stuart's medium.
- Culture on Blood agar, chocolate agar and Mueller-Hinton starch casein hydrolysate agar are the media commonly used for culturing meningococci.
- Modified Thayer-Martin (with vancomycin, colistin and nystatin) is a useful selective medium.
- Presumptive diagnosis of meningococcal meningitis is made earliest by Latex agglutination.

> - PCR is a **rapid** method for making diagnosis of meningococcal meningitis.
> - PCR amplification of DNA in CSF is the most sensitive method for diagnosis.
> - But, the most commonly used method for diagnosis is isolation on culture from specific specimen.

Vaccine

- Meningococcal vaccine is prepared from Capsular polysaccharide.
- Vaccines available for group A, C, Y and W-135. Bivalent (A, C), trivalent (A, C, W135) and tetravalent (A,C,Y,W135) vaccines available.
- Meningococcal group B vaccine was not available for last two decades. Recently, group B vaccine has also been developed in many countries (UK, Ireland) and is a part of routine immunization schedule.
- But, meningococcal group B vaccine is not derived from capsular polysaccharide.

> - Meningococcal group-B capsular polysaccharide is poorly immunogenic, therefore its vaccine is not prepared from polysaccharide (unlike group A, C, Y, W135)
> - *Its vaccine is developed from surface proteins*:
>   - Factor H Binding protein (fHbP)
>   - Neisseria Heparin binding protein (NHBA)
>   - Neisseria Adhesion A (NadA).

64. Gonococci have affinity for:

a. Vaginal mucosa
b. Epithelium of urethra
c. Testis
d. All of the above

Ans. is 'b' Epithelium of urethra

65. Petechiae are seen in infection with:

a. Pneumococci
b. *N. meningitidis*
c. *Pseudomonas*
d. *Yersinia*

Ans. is 'b' *N. meningitidis*

66. True about meningococcal vaccine:

a. Group B vaccine not available
b. Derived from capsular polysaccharide
c. Bivalent vaccine contains A, W-135
d. All are true

Ans. is 'b' Derived from capsular polysaccharide

67. A child presented with fever, neck rigidity and generalised rash as shown in the figure. Later he developed shock and hemorrhage. Gram stain revealed gram negative diplococci. What is the likely agent? *(NEET 2020)*

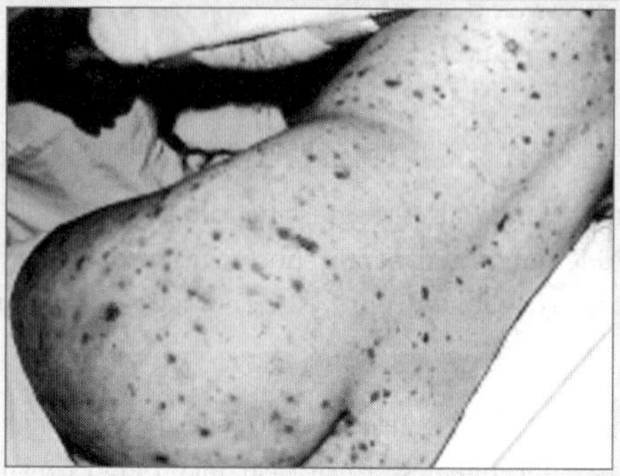

a. L.monocytogenes
b. H.influenza
c. N.meningitidis
d. S.pneumoniae

Ans. is 'c' N.meningitidis

CORYNEBACTERIUM DIPHTHERIAE

- It is club-shaped, irregularly stained gram-positive pleomorphic rod that shows Chinese letter or cuneiform arrangement with metachromatic granules (stained with Albert's stain).
- It causes diphtheria, which is typically spread through aerosol route or person-to-person contact or through contact with objects that have the bacteria on them.
- Even if an infected person does not show any signs or symptoms of diphtheria, they are still able to transmit the bacterial infection for up to six weeks after the initial infection.
- The bacteria most commonly infect nose and throat. Toxins released by this bacteria spread through bloodstream and often cause a thick, gray coating in nose, throat, lungs.
- Patient should be kept in isolation room and all the steps of droplet precaution should be followed for the prevention of transmission of it in hospitals.

68. Contact isolation is done for: *(NEET 2019)*

a. MRSA
b. Mumps
c. Diphtheria
d. Asthma

Ans. is 'c' Diphtheria

BURKHOLDERIA

- *B. mallei* is a non-motile gram negative bacilli (in contrast to *B. pseudomallei* which is motile).
- *Burkholderia mallei* → Glander's disease
- *Burkholderia pseudomallei* → Melioidosis.

Burkholderia *Pseudomallei*

- It is also known as Whitmore bacillus.
- It is aerobic gram negative bacillus.
- It is motile which differentiate it from nonmotile *B. mallei.*
- It shows typical bipolar 'safety pin' appearance with methylene blue stain.
- It is free living saprophyte normally found in soil, ponds and rice paddies and on products from endemic areas.
- It produces two heat labile toxins, one lethal and other necrotizing.
- It causes melioidosis. Most common manifestation of melioidosis is acute pulmonary manifestation. Other manifestations are acute septicemia, localized skin infections, suppurative parotitis and chronic infections.

- Virtually every organ can be affected and hence melioidosis has been called the "great imitator" of other infectious disease.
- Isolation of organism on selective medium is diagnostic.
- Ceftazidime is the drug of choice. Carbapenems (imipenem, meropenem) are also first line drugs. Melioidosis is also known as Vietnam Time-Bomb disease.

Burkholderia *Mallei*

- It is a non-motile gram negative bacilli (in contrast to *B. pseudomallei* which is motile).
- Mallein test is a skin test (like tuberculin test) for *B. mallei*.
- It causes Glanders and Farcy.
- *Strauss reaction*: Intraperitoneal injection in male guinea pig causes testicular swelling.
- It is a category 'B' bioterrorism agent.

Burkholderia Cepacia Complex

- It is an environmental organism that in habits moist environments, detergents and IV fluids.
- It has been recognized as a plant pathogen causing onion rot (cepia, latin for onion).
- **Cepacia syndrome:** Characterized by a rapidly fatal respiratory infection and septicemia in patients with cystic fibrosis.
- It is resistant to multiple antibiotics, hence has been emerging as an important nosocomial pathogen in ICUs causing pneumonia, wound infections, etc.
- *Burkholderia cepacia* complex strains are intrinsically resistant to a wide range of antimicrobial agents including aminoglycoside, polymyxin, first and second generation cephalosporins and carboxypenicillins.
- Antimicrobial agents that are effective against *B. cepacia* complex in vitro include trimethoprim/sulfamethoxazole, ceftazidime, carbapenems, ureidopenicillin, fluoroquinolone, minocycline and chloramphenicol.

69. Which *Burkholderia* is non-motile?

a. *B. mallei*
b. *B. pseudomallei*
c. Both are motile
d. Both are non-motile

Ans. is 'a' *B. mallei*

70. Which of the following causes Melioidosis?

a. *Burkholderia mallei*
b. ***Burkholderia pseudomallei***
c. *Burkholderia cepacia*
d. None

Ans. is 'b' *Burkholderia pseudomallei*

71. *Burkholderia cepacia* is intrinsically resistant to: *(NEET 2018)*

a. Ceftazidime
b. Trimethoprim/sulfamethoxazole
c. Temocillin
d. Cefotetan

Ans. is 'd' Cefotetan

YERSINIA PESTIS

- Gram negative, non-motile coccobacillus shows pleomorphism.
- Surrounded by a slim layer (envelope or capsule).
- Wayson or Giemsa or methylene blue stains shows typical bipolar staining with **safety pin appearance.**

Culture Characteristics

- The optimum temperature for growth is 27°C (unlike most pathogens).
- In **Ghee broth** a characteristic growth occurs which hangs down into broth from the surface resembling stalactites—**Stalactite growth.**
- On blood agar, dark colonies due to heme pigment.
- Growth of *Yersinia* occurs fastest at 30°C.

72. Stalactite growth is seen characteristically in:

a. *H. influenzae*
b. *C. diphtheriae*
c. *Y. pestis*
d. *T. pallidum*

Ans. is 'c' *Y. pestis*

RICKETTSIAL DISEASES

Disease	Agent	Insect vector	Mammalian reservoir
• Typhus group – Epidemic typhus – Murine typhus (Endemic typhus) – Scrub typhus	 R. prowazekii R. typhi R. tsutsugamushi	 Louse Flea Mite	Humans, Rodents
• Spotted fever group – Indian tick typhus – Rocky mountain spotted fever – Rickettsial pox	 R. conori R. rickettsiae R. akari	 Tick Tick Mite	Rodents, dogs, Mice
• Others – Q fever – Trench fever	 Coxiella burnetii Bartonella quintana	 Nil Louse	Cattle, sheep, goats, Humans

Diagnosis

- Both epidemic typhus and endemic typhus are positive for OX-19 antigen. Thus Weil-Fleix reaction differentiate between the two.
- Serological diagnosis of Rickettsial infection may be made by:
  - Heterophile Weil-Felix reaction
  - Specific tests using rickettsial antigens.

Weil-Felix Reaction

- This reaction is an agglutination test in which sera are tested for agglutinins to O antigens of certain non-motile proteus strains OX-19, OX-2 and OX-K.
- The basis of the test is the sharing of an alkali—stable carbohydrate antigen by some rickettsia and by certain strains of proteus, *P. vulgaris* OX-19 and OX- and *P. mirabilis* OX-K.
- The test is usually done as a tube agglutination, though rapid slide agglutination methods have been employed for screening.
  - Scrub typhus is positive with OX-K
  - Epidemic typhus and endemic typhus are positive for OX-19.
  - Rocky mountain spotted fever is positive with OX-19 and OX-2.
  - Q fever, trench fever and rickettsial pox do not show positive test with any of the three antigens. Thus, Weil-Felix test is not useful in these diseases.

Disease	OX-19	OX-2	OX-K
Rocky mountain spotted fever	+	+	–
Rickettsial pox	–	–	–
Epidemic typhus	+	–	–
Bril-Zinsser disease	+/–	–	–
Scrub typhus	–	–	+
Endemic typhus	+	–	–
Trench fever	–	–	–
Q fever	–	–	–

- ***Cat scratch disease** is caused by*: (i) *Bartonella henselae* (most common) (ii) *Afipia felis* is which is believed to be spread by the cat's saliva. Young cats pose a greater risk than older cats. Occasionally dog scratches or bites may be involved. Diagnosis is generally based on symptoms. Confirmation is possible by blood tests. *Bartonella henselae* is a fastidious, intracellular, Gram-negative bacterium.

73. Rocky mountain spotted fever is caused by:

a. *Rickettsia rickettsii* b. *Rochalimaea quintana*
c. *Rickettsia tsutsugamushi* d. *Coxiella burnetii*

Ans. is 'a' *Rickettsia rickettsii*

74. Causative agent of Q fever:

a. *Rickettsia rickettsii* b. *Rochalimae aquintana*
c. *Rickettsia tsutsugamushi* d. *Coxiella burnetii*

Ans. is 'd' *Coxiella burnetii*

75. Epidemic typhus is caused by:

a. Mite
b. Louse
c. Flea
d. Tick

Ans. is 'b' Louse

76. Scrub typhus is caused by:

a. *R. typhi*
b. *R. prowazeki*
c. *R. rickettsia*
d. *R. tsutsugamushi*

Ans. is 'd' *R. tsutsugamushi*

77. Which test cannot differentiate endemic and epidemic typhus?

a. Weil-Felix reaction
b. Complement fixation test
c. Immunofluorescence
d. Radio precipitation

Ans. is 'a' Weil-Felix reaction

78. True about Weil-Felix reaction are all *except*:

a. Agglutination test
b. OX-19 of *Proteus vulgaris*
c. Q- fever is positive for OX-19
d. All of the above

Ans. is 'c' Q- fever is positive for OX-19

79. Cat scratch disease is caused by:

a. *Streptobacillus moniliformis*
b. *Spirillum minus*
c. *B. henselae*
d. *R. tsutsugamushi*

Ans. is 'c' *B. henselae*

FOOD POISONING

Incubation period	Organism	Symptoms	Food source
1–6 hours	• Staph. aureus • *Bacillus cereus* (emetic type)	Diarrhea, vomiting, no fever Vomiting, diarrhea, no fever	Meat, dairy and poultry product Fried rice
8–16 hours	• *Bacillus cereus* (diarrheal type) • Cl. perfringens	Diarrhea, no vomiting, no fever, diarrhea, no vomiting, no fever	Wide range of food, meat vegetables, cereals
>16 hours	• V. cholerae • *V. parahaemolyticus* • *Salmonella* species • *Campylobacter jejuni*	Diarrhea, vomiting, no fever Diarrhea, vomiting, fever Diarrhea, fever, rarely vomiting Diarrhea, fever, no vomiting	Wide range of food, Sea food Beef, poultry, eggs, dairy products Potato or egg salad, raw vegetables Poultry raw milk

❖ *Staph. aureus* and *B. cereus* can cause gasteroenteritis within 6 hours.
- *Staph. aureus* food poisoning—caused by dairy products and causes diarrhea.
- *Bacillus cereus* food poisoning—caused by fried rice and causes emetic type (not diarrheal type)

80. Food poisoning with shortest incubation period is caused by:

a. *Salmonella*
b. *Cl. perfringens*
c. *V. cholerae*
d. *Bacillus cereus*

Ans. is 'd' *Bacillus cereus*

81. A child has developed diarrhea 4 hours after eating ice-cream. The causative agent is:

a. *Staph. aureus*
b. *Bacillus cereus*
c. *Salmonella*
d. *Vibrio*

Ans. is 'a' *Staph. aureus*

82. Which of the following can present as food poisoning within 3 hours of food intake? *(NEET 2020)*

a. *S.enteritidis*
b. *S.aureus*
c. *C.perfringes*
d. *V.parahemolyticus*

Ans. is 'b' *S.aureus*

IMPORTANT BACTERIAL TOXINS

Toxins	Mechanism of action
Botulinum toxin	• Acts on the peripheral nervous system (i.e. neuromuscular junctions) by inhibiting myoneural junction acetylcholine release and cause flaccid paralysis (many strains of *Clostridium botulinum* synthesized C2 toxin, that ADP-ribosylates actin, thereby inhibiting its polymerization, affecting the shape of target cells, and resulting in enterotoxin activity in vivo).
Diphtheria toxin	• Inhibits protein synthesis in target cells by catalyzing the ADP-ribosylation of an amino acid (diphthamide) on elongation factor 2a, a host protein involved in translation of mRNA.
Pertussis toxin	• Acts by ADP ribosylation of several members of the family of guanine nucleotide-binding (G) proteins involved in signal transduction.
Heat stable toxin (ST) of *E. coli*	• Activates guanylyl cyclase to increase GMP.
V. cholerae toxin Heat labile toxin (LT) of *E. coli*	• Activates adenylate cyclase of the intestinal epithelial cell by ADP ribosylation of the stimulatory G protein. ↑ CAMP.
Shiga toxin	• Inhibits protein synthesis by enzymatic inactivation of the 28 sRNA
Verocytotoxin of *E. coli* toxin)	• Inhibits protein synthesis by inhibiting ribosomal function (same as shiga toxin)

83. Mechanism of action of diphtheria toxin:

a. ADP ribosylation
b. Activation of adenylyl cyclase
c. Activation of guanylyl cyclase
d. Inhibition

Ans. is 'a' ADP ribosylation

HACEK GROUP

❖ HACEK organisms are a group of fastidious, slow growing, gram negative bacteria whose growth requires on atmosphere of carbon dioxide.

❖ Normally reside in the oral cavity as commensal, but occasionally have been associated with local infections of mouth and systemic infections such as bacterial endocarditis.

❖ Species belonging to this group include:
- *Haemophilus* species (*H. parainfluenzae, H. haemolyticus, H. parahaemolyticus*)
- *Aggregatibacter actinomycetemcomitans; Aggregatibacter aphrophilus*
- *Cardiobacterium hominis*
- *Eikenella corrodens*
- *Kingella kingae.*

84. Which is not included in HACEK group:

a. *Haemophilus*
b. *Actinobacillus*
c. *Cardiobacterium*
d. *Klebsiella*

Ans. is 'd' *Klebsiella*

CHLAMYDIA

❖ Chlamydiae were once considered viruses due to their filterability through 0.45 μm filter and due to their failure to grow in cell-free media. However, the chlamydia shows the following properties of bacteria by which they differ from viruses:
- They contain both DNA and RNA.
- Possess cell wall as that of Gram-negative bacteria.
- Contain prokaryotic ribosomes.
- Multiply by binary fission.
- They produce and synthesize their own nucleic acid, lipid and proteins.
- Susceptible to a wide range of antibiotics, such as tetracyclines, erythromycin, macrolides, and rifampicin.

Chlamydiae were thought to be viruses because (like viruses) they:
- Pass through 0.45 μm filters.
- Are obligate intracellular parasite - cannot be grown in cell free media.

❖ *Chlamydia trachomatis* is classified into two broad biological variants which cause trachoma, inclusion conjunctivitis (TRIC) and lymphogranuloma venerum (LGV).

❖ The TRIC biovar has been classified into 12 serovars—A, B, Ba, C causing blinding trachoma in endemic areas and serovars D to K associated with the less serious ocular infections, inclusion conjunctivitis and with various genital infections.

❖ Serovars L1, L2, and L3 cause LGV and hemorrhagic proctitis.

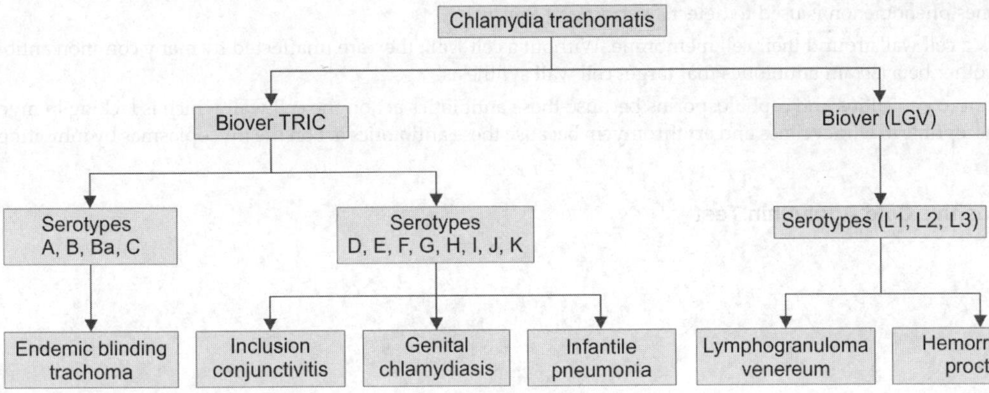

❖ Serovars D-K genital chlamydiasis cause:
- *In man*: Urethritis (NGU), epididymitis, proctitis, conjunctivitis, Reiter's syndrome.
- *In women*: Cervicitis, salpingitis, PID, infertility, Reiter's syndrome, perihepatitis (Fitz-Hugh Curtis syndrome).

85. *Chlamydia* is similar to bacteria in:

a. Filterable through filter
b. Ability to grow in cell free media
c. **Contains both DNA and RNA**
d. All of the above

Ans. is 'c' Contains both DNA and RNA

86. Similarity between *Chlamydia* and virus is:

a. Filterable through filter
b. Ability to grow in cell free media
c. Contains both DNA and RNA
d. All of the above

Ans. is 'a' Filterable through filter

87. Swimming pool conjunctivitis is caused by:

a. *Pseudomonas*
b. *Coxsackie virus*
c. *Chlamydia*
d. *Mycoplasma*

Ans. is 'c' *Chlamydia*

88. LGV is caused by:

a. *Neisseria gonorrhoeae*
b. *Chlamydia trachomatis*
c. *Trichomonas vaginalis*
d. *Haemophilus ducreyi*

Ans. is 'b' *Chlamydia trachomatis*

89. Best test to diagnose chlamydial infection:

a. Direct fluorescent antibody test
b. Enzyme immunoassay
c. Polymerase chain reaction
d. Culture on irradiated McCoy cells

Ans. is 'c' Polymerase chain reaction

90. Not caused by *Chlamydia trachomatis*:

a. Reiter's syndrome
b. Infertility
c. Conjunctivitis
d. Adult pneumonia

Ans. is 'd' Adult pneumonia

MYCOPLASMA

- ❖ May be cultivated in liquid or solid media. Generally facultative anaerobes.
- ❖ *Mycoplasma* and *Ureaplasma* do not produce turbidity in liquid medium.
- ❖ Grow in heart infusion peptone broth with 2% agar (PH 7.8) (P.P.L.O. broth) with fresh yeast extract and horse serum.
- ❖ For enrichment, 30% human ascitic fluid or animal serum (horse, rabbit) are added to the medium. (Serum acts as a source of cholesterol).
- ❖ Most mycoplasma colonies are hemolytic (β-hemolysis) due to production of hydrogen peroxide. The colony gives **'fried egg' appearance**.
- ❖ Colonies are best studied after staining by **Diene's method**- A block of agar containing the colony is cut and placed on a slide. It is covered with a cover slip on which an alcoholic solution of methylene blue and azure has been dried. Slide is then observed under a microscope.

(*Remember:* Dienes phenomenon is used to detect swarming of *Proteus)*

- *Mycoplasma* lack a cell wall around their cell membrane. Without a cell wall, they are unaffected by many common antibiotics such as penicillin or other beta lactam antibiotics that target cell wall synthesis.
- They are resistant to penicillins and cephalosporins because these antibiotics act on the cell wall which is lacking in mycoplasmas. They remain susceptible to tetracyclines and erythromycin because these antibiotics act on the mycoplasmas by inhibiting synthesis of protein.

Infections with Positive Cold Agglutinin Test

- *Mycoplasma*
- CMV
- Influenza
- EBV (IMN).

Cold Agglutinin Type Hemolytic Anemia

This form of immunohemolytic anemia is caused by IgM antibodies that bind red cells avidly at low temperatures (0–4°C). It is less common than warm antibody immune hemolytic anemia, accounting for 15% to 30% of cases. Cold agglutinin antibodies sometimes appear transiently following certain infections, such as with *Mycoplasma pneumoniae,* Epstein-Barr virus, cytomegalovirus, influenza virus, and human immunodeficiency virus (HIV). In these settings the disorder is self-limited, and the antibodies rarely induce clinically important hemolysis. Chronic cold agglutinin immunohemolytic anemia occurs in association with certain B-cell neoplasms or as an idiopathic condition.

91. Fried Egg colony is seen in culture of:

a. *Mycoplasma* b. *Legionella*
c. Trachoma d. *Haemophilus*

Ans. is 'a' *Mycoplasma*

92. Diene's stain is used for:

a. *Compylobacter* b. *Helicobacter*
c. *Rickettsiae* d. *Mycoplasma*

Ans. is 'd' *Mycoplasma*

93. Cold agglutinin test is positive in infection with:

a. *Mycoplasma* b. *Rickettsiae*
c. *Candida* d. All of the above

Ans. is 'a' *Mycoplasma*

94. *Mycoplasma* is inherently resistant to:

a. Doxycycline b. Azithromycin
c. Ceftriaxone d. Ciprofloxacin

Ans. is 'c' Ceftriaxone

Pathogenic spirochetes belong to three genera: *Treponema, Borrelia* and *Leptospira.*

Spirochete	Species	Disease
Treponema	*Pallidum* *Endemicum* *Pertunae* *Carateum*	Syphilis Bejel Yaws Pinta
Borrelia	*Burgdorferi* *Recurrentis* *Vincentii*	Lyme disease Relapsing fever Vincent angina
Leptospira	*Interrogans*	Weil's disease

95. Borrelia causes which of the following?

a. Weil's disease b. Bejel
c. Vincent angina d. Yaws

Ans. is 'c' Vincent angina

96. Lyme disease caused by:

a. *Leptospira* b. *Borrelia*
c. *Treponema* d. *Bordetella*

Ans. is 'b' Borrelia

- **Neurosyphilis** is generally considered as a part of late syphilis, invasion of CNS occurs early within first week of infection, which is followed by years of asymptomatic period.
- Diagnosis by examination of CSF for pleocytosis, increase protein concentration, VDRL reactivity.
- A positive CSF VDRL makes the diagnosis of neurosyphilis.
- The quantitative estimation of reaginic antibodies (e.g. by VDRL) is a good prognostic marker used for treatment of syphilis.
- A four-fold decrease in titer following therapy suggests adequate therapy, whereas a four-fold increase in titer of reaginic antibodies following therapy suggests reinfection or relapse.
- If both test i.e. VDRL and FTA- ABS IgM (specific) test are positive in the infant then congenital syphilis should be strongly suspected and the child should be treated.
- A positive test confirms neurosyphilis but a negative result does not rule out neurosyphilis. Due to the low sensitivity of the CSF -VDRL, fluorescent treponemal antibody absorption test (FTA-ABS) can be used to supplement VDRL.
- VDRL test is also used for monitoring the treatment response.
- VDRL has to be done at 3 months' intervals for at least 1 year.

97. Diagnostic test for neurosyphilis: *(NEET 2019)*

a. VDRL
b. RPR
c. TPI
d. FTA-ABS

Ans. is 'a''VDRL

98. Most effective test for prognosis of syphilis is:

a. VDRL b. FTA-ABS
c. TP-PA d. CFT

Ans. is 'a' VDRL

- ***Leptospira interrogans*** belongs to spirochetes, causes leptospirosis a zoonotic infection.
- The 3 important epidemiological determinants for leptospirosis include exposure to rodents, rainfall and rice field.
- **Weil's disease** (Hepato-renal-hemorrhagic syndrome), a severe form of icteric illness occurs in 10% patients.
- **Specimens for diagnosis:** CSF, blood and urine
- Dark-field microscopy or by immunofluorescence or light microscopy after silver impregnation staining used for diagnosis of leptospirosis.
- EMJH (Ellinghausen, McCullough, Johnson, Harris) medium, Korthof's and Fletcher's media used for culture.
- **Microscopic agglutination test [MAT]** (Gold Standard and reference test) detects antibodies against specific serovars of *L. interrogans* and also Macroscopic agglutination test used for diagnosis.
- Treatment with Doxycycline and Penicillin.

99. Microbiological test used for diagnosing *Leptospira* infection: *(NEET 2019)*

a. Cold agglutination
b. Standard agglutination
c. Microscopic agglutination
d. None of these

Ans. is 'c' Microscopic agglutination

MYCOBACTERIUM

Mycobacterium. tuberculosis discovered by Robert Koch. It is gram-positive, obligate aerobe, acid-fast, straight or slightly curved bacilli. Electron microscopy shows thick cell wall.

- Generation time of tubercle bacillus—14 hours.
- Generation time of lepra bacillus—12–13 days.
- Fish tank granuloma, also called 'swimming pool granuloma' is caused by *M. marinum.*

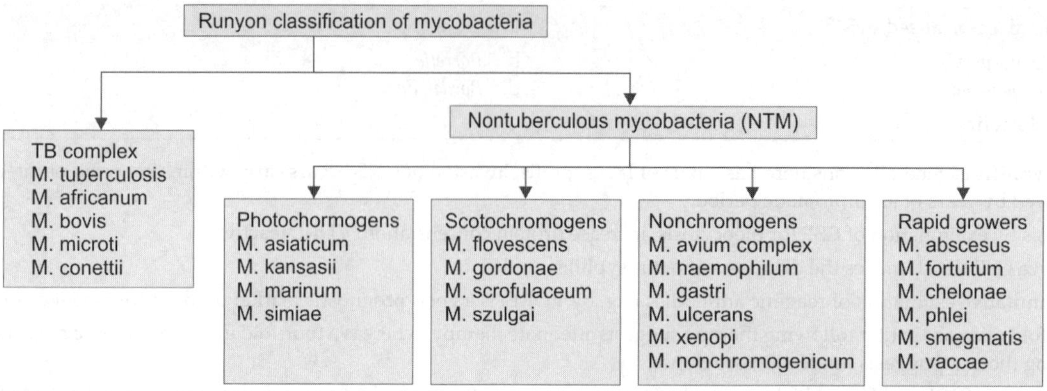

100. Not true about tubercular bacilli:

a. Facultative anaerobe
b. Discovered by Robert Koch
c. Gram positive
d. Has thick cell wall

Ans. is 'a' Facultative anaerobe

101. Generation time for *M. tuberculosis*:

a. 10–15 minutes
b. 10–15 hours
c. 10–15 days
d. 5–10 days

Ans. is 'b' 10–15 hours

102. Which is a photochromogens?

a. *M. marinum*
b. *M. tuberculosis*
c. *M. ulcerans*
d. *M. xenopi*

Ans. is 'a' *M. marinum*

103. Swimming pool granuloma is caused by:

a. *M. fortuitum*
b. *M. kansasii*
c. *M. marinum*
d. *M. leprosy*

Ans. is 'c' *M. marinum*

DRUGS OF CHOICE FOR CHEMOPROPHYLAXIS

Infection	Drug of choice for chemoprophylaxis
• Cholera	• Tetracycline
• Plague	• Tetracycline
• *P. jirovecii* infection	• Cotrimoxazole
• Whooping cough	• Erythromycin
• Toxoplasmosis	• Cotrimoxazole
• Influenza	• Amantadine
• Rickettsia	• Tetracyclines
• Bird flu	• Oseltamivir
• Gonorrhea/syphilis	• Procaine penicillin
• Meningococci	• Rifampicin (sulfadiazine if strain is sensitive)
• Diphtheria	• Erythromycin
• Flacterial conjuctivitis	• Erythromycin ointment
• TB	• INH
• MAC	• Clarithromycin/Azithromycin
• Malaria	• Chloroquine
• Surgical prophylaxis	• Cefazolin

104. Which of the following is the drug of choice for chemoprophylaxis of cholera?

a. Tetracycline
b. Doxycycline
c. Furazolidone
d. Cotrimoxazole

Ans. is 'a' Tetracycline

VIROLOGY

STRUCTURE OF VIRUS

- The extracellular infectious virus particle is called as the virion.
- The virion consists of a nucleic acid surrounded by a protein coat, the capsid. Capsid is composed of repeating units called capsomeres. The protein making up the capsomere is determined by viral nucleic acid.
- The capsid with the enclosed nucleic acid is known as the nucleocapsid.
- Two kinds of symmetry are encountered in the capsid:
  - Icosahedral (cubical)
  - Helical
- Virion may be enveloped or non-enveloped (naked).
- Envelope is lipoprotein in nature, lipid is derived from host cell, while protein is virus coded.

105. Capsid of virus is coded by:

a. Viral nucleic acid b. Host cell nucleic acid
c. Bacteriophage genome d. Any of the above

Ans. is 'a' Viral nucleic acid

GENERAL PROPERTIES OF DIFFERENT FAMILIES OF VIRUSES

Nucleic acid core	Capsid symmetry	Virion: enveloped or naked	Physical type of nucleic acid	Virus family
DNA	Icosahedral	Naked	ss	Parvoviridae
			ds circular	Polyomaviridae
			ds circular	Papillomaviridae
			ds	Adenoviridae
		Enveloped	ds circular	Hepadnaviridae
			ds	Herpesviridae
	Complex	Enveloped	ds	Poxviridae
RNA	Icosahedral	Naked	ss	Picornaviridae
			ss	Astroviridae
			ss	Caliciviridae
			ds segmented	Reoviridae
		Enveloped	ss	Togaviridae
			ss	Flaviviridae
			ss diploid	Retroviridae
			ss	Coronaviridae
			ss segmented	Arenaviridae
			ss segmented	Orthomyxoviridae
	Helical	Enveloped	ss segmented	Bunyaviridae
			ss	Birnaviridae
			ss	Rhabdoviridae
			ss	Paramyxoviridae
			ss	Filoviridae

- All DNA viruses have linear DNA, except:
  - Papovaviridae and
  - Hepadnaviridae, which have circular DNA.
- All DNA viruses have double stranded DNA, except Parvovirus which has single stranded DNA.
- All RNA viruses have linear RNA, except
  - Arenaviridae and
  - Bunyaviridae, which have circular RNA
- All RNA viruses have single stranded RNA, except reoviridae (Rotavirus) which has double stranded RNA.

106. Single stranded DNA virus:

a. Papilloma virus
b. Parvovirus
c. Hepadna virus
d. Herpesvirus

Ans. is 'b' Parvovirus

107. Nonenveloped RNA virus:

a. Rotavirus
b. Togavirus
c. Herpesvirus
d. Chickenpox

Ans. is 'a' Rotavirus

CLASSIFICATION OF VIRUSES

DNA viruses	
Poxviridae	Variola, vaccinia, cowpox, monkey pox, tanapox, Molluscum contagiosum
Herpesviridae	HSV-1, HSV-2, varicella-zoster, EBV, CMV, HTLV-1, RK-virus
Adenoviridae	Adenovirus
Parvoviridae	Parvovirus, adenosatellovirus, densovirus
Papillomaviridae	Papilloma virus (HPV)
Polyomaviridae	Polyomavirus, JC virus, BK virus, Merkel cell polyomavirus
Hepadnaviridae	Hepatitis-B virus

RNA viruses	
Picornaviridae	Poliovirus, coxsackie virus, echovirus, enterovirus, rhinovirus, Hepatitis A virus
Caliciviridae	Norwalk virus, Hepatitis E virus
Togaviridae	Rubella virus, Eastern equine encephalitis virus, Western equine encephalitis virus
Flaviviridae	Yellow fever virus, Dengue virus, St. Louis encephalitis virus, West Nile virus, Hepatitis C virus, Hepatitis G virus
Coronaviridae	Coronaviruses
Rhabdoviridae	Rabies virus, Vesicular stomatitis virus
Filoviridae	Marburg virus, Ebola virus
Paramyxoviridae	Parainfluenza virus, Respiratory syncytial virus, Newcastle disease virus, Mumps virus, Rubeola (measles) virus
Orthomyxoviridae	Influenza virus
Reoviridae	Rotavirus, Reovirus, Colorado tick fever virus
Retroviridae	HIV, HTLV (Human T lymphotropic virus)
Bunyaviridae	Hantavirus, Sand fly fever virus

108. Rubella virus belongs to which family? *(NEET 2019)*

a. Rheovirus
b. Togavirus
c. Picornavirus
d. Orthomyxovirus

Ans. is 'b' Togavirus

109. Molluscum contagiosum is caused by:

a. Poxvirus
b. Picornavirus
c. Bunyaviridae
d. Togaviridae

Ans. is 'a' Poxvirus

110. Ebola virus belongs to:

a. Picornaviridae
b. Togaviridae
c. Flaviviridae
d. Filoviridae

Ans. is 'd' Filoviridae

111. Virus which belongs to Rhabdoviridae:

a. West Nile virus
b. Vesicular stomatitis virus
c. Newcastle disease virus
d. Rhinovirus

Ans. is 'b' Vesicular stomatitis virus

112. Influenza is caused by which virus?

a. Paramyxovirus
b. Orthomyxovirus
c. Bunyaviridae
d. Togaviridae

Ans. is 'b' Orthomyxovirus

113. Which flavivirus causes hepatitis?

a. Hepatitis A
b. Hepatitis B
c. Hepatitis E
d. Hepatitis C

Ans. is 'd' Hepatitis C

114. Which of the following is Hepadna virus?

a. HAV
b. HBV
c. HCV
d. HDV

Ans. is 'b' HBV

ONCOGENIC VIRUSES

Many viruses have been implicated in the causation of cancers:

- RNA viruses
  - All oncogenic RNA viruses belong to family retroviridae.
  - Human T-cell lymphotropic virus (causing Adult T-cell lymphoma).
- DNA viruses
  - *DNA viruses causing cancers are*:
    - *Papillomaviridae (HPV)*: Causes cervical carcinoma, SCC and oropharyngeal carcinoma.
    - *Herpesviridae*: These viruses are:
      - *EBV*: Causes nasopharyngeal carcinoma and Burkitt's lymphoma.
      - *HHV-8*: It causes Kaposi's sarcoma.
    - *Hepadnaviridae (HBV)*: It causes hepatocellular carcinoma.
    - *Flaviviridae (HCV)*: It causes hepatocellular carcinoma
    - *Merkel cell polyomavirus:* It causes Merkel cell carcinoma.

115. Not a DNA oncovirus:

a. HSV-2
b. HPV
c. HTLV
d. HBV

Ans. is 'c' HTLV

EBV ASSOCIATED MALIGNANCIES

- Burkitt's lymphoma
- Hodgkin's disease (mixed cellularity type)
- T cell lymphoma
- Gastric carcinoma
- Angiocentric nasal NK/T cell immunoproliferative lesions
- Angioimmunoblastic lymphadenopathy
- Nasopharyngeal carcinoma
- Tonsillar carcinoma
- Thymoma
- CNS lymphoma in AIDS and transplant recipient
- Leiomyosarcoma.

Other Associated Non-Malignant Conditions

- Oral hairy leukoplakia in AIDS patients
- Chronic fatigue syndrome
- X-linked lymphoproliferative syndrome (Duncan's disease).

116. EBV causes which of the following?

a. Burkitt's lymphoma
b. Hodgkin's lymphoma
c. Nasopharyngeal carcinoma
d. All of the above

Ans. is 'd' All of the above

117. Oral hairy leukoplakia is caused by:

a. HSV
b. EBV
c. CMV
d. HPV

Ans. is 'b' EBV

INCLUSION BODIES

Intracytoplasmic	Acidophilic	Negri bodies	Rabies
		Guarnieri bodies Bollinger bodies Henderson-Peterson bodies Paschen Halber Staedter Prowazek (HD body)	Variola, vaccinia Fowlpox Molluscum contagiosum Smallpox Chlamydia trachomatis
	Basophilic	Levinthal Cole Lillie (LCL Body)	Chlamydia psittaci
Intra nuclear	Acidophilic	Cowdry type A (granular)	Herpes, Chickenpox, CMV, Yellow fever
		Torres bodies	Yellow fever
		Cowdry type B	Polio virus
	Basophilic	Cowdry type B	Adenovirus
Both intracytoplasmic and intranuclear		Warthin Finkeldey	Measles

Note: CMV produces intranuclear 'owl's eye inclusion body.

118. All viruses are associated with specific inclusion body, *except*:

a. CMV
b. Molluscum contagiosum
c. EBV
d. Yellow fever

Ans. is 'c' EBV

119. Inclusion body of CMV is:

a. Cowdry type A
b. Cowdry type B
c. Intranuclear
d. Cytoplasmic

Ans. is 'c' Intranuclear

120. Both intranuclear and cytoplasmic inclusion is seen in:

a. Poxvirus
b. Herpes virus
c. Measles virus
d. Mumps virus

Ans. is 'c' Measles virus

CULTIVATION OF VIRUSES

- As viruses are obligate intracellular parasites they cannot be grown on any inanimate culture medium.

Three methods are employed for cultivation of viruses:

1. Animal inoculation

- Mice are most widely employed animals. Other animals used are guinea pigs, rabbits and ferrets.
- Usually adult mice are used, but for coxsackie virus, suckling mice are used as adult mice are not susceptible.

2. Embryonated eggs:

- Sites of inoculation are:
  - Chorioallantoic membrane—visible pocks are produced—HSV, Vaccinia, Smallpox, Cowpox, Camel pox.
  - Amniotic sac—Influenza, mumps.
  - Allantoic cavity—Influenza, Some paramyxoviruses
  - Yolk Sac—some viruses, Chlamydia, Rickettsia.

3. Tissue culture:

Most important method for virus isolation.

Three types of tissue culture are available:

- ❖ Organ culture
- ❖ Explant culture
- ❖ Cell culture (routinely employed).

Cell Culture

It is the most commonly employed method for virus isolation. It is of following types:

Primary cell culture: Cannot be maintained in serial cultures. Examples are Rhesus monkey kidney, Human amnion, chick embryo fibroblast and human embryonic kidney.

Diploid cell strains: Can be maintained in serial culture for a limited number of times (about 50 passages). Examples are WI-38, HL-8 and human diploid fibroblast.

Human diploid fibroblasts cell line is used for cultivation of coxsackie-A 7,9,16; CMV; Echovirus enteroviruses; HSV-1, 2; Poliovirus; parainfluenza virus, rhinovirus and VZV.

Continuous cell line: Can be maintained in serial culture indefinitely. Examples are HeLa, HEp-2, McCoy, Vero cells, BHK and Detroid-6.

121. HeLa cell line belongs to:

a. Primary cell culture b. Diploid cell strains
c. Continuous cell line d. Tissue culture

Ans. is 'c' Continuous cell line

CHICKENPOX

- ❖ Varicella zoster virus (VZV) is Herpes simplex virus type III (HSV-III) causative agent of **chickenpox** and **herpes-zoster (Shingles)**.
- ❖ It is an acute respiratory infection with incubation period 10–21days.
- ❖ Infection is acquired through respiratory tract via air droplets or rarely from conjunctiva.
- ❖ Infectious period (communicable period) for chickenpox is 2 days prior to 5 days after onset of rash, with a very high secondary attack rate of 90%.
- ❖ Chickenpox usually affects children of age group 5–9 years.
- ❖ Clinical features of chickenpox have two stages:
  1. Pre-eruptive stage
     - Characterized by fever, back pain, malaise and shivering.
  2. Eruptive stage
     - It is characterized by a characteristic rash with following features (which must be differentiated from rash of smallpox):
- ❖ Superficial and unilocular (rash of smallpox is deep seated and multilocular).
- ❖ Symmetrical, mostly on flexor surface (rash of smallpox usually affect extensor surface).
- ❖ **Centripetal** distribution (rash of smallpox has centrifugal distribution).
- ❖ Affects axilla but spares palms and soles (rash of smallpox affects palms and soles but spares axilla).
- ❖ Pleomorphic, with appearance of all stages of rash simultaneously (rash is monomorphic in nature in smallpox).
- ❖ Dew-drop on rose petal appearance (rash of smallpox has often umbilicated appearance).
- ❖ Area of inflammation around the rash (in smallpox there is no inflammation around the rash).
- ❖ Evolution of rash is rapid, scabs begin to form 4–7 days after rash (evolution is slow, scabs begin 10–14 days after rash).
- ❖ The chickenpox rash first appears on the **face** or trunk before spreading to other part of body. Though the disease affects children commonly, it is more severe in adults than in children.
- ❖ Primary infection with VZV causes chickenpox. Once chickenpox has resolved, the virus may remain inactive in nerve cells.
- ❖ Virus remains dormant in sensory ganglion of trigeminal nerve and reaches the eye along branches of the **ophthalmic division of the 5th nerve**—Most common nerve involved.
- ❖ Reactivation of latent VZV, when immunity has fallen to ineffective levels causes—**Herpes zoster.**
- ❖ When it reactivates, it travels from the nerve body to the endings in the skin, producing blisters. Risk factors for reactivation include old age, poor immune function.
- ❖ Shingles is characterized by a painful skin rash with blisters in a localized area. Head, neck and trunk are the most common affected sites.
- ❖ Giemsa staining of the scrapings from the ulcer base (Tzanck smear) reveals cytopathological changes similar to that of HSV infections, such as formation of multinucleated giant cells.
- ❖ For treatment, acyclovir, famciclovir or valacyclovir are the agents of choice.

122. Varicella–zoster virus is not associated with:

a. Latent infection
b. Chickenpox
c. Centrifugal rash
d. Thrombocytopenia

Ans. is 'c' Centrifugal rash

123. Identify the image: *(NEET 2019)*

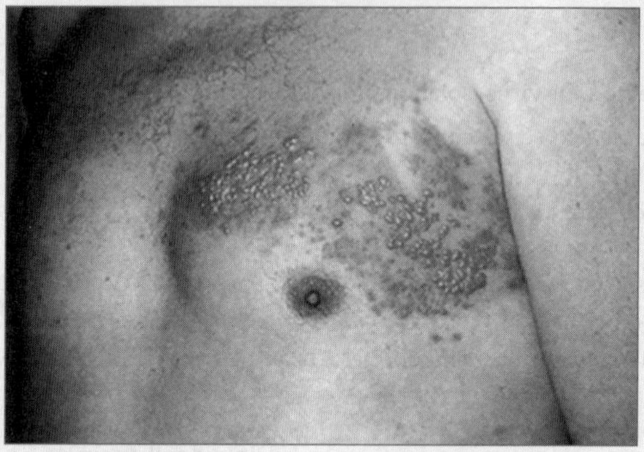

a. Herpes Zoster
b. Small pox
c. Chicken pox
d. Atopic dermatitis

Ans. is 'a' Herpes Zoster

RUBELLA

Rubella virus an enveloped ssRNA virus is the only member of the genus Rubivirus and belongs to the family of Togaviridae, which causes rubella, and congenital rubella syndrome when infection occurs during the first trimester of pregnancy.

Postnatal Rubella

- Rubella spread person-to-person by respiratory droplets via upper respiratory mucosa as it replicates locally in the nasopharynx.
- Incubation period: 14 days (12–23 days).
- Rashes are often first manifestations in children, but in older children and adults, 1 to 5 day prodrome often precedes the rash, which includes low-grade fever, malaise, and upper respiratory symptoms.
- Rashes are generalized and maculopapular in nature, start on the face, extend to trunk and extremities, and disappear in 3 days.
- **Forchheimer spots** may be seen in some cases. Pin head petechiae develop on the soft palate and uvula.
  Classical triad of congenital rubella syndrome:
  - Salt-and-pepper retinopathy and Cataract
  - Deafness (Sensorineural deafness ~58%)
  - Congenital heart defects (Patent ductus arteriosus ~50%).
- CNS defects: microcephaly, mental retardation, motor delay and autism.
- Transient changes such as hepatosplenomegaly, bone lesion, IUGR and thrombocytopenia with petechiae **(Blueberry Muffin syndrome)** may be seen.
- Outcome in the fetus may be miscarriage, fetal death, or premature birth with congenital defects.
- IgM antibodies do not cross placenta; their presence in a neonate is diagnostic of congenital rubella infection.

124. True about triad of congenital rubella syndrome: *(NEET 2019)*

a. PDA, cataract and deafness is seen
b. Hepatosplenomegaly, mental retardation, deafness
c. Chorioretinitis, multiorgan failure, pneumonitis
d. None of these

Ans. is 'a' PDA, cataract and deafness is seen

INFLUENZA VIRUS

- *Orthomyxoviruses*: Enveloped, negative-ssRNA viruses with 8-segment genome.
- Contain hemagglutinin (binds sialic acid and promotes viral entry) and neuraminidase (promotes progeny virion release) antigens. Patients at risk for fatal bacterial superinfection, most commonly *S aureus*, *S pneumoniae*, and H *influenzae*.

- *Genetic/Antigenic shift*: Causes pandemics. Reassortment of viral genome segments, such as when segments of human flu A virus reassort with swine flu A virus. Within the past one hundred years, four pandemics have resulted from the emergence of a novel influenza strain for which humans possessed little or no immunity: The H1N1 Spanish flu (1918), the H2N2 Asian flu (1957), the H3N2 Hong Kong flu (1968), and the H1N1 swine flu (2009).
- *Genetic/Antigenic drift*: Causes epidemics. Minor (antigenic drift) changes based on random mutation in hemagglutinin or neuraminidase genes
- Reformulated vaccine ("the flu shot") contains viral strains most likely to appear during the flu season, due to the virus' rapid genetic change. Killed viral vaccine is most frequently used. Live attenuated vaccine contains temperature-sensitive mutant that replicates in the nose but not in the lung; administered intranasally.

125. Which is the latest pandemic strain of influenza? *(NEET 2020)*

a. H1N1
b. H5N7
c. H5N1
d. H7N9

Ans. is 'a' H1N1

HEPATITIS VIRUSES

	HAV	HBV	HCV	HDV	HEV
Common name	Infectious hepatitis	Serum hepatitis	Non A non B or post transfusion hepatitis	Delta agent	Non A non B enteric transmitted
Family	Picorna (Entero 72)	Hepadnaviridae	Flaviviridae	Viroid like	Caliciviridae
Age	Children, young adults	Young, adults, babies, toddlers	Any age but more common in adults	Any age (similar to HBV)	Young adult (20–40 years)
Route	Feco-oral (mc), blood (+/–) sexual (+/–)	Blood (mc), sexual, vertical	Blood (mc), sexual (+/–) vertical (+/–)	Blood (mc), sexual (++) Vertical (+)	Feco-oral
I.P (days)	15–45, mean 30	30–180, mean 60–90	15–160, mean 50	30–180, mean 60–90	10–60, mean 40
Onset	Acute	Insidious	Insidious	Insidious	Acute
Fulminant	0.1%	0.1–1%	0.1%	5–20%	Usually 1–2% and pregnancy 20–40%
Carrier	None	Occasional (90% of neonates)	Common (85%)	Common	None
Oncogenic	Nil	Present (neonate)	Present	+/–	Nil
Associated other feature	Secondary attack rate 10–20%	HCC, cirrhosis, autoimmune disorder like AGN, arthritis PAN	HCC, cirrhosis, autoimmune- AGN arthritis, cryoglobulinemia	HCC, cirrhosis fulminant hepatitis	Secondary attack rate 1–2% not seen western countries
Prognosis	Excellent	Worse with age, debility	Moderate	Acute-good chronic-poor	Good
Prophylaxis	IG, inactivated vaccine	HBIG, recombinant vaccine	None	HBV vaccine (none for HBV carriers)	Recombinant
Therapy	None	Interferon, lamivudine, adefovir, entecavir	Pegylated interferon plus boceprevir	Interferon ± ribavirin telaprevir	None

Hepatitis A Virus (HAV)

- HAV is responsible for acute hepatitis only. Often, this is an anicteric illness, with clinical symptoms indistinguishable from other forms of viral gastroenteritis, particularly is in young children.
- The illness is much more likely to be symptomatic in older adolescents or adults, in patients with underlying liver disorders, and in those who are immunocompromized. It is characteristically an acute febrile illness with an abrupt onset of anorexia, nausea, malaise, vomiting and jaundice.
    - *In young children*: Mild anicteric gastroenteritis
    - *In older adolescents or adults*: Acute icteric febrile illness.

126. True about hepatitis A virus:

a. Transmitted by percutaneous route
b. Is Enterovirus -70
c. Causes acute hepatitis
d. Mostly affects adult age group

Ans. is 'c' Causes acute hepatitis

Microbiology

Hepatitis B Virus (HBV)

- A dsDNA virus belongs to hepadnaviridae family. The virus particle (size 30–42 nm) consists of an outer lipid envelope and an icosahedral nucleocapsid core composed of protein.
- The 42 nm virions, which are capable of infecting hepatocytes are referred to as **'Dane particles' (**first demonstrated by Dane in 1970).
- By electron microscopy three types of particles can be seen in the serum from patients with hepatitis B. These are:
  - Spherical particles measuring 22 nm in diameter
  - Filamentous or tubular particles with a diameter of 22 nm and of varying length
  - Double-walled, spherical structures measuring 42 nm in diameter. The former two particles are antigenically identical and are known as hepatitis B surface antigen, or HBsAg. The latter particle is the complete hepatitis viral particle known as **Dane particle.**

Virion (Dane particle)

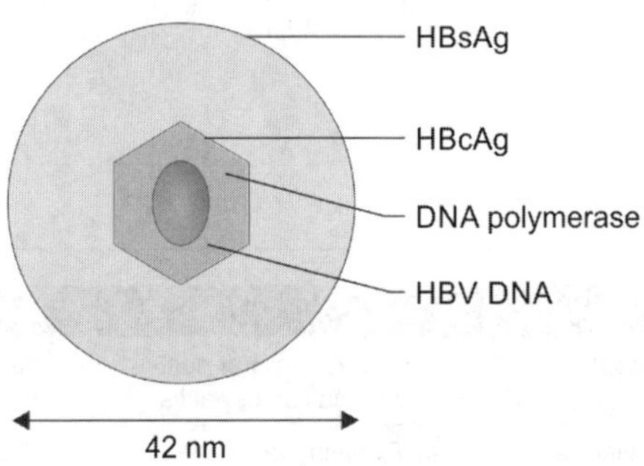

HBsAg particles

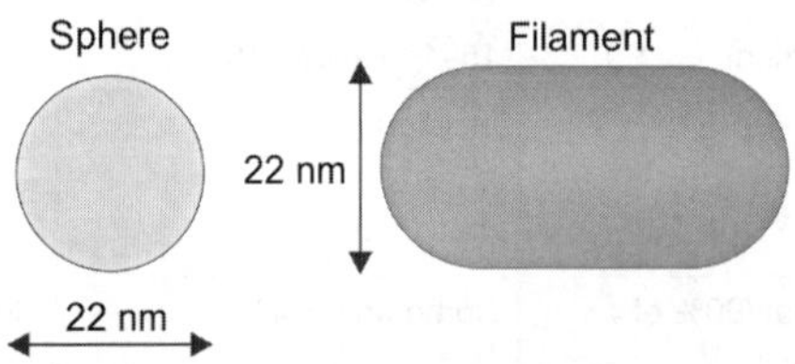

- There are four known genes encoded by genome—C, X, P, S.

Genes	Regions	Gene products	
S	S	Major protein (S)	HBsAg
	S + pre-S2	Middle protein (M)	HBsAg
	S + pre-S1 and S2	Large protein (L)	HBsAg
C	C	HBc Ag	
	C + preC	HBe Ag	
P	DNA Polymerase	DNA Polymerase	
X	HBx Ag	HBx Ag	

- P gene is the largest gene.
- X-gene codes for HBx Ag, which can transactivate the transcription of cellular and viral genes and may contribute to carcinogenesis. HBx Ag and its antibody are present in patients with severe chronic hepatitis and hepatocellular carcinoma.

> - P-gene encodes for DNA polymerase which has two activities:
>   – (i) DNA dependent DNA polymerase and (ii) Reverse transcriptase.

127. What is Dane particle? *(NEET 2018)*

a. HBVDNA
b. HBsAg + HBV DNA
c. HCV
d. HBeAg

Ans. is 'b' HBsAg + HBV DNA

128. Core antigen (HBc) in HBV is encoded by which gene? *(NEET 2018)*

a. S
b. C
c. P
d. X

Ans. is 'b' C

Microbiology

COXSACKIE VIRUSES

- *Coxsackie A (Serotypes 1 to 24)*: Cause aseptic meningitis (especially A7 and A9), Herpangina, febrile illness, acute hemorrhagic conjunctivitis (by A-24, enterovirus 70), and Hand-foot-mouth disease.
- *Coxsackie B (Serotypes 1 to 6)*: Cause a septic meningitis (all serotypes), neonatal disease, Bornholm disease (pleurodynia or epidemic myalgia), myocarditis, hepatitis, pancreatitis leading to juvenile diabetes mellitus (serotype B4), and pneumonia.
- *Hand, foot and mouth disease (HFMD)*: It is characterized by oral and pharyngeal ulcerations and vesicular rashes of the palms and soles which heal without crusting. It is particularly associated with **Coxsackievirus A-16** and Enterovirus 71.
- **Acute hemorrhagic conjunctivitis** is caused by Coxsackievirus A-24 and Enterovirus 70. It is a highly contagious ocular infection which can cause large-scale epidemics.

129. Coxsackievirus A-16 causes: *(NEET 2019)*

a. Yellow fever
b. Hand-foot-mouth disease
c. Rocky mountain spotted fever
d. Encephalomyocarditis

Ans. is 'b' Hand-foot-mouth disease

130. Acute hemorrhagic conjunctivitis is caused by which enterovirus? *(NEET 2018)*

a. Enterovirus 70
b. Enterovirus 71
c. Adenovirus
d. Enterovirus 69

Ans. is 'a' Enterovirus 70

131. Hand-foot-mouth disease is caused by: *(NEET 2018)*

a. Enterovirus-70
b. Coxsackie-A virus
c. Coxsackie-B virus
d. Enterovirus

Ans. is 'b' Coxsackie-A virus

132. Herpangina is caused by: *(NEET 2018)*

a. Adenovirus
b. Enterovirus–72
c. Coxsackie virus A
d. Coxsackie virus B

Ans. is 'c' Coxsackie virus A

HERPES SIMPLEX VIRUS

- There are two types of HSV; HSV-1 and HSV-2.
- Both HSV-1 and 2 have been isolated nearly all mucocutaneous sites and viscera.
- HSV-1 usually produces lesions above the waist (most common site- around mouth) and HSV-2 usually produces lesion below the waist (most common site- genital area).
- HSV-1: undergoes latency in trigeminal ganglia
- HSV-2: undergoes latency in sacral ganglia

Herpes simplex virus (HSV)	
HSV Type 1	***HSV Type 2***
Cause lesion in and around mouth	Cause lesion around genital area
Transmitted by direct contact or droplet spread	Usually transmitted sexually
Replicate poorly in chick embryo fibroblast cell	Replicate well
HSV Type 1	***HSV Type 2***
Relatively sensitive to antiviral agents	Resistant
Less neurovirulent	More neurovirulent
Infectivity is less temperature sensitive	More temperature sensitive
Site of latency –trigeminal ganglia	Sacral ganglia
On chick embryo CAM, form smaller pock	Form larger pock

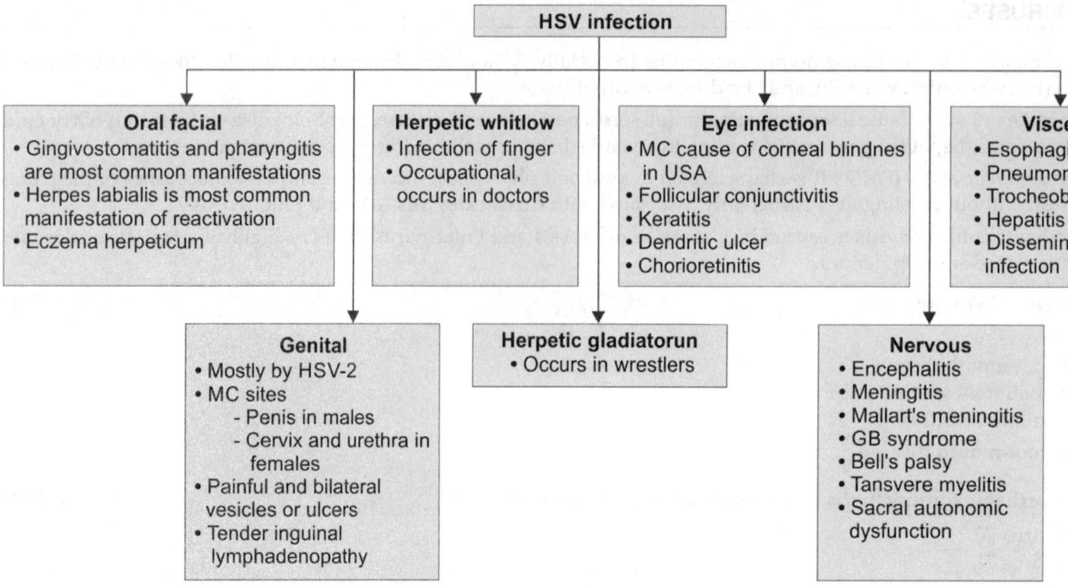

133. A patient presents with recurrent painful lesions as shown below. What is the diagnosis? *(NEET 2020)*

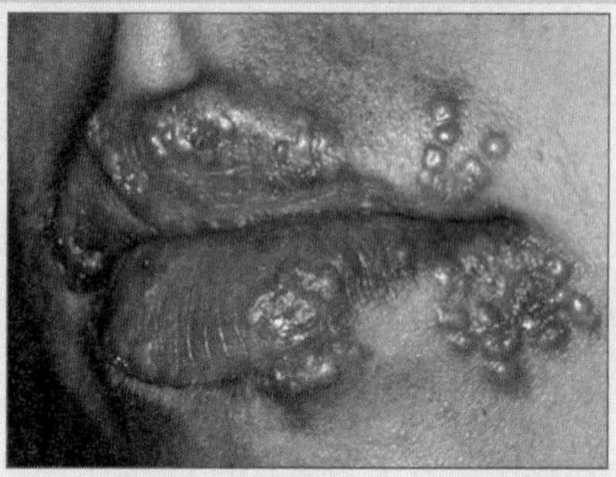

a. Herpangina
b. Ludwig angina
c. Herpes labialis
d. Trench mouth

Ans. is 'c' Herpes labialis

134. HSV-2 predominantly affects which part of body?

a. Face
b. Chest
c. Genital area
d. Back

Ans. is 'c' Genital area

135. HSV-2 causes latent infection in which nerve plexus/ganglia?

a. Trigeminal ganglion
b. Otic ganglion
c. Sacral ganglion
d. Ciliary ganglion

Ans. is 'c' Sacral ganglion

136. All infections are caused by HSV *except*:

a. Whitlow
b. Pharyngitis
c. Condyloma
d. Meningitis

Ans. is 'c' Condyloma

CYTOMEGALOVIRUS (CMV)

- Largest virus amongst herpesviruses, also known as salivary gland virus.
- They are characterized by enlargement of infected cells (cytomegalic cells) and intranuclear inclusions.
- Intranuclear inclusion is eccentrically placed and is surrounded by a halo—owl's eye appearance.
- Once infected an individual carries CMV for life.
- CMV is the most common organism causing intrauterine infection.
- CMV is the most common pathogen complicating organ transplantation.

Clinical Manifestations

- Most of the infections in immunocompetent persons are asymptomatic.
- Clinical features are divided into:
  1. **Congenital infection:**
     - Infection is acquired in pregnancy.
     - Cytomegalovirus infection is a common cause of congenital infections. Infections acquired in utero may take many forms. In approx. 95% of cases, it is asymptomatic. However, sometimes when virus is acquired from a mother with primary infection (who does not have protective immunoglobulins), classic **cytomegalic inclusion disease** (CID) develops.
     - CID resembles **Erythroblastosis fetalis**. Most common presentation is petechiae, hepatosplenomegaly and jaundice. Other features are microcephaly, cerebral calcification, chorioretinitis, IUGR, prematurity and thrombocytopenia.
  2. **Perinatal infection:**
     - Infection is acquired during delivery or postnatally by breastfeeding. Most patients are asymptomatic.
  3. **Beyond neonatal period:**
     - Most common presentation is heterophile antibody-negative mononucleosis (CMV mononucleosis).
  4. **Immunocompromised host:**
     - It causes retinitis, colitis, gastritis, esophagitis, pneumonitis, fever, leukopenia and hepatitis.
     - Maximum risk of infection after kidney transplant is between 1–4 months after transplantation. Most common presentation is fever, leukopenia and hepatosplenomegaly.
     - Most common presentation after bone marrow transplantation is interstitial pneumonia.

Laboratory Diagnosis

- Definitive diagnostic test (most specific test) is isolation of virus from urine, saliva, blood or bronchoalveolar washing.
- Most sensitive testis PCR for viral genome (DNA) detection in blood or intraocular fluid (in CMV retinitis).
- Serology (IgM or IgG) is not very useful.

Treatment

- Ganciclovir or valganciclovir are drugs of choice. Foscarnet is used for CMV retinitis.

137. Which of these infections resembles erythroblastosis? *(NEET 2019)*

a. EBV
b. CMV
c. HSV
d. *Staphylococcus*

Ans. is 'b' CMV

PARVOVIRUS B-19

- Parvovirus are nonenveloped ssDNA viruses.
- Only DNA virus which has single stranded DNA
- Smallest virus with smallest genome
- Only one medically important human parvovirus—Parvovirus B19
- Transmission is by respiratory route and through blood
- Infection is commonly acquired in childhood (5–10 years)
- Most of the infections are asymptomatic
- Most common presentation is respiratory infection with an erythematous maculopapular rash and arthralgia—**Erythema infectiosum** or **Fifth disease**
- Starts with prominent erythema of cheeks—**slapped cheek disease**
- Parvovirus B19 induces aplastic crisis in children with chronic hemolytic anemias, as in sickle cell disease
- Parvovirus B19 infection during second or third trimester of pregnancy may result in nonimmune fetal hydrops.

138. Erythema infectiosum is caused by:

a. Parvovirus B19
b. JC virus
c. Rota virus
d. Mumps

Ans. is 'a' Parvovirus B19

RABIES VIRUS

- *Rhabdoviridae contains two genera*:
  - *Vesiculoviruses*: Vesculo-stomatitis virus, Chandipura virus.
  - *Lyssavirus*: Rabies virus.
- It is an enveloped, bullet shaped, negative sense ssRNA virus.

- Rabies virus is sensitive to ethanol, iodine preparations, soap, quaternary ammonium compound, detergents and lipid solvents (like ether, chloroform). It is inactivated by phenol, beta-propiolactone (BPL), formalin, Sun light, UV irradiation, and by heat.
- Rabies is primarily a zoonotic disease of warm-blooded animals, particularly carnivorous such as dogs, cats, jackals and wolves.
- It is transmitted to man usually by bites or licks of rabid animals.
- It is the communicable disease which is always fatal.
- It is dead end infection in man.
- The characteristic histopathological picture in rabies is the intracytoplasmic inclusion body (Negri body) in the neurons, most abundant in the **Cerebellum and Hippocampus**.
- Demonstration of Negri bodies is still the most commonly used method as facilities for immunofluorescence are not available in many laboratories.
- Impression smears of the brain are stained by Seller's technique (basic fuchsin and methylene blue in methanol).
- **Negri bodies** are intracytoplasmic, round to oval, purplish pink structures with characteristic basophilic inner granules.

139. True about rhabdoviridae are all *except*:

a. Includes vesicular stomatitis virus
b. Rabies virus is inactivated by formalin
c. Rabies virus is negative sense double stranded RNA virus
d. All of the above correct

Ans. is 'c' Rabies virus is negative sense double stranded RNA virus

140. Most common site of Negri bodies in rabies:

a. Hypothalamus b. Thalamus
c. Midbrain d. Cerebellum

Ans. is 'd' Cerebellum

JAPANESE ENCEPHALITIS

Japanese encephalitis (JE) is caused by Japanese encephalitis virus (JEV), a leading cause of encephalitis in Asia, including India. It is spread by Culex mosquitoes. Pigs and wild birds serve as a reservoir for the virus.

Transmission Cycle

- Pigs→ *Culex* →Pigs.
- Ardeid birds→ *Culex* →Ardeid birds.

Pigs are considered as **amplifier host** for JE.

Humans are considered as dead end, there no man-mosquito-man cycle (unlike in dengue).

- In India, JE is endemic in many states, Gorakhpur district (UP) accounted for the largest burden.
- Incubation period 5–15 days. Symptoms may include headache, vomiting, fever, confusion, and seizures.
- Lab diagnosis by IgM capture antibody ELISA and Reverse transcriptase PCR for E gene.
- *Vaccine:* Live attenuated SA 14-14-2 vaccine give subcutaneously.

141. Identify the organism with similar life-cycle as shown in the image: *(NEET 2019)*

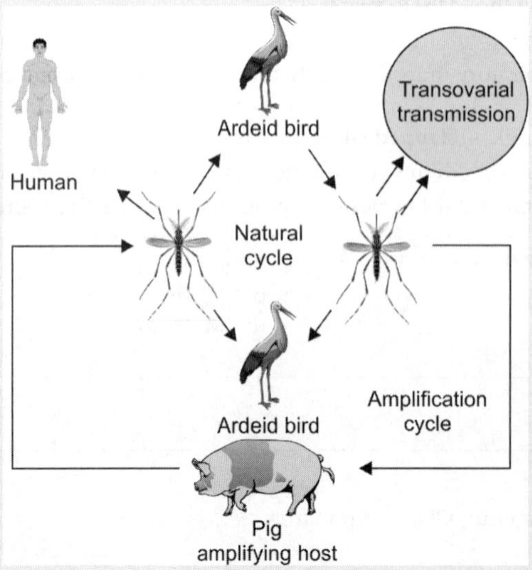

a. Malaria
b. Plague
c. Japanese encephalitis
d. Paragonimus

Ans. is 'c' Japanese encephalitis

142. All are true for Japanese encephalitis *except*: *(NEET 2020)*

a. Pigs are amplifier host
b. Humans are reservoir of infection
c. Vaccination of pigs is an effective control measure
d. Vector is culex vishnuii

Ans. is 'b' Humans are reservoir of infection

YELLOW FEVER

- Caused by Yellow fever virus of Flaviviridae family of hemorrhagic group of arboviruses.
- Its major vector is *Aedes aegypti.*
- *Reservoir of infection are:*
  - Monkeys and forest mosquitoes (forest/sylvian cycle)
  - Man and *Aedes aegypti* (urban cycle).
- Clinical incubation period is 3–6 days. One clinical attack provides lifelong immunity. Infants born of immune mothers have antibodies up to 6 months.
- Presence of fever, chills, headache, dizziness, myalgia, and backache followed by nausea, vomiting, and relative bradycardia, in severe cases hemorrhagic manifestations.
- Lab diagnosis by IgM ELISA and RT-PCR targeting NS5 antigen.
- Yellow fever 17D vaccine: live attenuated, in India prepared in CRI Kasauli; previously used Dakar vaccine derived from mouse brain was encephalitogenic.

143. Vector of yellow fever:

a. *Culex*
b. *Aedes*
c. *Tsetse* fly
d. *Anopheles*

Ans. is 'b' *Aedes*

HIV

- Subtype A is most prevalent worldwide.
- Subtype C is most prevalent in India.

The cells affected are:

- CD4 T Cells (major target)
- B lymphocytes
- Monocytes and macrophages
- Langerhans cells in dermis
- Microglia in the CNS
- Follicular dendritic cells from tonsils can be infected by HIV without the involvement of CD4.

The most common of the opportunistic infections that cause diarrhea in patients with AIDS are CMV infection, cryptosporidiosis, microsporidiosis, and MAC infection. CMV infection is the most common opportunistic viral infection in the GI tract of HIV-infected patients and can cause problems from the mouth to the anus. It most frequently causes a colitis associated with fever, crampy abdominal pain, and frequent (often bloody) stools.

"Cryptosporidium and Cystoisospora are the common causes of prolonged **watery** diarrhea in AIDS patients''.

- Important causes of diarrhea in AIDS patients:
  - *Bacteria*: *Salmonella, Shigella, Campylobacter,* and *Mycobacteria avium intracellulare.*
  - *Fungal*: *Histoplasma, Coccidioides, Penicillium.*
  - *Other*: CMV, *Microsporidia, Cystoisospora belli,* and *Cryptosporidia.*

Resistance to HIV Infection

Many individuals of Eurasian descent (up to 14% in some ethnic groups) have a deletion mutation, called CCR5 delta 32, in the gene encoding CCR5 is a coreceptor found on the surface of T cells that is necessary for many strains of the virus to enter the host cell. The mutation leads to the production of a receptor to which HIV cannot effectively bind and thus blocks viral people homozygous for this mutation have greatly reduced susceptibility to HIV infection, and those who are heterozygous have some protection from infection as well.

144. Which HIV virus is commonest in India subcontinent?

a. A
b. B
c. C
d. D

Ans. is 'c' C

145. CCR5 mutation is related to which condition?

a. Resistance to HIV infection
b. Susceptibility to HIV infection
c. Resistance to HBV infection
d. Susceptibility to HBV infection

Ans. is 'a' Resistance to HIV infection

146. HIV primarily replications in which cells?

a. CD4 T-cells
b. CD8 T-cells
c. Neutrophils
d. Follicular dendritic cells

Ans. is 'a' CD4 T-cells

147. Bloody diarrhea in HIV infected patient is mostly due to:

a. *Cryptosporidium*
b. *Isospora*
c. CMV
d. *Salmonella*

Ans. is 'c' CMV

148. An AIDS patient is presenting with watery diarrhea. What could by the causative organism?

a. *Candida*
b. *Vibrio cholerae*
c. ETEC
d. *Cryptosporidium*

Ans. is 'd' *Cryptosporidium*

ZIKA VIRUS (ZIKV)

- Zika virus (ZIKV) is a flavivirus related to yellow fever virus.
- It is transmitted by *Aedes* mosquito.
- Most common symptoms of Zika are fever, rash, joint pain, and conjunctivitis (red eyes).
- Zika virus infection during pregnancy can cause a serious birth defect called microcephaly as well as other severe fetal brain defects. Once a person has been infected, he or she is likely to be protected from future infections.

149. Zika virus causes:

a. Hepatitis
b. Myocarditis
c. Conjunctivitis
d. Nephritis

Ans. is 'c' Conjunctivitis

150. Vector of zika virus: *(NEET 2020)*

a. Anopheles
b. Culex
c. Aedes
d. Sandfly

Ans. is 'c' Aedes

ROTAVIRUS

- Rotavirus belongs to reoviridae — segmented dsRNA.
- Norwalk virus belongs to calciviridae — nonsegmented ssRNA.
- Both Rotavirus and Norwalk virus are causes of viral gastroenteritis.

Rotavirus Vaccine

- The Rotavirus vaccines are live-attenuated vaccines given orally.
- *Two new vaccines are now in use:*
  - RV5 oral pentavalent vaccine (Rotateq) contains five reassortant rotaviruses developed from S human strains on bovine rotavirus background [These five strains are GI, G2, G3, G4 and P(8)]
  - RV1 monovalent vaccine (Rotarix) contains one live attenuated rotavirus strain [the strain is G1 P(8)]
- Administration of Rotarix (2 doses) and Rotateq (3 doses) needs to be completed by 32 weeks of age to minimize any potential risk of intussusception.

151. What is similar between Rotavirus and Norwalk virus?

a. Both belong to same family
b. Both have segment genome
c. Both have single stranded RNA
d. Both are cause of viral gastroenteritis

Ans. is 'd' Both are cause of viral gastroenteritis

152. Rotateq oral vaccine for rotavirus contains:

a. 2 reassorted rotaviruses
b. 3 reassorted rotaviruses
c. 4 reassorted rotaviruses
d. 5 reassorted rotaviruses

Ans. is 'd' 5 reassorted rotaviruses

RESPIRATORY SYNCYTIAL VIRUS (RSV)

- ssRNA virus from Paramyxoviridae family.
- Respiratory syncytial virus (RSV) is one of the most common diseases of childhood.
- RSV can progress to bronchiolitis and/or pneumonia with an increased chance of significant morbidity or death.
- RSV completes its replication and assembly in the cytoplasm, with no involvement of the host cell nucleus.
- The first step in RSV application is attachment of virus particle to host cell mediated by G protein.
- RSV enters the cell by fusion with plasma membrane mediated by F protein (fusion protein).
- Virus replication and transcription, then occurs in the cytoplasm.
- There is assembly of virus in the cytoplasm which is followed by release of virus.

153. True about respiratory syncytial virus replication:

a. Replicate in the nucleus
b. Attaches to host cell surface by G protein
c. Fusion of host viral cell membrane by G protein
d. All are correct

Ans. is 'b' Attaches to host cell surface by G protein

PRION DISEASE

- Prions are infectious particle which contains protein only.
- They do not have nucleic acid.

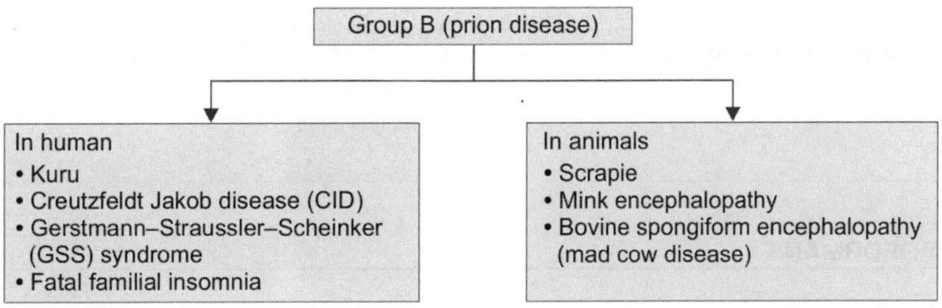

154. Prion structure contains primarily:

a. Protein
b. DNA
c. RNA
d. Both DNA and RNA

Ans. is 'a' Protein

155. Prion disease seen in human:

a. Bovine spongiform encephalopathy
b. Mad cow disease
c. Mink encephalopathy
d. Gerstmann-Straussler-Scheinker syndrome

Ans. is 'd' Gerstmann-Straussler-Scheinker syndrome

BIOTERRORISM AGENTS

- Bioterrorism agents can be separated into three categories, depending on how easily they can be spread and the severity of illness or death they cause.
- Bioterrorism agents of Category A are considered the highest risk and Category C agents are those that are considered emerging threats for disease.
- Important organisms in different categories are:

- *Category A*: Smallpox, Anthrax, Botulism, Plague, tularemia, viral hemorrhagic fever (yellow fever, KFD, Ebola, Marburg, Lassa).
- *Category B*: *Brucella, C. perfringens* (epsilon toxin), *Salmonella, Shigella, E. coli* O157: H7, Staphylococcus (enterotoxin-B), *V. cholerae*, Q fever, Typhus, fever, psittacossis, glanders, Melioidosis.
- *Category C*: Emerging infections like Nipah, Hanta virus, SARS corona virus.

156. Category A Bioterrorism agent:

a. *Brucella*
b. Melioidosis
c. Hanta virus
d. Ebola virus

Ans. is 'd' Ebola virus

157. Which of the following is a class A bioterrorism agent? *(NEET 2020)*

a. *C.Burnetti*
b. *B.anthracis*
c. *Nipah virus*
d. *B.pseudomallei*

Ans. is 'b' *B.anthracis*

MYCOLOGY

CULTURE OF FUNGI

- *Culture media used in mycology are*:
  - Sabouraud's dextrose agar (most common)
  - Czapek-Dox medium
  - Corn meal agar
- Culture media are supplemented with chloramphenicol and Gentamicin to minimize bacterial contamination and cycloheximide to reduce contamination with saprophytic fungi.
- Cultures are incubated at 22–30°C and 37°C.

158. Sabouraud's dextrose agar is used for isolation of:

a. *Pseudomonas*
b. *B. anthracis*
c. Fungi
d. *Ancylostoma*

Ans. is 'c' Fungi

CRYPTOCOCCUS NEOFORMANS

- Four capsular serotypes A, B, C and D
- It has **polysaccharide capsule**
- Most infections in immunocompromised patients are caused by serotype A
- Pigeon droppings commonly contains serotype A and D
- Eucalyptus tree contain serotype B
- *Cryptococcus* is a unique fungus that has a neurotrophic behavior and often causes CNS disease
- *Cryptococcus* is the most common cause of meningitis in HIV infected patients.

Lab Diagnosis

- Specimens include CSF, tissue, exudates, sputum, blood, cutaneous scrapings, and urine.
- Direct microscopy, specimens are often examined in wet mounts, both directly and after mixing with India ink, which delineates the capsule.
- **Mucicarmine** is special stain for *Cryptococcus*. ***Mucicarmine stains*** the mucopolysaccharide of the ***cryptococcal*** capsules.
- Colonies develop within a few days on most media at room temperature or 37°C. Media with cycloheximide inhibit *Cryptococcus* and should be avoided. Cultures can be identified by growth at 37°C and detection of **urease**. Alternatively, on an appropriate diphenolic substrate, the phenol oxidase (or laccase) of *C. neoformans* and *C. gattii* produces melanin in the cell walls and colonies develop a brown pigment.
- Serological tests for capsular antigen, can be performed on CSF, serum, and urine. The latex slide agglutination test or enzyme immunoassay (EIA) for cryptococcal antigen is positive in 90% of patients with cryptococcal meningitis.

159. Special stain for *Cryptococcus*: *(NEET 2019)*

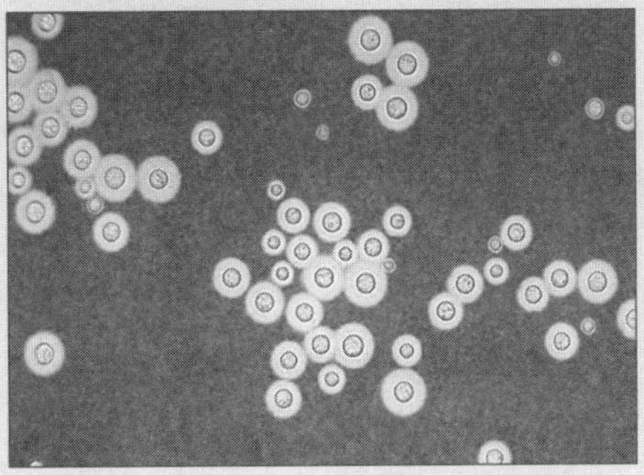

a. ZN stain
b. Gram stain
c. Mucicarmine
d. Malachite green

Ans. is 'c' Mucicarmine

160. An HIV infected patient is presenting with fever, neck rigidity and convulsions. Isolated organism from CSF is showing polysaccharide capsule. The likely causative agent:

a. Cryptococcus
b. Pneumococcus
c. Toxoplasmosis
d. *Neisseria meningitidis*

Ans. is 'a' Cryptococcus

IMPORTANT NEUROTROPIC FUNGI

- *Cryptococcus neoformans*
- *Cladophialophora bantiana*
- *Exophiala dermatitidis*
- *Ramichloridium mackenziei*
- *Ochroconis gallopava*
- *Histoplasma capsulatum.*

161. Neurotropic fungus is:

a. *Trichophyton*
b. *Microsporum*
c. *Cryptococcus*
d. *Sporothrix schenckii*

Ans. is 'c' *Cryptococcus*

ASPERGILLUS

- *Aspergillus* is a mould with septate branching hyphae.
- Ability of *A. fumigatus* to grow at 45°C helps to distinguish it from other species.
- Mode of transmission - Inhalation of *Aspergillus* spores (Conidia) into lungs.
- *Aspergillus fumigatus* is the most common cause of aspergillosis.

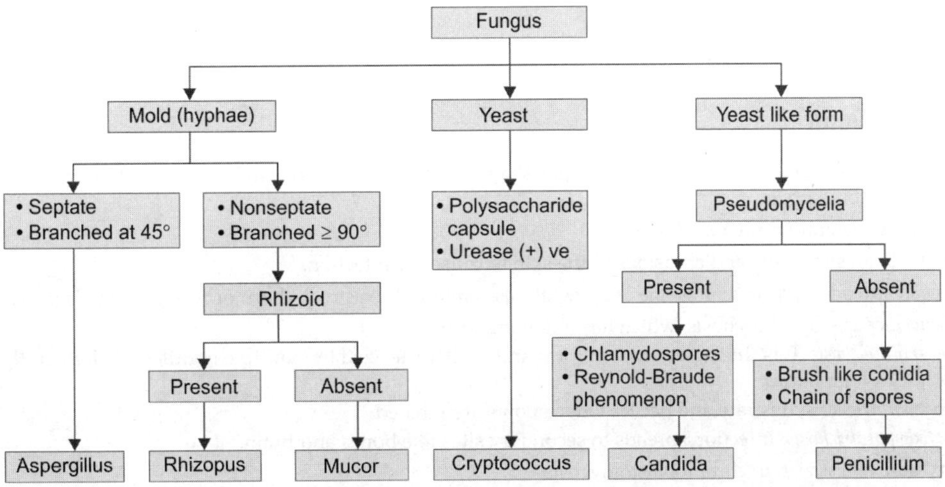

162. *Aspergillus fumigatus* is differentiated from other fungi by:

a. Showing septate hyphae
b. Grow at 45°C
c. Cause respiratory tract infection
d. Most common endemic mycosis

Ans. is 'b' Grow at 45°C

163. *Aspergillus* hyphae branch at what angle?

a. 45°
b. 60–90°
c. 90–120°
d. None

Ans. is 'a' 45°

HISTOPLASMA

- *Histoplasma capsulatum* is a dimorphic fungus.
- It is non-capsulated (Only medically important capsulated fungus is *Cryptococcus*).
- Infectious form is microconidia (small spores) and mode of transmission is inhalation of dust contaminated with bird or bat dropping.
- It causes intracellular infection of reticuloendothelial system.
- Most of the infections are asymptomatic.
- *Histoplasma capsulatum* causes Histoplasmosis also called as Darling's disease or Cave's disease or Caver's disease. Which many manifests as:
  - Acute pulmonary histoplasmosis: Pneumonitis, hilar adenopathy with erythema nodosum and erythema multiforme.

  Caseation necrosis and calcification may mimic tuberculosis
  - Chronic pulmonary histoplasmosis: Fibronodular apical infiltrates.
  - Disseminated infection: Fever, emaciation, lymphadenopathy, hepatosplenomegaly, endocarditis, meningitis.
  - Presumed ocular histoplasmosis syndrome (POHS).

164. Which of the following fungus is exclusively seen in reticuloendothelial cells?

a. Cryptococcus
b. *Candida*
c. *Aspergillus*
d. *Histoplasma*

Ans. is 'd' *Histoplasma*

HAIR PERFORATION TEST

- Hair perforation test is used to distinguish isolates of dermatophytes, particularly *T. mentagrophytes* and its variants.
- *T. mentagrophytes* perforates hair (unlike *T. rubrum*), a feature that is used to distinguish between two species.
- *T. mentagrophytes* produces wedge-shaped areas on hair perforation test.

165. Wedge shaped defect in hair perforation test is seen in:

a. T. rubrum
b. *T. mentagrophytes*
c. *T. tonsurans*
d. All of the above

Ans. is 'b' *T. mentagrophytes*

SPOROTHRIX SCHENCKII

- It is a dimorphic fungus, usually described as tiny, cigar-shaped bodies, 3–5 microns in length, which bear from one to three small oval buds at either or both poles.
- Occasionally a larger asteroid body may be seen.
- Fungus enters through small cuts and abrasions in the skin to cause the infection.
- Because roses can spread the disease, it is one of a few diseases referred to as rose-thorn or rose gardener's disease.
- *Sporothrix schenckii* causes sporotrichosis, which has following forms:
  - *Cutaneous sporotrichosis*: It is the most common form and is characterized by multiple nodules or ulcers at the entry point and along the line of lymphatics.
  - *Pulmonary sporotrichosis*: It is rare and occurs when spores are inhaled.
  - *Disseminated sporotrichosis:* Infection spreads to secondary sites like bones and brain.
- **Copper penny bodies** are seen in chromoblastomycosis.

166. Not true about *Sporothrix schenckii*:

a. Dimorphic fungus
b. Asteroid bodies
c. Copper penny bodies
d. Common in gardners

Ans. is 'c' Copper penny bodies

167. Which of the following fungal infection follows traumatic inoculation? *(NEET 2020)*

a. Blastomycosis
b. Coccidiodes
c. Paracoccidiodes
d. Sporothrix

Ans. is 'd' Sporothrix

TINEA CAPITIS

- Tinea capitis is dermatophytic infection of scalp and scalp hair.
- Occurs commonly in children. It is uncommon in adults (in contrast, T. crusis, T. manuum and T. unguium are common in adults).
- Caused by genera trichophyton or microsporum.
- As epidermophyton does not affect the hair, Epidermophyton does not cause T. capitis.
- Two most common species causing T. capitis are *M. canis* and *T. tonsurans*. Tinea capitis may be two types.
  - *Endothrix*: Invasion of hair shaft by fungus. It is caused by *T. tonsurans* (MC), *T. violaceum, T. schoenleinii.*
  - *Ectothrix*: Fungal invasion is restricted to the outer most cuticle of hair. It is caused by *M. canis* (MC), *M. audouini, T. mentagrophytes.*
- As ectothrix is the commonest type of T. capitis, *Microsporum canis* is the most common cause of T. capitis.

168. Ectothrix is caused by:

a. *T. tonsurans*
b. *T. violaceum*
c. *Microsporum canis*
d. All of the above

Ans. is 'c' *Microsporum canis*

MALASSEZIA FURFUR

- *Malassezia furfur* is a lipophilic fungus that is found in areas of the body that are rich in sebaceous glands, such as neck, chest, or upper arm.
- It causes **tinea versicolor** (pityriasis versicolor).
- Characterized by flat-round scaly patches of hypo- to hyperpigmentation of skin.
- Lesions are non-inflammatory and non-pruritic.
- Examination of skin scrapings shows an abundance of yeast like cells and short, branched filaments.
- The fungus can be grown on Sabouraud's dextrose agar, covered with a layer of olive oil.
- *Seborrheic dermatitis*: another manifestation of *Malassezia furfur*, manifests as erythematous pruritic scaly lesions called dandruff in adults and cradle cap in babies.

169. Lipophilic fungus is:

a. Malassezia furfur
b. Candida
c. Cryptococcus
d. Histoplasma

Ans. is 'a' Malassezia furfur

PARASITOLOGY

ENTAMOEBA HISTOLYTICA

- It is intestinal amoeba, inhabitat in the large intestine of humans and animals.
- Commonly causes amoebic dysentery and amoebic liver abscess.
- Transmitted by feco-oral route.
- Infective form is mature quadrinucleated cyst.
- In stool sample need to differentiate with *Entamoeba coli*, as it is a non-pathogenic amoeba that colonizes the large intestine.

Differences between *Entamoeba histolytica* and *Entamoeba coli*

	Entamoeba histolytica	Entamoeba coli
Trophozoite		
Size	15–20 μm	20–25 μm
Motility	Very active and unidirectional purposeful motility Pseudopodia with finger like projection	Sluggish, non-purposeful and aimless motility in any direction Blunt pseudopodia
Cytoplasm	Clearly differentiated to ectoplasm and endoplasm	Not differentiated
Cytoplasmic inclusions	RRC, leucocytes, tissue debris and bacteria	Same except it does not contain RBC
Nulceus	Karyosome is small and central Nuclear membrane is thin and lined by fine chromatin granules	Karyosome is large and eccentric Nuclear membrane is thick and lined by coarse chromatin granules
Precyst		
	10–20 μm size, oval, no food vacuoles and nucleus and nucleus same as trophozoite	Same as *E. histolytica* except size is 20 μm
Cyst		
Size	12–15 μm	12–25 μm
Nucleus	Same as trophozoite	Same as trophozoite
Number of nuclei	1–4	1–8
Chromatoid body	Thick bars with rounded ends	Filamentous and thread like ends

- Flask shaped ulcers are seen in *Entamoeba histolytica.*
- Disease occurs when amoeba comes in contact with the cells lining of intestine.
- Adherence of *E. histolytica* to colonic mucosa is mediated by Lectin.
- Parasite then induces apoptosis of epithelial cells through a channel forming pore protein
- This process can lead to penetration and digestion of human tissues, resulting *flask-shaped ulcerations* on the intestinal mucosa.
- *Entamoeba histolytica* ingests the destroyed cells by phagocytosis and is often seen with red blood cells (a process known as erythrophagocytosis) inside when viewed in stool samples

170. Flask shaped ulcers are seen in: *(NEET 2019)*

a. *Giardia* b. *Entamoeba histolytica*
c. *H. pylori* d. *Enterobius*

Ans. is 'b' *Entamoeba histolytica*

171. *Entamoeba coli* is differentiated by *Entamoeba histolytica* by presence of:

a. Very active movement b. Thin nuclear membrane
c. Cyst with 1–4 nuclei d. Blunt pseudopodia

Ans. is 'd' Blunt pseudopodia

MICROSCOPIC EXAMINATION OF STOOL

- Concentration techniques for stool processing:
  - Sedimentation technique
  - Floatation technique
- *Sedimentation techniques*: Eggs and cysts settle down at bottom following centrifugation. Most commonly used method is Formalin-ether concentration technique.
- *Floatation techniques*: Eggs and cysts float at the surface due to specific gravity gradient.

Organisms	Technique
• Cyst of G. lamblia • Cyst of E. histolytica • Eggs of Trichuris trichura	Zinc sulphate floatation technique
• Fertilized eggs of Ascaris • Eggs of Ankylostoma duodenale • Eggs of H. nanu • Eggs of Enterobius	Sodium chloride floatation technique
• Oocysts of cryptosporidium • Oocysts of Isospora belli	Sugar floatation technique

Floatation technique is not useful in:
- Unfertilized eggs of *Ascaris*
- Eggs of *T. saginata and T. solium*
- Eggs of all intestinal flukes
- Larvae of *Strongyloides stercoralis*

172. Floatation technique is useful for:

a. Eggs of *Taenia solium*
b. Fertilized eggs of *Ascaris*
c. Eggs of intestinal flukes
d. Larvae of *Strongyloides*

Ans. is 'b' Fertilized eggs of *Ascaris*

LIFE CYCLE OF A PARASITE

- The sequential stages in growth, development and multiplication constitute its life cycle.
- *The life cycle of a parasite may be*:
  - Simple: Requires a single host
  - Complex: Requires more than one host.

Parasite with a simple life cycle	
Parasite	***Host***
Protozoal parasites	
Entamoeba histolytica	Human beings
Giardia lamblia	Human beings
Trichomonas vaginalis	Human beings
Balantidium coli	Pigs and human beings
Helminths (nematodes)	
Ascaris lumbricoides	Human beings
Enterobius vermicularis	Human beings
Strongyloides stercoralis	Human beings
Trichuris trichiura	Human beings
Ancylostoma duodenale	Human beings
Necator americanus	Human beings

Parasites with a complex life cycle with two hosts		
Parasite	***Definitive host***	***Intermediate host***
Protozoal parasites		
Plasmodium spp.	Mosquitoes	Human beings
Leishmania donovani	Rodents, dogs, human beings	Sand flies
Toxoplasma gondii	Cats	Rodents, human beings
Trypanosoma cruzi Trypanosoma brucei	Human beings, animals Human beings, animals	Tritominine bugs Tsetse flies
Cestodes		
Taenia solium	Human beings	Pigs
Taenia saginata	Human beings	Cattle
Echinococcus granulosus	Dogs, other canine animals	Human beings herbivorous animals
Trematodes		
Fasciolopsis buski	Human beings, pigs	Snails
Fasciola hepatica	Human beings, animals	Snails
Schistosoma spp.	Human beings, animals	Snails
Nematodes		
Trichinella spiralis	Human being, pigs	Same animal as intermediate host
Wuchereria bancrofti	Human beings	Mosquitoes
Brugia malayi	Human beings, animals	Mosquitoes
Loa loa	Human beings	Deer flies
Onchocerca volvulus	Human beings	Black flies
Dracunculus medinensis	Human beings	Cyclops

Parasites with a complex life with three hosts			
Parasite	***Definitive host***	***First intermediate host***	***Second intermediate host***
Cestodes Diphyllobothrium (fish tapeworm)	Human beings, animals	Cyclops	Fish
Trematodes Clonorchis sinensis Paragonimus westermani	Human beings, animals Human beings	Snails Snails	Fish Crabs, crayfish

173. Intermediate host is not required for which parasite?

a. *Toxoplasma*
b. *Schistosoma*
c. *Ancylostoma*
d. Fish tapeworm

Ans. is 'c' *Ancylostoma*

LOCALIZATION OF PARASITE IN HUMAN BODY

Organ/tissue	Protozoan parasites	Helminthes
Muscle	*Toxoplasma gondii*	• Trichinella spiralis • Gnathostoma spinigerum • Spirometra • Echinococcus • Taenia solium (cysticercus cellulosae)
Brain	*Acanthamoeba spp.* *Entamoeba histolytica* *Naegleria fowleri* *Plasmodium falciparum* *Trypanosoma brucei* *Trypanosoma cruzi* *Toxoplasma gondii*	• Angiostrongylus cantonensis (larvae) • Echinococcus granulosus (Hydatid cyst) • Gnathostoma spinigerum (larvae) • Paragonimus westermani (adult) • Schistosoma japonicum (egg) • Spirometra spp. (larva) • Toxocara spp. (larva) • Taenia multiceps • Taenia solium (cysticercus cellulosae)
Eyes	*Acanthamoeba*	• Gnathostoma spinigerum (larva) • Loa-Loa (adult) • Oncocercaria (microfilaria) • Echinococcus (hydatid cyst) • *Toxocara (larva)*
Heart	*Trypanosoma cruzi*	• *Echinococcus* (hydatid cyst) • *Toxocara* (Larva)
Lymph nodes	*Trypanosoma brucei* *Toxoplasma gondii*	• B. malayi • W. bancrofti
Liver	*E. histolytica* *Leishmania donovani* *Plasmodium*	• *Ascaris* (larva) • *Echinococcus* (hydatid cyst) • *Fasciola hepatica* • *Clonorchis sinensis* • Opisthorchis viverrini • Opishorchis felineus • Toxocara
Lung	*E. histolytica* *Leishmania donovani* *Trypanosoma cruzi*	• *Ascaris lumbricoides* (larvae) • *Echinococcus granulosus* (hydatid cyst) • *Ancylostoma duodenale* (larvae) • *Necator americanus* (larvae) • *Strongyloides stercoralis* (larvae) • *Toxacara* (larvae) • *Paragonimus westermani* (lung fluke)
Spleen	*Leishmania donovani* *Plasmodium falciparum*	• *E. granulosus* (hydatid cyst).

174. Lung cysts are caused by which parasite?

a. *Ascaris*
b. *Toxocara*
c. *Trypanosoma*
d. *Echinococcus*

Ans. is 'd' *Echinococcus*

175. Lung fluke is:

a. *Echinococcus*
b. *Paragonimus*
c. *Trichinella*
d. *Fasciola*

Ans. is 'b' *Paragonimus*

PARAGONIMUS WESTERMANI

- Paragonimiasis is a food-borne parasitic zoonosis caused by the genus *Paragonimus*. Fresh water snails, crabs, and crayfish are the first and second intermediate hosts, respectively. Humans acquire this infection by ingesting uncooked/undercooked crustaceans.
- The **most important endemic areas** are in the Far East, principally Korea, Japan, Taiwan, the highlands of China, and the Philippines.
- During invasion and migration of the flukes, diarrhea, abdominal pain, fever, cough, urticaria, hepatosplenomegaly, pulmonary abnormalities, and eosinophilia may develop.
- Unembryonated eggs are passed in the sputum of a human, also called Lung fluke.
- During the chronic phase, the lungs are damaged most, but other organs may be involved.
- The clinical picture resembles and is often confused with TB.
- Laboratory diagnosis of Paragonimiasis is done by demonstration of ova in the sputum/feces/pleural fluid or by serology.
- Praziquantel is the treatment of choice.

176. A 36-year-old male patient presents with h/o fever, cough, rusty sputum, sputum negative for TB, H/o travel to China and eaten crab. Name the infection: *(NEET 2019)*

a. *Paragonimus westermani*
b. *Fasciola hepatica*
c. *Fascilopsis buski*
d. *Entamoeba histolytica*

Ans. is 'a' *Paragonimus westermani*

177. Eggs seen in sputum and stools:

a. *Paragonimus*
b. *Fasciola*
c. *Clonorchis*
d. *P. jirovecii*

Ans. is 'a' *Paragonimus*

ECHINOCOCCUS/DOG TAPEWORM

- Trunk – 3 proglottids
- Egg undistinguishable from *Taenia*
- Dog–definite host
- Sheep–intermediate host
- Man–Accidental/Intermediate host

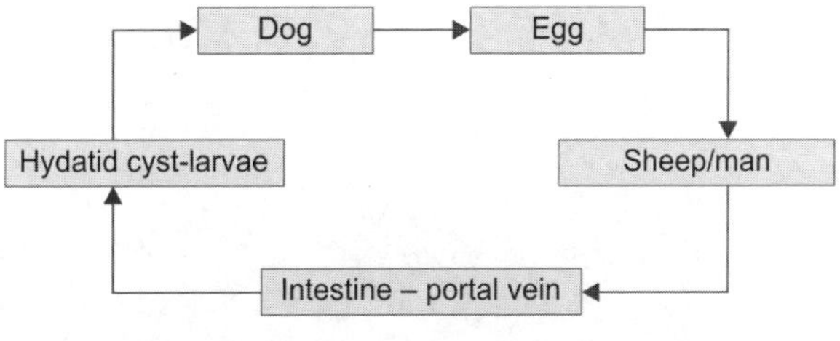

- *Outer pericyst*:—fibrous host reaction–calcification seen
- Ectocyst–acellular—chitin lamellated
- Endocyst—germinal layer
- Hydatid fluid—acidic hydatid sand–brood capsule
- Casoni's intradermal test—type 1 hypersensitivity
- USG—**water lily sign**—detached endocyst floating

- PAIR (Puncture, aspiration, injection, reaspiration)– indications:
    - Cyst communicating bite duct
    - Multiple internal septations
    - Superficial
    - TOC- surgery- pericystectomy.

178. Adult form of echinococcus granulosus has definite host as: *(NEET 2018)*

a. Dog
b. Cat
c. Cattle
d. Pig

Ans. is 'a' Dog

TRICHURIS TRICHIURA (WHIP WORM)

- Eggs are barrel shaped surrounded by a shell, bear mucus plug at both the poles. Bile stained elongated, floats in saturated salt solution.
- It can cause gastrointestinal problems, such as abdominal pain, diarrhea, mucous or bloody stools, weight loss, and weakness.
- Rectal prolapse is a hallmark, albeit rare, symptom of a heavy *T. trichiura* infection that occurs in children more frequently than adults. When rectal prolapse occurs, worms can often be identified on the edematous rectum.
- In a whipworm infection, the rectum loses its internal support because the worms bury their thin heads into the intestinal lining, loosening the elastic epithelium and weakening the surrounding muscles.
- Treatment with albendazole 400 mg and ivermectin 200 mg daily for 3 days.

179. A patient is having gastrointestinal problems including abdominal pain and distension, bloody or mucus-filled diarrhea, and tenesmus, with rectal prolapse, A stool, ova and parasites exam reveals the presence of typical Barrel- shaped eggs, possible causative agent is: *(NEET 2019)*

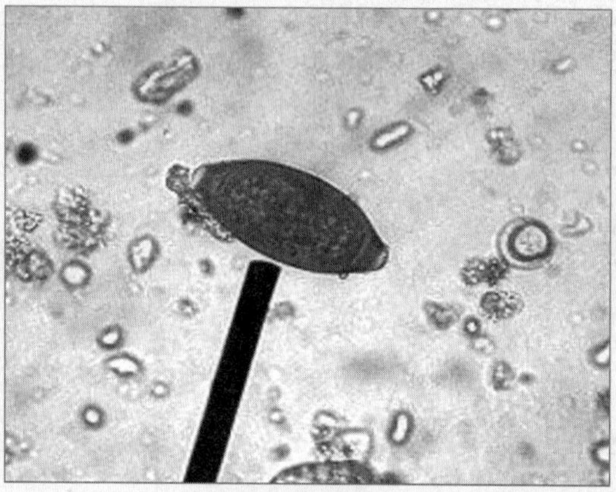

a. *Campylobacter*
b. *Clostridium difficile*
c. *Giardia lamblia*
d. *Trichuris*

Ans. is 'd' *Trichuris*

180. Identify the given organism: *(NEET 2020)*

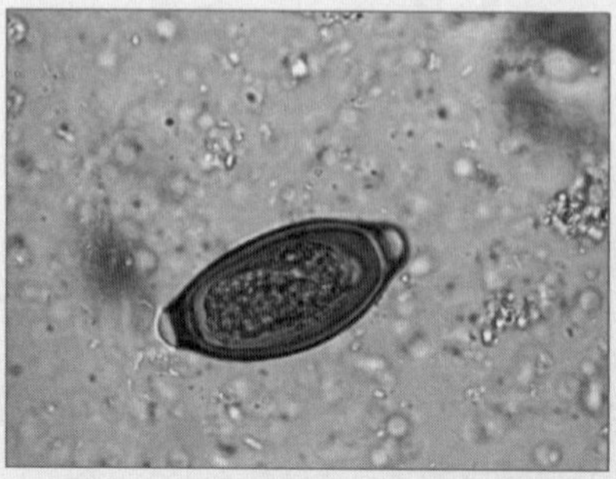

a. *D.latum*
b. *T.trichura*
c. *S.hematobium*
d. *A.duodenale*

Ans. is 'b' *T.trichura*

Microbiology

SCOLEX AND HOOKLETS

- Scolex is pear-shaped or knoblike head of cestodes (tapeworms).
- Scolex is covered with suckers and hooks:
  - *Taenia solium*: Scolex contains four suckers and rostellar hooks (rostellum with hooks).
  - *Taenia saginata*: Scolex contains four suckers but **no hooks**/rostellum (hookless).
  - *H. nana*: Scolex contains four suckers and rostellum of hooks.
  - *H. diminuta*: Scolex contains four suckers but **no hooks** (hookless).
  - *Echinococcus*: Scolex contains suckers and rostellum of hooks.
  - *Diphyllobothrium latum*: Scolex has two elongated sucking grooves (instead of suckers). There are **no hooks** (hookless).

181. Cyst with scolex and hooks is seen in: *(NEET 2018)*

a. *T. saginata* b. Fish tapeworm
c. Echinococcus d. *H. diminuta*

Ans. is 'c' Echinococcus

TOXOPLASMA GONDII

- It is an obligate intracellular parasite.
- It exists in 3 morphological forms:
  - 2 asexual forms (tachyzoite and bradyzoite/tissue cyst)
  - Sexual form is oocyst.
- Tachyzoite is a crescent shaped, actively multiplying form usually seen in acute infection.
- *Definitive host:* cat and other felines.
- *Intermediate host:* man, goat, sheep, cattle.
- Transmitted by ingestion of sporulated oocysts (infective form) from contaminated soil, food, or water. Also by blood transfusion, organ transplantation where tachyzoites are infective form.
- Acute toxoplasmosis in the immunocompetent host is usually asymptomatic and self-limited.
- Cervical lymphadenopathy is most common manifestation in acute disease.
- In immunocompromised host (patients associated with HIV, malignancies) or in fetus causes *Toxoplasma* encephalitis, pulmonary infections and chorioretinitis.

Congenital Toxoplasmosis

- Mother acquiring *Toxoplasma* infection in pregnancy is usually asymptomatic. However, she can transmit the infection to fetus.
- If mother infected in **first trimester**, transplacental incidence is lowest (15%), but the disease in neonate is most severe.
- In third trimester, transplacental incidence is maximum (65%), but the infant is usually asymptomatic at birth.
- If mother is infected before pregnancy, then the fetus is mostly uninfected except when the mother is immunocompromised.
- **Manifestations: hydrocephalus**, diffuse **cerebral calcification**, hepatosplenomegaly, mental retardation, myocarditis, lymphadenitis, microcephaly, myocarditis, **chorioretinitis**, pneumonitis and multiorgan failure.
- **"TORCH" infection:** *Toxoplasma* infection (T), Rubella (R), CMV (C), HSV (H), others (O) which includes syphilis, Varicella, etc.
- Chorioretinitis is usually treated with a combination of corticosteroids and antibiotics.

Lab Diagnosis

- Direct microscopy: detects tachyzoites in blood and bradyzoites in tissue biopsy.
- ELISA: detection of IgG, IgM, and *Toxoplasma* antigen in serum.

Sabin-Feldman Dye Test

- It is a serological neutralization test used for diagnosis of toxoplasmosis.
- Test is based on the presence of certain antibodies that prevent methylene blue dye from entering the cytoplasm of *Toxoplasma* organisms.
- Patient serum is treated with toxoplasma trophozoites and complements as activator and then incubated. After incubation, methylene blue dye is added.
- If anti-toxoantibodies are present in the serum, because these antibodies are activated by the complements and lyse the parasite membrane. *Toxoplasma* trophozoites are not stained (positive result); if there are no antibodies, trophozoites with intact membrane are stained and appear blue under microscope (negative result).

182. All are true about congenital Toxoplasmosis *except*: *(NEET 2019)*

a. Chorioretinitis b. Conjunctivitis
c. Hydrocephalus d. Cerebral calcifications

Ans. is 'b' Conjunctivitis

183. Sabin-Feldman dye test is done for: *(NEET 2018)*

a. Toxoplasmosis
b. Echinococcosis
c. Chagas disease
d. Sleeping sickness

Ans. is 'a' Toxoplasmosis

COCCIDIAN PARASITES

Property	Cryptosporidium	Cyclospora	Cystoisospora
Infective form	Sporulated oocyst • Thick walled oocyst (80%) by contaminated food and water • Thin walled (20%) Autoinfection	Sporulated oocyst (contaminated food and water)	Sporulated oocyst (contaminated food and water)
Sporulated oocyst	4–6 µm, **round** contains four sporozoites	8-12 µm, **round** contains 2 sporocysts, each having two sporozoites	23-26 µm, **oval** contains 2 sporocyst, each having four sporozoites
Acid fastness Detection limit >50,000 oocyst/ mL stool	Uniformly acid fast	Variable acid fast	Uniformly acid fast
Auto-fluorescence	No, but can be stained with fluorescent dye	Auto fluorescence ++	Auto fluorescence +/-
Sporulation of the oocyst	Occurs inside the host cells (enterocytes)	Occurs In soil (environment)	Occurs in soil (environment)
Diagnostic form	Sporulated oocyst	Unsporulated oocyst	Unsporulated oocyst
Autoinfection	Seen	Not seen	Not seen
Treatment	Nitazoxanide	Co-trimoxazole	Co-trimoxazole
Outbreaks	Common	Common	Less
Microscopic appearance	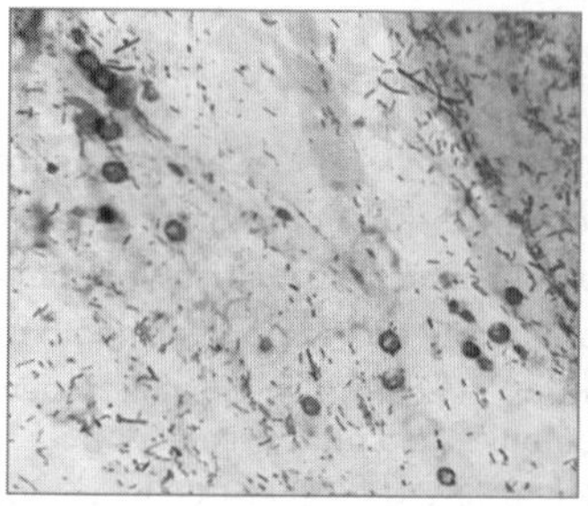	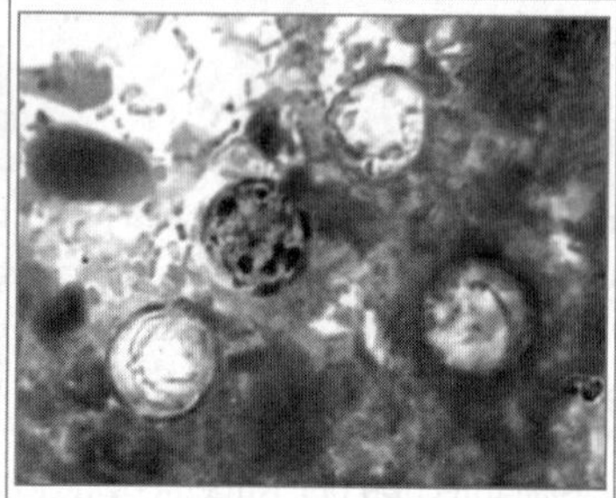	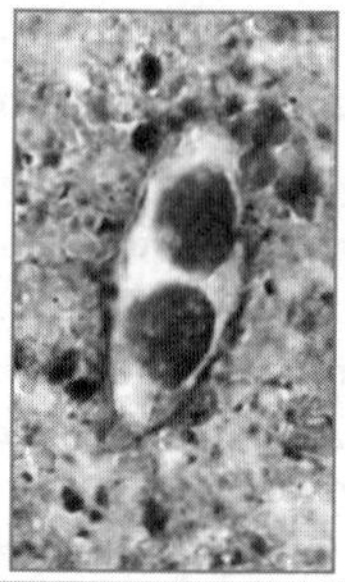

184. DOC for shown organism: *(NEET 2019)*

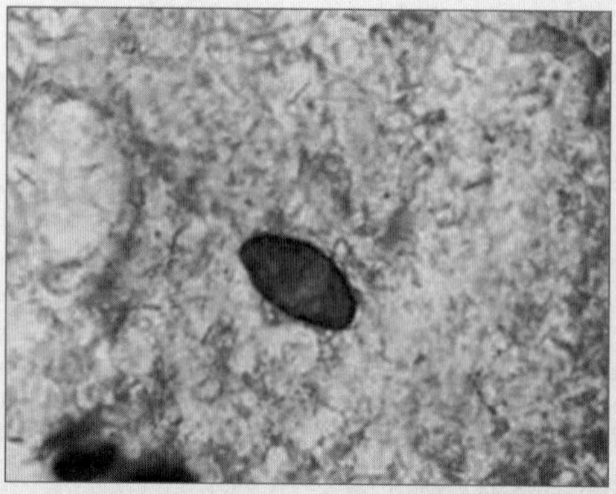

a. Penicillin G
b. Benzathine penicillin
c. Co-trimoxazole
d. Albendazole

Ans. is 'c' Co-trimoxazole

185. HIV patient presents with chronic watery diarrhea. Colonoscopic biopsy is shown below. What is the diagnosis? *(NEET 2020)*

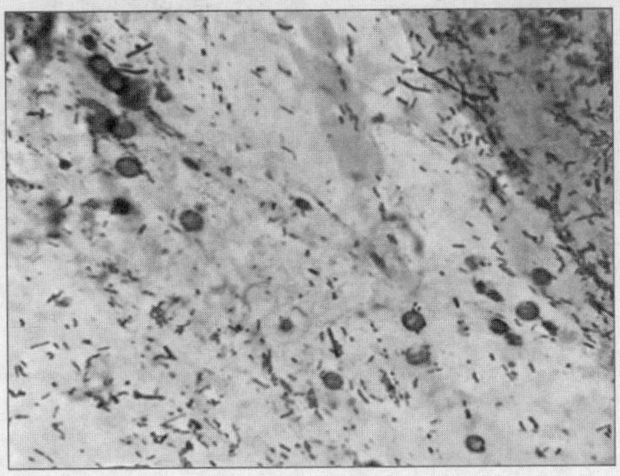

a. CMV
b. Microspora
c. Giardia
d. Cryptosporidium

Ans. is 'd' Cryptosporidium

MALARIA

Characteristic features of different species:

	P. vivax	P. falciparum	P. malariae	P. ovale
Hypnozoites	**Yes**	**No**	**No**	**Yes**
Erythrocyte preference	Reticulocyte (young erythrocytes)	Young erythrocytes, but can infect all stages	Old erythrocytes	Reticulocytes (young erythrocytes)
Stages found in peripheral blood	Rings, trophozoites, schizonts gametocytes	Only rings and gametocytes	As in vivax	As in vivax
Ring stage (early trophozoite)	Large 23 µm usually single, prominent chromatic	Dedicate small, 1.5 µm double chromatin and multiple rings, Accole forms (ring forms on the edge of RBCs) found	Similar to vivax, but thicker	Similar to vivax, more compact
Late trophozoite	Large irregular, actively amoeboid prominent vacuole	Compact, seldom seen in blood smear	Band from characteristic	Compact coarse pigment
Schizont	Large filling red cell	Small, compact. Seldom seen in blood smear	Medium size	Medium size
Number of merozoites	12–24 irregular grape-like cluster	8–24 in grape-like cluster	6–12 in daisy-head or rosette pattern	6–13 irregularly arranged
Microgametocyte	Spherical, compact pale blue cytoplasm diffuse nucleus	Sausage or banana shaped pale blue or pink cytoplasm. Large diffuse nucleus	As in vivax	As in vivax
Microgametocyte	Large, spherical, deep blue cytoplasm, compact nucleus	Crescentic, deep blue cytoplasm, compact nucleus	As in vivax	As in vivax
Infected erythrocyte	Enlarged pale, with Schuffner's dots	Normal size, Maurer's clefts, sometimes basophilic stippling	Normal occasionally Ziemann's stippling	Enlarged, oval fimbriated, prominent Schuffner's dots
Pigment color	Yellow brown	Dark brown	Brown black	Black
Duration of erythrocytic cycle	48 hours	36–48 hours	72 hours	48 hours
Appearance of parasite in thick smear	12th day after infection	10th day after infection		
Gametocyte appears in blood	16th day of infection (4days after appearance of sexual parasite)	21st day of infection (10 days after appearance of sexual parasite)		

186. A pregnant female presents with chills, rigors and fever. PBS is shown below. What is the likely agent? *(NEET 2020)*

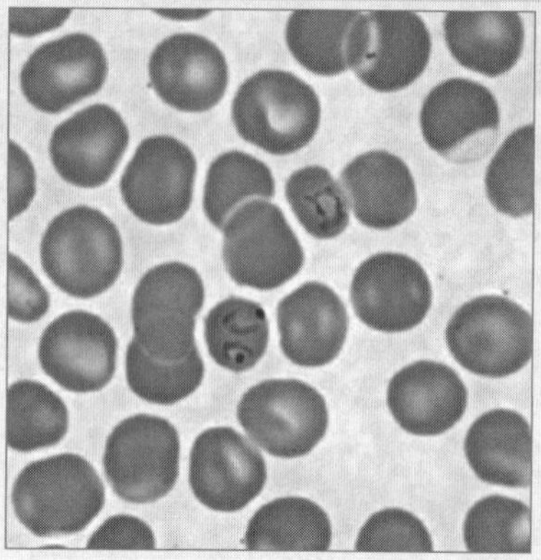

a. *P.vivx*
b. *P.falciparum*
c. *P.ovale*
d. *P.malariae*

Ans. is 'b' *P. falciparum*

Explanation: Peripheral blood smear shows accole forms characteristic for *P.falciparum*.

187. Stage of *P. falciparum* not seen in peripheral blood:

a. Schizont
b. Gametocyte
c. Ring form
d. Double ring

Ans. is 'a' Schizont

188. Maurer's dots are seen in which species of plasmodium?

a. *P. ovale*
b. *P. vivax*
c. *P. falciparum*
d. *P. malariae*

Ans. is 'c' *P. falciparum*

BABESIOSIS

- Babesia is an intraerythrocytic protozoa of animals, causes tick born malaria like illness in cattle and sheep.
- It rarely affects humans causing opportunistic infection.
- Ticks transmit the human strain of babesiosis.
- Definitive host: *Ixodid* ticks (hard ticks).
    - *Intermediate host*: Man or other mammals.
    - *Infective form*: Sporozoites are the infective form for humans.
    - *Mode of transmission*: Infection in vertebrate occurs through bite of the nymphal stage of Ixodid ticks.
- Babesia parasites reproduce in red blood cells where they can be seen as cross-shaped inclusions (four merozoites asexually budding, but attached together forming a structure looking like a **'Maltese cross'**) and cause hemolytic anemia, quite similar to malaria.
- 'Maltese cross formations' on the blood film are diagnostic (pathognomonic) of babesiosis, since they are not seen in malaria, the primary differential diagnosis.
- Rings of Babesia spp. have delicate cytoplasm and are often pleomorphic. Infected red blood cells (RBCs) are not enlarged; multiple infections of RBCs can be common. Rings are usually vacuolated and do not produce pigment.

189. Slide of peripheral blood smear of a patient suffering with fever and chills is shown. Vector for the disease shown in the image in: *(NEET 2018)*

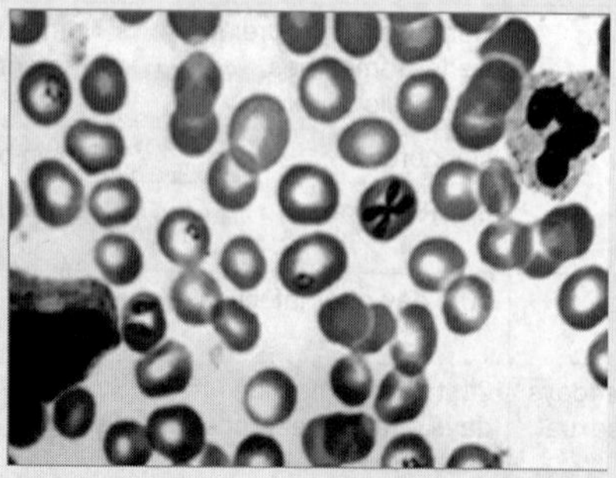

Microbiology

a. Hard tick
b. *Anopheles*
c. *Culex*
d. Tsetsefly

Ans. is 'a' Hard tick

190. Maltese cross on microscopy is seen in: *(NEET 2018)*

a. *Cryptococcus neoformans*
b. *Babesia microti*
c. Blastomycosis
d. *Penicillium marneffei*

Ans. is 'b' *Babesia microti*

LEISHMANIA

- Visceral leishmaniasis (Kala azar)—*L. donovani*
- Cutaneous leishmaniasis
  - Oriental sore—*L. tropica*
  - Mucocutaneous leishmaniasis (Espundia)—*L. braziliensis*
- There are 2 morphological forms of Leishmania, promastigote and amastigote.
- The promastigote is found in the vectors of leishmaniasis, female sand flies of the general *Lutzomyia* and *Phlebotomus.*
- Leishmania parasites are acquired by the fly in the amastigote form during the taking of a blood meal.
- The first developmental event observed is the transformation of the amastigote to the promastigote form.
- Approximately 3 days after feeding, the promastigotes begin to escape from the peritrophic membrane of midgut epithelium and spread toward the anterior portion of the midgut.
- At this point, promastigotes are commonly seen attached to the midgut epithelium or with their flagella inserted between microvilli.
- From day 5 onwards, increasing numbers of slender, non-replicating, rapidly moving promastigotes can be observed in the lumen of the anterior midgut and foregut.
- It is this highly infectious metacyclic form of promastigotes which is delivered to the vertebrate host.
- Upon delivery to the vertebrate host, the promastigotes are quickly taken up by tissue phagocytes, and by monocytes and neutrophils brought to the site due to the damage created by sand fly feeding.
- Within macrophages, promastigotes lose their flagellum and transform into non-motile amastigotes.
- The amastigote survives and replicates within the acidic environment of the phagolysosome, eventually lysing the infected cell, freeing amastigotes to infect nearby cells. When a sand fly acquires a blood meal from an infected host, it acquires either free amastigotes, or amastigote-infected mononuclear cells, and the life-cycle continues.

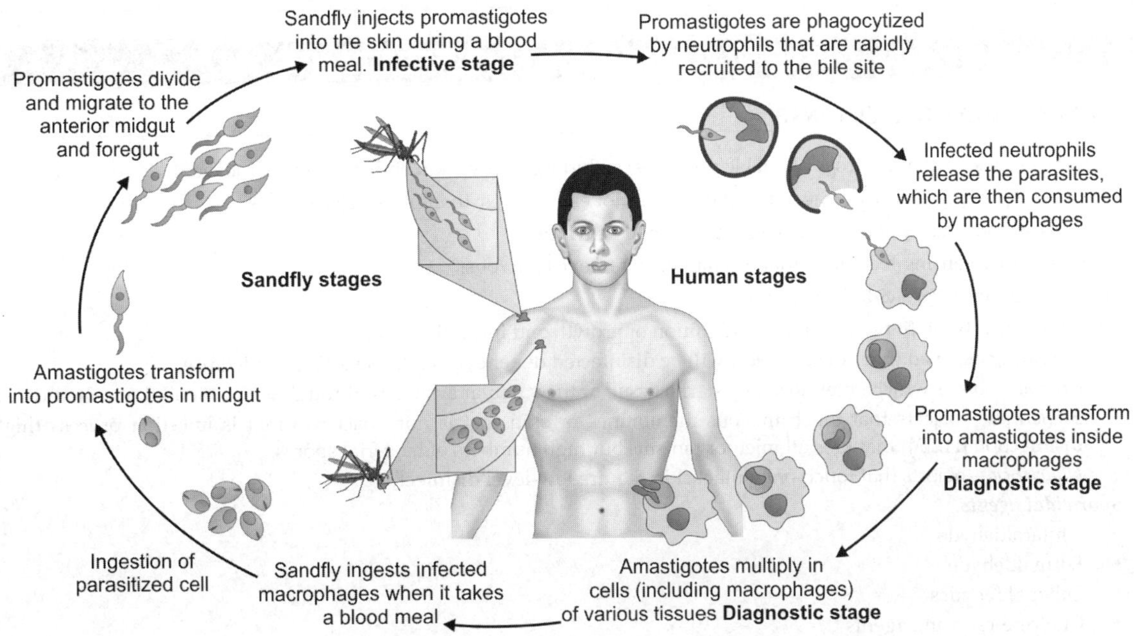

191. Visceral leishmaniasis is caused by:

a. *L. braziliensis*
b. *L. tropica*
c. *L. donovani*
d. *L. orientalis*

Ans. is 'c' *L. donovani*

192. Promastigote form of Leishmania in vector is seen in:

a. Hindgut
b. Foregut
c. Coelomic cavity
d. Any of the above

Ans. is 'b' Foregut

193. Promastigote forms of Leishmania are formed in which of the following body parts of sand fly:

a. Hindgut
b. Foregut
c. Coelomic cavity
d. Midgut

Ans. is 'd' Midgut

LARVA MIGRANS

Nonhuman *Ancylostoma* species cause cutaneous larvae migrans. It is a serpiginous skin eruption caused by burrowing larvae of animal hookworms. After larvae penetrate the skin, erythematous lesions form along the tortuous tracks of their migration. It is also known as creeping eruption.

- **Cutaneous larva migrans** (creeping eruption), common causes are:
  - *Ancylostoma braziliense* (most common)
  - *A. caninum*
  - *Uncinaria stenocephala*
  - *Gnathostoma spinigerum*
  - *Bunostomum phlebotomum*
- **Visceral larva migrans**, common causes are:
  - *Toxocara canis* (most common)
  - *T. catii*
  - *Angiostrongylus cantonensis*
  - *Angiostrongylus costaricensis*
  - *Anisakis* spp.

194. Cutaneous larva migrans caused by: *(NEET 2018)*

a. *Nector americanus*
b. *Ancylostoma duodenale*
c. *Ancylostoma braziliense*
d. *Ancylostoma caninum*

Ans. is 'c' *Ancylostoma braziliense*

STERILIZATION AND DISINFECTANTS

STERILIZATION AND DISINFECTANTS

- Sterilization—a process that destroys all viable microbes, including viruses and endospores; microbicidal.
- Disinfection—a process to destroy vegetative pathogens, not endospores; inanimate objects.
- Antiseptic—disinfectants applied directly to exposed body surfaces.
- Sanitization—any cleansing technique that mechanically removes microbes.
- Bactericidal (microbicidal)—cidal means kill.
- Bacteriostatic (microbiostatic)—static means inhibition of growth and multiplication.
  - EH Spaulding believed that how an object will be disinfected depended on the object's intended use.
    - *Critical*—objects which enter normally sterile tissue or the vascular system or through which blood flows should be sterile.
    - *Semicritical*—objects that touch mucous membranes or skin that is not intact required is infection process (high-level disinfection [HLD]) that kills all microorganisms but high numbers of bacterial spores.
    - *Noncritical*—objects that touch only intact skin require low-level disinfection.
  - ***Sporicidal agents***:
    - Glutaraldehyde
    - Formaldehyde
    - Other aldehydes
    - Chlorine-releasing agents

- Iodine and iodophores
- Peroxygens
- Ethylene oxide
- P-Propiolactone

- *Physical methods*:
  - Pasteurization (Pasteurization is done to destroy the pathogens in milk. It kills nearly 90% of bacteria in milk, including more heat resistant tubercular bacilli and Q-fever organism. However, thermoduric bacteria and spores are not killed.
    - *First used with milk*: 72°C for 20 seconds
    - Heating to 80°C for 1 minute will kill most vegetative organisms
    - *Examples*: Bed-pan washer, proctoscope

❖ There are following methods of **pasteurization**:

- *Holder method (Vat method)*: Milk is kept at 63–66°C for 30 minutes and then rapidly cooled to 5°C.
- High temperature short time (HTST) method
  It is also called **Flash method**. Milk is heated to 72°C for 15 seconds and then rapidly cooled to 4°C.
  It is now the most widely used method.
- **Ultra-high temperature (UHT) method**
  - Milk is rapidly heated in two stages to 125°C for few seconds, 2nd stage being under pressure. It is then rapidly cooled.
  - Dry heat (hot air oven): used on waxes, oils (wet heat usually preferred).
  - Incineration
    - The ultimate sterilization
    - Used for disposal of hospital waste.
  - Wet heat
    - Boiling
    - Limited use as spores may be resistant, boilers may be misused
    - Low temperature steam disinfection (75°C for 30 minutes)
    - Used for, e.g. ventilator tubing
    - Autoclaving
    - High-temperature steam plus pressure (same principle as pressure cooker)

Method	Temperature (°C)	Holding time (in minutes)
Autoclave	121	15
	126	10
	134	3
Hot air oven	160	45
	170	18
	180	7.5
	190	1.5

Methods of Disinfection and Sterilization

Method	Activity level	Spectrum	Uses/comments
Heat			
Autoclave	Sterilizing	All	General
Boiling	High	Most pathogens, some spores	General
Pasteurization	Intermediate	Vegetative bacteria	Beverages, plastic hospital equipment
Ethylene oxide gas	Sterilizing	All	Potentially explosive; aeration required
Radiation			
Ultraviolet	Sterilizing	All	Poor penetration
Ionizing	Sterilizing	All	General, food
Chemicals			
Alcohol	Intermediate	Vegetative bacteria, fungi, some viruses	
Hydrogen peroxide	High	Viruses, vegetative bacteria, fungi	Contact lenses; inactivated by organic matter
Chlorine	High	Viruses, vegetative bacteria, fungi	Water; inactivated by organic matter
Iodophors	Intermediate	Viruses, vegetative bacteria, a fungi	Skin disinfection; inactivated by organic matter
Phenolics	Intermediate	Some viruses, vegetative bacteria, fungi	Handwashing
Glutaraldehyde	High	All	Endoscopes, other equipment
Quaternary ammonium compounds	Low	Most bacteria and fungi, lipophilic viruses	General cleaning; inactivated by organic matter

PROCEDURE OF STERILIZATION OF SOME IMPORTANT MATERIALS

Material	Methods
Inoculating loop or wire, the tip of forceps and searing spatulas	Flaming
Contaminated animal carcasses and pathological material	Incineration
Glassware, syringes, petri dishes, test tubes, Flasks, surgical instruments	Hot air oven
Most of the culture media	Autoclaving or membrane filter
Sharp instruments	5% cresol or hot air oven
Clinical thermometer	Savlon
Cystoscopes, bronchoscopes and other endoscopes, corrugated rubber anesthetic tubes, face masks, plastic endotracheal tubes	Glutaraldehyde
Milk	Pasteurization
Suture material except catgut	Autoclaving
Catgut	Ionizing radiation
Bacterial vaccines	Vaccine bath
Dressing, aprons, gloves, catheters surgical instruments except sharp instruments	Autoclaving
Heat sensitive catheters, wards fumigation, laboratories, sick rooms, operation theaters	Formaldehyde gas or UV rays
Prepacked items such as syringes and catheters	Infrared radiation
Culture media containing gelatin or sugar	Tyndallization

Type of sterilization	Spore used
Moist heat (autoclave)	*Bacillus stearothermophilus* (now called *Geobacillus stearothermophilus*)
Dry heat (hot air oven)	Bacillius subtilis
Ionizing radiation	Bacillus pumilus
Gas sterilization (ethylene oxide)	Bacillus subtilis
Plasma sterilization	Geobacillus stearothermophilus

195. Cold sterilization is done by:

a. Liquid nitrogen
b. Glutaraldehyde
c. H_2O_2
d. ϒ-rays

Ans. is 'd' ϒ-rays

196. Glassware is sterilized in hot air oven at what temperature?

a. 70°C for 30 minutes
b. 50°C for 1 hour
c. 121°C for 15 minutes
d. 160°C for 45 minutes

Ans. is 'd' 160°C for 45 minutes

197. Which of the following is a method of Pasteurization?

a. Vat method
b. Pasteur method
c. Billing method
d. Flash method

Ans. is 'a' Vat method; 'd' Flash method

198. Temperature in Flash method of Pasteurized:

a. 66°C
b. 72°C
c. 100°C
d. 125°C

Ans. is 'b.' 72°C

199. Holder method of pasteurization does not kill:

a. *Mycobacteria*
b. *Brucella*
c. *Salmonella*
d. *Coxiella burnetii*

Ans. is 'd' *Coxiella burnetii*

200. Method of sterilization of syringes:

a. Hot air oven
b. Autoclaving
c. Irradiation
d. Ethylene dioxide

Ans. is 'a' Hot air oven

201. Laparoscope is sterilized by:

a. Glutaraldehyde
b. Formalin
c. Autoclaving
d. Boiling

Ans. is 'a' Glutaraldehyde

202. Autoclaving is used for sterilization of:

a. Culture media
b. Catgut suture
c. Endoscope
d. Heat labile instruments

Ans. is 'a' Culture media

203. Temperature in ultra-high temperature (UHT) method of pasteurization:

a. 65°C for 30 minutes
b. 72°C for 15 seconds
c. 68°C for 30 minutes
d. 125°C for few seconds

Ans. is 'd' 125°C for few seconds

204. Which of the following has sporicidal activity?

a. 2% Glutaraldehyde
b. 2% cresol
c. Chlorhexidine
d. Isopropyl alcohol

Ans. is 'a' 2% Glutaraldehyde

205. *Bacillus stearothermophilus* is used as an indicator for:

a. Hot air oven
b. Radiation
c. Gas sterilization
d. Autoclaving

Ans. is 'd' Autoclaving

206. Heat sensitive articles are sterilized by:

a. Absolute alcohol
b. Ultraviolet rays
c. Chlorine releasing compounds
d. Ethylene oxide gas

Ans. is 'd' Ethylene oxide gas

207. Cutaneous larva migrans caused by: *(NEET 2018)*

a. *Nector americanus*
b. *Ancylostoma duodenale*
c. *Ancylostoma braziliense*
d. *Ancylostoma caninum*

Ans. is 'c' *Ancylostoma braziliense*

CHLORINATION

- Chlorination is one of the greatest advances of water purification. It is a supplement not a substitute to sand filtration. Chlorine kills pathogenic bacteria, but it has no effect on spores and certain viruses (e.g. polio, viral hepatitis) except in high doses. Apart from its germicidal effect, chlorine has several important secondary properties of value in water treatment: It oxidizes iron, manganese and hydrogen sulfide; it destroys some taste and odor producing constituents; it controls algae and slime organisms; and aids coagulation.
- *Action of chlorine*: When chlorine is added to water, there is a formation of hydrochloric and hypochlorous acids. The hydrochloric acid is neutralized by the alkalinity of the water. The hypochlorous acid ionizes to form hydrogen ions and hypochlorite ions.
- The disinfecting action of chlorine is mainly due to the hypochlorous acid, and to a small extent due to the hypochlorite ions. The hypochlorous acid is the most effective form of chlorine for water disinfection. It is more effective (70–80 times) than the hypochlorite ion. Chlorine acts best as a disinfectant when the pH of water is around 7 because of the predominance of hypochlorous acid. When the pH value exceeds 8.5 it is unreliable as a disinfectant because about 90% of the hypochlorous acid gets ionized to hypochlorite ions. It is fortunate that most waters have a pH value between 6–7.5.

208. Active disinfectant property of Bleaching powder is mainly due to formation of: *(NEET 2020)*

a. Hydrogen chloride
b. Hypochloric acid
c. Hypochlorous acid
d. Chloramines

Ans. is 'c' Hypochlorous acid

Explanation: In an acidic environment, bleaching powder (calcium hypochlorite) produces chlorine which is responsible for its disinfectant property.

DETERMINING THE EFFICIENCY OF A DISINFECTANTS

Rideal-Walker Test

- Phenol is taken as the standard – Phenol coefficient.
  Suspensions containing equal number of typhoid bacilli are submitted to action of varying concentrations of phenol and of the disinfectant to be tested. The dilution of the test disinfectant which sterilizes the suspension in a given time, divided by the corresponding dilution of phenol, is stated as the phenol coefficient of the disinfectant.

Chick-Martin Test

In this test, the disinfectant acts in the presence of organic matter (dried yeast or feces), hence is superior to Rideal-Walker test as it reflects natural conditions.

209. Rideal-Walker coefficient is related with:

a. Disinfecting power
b. Parasitic clearance
c. Dietary requirement
d. Statistical correlation

Ans. is 'a' Disinfecting power

BIOMEDICAL WASTE MANAGEMENT

Category	Type of waste	Bag/container	Treatment and disposal options
Yellow	(a) Human anatomical waste (b) Animal anatomical	Yellow non-chlorinated plastic bags	Incineration/plasma pyrolysis/deep burial
	(c) Soiled waste		Incineration/plasma pyrolysis/deep burial or autoclaving / microwaving/hydroclaving Then Shredding/mutilation
	(d) Expired/discarded medicines (e) Chemical waste	Yellow non-chlorinated plastic bags or containers	Incineration/encapsulation/plasma pyrolysis
	(f) Chemical liquid waste	Separate collection system leading to effluent treatment system	Pretreatment Then Drain
	(g) Discarded linen, mattresses, beddings contaminated with blood or body fluid	Non-chlorinated yellow plastic bags or suitable packing material	Non-chlorinated chemical disinfection Then Incineration/Plasma pyrolysis/Energy recovery or shredding mutilation
	(h) Microbiology, Biotechnology Clinical laboratory waste	Autoclave safe plastic bags or containers	Pre-treat with Non-chlorinated chemicals Then Incineration
Red		Red non-chlorinated plastic bags or containers	Autoclaving/microwaving/hydroclaving Then Shredding/mutilation Then Energy recovery/plastics to diesel or fuel oil/road making
White (translucent)		Puncture proof, leak proof, tamper proof containers	Autoclaving/dry heat Then Shredding/mutilation/encapsulation Then Iron foundries/sanitary landfill/waste sharp pit
Blue	(a) glassware (b) metallic body implants	Cardboard boxes with blue colored making	Sodium hypochlorite/autoclaving/microwaving/ hydroclaving Then Recycling

210. which of the following BMW is disposed in yellow bags as per current guidelines? *(NEET 2020)*

a. Broken glass pieces
b. Blood-bags
c. Metallic sharps
d. Urine-bags

Ans. is 'b' Blood-bags

211. Chemical liquid waste is disposed in which bag? *(NEET 2020)*

a. Red
b. Yellow
c. Blue
d. Black

Ans. is 'b' Yellow

CLINICAL MICROBIOLOGY

Sexually transmitted infections

Disease	*Clinical features*	*Organism*
AIDS	Opportunistic infections, Kaposi sarcoma, lymphoma	HIV
Chancroid	Painful genital ulcer with exudate, inguinal adenopathy	Haemophilus ducreyi (it is so painful, you "do cry")
Chlamydia	Urethritis, cervicitis, epididymitis, conjunctivitis, reactive arthritis, PID	Chlamydia trachomatis (*D–K*)
Condylomata acuminata	Genital warts, koilocytes	HPV-6 and -II
Genital herpes	Painful penile, vulvar, or cervical vesicles and ulcers; can cause systemic symptoms such as fever, headache, myalgia	HSV-2 less commonly HSV-1
Gonorrhea	Urethritis, cervicitis, PID, prostatitis, epididymitis, arthritis, creamy purulent discharge	*Neisseria gonorrhoeae*
Granuloma inguinale (Donovanosis)	Painless, deefy red ulcer that bleeds readily on contact Uncommon in US	*Klebsiella (Calymmatobacterium)* granulomatis; cytoplasmic Donovan bodies (bipolar staining seen on microscopy)
Hepatitis B	Jaundice	HBV
Lymphogranuloma venereum	Infection of lymphatics; painless genital ulcers, painful lymphadenopathy (i.e., buboes)	*C trachomatis* (L1-L3)
Primary syphilis	Painless chancre	*Treponema pallidum*
Secondary syphilis	Fever, lymphadenopathy, skin rashes, condylomata lata	
Tertiary syphilis	Gummas, tabes dorsalis, general paresis, aortitis, Argyll Robertson pupil	
Trichomoniasis	Vaginitis, strawberry cervix, motile in wet prep Urethritis	*Trichomonas vaginalis*

212. A young male presented with complaints of urethritis. Which organism cannot cause this presentation? *(NEET 2020)*

a. *C.trachomatis*
b. *H.ducreyi*
c. *N.gonorrhea*
d. *T.vaginalis*

Ans. is 'b' *H. ducreyi*

213. A young female presents with whitish discharge per vaginum. On examination, the cervix was covered with punctate red dots resembling a strawberry. What is the diagnosis? *(NEET 2020)*

a. Garednerella vaginalis
b. Candida albicans
c. Trichomonas vaginalis
d. Herpes genitalis

Ans. is 'c' Trichomonas vaginalis

214. Causative agent for donovanosis is: *(NEET 2020)*

a. *C.trachomatis*
b. *K.granulomatis*
c. *L.donovani*
d. *H.ducreyi*

Ans. is 'b' *K. granulomatis*

NOCARDIA

- Gram-positive pleomorphic rods which show branching and beaded staining patterns.
- *Nocardia asteroides* is the most common species.
- Infection usually occurs in immunocompromised patients.

Clinical Features

- Most commonly presents with pneumonia—cough, dyspnea and fever.
- *Nocardia* species are deeply involved in the process of endocarditis as one of its main pathogenic effects.
- CNS may be involved—encephalitis or brain abscess formation.
- Actinomycetoma, lymphocutaneous disease, cellulitis, or subcutaneous abscesses may form.

Diagnosis

- Microscopy—crooked, branching, beaded, gram-positive filaments.
- Fast in modified Kinyoun, Ziehl-Neelsen, and Fite-Faraco methods.

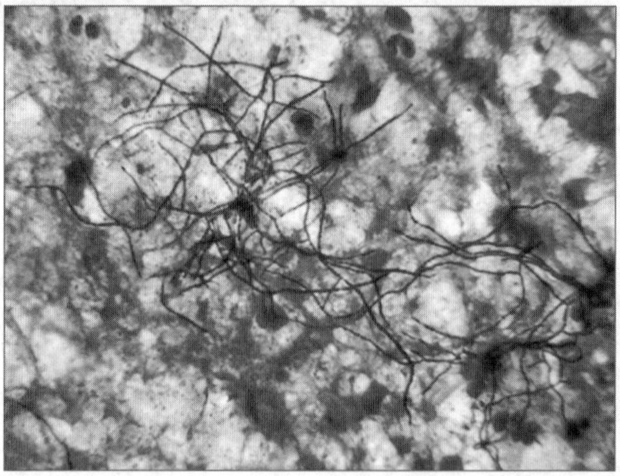

- Culture using selective media—colistin-nalidixic acid agar, modified Thayer-Martin agar, or buffered charcoal-yeast extract agar.
- Among the given options only *Nocardia asteroides* is acid fast. *Nocardia* is strict aerobe, acid fast, Gram positive and branching beaded filamentous. Most common clinical manifestation of *Nocardia* is pneumonia.

215. A patient is having pneumonia. Sputum examination shows partially acid fast, gram positive aerobic branching filaments. The causative organism is:

a. *Actinomyces israelii* b. *Nocardia asteroides*
c. *Aspergillus fumigatus* d. *Staphylococcus aureus*

Ans. is 'b' *Nocardia asteroides*

PNEUMOCYSTIS PNEUMONIA (PCP)

- *P. jirovecii* pneumonia produces a diffuse, symmetric, fine-to-medium reticulonodular pattern.
- Reticulonodular shadow is seen in interstitial pneumonia.
- The risk of PCP is greatest among those who have experienced a previous bout of PCP and those who have CD4 T cell counts of <200/μL.
- Recurrent fever, night sweats, thrush, and unexplained weight loss also are associated with an increased incidence of PCP. For these reasons, it is strongly recommended that all patients with CD4 T cell counts <200/μL (or a CD4 percentage <15) receive some form of PCP prophylaxis.

Diagnosis of *P. jirovecii*

- Best specimen is bronchoscopy with **BAL** (bronchoalveolar lavage) fluid. Sputum can also be used.
- *Following are methods for diagnosis*:
  - *Histopathologic staining for cysts and other stages*: It is most commonly used method for diagnosis. Methenamine silver, toluidine blue and crystal violet stain the cyst wall. Wright Giemsa stains all development stages.
  - Immunofluorescence with monoclonal antibodies.
  - *PCR*: It is most sensitive.

216. A 30-year-old male is having productive cough with dyspnea. Blood gas analysis shows low PaO_2. Chest X-ray is showing reticulonodular pattern. The causative agent is:

a. *Staph. aureus* b. *Pneumococcus*
c. *P. jirovecii* d. *Pseudomonas*

Ans. is 'c' *P. jirovecii*

Microbiology

217. Best specimen for diagnosis of *Pneumocystis jirovecii* pneumonia:

a. Sputum
b. BAL fluid
c. Bronchial biopsy
d. Alveolar biopsy

Ans. is 'b' BAL fluid

MYCETOMA

- It is a localized chronic granulomatous involvement of the subcutaneous and deeper tissues, commonly affecting the foot and less often the hand and other parts.
- Presenting as a subcutaneous swelling with multiple discharging sinuses.
- Sinuses discharge seropurulent fluid containing granules.
- These granules are microcolonies of the etiological agents.
- Mycetoma can be caused by both fungus and bacteria.

A. Eumycetoma (Mycetoma caused by fungus):

- It is caused by subcutaneous infection of fungi. Based on the color of granules in discharge these may be divided into:
  - *Black grain mycetoma*: Caused by *Madurella mycetomatis, Madurella grisea, Exophiala jeanselmia curvularia geniculata.*
  - *White grain mycetoma*: Caused by *Pseudallescheria boydii, Aspergillus nidulans, Fusarium, Acremonium*

B. Actinomycetoma (Mycetoma caused by bacteria)

- It is caused by *Actinomedura madurae* (most common cause in India), *Actinomyces, nocardia, Streptomyces* and *Allescheria boydii.*
- Color of granules is white to yellow.
- *Actinomadura pelletieri* produces red granules.

218. A 60-year-old farmer has developed swelling on the sole of foot with discharging yellow granules. The diagnosis is:

a. Fungal mycetoma
b. Eumycetoma
c. Actinomycosis
d. Candidiasis

Ans. is 'c' Actinomycosis

HOSPITAL-ACQUIRED INFECTION (HAI)

- Hospital-acquired infection or nosocomial infection are applied to infections developing in hospitalized patients, not present or in incubation at the time of their admission.
- Such infections may become evident during their stay in hospital or, sometimes, only after their discharge.
- Infections are considered nosocomial if they first appear after **48 hours or more of** hospital admission or **within 30 days** after discharge.

219. Definition of nosocomial infection includes:

a. Infection within 24 hours of admission
b. Infection within 48 hours of admission
c. Infection 40 days after discharge
d. Infection within 30 days after discharge

Ans. is 'd' Infection within 30 days after discharge

PARASITES ASSOCIATED WITH MALIGNANCY

- *Clonorchis sinensis*: Liver bile duct (cholangiocarcinoma)
- *Opisthorchis viverrini*: Bile duct (cholangiocarcinoma)
- *Schistosoma haematobium*: Urinary bladder (squamous cell Ca)
- *Fasciola hepatica*: Cholangiocarcinoma.

220. Cholangiocarcinoma is caused by:

a. *Clonorchis sinensis*
b. *Opisthorchis viverrini*
c. *Fasciola hepatica*
d. All of the above

Ans. is 'd' All of the above

PARASITES CAUSING ANEMIA

- *Ancylostoma duodenale*: Iron deficiency anemia (microcytic hypochromic)
- *Necator americanus*: Iron deficiency anemia (microcytic hypochromic)
- *Babesia*: Hemolytic anemia

- *Diphyllobothrium latum*: Megaloblastic (Vit B12 def. anemia)
- *Leishmania donovani*: Autoimmune hemolytic anemia
- *Plasmodium* spp.: Autoimmune hemolytic anemia
- *Trichuris trichiura*: Iron deficiency (microcytic hypochromic).

221. Megaloblastic anemia is caused by:

a. Diphyllobothrium latum
b. Schistosoma haematobium
c. Echinococcus granulosus
d. Taenia solium

Ans. is 'a' Diphyllobothrium latum

- ***Important causes of Traveler's diarrhea***:
  - ***Bacteria***: ETEC (most common), Enteroaggregative *E. coli* (2nd mc), EIEC, *Shigella, Salmonella, Campylobacter, V. cholerae.*
  - ***Viruses***: Rotavirus, Norwalk like virus.
  - ***Parasites***: *E. histolytica, Giardia lamblia, Cryptosporidium, Cyclospora*

222. Not a cause of Traveler's diarrhea:

a. ETEC
b. *Shigella*
c. *V. cholerae*
d. *Staphylococcus*

Ans. is 'd' *Staphylococcus*

IMPORTANT CAUSES OF ATYPICAL PNEUMONIA

- *Mycoplasma pneumoniae* — most common cause
- Viruses—Influenza, RSV, Adenovirus, Rhinovirus, Coronavirus.
- *Legionella*
- *Chlamydia*
- *Coxiella burnetii*
- *P. jirovecii.*

223. Which of the following causes atypical pneumonia:

a. Pseudomonas
b. Coronavirus
c. *Listeria*
d. Pneumococcus

Ans. is 'b' Coronavirus

Pulmonary Eosinophilia is caused by

- *Ascaris*
- *Strongyloides stercoralis*
- *Ancylostoma (hookworm)*
- *Wuchereria bancrofti or Brugia malayi*
- *Toxocara*

One of the very few non-parasitic infections that regularly cause eosinophilia is **Coccidioidomycosis**, a fungal infection.

224. Pulmonary eosinophilia is found in infection with:

a. Babesiosis
b. Malaria
c. Strongyloidiasis
d. Trypanosomiasis

Ans. is 'c' Strongyloidiasis

225. Non-parasitic eosinophilia is caused by infection with:

a. *Staphylococcus*
b. *Ehrlichia*
c. Coccidioidomycosis
d. Candidiasis

Ans. is 'c' Coccidioidomycosis

CANDIDA ALBICANS

- Dimorphic; forms pseudohyphae (branching filamentous cells that exist as elongated and constricted chains of yeast cells) and budding yeasts at 20°C, germ tubes at 37°C

- ❖ Systemic or superficial fungal infection. Causes oral and esophageal thrush in immunocompromised (neonates, steroids, diabetes, AIDS), vulvovaginitis (diabetes, use of antibiotics), diaper rash, endocarditis (IV drug users), disseminated candidiasis (especially in neutropenic patients), chronic mucocutaneous candidiasis.
- ❖ *Treatment*: Oral fluconazole/topical azole for vaginal; nystatin, Auconazole, or echinocandins for oral/esophageal; fluconazole, echinocandins, or amphoteric in B for systemic.

226. Culture obtained from the lesion shown below demonstrates branching with narrowed ends. What is the diagnosis? *(NEET 2020)*

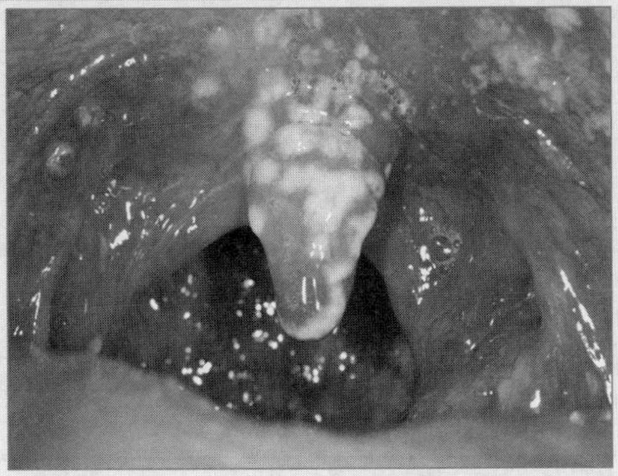

a. C.diphtheria b. *C.albicans*
c. CMV d. HSV

Ans. is 'b' *C. albicans*

Explanation: The image shows candida thrush – white cheesy exudates on erythematous mucosa in posterior oropharynx.

Candidal infections are identified by their location on the body as follows:

- ❖ Axillae, under pendulous breasts, groin, intergluteal folds: intertrigo
- ❖ *Glans penis*: balanitis
- ❖ *Follicular pustules*: candidal folliculitis
- ❖ *Nail folds*: candidal paronychia
- ❖ *Mouth and tongue*: oral candidiasis (thrush)
- ❖ Area included under diaper-diaper dermatitis.

227. Candiasis of penis is:

a. Thrush b. Leukoplakia
c. Balanitis d. None

Ans. is 'c' Balanitis

DIABETIC ULCERS

Etiology and Pathogenesis

- ❖ Peripheral neuropathy, pressure, and trauma are felt to play prominent roles in the development of diabetic ulcers.
- ❖ Neuropathy (associated with uncontrolled hyperglycemia) is one of the major predictors of it.
- ❖ Ill-fitting shoes and socks were the most common reasons for foot ulcers in diabetic patients.
- ❖ Once an ulcer develops, peripheral vascular disease and intrinsic wound healing disturbances contribute to adverse outcomes.

Clinical Findings

Callus formation precedes necrosis and breakdown of tissue over bony prominences of feet, usually on great toe and sole, over first and/or second metacarpophalangeal joints. Ulcers are surrounded by a ring of callus and may extend to underlying joint and bone. Complications are soft tissue infection and osteomyelitis.

"A mixture of gram-positive cocci and gram-negative aerobes and anaerobes is often implicated in cellulitis surrounding diabetic and decubitus ulcers".

228. Cellulitis surrounding diabetic ulcer is mostly caused by:

a. Streptococcus pyogenes b. Staphylococcus
c. Mixed organisms d. Pseudomonas

Ans. is 'c' Mixed organisms

OPPORTUNISTIC INFECTIONS IN IMMUNODEFICIENCY DUE TO DEFECT IN MYELOID CELLS

- *Staph. aureus*
- *E. coli*
- *Klebsiella*
- *Neisseria*
- *Pneumococcus*
- *Candida.*

Conditions causing defect in myeloid cells are:

- Chronic granulomatous disease
- G6PD and **pyruvate kinase** deficiency
- Chediak-Higashi syndrome
- Myeloperoxidase deficiency

229. *E. coli* infection occur in which enzyme defect?

a. Lactase
b. Pyruvate kinase
c. Pepsin
d. Trypsin

Ans. is 'b' Pyruvate kinase

Previously Asked Facts

- Periplasmic space is a narrow space between cytoplasmic membrane (plasma membrane) and cell wall, which is seen in Gram negative bacteria.
- Involution forms are seen in death/decline phase of bacterial growth.
- There are two general patterns of cell division in microorganisms:
  - In eukaryotes (protozoa, fungi, unicellular algae) → Process of mitosis.
  - In prokaryotes (bacteria) → Process of binary fission.
- Resolving power of electron microscope is 1–5 A°.
- Iron helps in virulence of *Staphylococcus aureus.*
- Culture media containing potassium tellurite- Monsur's GTTA medium for *V. cholerae* and Tellurite blood agar for *Corynebacterium* spp.
- Monsur's gelatin taurocholate trypticase tellurite agar (GTTA) medium (pH 8.5): High pH of the medium and presence of potassium tellurite in this medium inhibits most of Gram-positive bacteria and enteric bacteria with exception of Proteus species.
- Initially *Enterobacteriaceae* was classified on the bases of their lactose fermenting ability on MacConkey's medium, the most popular medium for the isolation of fecal bacilli.
- Lactose fermenters produce pink/bright red colonies on MacConkey's agar, while lactose non-fermenters produce pale colonies:
  - *Lactose fermenters (rapid)*: These are Coliforms, e.g. *Escherichia, Klebsiella* and *Enterobacter* species.
  - *Late lactose fermenters (slow)*: These are *Shigella sonnei, Serratia, Citrobacter, Providencia* and *Erwinia.*
  - *Non-lactose fermenters*: *Shigella* except *Shigella sonnei, Salmonella, Proteus.*
- Generation time of coliform bacilli – 20 minutes.
- Most common organism causing UTI after transurethral resection of prostate (TURP) is *E. coli.*
- Schick test is a neutralization test. A test for previously acquired immunity to diphtheria.
- Diphtheria toxin binds to specific receptors (HB-EGF receptors) present on cell membrane of susceptible cells and enters by receptor mediated endocytosis.
- Diphtheria toxin acts by inhibiting protein synthesis. It inhibits polypeptide chain elongation in the presence of NAD by inactivating elongation factor, EF-2.
- The strain almost universally used for toxin production is the "Park-Williams 8 strain".
- Erythrasma, a localized infection of the stratum corneum usually affecting the axilla and groin, is caused by *Corynebacterium minutissimum.*
- Dark ground (dark field) microscopy is used for Spirochetes and Flagella.
- *T. pallidum* (causative agent of syphilis) is a spirochete.
- Silver impregnation staining technique used for spirochetes (*Treponema, Borrelia, Leptospira*).
- Capsule of *Bacillus anthracis* is stained by Methylene blue.
- Cutaneous anthrax, also known as Hide porter's disease, is when anthrax occurs on the skin.
- Most common type of actinomycosis Cervicofacial.
- Cervicofacial actinomycosis presents as a swollen, erythematosus process in the jaw area (known as "lumpy jaw") which progresses into fistulas.

- **Immunoglobulins:**
  - All immunoglobulins are heat stable, except—IgE (only heat labile Ig)
  - Only immunoglobulin secreted by sero-mucinous glands— IgA
  - Immunoglobulins present in milk—IgA and IgG
  - Immunoglobulin to fix complement via alternate pathway - IgA & IgD & IgG (G4)
  - Immunoglobulin to fix complement via classical pathway—IgG and IgM
  - Immunoglobulin with maximum serum concentration - IgG
  - Immunoglobulin with maximum molecular weight—IgM
  - Immunoglobulin with maximum sediment coefficient—IgM
  - Immunoglobulin with shortest half-life—IgE
  - Immunoglobulin with least carbohydrate—IgG
  - Immunoglobulin with maximum carbohydrate—IgE
  - Immunoglobulin with maximum half-life—IgG
  - Immunoglobulin with minimum half-life–IgE
- Pentameric immunoglobulin- IgM
- Bacteriophages are viruses that infect bacteria.
- Polio virus in stools is isolated by Tissue culture method.
- Isolation of poliovirus from clinical specimen (feces, throat swab) by tissue culture is the most specific method in the diagnosis of poliomyelitis.
- Human immunodeficiency virus (HIV) was isolated in 1983 from a patient with lymphadenopathy, and by 1984 it was demonstrated clearly to be the causative agent of AIDS.
- Incubation period of Ebola virus is: 5–20 days.
- Classical infectious mononucleosis is caused of Epstein-Barr virus (EBV).
- CMV can also cause infectious mononucleosis called CMV mononucleosis or heterophile negative mononucleosis.
- Other diseases which can cause heterophile-negative mononucleosis are: Toxoplasmosis.
- Most common cause of seizures: *Toxoplasma*
- MC cause of focal neurological deficit: *Toxoplasma*
- Most common cause of meningitis: *Cryptococcus*
- *Schistosoma haematobium* is a well-known cause of urinary bladder cancer.
- Calabar swelling is due to adult worms of *Loa loa* (African eye worm).
- *The diseases in which human acts as dead end host*:
  - Japanese encephalitis
  - Echinococcosis (hydatid disease)
  - Trichinosis
  - Tetanus
  - Bubonic plague
- Savlon contains chlorhexidine gluconate (hibitane) and cetrimide (cetavlon) in various percentages. It is used as skin disinfectant (antiseptic).
- **Tyndallization (Intermittent Sterilization):**
  - Media containing sugar or gelatin are sterilized by heating at 100°C for 20 minutes on 3 successive days.
  - First exposure kills all vegetative bacteria.
  - Spores germinate are killed on subsequent exposures.

CHAPTER 7

Forensic Medicine

IDENTIFICATION

DETERMINATION OF BONE AGE

Ossification of carpal bones			
Bone	***Ossification time***	***Bone***	***Ossification time***
Capitate	2 months	Scaphoid	5 years
Hamate	3 months	Trapezium	6 years
Triquetral	3 years	Trapezoid	7 years
Lunate	4 years	Pisiform	8–12 years

Ossification centres before Birth	
2 months Intrauterine life	Center appears for mandible, clavicle, ribs, vertebrae, frontal and parietal bones
3 months Intrauterine life	Center appears for sacrum
4 months Intrauterine life	Center appears for temporal and occipital bones
5 months Intrauterine life	Center appears for calcaneum
6 months Intrauterine life	Center appears for sternum
7 months Intrauterine life	Center appears for talus
9 months Intrauterine life	Center appears for lower end of femur
At birth	Center appears for upper end of tibia and head of humerus

Age	Appearance of epiphyseal centres	Union of epiphysis with diaphysis
5th year	Head of radius	Greater tubercle fuses with head of humerus
6th year	Lower end of ulna	—
6th to 7th year	Medial epicondyle of humerus	—
9th year	Olecranon	—
9th to 11th year	Trochlea of humerus	—
11th year	Lateral epicondyle of humerus	—
13th year	Separate centres in triradiate cartilage of acetabulum	—
12th to 14th year	Lesser trochanter of femur	—
14th year	Iliac crest; head & tubercles of ribs	Medial epicondyle of humerus; lateral epicondyle with trochlea; patella complete.
15th year	Acromion process	Coracoid with scapula; triradiate cartilage of acetabulum
16th year	Ischial tuberosity	Lower end of humerus; olecranon to ulna; upper end of radius; metacarpals; proximal phalanges
17th to 18th year	—	Head of femur; lesser greater trochanter of femur; acromion process; lower end of ulna
18th to 19th year	Medial end of clavicle	Lower end of femur; upper end of tibia & fibula; head of humerus; lower end of radius
20th to 21st year	—	Iliac crest; medial end of clavicle; ischial tuberosity, head of ribs

1. First carpal bone to appear is:

a. Trapezium
b. Capitate
c. Pisiform
d. Lunate

Ans. is 'b' Capitate

2. Four carpal bones are present at what age?

a. 2 years b. 4 years
c. 6 years d. 8 years

Ans. is 'b' 4 years

3. Ossification center to appear before birth:

a. Medial epicondyle of humerus b. Olecranon
c. Clavicle d. Pisiform

Ans. is 'c' Clavicle

Differences between Male and Female Pelvis

Trait	*Male*	*Female*
1. Bony framework	Massive, rougher, marked muscle sites Stands higher and more erect	Less massive, slender, smoother Less muscle marking.
2. General	Deep funnel	Flat bowl
3. Ilium	Less vertical; curve of iliac crest reaches higher level and is more prominent	More vertical; distance between iliac crests is less; iliac fossae shallow; curves of crest well marked
4. Preauricular sulcus attachment of anterior sacroiliac ligament)	Not frequent; narrow, shallow	More frequent, broad and deep
5. Acetabulum	Large, 52 mm in diameter directed laterally	Small, 46 mm in diameter directed anterolaterally
6. Obturator foramen	Large often, oval with base upwards	Small, triangular with apex forwards
7. Greater sciatic notch	Smaller, narrower, deeper	Larger, wider, shallower
8. Iliopectineal line	Well marked and rough	Rounded and smooth
9. Ischial tuberosity	Inverted	Everted; more widely separated
10. Body of pubis	Narrow, triangular, thick; short ischial ramus	Broad, square, ischial ramus is lengthened and narrowed, pits on posterior surface if borne children
11. Ramus of pubis	It is like continuation of body of pubis	Has a constricted or narrowed appearance and is short and thick
12. Ischiopubic rami	More everted, thicker and rougher	Less everted thinner and smoother
13. Symphysis	Higher, bigger and narrow in width Margins of pubic arch everted	Lower, wider and rounded, margins of pubic arch not everted; distance between two pubic tubercles greater. The dorsal border is irregular and shows depressions or pits (scars of parturition)
14. Subpubic angle	V-shaped, sharp angle 70° to 75°	U-shaped, rounded, broader angle 90° to 100°
15. Pelvic brim or inlet	Heart-shaped	Circular or elliptical; more spacious diameters longer
16. Pelvic cavity	Conical and funnel-shape	Broad and round
17. Pelvic outlet	Smaller	Larger
18. Sacroiliac articulation	Large, extends to 2 ½ to 3 vertebrae	Small oblique extends to 2 to 2 ½ vertebrae
19. Sacroiliac joint surface	Large and less sharply angulated	L-shaped and elevated anteriorly
20. Sacrum	Longer, with more distributed curvature; promontory well marked. Body of first sacral vertebra larger	Short wider; upper half almost straight, curve forward in lower half; promontory less marked. Body of first sacral vertebra small
21. Coccyx	Less movable	More movable
22. Ischiopubic index Public length in mm × 100 Ischial length in mm	73 to 94	91 to 115
23. Sciatic notch index Width of notch index × 100 Depth of sciatic notch	4 to 5	5 to 6
24. Pubic ramus ratio	1:1	2:1 or greater

4. Subpubic angle in female is:

a. 70 degrees b. 90 degrees
c. 120 degrees d. 180 degrees

Ans. is 'b' 90 degrees

DACTYLOGRAPHY (DERMATOGLYPHICS, DACTYLOSCOPY, GALTON SYSTEM, FINGERPRINT STUDY)

Fingerprint identification is the method of identification using the impressions made by the minute ridge formations or patterns found on the fingertips. No two persons have exactly the same arrangement of ridge patterns, and the patterns of any one individual remain unchanged throughout life.

Classifications of Fingerprint Pattern

Sir Henry Galton (1892), depending on the arrangement of papillary ridges classified the fingerprints into four major or primary types .

1. Loop (65% of population)
2. Whorl (25% of population)
3. Arch (7% of population)
4. Composite/compound is a mixed picture of all three patterns above (2-3% of population).

Medicolegal Importance of Fingerprint

- Visible fingerprints: Fingers when smeared with blood, grease, etc. will leave their prints/impression on the weapon used for the crime/ furniture or such other articles that may be touched by criminal at the scene of crime unintentionally and can give clue for identifying the criminals. Such fingerprints constitute visible fingerprints.
- Latent fingerprints (invisible fingerprints): Fingerprint experts can render a faint and invisible/latent fingerprint visible by special techniques using some developing agents which are chemical powders and liquids. When these latent fingerprints are obtained at the crime scene by chance, these prints are termed as the chance fingerprints.
- Plastic fingerprints: These are prints of the finger left on soft materials such as wax, soap, dust, etc.
- Fingerprints from dead body: Tip of the finger may get shriveled in a dead body and then may mask the picture. So to avoid this, soak the fingers in alkaline solution first and then take the print. Fingerprint may be even taken from putrefied body where the cuticle of fingerball is pealed off from dermis, which will have the ridge pattern still intact.
- Identical twins have the same DNA but their fingerprints are still different.

Conditions Modifying Fingerprints

- *Temporary modification*: It may be due to:
  - Moderate ridge atrophy (± loss of pattern): Coeliac disease
  - Incomplete ridge atrophy or alteration: Acanthosis nigricans dermatitis, dry atrophic skin, scleroderma
  - Distance between ridges change (no change in pattern): Rickets, acromegaly, infantile paralysis.
  - Modification by applying physical agents (by criminals): CO_2, snow, corrosives, burns, eroding agent.
- *Permanent modification*: It occurs in leprosy, radiation, electric injury, by skin grafting and by complete destruction of skin.

5. Finger pattern may be impaired permanently in case of:

a. Acanthosis nigricans
b. Leprosy
c. Scleroderma
d. Snow exposure

Ans. is 'b' Leprosy

6. Identical twins will not have same: *(NEET 2019)*

a. Fingerprints
b. DNA copies
c. Iris color
d. Blood group

Ans. is 'a' Fingerprints

TATTOO MARKS

Mode of production: Tattoo marks are designs made in the skin by multiple small puncture wounds with needles or an electric vibrator dipped in coloring matter. The dyes commonly used are Indian ink, carbon (black), cinnabar or vermilion (mercuric sulphide) red, chromic acid (green), indigo, cobalt, Prussian blue (ferric ferrocyanide), ultramarine (blue). Techniques and dyes vary from country to country. Most of the marks are found on the arms, forearms and chest, but may be present on any part of the body.

Natural disappearance: If the pigment has been deposited below the epidermis, it will very slowly become fainter and certain pigments, such as vermilion, and ultramarine may disappear after about ten years. If the dye is deposited into deeper layers of dermis, it will be removed by phagocytes. The rate of fading depends not only on the composition of the pigment. But also on the depth to which it penetrates the skin, and the site which is tattooed. Tattoos on the hands disappear early due to constant friction. A faded tattoo mark becomes visible by the use of ultraviolet lamp or rubbing the part and examining with magnifying lens. Infrared photography makes old tattoos readily visible. Lymph nodes near a tattoo mark show a deposit of a pigment. The color, design, size and situation of tattoo marks should be noted.

7. During autopsy of a person, the relatives claimed that the deceased had a tattoo, however it was not visible on the body. Which sample should be dissected to get the evidence of tattoo? *(NEET 2020)*

a. Skin
b. Lymph nodes
c. Nerves
d. Blood vessels

Ans. is 'b' Lymph nodes

THANATOLOGY

LIVOR MORTIS

Livor mortis, also known as hypostasis/postmortem staining/suggillation/Vibices, is the discoloration of the skin due to the pooling of blood in the dependent parts of the body following death. The blood pools because the heart can no longer circulate the blood. Gravity will make the blood settle and the areas where it settles turns to a dark blue or purple color, which is termed 'lividity'.

The blood begins to pool immediately following death and is visible within a couple of hours. After the first two hours, the skin is bluish and blotchy. After five or six hours, the blotches become confluent and the skin will turn white when applied with pressure. After ten to twelve hours, the livid color remains even when pressed. Fixation of lividity is due to stagnation of blood in distended capillaries and venules.

It is important to note that the blood will migrate to the lowest point in the body that it can travel. This may not necessarily be the lowest part of the body. For instance, if the victim was a hanging victim, the lividity will show in the feet, fingertips and earlobes. If the body is found in a supine position, the lividity will be found in the parts of the body touching the ground. Being able to identify the discoloration can be very useful in determining if a body has been moved after death. If the position of body is changed after development of lividity but before it becomes fixed, these patches will disappear and fresh ones will develop in the new dependent areas but lividity to a slight degree will remain in the original area due to staining of tissue by hemolysis.

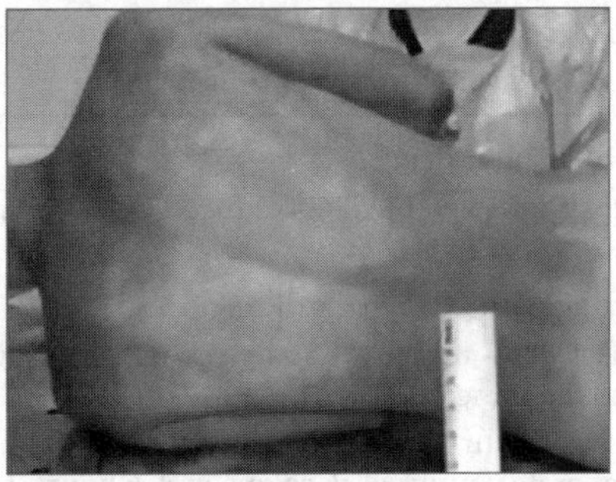

Postmortem Lividity

Color of postmortem staining in various poisonings:

Poison	Color
Carbon monoxide	Cherry red
HCN, burns	Bright red
Nitrites, potassium chlorate, potassium bicarbonate, nitrobenzene, aniline (causing methaemoglobinuria)	Chocolate or copper brown
Phosphorous	Dark brown or yellow
Hydrogen sulphide	Bluish green

8. Suggillation is due to which of the following?

a. Gravity leading to pooling of blood
b. Escape of blood from microvasculature
c. Molecular death leading to stiffening of muscles
d. Autolysis of enzymes

Ans. is 'a' Gravity leading to pooling of blood

9. Which of the following is present in postmortem staining?

a. Seen on dependent parts of body
b. Extravasation of blood from capillaries
c. Lividity is greatest on the pressure points
d. Develop rapidly in running water

Ans. is 'a' Seen on dependent parts of body

10. Cherry red postmortem staining is seen in:

a. Cyanide
b. Carbon monoxide
c. Nitrites
d. Phosphorus

Ans. is 'b' Carbon monoxide

Antemortem vs postmortem wound

Feature	*Antemortem wound*	*Postmortem wound*
Hemorrhage	• Arterial • Blood clotted and the clot is laminated • Firmly adherent to the lining of endothelium • Firm, rubbery and variegated • Copious • Deep staining of edges which cannot be washed away	• Venous • Blood usually not clotted and if clotted it is non-laminated • Weakly adherent to the lining of endothelium • Soft friable chicken fat (yellow) or Currant Jelly (red) appearance • Homogenous • Slight • Staining is superficial and can be washed away
Wound edges	Gaping, everted swollen	Apposed, not swollen
Vital reaction	Signs of inflammation, infection (pus, slough) and healing (granulation tissue) present	Not present
Wound serotonin & histamine content	Increased	No increase
Microscopy	• Clot has platelets • Leucocyte & RBC infiltration in between muscle fibres	• Clot lacks platelets • No infiltration

11. Postmortem wound is differentiated from antemortem wound by:

a. Wound serotonin content
b. Blood clot
c. Wound edges
d. All of the above

Ans. is 'd'All of the above

RIGOR MORTIS

- Rigor mortis refers to the stiffening of the body after death.
- It occurs due formation of actin-myosin cross links when ATP is reduced to less than 85% of normal.
- Nysten's law deals with the progression of rigor mortis
- It first affects the involuntary muscles starting with the myocardium
- The order of appearance in voluntary muscles is – upper eyelids, neck muscles, jaw, facial muscles, upper limbs, trunk muscles, lower limbs. Order of disappearance is also the same.
- In tropical countries (e.g. India), it begins 1–2 hours after death, takes further 2 hours to develop, and lasts for 18–36 hours in summer and 24–48 hours in winter. In temperate countries, it begins in 3–6 hours, takes further 2–3 hours to develop and lasts for 2–3 days.
- Causes of faster onset of rigor mortis - extremes of age, malnutrition, immersion in water.
- Onset is delayed in pneumonia, myasthenia gravis.

ADIPOCERE FORMATION AND MUMMIFICATION

Adipocere is a spontaneous form of partial preservation by the hydrolysis or saponification of body fat. It is therefore more commonly seen and is more prominent in women and in young, well-nourished children. The hydrolysed fat is at first yellowish-brown in color and of firm consistency; as time passes, it becomes white and friable. It has an offensive, pervasive and persistent odor. When ignited, it burns with a smoky yellow lambent flame. Its formation is dependent upon the presence of adequate moisture (for example, immersion in water or burial in a bog). Acidity is also an important factor. Bodies buried in peat bogs, which are highly acid, or interred in coffins with oak shavings rich in thiamine, may be preserved for hundreds, or even thousands, of years.

Mummification is uncommon in temperate climates. The drying out and hardening of the tissues associated with this condition require temperatures far higher than those normally achieved. It proceeds from exterior to interior. Therefore, first to be involved is skin, especially of exposed body parts like lips, nose tip, hands (fingers) and feet (toes). The skin becomes dry, brittle and shrunken. It is usually of dark brown color. The tips of the fingers and toes may be lost. The hair, irrespective of its color in life, is usually foxy red. The internal organs are also dry and shrunken, but may be sufficiently well preserved for a naked eye diagnosis to be made. Microscopy is unrewarding, both in mummified and adipocerous bodies. Features of the body are preserved. A mummified body is odorless.

PUTREFACTION

- Putrefaction is the last stage in resolution of body from the inorganic to organic state and is a certain sign of death.
- Two factors are responsible for putrefaction:
  - Bacterial enzymes from colon
  - Autolysis (Release of cytoplasmic enzymes)

- Three conditions are necessary for putrefaction: (i) warmth (10-45° celsius), (ii) moisture (humidity) and (iii) air. If air is absent, adipocere formation (saponification) occurs, and in the absence of moisture, mummification occurs.
    - Moisture present, warmth present, air present → Putrefaction.
    - Moisture present, warmth present, air absent, i.e. warm humid climate → Adipocere formation (saponification).
    - Moisture absent, warmth present, air present, i.e. hot dry climate → Mummification
- **Characteristic features:**
    - *Color changes*: First visible external evidence of putrefaction; greenish discoloration of the skin over right iliac fossa
    - *Marbling*: Staining of the walls of the superficial veins following hemolysis of red cells; prominent in 36 to 48 hours.
    - Development of foul smelling gases.
- **Organs show putrefactive changes in the following order**
    - Larynx and trachea > Stomach and Intestines > Spleen > Liver > Brain > Heart and Lungs > Kidneys and Bladder > Uterus (last organ to putrefy in females); Prostate (last organ to putrefy in males)
- **Putrefaction is delayed in**: Death due to wasting diseases or anemia, and poisoning by Carbolic acid, Zinc chloride, Strychnine and chronic heavy metal poisoning.
- **Casper's dictum:** It is the effect of medium (in which body lies) on rate of putrefaction. Casper's dictum states that a body decomposes in air twice as rapidly as in water and eight times as rapidly in earth.

12. First affected in rigor mortis? *(NEET 2019)*

a. Eyelids
b. Myocardium
c. Jaw
d. Neck

Ans. is 'b' Myocardium

13. Ideal condition for Adipocere formation includes:

a. Warm humid weather
b. Dry hot air
c. Cold humid air
d. Cold dry weather

Ans. is 'a' Warm humid weather

14. Among the following, which is the earliest organ to putrefy?

a. Brain
b. Kidney
c. Heart
d. Prostrate

Ans. is 'a' Brain

15. Mummified body smells like:

a. Odorless
b. Fishy
c. Bitter almond
d. Sweetish

Ans. is 'a' Odorless

16. According to Casper's dictum, decomposition is the fastest when the body is in which of the following?

a. Air
b. Water
c. Earth
d. Soil

Ans. is 'a' Air

17. Rigor mortis occurs due to:

a. Breakdown of enzymes in the body
b. Depletion of ATP
c. Accumulation of blood in dependent areas
d. Loss of heat

Ans. is 'b' Depletion of ATP

18. A dead body was received for autopsy. It was bloated, with swollen tongue and blisters spread on entire body. What is the reason possible? *(NEET 2020)*

a. Decomposition
b. Scalds
c. Burns
d. Electrocution

Ans. is 'a' Decomposition

Explanation: The terms decomposition and putrefaction are used as synonyms

INJURIES

CARTRIDGE

- Cartridge is the ammunition used in firearms.
- Cartridge consists of:

- **Cartridge case:** It is the outer covering of the cartridge. In shotgun it is cylindrical. In rifled weapons, it is tapering. Center of base has percussion cap (detonator cap) which has sensitive composition, i.e. prime, consisting of potassium chlorate, antimony sulphide, mercury fulminate, barium nitrite, lead peroxide or tetrazine. In all weapons, after firing, the cartridge case remains in the barrel and it is to be taken out manually (shotgun, revolvers, rifle) or it is ejected out automatically, e.g. in pistols.
- **Propellant (gunpowder):** It is composed of black powder or smokeless powder in the form of grains, pellets, thin cylindrical cords or flakes. Its ignition results in formation of expanding hot gases under pressure which (gas pressure) propels the projectile by providing it necessary muzzle velocity and striking energy. The classical gun powder is known as black powder, consists of charcoal (15%), Sulphur (10%), and potassium nitrate (75%).
- **Projectile (missile):** Projectile is an object propelled by force of rapidly burning gases. In shotgun these are lead shots and pellets and in rifled weapons (pistol, rifle, revolver), these are bullets.
- **Wads:** Wads are present only in the cartridge of a shotgun. Wad can be made of paper, left, card board, or plastic. These are circular disc of various thicknesses, used to adjust the contents of a shotgun cartridge.

VARIETIES OF BULLETS

- **Incendiary (igniting) bullet:** The tip of bullet contains self-igniting material, e.g. barium nitrate and powdered aluminum and magnesium, so that it catches fire on hitting the target.
- **Explosive bullet:** The tip contains a detonator or lead azide, so that the bullet explodes on hitting the target.
- **Dum-dum bullet (expanding bullet):** It is a jacketed bullet with its nose tip chiseled or cut off. It is designed to increase in diameter and expand upon striking the target, thus producing larger diameter wounds of limited penetration and in order to stop it from leaving the body. Compared to regular bullets, dum-dum bullets are intended to cause maximum tissue damage.
- **Tandem bullet (Piggy tail bullet):** It is called one-behind-other bullet because two bullets are ejected one after the other, when first bullet failed to leave the barrel and is ejected by subsequently fired bullet.
- **Ricochet bullet:** Ricocheting of bullet is defined as deviation in the direction or path of bullet because of striking of bullet to an intermediary object. External ricocheting results from the bullet hitting an object before entering the body, e.g. door, wall or furniture etc. Internal ricocheting results from bullet hitting the bone inside the body.
- **Tumbling bullet:** One that rotates in end on end during its motion.
- **Souvenir bullet:** A bullet left in body for long time and is surrounded by fibrous tissue.

19. Bullet fixed from a gun is not released. It is ejected out with subsequent shot. Such a bullet is called as:

a. Tandem bullet
b. Dum-dum bullet
c. Incendiary bullet
d. Tumbling bullet

Ans. is 'a' Tandem bullet

20. Which of the following causes maximum damage?

a. Tandem
b. Dum-dum
c. Souvenir
d. Piggy

Ans. is 'b' Dum-dum

21. Compound used as primer in weapon is:

a. Potassium chlorate
b. Sulphur
c. Potassium nitrate
d. Nitrocellulose

Ans. is 'a' Potassium chlorate

22. Ricochet bullet is:

a. Bullet producing a key hole entry wound
b. Bullet with nose tip chiseled off
c. Deviation in the direction or path of bullet
d. Bullet containing igniting material

Ans. is 'c' Deviation in the direction or path of bullet

FEATURES OF FIREARM INJURIES AT VARIOUS RANGES

Hard Contact

Over Soft Tissues

- Circular hole
- Abrasion collar
- Bruising
- Local reddening (heat and CO)
- Little or no surface burning
- Little or no propellant soiling/powder tattooing
- +/– muzzle impression

Over Bone

- ❖ Split/cruciate wound
- ❖ Local reddening
- ❖ Bruising
- ❖ Little or no surface burning/propellant soiling
- ❖ Abrasion collar partially lost on skin tags

Close Range: <15 cm

- ❖ Circular hole and abrasion collar
- ❖ Flame burn on skin
- ❖ Burnt hairs
- ❖ Soot/smoke soiling
- ❖ Punctate propellant tattooing marks
- ❖ Unburnt propellant flakes
- ❖ Little/no CO in tissues

Intermediate Range: 15–30 cm

- ❖ No soot
- ❖ +/– tattooing
- ❖ No CO
- ❖ Rarely flame burns

Distant Range: >40–60 cm

- ❖ Circular hole with abrasion collar
- ❖ No burning/soiling
- ❖ No burnt hairs
- ❖ No CO

'Far Distant' (At Limit of Range)

- ❖ Larger irregular hole
- ❖ Irregular abrasion collar
- ❖ Irregular abrasion rim ('tumbling bullet')

23. In alleged history of gunshot injury, there is burning, blackening and tattooing around the wound with dirt collar. The injury is: *(NEET 2019)*

a. Close shot entry wound
b. Close shot exit wound
c. Distant shot entry wound
d. Distant shot exit wound

Ans. is 'a' Close shot entry wound

TYPES OF INJURIES

Features	Incision	Laceration	Stab wound
Mode of injury	By sharp objects or weapons	By blunt objects or weapons	By pointed sharp or blunt weapons
Site	Anywhere in the body	Usually over bony prominences	Anywhere in the body; usually in the trunk
Margins	Smooth, clean cut & everted edges	Irregular & undermined edges	Clean-cut, parallel edges Irregular edges if blunt weapon is used
Surrounding abrasions and bruising	Absent	Usually present	Absent
Shape	Linear	Usually irregular	Linear or irregular
Dimensions	Usually longer than deep; often gaping	Usually longer than deep	Depth greater than length & breadth
Depth of wound	Structures cleanly cut to the depth of wound	Small strands of tissue at the bottom bridge across margins	Structures cleanly cut
Hemorrhage	Usually profuse & external spurting of blood may be seen	Slight except scalp & external	Varies; usually internal
Hair bulbs	Cleanly cut	Crushed or torn	Usually clean cut

Contd...

Contd...

Features	Incision	Laceration	Stab wound
Bones	May be cut	May be fractured	May be punctured
Foreign bodies	Absent	Present	Absent
Clothes	May be cut	May be torn	May be cut

- Blunt force on areas where the skin is close to rigid structures like bone with scanty subcutaneous tissue, may produce a laceration that by linear splitting of tissue may look like incised wound, i.e. incised-like wound. Examples of such area are scalp, eyebrows, cheek bones (zygomatic), lower jaw, iliac crest, perineum and skin. A wound produced by a fall on knee or elbow with limb flexed and by a sharp stone also simulates incised wound.

Heat Ruptures (Heat Splits or Fissure)

- In severe burns, skin splits frequently especially over extensor surfaces (e.g. thigh, back of arm) and joints.
- These are multiple and may be several centimeters in length. They may be confused with incised wounds.
- Differentiating features of heat rupture are:
  - Presence of intact nerves, blood vessels and connective tissue in the floor of rupture
  - Absence of bleeding in the wound, since heat coagulates the blood in vessels
  - Irregular margins
  - Absence of bruising or other vital reactions in margin.

Degloving Injury

- The clinical entity of degloving injury means that the skin has been lost, but the musculoskeletal unit is intact, and hence, the movements of the part have been preserved.
- Degloving, also called avulsion, is a type of severe injury that happens when the top layers of skin and subcutaneous tissue are ripped from the underlying muscle, connective tissue, or bone. It can affect any body part, but it is more common in the legs.
- Depending on the angle that the tire pulls across the extremity, the skin and subcutaneous tissue may be pulled or sheared off on leading edge of extremity.

24. Degloving injury involves removal of: *(NEET 2019)*

a. Skin, subcutaneous tissue, fascia, muscle
b. Skin, subcutaneous tissue, fascia
c. Skin only
d. Skin and subcutaneous tissue

Ans. is 'd' Skin and subcutaneous tissue

25. Laceration at which site looks like an incision:

a. Scalp
b. Eyebrows
c. Lower jaw
d. All of the above

Ans. is 'd' All of the above

26. Characteristic of heat rupture:

a. Lacerated nerves, blood vessels
b. Profuse bleeding
c. Regular margins
d. Absence of bruising in the margin

Ans. is 'd' Absence of bruising in the margin

PUGILISTIC ATTITUDE

Pugilistic attitude aka heat rigor or heat stiffening is the characteristic attitude attained by the dead body which suffered from severe burns.

It is similar to the defensive position adopted by boxers and consists of flexion at the elbows, knees, hip & neck and clenching of hand into a fist.

Mechanism

- Pugilistic attitude is due to heat induced coagulation of muscle proteins resulting in contractures.
- High temperatures > 50°C are required; well established at 75°C
- Contraction of paraspinal muscles causes a marked opisthotonos.

Characteristic Features

- The posturing is stronger than that produced by rigor mortis. It is irreversible.

Interpretation

- It is seen in both antemortem and postmortem burns, hence it cannot be used to ascertain burns as the cause of death.
- Pugilistic attitude is never seen in living victims.

27. Which of the following is not true about pugilistic attitude?

a. Occurs due to rigor mortis
b. Due to extensive heat [>65° C]
c. Permanent change
d. Coagulation of proteins

Ans. is 'a' Occurs due to rigor mortis

BLAST INJURIES

- Primary blast injuries occur due to the shock waves produced by an explosion
- Sudden changes in barometric pressure are propelled from the point of detonation
- Air filled hollow organs including ear, lungs & GIT are most commonly injured due to the rapid change in pressure.
- Damage to the lungs is the most common life-threatening injury.

Injuries may occur due to various mechanisms:

Primary injury: Due to rapid increase in pressure. It damages hollow organs.

Secondary injury: Caused by airborne debris. It results in Marshall's triad injuries- bruises, abrasions & puncture lacerations.

Tertiary injury: Caused by the blast wind due to which victim is thrown in the air and hits other objects leading to trauma

Quaternary injury: Injuries due to any complications other than those mentioned above, e.g. burns, crush injuries, histotoxic anoxia.

Most commonly affected organs:

- Air blast: Tympanic membrane
- Underwater blast (when fully submerged): Tympanic membrane
- Underwater blast (when head is out of water): GIT

Most severely affected organs:

- Air blast: lungs
- Underwater blast: GIT

28. Least common organ affected in blast injury is:

a. Lung
b. Eardrum
c. Muscles
d. GIT damage

Ans. is 'c' Muscles

BATTERED BABY SYNDROME (CAFFEY'S SYNDROME/ INFANTILE WHIPLASH SYNDROME)

- Battered baby is a child who has received non-accidental physical injuries repeatedly from the parent.
- The child is usually an unwanted baby less than 3 years of age.

Classical Features

- Discrepancy between the examination findings and history provided by the parents
- Delay between time of injury & seeking medical care.
- Injuries of varying duration and severity.

Pattern of Injuries

- *Most common method of injury*: Direct manual violence
- *Most characteristic lesion*: Laceration of mucosa of upper lip with tear of frenulum & alveolar margins of gums.
- Burns, lacerations, retinal & subhyaloid hemorrhage, rib fractures, spiral fractures of long bones & displaced epiphysis, subperiosteal hematoma are also seen.
- Violent shaking causes subdural hematoma and intraocular bleeding- known as infantile whiplash syndrome
  - Multiple bruises of different ages are seen
- Skull fracture or subdural hematoma is the most common cause of death followed by liver or mesenteric injury.
- Fracture of ribs, acromion process, sternum of spinous process of vertebrae may occur, which is otherwise uncommon in children.
- Violent movements of limbs results in typical 'corner' or 'bucket-handle'-fractures in metaphyseal region, which is highly specific.
- Multiple 'eggshell' fractures of the skull are also seen.

29. Battered baby syndrome is identified by: *(NEET 2019)*

a. Stab wound
b. Gunshot wound
c. Bruises of different ages
d. None of the above

Ans. is 'c' Bruises of different ages

Previously Asked Facts

- X-ray of choice for age detection at around 16–17 years of age is Wrist.
- Pelvis is the best bone for sex determination.
- Crural Index = Length of femur/Length of tibia × 100; used for race determination.
- Rule of Hasse is used to estimate the age of fetus from its crown-heel length in cm. During first five months, age in lunar months = √CHL in cm; At age of > 5 months, Age in lunar months = CHL/5.

Feature of Mandible	Infancy	Adult	Old age
Angle of mandible	Obtuse angle	Right angle	Obtuse angle
Mental foramen	Near lower border	Midway b/w upper and lower border	Looks apparently nearer the upper border d/t loss of teeth

- At 3 years all the temporary teeth are present → 20 in number.
- First temporary tooth to erupt is lower central incisors and last temporary tooth to erupt is 2nd molar. The sequence of eruption is lower central incisor> upper central incisor> upper lateral incisor >lower lateral incisor>1st molar> Canine > 2nd molar. Therefore, eruption of temporary teeth is completed by eruption of 2nd molar at 2 years.
- First permanent tooth to erupt is 1st molar and last to erupt is 3rd molar. The sequence of eruption is 1st molar> central incisor> lateral incisor > 1st premolar > 2nd premolar > canine >2nd molar > 3rd molar. Eruption of permanent teeth is completed by eruption of 3rd molar between 17–25 years.
- *Locard exchange principle*: Whenever two objects come in contact with each other, there is a mutual transfer of material from one object to the other. This is the basis of all crime detection.
- Forensic entomology is the use of insects and other arthropods in legal investigations. The forensic entomologist may estimate a portion of the postmortem interval based on the age of the insect present.
- Lecithinase is an enzyme produced by *Clostridium welchii,* which hydrolyses the lecithin present in all the cell membranes including blood cells and thus is responsible for producing postmortem hemolysis.
- Exhumation is lawful digging out of a dead body from the grave for the purpose of identification or determination of cause of death. Only a magistrate (executive magistrate) can order for exhumation. In India, there is no time limit for exhumation, i.e. can be done at any time after death.
- Normally, temperature falls after death. But in some situations, for initial 2–3 hours the dead body may heat, i.e. postmortem caloricity. This may occur due to disturbed heat regulation (heat stroke, pontine hemorrhage); heat production by muscular activity (tetanus, strychnine poisoning, asphyxial death); Acute infections (pneumonia, septicemia) or very high atmospheric temperature.
- Tissue damage (or destructive power of bullet) is dependent on striking (kinetic) energy of bullet, which is proportional to its mass and square of velocity ($KE = \frac{1}{2} mv^2$).
- Most common organ injured in direct stab injury is Liver.
- Hesitation, or tentative, wounds are defined either as any cut or wound that is self-inflicted after a decision is made not to commit suicide, or any tentative cut or wound that is made before attempting the final, fatal wound. Such wounds are usually superficial, sharp, forced skin cuts found on the body of victims.
- Coup injury is defined as the injury of skull and/or brain at the site of impact. Contrecoup injury is defined as an injury to the skull or brain, on opposite (contralateral) side of the area of impact. It is caused when moving head is suddenly decelerated by hitting a firm surface.
- *Cafe coronary*: It refers to accidental chocking by bolus of food obstructing larynx. Death is mostly due to asphyxia, or due to reflex cardiac arrest caused by stimulation of laryngeal nerve endings.
- Homicide by constriction of neck with rods is known as Bansdola.
- Diatom test is used to diagnose death due to Drowning. Diatoms are unicellular algae, suspended in water.
- The age of consent in India has been increased to 18 years, which means any sexual activity irrespective of presence of consent with a woman below the age of 18 will constitute statutory rape.
- Sexual Perversions
  - *Sadism*: Sexual gratification is obtained or increased from acts of physical cruelty or infliction of pain on partner
  - *Masochism*: Sexual gratification is obtained or increased by the suffering of pain
  - *Necrophilia*: Desire for sexual intercourse with dead bodies.
  - *Transvestism (Eonism)*: Desire of being identified with the opposite sex
  - *Fetishism*: A fetish is an abnormal stimulus or object of sexual desire. Fetishism means the use of such objects of sexual gratification leading to orgasm.
  - Buccal coitus (Sin of Gomorrah): In this, the male organ is introduced into mouth, usually of a young child.
  - Tribadism (Lesbianism or female homosexuality): Sexual gratification of a woman is obtained by another woman by kissing, body contact, manipulation of breast and genitalia. Active partner is called dyke or butch and the passive agent is called femme. This is not an offence in India.
- Most common hymen tear in sexual assault is posterolateral.

FETICIDE AND INFANTICIDE

TESTS USED IN INFANTICIDE

Ploucquet Test

- Weight of lung is measured in relation to body weight. Before birth weight of lung is 1170 of body weight and after respiration it becomes 1/35 of body weight due to increased blood flow in lung beds.

Static Test or Fodere Test

- The average weight of both lungs before respiration is 30-40 gm and after respiration is 60–0 cm.

Hydrostatic Test (Raygat Test, Breslau's 1st Life Test)

- The specific gravity of a non-respired lung is 1040-1050 and of a respired lung is 940-950, so, after respiration lung floats on water (specific gravity of water is 1000).
- False positive hydrostatic test may occur, i.e. non-respired lung may float) in decomposition and in attempted artificial respiration.
- False negative hydrostatic test (i.e. respired lung may sink down) may occur in atelectasis, pulmonary oedema, bronchopneumonia and congenital syphilis.

Breslau's Second Life Test

- It assumes that a live born child would respire and therefore, would also swallow some air into the stomach and bowel.
- Hence they float on water. This test is falsely positive in putrefaction (due to putrefied gases) or in cases of attempted artificial respiration.

Wredin Test

Before birth middle ear contains gelatinous embryonic tissue which is replaced by air after respiration.

30. Which of the following is the test done to confirm live born fetus after fetal death?

a. Mirror test
b. Breslau test
c. Magnus test
d. Paraffin test

Ans. is 'b' Breslau test

31. Which of the following tests requires specific gravity of lungs to assess live birth?

a. Breslau test
b. Fodere test
c. Raygat test
d. Ploucquet test

Ans. is 'c' Raygat test

EVIDENCE

TESTS FOR IDENTIFICATION OF BLOOD STAINS

- **Routine (screening) tests**: Most of these tests rely on the activity of peroxidase enzymes in blood to react with a chemical stain causing it to change color, or in the case of luminol, glow in the dark. Examples for such tests are:
  - Benzidine test—most reliable, but not done since benzidine is carcinogenic. Dark blue is seen if blood is present.
  - Leucomalachite green—gives peacock blue color
  - Phenolphthalein test or Kastle Meyer's test—gives pink color
  - Ortho toluidine—gives blue color
  - Tetra-methyl benzidine
  - Luminol spray
- **Confirmatory tests**: include several tests namely, microchemical tests, microscopic examination, spectroscopic examination, etc.
  - Microchemical tests— These tests are based on the property of haem (iron) part of haemoglobin to form characteristic colored crystals with certain reagents, and these crystals can be seen only microscopically.
    - Haemin crystal (Teichmann test)—brown rhomboid crystals of hemin are produced.
    - Hemochromogen crystal (Takayama test) test—pink feathery crystals of hemochromogen are produced.
  - Microscopic examination: This is possible only with a fresh stain and one can clearly identify the RBCs and WBCs, which helps in confirming the stain as blood.
  - Spectroscopic examination: This is a more reliable test for both old and fresh blood stains. The test needs only a very small quantity of stain. This test depends on property of the translucent colored fluid to absorb certain rays from the solar spectrum. However, this needs the use of equipment called spectroscope.

Detection of species (whether the blood has come from human or animal)

For detection of species, serological (immunological) tests are used. These tests are:

- Precipitin test
- Haemaglutination inhibition test (antiglobulin consumption test or absorption inhibition test)
- Gel diffusion test
- Double diffusion test
- Precipitation electrophoresis
- Latex agglutination test
- Isoenzyme method (enzymological test)

32. Blood stains on body and clothing can be made visible by:

a. Phenolphthalein test
b. Harrison and Gilroy test
c. Florence test
d. Barberio test

Ans. is 'a' Phenolphthalein test

33. Test for species differentiation of blood:

a. Blood grouping
b. Precipitin test
c. Benzidine test
d. Amidopyridine test

Ans. is 'b' Precipitin test

TESTS TO DETECT SEMEN

- **Chemical tests:**
  - Microchemical tests: Florence test (produces brown crystals of choline periodide), and Barberio's test (produces yellow crystals of spermine picrate by picric acid)
  - Enzyme tests: Acid phosphatase, creatinine phosphokinase (> 400 units) and specific glycoproteins (P30 or MHS-5).
  - Ammonium molybdate test: It gives deep yellow color, due to presence of phosphorus.
- **Microscopic examination:**
  - It is done to demonstrate the presence of spermatozoa in the vaginal fluid or in stain.
- **Biological examination:**
  - Precipitin test: To know the species to which semen belongs.
- **UV light:**
  - Invisible, softened and dry semen stains of the clothes can be rendered distinct by the filtered UV light, which produces bluish fluorescence.
- **Testes for determination of specific protein component (e.g. LDH isoenzyme)**
  - These are immune electrophoresis, gel diffusion precipitation, gel electrophoresis, immune diffusion, isoelectric focusing and TLC (thin layer chromatography).

34. Test to detect spermine in semen is:

a. Barberio test
b. Ammonium molybdate test
c. Acid phosphatase test
d. Florence test

Ans. is 'a' Barberio test

35. A child with rectal bleeding was suspected to be sexually abused. Anal swabs were taken and reaction with picric acid revealed formation of crystals. What test is performed? *(NEET 2020)*

a. Barberio's test
b. Florence test
c. Acid phosphatase test
d. Ammonium molybdate test

Ans. is 'a' Barberio's test

TOXICOLOGY

CHRONIC LEAD POISONING (PLUMBISM/SATURNISM)

Clinical Features

- Facial pallor—earliest sign
- Lead line/Burtonian lines in gums
- Colicky abdominal pain and constipation

- Sterility in males and females
- Wrist drop & foot drop – Motor nerve palsies
- Lead encephalopathy in children.

Diagnosis

- >200 punctate basophilic stippled cells /mm^3 is diagnostic
- Zinc protoporphyrin & free erythrocyte protoporphyrin > 50 mg/100 mL
- Increased lead & aminolevulinic acid (>25 mg/100 mL)
- Increased urinary coproporphyrin and ALA levels.
- Presence of 0.25 mg lead /liter of urine is diagnostic.

X-ray Findings in Lead Poisoning

- Radio-opaque bands /lines at metaphysis of long bones in children.

Treatment

- Gastric lavage with 1% solution of sodium or magnesium sulphate
- Chelating agent: BAL, DMSA
- Most effective antidote: Calcium Disodium Versenate
- Intravenous calcium chloride causes deposition of lead in skeleton from blood
- Dialysis

36. Pure motor palsy seen in poisoning of:

a. Lead poisoning
b. Arsenic poisoning
c. Cocaine poisoning
d. Cannabis poisoning

Ans. is 'a' Lead poisoning.

MERCURY POISONING

Metallic mercury is not poisonous on ingestion, as it is not absorbed. But its vapours are poisonous. Mercuric compounds are more poisonous than mercurous compounds. Mercuric chloride (HgCI2), also called corrosive sublimate is most poisonous salt of mercury.

- Acute poisoning presents with syncope, convulsions general instability and nephrotoxicity (proximal tubular). The mouth, tongue and fauces become corroded and appears grayish white.

Chronic Mercury Poisoning

- Excessive salivation, metallic taste, loosening of teeth, and blue black lining on gums (similar to lead poisoning).
- Diphtheria like membranous colitis and dysentery.
- Anorexia, insomnia, sweating, nausea, irritability and photophobia.

Special features are:

- **Mercuria lentis**: Brownish deposition of mercury on anterior lens capsule.
- **Tremors**: There are moderately coarse, intentional tremors starting in fingers and hands, and legs. They are also called Danbury tremors or hatter's shake or glass blower's shake.
- **Erethism** (neuropsychiatric changes): The personality disturbance is characterized by shyness, irritability tremors, loss of memory and insomnia. There may be depression, delusion and hallucination.
- **Acrodynia** (Pink disease): This is idiosyncratic hypersensitivity reaction with a generalized pinkish rash described as 5 P's: pinkish, puffy, painful, paraesthetic hands and peeling of skin.
- **Minamata disease**: It is due to organic mercury poisoning due to eating fish poisoned by mercury.
- **Membranous glomerulopathy**

37. Hatter's shake is seen in:

a. Phosphorus poisoning
b. Mercury poisoning
c. Arsenic poisoning
d. Lead poisoning

Ans. is 'b' Mercury poisoning

ACID POISONING

- Acids are potent desiccants and produce immediate coagulative necrosis of tissues.
- Hydrofluoric acid (HF) is an exception, because it produces liquefactive necrosis.
- An eschar is formed at the site of exposure, which then limits further damage.

- Mechanism of eschar formation: When a strong acid is mixed with a solvent, large amount of heat is produced. This thermochemical reaction results in eschar formation.
- Stronger acid solutions with lower pH (higher H^+ content) are more corrosive.
- Acid causes greater damage to gastric mucosa than esophageal mucosa because squamous epithelium is more resistant to acid exposure. However, when exposed to alkali, esophageal mucosa is more severely damaged.
- Antrum and pylorus are most commonly affected parts of the stomach.
- Magenstrasse is the term applied to the pathway acidic agents follow in stomach. The pathway of acids and alkalis follows a tubular portion adjacent to the lesser curvature from the cardia to gastric outlet, which is why it is the location of greatest damage in acid poisoning.
- There are highest chances of perforation of stomach with H_2SO_4, among all mineral acids.
- 'Vitriolage' is throwing of any corrosive on another person.

38. True about acid poisoning is:

a. Greatest damage is along the lesser curvature
b. Corrosives cause vaporization of tissues
c. Vitriolage means ingestion of acid in empty
d. Highest chance of perforation is with nitric acid

Ans. is 'a' Greatest damage is along the lesser curvature

POSTMORTEM IMBIBITION OF ARSENIC

- In exhumations, the possibility of imbibition of arsenic from the stomach into neighbouring viscera and also contamination from the surrounding earth should be remembered.
- If nails, hair and bones contain more arsenic than that of the soil present around the body, it indicates poisoning by arsenic.
- If arsenic is introduced into the stomach after death, the transudation occurs into the organs of the left side before those of the right and signs of inflammation and ulceration are absent.

39. The poison detected in exhumed bodies is: *(NEET 2020)*

a. Arsenic
b. Azide
c. Carbon dioxide
d. Hydrogen sulphide

Ans. is 'a' Arsenic

SNAKE BITE

Features	Elapids (cobra, krait)	Vipers	Sea snakes
Type of venom	Neurotoxic	Hemotoxic	Myotoxic
Site of action	Motor neurons; effect similar to curare	Endothelial cells & RBCs; causes hemolysis	Muscles
Local symptoms at the site of bite	Minimal	Severe (severe swelling, oozing of blood & cellulitis)	Minimal
Clinical presentation	Weakness of muscles legs & face	Features of coagulopathy	Generalized muscle pain and weakness, myoglobinuria

40. Sea snake is:

a. Neurotoxic
b. Vasculotoxic
c. Myotoxic
d. All of the above

Ans. is 'c' Myotoxic

CHELATING AGENTS

Chelating agents are used in heavy metal poisoning. They form complex with metal which is more soluble in water than the metal itself, resulting in higher renal excretion of complex. Important chelating agents are:

- **Dimercaprol (BAL):**
  - It is used in poisoning by Gold (Au), Copper (Cu), Bismuth (Bi), Nickel (Ni), Arsenic (As), Antimony (Sb) and Mercury (Hg).
  - It is used as adjuvant to calcium disodium edetate in lead poisoning and adjuvant to penicillamine in copper poisoning (or Wilson's disease).
  - It is contraindicated in iron (Fe) and cadmium (Cd) poisoning.
- **Calcium disodium edetate ($CaNa_2EDTA$):**
  - Most important use is lead poisoning and it is also useful in Zn, Mn, Fe, Cu and radioactive metal.
  - It has no role in mercury poisoning.

- ❖ **Penicillamine**
  - It is the drug of choice for copper poisoning and Wilson's disease. It is also used as an adjuvant to EDTA in lead poisoning and to BAL in mercury poisoning.
- ❖ **Desferoxamine:** It is the drug of choice for acute iron poisoning.
- ❖ **Deferipone:** It is the drug of choice for transfusion siderosis

41. BAL is used as an antidote of poisoning by:

a. Mercury
b. Manganese
c. Copper
d. Iron

Ans. is 'a' Mercury

GASTRIC LAVAGE

- ❖ Indicated for ingested poisons
- ❖ Useful within 2-4 hours (max 6–8 hours) after ingestion of poison
- ❖ In poisoning with salicylates, phenothiazines, TCAs and anti-histamines, lavage can be done up to 12–18 hours after ingestion of poison.

Contraindications

- ❖ The only absolute contraindication is corrosive (acids and alkalis) poisoning – Except Carbolic Acid.
- ❖ Relative contraindications include – Comatose patients, convulsions, pregnancy and children.

Solutions used for Gastric Lavage

Poison	*Solutions*
Most poisons – known or unknown	Water or saline
Oxidizable poisons (salicylates)	Potassium permanganate ($KMnO_4$)- 1:5000 or 1:10000 solution
Cyanides	Sodium thiosulfate 25%
Carbolic acid	Castor oil and warm water
Oxalates	Calcium gluconate
Iron	Desferrioxamine

42. Gastric lavage is not contraindicated after ingestion of which acid? *(NEET 2019)*

a. HCl
b. H_2SO_4
c. Carbolic acid
d. Nitric acid

Ans. is 'c' Carbolic acid

VISCERA PRESERVATION FOR CHEMICAL ANALYSIS

Routinely five bottles are sent for analysis and is sufficient in cases where the poison is suspected to be ingested. When the mode of administration is not by ingestion, then additional viscera has to be preserved depending on mode of exposure.

- ❖ Bottle No 1 – Stomach with its contents
- ❖ Bottle No 2 – Upper 30 cm of the duodenum with its contents
- ❖ Bottle No 3 – 500 g of liver and half of each kidney
- ❖ Bottle No 4 – 100 mL of blood with sodium fluoride as preservative
- ❖ Bottle No 5 – 100 mL of the preservative used—Saturated solution of sodium chloride is used as a preservative in most cases.

Additional viscera in special circumstances

Viscera	*Poison*
Brain	Volatile and anesthetic poisons
CSF and brain	Alcohol
Heart	Cardiac poisons (aconite, digitalis)
Spinal cord	Nervous poisons (strychnine)
Bile	Morphine and salicylates poisoning
Hair, nail and long bones	Heavy metal poisoning (arsenic)
Skin and subcutaneous tissues	Injected poisons, drugs and venoms
Blood with liquid paraffin on the top	Volatile poisons, mainly CO and sewer gas

43. Viscera in toxicology are stored in: *(NEET 2019)*

a. Glycerine
b. Rectified spirit
c. Formalin
d. Saturated salt solution

Ans. is 'd' Saturated salt solution

MEDICAL JURISPRUDENCE

IMPORTANT SECTIONS RELATED TO CONSENT

- Section 53 (1) CrPC: The accused in criminal cases can be examined by the doctor without his consent and even using force, if the application for examination is from a person not below the rank of sub-Inspector.
- Section 54 CrPC: An arrested person can also request to be examined by a doctor to detect any evidence, which he feels is good for him.
- Section 87 IPC: A person >18 years of age can give consent to suffer any harm if the act is not intended & not known to cause death or grievous hurt.
- Section 89 IPC: A child <12 years of age or a person of unsound mind cannot give consent to suffer any harm for an act which may cause grievous hurt or death even if done in good faith, but the consent has to be obtained from the guardian of the child or a sane person.
- Section 90 IPC: Consent given by an insane person or given under fear of injury, death etc. or due tomisconception of a fact is invalid.
- Section 92 IPC: Any harm caused to a person in good faith even without the person's consent is not an offence if the circumstances were such that it was impossible to obtain the consent of the person or his lawful guardian at that material time for that thing to be done for the benefit of the person.
- Person above 18 years with sound mind can give consent for organ donation.

44. Minimum age for giving consent for organ donation in India is:

a. 12 years
b. 15 years
c. 18 years
d. 21 years

Ans. is 'c' 18 years

IMPORTANT SECTIONS OF IPC

44 IPC	Definition of injury (any harm caused to a person in body, mind, reputation or property)
53 IPC	An accused can be examined by a medical practitioner at the request of police, even without his consent and by use of force
82 IPC	A child under the age of seven is incapable of committing an offence
84 IPC	Insanity & criminal responsibility (McNaughten's rule)
85 IPC	Criminal responsibility of a person incapable of judgment by reasons intoxicated against his will
191 IPC	Defines perjury
193 IPC	Punishment for perjury
197 IPC	Punishment for doctors for submitting false medical certificates
202 IPC	Intentional omission to give information of offence by person bound to inform
228A IPC	Disclosure of identity of victim of certain offences under section 376 rape
269 IPC	Negligent act likely to spread infection or disease dangerous to life
270 IPC	Malignant act likely to spread infection or disease dangerous to life
294 IPC	Punishment for obscene acts or words in public (the law does not clearly define what constitutes an obscene act)
299 IPC	Culpable homicide
300IPC	Definition of murder
302 IPC	Punishment for murder
304A IPC	Causing death by negligence, punishment up to 2 years (medical negligence)
304B IPC	Dowry death, punishment 7 years to life imprisonment
306 IPC	Abetment of suicide
307 IPC	Attempt to murder
308 IPC	Abetment to commit culpable homicide
312 IPC :	Causing illegal miscarriage with woman's consent
313 IPC	Causing illegal miscarriage without woman's consent

Contd...

Contd...

314 IPC	Death of mother caused by act done with intent to cause miscarriage
315 IPC	Act done with intent to prevent child being born alive or to cause it to die after birth
316 IPC	Causing death of quick unborn child by act amounting to culpable homicide
317 IPC	Exposure & abandonment of child under 12 years
318 PC	Concealment of birth by secret disposal of dead body
319 IPC	Definition of Hurt (whoever causes bodily pain, disease, or infirmity to any person is said to cause hurt)
320 IPC	Grievous hurt definition
321 IPC	Voluntarily causing hurt
322 IPC	Voluntarily causing Grievous hurt
323 IPC	Punishment for voluntarily causing hurt
324 IPC	Voluntarily causing hurt by dangerous weapons or means
325 IPC	Punishment for voluntarily causing grievous hurt (7 years imprisonment +/- fine)
326 IPC	Voluntarily causing grievous hurt by dangerous weapons or means (10 years imprisonment +/- fine)
330 IPC	Voluntarily causing hurt to extort confession or to compel restoration of property
331 IPC	Voluntarily causing grievous hurt to extort confession or to compel restoration of property
351 IPC	Deals with assault
354 IPC	Assault or criminal force to woman with intent to outrage her modesty
375 IPC	Defines rape
376 IPC	Punishment of rape
377 IPC	Unnatural sexual offences
497 IPC	Adultery
498A IPC	Punishment for cruelty by husband or his relatives

IMPORTANT SECTIONS OF IPC RELATED TO EVIDENCE

- Sec 179 IPC—Omission to give notice or information to public servant by person legally bound to give it
- Sec 177 IPC—Furnishing false information
- Sec 191 IPC—Give false evidence
- Sec 192 IPC—Fabricating false evidence
- Sec 193 IPC—Punishment for false evidence
- Sec 194 IPC—Giving false evidence/intent to procure conviction of capital offence
- Sec 194 IPC—Giving false evidence/intent to procure conviction of offence punishable with imprisonment for life
- Sec 197 IPC—Issuing/signing false certificate.

McNaughten's rule (aka right or wrong test/legal test): Insanity was a defense to criminal charges only if at the time of the committing the act, the party accused was labouring under such a defect of reason, from a disease of the mind, as not to know the nature and quality of the act he was doing; or, if he did know it, that he did not know he was doing what was wrong. This has been accepted in India under IPC section 84.

45. Use of dangerous weapon is related to which section of IPC?

a. 304
b. 319
c. 322
d. 324

Ans. is 'd' 324

46. Punishment for perjury falls under which section of IPC? *(NEET 2019)*

a. 190
b. 191
c. 192
d. 193

Ans. is 'd' 193

Perjury is the offence of willfully telling an untruth or making a misinterpretation under oath (false evidence).

47. At what age person is held responsible for criminal activity:

a. 7 years
b. 12 years
c. 16 years
d. 18 years

Ans. is 'a' 7 years

48. Dowry death is described in which section of IPC?

a. 174
b. 304
c. 498
d. 375

Ans. is 'b' 304

49. Which section of IPC is related to criminal abortion?

a. 307
b. 313
c. 323
d. 304

Ans. is 'b' 313

50. Outraging modesty of women is which section of IPC?

a. 375
b. 354
c. 195
d. 304

Ans. is 'b' 354

51. Punishment for causing grievous hurt includes how many years of imprisonment?

a. 1 year
b. 3 years
c. 7 years
d. 10 years

Ans. is 'c' 7 years

52. Exhibitionism comes under which section of IPC? *(NEET 2019)*

a. 290
b. 294
c. 230
d. 291

Ans. is 'b' 294

MEDICAL NEGLIGENCE

- Professional negligence is defined as 'omission to do something which a reasonable competent man would do or doing something which a prudent reasonable man would not do, either of these results in direct damage or death of the patient.
- Medical negligence arises when the standard of care exhibited by the doctor while doing a procedure or treatment was below the prescribed standard.
- Negligence results either from the doctor's lack of knowledge and skill or failure to excise reasonable degree of care and skills while performing the procedure/act.
- When a patient dies during the treatment due to alleged medical negligence, the doctor is booked under section 304 (A) of IPC.

Components of Negligence Suit

- For the charge of negligence to be established against a doctor, the following components have to be proved beyond any reasonable doubt.
  - Existence of a duty of care
  - Dereliction of such duty
  - Damage
  - Direct cause: The resultant damage should be a direct effect of such dereliction. Also, it has to be proved that the resultant damage was reasonably foreseeable (commonly expected)
- Even if it is proved that the doctor was negligent but such an act did not cause any damage to the patient, then the doctor cannot be held liable for any compensation.
- Burden of Proof: The patient should prove all four elements of negligence by a preponderance of the evidence. It requires enough proof to show that is more likely than not, that each of the 4 elements of a negligent claim is true.

53. If a person willingly produces false evidence under oath, he is punishable under: *(NEET 2020)*

a. Section 191 IPC
b. Section 193 IPC
c. Section 197 IPC
d. Section 198 IPC

Ans. is 'b' Section 193 IPC

54. In a civil case of medical negligence against a doctor, the onus of proof lies upon: *(NEET 2020)*

a. Doctor
b. Patient
c. Judicial magistrate
d. Police rank not less than sub-inspector

Ans. is 'b' Patient

HYMEN

- Rupture of the hymen occurs with the first sexual intercourse.
- Tearing usually occurs in 4 or 8 o'clock position or in the middle. Soon after the act, the margins of the torn hymen are sharp and red, which bleed on touch.
- By 3-4 days, the edges are congested and swollen, which heal completely in 1 week.
- Rupture of the hymen due to sudden stretching can be caused by agents other than the penis, such as fingers. And, therefore evidence of local injury us not a proof of penetration.
- Frequently, in the absence of frank hymenal tearing, there is abrasion and bruising of hymen, vaginal orifice and vaginal canal.
- **Rape on children:** In young children, there are few or no signs of general violence, for the child usually has no idea of what is happening and also incapable of resisting. The hymen is deeply situated and as the vagina is very small, it is impossible for the penetration of adult organ to take place. As such, the hymen is usually intact and there may be little redness and tenderness of the vulva.

55. During the rape of a child, which of the following is true with respect to hymen? *(NEET 2020)*

a. Remains intact because it is elastic
b. Remains intact because it is deeply seated
c. Ruptures because it is superficially seated
d. Ruptures because it is thin

Ans. is 'b' Remains intact because it is deeply seated

Magnitude of Substance Use in India (*Reference*: http://socialjustice.nic.in/writereaddata/UploadFile/Magnitude_Substance_Use_India_REPORT.pdf)

- Alcohol is the most common psychoactive substance used by Indians. Nationally, about 14.6% of the population (between 10 and 75 year of age) uses alcohol.
- After Alcohol, Cannabis and Opioids are the next commonly used substances in India. About 2.8% of the population (3.1 crore individuals) reports having used any cannabis product within the previous year.
- About 2.1% of the country's population (2.26 crore individuals) use opioids which includes Opium (or its variants like poppy husk known as doda/phukki), Heroin (or its impure form – smack or brown sugar) and a variety of pharmaceutical opioids.
- Other categories of drugs such as, Cocaine (0.10%) Amphetamine Type Stimulants (0.18%) and Hallucinogens (0.12%) are used by a small proportion of country's population.

56. The most widely used dependence causing substance is: *(NEET 2020)*

a. Cocaine
b. Cannabis
c. Heroin
d. Amphetamine

Ans. is 'b' Cannabis

Previously Asked Facts

- Maceration of fetus is a process of aseptic autolysis. It occurs when a dead fetus remains in the uterus surrounded by liquor amnii but with exclusion of air. The earliest sign of maceration is skin slippage. The earliest radiological sign is Robert sign (gas in great vessels; occurs after 12 hours). Spalding sign (overlapping of fetal skull bones) occurs after 4-7 days.
- The characteristic finding in lightening burns is filigree burns/arborescent burns/arborescent marking litchenberg flower. In this burns are seen as colored branching patterns, especially on shoulder and flanks.
- Strychnine poisoning mimics Tetanus.
- Strychnine seeds contain active principles strychnine, brucine, and loganin.
- Amyl nitrite is used as an antidote in poisoning of hydrocyanic acid (cyanide). Nitrates generate methaemoglobin which has high affinity for cyanide and forms cyanmethaemoglobin. Cyanmethaemoglobin may again dissociate to release cyanide therefore, sodium thiosulfate is given to form sod thiocyanate which is poorly dissociable and is excreted in urine.
- Datura seeds are large, thick, dark yellow in color, kidney-shaped, have numerous small depressions on surface, odorless and bitter in taste.
- Chloral hydrate is a colorless, crystalline substance having peculiar pungent odour and pungent bitter taste. In larger doses, depresses CNS and paralyses vital centers. It is given in food or drink to make person helpless, called knock out drops. Chloral hydrate is also called dry wine.
- Cannabis, also known as marijuana, is obtained from the Indian Hemp plant or Cannabis indica (Cannabis sativa). All parts of the plant, male or female, contain the active material, except stem, root and seeds. The highest concentration of active principles of Cannabis are contained in its resin.
- Symptoms of opioid withdrawal – Lacrimation, goose flesh (Piloerection), anxiety & fear, Mydriasis (dilated pupil), sweating, insomnia, abdominal colic, muscle cramps & body pain.
- Activated charcoal is a mechanical (physical) antidote, which absorbs poisons and thus prevent their absorption. It is best used in poisoning with amphetamines, antidepressants, antiepileptics, atropine, antihistaminics, barbiturates, opium, theophylline, strychnine, quinine and chloroquine. Activated charcoal is contraindicated in poisoning with phenol, corrosives, cyanides, heavy metals and hydrocarbons.

- 'Cold Turkey' means abrupt and complete cessation of taking a drug to which one is addicted.
- Specific antidote of Paracetamol poisoning is N-acetylcysteine (NAC)
- Symptoms of acute phosphorus poisoning – Garlic smell in breath, smoky stools (fumes emanating from the stool), manifestations of liver failure.
- Calotropis gigantea contains active principle named gigantin.
- Burtonian line is a blue line, which is seen on upper gums in lead poisoning. Similar blue line (but not called Burtonian line in these cases) is also seen in poisoning with Mercury (Hg) and Copper (Cu).
- Rave drugs or Party drugs are ecstasy (MDMA), gamma hydroxybutyrate and rohypnol.

Form of Cannabis	Part of cannabis plant from which it is obtained
Bhang	Dried leaves and fruit shoots
Ganja	**Dried flowering tops of female plant**
Charas (hashish)	**Resinous exudates from leaves and stem of plant**

- A cocaine and cocaine metabolite test system is a device intended to measure cocaine and a cocaine metabolite (benzoylecgonine) in serum, plasma and urine. Measurements obtained by this device are used in the diagnosis and treatment of cocaine use or overdose.
- Marking nut is Semecarpus anacardium. Juice applied to skin produces irritation, painful blisters followed by itching and eczema. Therefore it is used to produce artificial bruises.
- Expert witness is a person who has been trained or is skilled in technical or scientific subject, and capable of drawing opinions and conclusions from the facts observed by himself, or noticed by others, e.g., doctor, firearms expert. Fingerprints expert, handwriting expert. etc. Described under Section 45, IEA.
- Magistrate's inquest is done under sec 176 CrPC is case of:
    - Death in prison, reformatories, Borstal school
    - Death in police custody while under police interrogation.
    - Death in psychiatry hospital.
    - Dowry death; i.e. death of a married female less than 30 years of age or death within 7 years of marriage
    - Death due to police firing.
    - Exhumation.
    - Custodial rape
- Holograph will is one which is written by the testator in his own handwriting.
- Res ipsa loquitur – means 'The thing or fact speaks for itself too'
- International Death Certificate - The certificate has two parts (Part I and Part II) and a section to record the time interval between the onset of each condition and the date of death.
    - Part I → To record diseases or conditions related to the sequence of events leading directly to the death.
    - Part II → To record conditions that have no direct connection with the events leading to death but which, by their nature, contributed to the death
- The Indian Evidence Act, under section 108 provides 7 years from the date whence a person is declared to be missing and his whereabouts are not known for presuming a person to be dead (Death in absentia).
- Adulteration of drug is punishable under section 274 of IPC

CHAPTER 8

Orthopedics

IMAGING IN ORTHOPEDICS

PERIOSTEAL RESPONSE

Continuous Solid (Thick and irregular)	Benign; seen in Osteoid Osteoma, Chronic Osteomyelitis
Multilamellar (ONION PEEL appearance)	Aggressive; seen in Ewing's Sarcoma, Osteomyelitis (Alternating periods of rapid and slow growth)
SPICULATED (Sunburst appearance)	Aggressive; Seen in Osteosarcoma

CODMAN's ANGLE – Interrupted periosteal response; Aggressive; Osteosarcoma, Can be seen in both benign and malignant lesions.

1. Which of the following is not an aggressive periosteal reaction?

a. Spiculated
b. Laminated
c. Thick and irregular
d. Interrupted

Ans. is 'c' Thick and irregular

RADIOLOGICAL ANGLES

Bohler's Angle (Tuber Joint Angle)

- It measures the angular relationship between talus and calcaneum line
- Normally this angle ranges between 20 and 40 degree.
- Flattening of this angle is a classic X-ray sign of depressed fracture of calcaneum.

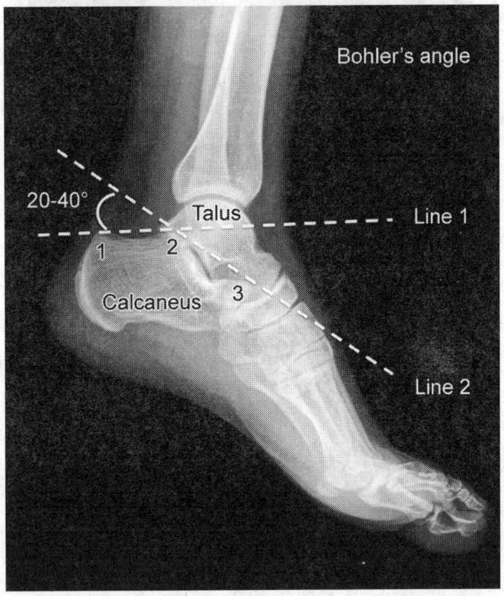

Crucial Angle of Gissane

- This angle is formed between downward and upward portion slopes of calcaneum superior surface.
- Normal angle of Gissane is approximately 100 degree.
- An increase in the angle of Gissane indicates intra-articular fracture of calcaneum (by axial compressive force).

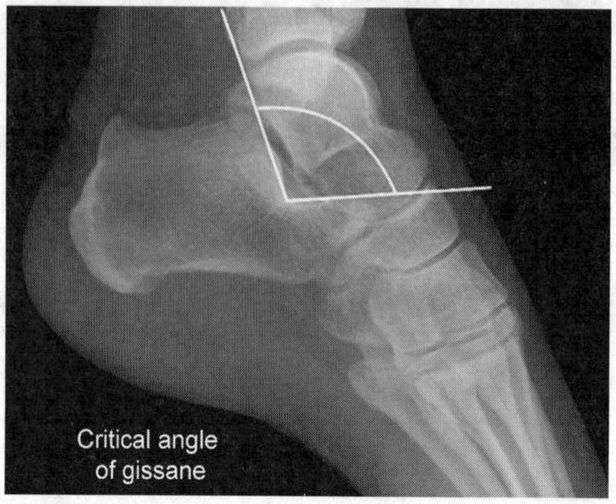

2. Bohler's angle is decreased in fracture of:

a. Calcaneum
b. Lisfranc
c. Scaphoid
d. Lunate

Ans. is 'a' Calcaneum

KITE'S ANGLE

- Angle formed by the intersection of a line bisecting the head and neck of the talus and a line running parallel with the lateral surface of the calcaneus.
- Normal range–15–30°
- <15° in hindfoot varus; >30° in hindfoot valgus

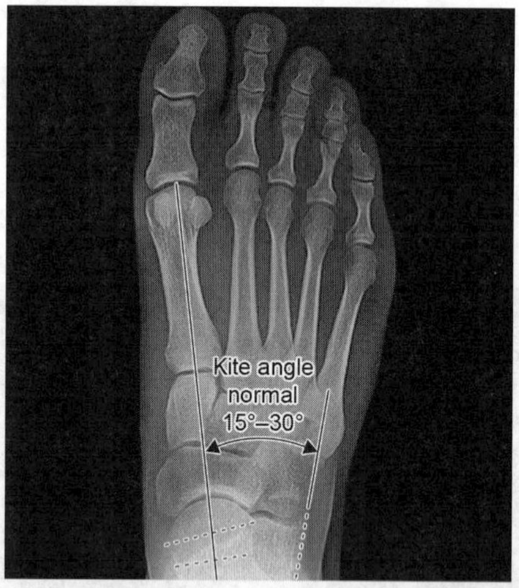

COBB'S ANGLE

Most widely used measurement to quantify the magnitude of spinal scoliosis, on plain radiographs.

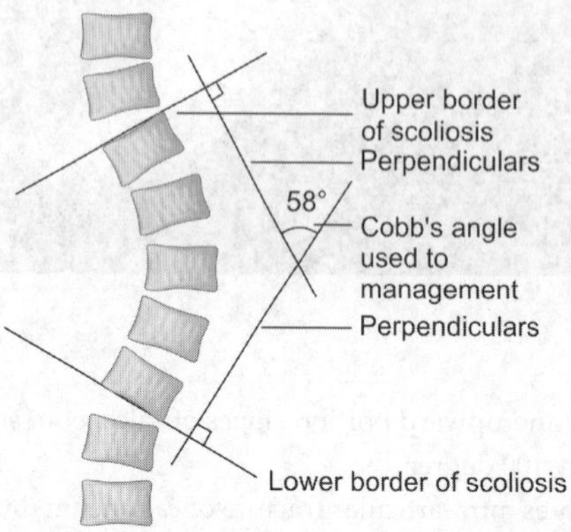

3. Identify the angle of scoliosis shown in the image: *(NEET 2020)*

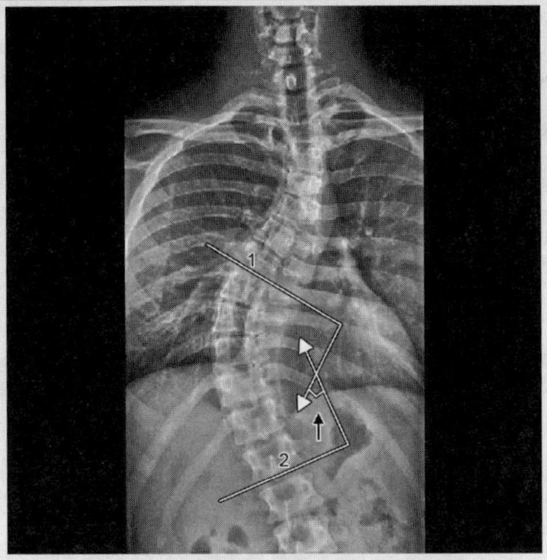

a. Kite's angle
b. Cobb's angle
c. Bohler's angle
d. Gissane angle

Ans. is 'b' Cobb's angle

Explanation: This X-ray of spine shows lateral curvature (scoliosis) and angle marked is for its measurement—Cobb's angle.

INFECTIONS

CHRONIC OSTEOMYELITIS

Presenting Complaints

A chronic discharging sinus is the commonest presenting symptom. The onset of sinus may be traced back to an episode of acute osteomyelitis during childhood. Often sinuses heal for short periods, only to reappear with each acute exacerbation. Quality of discharge varies from seropurulent to thick pus. There may be a history of extrusion of small bone fragments from the sinus. Pain is usually minimal but may become aggravated during acute exacerbations. Generalized symptoms of infection such as fever etc., are present only during acute exacerbations.

Radiological Features

- Thickening and irregularity of the cortices
- Patchy sclerosis
- *Bone cavity*: This is seen as an area of rarefaction surrounded by sclerosis
- *Sequestrum*: Sequestrum is a piece of dead bone, surrounded by infected granulation tissue. This appears denser than the surrounding normal bone because the decalcification which occurs in normal bone, does not occur in dead bone. Granulation tissue surrounding the sequestrum gives rise to a radiolucent zone around it. A sequestrum maybe visible in soft tissues.
- Involucrum is the dense sclerotic bone overlying a sequestrum. There may be some holes in the involucrum for pus to drain out. These holes are called cloacae.

Treatment

Treatment of chronic osteomyelitis is primarily surgical. Antibiotics are useful only during acute exacerbations and during postoperative period.

Various surgical options are:

- Sequestrectomy
- Saucerisation
- Curettage
- Excision of an infected bone
- Amputation

Multifocal Nonsuppurative Osteomyelitis

Focal sterile inflammatory disease with prolonged, self-limiting and recurring episodes. It has been seen to be associated with SAPHO syndrome (Synovitis, Acne, Pustulosis, palmo-plantar Hyperostosis and Osteitis). Despite the local and systemic signs of inflammation, there is no purulent discharge and microbes are seldom isolated. This is a diagnosis of exclusion.

4. X-ray appearance of sequestrum is:

a. Unnatural radiodense fragments
b. Osteopenic fragment
c. Fragment with honeycomb loculated appearance
d. Radiolucent area with speckled calcification

Ans. is 'a' Unnatural radiodense fragments

5. A 25-year-old male having pain and deformity of the tibia as shown in X-ray. He had history of trauma 2 years back. What is the most probable diagnosis? *(NEET 2018)*

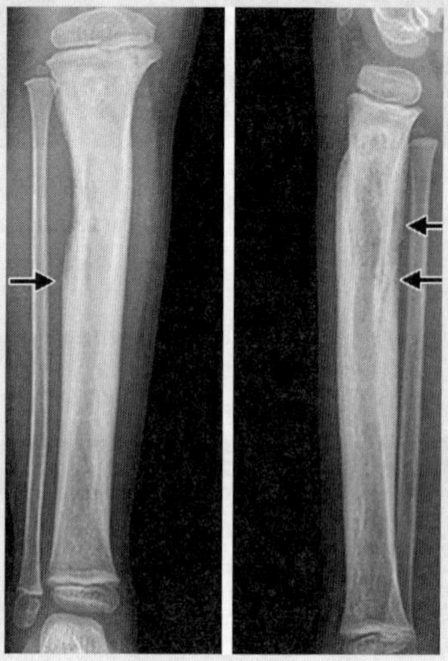

a. Ewing's sarcoma
b. Chronic osteomyelitis
c. Osteosarcoma
d. Stress fracture tibia

Ans. is 'b' Chronic osteomyelitis

6. Multifocal non-suppurative osteomyelitis is characterized by: *(NEET 2018)*

a. Inflammation with purulent discharge
b. No inflammation with purulent discharge
c. Inflammation without purulent discharge
d. No inflammation, no purulent discharge

Ans. is 'c' Inflammation without purulent discharge

POTT'S SPINE

- Spine is the most common site of skeletal tuberculosis (50% cases).
- *Regional distribution of involvement*: Lower thoracic > Lumbar > Upper Thoracic > Cervical and Sacral region. So dorsolumbar region (not dorsolumbar junction) is the most commonly involved segment.
- Most common type is infection in paradiscal region and least common is in the posterior area. Paradiscal type (MC) > Central type (central part of vertebral body) > Anterior type (anterior surface of vertebral body) > appendiceal type (involving pedicle, lamina and less commonly transverse process).

Imaging Features

- Earliest X-ray feature is loss of curvature due to paravertebral spasm.
- Next radiological feature is reduction of intervertebral disc space and osteoporosis of two adjacent vertebrae with fuzziness of endplates.
- Paraspinal abscess appears as fusiform shadow along vertebral column.
- X-rays can show scalloping effect or aneurysmal appearance or sawtooth appearance due to erosions by abscess.
- MRI is the best radiological investigation for Pott's spine (showing soft-tissues, cartilage and marrow changes).
- Radiological picture always lags behind the biological process which is already progressive.

Treatment

Conservative Treatment

- Chemotherapy (ATT) is the mainstay of conservative treatment.
- Immobilization by traction (in cervical spine) or brace (in dorsal region).

Surgical Treatment

Following are the main indications for surgery:

- Deterioration in neural or clinical status on treatment
- No improvement in neural or clinical status after conservative trial of 3-4 weeks or
- Bowel-bladder involvement.

Surgical options for most of the cases are—Anterior decompression + bone grafting or Anterolateral decompression + bone grafting and both have similar success rates.

Posterior structures like lamina are never removed because disease destroys anteriorly and if surgeon destroys posteriorly, then there will be instability.

7. Which of the following is not true about the management of Pott's paraplegia?

a. Chemotherapy is the mainstay of conservative management
b. Paraplegia not improving with conservative treatment even after 3–6 months is an indication for operative intervention
c. Decompression via anterolateral approach is most preferred
d. Posterior fusion and instrumentation can be used to correct the deformity

Ans. is 'd' Posterior fusion and instrumentation can be used to correct the deformity

8. Both bone and disc spaces are involved in which spine disease?

a. Tuberculosis
b. Osteoporosis
c. Osteoid osteoma
d. Eosinophilic granuloma

Ans. is 'a' Tuberculosis

Explanation: Pott's spine involves – 2 vertebra + disc (cartilage) – Paradiscal disease

TUBERCULOSIS OF KNEE

- Initial focus is in synovium.
- Tubercular arthritis is insidious in onset and often monoarticular in involvement. It is the most common cause of monoarticular arthritis in children.
- Tubercular arthritis is a synovial disease, so peripheral destruction of joint occurs earlier than the central part and movements are lost gradually.
- At times with tubercular arthritis both sides of joint are involved and two foci of tuberculosis will be directly opposite each other (Kissing arthritis).
- Affected joint will be stiff and soon the night cries develop, because irritation from the process is low grade, muscle spasm protects the part quite satisfactorily during the day, but when the child is asleep, the protective action of muscle is lost and on motion pain is produced.
- Synovial fluid shows elevated TLC, lowered sugar level and poor mucin clot formation.
- Tuberculosis of the knee is the classical cause of triple deformity, which includes posterior subluxation of tibia, external rotation of tibia and flexion of knee (PERF).
- It can be treated by ATT and joint replacement/arthrodesis (Charnley method). Wilkinson joint debridement procedure is done for tuberculosis of knee in early stages.

9. A 20-year-old male presents with history of gradual onset pain and swelling in left knee since 6 months. Now since last 1 month patient has started limping while walking and also has flexion deformity of knee. Ultrasonography shows presence of synovial thickening. What is the most probable diagnosis?

a. Tuberculosis of knee
b. Pigmented villonodular synovitis
c. Synovial sarcoma
d. Hemarthrosis

Ans. is 'a' Tuberculosis of knee

SEPTIC (PYOGENIC) ARTHRITIS

Etiology

- Hematogenous route of infection is the most common route in all age groups.
- *Staphylococcus aureus*: Most common organism.

Orthopedics

Diagnosis

- X-rays are usually normal. MRI may show effusion, synovitis or cartilage destruction.
- Aspiration of joint fluid helps to confirm the diagnosis by culture and also helps to differentiate from transient synovitis.
- Order of investigations done – X-ray → MRI → Aspiration

Clinical Presentation

- Absent movements of a joint after ruling out trauma in pediatric population is septic arthritis until proven otherwise.
- *Knee*: Most commonly affected joint; position is flexion
- *Hip*: Position is flexion, abduction and external rotation.

Treatment

- Arthrotomy (opening the joint capsule), surgical drainage (decompression), synovectomy and antibiotics.
- Non-operative treatment is not considered in septic arthritis as cartilage destruction occurs very rapidly and can cause permanent joint destruction.

Tom-Smith arthritis is septic arthritis of hip in infants which may destroy the cartilaginous femoral head rapidly and completely (chondrolysis). So, child presents with limp, unstable gait, shortening of limb and increased hip movements in all directions. Treatment includes procedures to stabilize the hip.

10. Most common joint involved in septic arthritis is: *(NEET 2019)*

a. Knee b. Hip
c. Shoulder d. Elbow

Ans. is 'a' Knee

11. Tom-Smith arthritis destroys: *(NEET 2018)*

a. Acetabular roof b. Femoral capital epiphysis
c. Femoral neck d. Greater trochanter

Ans. is 'b' Femoral capital epiphysis

BRODIE'S ABSCESS

- It is a long standing localized pyogenic abscess in the bone (long standing because of strong defence mechanism of body)
- Seen in immunocompetent host
- It usually involves long bones (metaphysis or diaphysis); e.g. Upper end of tibia
- Classical Brodie's abscess looks like a small walled off (sclerotic margins) cavity in bone with little or no periosteal reaction.
- Usual isolated organism is *Staphylococcus aureus* (although most cultures are negative)
- *Treatment*: Trial of injectable antibiotics is given; if it fails curettage of the cavity is carried out.

12. Identify the condition: *(NEET 2019)*

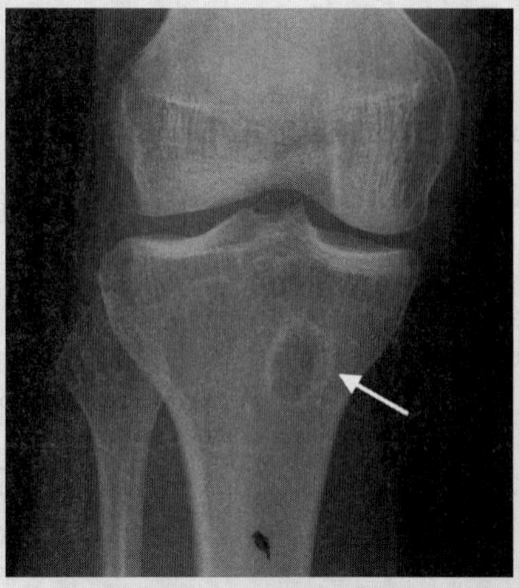

a. Brodie's abscess b. Osteoid osteoma
c. Intracortical hemangioma d. Chondromyxoid fibroma

Ans. is 'a' Brodie's abscess

ORTHOPEDIC ONCOLOGY

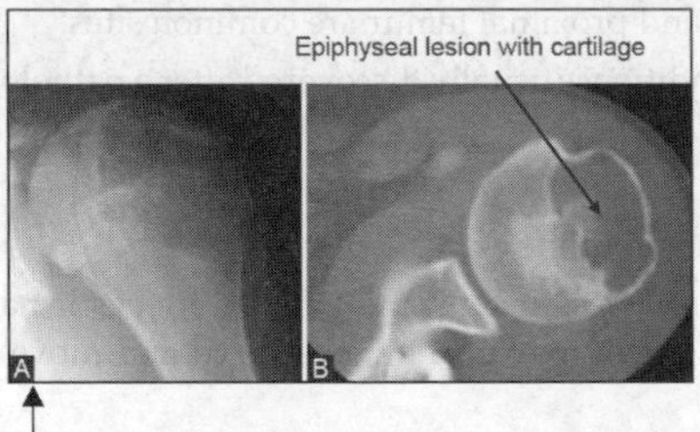

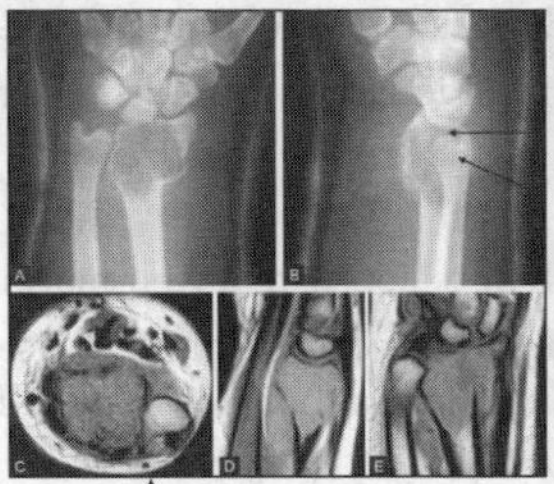

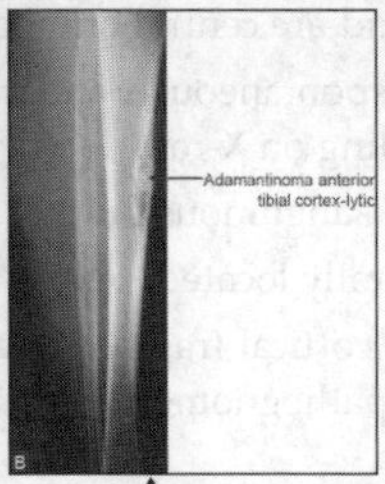

*

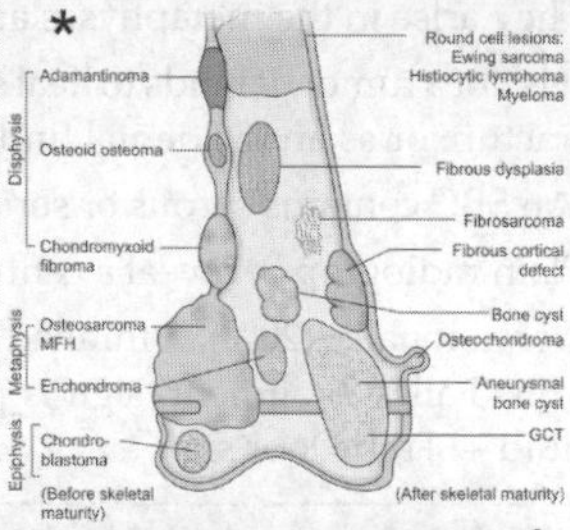

* Benign tumors have well defined margins and uniform consistency malignant tumors have all defined margins and variable consistency **In Questions middle of a bone means diaphysis and ends of a bone means epiphysis or metaphysis**

* Initial investigation X-ray followed by MRI for most of the Tumors for multiple metastasis investigation is PET-CT > Bone scan Biopsy is always the gold standard for all the Tumors Becareful not to select the answer on the basis of periosteal reaction as they are non specific

Presentation → Swelling

- **Well defined margins uniform consistency** → Benign
  - **Epiphyseal before skeletal maturity calcified masses** → Chondroblastoma → Extended Curettage
  - Metaphyseal
    - Bony growth away from joint large to feel Small on X-ray → Osteochondroma → Extra-periosteal resection
    - 1st Decade single cavity Expansile Cyst → * Proximal Humerus fallen leaf or trap door sign → Unicameral Bone Cyst → Curettage + Bone Graft
    - * 2nd Decade eccentric multiloculated lower limb → Aneurysmal Bone Cyst → Extended curettage + Bone Graft
  - Diaphyseal night pain relived on taking salicylates nidus → Osteoid Osteoma → Excision along with nidus or Radio frequency ablation
    - * **Lvory Osteoma or compact osteoma or eburnated osteoma is seen in skull**
- **Intermediate Aggressive**
  - Epiphyseal Soap Bubble Appearance. After Skeletal maturity → * **GCT (closest differential is non-ossifying fibroma)** → Excision/Extended curettage
  - Diaphyseal Soap Bubble appearance → Anterior cortex tibia → Adamantinoma → Wide local excision
- **Ill defined margins variable consistency** → Malignant → Metaphyseal → Calcification → Chondrosarcoma → Surgery
- **Infection (Fever, Pain, Local, Temperature raised)**
  - Diaphyseal 1st decade → Onion peel or Codmans Δ or Sunray appearance → * Ewing Sarcoma round Cell Tumor, Glycogen positive, Mic2 Positive → * Neo-adjuvant CT, Adjuvant CT, Surgery, **Fever Metastasis and chemo-resistance poor prognostic factors**
  - Metaphyseal 2nd decade → * Onion peel or Codmans Δ or Sunray appearance **pulsatile** → Osteosarcoma → * **Neo-adjuvant CT, Adjuvant CT, Surgery, T10 Protocol (Etoposide is not used)**

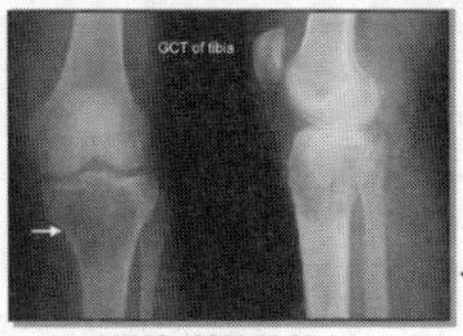

AIIMS NOV 2015 *

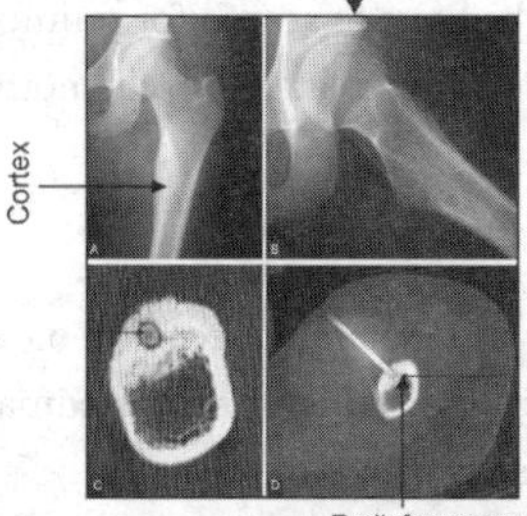

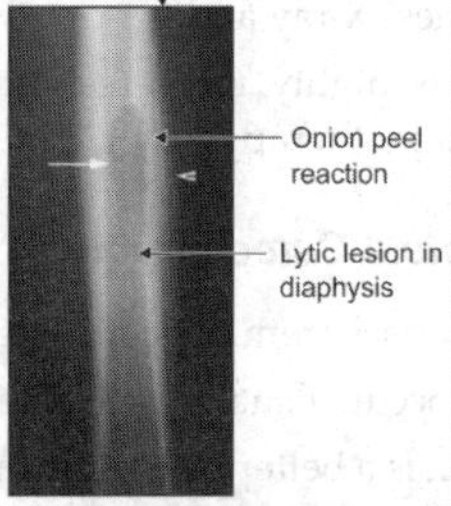

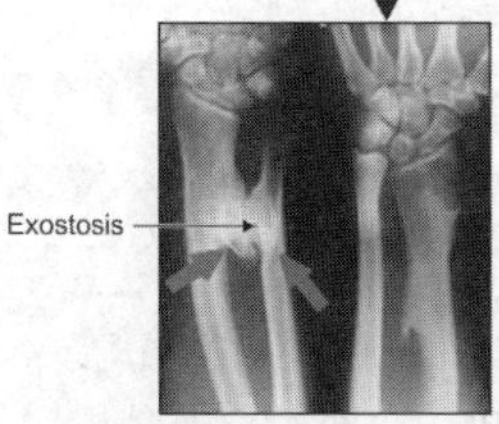

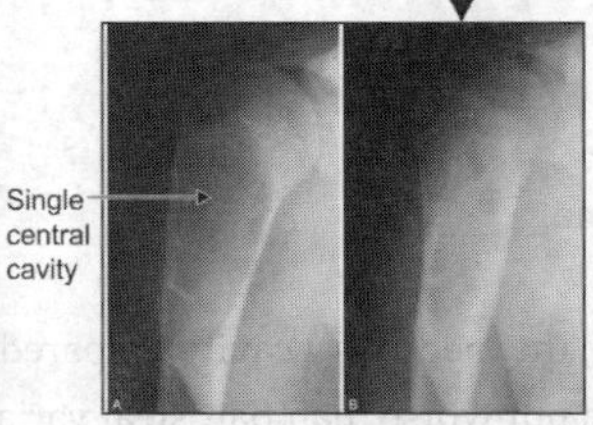

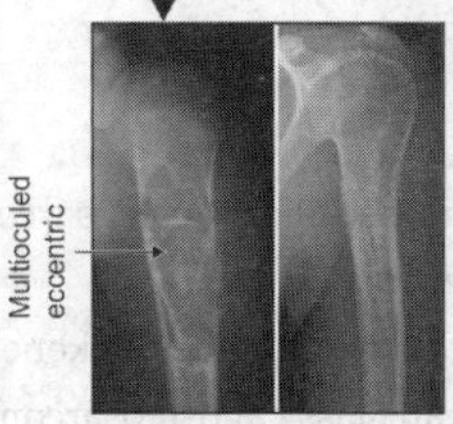

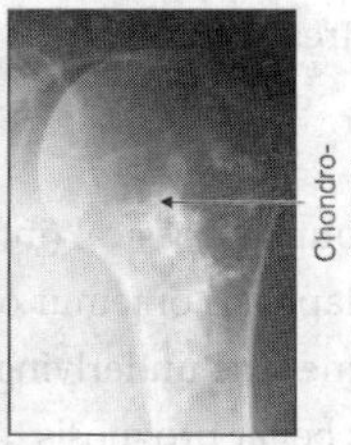

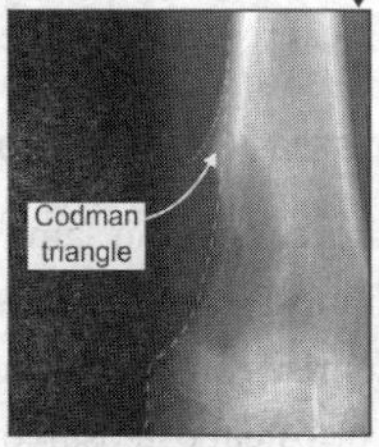

* **Latest Questions**

SIMPLE BONE CYST

- Also known as unicameral bone cyst and affects children in the first and second decade.
- They arise in the metaphyses and are central or medullary. The proximal humerus and proximal femur are common sites.
- It is not a tumor, it tends to heal spontaneously and it is seldom seen in adults. The condition is usually discovered after a pathological fracture or as an incidental finding on X-ray.
- An SBC contains serous or serosanguinous fluid.
- Plain radiographs reveal a centrally located, purely lytic lesion with a well-marginated outline.
- Occassionally (20%), a thinned cortical fragment fractures and falls into the base of the lesion confirming its empty cystic nature. This 'Fallen Fragment' sign is pathognomonic of a unicameral bone cyst. Bone fragment may also hinge around and move with fluid – 'Trap Door sign'

13. Fallen fragment sign is characteristic of: *(NEET 2018)*

a. Aneurysmal bone cyst
b. Simple bone cyst
c. Giant cell tumor
d. Ewing's sarcoma

Ans. is 'b' Simple bone cyst

OSTEOSARCOMA

- Tumor characterized by production of osteoid matrix by malignant cells.
- This is predominantly a tumor of childhood or adolescence, occurring most commonly in the 10–25 years.
- The most common site of involvement is metaphysis of long bone around knee:
  - Lower end of femur (45%)
  - Upper end of tibia (25%)
  - Other sites of involvement are proximal humerus (9%), and very rarely radius and fibula.
- The usual presentation is local pain associated with gradually increasing swelling.
- About 15% of patients have pulmonary metastasis by the time they are diagnosed.

Variants

Classic (intramedullary) Osteosarcoma

- It is a highly malignant tumor arising within the bone and spreading rapidly outwards to the periosteum and surrounding soft tissue.
- On a plain radiograph, periosteal reaction may take the form of 'Codman's triangle' or it may have a 'sunburst' or 'hair-on-end' appearance.
- MRI is the best investigation to measure the extent of the tumor within the bone and soft-tissue and to determine the relationship of tumor to nearby anatomical structures.
- Chest X-ray and CT chest should be done to search for pulmonary metastases; the lungs are the most common sites of metastases.
- It is highly radio-resistant and ideally treated by chemotherapy followed by limb salvage surgery/amputation followed by chemotherapy.

Parosteal Osteosarcoma

- It arises from the cortex of a bone and generally occurs in older individuals (3rd–4th decade).
- It occurs usually at the metaphysis of distal femur or proximal tibia.
- It has a better prognosis than classical osteosarcoma.
- X-ray shows a dense bony mass on the surface of the bone; the cortex is not eroded and usually a thin gap remains between cortex and tumor.
- Local resection is the usual treatment.

Periosteal Osteosarcoma

- It occurs in the same age group as classical (intramedullary) osteosarcoma.
- It most often involves the diaphysis of femur or tibia.
- It arises on the surface of bone. The underlying cortex may be thickened; the medullary cavity is spared.
- Periosteal osteosarcoma has better prognosis than classical osteosarcoma but worse than parosteal variant.
- Treatment is same as for classical (intramedullary) osteosarcoma.

14. Which is intramedullary tumor among carcinoma of bone?

a. Classical osteosarcoma
b. Parosteal osteosarcoma
c. Periosteal osteosarcoma
d. None of the above

Ans. is 'a' Classical osteosarcoma

15. A 22-year-old male presents with bony mass in the metaphyseal region of right knee with: Typical sun-ray appearance and CT Scan of the chest reveals osteoblastic metastases. What is the most probable diagnosis?

a. Osteosarcoma
b. Chondrosarcoma
c. Ewing's sarcoma
d. Osteochondroma

Ans. is 'a' Osteosarcoma

16. A 33-year-old female presents with a slow growing bony mass along the distal femur cortex in the metaphyseal region with an appreciable gap between the cortex and tumor without any cortical invasion. What is the usual treatment for the same?

a. Local resection
b. Amputation
c. Chemotherapy
d. Radiotherapy

Ans. is 'a' Local resection

Explanation: Slow growing bony mass along the distal femur cortex in the metaphyseal region with an appreciable gap between the cortex and tumor without any cortical invasion in an individual in the 3rd or 4th decade of life is suggestive of parosteal osteosarcoma.

GIANT-CELL TUMOR (OSTEOCLASTOMA)

- It is bone lesion of uncertain origin, most commonly seen in distal femur, proximal tibia, proximal humerus and distal radius.
- Most commonly seen in 20-40 years of age, after epiphyseal fusion.
- *Histology:* Multinucleated giant cells are seen on a background of stromal cells with little or no visible intercellular tissue. The nuclei of the mononuclear cells are identical to the nuclei of giant cells—a feature that helps to distinguish giant cell tumor from other tumors that may contain giant cells.

Clinical Features

- Most commonly presents with pain, with or without swelling.
- Pathological fracture occurs in 10-15% of cases.
- Pulmonary metastasis occurs in 4% of cases, but they usually regress spontaneously.

Radiological Features

- Eccentric lytic lesion at epiphyseal region with distinct margins, bounded by subchondral bone plate, with soap bubble appearance.

Treatment

- Curettage and 'stripping' of the cavity, followed by swabbing with hydrogen peroxide or by the application of liquid nitrogen.
- More aggressive tumors and recurrent lesions: Excision followed by bone grafting.

17. Which statement is incorrect about the pathology shown? *(NEET 2019)*

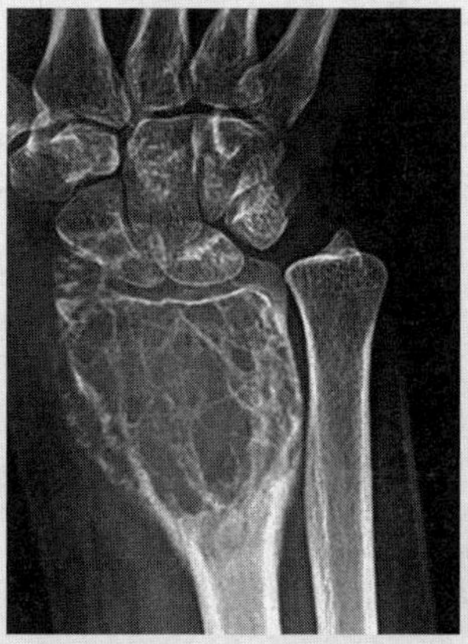

a. Tumor arises from epiphyseal region
b. Tumor has distinct margins
c. Eccentric lesion
d. Chemotherapy is the treatment of choice

Ans. is 'd' Chemotherapy is the treatment of choice

18. A 30-year-man presents with swelling over knee joint. Biopsy reveals mononuclear and giant cells. What is the diagnosis? *(NEET 2020)*

a. Chondrosarcoma
b. Osteoclastoma
c. Osteosarcoma
d. Chondroblastoma

Ans. is 'b' Osteoclastoma

Explanation: Lesion with giant cells and mononuclear cells in skeletally mature patient, GCT is the best answer

COMMON ORTHOPEDIC INJURIES

Common Fracture Eponyms

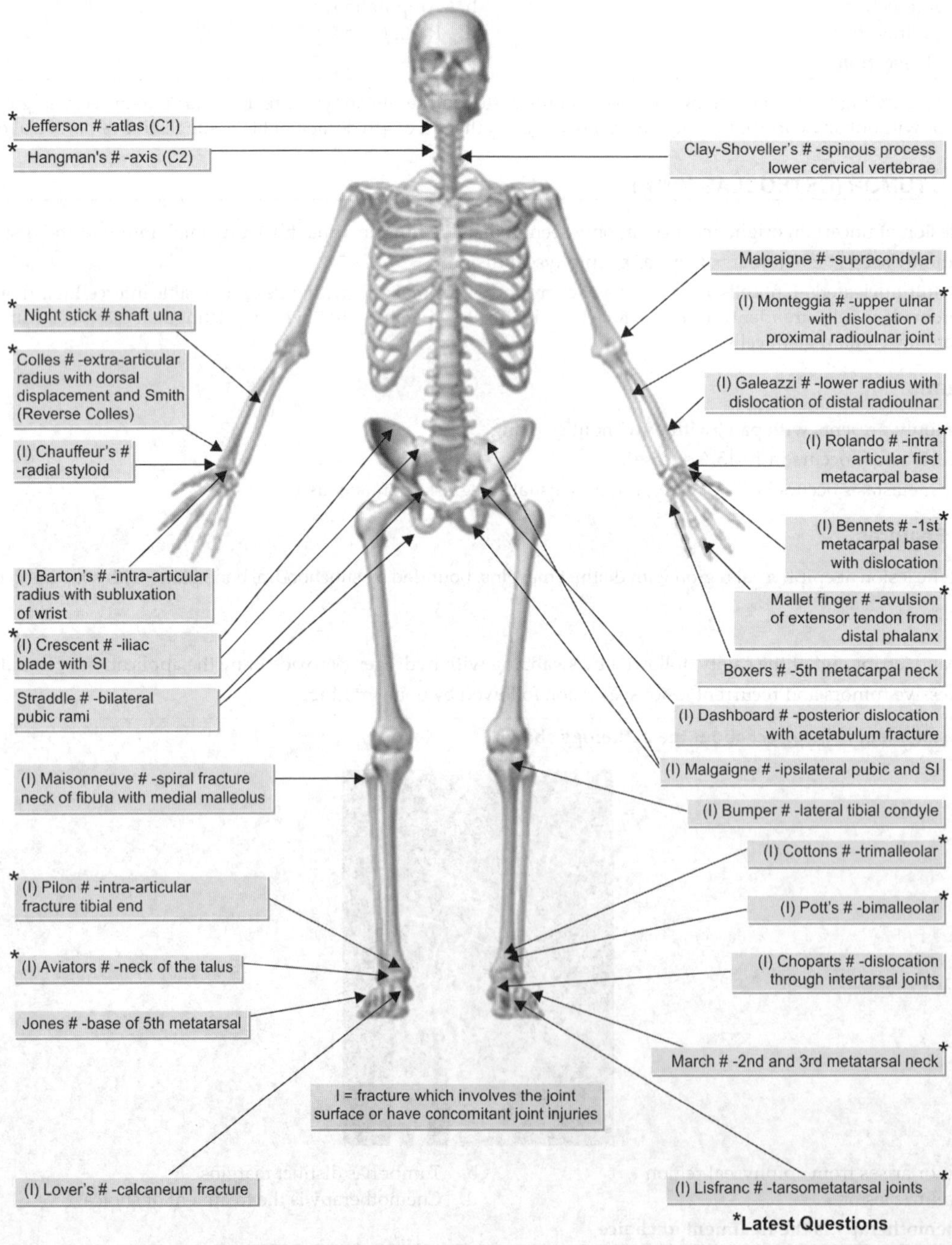

***Latest Questions**

19. Trimalleolar fracture of ankle is:

a. Cotton's fracture
b. Barton fracture
c. Malgaigne fracture
d. Smith's fracture

Ans. is 'a' Cotton's fracture

20. Mallet finger is due to:

a. Avulsion of extensor tendon from base of distal phalanx
b. Avulsion of flexor tendon from base of distal phalanx
c. Avulsion of extensor tendon from base of proximal phalanx
d. Avulsion of flexor tendon from base of proximal phalanx

Ans. is 'a' Avulsion of extensor tendon from base of distal phalanx

21. Which bone is most likely to fracture by fall on an outstretched hand? *(NEET 2018)*

a. Radius
b. Ulna
c. Scaphoid
d. 1st metacarpal

Ans. is 'a' Radius

Explanation: Most common fracture around the wrist and most common fracture caused by fall on outstretched hand is distal end of radius. Scaphoid fracture is the second commonest fracture caused by fall on outstretched hand.

NERVE INJURY

Most common nerves injured various fractures are given below:
- Surgical neck of humerus—Axillary nerve
- Shaft of humerus—Radial nerve
- Medial condyle of humerus—Ulnar nerve
- Volkmann's ischemic contracture—Anterior interosseous nerve
- Monteggia fracture dislocation—Posterior interosseous nerve
- Lunate dislocation—Median nerve
- Hip dislocation—Sciatic nerve

22. Nerve commonly damaged in fracture shaft humerus is:

a. Axillary nerve
b. Radial nerve
c. Ulnar nerve
d. Median nerve

Ans. is 'b' Radial nerve

IMPINGEMENT SYNDROME

- Tendinitis of the rotator cuff is the major cause of a painful shoulder.
- The rotator cuff consists of the tendons of the supraspinatus, infraspinatus, subscapularis, and teres minor muscles, and inserts on the humeral tuberosities.
- The supraspinatus tendon is the most often affected, probably because of its repeated impingement between the humeral head and the undersurface of the anterior third of the acromion and coracoacromial ligament above as well as the reduction in its blood supply that occurs with abduction of the arm. This phenomenon is described as impingement syndrome.
- The process begins with edema and hemorrhage of the rotator cuff which evolves to fibrotic thickening and eventually to rotator cuff degeneration with tendon tears and bone spurs.
- Subacromial bursitis also accompanies this syndrome.
- Symptoms usually appear after injury or overuse, especially with activities involving elevation of the arm with some degree of forward flexion.
- Impingement syndrome occurs in persons participating in baseball, tennis, swimming, or occupations that require repeated elevation of the arm.
- Severe pain is experienced when the arm is actively abducted into an overhead position. The arc between 60° and 120° (mid-range abduction) is especially painful. This is also described as "painful arc syndrome".
- NSAIDs, local glucocorticoid injection, and physical therapy may relieve symptoms.
- Surgical decompression of the subacromial space may be necessary in patients refractory to conservative treatment.

23. Which of the following shoulder movements is/are weak in patients of supraspinatus tear?

a. Abduction
b. Adduction
c. External rotation
d. Internal rotation

Ans. is 'a' Abduction

24. Which of the following is not true about impingement syndrome?

a. It is the tendinitis caused by inflammation of the rotator cuff tendons
b. Supraspinatus tendon is most often involved
c. Shoulder abduction in the arc of 60–120° is particularly painful
d. Surgical decompression of the subacromial space is frequently indicated

Ans. is 'd' Surgical decompression of the subacromial space is frequently indicated

25. Painful arc syndrome is seen in: *(NEET 2019)*

a. Mid-abduction
b. Initial abduction
c. Full range of abduction
d. Overhead abduction

Ans. is 'a' Mid-abduction

DISLOCATION OF THE SHOULDER

This is the commonest joint in the human body to dislocate. It occurs more commonly in adults, and is rare in children. Anterior dislocation is much more common than posterior dislocation.

Classification

a. *Anterior dislocation*: The head of the humerus comes out of the glenoid cavity and lies anteriorly. It may be further classified into three subtypes depending on the position of the dislocated head.
   - *Preglenoid*: The head lies in front of the glenoid.
   - *Subcoracoid*: The head lies below the coracoid process. Most common type of dislocation.
   - *Subclavicular*: The head lies below the clavicle.

b. **Posterior dislocation:** In this injury, the head of the humerus comes to lie posteriorly, behind the glenoid.

c. **Luxatio erecta (inferior dislocation):** This is a rare type, where the head comes to lie in the subglenoid position.

Presenting complaints: In case of anterior shoulder dislocation, the patient enters the casualty with his shoulder abducted and the elbow supported with opposite hand. There is a history of a fall on an out-stretched hand followed by pain and inability to move the shoulder. There may be a history of similar episodes in the past.

On examination: The patient keeps his arm abducted. The normal round contour of the shoulder joint is lost, and it becomes flattened. On careful inspection, one may notice fullness below the clavicle due to the displaced head. This can be felt by rotating the arm.

- **Dugas' test**: Inability to touch the opposite shoulder.
- **Hamilton ruler test:** Because of the flattening of the shoulder, it is possible to place a ruler on the lateral side of the arm. This touches the acromion and lateral condyle of the humerus simultaneously.

  Posterior dislocation usually occurs following a convulsion. There are few symptoms and signs.

Early complications: Injury to the axillary nerve may occur after anterior shoulder dislocation resulting in paralysis of the deltoid muscle with a small area of anaesthesia over the lateral aspect of the shoulder. The diagnosis is confirmed by asking the patient to try to abduct the shoulder. Though shoulder abduction may not be possible because of pain, one can feel the absence of contraction of the deltoid. Treatment is conservative, and the prognosis is good.

Late complications: The shoulder is the commonest joint to undergo recurrent dislocation. This results from the following causes: (i) anatomically unstable joint, e.g. in Marfan's syndrome; (ii) inadequate healing after the first dislocation, or (iii) an epileptic patient.

Treatment: In cases of acute dislocation, reduction is done under GA. Kocher's maneuver or Hippocrates maneuver may be used. Recurrent dislocations require surgical repair.

Recurrent Shoulder Dislocation

Bankart lesion and Hill-Sachs lesion are two important lesions associated with recurrent anterior shoulder dislocation. Bankart has an anterior tear of the glenoid labrum whereas Hill-Sachs is posterolateral defect of the humeral head.

26. Bankart's lesion occurs in patients with:

a. Recurrent anterior shoulder dislocation
b. Recurrent posterior shoulder dislocation
c. Posterior elbow dislocation
d. Posterior hip dislocation

Ans. is 'a' Recurrent anterior shoulder dislocation

27. Most common dislocation of shoulder causing axillary nerve injury is:

a. Anterior dislocation
b. Posterior dislocation
c. Recurrent instability
d. Inferior dislocation

Ans. is 'a' Anterior dislocation

SUPRACONDYLAR FRACTURE OF THE HUMERUS

This is one of the most serious fractures in childhood as it is often associated with complications. It usually occurs in children aged 5-7 years.

Mechanism

The fracture is caused by a fall on an out-stretched hand. As the hand strikes the ground, the elbow is forced into hyperextension resulting in fracture of the humerus above the condyles.

Pathoanatomy

The fracture line extends transversely through the distal metaphysis of humerus just above the condyles.

Types

A supracondylar fracture may be of extension or flexion type, depending upon the displacement of the distal fragment. The extension type is the more common of the two. In this, the distal fragment is extended (tilted backwards) in relation to the proximal fragment. In the flexion type, the distal fragment is flexed (tilted forwards) in relation to the proximal fragment.

Gartland Classification of extension type fractures:

- *Type I*: undisplaced or minimally displaced
- *Type II*: displaced but with intact cortex
- *Type III*: completely displaced

Three point bony relationship around the elbow is not disturbed in Supracondylar fracture of humerus. (The three prominent bony points around elbow are medial epicondyle, lateral epicondyle and tip of the olecranon).

Complications

Nerve injury: Anterior interosseous nerve is most commonly injured followed by radial and ulnar nerves.

Vessel injury: Brachial artery

Malunion: It is the commonest complication of supracondylar fracture and results in cubitus varus (Gun stock deformity).

28. Most common complication of supracondylar fracture of humerus is:

a. Malunion
b. Median nerve injury
c. Myositis ossificans
d. Volkmann's ischemic contracture

Ans. is 'a' Malunion

MONTEGGIA AND GALEAZZI FRACTURES

	Monteggia Fracture	Galeazzi Fracture
Location	Fracture of proximal 1/3rd of ulna along with dislocation of proximal radioulnar joint	Fracture of distal 1/3rd of radius along with dislocation of distal radioulnar joint
Mechanism of injury	Fall on hand, especially if pronation occurs during the fall; may also occur due to hyperextension	Fall on hand, especially if associated with rotation force
Clinical features	Marked pain and swelling, especially on the lateral aspect of elbow	Pain and tenderness over lower end of ulna; piano key sign-instability on ballottement of lower end of ulna
Radiological findings	Fracture of upper third of ulna with forward bowing, with forward dislocation of radial head	Fracture of lower third of radius, with angulation. The distal radio-ulnar joint is subluxated or dislocated.
Treatment	Open reduction and external fixation	*Children*: Closed reduction is often successful; *Adults*: Open reduction and external fixation

Monteggia Fracture Dislocation

- Two main categories depending upon the angulation of the ulna fracture—extension and flexion type. The extension type, is the commoner of the two, where the ulna fracture angulates anteriorly (extends) and the radial head dislocates anteriorly. The flexion type is where the ulna fracture angulates posteriorly (flexes) and the radial head dislocates posteriorly.
- This is a very unstable injury, frequently re-displacing even if it has been reduced once. In case, the reduction is not possible or if re-displacement occurs, an open reduction and internal fixation using a plate is performed. The radial head automatically falls into position, once the ulna fracture is reduced.
- Malunion occurs commonly in cases treated conservatively, because of an undetected re-displacement within the plaster.

29. Which of the following is not true about Monteggia fracture dislocation?

a. Fracture of proximal third of ulna with dislocation of radial head
b. Extension type is a commoner type
c. Ulna angulates posteriorly in the extension type
d. Malunion occurs commonly in conservatively managed patients

Ans. is 'c' Ulna angulates posteriorly in the extension type

SCAPHOID FRACTURE

- Scaphoid is the most commonly fractured bone in the carpus, in adult as well as children. Scaphoid fracture is seen most commonly in males between the ages of 15 and 30. Middle third (Waist) fractures are most common accounting for 70% of scaphoid fractures > proximal pole fracture (20%) > distal pole fracture (10%), in adults and adolescents. Distal pole avulsion type fracture is most common fracture type in children.
- Most of the blood supply to the scaphoid enters distally, so blood supply of scaphoid diminishes proximally. This accounts for the fact that 1% of distal third, 20% of middle third, 40% of proximal third and 100% of proximal pole fractures result in avascular necrosis or nonunion of the proximal fragment.
- A delay in diagnosis and treatment of this fracture may alter the prognosis for union.
- A wrist sprain that is sufficiently severe to require radiographic examination initially should be treated as a possible fracture of the scaphoid, and radiographs should be repeated in 2 weeks even though initial radiographs may be negative.
- Fullness and tenderness in anatomical snuff box. Proximal pressure along the axis of the thumb may be painful.
- Recent fracture shows only in the oblique view.
- MRI can diagnose occult fractures.
- MRI, especially with gadolinium enhancement, also is useful in assessing the vascularity of a fractured scaphoid.
  Nondisplaced, Stable Scaphoid Fractures: Scaphoid Glass Holding Cast
  Displaced, Unstable Scaphoid Fractures: Headless Screw (Herbert) is used

Complication: Nonunion > Avascular Necrosis.

30. Treatment of scaphoid fracture:

a. Conservative
b. Compression screws
c. Compression plating
d. Traction

Ans. is 'a' Conservative

31. Which part of scaphoid is most susceptible to avascular necrosis? *(NEET 2019)*

a. Distal 1/3 rd
b. Middle 1/3 rd
c. Proximal 1/3 rd
d. Scaphoid tubercle

Ans. is 'c' Proximal 1/3 rd

WRIST DISLOCATION

- Lunate dislocation
  - Lunate dislocates anteriorly but the rest of the carpals remain in position.
- Perilunate dislocation
  - Lunate remains in position and the rest of the carpals dislocate dorsally
  - Perilunate dislocation is more common
  - Complications may be AVN, osteoarthritis and median nerve injury
  - The most common type of perilunate instability is trans-scaphoid perilunate fracture dislocation
  - Median nerve is most commonly injured nerve
  - The most commonly used method for closed reduction is Tavernier's maneuver.

32. Perilunate dislocation is defined as: *(NEET 2018)*

a. Lunate at place while others dislocate
b. Lunate is displaced while other are at place
c. Capitate dislocates volarly
d. Lunate is displaced volarly while carpus dislocate dorsally

Ans. is 'a' Lunate at place while others dislocate

ODONTOID FRACTURES

Anderson and D'Alonzo Classification

- *Type 1*: Avulsion of tip (by alar ligaments). Unites conservatively.
- *Type 2*: Fracture at junction of odontoid process and axis; most dangerous type. Treatment is screw fixation.
- *Type 3*: Fracture through body of axis. Conservative management.

33. Most dangerous type of odontoid fracture as per Anderson and D' Alonzo classification and its respective management is:	
a. Type I—immobilization in rigid collar	b. Type II—screw fixation
c. Type III—halo vest immobilization	d. Type IV—open reduction internal fixation
Ans. is 'b' Type II—screw fixation	

TRENDELENBURG TEST

- It tests the stability of the hip; particularly of the abductor mechanism of the limb on which the patient is standing.
- Principle of the test:
  - Normally when one leg is raised from the ground the pelvis tilts upwards on that side, through the action of hip abductors of the standing limb. If the abductors are inefficient they are unable to sustain the pelvis against the body weight and it tilts downwards instead of rising up on the side of the lifted leg. Note that the test is performed with the patients standing on the affected leg.

Causes of Positive Trendelenburg Test

- Any failure of abductor mechanism causes dipping of the pelvic (ASIS) on the normal side.
- There are three fundamental causes:
  - Paralysis of the abductor muscles
    - Polio
    - Paralysis of superior gluteal nerve (Supplies gluteus medius and minimus).
  - Marked approximation of the insertion of the abductor muscles to their origin by upward displacement of the greater trochanter; so that the muscles are slack.
    - Severe coxa vara
    - Dislocation of hip
  - Absence of stable fulcrum and lever arm about which the abductor muscles can act.
    - Neck femur fracture
    - Dislocation of hip
    - Destruction of head as in Perthes disease.

34. Trendelenburg test is positive in:	
a. Dislocation of hip	b. Fracture neck of femur
c. Coxa vara	d. All of the above
Ans. is 'd' All of the above	

LIGAMENT INJURIES OF THE KNEE JOINT

ACL	PCL (stouter ligamentous structure)
• It is intracapsular, extrasynovial • It is major stabilizer of knee. Its mechanism is to stabilize internal rotation and extension of tibia on femur. Its function is multiple in that it limits forward gliding of tibia on femur and limits hyperextension. It makes a significant contribution to lateral stability and limits antero-lateral rotation of tibia on femur. It is injured by occurrence of excessive movements which it limits.	• It is intracapsular, extrasynovial • It limits backward glide of tibia on femur (posterior translation) and checks hyperextension only after the ACL is ruptured. PCL restricts external rotation as well. Classically injured by high velocity trauma with posterior dislocation of tibia on a flexed knee as in a 'dash board impact' in a motor car. (Remember Dash Board Injury is posterior dislocation of hip also.) Posterior cruciate ligament is active in all knee movements.
• Anterior cruciate ligament (ACL) is most important for walking downhill.	• Posterior cruciate ligament (PCL) is most important for walking uphill
• Anterior Cruciate Ligament: Lachman's test (most sensitive done at 20° knee flexion) Anterior drawer test (done at 90° of knee flexion) • Pivot shift test: Flexion rotation drawer test (2nd best) Test for ACL in decreasing order of sensitivity and specificity: Lachman's test> flexion rotation drawer test> anterior drawer test> pivot shift phenomenon tested by lateral pivot shift test of macintosh or jerk test of Hughston and loose.	• Posterior Cruciate Ligament: Posterior tibial sag Posterior drawer test Reverse pivot shift test Quadriceps active test
• Treatment of ACL tear—Arthroscopic ACL reconstruction with hamstring graft (Remember ligaments are usually reconstructed not repaired).	• Treatment is Arthroscopic reconstruction.

35. Anterior gliding of tibia on femur prevented by:

a. Anterior cruciate ligament
b. Posterior cruciate ligament
c. Ligament of Humphrey
d. Ligament of Wriesberg

Ans. is 'a' Anterior cruciate ligament

IMPORTANT CLASSIFICATIONS OF VARIOUS FRACTURES

1. Allman's: Fracture clavicle
2. Campbell's Rockwood: AC joint
3. Neers: Proximal Humerus
4. Gartland: supracondylar Humerus
5. Milch: Lateral Condyle Humerus
6. Masons: Head Radius
7. Bado's: Monteggia
8. Frykmann's/Fernandez: Colles
9. Dennis: 3 Columns of spine
10. Young and Burges/Tiles: Pelvis
11. Judet and Letournel: Acetabulum
12. Thompson and Epstein: Posterior dislocation of hip
13. Pipkins: Head of femur
14. Gardens/Pauwels: Neck Femur
15. Boyd and Griffin/Evans: Intertrochanteric fracture
16. Winquist and Hansen's: Shaft femur
17. Schatzkers: Proximal tibia
18. Ruedi and Allgower: Distal tibia
19. Hawkins: Neck talus
20. Essex Lopresti (X-ray)/Sanders (CT Scan): Calcaneum
21. Gustilo Anderson: Open fracture
22. Tscherne: Soft tissue injury in closed fracture

Pipkin Classification of Femoral Head Fracture

- *Type I*: Femoral head fracture inferior (caudal) to fovea.
- *Type II*: Femoral head fracture superior (cephalad) to fovea.
- *Type III*: Femoral head fracture with associated femoral neck fracture.
- *Type IV*: Type I, II or III with associated acetabular fracture.

36. Patient with femur head fracture with associated fracture of acetabulum will fall into Pipkin type:

a. I
b. II
c. III
d. IV

Ans. is 'd' IV

INTRACAPSULAR FEMORAL NECK VS EXTRACAPSULAR INTERTROCHANTERIC FRACTURE

Features	Fracture neck of femur (Intracapsular)	Intertrochanteric fracture (Extracapsular)
Age	Elderly (65–75 years)	More elderly (10–12 years more elder)
Shortening	Minimum	Gross
External rotation	Minimum	Gross
Tenderness	Over anterior joint line	Over greater trochanter
Greater trochanter	Normal	May be broadened and deformed
Surgery	Fixation is not as successful	Fixation is often successful
Complication	AVN, nonunion	Malunion

37. Which of the following is not true about intracapsular fracture of femur neck?

a. Displacement is less common than extracapsular fractures
b. Malunion is common complication
c. Contour of greater trochanter is normal
d. Tenderness is mainly present over the anterior joint line

Ans. is 'b' Malunion is common complication

FRACTURE OF NECK OF FEMUR

Garden's Classification

Garden Classification of Hip Fracture

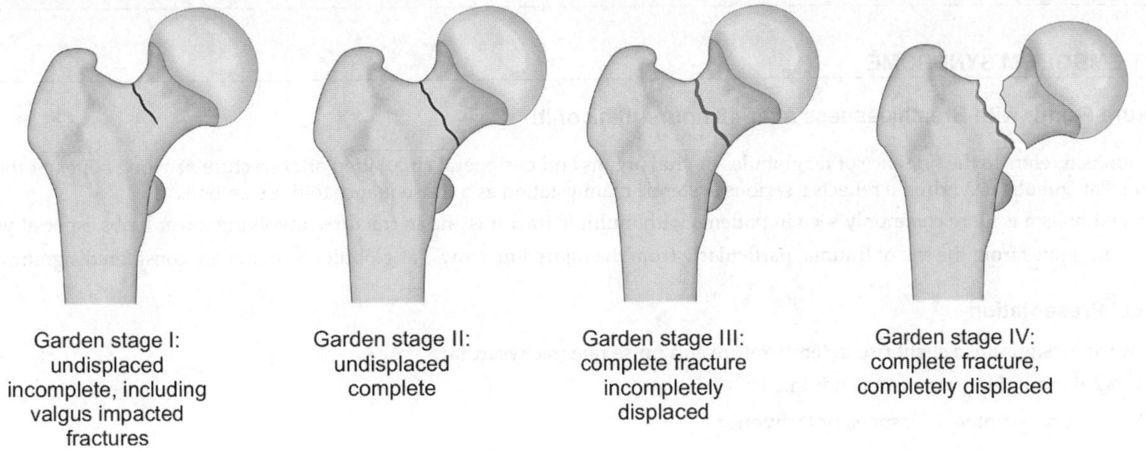

Pauwel's Classification

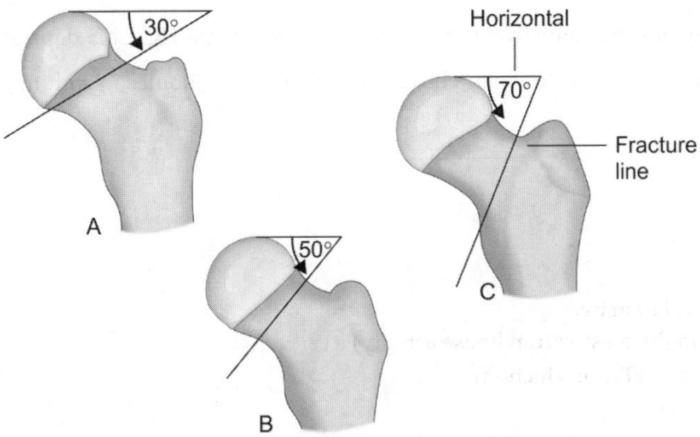

Clinical features: Occasionally, a patient with an impacted fracture may arrive walking; the only complaint being a little pain in the groin. More often, the patient is an elderly, brought to the casualty department with complaints of pain in the groin and inability to move his limb or bear weight on the limb following a 'trivial' injury like slipping on the floor, missing a step etc. There is little pain or swelling. Often, the injury is trivial, and pain and swelling almost absent. In such cases, the fracture diagnosis is missed for days or weeks. Careful examinations reveals the following:

- External rotation of the leg, the patella facing outwards.
- Shortening of the leg, usually slight.
- Tenderness in the groin.
- Attempted hip movements painful, and associated with severe spasm.
- Active straight leg raising not possible.

Treatment

- < 65 years, ≤ 3 weeks fracture—closed reduction and internal fixation with multiple screw is the treatment of choice. In basicervical fracture Dynamic Hip Screw can be done. If closed reduction is not possible open reduction and screw fixation is indicated.
- <65 years, >3 week fracture—osteotomy/Bone grafting + fixation.
- ≥ 65 years- No pre-existing arthritis—hemiarthroplasty
- Pre-existing arthritis (any age)—total hip replacement

  Complications are Osteonecrosis > Nonunion > Osteoarthritis

38. All of the following are complication of fracture neck of femur *except*:

a. Nonunion
b. Sciatic nerve injury
c. Avascular necrosis
d. Osteoarthritis

Ans. is 'b' Sciatic nerve injury

FAT EMBOLISM SYNDROME

Fracture Femur with Breathlessness after 48 hours think of it!

Fat embolism refers to the presence of fat globules in vital organs and peripheral circulation after fracture of a long bone or other major trauma. Fat embolism syndrome reflects a serious systemic manifestation as a consequence to these emboli.

Fat embolism is more commonly seen in patients with multiple fractures and in fractures involving lower limbs especially femur.

Fat originates from the site of trauma, particularly from the injured marrow. Fat globules > 10 mm are considered significant.

Clinical Presentation

Early warning signs are a slight rise in temperature and pulse rate (tachycardia)

The classical triad of fat embolism syndrome is:

1. Respiratory symptoms: Dyspnea or tachypnea.
2. Neurological symptoms: Confusion or disorientation.
3. Petechial rash: In axilla, neck, periumbilical area, conjunctiva of lower lid, front and back of chest, shoulder.

Diagnostic Criterion for Fat Embolism

Gurd's Major Criteria (4): Axillary or subconjunctival petechia, PaO_2 below 60 mm Hg, CNS depression, Pulmonary oedema

Gurd's Minor Criteria (8): Tachycardia, Fever, Anemia, Thrombocytopenia, Fat globules in sputum, Fat globules in urine (Gurd Test), Increasing ESR, Retinal emboli

1 major + 4 minor = fat embolism

Prevention

- Fracture stabilization
- Removing fat emboli from circulation by:
  - Lipolytic agents as heparin (increase serum lipase activity)
  - Hypertonic glucose (decrease FFA production)
- Offset its effect by:
  - Dextran (expand plasma volume, reduces RBC aggregation and platelet adherence)
  - Aprotinin (protease inhibitor)-decreases platelet aggregation and serotonin release
  - Alcohol has vasodilator and lipolytic effect.

Treatment

The aim of treatment is maintaining adequate oxygen level in the blood. If necessary, by using intermittent positive pressure ventilation. Oxygen is the only therapeutic tool of proven use.

It should be administered in sufficient amount to maintain arterial PO_2 > 80 mm Hg. O_2 toxicity (pneumonitis) is avoided by using O_2 conc. below 40%.

Steroids are given to Avoid Pneumonitis

39. A child brought to EM with multiple injuries which included a femur fracture as well. He was confused with dyspnea and rash over the body. What is the diagnosis?

a. Fat embolism
b. Air embolism
c. Pulmonary embolism
d. DIC

Ans. is 'a' Fat embolism

Explanation: Fat embolism although should be diagnosed with trauma to long bone, usually Femur and clinical presentation of pulmonary involvement, CNS depression and skin involvement (Petechiae). The diagnosis is considered usually after 48 hours. But out of given options Fat embolism is the best possible answer.

PEDIATRIC ORTHOPEDICS

SALTER-HARRIS CLASSIFICATION FOR EPIPHYSEAL INJURIES

Salter-Harris types	Features
I	Fracture line is entirely within physis causing epiphyseal slip
II	Fracture line extends from physis into metaphysis (Thurston-Holland's fragment sign); most common epiphyseal injury
III	Fracture line extends from physis into epiphysis causing epiphyseal split
IV	Fracture line extends across epiphysis (articular surface), physis and metaphysis
V	Crush injury of physis with initially normal X-rays

40. Which of the following is false regarding Salter Harris classification?

a. Classifies epiphyseal injuries
b. Type II is the most common type of epiphyseal injury
c. Type IV includes injury through epiphysis, physis, metaphysis
d. Type V is the perichondrial ring injury

Ans. is 'd' Type V is the perichondrial ring injury

DEVELOPMENTAL DYSPLASIA OF HIP (DDH)

- This is a spontaneous dislocation of the hip occurring before, during or shortly after birth.
- More common in girls usually seen on left side.

Etiology and Pathogenesis

- Hereditary predisposition
- Hormonal factors—high levels of maternal estrogen, progesterone and relaxin in the last few weeks of pregnancy may aggravate ligamentous laxity in the infant
- Breech malposition favors dislocation
- It is associated with higher incidence of plagiocephaly and congenital torticollis.

Clinical Features

Various tests for diagnosis of DDH are listed below:

Barlow's test

- 1st part: In position of 90° flexion of hips and knees, the hip is adducted and pushed. This will lead to dislocation of hip.
- 2nd part: Now the hip is abducted and pulled. This will cause 'clunk' indicating reduction of hip.

Ortolanis test: This test is similar to the second part of Barlow's test. The hips and knees are held in a flexed position and gradually abducted. A 'click of entrance' will be felt as the femoral head slips into the acetabulum from the position of dislocation.

Galeazzi sign: The level of the knees are compared in a child lying with hip flexed to 70°and knees flexed. There is a lowering of the knee on the affected side.

Vascular sign of Narath: Femoral artery pulse is palpated against the femoral head.

- If very readily palpated: Possible unreduced anterior hip dislocation.
- If palpated with great difficulty, it implies femoral head displaced from the hip joint due to hip dislocation, most commonly posterior hip dislocation.

Imaging

- Ultrasonography: It is widely used as a screening test for DDH. It has the advantage of demonstrating acetabulum and the non-ossified femoral head.
- Plain Radiograph:
  - Delayed appearance of the ossification centre of the head of the femur.
  - Retarded development of the ossification centre of the head of the femur.
  - Sloping acetabulum.
  - Lateral and upward displacement of the ossification centre of the femoral head.
  - A break in Shenton's line: On an anteroposterior X-ray of pelvis with both hips, Shenton's line normally appears continuous from the inferior border of the femoral neck to the inferior border of the pubic ramus; any interruption in the line suggests an abnormal position of the femoral head.

41. Shenton's line is seen in X-ray of:

a. Anteroposterior pelvis with both hips
b. Anteroposterior shoulder
c. Lateral cervical spine
d. Lateral lumbosacral spine

Ans. is 'a' Anteroposterior pelvis with both hips

42. Which of the following is not true about the tests for hip instability in neonates?

a. Ortolani test has two parts
b. They are performed at 2–3 days of birth
c. In Ortolani test examiners fingers rest on the greater trochanter
d. In Barlow test examiners thumb is placed in the groin

Ans. is 'a' Ortolani test has two parts

INFANTILE COXA VARA

This is coxa vara resulting from some unknown growth anomaly at the upper femoral epiphysis. It is noticed as a painless limp in a child who has just started walking. In severe cases, shortening of the leg may be obvious. On examination, abduction and internal rotation of the hip are limited and the leg is short. X-rays will show a reduction in neck-shaft angle.

The epiphyseal plate may be too vertical. There may be a separate triangle of bone in the inferior portion of the metaphysis, called Fairbank's triangle. Treatment is by a subtrochanteric corrective osteotomy.

43. Fairbanks triangle is seen in:

a. Infantile coxa vara
b. SCFE
c. Perthes disease
d. DDH

Ans. is 'a' Infantile coxa vara

SLIPPED CAPITAL FEMORAL EPIPHYSIS (SCFE)

- SCFE is the separation of proximal femoral capital epiphysis (head) at growth plate.
- Most of the time, the epiphysis slips backward, i.e. posteromedially, resulting in coxa vara.
- Occurs during adolescent period (11–15 years) when the growth plate is weak due to accelerated growth.
- Obese males are affected more frequently than females.
- SCFE is commonly associated with endocrinopathies, e.g. hypothyroidism, hypogonadism, increased growth hormone (acromegaly, pituitary adenoma).

Clinical Features

- There may be history of trauma (history of fall).
- Pain in the groin often radiates to thigh and knee.
- Limp (antalgic gait)
- Movements are restricted particularly abduction and internal rotation.
- Flexion is also restricted and extension is increased. And this clinical feature differentiates SCFE with all other hip pathologies because most of the hip pathologies have opposite deformity, i.e. flexion deformity with restricted extension.
- External rotation is increased along with extension.
- When hip is flexed it goes into external rotation, i.e. obligatory external rotation. It is a very important sign of SCFE.
- Waddling gait is present.
- Trendelenburg's test is positive

44. Which of the following is not true about SCFE?

a. Males are affected more frequently
b. Extension is restricted
c. Commonly occurs during adolescence
d. Varus, adduction and external rotation deformities are present

Ans. is 'b' Extension is restricted

PERTHES' DISEASE/COXA PLANA

- Perthes' disease is an osteochondritis of the epiphysis of the femoral head (capital femoral epiphysis).
- In the disease, the femoral head becomes partly or wholly avascular and deformed.
- The disease occurs commonly in males in the age group of 5–10 years.

- Perthes' disease is the most common form of osteochondrosis (osteochondrosis are characterized by avascular necrosis (AVN) and defective endochondral ossification of primary or secondary ossification centers).
- The etiology remains unknown, but is currently accepted that the disorder is caused by an interruption of the blood supply to the capital femoral epiphysis, causing avascular necrosis.
- Clinical features of Perthes' disease:
  - Perthes' disease is common in male of age group 5–10 years.
  - Pain in the hip, often radiating to knee
  - Limp (antalgic limp)
  - Abduction, internal rotation and flexion of hip are restricted
  - Shortening of limb
  - Positive Trendelenburg test
  - During the disease process, bone age is 1–3 years lower than the normal. After healing, bone age returns to normal.

45. Which of the following is not true about Perthes' disease?

a. It is also called coxa plana
b. Occurs more commonly in females
c. It is caused by interruption in the blood supply of the capital femoral epiphyses
d. Abduction, internal rotation and flexion of hip are restricted

Ans. is 'b' Occurs more commonly in females

CONGENITAL TALIPES EQUINO VARUS (CTEV)

- CTEV is the commonest and most important congenital deformity of the foot. CTEV is more common in males than in females (male to female ratio 2.5 : 1). In half of the cases CTEV is bilateral. Right and left foot are equally affected.

Bone and Joints

- Calcaneus is in varus position.
- Talus displaced medial and plantar wards.
- Navicular medially displaced and rotated.
- Cuboid displaced medially and articulates with the non-articular surface of the calcaneus (known as cuboid sign or locked cuboid).
- Metatarsals deviates medially at tarsometatarsal joints.

Treatment

- The most widely accepted practice is to rely upon conservative treatment by correction and splintage during the first year of life, often using the so-called Ponseti technique. Beyond that, if casting and splintage fail to correct the position then operative correction is carried out.
- Serial manipulation and above knee plaster casting is done weekly for the first 6 weeks. After that, it is done every 2 weeks until the correction is achieved. Two methods for sequential manipulation of deformities have been described:
  - *Kites method*: The deformities are corrected sequentially in following order: Adduction followed by inversion and finally equinus. By this method, correction is achieved in 30% (success rate 30%) of cases, rest need surgery.
  - *Ponseti's technique*: This involves first correcting the cavus deformity, then the adduction and heel varus and finally the equines deformity. This technique is now mostly accepted technique for CTEV correction as it is based on better understanding of the pathoanatomy of the deformed foot. The success of reduction is 90–98%.

Treatment of Neglected or Relapsed Cases

- *Neglected CTEV*: Neglected CTEV are those, who have not taken any treatment for CTEV.
- *Relapsed cases*: Relapsed cases are those, who had achieved full correction initially but the deformities have relapsed now.
- All these require surgical correction and the surgery depends upon the age of the patient.
  - *< 4 years of age*: Posteromedial soft tissue release.
  - *> 4 years*: Posteromedial soft tissue release with a bony procedure:
    - *4–8 years*: Dilwyn- Evans procedure (resection and fusion of calcaneocuboid joint)
    - *8–10 years*: Wedge tarsectomy.
    - *> 10 years*: Triple arthrodesis (subtalar, calcaneo-cuboid, and talonavicular joints).

Characteristics of CTEV Shoes

- It has straight inner (medial) border which helps prevent forefoot adduction.
  - It has outer shoe raise which helps prevent forefoot inversion.
  - There is no heel which helps prevent equinus.

46. CTEV shoe true is:

a. It is the same as normal shoe
b. It has straight medial border
c. It has medical shoe raise
d. It has heel with extra length

Ans. is 'b' It has straight medial border

47. Which of the following is true about CTEV?

a. It is more common in females
b. Right foot is usually more affected than the left
c. Talus is displaced medial and plantar wards
d. Tibia usually shows lateral torsion

Ans. is 'c' Talus is displaced medial and plantar wards

PULLED ELBOW/NURSE MAID'S ELBOW

It is subluxation of radial head or more accurately subluxation of the annular (orbicular) ligament which slips up over the head of radius into the radiocapitellar joint.

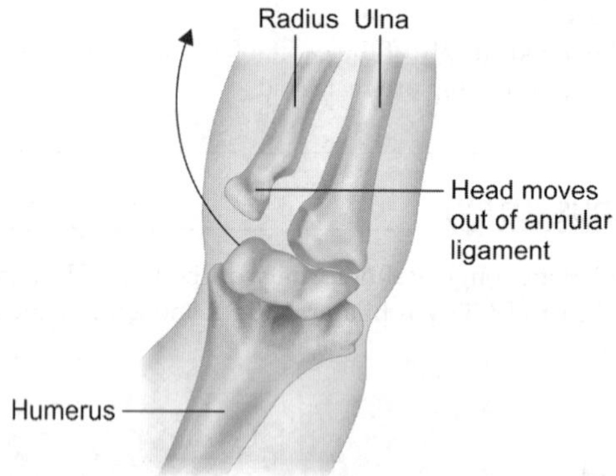

Fig. Pulled elbow

Mechanism of Injury: Traction to elbow.

Clinical Features

- Maximum incidence in 1–4 years age group.
- The child holds the elbow in slight flexion with the forearm pronated.
- X-rays are normal

Treatment

- Reduced by flexing the elbow to 90° and rapidly and firmly rotating the forearm into full supination on outdoor basis without anaesthesia. Immobilization is not necessary.
- Supination is a gravity assisted movement and pulled elbow may be reduced spontaneously by gravity, but this may take time.

48. A small child was playing with her maid where she rotated him by holding from arms. Immediately after, the child started crying. On examination, his arm was pronated. What is the likely diagnosis? *(NEET 2020)*

a. Dislocation of elbow
b. Pulled elbow
c. Fracture head of radius
d. Fracture coronoid process

Ans. is 'b' Pulled elbow

Explanation: History of traction on elbow with forearm pronated is classical of pulled elbow.

BONE AGE

- Left hand and wrist X-ray PA view – most commonly used for bone age assessment
- Based on appearance of carpal bones
- First to appear is Capitate, then in a counter-clockwise fashion except pisiform which is the last carpal bone to appear

Capitate	1-3 months
Hamate	2-4 months
Triquetrum	3 years
Lunate	4 years

Contd...

Contd...

Scaphoid	5 years
Trapezium	5 years
Trapezoid	5 years
Pisiform	12 years

49. Identify the most probable age of the child under POCSO (Protection of Children from Sexual Offences Act) by looking at the X-ray below: *(NEET 2020)*

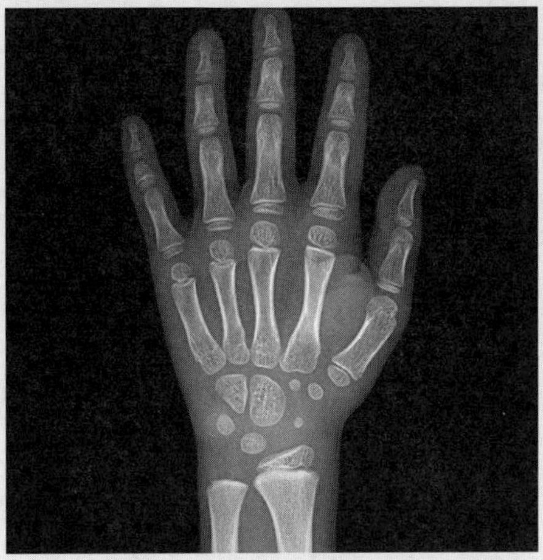

a. 4 years
b. 7 years
c. 10 years
d. 13 years

Ans. is 'b' 7 years

The X-ray shows 7 Carpal bones. Thus, minimum age is 5 here. Also, pisiform is not seen. Hence, the age is between 5 - 12. The best answer is 7 years as the normal age range for appearance of pisiform is 8-12 years.

MISCELLANEOUS

DE QUERVAIN'S TENOSYNOVITIS

The abductor pollicis longus and extensor pollicis brevis tendons may become inflamed beneath the retinacular pulley at the radial styloid within the first extensor compartment.

Finkelstein's test is pathognomonic. The examiner places patients' thumb across the palm in full flexion, and then holding the patient's hand firmly, turns the wrist sharply into adduction. In positive test this is acutely painful; repeating the movement with the thumb left free is relatively painless.

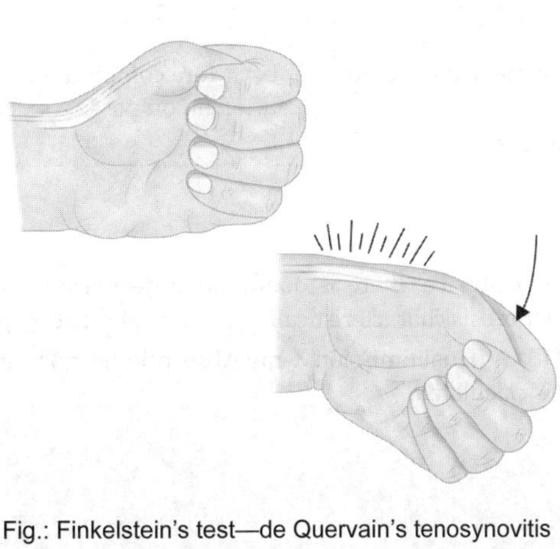

Fig.: Finkelstein's test—de Quervain's tenosynovitis

Differential diagnosis includes scaphoid non-union, arthritis at the base of thumb and intersection syndrome.

Treatment includes NSAIDs with splint: If it fails, then steroid injection into tendon sheath and if not relieved then treatment consists of splitting the thickened tendon sheath.

ACUTE SUPPURATIVE TENOSYNOVITIS

- It is purulent infection of synovial flexor sheath
- Most common organism – Staphylococcus aureus
- Most common digits involved – Ring, middle and index fingers
- Kanavel's cardinal signs
  - Flexed involved digit
  - Tenderness over tendon sheath
  - Severe pain on passive extension of involved digit
  - Fusiform swelling of involved digit
- Treatment
  - Established pyogenic tenosynovitis is a surgical emergency—prompt surgical drainage along with antibiotics.

50. Which tendons are involved in the test shown below? *(NEET 2020)*

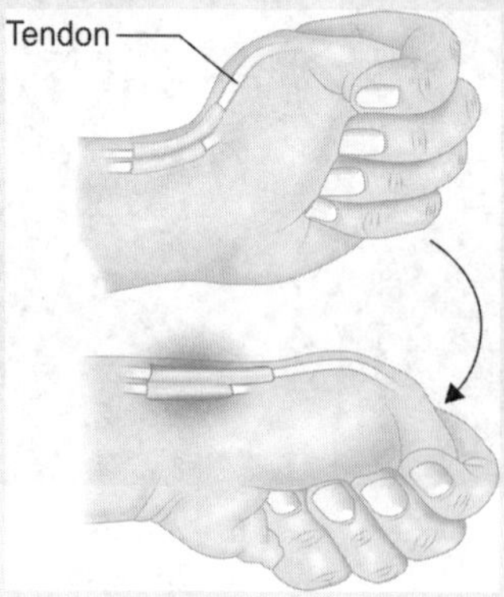

a. EPL and EPB
b. APL and EPB
c. APL and APB
d. APL and EPL

Ans. is 'b' APL and EPB

Explanation: Finkelstein test has been shown which helps to diagnose de Quervain's tenosynovitis (Inflammation of Abductor Pollicis Longus and Extensor Pollicis brevis).

51. de-Quervain's tenosynovitis involves tendon sheath of which two muscles? *(NEET 2018)*

a. Abductor pollicis longus and extensor pollicis brevis
b. Abductor pollicis longus and extensor pollicis longus
c. Abductor pollicis brevis and extensor pollicis longus
d. Abductor pollicis brevis and extensor pollicis brevis

Ans. is 'b' Abductor pollicis longus and extensor pollicis longus

52. True about acute tenosynovitis is: *(NEET 2018)*

a. Conservative management is the mainstay therapy
b. More commonly involves thumb
c. Posture of finger is in extension
d. Pain on passive extension of finger

Ans. is 'd' Pain on passive extension of finger

OSTEOPOROSIS

Osteoporosis is reduction in bone mass (density) i.e. there is quantitative decrease of units of bone formation but each unit has qualitatively normal configuration. So, osteoporosis characteristically has normal calcium, phosphate and alkaline phosphatase levels.

Bone Mineral Density is measured by DEXA (Dual Emission X-ray Absorptiometry) Scan and it is matched to DEXA scan of 30-year old individual of the same sex and T score is calculated.

WHO Classification

- T score 0 to –1 is normal
- T score –1 to –2.5 is osteopenia
- T score less than –2.5 is osteoporosis
- Osteoporosis with a fracture is severe osteoporosis

Etiologies of Osteoporosis

- Inherited, e.g. osteogenesis imperfecta, Marfan syndrome.
- Nutritional, e.g. malnutrition, malabsorption
- Drugs, e.g. Anticonvulsants, Alcohol, Heparin, Lithium, aluminium, cytotoxic drugs, excessive thyroxine.
- Endocrinal disorders, e.g. hyperparathyroidism, thyrotoxicosis IDDM, Cushing syndrome
- Rheumatological disorders: Rheumatoid arthritis, Ankylosing spondylitis

Imaging

- Radiological features are loss of vertical height of vertebrae (collapse) and codfish appearance (concave superior and inferior surfaces) of vertebrae.
- Singh's Index is used for osteoporosis grading.

Treatment: Drugs used in osteoporosis:

1. Inhibit resorption: Bisphosphonates (drug of choice), Denosumab, calcitonin, estrogen, SERMS, gallium nitrate.
2. Stimulate formation: Teriparatide (PTH analogue), calcium, calcitriol, fluorides.
3. Both actions: Strontium ranelate.

53. An old lady complains of chronic backpain since a few months. X-ray is shown below. What is the probable diagnosis? *(NEET 2020, 2019)*

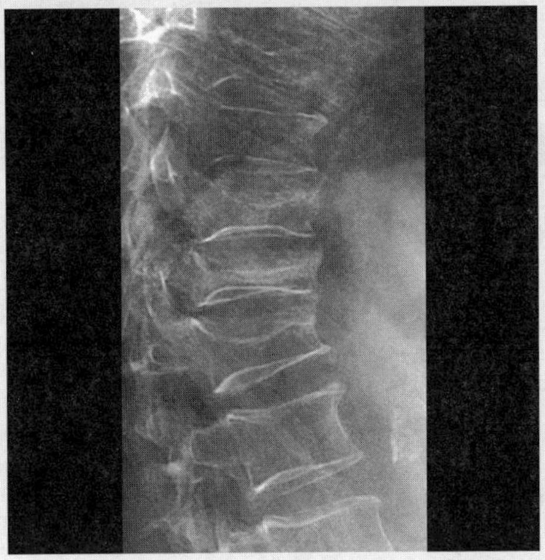

a. Osteoporosis
b. Spondylolysis
c. Spondylolisthesis
d. Osteopetrosis

Ans. is 'a' Osteoporosis

Explanation: The image shows Codfish Vertebra seen in Osteoporosis.

54. Which drug is used as a first line management for postmenopausal female with osteoporosis? *(NEET 2020)*

a. Bisphosphonates
b. Raloxifene
c. Estrogen
d. Combined OC pills

Ans. is 'a' Bisphosphonates

SPLINTS

Name	Use
Cramer-wire splint	Emergency immobilization
Thomas splint	Fracture femur-anywhere
Bohler-Braun splint	Fracture femur-anywhere
Aluminium splint	Immobilization of fingers
Dennis Brown splint	CTEV
Cock-up splint	Radial nerve palsy
Knuckle-Bender splint	Ulnar nerve palsy

Contd...

Contd...

Name	Use
Toe-raising splint	Foot drop
Volkmann's splint	Volkmann's ischaemic contracture (VIC)
Four-post collar	Neck immobilization
Aeroplane splint	Brachial plexus injury
SOMI brace	Cervical spine injury
Anterior spinal hyperextension (ASHE)	Dorso-lumbar spinal injury
Taylor's brace	Dorso-lumbar immobilization
Milwaukee brace	Scoliosis
Boston brace	Scoliosis
Lumbar corset	Backache

55. Knuckle bender splint is used in management of:

a. Radial nerve palsy
b. Ulnar nerve palsy
c. Median nerve palsy
d. Peroneal nerve palsy

Ans. is 'b' Ulnar nerve palsy

ARTICULAR VS NON-ARTICULAR PAIN

Articular pain	Non-articular pain
Deep or diffuse pain	Point or local tenderness
Painful or limited range of movement—both active and passive	Painful active movements, but not on passive
Swelling of joint	Physical findings are remote from joint capsule
Crepitation and joint instability	Swelling, crepitation, joint instability and deformity are rare

56. Non-articular bone pain differentiated from articular bone pain by: *(NEET 2018)*

a. Pain in both active and passive movements
b. Pain in only active movements
c. Crepitus
d. Swelling

Ans. is 'b' Pain in only active movements

FEATURES OF INFLAMMATORY ARTHRITIS

Presence of Some or all Four Cardinal Signs of Inflammation

- Erythema
- Pain
- Warmth
- Swelling

Systemic Symptoms

- Prolonged morning stiffness, often lasting for several hours (Non-inflammatory arthritis are associated with intermittent stiffness, stiffness usually lasts less than 1 hour)
- Fatigue
- Fever and weight loss.

Laboratory Evidence of Inflammation

- Elevated ESR
- Elevated C reactive protein
- Thrombocytosis
- Anemia of chronic disease.

X-ray

- X-ray feature of inflammatory arthritis shows rarefaction while X-ray features in non-inflammatory arthritis reveals sclerosis.

57. Which of the following is not true regarding inflammatory arthritis?

a. Presence of morning stiffness
b. Sclerosis on X-ray
c. Anemia of chronic disease
d. Presence of fever, weight loss and elevated ESR

Ans. is 'b' Sclerosis on X-ray

ANKYLOSING SPONDYLITIS

- Also known as Marie-Strumpell or Bechterew's disease.
- It is a chronic inflammatory disease affecting the spine and sacroiliac joints.
- HLA B27 is positive in 90% patients.
- Sacroilitis is the earliest manifestation with features of both enthesitis and synovitis.

Joints Involved in Ankylosing Spondylitis

- Primarily affects axial skeleton.
- The disease usually begins in the sacroiliac joints and usually extends upwards to involve the lumbar, thoracic, and often cervical spine.
- Hip joint is the most commonly affected peripheral joint. Rarely knee and ankle are also involved.

Clinical Presentation

- It is most commonly seen in young males aged 15–25 years.
- Most common symptom is dull backache, insidious in onset, associated with morning stiffness and improves with activity.
- Anterior uveitis is the most common extra-articular manifestation.

Spine Radiograph Findings

- Haziness of sacroiliac joint margins is the earliest change.
- Later on, SI joints show irregular subchondral erosions, sclerotic articular margins, joint space widening and eventually bony ankylosis.
- Calcification of supraspinous and interspinous ligaments (Dagger sign) and that of sacroiliac and sacrotuberous ligament.
- Enthesopathy: Calcification at the attachment of muscles, tendons and ligaments.
- Trolley/tram track sign: Three linear radiopaque lines due to ligament calcification.
- Squaring of vertebra, loss of lumbar lordosis and syndesmophytes are seen. Bamboo spine appearance is due to syndesmophytes.
- MRI is the most sensitive examination for sacrolitis

58. All are true about Marie-Strumpell disease *except*:

a. Most commonly involves the sacroiliac joints
b. Enthesitis is common
c. More common is males
d. Roentgenogram is the most sensitive investigation

Ans. is 'd' Roentgenogram is the most sensitive investigation

DISEASES AND USUAL JOINTS AFFECTED

Septic	Knee
Syphilitic arthritis*	Knee
Gonococcal arthritis*	Knee
Gout	MTP joint of Great toe
Pseudogout*	Knee
Rheumatoid arthritis	Metacarpophalangeal joint
Ankylosing spondylitis*	Sacroiliac joint
Diabetic charcot joint*	Foot joint (midtarsal)
Senile osteoporosis*	Vertebra
Paget's disease*	Pelvic bones > Femur > Skull > Tibia
Osteochondritis dissecans*	Knee > elbow
Actinomycosis*	Mandible
Hemophilic arthritis*	Knee (children-ankle)
Acute Osteomyelitis*	Lower end of femur (Metaphysis)
Brodie's abscess*	Upper end of tibia

Characteristic Joint involvement in HANDS in various Arthritis

Joint involved	Arthritis
Distal Interphalangeal joint	Osteoarthritis, Psoriasis
Proximal Interphalangeal joint	Osteoarthritis, Rheumatoid Arthritis
Metacarpophalangeal joint	Rheumatoid Arthritis, Hemochromatosis
1st Carpometacarpal joint	Osteoarthritis
Wrist	Rheumatoid Arthritis
Joint spared	**Arthritis**
Wrist, Metacarpophalangeal joint	Osteoarthritis
Distal Interphalangeal joint	Rheumatoid arthritis

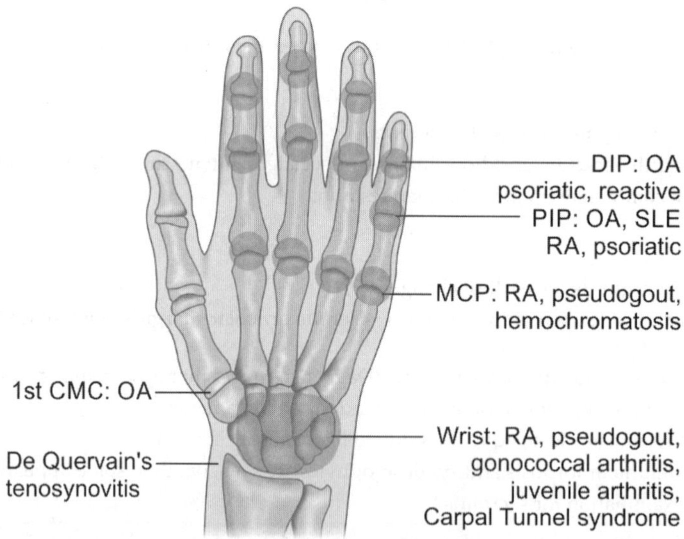

The hand (to diagnose arthritis)

59. Involvement of PIP, DIP and 1st CMC with sparing of wrist and MCP is seen in? *(NEET 2020)*

a. Rheumatoid arthritis
b. Osteoarthritis
c. Psoriatic arthropathy
d. Jaccoud arthropathy

Ans. is 'b' Osteoarthritis

Explanation: Sparing of wrist and MCP is a feature of Osteoarthritis. RA spares DIP and involves PIP, MCP and Wrist.

CHARACTERISTIC DEFORMITIES OF HAND AND FOOT IN RA

- 'Z-deformity', i.e. radial deviation of the wrist with ulnar deviation of the digits, often with palmar subluxation of proximal phalanges.
- 'Swan-neck deformity', i.e. hyperextension of PIP joints with compensatory flexion of the DIP joints.
- Boutonniere deformity, i.e. flexion contracture of PIP joints and hyperextension of DIP joints. It is due to rupture of extensor tendon.
- Hyperextension of 1st interphalangeal joint and flexion of MP joint with a consequent loss of thumb mobility and pinch—Swan Neck deformity of thumb.
- Eversion at hindfoot (subtalar joint), plantar subluxation of metatarsal heads, widening of forefoot, hallux valgus, and lateral deviation and dorsal subluxation of toes; hammer toe (flexion of PIP).
- Wind swept deformities of toes, i.e. valgus deformities of toes in one foot and varus in other (as wind sweeps all the structure in one direction).

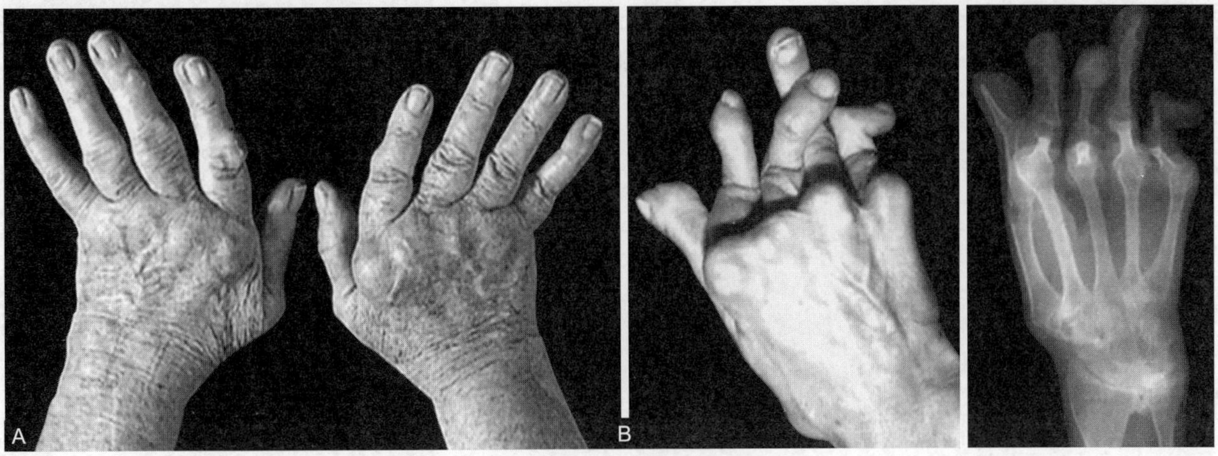

Deformities of hand in RA: (A) Ulnar deviation of fingers; (B) Arthritis mutilans

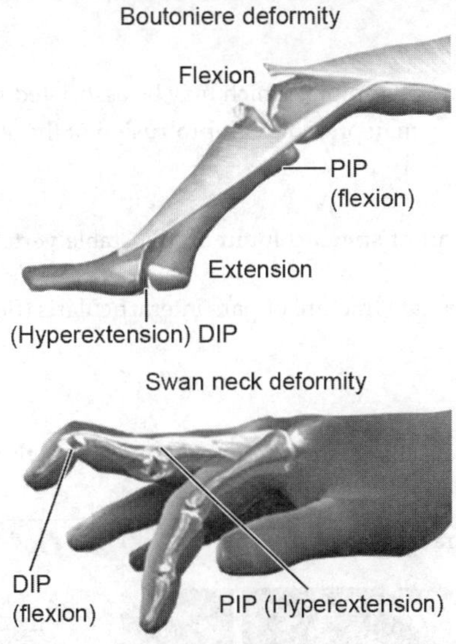

Finger deformities in RA

60. A female presents with pain and swelling over multiple peripheral small joints and deformity shown below. What is the likely diagnosis? *(NEET 2020)*

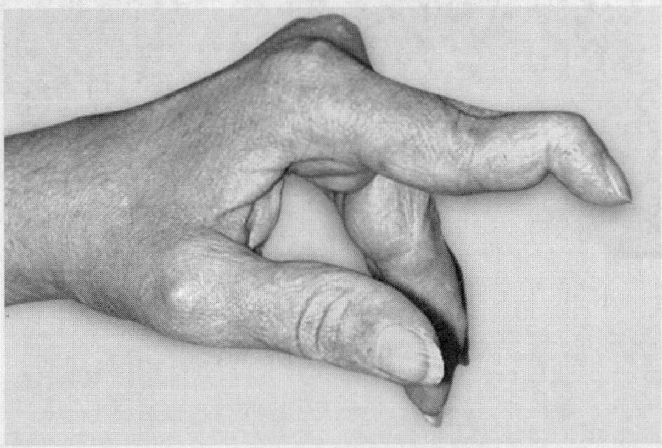

a. RA
b. Psoriatic arthropathy
c. Osteoarthritis
d. Scleroderma

Ans. is 'a' RA

Explanation: The image shows swan neck deformity seen in RA.

SPONDYLOLISTHESIS

- Spondylolisthesis involves forward displacement of one vertebra over another.
- Most commonly involves L4-L5 and L5-S1.

Types

- Dysplastic (20%)
- Lytic or isthmic (50%)
- Degenerative (25%)
- Post-traumatic
- Pathological
- Postoperative

Pathology

- In lytic type, the pars interarticularis is disrupted on both sides (spondylolysis), separating the posterior neural arch from vertebral body; gap is later filled by fibrous tissue.
- The vertebral body undergoes anterior dislocation under stress.

Clinical Features

- Low backache is the most common presenting symptom, which may be associated with sciatic pain.
- The condition is painless in children, but they may present with protrusion of the abdomen and abnormal stance.

Radiological Features

- Lateral view: Forward shift of the upper part of spinal column on the stable vertebra below; elongation of the arch or defective facets may be seen.
- Oblique views are needed to clearly demonstrate fracture of pars interarticularis (Beheaded Scottie dog sign)

Treatment

- Conservative treatment is suitable for most patients.
- Operative treatment: If the symptoms are disabling and interfere significantly with work and recreational activities; if the slip is >50% and progressing; if neurological compression is significant.

61. What is the diagnosis in the following radiograph? *(NEET 2019)*

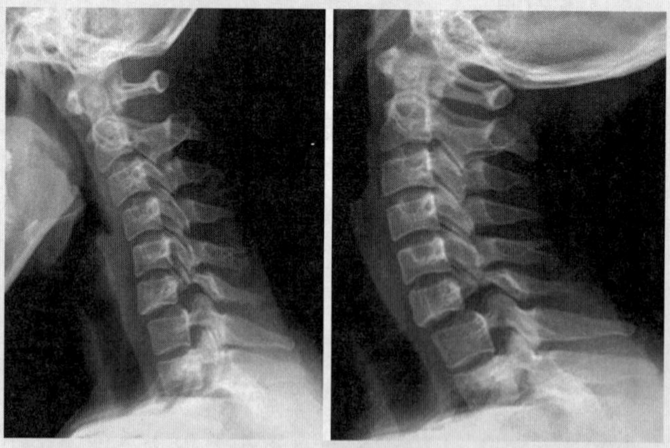

a. Osteoporosis
b. Spondylolisthesis
c. Spondylolysis
d. Discitis

Ans. is 'b' Spondylolisthesis

POPEYE SIGN

The rupture of the biceps tendon usually occurs when a sudden eccentric biomechanical load is applied with the forearm flexed and supinated, which can cause the rupture of either the proximal or the distal tendon junctions. Risk factors include older age, smoking habit, the use of certain drugs (corticosteroids, statins), and shoulder overuse (sports or work-related activities).

Typical finding on physical examination is known as Popeye sign or Popeye deformity, which is caused by bulging of the biceps muscle belly after rupture of the biceps tendon.

62. Identify the given sign: *(NEET 2020)*

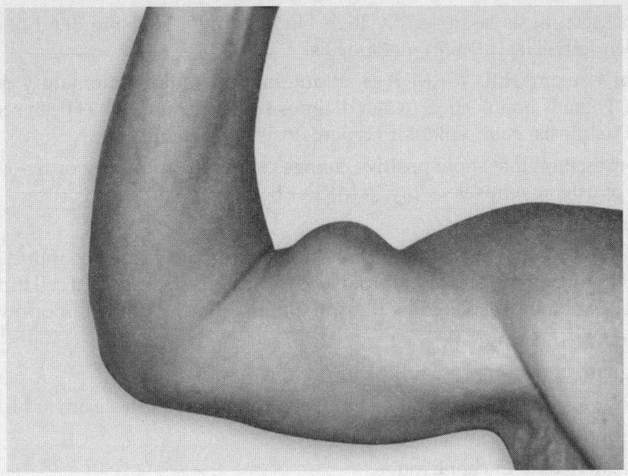

a. Popeye sign
b. Inverted champagne bottle sign
c. Biceps hematoma
d. Biceps palsy

Ans. is 'a' Popeye sign

Explanation: This image shows bulging biceps due to ruptured tendon. The Popeye is a cartoon character with bulging muscles. Hence his name.

Intrinsic Muscles of Hand		
Muscle	***Nerve Supply***	***Function***
Thenar muscles		
Abductor pollicis brevis	Median nerve	Abducts thumb
Flexor pollicis brevis	Median nerve–superficial head Deep branch of Ulnar nerve–deep head	Flexes thumb
Opponens pollicis	Median nerve	Opposes thumb to other digits
Adductor pollicis	Deep branch of Ulnar nerve	Adducts thumb
Hypothenar muscles		
Palmaris brevis	Superficial branch of Ulnar nerve	Wrinkles skin on medial side of palm
Abductor digiti minimi	Deep branch of Ulnar nerve	Abducts little finger
Flexor digiti minimi brevis	Deep branch of Ulnar nerve	Flexes little finger
Opponens digiti minimi	Deep branch of Ulnar nerve	Opposes little finger to thumb
Central muscles		
Lumbricals (4) 1st and 2nd–Unipennate 3rd and 4th–Bipennate	**Median nerve–First and Second** Deep branch of Ulnar nerve–third and fourth	**Flex Metacapophalangeal joints and extend Interphalangeal joints of fingers**
Palmar interossei (4) All are unipennate	Deep branch of Ulnar nerve	Adducts digits, flex Metacarpophalangeal joints and extend Intephalangeal joints
Dorsal interossei (4) All are bipennate	Deep branch of Ulnar nerve	Abducts digits, flex Metacarpophalangeal joints and extend Intephalangeal joints

63. Hyperextension at MCP joint and flexion at IP joint occurs due to involvement of which muscle? *(NEET 2020)*

a. Lumbricals and interossei
b. Palmar interossei
c. Dorsal interossei
d. Adductor pollicis

Ans. is 'a' Lumbricals and interossei

Explanation: The Lumbricals (+ interossei) paralysis causes claw hand (MCP hyperextension and IP joint flexion)

Previously Asked Facts

- *Staphylococcus aureus* is the most common organism causing acute osteomyelitis in all age groups. Salmonella is the most common organism in sickle cell anemia patients.
- Acute osteomyelitis starts in Metaphysis because of – Rich blood supply, Hair-pin bend of metaphyseal vessels (leading to stasis), and depleted reticuloendothelial system in metaphysis.
- Chronic Recurrent Multifocal Osteomyelitis (CRMO) is an autoimmune/autoinflammatory disease involving multiple bones with inflammation and pain. There is no infection. It is a diagnosis of exclusion. It has been seen to be associated with SAPHO syndrome (Synovitis, Acne, Pustulosis, palmo-plantar Hyperostosis and Osteitis)
- In osteomyelitis, order of investigation that show positive changes are in the following order- MRI → Bone scan → X-ray. Order of investigation done in case of osteomyelitis is- X-ray → MRI → Bone scan.
- Felon is an infection of pulp space in hand.
- Oncogenic osteomalacia—Hypophosphatemic vitamin D resistant osteomalacia may be induced by certain tumors, particularly vascular tumors like hemangiopericytomas, and also fibrohistiocytic lesions such as giant cell tumors and pigmented villonodular synovitis. The condition is believed to be mediated by phosphatonin. Removal of the tumor reverses the bone changes.
- Most common bone malignancy – Metastases
- Most common primary malignant bone tumor – Multiple myeloma
- Most common benign bone lesion – Fibrous cortical defect > Osteochondroma (These are not true tumors)
- Most common benign bone tumor – Osteoid osteoma
- Most common tumor in bones of hand – Enchondroma
- Tumor Matrix Mineralization.

	Osteoid matrix (dense homogenous)	Chondroid matrix (calcified rings and arcs)
Benign	Osteoid, osteoma, osteoblastoma, bone islands	Osteochondroma, chondroblastoma, endochondroma, chondromyxoid fibroma
Malignant	Osteosarcoma	Chondrosarcoma

- Stress fracture is due to imbalance between load and resistance of bone. It is of 2 types. Fatigue fracture is caused by application of abnormal stress on normal bone. Insufficiency fracture is caused by normal activity on weak bone. Most common site of stress fracture is 2nd and 3rd metatarsal neck. MRI is investigation of choice for stress fractures.
- de Quervain's tenosynovitis involves inflammation of Extensor pollicis brevis and abductor pollicis longus.
- Deformities caused by fractures

Deformity	Fracture
Gun stock deformity (cubitus varus)	Supracondylar fracture of the humerus
Cubitus valgus	Fracture of lateral condyle of humerus
Dinner fork deformity	Colles fracture
Mallet finger	Avulsion of the extensor tendon from base of distal phalanx
Coxa vara	Inter-trochanteric fracture
Genu valgum	Condylar fractures of tibia (e.g. bumper fracture)

- Jefferson's fracture is burst fracture of ring of atlas (C1) vertebra. It is most common fracture of Atlas. There is 50% association of concomitant injury in cervical spine elsewhere.
- Special tests for Tennis elbow (Lateral Epicondylitis)
  - Cozen's test: With the forearm pronated, ask the patient to make a tight fist. The examiner now holds the fist and palmar flexes the wrist. Pain will be felt at the lateral epicondyle in a case of tennis elbow.
  - Wringing test: When the patient is asked to wring a towel, pain is felt at the lateral epicondyle in tennis elbow.
- Green stick fracture is Incomplete transverse fracture pattern in children. The cortex in tension fractures completely while the cortex in compression remains intact but frequently undergoes plastic deformation.
- Posterior dislocation is the commonest type of elbow dislocation.
- Most common site for fracture in children—Distal radius/ulna
- 2nd most common site for fracture in children—Clavicle
- Most common fracture around elbow in children—Supracondylar fracture
- Tenderness in anatomical snuffbox is a hallmark of scaphoid fracture and/or scapholunate ligament injury
- *Sprengel deformity*: The shoulder on the affected side is elevated; the scapula is abnormally high, smaller than usual and somewhat prominent. The neck appears shorter than usual. Shoulder movements are painless but abduction and elevation may be limited. X-rays show the elevated scapula and any associated vertebral anomalies; sometimes there is also a bony bridge between the scapula and the cervical spine (the omo vertebral bar).

- Milwaukee brace is used for management of Scoliosis.
- Most common site for osteoporotic vertebral wedge compression fracture is Dorsolumbar spine
- Most mobile segment of vertebral column is Cervical spine
- Most common type of hip dislocation is Posterior.
- Normally femoral pulse is felt in the groin against head of the femur. In posterior dislocation of hip the vessels fall back unsupported, so femoral arterial pulsation, which is felt against the head of the femur will be feeble or may not be palpable – Vascular sign of Narath.
- Posterior hip dislocation – Hip is flexed, adducted and internally rotated and leg is shortened. Anterior hip dislocation – Hip is flexed, abducted and externally rotated; leg is lengthened. Palpable femur head on per rectal exam is a feature of Central hip dislocation.
- Jumper's knee (Patellar tendinitis) - Apophysitis (inflammation) of the patellar tendon as it inserts into the patella.
- Iliotibial band contracture in patients of poliomyelitis can lead to Flexion, abduction and external rotation deformity at hip (most common) and flexion and valgus at knee.
- Patellar alignment can be assessed by measuring the Q-angle (quadriceps angle). This is the angle subtended by a line drawn from the anterior superior iliac spine to the center of the patella and another from the center of the patella to the tibial tubercle. It normally averages about 14° in men and 17° in women. Limbs with larger Q-angles have a greater tendency for lateral patellar subluxation.
- Primary dynamic stabilizer of patella against the lateral pull of vastus lateralis is Vastus medialis obliquus.
- Sudden inversion of foot leads to Lateral collateral ligament injury (anterior talofibular > calcaneofibular > posterior-talofibular ligament) in ankle.
- Most common complication of fractures of tibia is non-union or Delayed union.
- Examples of irritative bursitis:

Prepatellar bursitis	Housemaid's knee
Infrapatellar bursitis	Clergyman's knee
Olecranon bursitis	Student's elbow
Ischial bursitis	Weaver's bottom
On lateral malleolus	Tailor's ankle
On great toe	Bunion

- K-nail is used for transverse or short oblique fracture of femur, especially in ischemic area. K-nail (Kuntscher cloverleaf intramedullary nail) provides three points fixation due to elastic deformation. These three points of fixation are both ends of bone (2 points) and isthmus (3 points)
- Dunlop's traction is used in management of fracture humerus. It is a skin traction applied to the arm with the child supine.
- For shaft of femur fracture; In children, conservative treatment is given by:
  - *0–2 years*: Plaster spica or modified Bryant or Gallow's traction or Pavlik harness (< 6 month of age).
  - *2–10 years*: Split Russel traction
  - *10–15 years*: 90–90 degree femoral skeletal traction.
- Cobra head plate is used for Hip Arthrodesis.
- Brisk percussion along the course of an injured nerve from distal to proximal direction may elicit a tingling sensation in the distal distribution of the nerve. This is described as Tine's sign used to assess nerve regeneration. The point of hypersensitivity marks the site of abnormal nerve sprouting: if it progresses distally at successive visits this signifies regeneration; if it remains unchanged this suggests a local neuroma.
- Neurological signs in Prolapsed Vertebral Disc.

Level	Nerve root affected	Motor weakness	Sensory	Reflexes
LS-S1	S1 root	Weakness of plantar flexors of root	Over lateral side of foot	Ankle jerk sluggish or absent
L4-L5	L5 root	Weakness of EHL and dorsiflexors of foot	Over dorsum of foot and lateral side of leg	Ankle jerk normal
L3-L4	L4 root	Weakness of extensors of knee	Over great toe and Medial side of leg	Knee jerk Sluggish or absent

- Intermittent administration of low-dose PTH enhances osteoblast activity and bone formation. Two PTH peptides have been approved for the treatment of osteoporosis: teriparatide (PTH 1–34) and PTH 1–84
- In fasciotomy for compartment syndrome, structures released are—Skin, subcutaneous tissue, superficial fascia and deep fascia.

CHAPTER 9 Ophthalmology

EYELIDS

Trichiasis refers to an acquired condition in which eyelashes emerging from their normal anterior origin are curved inward toward the cornea. Most cases are probably the result of subtle cicatricial entropion of the eyelid margin. Trichiasis can be idiopathic or secondary to chronic inflammatory conditions.

Distichiasis is a congenital (often autosomal dominant) or acquired condition in which an extra row of eyelashes emerges from the ducts of meibomian glands. These eyelashes can be fine and well tolerated or coarser and a threat to corneal integrity.

Madarosis is a terminology that refers to loss of eyebrows or eyelashes.

Tylosis (hyperkeratosis palmaris et plantaris) is characterized by focal thickening of the skin of the hands and feet and is associated with a very high lifetime risk of developing squamous cell carcinoma of the oesophagus.

1. Extra set of eyelashes emerging from posterior margin of eyelid is known as: *(NEET 2020)*

a. Distichiasis
b. Trichiasis
c. Tylosis
d. Madarosis

Ans. is 'a' Distichiasis

SYMPATHETIC OPHTHALMITIS

Sympathetic Ophthalmia is a bilateral, granulomatous uveitis that occurs **after trauma** to the eye. The disease is vision-threatening and many patients still end up with significant vision loss especially if treatment is not instituted quickly. The onset can be insidious and slow or acute. Patients usually present with blurry vision, a red eye, and decreased vision. The clinical examination is significant for mutton fat keratic precipitates, serous retinal detachments and pinpoint hyperfluorescence seen on fluorescein angiography. Prevention is limited to urgent closure of the traumatized eye and enucleation within 10 days to 2 weeks after the traumatic event. Treatment is limited to corticosteroids and immunomodulators. The etiology is thought to be autoimmune but many questions still remained unanswered.

2. The triggering factor that is a must for sympathetic ophthalmia to occur is: *(NEET 2020)*

a. Penetrating trauma
b. Blunt trauma
c. Autoimmune response
d. Allergic exposure

Ans. is 'a' Penetrating trauma

CAVERNOUS SINUS THROMBOSIS

Cavernous sinus thrombosis (CST) is unilateral to start with, but rapidly involves the opposite eye as well due to free venous communications between the cavernous sinuses of both sides. Since 6th nerve lies within the substance of cavernous sinus, it is usually the first one to get involved. Bilateral 6th nerve palsy is suggestive of CST.

Orbital cellulitis and retinoblastoma are unilateral in majority of cases. Thyroid ophthalmopathy does not cause 6th nerve palsy. It leads to restrictive squint due to muscle infilteration.

3. A patient presents with unilateral proptosis and bilateral 6th nerve palsy. What could be the possible cause? *(NEET 2020)*

a. Cavernous sinus thrombosis
b. Orbital cellulitis
c. Retinoblastoma
d. Thyroid ophthalmopathy

Ans. is 'a' Cavernous sinus thrombosis

THYROID EYE DISEASE

4. A euthyroid patient with chemosis, bilateral proptosis and diplopia. What can be the cause? *(NEET 2020)*

a. Thyroid ophthalmopathy
b. Orbital cellulitis
c. Orbital lymphoma
d. Orbital pseudotumor

Ans. is 'a' Thyroid ophthalmopathy

Explanation:

- All the 4 conditions given can have the presentation mentioned in question.
- Orbital cellulitis is usually unilateral so can be ruled out safely.

- ❖ Orbital pseudotumor is U/L >B/L and is a diagnosis of exclusion after ruling out thyroid ophthalmopathy and lymphoproliferative disorders.
- ❖ Orbital lymphoma usually have complaints of decreased vision and signs of anterior uveitis along with a palpable/visible orbital mass in addition to the given presentation.
- ❖ Thyroid ophthalmopathy is the MCC of bilateral inflammatory proptosis. But the confusing word here was "euthyroid". So to add to our knowledge, thyroid eye disease is usually a/w hyperthyroid state but can also be euthyroid or hypothyroid. Orbitopathy can progress irrespective of thyroid hormone levels of the body.
- ❖ So the best answer here would be thyroid ophthalmopathy (think of common things first!)

EXTRAOCULAR MUSCLES

Muscle	Nerve supply	Primary action	Secondary action	Tertiary action
MR	CN III	Adduction	–	–
LR	CN VI	Abduction	–	–
SR	CN III	Extorsion	Intorsion	Adduction
IR	CN III	Depression	Extorsion	Adduction
SO	CN IV	Intorsion	Depression	Abduction
IO	CN III	Extorsion	Elevation	Abduction

Yoke Muscles (Contralateral Synergists)

- ❖ It refers to the pair of muscles (one from each eye) which contract simultaneously during version movements.
- ❖ For example, right lateral rectus and left medial rectus act yoke muscles for dextroversion movements.
- ❖ Other pairs of yoke muscles are: Right MR and left LR, right LR and left MR, right SR and left IO, right IR and left SO, right SO and left IR and right IO and left SR

5. Yoke muscle of right superior oblique is:

a. Left superior rectus
b. Left inferior rectus
c. Right superior rectus
d. Left lateral rectus

Ans. is 'b' Left inferior rectus

6. Action of superior oblique muscle is:

a. Intorsion, abduction and depression
b. Adduction, intorsion and depression
c. Abduction, extorsion and depression
d. Elevation, intorsion and adduction

Ans. is 'a' Intorsion, abduction and depression

3RD NERVE PALSY

The moment shown in the image is adduction which is controlled by the medial rectus muscle innervated by the third cranial nerve.

Cranial nerve function and muscle innervation relative to eye movement

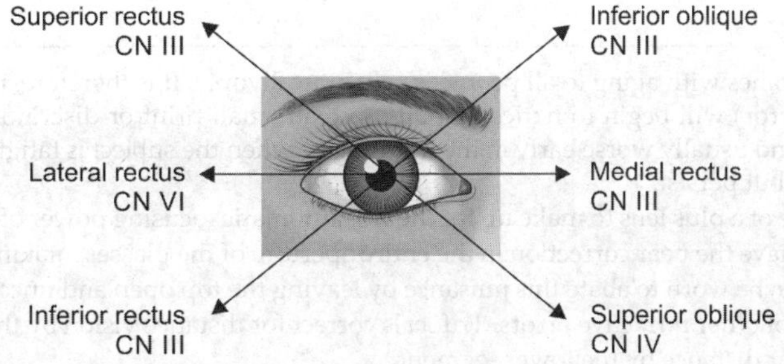

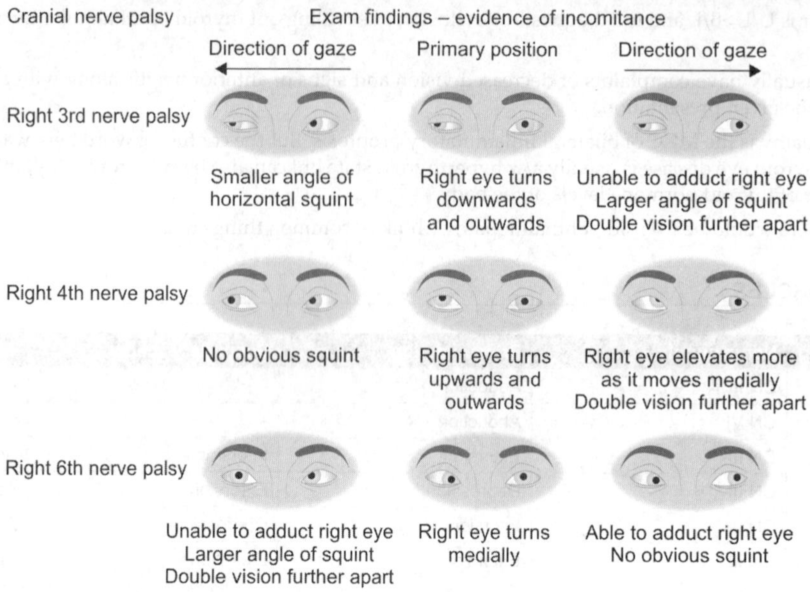

Interpretation of incomitance (that is, angle of squint varies with direction of gaze)

7. The following eye movement will be lost due to injury to: *(NEET 2020)*

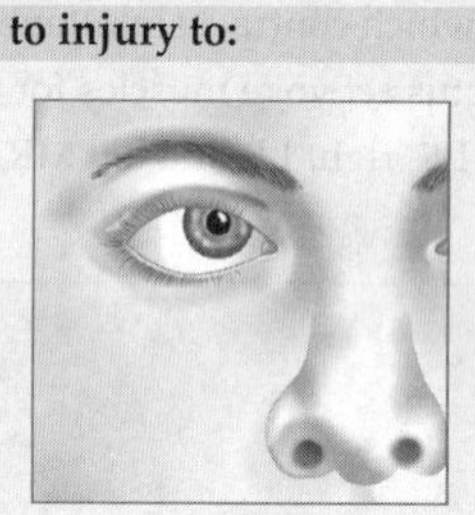

a. 3rd nerve
b. 4th nerve
c. 6th nerve
d. 7th nerve

Ans. is 'a' 3rd nerve

REFRACTIVE ERRORS

MYOPIA

When the image of distant objects focuses in front of the retina in the unaccommodated eye, the eye is myopic, or nearsighted. If the eye is longer than average, the error is called axial myopia. (For each additional millimeter of axial length, the eye is approximately 3 diopters more myopic.) If the refractive elements are more refractive than average, the error is called curvature myopia or refractive myopia. As the object is brought closer than 6 m, the image moves closer to the retina and comes into sharper focus. The point reached where the image is most sharply focused on the retina is called the "far point." One may estimate the extent of myopia by calculating the reciprocal of the far point. Thus, a far point of 0.25 m would suggest a 4-diopter minus lens correction for distance. The myopic person has the advantage of being able to read at the far point without glasses even at the age of presbyopia. A high degree of myopia results in greater susceptibility to degenerative retinal changes, including retinal detachment.

Concave spherical (minus) lenses are used to correct the image in myopia. These lenses move the image back to the retina.

PRESBYOPIA

The loss of accommodation that comes with aging to all people is called presbyopia. It is therefore, not a refractive error. A person with emmetropic eyes (no refractive error) will begin to notice inability to read small print or discriminate fine close objects at about age 44–46. This is worse in dim light and usually worse early in the morning or when the subject is fatigued. These symptoms increase until about age 55, when they stabilize but persist.

Presbyopia is corrected by use of a plus lens to make up for the lost automatic focusing power of the lens. The plus lens may be used in several ways. Reading glasses have the near correction in the entire aperture of the glasses, making them fine for reading but blurred for distant objects. Half-glasses can be worn to abate this nuisance by leaving the top open and uncorrected for distance vision. Bifocals do the same but allow correction of other refractive errors. Trifocals correct for distance vision by the top segment, the middle distance by the middle section, and the near distance by the lower segment.

ASTIGMATISM

Refractive Types of Astigmatism

1. Simple astigmatism, wherein the rays are focused on the retina in one meridian and either in front (simple myopic astigmatism) or behind (simple hypermetropic astigmatism) the retina in the other meridian.
2. *Compound astigmatism*: In this type, the rays of light in both the meridian are focused either in front or behind the retina and the condition is labeled as compound myopic or compound hypermetropic astigmatism, respectively.
3. Mixed astigmatism refers to a condition wherein the light rays in one meridian are focused in front and in other meridian behind the retina. Thus in one meridian eye is myopic and in another hypermetropic.

Treatment comprises prescribing appropriate cylindrical lens, discovered after accurate refraction. Spectacles with full correction of cylindrical power and appropriate axis should be used for distance and near vision. Surgical correction of astigmatism is quite effective.

Axis of the Principal Meridian

- *Regular astigmatism:* Principal meridians are perpendicular. (The steepest and flattest meridians of the eye are called principal meridians.)
  - With-the-rule astigmatism–the vertical meridian is steepest (a rugby ball or American football lying on its side)
  - Against-the-rule astigmatism–the horizontal meridian is steepest (a rugby ball or American football standing on its end)
  - Oblique astigmatism–the steepest curve lies in between 120 and 150 degrees and 30 and 60 degrees
- *Irregular astigmatism*: Principal meridians are not perpendicular.

In with-the-rule astigmatism, the eye has too much "plus" cylinder in the horizontal axis relative to the vertical axis (i.e., the eye is too steep along the vertical meridian relative to the horizontal meridian). Vertical beams of light focus in front (anterior) to horizontal beams of light, in the eye. This problem may be corrected using spectacles which have a "minus" cylinder placed on this horizontal axis. The effect of this will be that when a vertical beam of light in the distance travels towards the eye, the "minus" cylinder (which is placed with its axis lying horizontally–in line with the patient's excessively steep horizontal axis/vertical meridian) will cause this vertical beam of light to slightly "diverge", or "spread out vertically", before it reaches the eye. This compensates for the fact that the patient's eye converges light more powerfully in the vertical meridian than the horizontal meridian. Hopefully, after this, the eye will focus all light on the same location at the retina, and the patient's vision will be less blurred.

In against-the-rule astigmatism, a plus cylinder is added in the horizontal axis (or a minus cylinder in the vertical axis).

Axis is always recorded as an angle in degrees, between 0 and 180 degrees in a counter-clockwise direction. Both 0 and 180 degrees lie on a horizontal line at the level of the center of the pupil, and as seen by an observer, 0 lies on the right of both the eyes.

Irregular astigmatism, which is often associated with prior ocular surgery or trauma, is also a common naturally occurring condition. The two steep hemimeridians of the cornea, 180° apart in regular astigmatism, may be separated by less than 180° in irregular astigmatism (called *nonorthogonal* irregular astigmatism); and/or the two steep hemimeridians may be asymmetrically steep—that is, one may be significantly steeper than the other (called *asymmetric* irregular astigmatism). Irregular astigmatism is quantified by a vector calculation called topographic disparity.

The term "cylinder" means that this lens power added to correct astigmatism is not spherical, but instead is shaped so one meridian has no added curvature, and the meridian perpendicular to this "no added power" meridian contains the maximum power and lens curvature to correct astigmatism. The number in the cylinder column may be preceded with a minus sign (for the correction of nearsighted astigmatism) or a plus sign (for farsighted astigmatism). Cylinder power always follows sphere power in an eyeglass prescription.

8. Which is an example of the simple myopic astigmatism among the prescriptions given below?

a. Treatment with (+) spherical lens
b. Treatment will be cylinder/plano (–) lens
c. Treatment will be (–) spherical lens
d. (–)(+) (+)(–) on both 90 and 180 degree

Ans. is 'b' Treatment will be cylinder/plano (-) lens

Explanation: Combination of concave cylinder with plano sphere indicates myopia in one axis and normal neutralisation in other, the indicator of simple myopic astigmatism.

9. What is against the rule correction in astigmatism? *(NEET 2019)*

a. –1.25 cyl 90
b. –2 spherical 180
c. –3 cyl 180
d. +2 cyl 180

Ans. is 'a' –1.25 cyl 90

SNELLEN'S CHART

Snellen defined "standard vision" as the ability to recognize one of his optotypes when it subtended 5 minutes of arc. Thus the optotype can only be recognized if the person viewing it can discriminate a spatial pattern separated by a visual angle of 1 minute of arc. 6/60 vision means that the patient can see at 6 m what Snellen's assistant could see at 60 m. The essence of correct identification of the letters on the Snellen's chart is to see the clear spaces between the black elements of the letter. At exactly 6 meters distance from the patient, the letters on the 6/6 line shall subtend 5 minutes of arc (such that the individual limbs of the letters subtend 1 minute of arc)

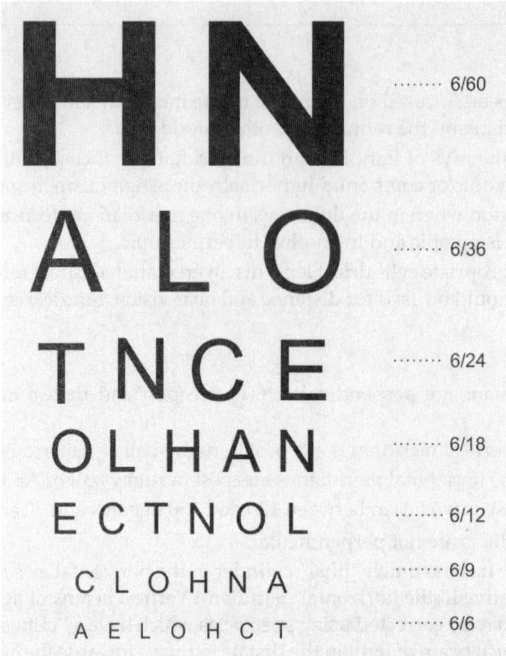

10. In Snellen's chart, eye subtends an angle of how many minute with letters on Snellen's chart?

a. 1 min of arc
b. 5 min of arc
c. 10 min of arc
d. 15 min of arc

Ans. is 'b' 5 min of arc

TECHNIQUES OF TONOMETRY

Method	Mechanism	Advantages	Disadvantages
Goldmann applanation Perkins tonometer	Applanation Tonometry (contact type), fixed area, variable force Malakoff, Posner tonometer, with fixed force variable area	Reference standard	Overestimation with too much fluorescein, very thick or steep corneas. Underestimation with too little fluorescein, corneal edema thin corneas. Affected by scleral rigidity scleral rigidity
Schiøtz indentation or Von Graefe tonometer	Indentation tonometry	Portable may be sterilized for use	Cannot be used upright (unless head tilted far back) Affected by corneal thickness irregular/scarred cornea, and risk of corneal abrasion if eye moves
Tono-Pen, Mackay-Marg tonometer	Mixed indentation and applanation mechanism	Highly portable, easy to use position–independent digital readout can use over bandage contact lens disposable covers (no need to sanitize)	Cost of covers and battery In some cases, readings can vary significantly from Goldmann
Non-contact (Airpuff)	Similar to Goldmann, except no applanation. Noncontact	No anesthesia of sterilization required	Most are not portable frequent maintenance needed CT may influence measurement more than Goldmann (except ocular response analyzer)
Pneumo tonometry	Cushion of air used to applanate (Mixed indentation and applanation mechanism)	Portable position independent	Expensive parts frequent maintenance needed sanitation is difficult
Rebound (iCARE tonometer)	Small, magnetized, ball-shaped probe is projected forward to bounce off the cornea at the push of a button: speed of deceleration is used to calculate pressure	Portable easy to use No anesthesia required Patient comfort disposable probes	Cost of disposable probes CT may influence measurement more than Goldmann
Dynamic contour tonometry (Pascal)	Concave-shaped plastic tip with a central pressure sensor is applied to the cornea at a constant force of 1g. No applanatin of or indentation	Digital readout Disposable covers (no need to sanitize) More independent of CT than Goldmann Accurate in thin eyes and post LASIK eyes Reports ocular pulse amplitude	Expensive cost of disposable covers Learning curve
Transpalpebral	Pressure measured mechanically or electronically (depending on device) through the upper eyelid, or by digital palpation	Only useful when conventional tonometry not possible—corneal prostheses, extremely irregular or scarred corneas, uncooperative patient	Readings vary significantly from Goldmann

11. What is the type of Goldmann tonometry?

a. Applanation tonometry
b. Dynamic contour tonometry
c. Rebound tonometry
d. Impression tonometry

Ans. is 'a' Applanation tonometry

DIRECT VS INDIRECT OPHTHALMOSCOPY

Features	Indirect ophthalmoscopy	Direct ophthalmoscopy
Examination distance	At an arm's length	As close to patient's eye as possible
Image	Real, inverted	Virtual, erect
Condensing lens	+ 20 D convex lens	Not required
Magnification	5x	15x
Area of field in focus	8 DD	2 DD
Stereopsis	Present	Absent
Accessible view	Up to ora serrate i.e. peripheral retina	peripheral retina not visualised
Examination through hazy media	Possible	Not possible
Patients position	Supine	Sitting
Ease	Difficult, require training	Easy procedure for visualization of posterior pole of retina

12. How much is image magnification on direct ophthalmoscope examination?

a. 1 time
b. 10 times
c. 15 times
d. 20 times

Ans. is 'c' 15 times

STRABISMUS

PARALYTIC SQUINT

Paralytic or incomitant squint occurs when there is an acquired defect of movement of an eye. The squint (and double vision) is maximally demonstrated by looking in the direction of action of the weakened muscle.

Paralytic squints occur due to disease of the III, IV and VI cranial nerves. A nerve palsy may be isolated or there may be multiple nerves involved. Each nerve may be affected at any point along its course from the brainstem to the orbit.

Differences

		Paralytic (incomitant)	Non-paralytic (comitatnt)
1.	Occurrence	Less common (15%)	More common (85%)
2.	Onset	Usually acquired and sudden; usually a sign of neurological or orbital disease; any age	Usually congenital
3.	Deviation	Secondary deviation >primary deviation	Primary deviation = secondary deviation
4.	Limitation of movement	+	–

13. Secondary deviation is more than primary deviation in: *(NEET 2020)*

a. Concomitant squint
b. Paralytic squint
c. Restrictive squint
d. Accommodative squint

Ans. is 'b' Paralytic squint

ESOTROPIA

Esotropia is an eye misalignment in which one eye is deviated inward, or nasally. The deviation may be constant or intermittent. The deviating eye may always be the same eye or may alternate between the two eyes.

Infantile Esotropia

An infant with an esotropia that is usually constant and presents within the first one year of life. It is associated with a large angle deviation, latent nystagmus, cross fixation, a normal accommodative convergence to accommodation ratio, and age-appropriate refractive errors.

Accommodative Esotropia

Occurs in children over 1 year of age. In general, this is associated with hypermetropia which reduces the angle and/or frequency of the esotropia when the hypermetropic correction is worn. Accommodative esotropia may also be associated with microtropia/monofixation syndrome.

Non-accommodative Esotropia

This subtype has an onset after 1 year of age, can be constant or intermittent, and is not affected by the level of accommodation.

Divergence Insufficiency Type Esotropia

This type of esotropia is found in the population 30 years of age and above. These patients have reduced fusional divergence amplitudes, the esotropia is worse at distance than near, and they may have trouble with driving or diplopia with distance fixation.

Microtropia/Monofixation Syndrome

This is characterized by patients with a central scotoma in one eye together with peripheral fusion, fusional amplitudes, and gross stereopsis.

14. Esotropia is commonly seen in: *(NEET 2020)*

a. Myopia
b. Hypermetropia
c. Astigmatism
d. Emmetropia

Ans. is 'b' Hypermetropia

MADDOX ROD TEST

The **Maddox rod** test can be used to subjectively detect and measure a latent, manifest, horizontal or vertical strabismus for near and distance. The test is based on the principle of diplopic projection. Dissociation of the deviation is brought about by presenting a red line image to one eye and a white light to the other, while prisms are used to superimpose these and effectively measure the angle of deviation (horizontal and vertical). The strength of the prism indicates the amount of deviation present. The Maddox rod is a handheld instrument composed of red parallel plano convex cylinder lens, which refracts light rays so that a point source of light is seen as a line or streak of light. Due to the optical properties, the streak of light is seen perpendicular to the axis of the cylinder.

The Maddox rod test should be used in cases of:

- Small to moderate (i.e.<25 pd) vertical deviations where there is simultaneous perception and normal retinal correspondence (NRC)
- Decompensated phorias.
- Acquired strabismus (rather than congenital or early onset)

15. Identify the instrument. *(NEET 2019)*

a. Maddox rod
b. Maddox wing
c. Maddox glass
d. Red glasses

Ans. is 'a' Maddox rod

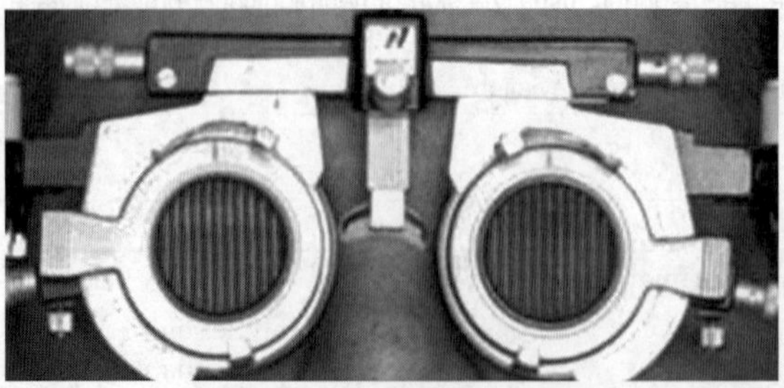

COVER-UNCOVER TEST

In the cover test, the child's attention is attracted to a target. The vision of one eye is then occluded. The tested (uncovered) eye is observed for movement from a deviated position to one that fixes on the target (a sign of tropia, also called manifest strabismus). The untested eye is then uncovered and the tested eye is observed again for any drift out of alignment.

Ophthalmology

In the cover-uncover test, a cover is placed over one eye for one to two seconds while the child's attention is called to the target. The cover is then removed rapidly, and the previously covered eye is observed for any movement from a deviated position back to fixation on the target (a sign of phoria, also called latent strabismus). Minimal phoria is a normal variant.

The alternate cover test can reveal a hidden phoria. The cover is held over one eye for a few seconds, then moved rapidly over the other eye and held for a few seconds, then moved back to cover the first eye. This is repeated several times, and each time the cover is moved, the previously covered eye is observed for any "refixation" from a deviated to a normal position.

The cover, cover-uncover, and alternate cover tests should be performed on both eyes, focusing first on a near object and then on a far object. The tests should be repeated three times to check for reproducibility. If any strabismus is detected, the patient should be referred. In some children, strabismus may be present only intermittently, especially when a child is tired. If the parent or caregiver reports eye deviation, the child should be referred for further evaluation, even if the deviation is not seen in the office.

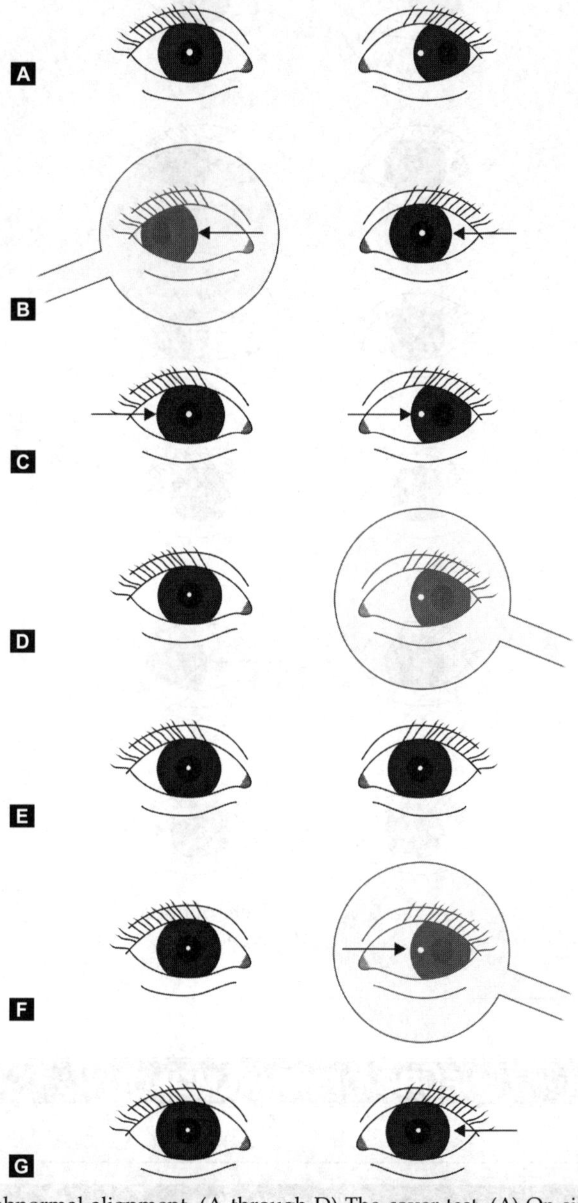

Figure above: Screening tests for abnormal alignment. (A through D) The cover test. (A) On simple observation, one eye (the tested eye, which is the patient's left eye in this illustration) appears to deviate. (B) The uncovered (tested) eye is observed for movement into alignment as the other eye is covered (in this illustration, an exotropia is exposed). This movement into alignment can come from any direction and is generally reproducible on repeat examinations. (C) When the opposite eye is uncovered, the tested eye is observed to return to its original location. (D) When the test eye is the normal eye (which is the patient's right eye in this illustration), it does not move when the opposite eye is covered or uncovered. (E through G) The cover-uncover test. (E) The tested eye (which is the patient's left eye in this illustration) is covered. On simple observation, before it is covered, the eye appears to be in alignment. (F) The tested eye is covered for a few seconds. (G) As the cover is rapidly removed, the tested eye is observed for movement back into alignment (in this illustration, an exophoria is exposed).

16. Following test is used to diagnose which ocular condition?

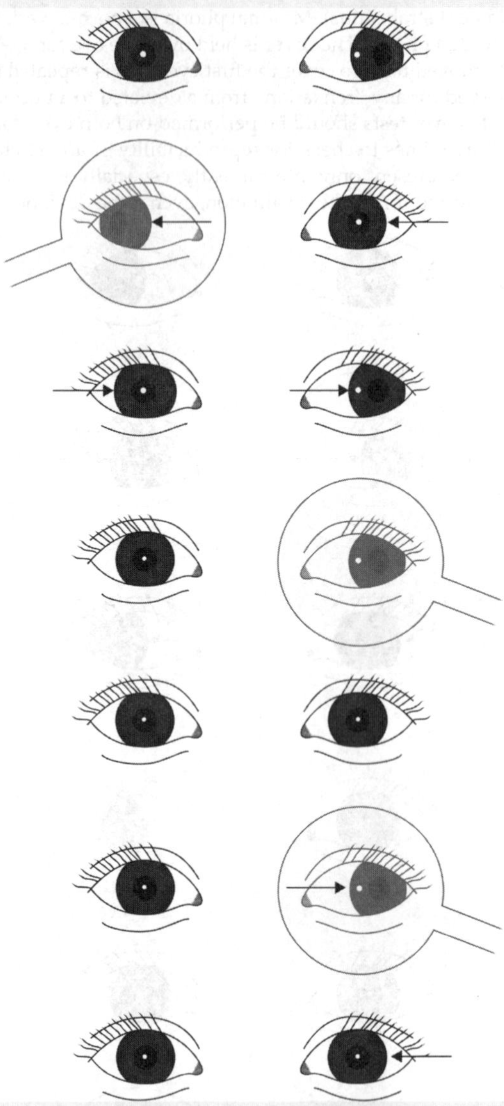

a. Strabismus
b. Heterophoria
c. Both a and b
d. None

Ans. is 'c' Both a and b

NEURO-OPHTHALMOLOGY

LESIONS OF OPTIC PATHWAY

Site of lesion	Visual field defect
Optic nerve	Blindness
Optic chiasma	Bitemporal hemianopia
Optic tract	Incongruent homonymous hemianopia
Lateral geniculate body	Homonymous hemianopia
Optic radiation (Total)	Homonymous hemianopia, sometimes with macular sparing

Contd...

Contd...

Site of lesion	Visual field defect
Optic radiation lower fibres (temporal lobe)	Homonymous upper quadrantanopia
Optic radiation upper fibres (parietal lobe)	Homonymous lower quadrantanopia
Visual cortex (anterior occipital cortex)	Homonymous hemianopia with macular sparing
Occipital cortex tip	Homonymous macular defect

17. Incongruous homonymous hemianopia with hemianopic pupil is seen in lesion of: *(NEET 2020)*

a. Optic nerve
b. Optic chiasma
c. Optic tract
d. Optic radiation

Ans. is 'c' Optic tract

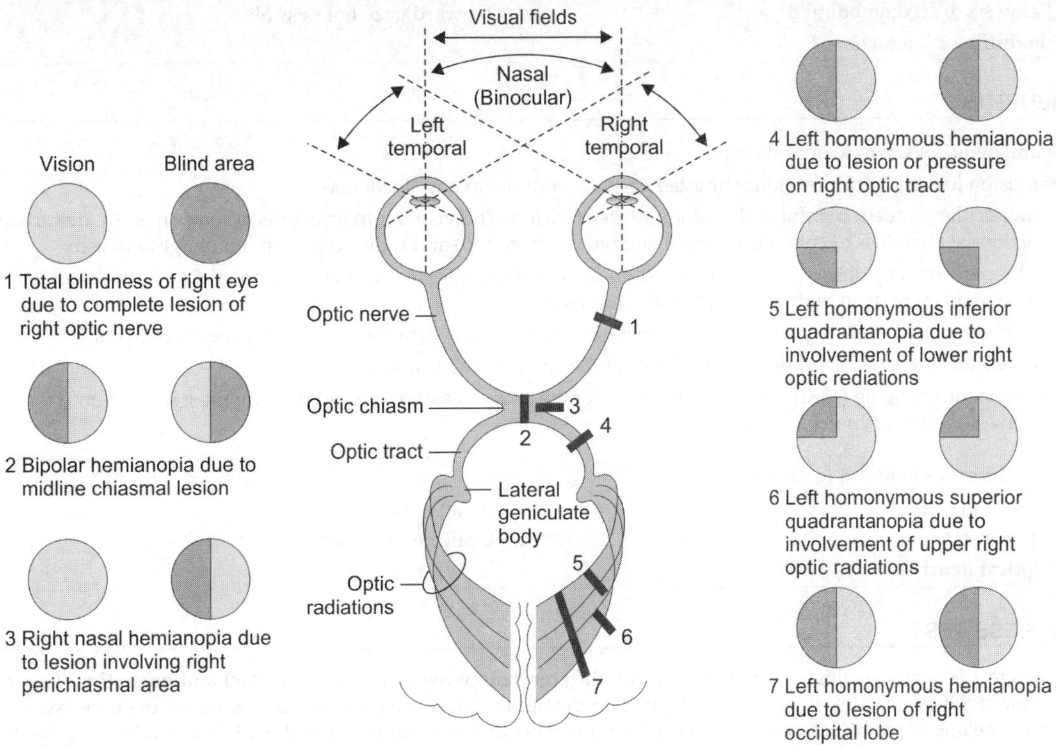

TYPES OF PUPILS

Type	Clinical findings	Anisocoria	Lesion
Marcus-Gunn pupil	A deafferented pupil which constricts to consensual but not direct light	Absent	CN II
Hutchinson pupil	A dilated pupil that does not respond to direct or consensual light	Present	CN II
Horner's syndrome	A small pupil with associated ipsilateral ptosis and decreased facial sweating	Present	Sympathetics
Adle's tonic pupil	A dilated pupil with an impaired light response and slow constriction to near vision	Present	Parasympathetics
Argyll Robertson pupil	A small, irregular pupil that constricts to near vision but not to light	Absent	Pretectum

18. Lesion in the optic chiasma causes:

a. Bitemporal hemianopia
b. Upper nasal
c. Lower nasal
d. Homonymous hemianopia

Ans. is 'a' Bitemporal hemianopia

19. Marcus Gunn pupil is seen in:

a. Retinitis pigmentosa
b. Retinal detachment
c. Diabetic retinopathy
d. Optic neuritis

Ans. is 'd' Optic neuritis

THIRD NERVE PALSY

- The primary symptom is diplopia caused by misalignment of the visual axes, and the pattern of image separation is the key to diagnosing which particular ocular motor cranial nerve (and extraocular muscle) is involved.
- With unilateral third cranial nerve palsy (i.e., oculomotor nerve palsy), the involved eye usually is deviated "down and out" (i.e., infraducted and abducted) due to unopposed action of superior oblique and lateral rectus.
- There may be partial ptosis (paralysis of levator palpebrae superioris). Both LPS and Muller's muscle function to retract the lid, hence only partial ptosis is seen in oculomotor nerve palsy due to intact sympathetic innervation of Muller's muscle.
- Pupillary dilatation (paralysis of sphincter papillae) can cause anisocoria, symptomatic glare in bright light. Loss of light reflex
- Accommodation deficit (paralysis of ciliary muscle) that may cause blurred vision for near objects

20. Oculomotor nerve palsy show all of the following *except*:

a. Ptosis	b. Inability of lateral gaze
c. Paralysis of accommodation	d. Upward gaze not possible

Ans. is 'b' Inability of lateral gaze

OPTIC NEURITIS

- Usually unilateral, except in toxic amblyopia.
- Profound vision loss and central vision is affected early (in contrast to papilloedema).
- There is monocular sudden, painful and profound loss of vision. The visual impairment is accompanied by disturbance of other visual functions such as loss of color vision (typically red desaturation) and reduced perception of light intensity.
- Occasionally patients may observe an altered perception of moving objects (Pulfrich phenomenon) or a worsening of symptoms with exercise or an increase in body temperature (Uhthoff sign).
- There is pain behind the eyeball, particularly in retrobulbar neuritis in which there is pain on eye movements.
- Visually evoked response (VER) shows reduced amplitude and delayed transmission time.
- Magnetic resonance imaging (MRI) is far more superior for the study of soft tissue and thus, for most neuro-ophthalmic conditions, MRI is the investigation of choice.

21. Painful eye movement is a feature of:

a. Optical neuritis	b. Papilloedema
c. Optic atrophy	d. Optic nerve hypoplasia

Ans. is 'a' Optical neuritis

PHOTOSTRESS TEST

The photostress test is a simple clinical technique that **can differentiate between retinal (macular) and postretinal (e.g. optic nerve) disease.** The test involves exposing the eye to the light from the ophthalmoscope for 10 s and measuring the time taken for acuity to return to within one line of pre-bleach acuity. Subject with normal healthy macular function should be able to read in the 50–60 s range. Patients with a macular problem may have recovery times lasting 1.5 to 3 min or longer. In car drivers with macular degeneration photostress effects from opposing cars may bleach retinal pigments and cause a dramatic drop in visual acuity. In patients with optic nerve disease the bleaching of the retina will have no effect on the recovery time. Photostress recovery time increases with age but is independent of pupil size and visual acuity.

22. Photostress test is used to differentiate: *(NEET 2020)*

a. Optic nerve and macular function	b. Retina and vitreous
c. Lens and cornea function	d. Cataract and glaucoma

Ans. is 'a' Optic nerve and macular function

Previously Asked Facts

- Medial wall of orbit is formed by the ethmoid, maxilla, lacrimal and sphenoid bones. The ethmoid bone separates the orbit from the ethmoid sinus.
- Gene for eye morphogenesis is Pax 6.
- Spasm of accommodation mimics Myopia
- Dispersive prism functions for splitting light into different wavelengths.
- Aniseikonia is difference in the size of image formed by the two eyes
- Inheritance of colour blindness is X-linked recessive

- ❖ In reduced schematic eye, the entire system (of eye) can be regarded as one lens with one optical centre which lies in the posterior part of crystalline lens. The diopteric power of reduced eye is + 60D, of which + 44D is contributed by cornea and + 16D by the crystalline lens.
- ❖ Occlusion of the blood flow in the central retinal artery leads to painless loss of vision.
- ❖ The cornea is a three dimensional prolate ellipsoid, like a bullet or a tulip. It is steeper in the centre and flatter in the periphery. After refractive surgeries like myopic LASIK, cornea is converted to oblate ellipsoid, which is steeper in the periphery and flatter in the centre.
- ❖ Perimetry is the systematic measurement of visual field function.
  - Static perimetry: A method of assessing fields, usually automated, in which the location of a stimulus remains fixed.
- ❖ *Kinetic (dynamic) perimetry*: A stimulus of constant intensity is moved from a non-seeing area to a seeing area at a standardized speed until it is perceived, and the point of perception is recorded on a chart; e.g.—Goldmann or Lister perimetry
- ❖ Degenerative myopia is characterized by progressive anteroposterior elongation of the scleral envelope associated with a range of secondary ocular changes. A pale tessellated (tigroid) appearance of retina is seen due to diffuse attenuation of the RPE. Foster Fuchs spot (subretinal hemmorhage at macula) is also seen.
- ❖ Purkinje image test is used in Pachymetry (measurement of corneal thickness)
- ❖ *Cycloplegic refraction*: Atropine ointment is used for 0–5 years of age, Cyclopentolate is used for 5–15 years of age and after 15 years, tropicamide is generally used
- ❖ Cross fixation is the use of the right eye to view the left visual field and the use of the left eye to view the right visual field. This behavior is very common in children with infantile esotropia.
- ❖ Divergent squint is also called as exotropia. It is less common than convergent squint (esotropia). 6th nerve palsy causes convergent squint.
- ❖ As the pupillomotor fibers in CN III travel outside the sheath of the IIIrd nerve, they avoid injury secondary to intrinsic ischemic damage in diabetes, resulting in normal pupillary reactions. Diabetic third nerve palsies are characteristically pupil-sparing and thus, both light and accommodation reflex are normal.
- ❖ Pupillary light reflex refers to constriction of pupil in response to light.
  - *Afferent*: Retina → Optic nerve → Optic chiasma → Optic tract → Pretectal nucleus → Internuncial neurons → EWN (Edinger Westphal nucleus).
  - *Efferent*: Edinger Westphal nucleus → Occulomotor (3rd) nerve → Ciliary ganglion → Short ciliary nerve → Sphincter pupillae.
- ❖ Some fibres decussate at optic chiasma and go to contralateral side which is responsible for consensual or indirect light reflex.
- ❖ *Corneal reflex-afferent*: The nasociliary branch of the ophthalmic branch (V1) of the cranial nerve V (trigeminal nerve) sensing the stimulus on the cornea, lid, or conjunctiva. *Efferent*: The temporal and zygomatic branches of the facial nerve initiating the motor response.
- ❖ Neuron order in optic pathway
  - Sensory organs–Photoreceptors (rods and cones)
  - First order neuron–Axon of Bipolar cells in retina
  - Second order neuron–Axon of ganglion cells (Optic nerve, chiasma, optic tracts)
  - Third order neuron–Axons from lateral geniculate ganglion (Optic radiation)
- ❖ Most common visual defect in papilloedema is Amaurosis fugax (recurring brief episodes of visual obscuration)

CATARACT

TYPES OF CATARACT

Disease	Type of cataract
Myotonic dystrophy	Christmas tree cataract, Blue dot cortical cataract, posterior subcapsular cataract.
Wilson's disease	Sunflower cataract (Petals of flower cataract)
Diabetes mellitus	Snowflake cataract or Snowstorm cataract
Down's syndrome	Snowflake cataract
Atopic dermatitis	Blue dot cortical cataract, posterior subcapsular cataract
Congenital rubella	Nuclear cataract
Galactosemia	Oil drop cataract
Complicated cataract (Iridocyditis, High myopia)	Posterior cortical breads' Crumb appearance
Blunt trauma	Vossius ring on anterior surface of lens, Rosette shaped cataract

23. Blue dot cataract is caused by:

a. Diabetes
b. Wilson's disease
c. Atopic dermatitis
d. Chalcosis

Ans. is 'c' Atopic dermatitis

POSTOPERATIVE COMPLICATIONS AFTER CATARACT SURGERY

Early

- Hyphema (collection of blood in anterior chamber)
- Iris prolapse
- Striate keratopathy
- Flat (shallow) anterior chamber
- Anterior uveitis
- Bacterial endophthalmitis

Late

- Cystoid macular edema (CME)
- Delayed chronic postoperative endophthalmitis
- Retinal detachment
- After cataract
- Glaucoma-in-aphakia and pseudophakia

Endophthalmitis

Endophthalmitis is the infection of the eye involving the vitreous. This can occur at any time following cataract surgery ranging from within 2 days to few months after surgery. Most common causative organism includes *Staphylococcus* epidermidis. Prolonged surgery (more than 60 minutes), vitreous loss and diabetes mellitus are risk factors for development of endophthalmitis.

Organisms depends upon the type of endophthalmitis:

A. Exogenous endophthalmitis
   - Postoperative
     - Acute postoperative (within 1–7 days after surgery): *S. epidermidis, S. aureus,* Strep negative bacilli
     - Delayed onset (a week to months after surgery): Propionibacterium acnes
   - Posttraumatic: *Bacillus, S.epidermidis,* fungi, *streptococcus spp.*

B. Endogenous endophthalmitis: Bacillus cereus (especially in IV drug abusers), *S. aureus, H. influenzae, meningococci, Mucor* and *Candida*
   - Generally present between 48 and 72 hours after surgery and include: Ocular pain, diminished vision, eyelid edema, exudates in pupillary area, hypopyon and diminished or absent red pupillary glow.

Treatment includes intravitreal antibiotics injection, frequent topical administration of fortified antibiotics, periocular antibiotics injection. Steroid therapy may be used concurrently with caution. Vitrectomy may be required in cases not responding to medical therapy to remove the infected vitreous and facilitate better penetration of the antibiotics.

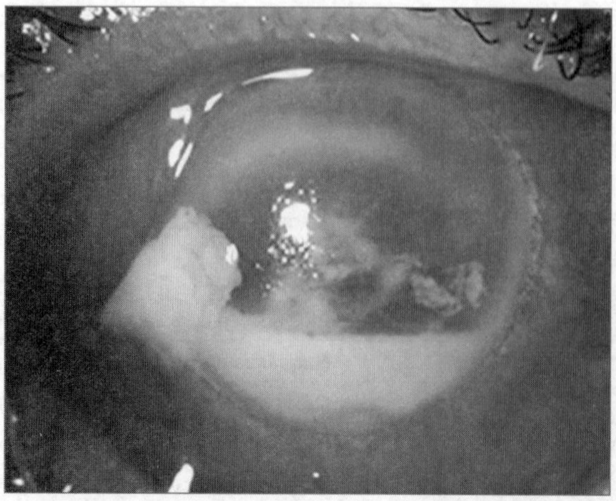

After-Cataract or Secondary Cataract or Posterior Capsular Opacification (PCO)

- Posterior capsular opacification (PCO) is seen after extra capsular cataract extraction (ECCE).
- Opacification of the posterior capsule is caused by postoperative proliferation of cells in the capsular bag and is the most common complication of ECCE.
- After-cataract may present as thickened posterior capsule, or dense membranous after cataract or Soemmering ring which refers to a thick ring of after cataract formed behind the iris, enclosed between the two layers of capsule or Elschnig's pearls in which the vacuolated subcapsular epithelial cells are clustered like soap bubble along the posterior capsule.
- After-cataract, if thin, can be cleared centrally by Nd:YAG laser capsulotomy. Thick membranous after-cataract needs surgical membranectomy.

24. A 70 years old lady 2 days following cataract surgery presents with eye complaints as shown in the image. Next step in its management is:

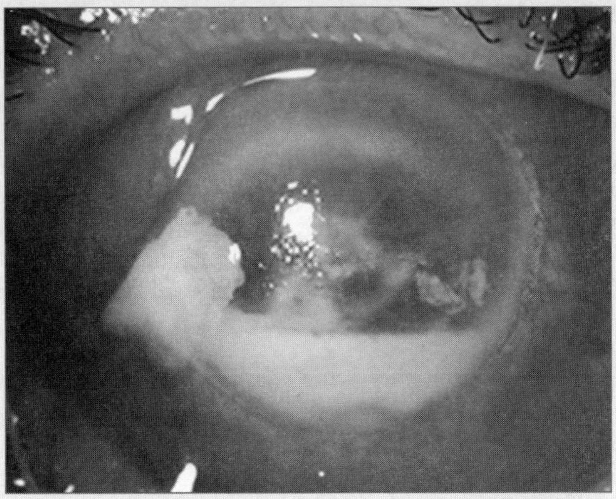

a. Intravitreal antibiotic
b. Intravitreal steroids
c. Eye patch and dressing
d. Intravitreal mannitol

Ans. is 'a' Intravitreal antibiotic

Explanation: The image shows hypopyon indicator of endophthalmitis.

25. Postoperative complications of cataract are all *except*:

a. After cataract
b. Endophthalmitis
c. Glaucoma
d. Scleritis

Ans. is 'd' Scleritis

26. Posterior capsule opacities are treated by:

a. Argon green laser
b. Lens explantation
c. Nd:YAG laser
d. Diode laser

Ans. is 'c' Nd:YAG laser

SURGERIES IN CATARACT

1. *Intracapsular cataract extraction (ICCE)*: Entire cataractous lens along with intact capsule is removed
2. *Extracapsular cataract extraction* (ECCE): Major portion of anterior capsule with epithelium, nucleus and cortex are removed; leaving behind intact posterior capsule.

Presently, ECCE techniques are surgery of choice for cataracts.

Phacoemulsification

- Phacoemulsification is an alternative approach to ECCE. With conventional ECCE, the entire nucleus of the lens is removed from the eye through a large (10 mm) incision. In phacoemulsification, ultrasound-driven needle emulsifies and aspirates the lens through a considerably smaller (3 to 4 mm) incision.
- Steps in phacoemulsification include: (i) Corneoscleral incision, (ii) Continuous curvilinear capsulorhexis, (iii) Hydrodissection and hydrodelineation, (iv) Emulsification and aspiration of nucleus and then cortex, (v) Foldable IOL implantation in posterior chamber.

- Recovery with phacoemulsification is fastest as incision is very small and no sutures are used.
- Trypan blue has been used as an adjunct for improving visualization of the anterior capsule during phacoemulsification of mature white cataracts for the past few years.

Femtosecond Laser

Mechanism of action: Photoionization of optically transparent tissues-like cornea, leading to generation of free electrons and ionized molecules.

- It has a wavelength of 1053 μm and a pulse duration of 10^{-15} seconds.
- *Advantage*: Low pulse duration results in minimal collateral tissue damage.

Uses

- Corneal refractive surgery: LASIK flap creation, Astigmatic keratotomy (AK)
- Presbyopia correction
- Laser-assisted anterior and posterior lamellar keratoplasty
- Customized trephination in penetrating keratoplasty
- Wound construction, capsulorrhexis and nuclear fragmentation in cataract surgery.

27. What is the new advance in cataract surgery?

a. Femtosecond laser
b. Neodymium laser
c. Nanosecond laser
d. Picosecond laser

Ans. is 'a' Femtosecond laser

28. Which of the following step is not done during phaco-emulsification surgery for cataract?

a. Aspiration of cortex
b. Continuous curvilinear capsulorrhexis
c. Foldable IOL implantation
d. Sclerocorneal tunnel

Ans. is 'd' Sclerocorneal tunnel

Explanation: Sutureless self-sealing valvular sclerocorneal tunnel incision is used for intraocular lens implantation in manual Small Incision Cataract Surgery (SICS)

CONGENITAL CATARACT

- Congenital cataract occurs in about 3 in 10,000 live births. Two thirds are bilateral.
- Autosomal dominant (AD) inheritance is the most common aetiological factor; others include chromosomal abnormalities, metabolic disorders and intrauterine infections.
- Isolated inherited congenital cataracts carry a better visual prognosis than those with coexisting ocular and systemic abnormality.

Management of Congenital and Developmental Cataract

- Treatment is not indicated in a developmental cataract unless vision is considerably impaired.
- If the opacity is large, the treatment of choice is extracapsular extraction of lens. Intracapsular cataract extraction in children is contraindicated because of vitreous traction and loss at the Wieger capsulohyaloid ligament.
- Timing of surgery is very crucial. The critical period for developing the fixation reflex in both unilateral and bilateral visual deprivation disorders is between 2–4 months of age. Any cataract dense enough to impair vision must be dealt with before this age and the earliest possible time is preferred.
- Method for extracapsular cataract extraction are:
  - Posterior capsulectomy and anterior vitrectomy (Procedure of choice)
  - Lens aspiration
  - Lensectony

29. False about treatment of cataract in children is:

a. ECCE is the treatment of choice
b. In case of bilateral cataract impairing vision surgery must be done by 4–6 weeks of age
c. Lensectomy is not one of the methods of extracapsular extraction
d. Intraocular lens implantation must be done only after 2 years of age

Ans. is 'c' Lensectomy is not one of the methods of extracapsular extraction

ECTOPIA LENTIS

Ectopia lentis refers to a hereditary or acquired displacement of the lens from its normal position. The lens may be completely dislocated, rendering the eye functionally aphakic (luxated), or partially displaced, remaining partly within the pupillary area (subluxated).

Causes

- Acquired
  - Trauma
  - Inflammation, e.g. chronic cyclitis, syphilis
  - Hypermature cataract
  - Large eye, e.g. high myopia, buphthalmos
- Congenital
  - Familial ectopia lentis
  - Aniridia
  - Marfan syndrome—Bilateral ectopia lentis (80%); subluxation is most frequently superotemporal
  - Weill-Marchesani syndrome—Ectopia lentis (50%). Subluxation is in an inferior direction and occurs in late childhood or early adulthood
  - Homocystinuria

30. Which is the syndrome not associated with lens dislocation?

a. Marfan's syndrome
b. Weill-Marchesani syndrome
c. Aniridia
d. Usher syndrome

Ans. is 'd' Usher syndrome

LOSS OF VISION

Sudden		Gradual	
Painful	***Painless***	***Painful***	***Painless***
• Acute congestive (angle closure) glaucoma • Acute iridocyclitis(uveitis) • Chemical and mechanical injury to eyeball • Endophthalmitis • Optic neuritis	• Macular edema • central retinal artery occlusion (CRAO) • central retinal vein occlusion (CRVO) • Central serous retinopathy • Retinaldetachment • Exudative age-related macular degeneration (ARMD) • Vitreous and retinal haemorrhage • Methyl alcohol amblyopia • Subluxation or dislocation of lens	• Corneal ulceration • Chronic simple glaucoma • Chronic iridocyclitis(uveitis)	• Progressive pterygium • Corneal dystrophy • Corneal degeneration • Cataract (development and senile) • Chorioretinal degeneration • Dry type—Age-related macular degeneration (ARMD) • Diabetic retinopathy • Refractive errors • Presbyopia

31. Sudden loss of vision is seen in all *except*:

a. Central retinal artery occlusion
b. Retinal detachment
c. Open angle glaucoma
d. Vitreous haemorrhage

Ans. is 'c' Open angle glaucoma

CONGENITAL GLAUCOMA

Clinical onset: at birth (intrauterine) or < 3 years.

Clinical Symptoms

- Photophobia is earliest symptoms due to corneal edema
- Lacrimation is most common.
- Blepharospasm

Clinical Sign

- *Earliest sign:* Corneal Haze/Ground glass appearance
- Haab's striae
- Blue eyes (Scleral thinning)
- Anisometric amblyopia

Treatment

Unlike adult glaucoma, the initial treatment for congenital glaucoma is often surgical. A drainage surgery is often recommended for congenital glaucoma.

- *Pharmacotherapy*: β-blocker + Carbonic anhydrase inhibitors (but not effective).

Surgical

- Trabeculotomy + Trabeculectomy–Treatment of choice
- *Goniotomy*: Treatment of choice if clear cornea.

32. The treatment of congenital glaucoma is:

a. Essentially topical medications
b. Trabeculoplasty
c. Trabeculotomy
d. Goniotomy

Ans. is 'c' Trabeculotomy

RETINA

EXUDATIVE RETINAL DETACHMENT (RD)

The characteristic feature of a significant **exudative retinal detachment** is the presence of **shifting** subretinal **fluid**. The **fluid shifts** to the most dependent location when patients change body position.

33. Shifting fluid sign is a hallmark feature of: *(NEET 2020)*

a. Rhegmatogenous RD
b. Tractional RD
c. Exudative RD
d. Retinal dialysis

Ans. is 'c' Exudative RD

LAYERS OF RETINA

- Pigment epithelium: Outermost layer; contains a single layer of cells containing pigment
- Layer of rods and cones
- External limiting membrane: Fenestrated membrane through which processes of rods and cones pass
- Outer nuclear layer: Contains nuclei of rods and cones
- Outer plexiform layer: Contains connections of photoreceptors with dendrites of bipolar and horizontal cells
- Inner nuclear layer: Contains cell bodies of bipolar cells, horizontal, amacrine and Muller's cells.
- Inner plexiform layer: Contains connections between axons of bipolar cells and dendrites of ganglion cells and processes of amacrine cells
- Ganglion cell layer: Contains cell bodies of ganglion cells
- Nerve fibre layer: Contains axons of ganglion cells
- Internal limiting membrane: Innermost layer; essentially a basement membrane

34. Cell bodies of Muller's cells are present in which layer of retina?

a. Inner nuclear layer
b. Outer nuclear layer
c. Re tinal pigment epithelium
d. Ganglion cell layer

Ans. is 'a' Inner nuclear layer

HYPERTENSIVE RETINOPATHY

Keith-Wagner-Barker classification of hypertensive retinopathy	
Grade I	Mild to moderate narrowing or sclerosis of arterioles
Grade II	• Moderate to marked narrowing or sclerosis of arterioles • 'S' shaped deflection of veins at AV crossing: Salus' sign
Grade III	• Retinal arteriolar narrowing and focal constriction • Prominent arteriovenous crossing changes with following signs – Banking of veins distal to AV crossing → Bonnet sign – Tapering of veins on either side of crossing → Marcus-Gunn sign (Gunn sign) – Right angle deflection at AV crossing → Salus' sign • Retinal edema, cotton-wool patches (soft exudate) • Superficial (flame shaped) hemorrhages
Grade IV	Grade III changes plus papilledema, macular star

35. Give the diagnosis.

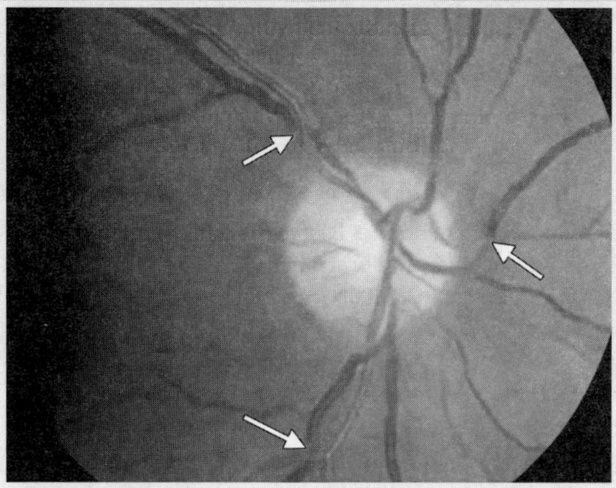

a. Non-proliferative diabetic retinopathy
b. Proliferative diabetic retinopathy
c. Hypertensive retinopathy
d. Central retinal artery occlusion

Ans. is 'c' Hypertensive retinopathy

Explanation: Arrows show deflection of veins at AV crossing.

RETROLENTAL FIBROPLASIA (RETINOPATHY OF PREMATURITY)

- Retinopathy of prematurity (ROP) affects immature retinal vasculature of premature babies.
- It may occur due to high exposure to oxygen in premature infants
- All babies weighing less than 1500 gm at birth or having a gestation period of less than 32 weeks should be screened with indirect ophthalmoscopy for ROM.
- Classification on the basis of severity:
  - Stage I—Appearance of thin, flat, white structure (demarcation line) at the junction of vascularized retina posteriorly and avascular retina anteriorly.
  - Stage II—the demarcation line develops into a pink or white elevation of thickened tissue.
  - Stage III—proliferation of vessels over the ridge and into vitreous
  - Stage IV—partial retinal detachment
    - Stage IVa—partial detachment with macular sparing
    - Stage IVb—partial detachment with macula involved
  - Stage V—total retinal detachment.

Management

- Most of the cases (approx 80%) of ROP resolve spontaneously, hence intervention is chosen according to the below given protocol. ROP is divided into threshold and prethreshold disease.
- Treatment of threshold disease is - Laser photocoagulation.
- Prethreshold disease is divided into 2 types: High risk or Type I - treatment is laser photocoagulation and Low risk or Type II - treatment is weekly or twice weekly observation.

36. Retrolental fibroplasia–which of the following is false?

a. Total retinal detachment is seen in stage V
b. Treatment of threshold disease is laser photocoagulation
c. Demarcation line is first seen is stage II
d. It may occur due to high exposure to oxygen in premature infants

Ans. is 'c' Demarcation line is first seen is stage II

Previously Asked Facts

- In Phacoemulsification, lens nucleus is emulsified using high frequency sound waves.
- Prolonged use of corticosteroid eye drops causes Posterior Subcapsular Cataract
- Oldest fibres of the lens are in the nucleus (central part). Cortex is the peripheral part containing the youngest fibres.
- Hemeralopia is the inability to see clearly in bright light (also known as day blindness) and is seen in posterior subcapsular cataract
- In aqueous humour, ascorbic acid is actively transported to a concentration some 15 times greater than that in plasma.

- Onion peel appearance cataract is seen in posterior polar cataract.
- Normal IOP range is 11–21 mm Hg. Mean normal IOP is 16 mm Hg.
- The damage to visual fields in glaucoma occurs in the order of superior-inferior-nasal-temporal-central.
- Open angle glaucoma
  - Treatment of choice-topical antiglaucoma drugs
  - Drug of choice-Beta blocker (timolol)
  - Surgery of choice-Argon or Diode laser trabeculoplasty
- Acute congestive glaucoma
  - Treatment of choice for acute congestive glaucoma → Laser iridotomy (patient choice), Peripheral iridectomy (2nd choice)
  - Drug of choice for acute congestive glaucoma → Pilocarpine
  - Initial drug used to lower IOP → Systemic mannitol or acetazolamide
- Angle closure glaucoma presents with–Edematous cornea, shallow anterior chamber, pupil is vertically oval and fixed, nonreactive to both light and accommodation, edematous and hyperemic optic disc and markedly raised IOP (40–70 mm Hg)
- 100 days glaucoma is seen in Central Retinal Vein Occlusion (CRVO)
- Long term side effect of phakic IOLs is chronic glaucoma.
- Glaucomatocyclitic crisis (Posner-Schlossman syndrome) is a unilateral recurrent non-granulomatous iritis associated with elevated ocular pressure during the attacks. Visual fields, the optic nerve head, and anterior chamber angle are normal.
- Vogt's triad may be seen in any type of post-congestive glaucoma. Characterized by:
  - Glaucomflecken (Anterior subcapsular lenticular opacity)
  - Patches of iris atrophy
  - Slightly dilated non-reacting pupil (due to sphincter atrophy)
- Brimonidine is alfa 2 agonist and is contraindicated in young children less than 2 years.
- Uveal tissue constitutes the middle vascular coat of the eyeball (inner coat is retina and outer coat is cornea and sclera). From anterior to posterior, it can be divided into three parts: Iris, ciliary body and choroid.
- Treatment of choice for all form of uveitis is corticosteroids.
  - Anterior uveitis (Iridocyclitis) → Topical corticosteroids.
  - Intermediate uveitis (Pars planitis) → Systemic corticosteroids.
  - Posterior uveitis (choroiditis) → Systemic corticosteroids
- Signs of trachoma
  - Conjunctival signs: Congestion, conjunctival follicles (boiled sago grain like), Papillary hyperplasia conjunctival scarring (Arlt's line)
  - Corneal signs: Superficial keratitis, Herbert follicles, Pannus, Corneal ulcer, Herbert pits, Corneal opacity
- Koeppe's nodules are small nodules seen at the inner margin of the iris in patients with granulomatous anterior uveitis, which occurs in conditions such as sarcoidosis and tuberculosis.
- Busacca's nodules occur on the peripheral part of anterior surface of iris. Also seen in Granulomatous anterior uveitis.
- Iris pearls are seen in uveitis due to Leprosy
- Subacute retinitis of Roth: It typically occurs in patients suffering from subacute bacterial endocarditis (SABE). It is characterized by multiple superficial retinal hemorrhages involving posterior part of the fundus. Most of the hemorrhages have a white spot in the center (Roth's spot).
- Bruch's membrane is the innermost layer of the choroid. It is also called the vitreous lamina, because of its glassy microscopic appearance. It is 2–4 μm thick. It lies between choroid and the retina.
- Angioid streaks are dark brown pigmented streaks that radiate from the peripheral retina into the macular and peripheral fundus. These are due to changes in the elastic tissue of Bruch's membrane and are frequently associated with more widespread degeneration of similar nature as in the elastic tissue of skin (pseudoxanthoma elasticum) or arterial walls.
- Causes of ring scotoma are:
  - Retinitis pigmentosa
  - High myopia,
  - Primary open angle glaucoma
  - Aphakic spectacle correction
  - Panretinal photocoagulation
- Causes of Soft Exudates (Cotton Wool Spots)
  - All types of severe hypertension (hypertensive retinopathy)
  - Diabetic retinopathy
  - Collagen vascular disorders
  - Infections: AIDS, septic retinitis (including SABE)
  - Microembolization: IV drug abuse, Post cardiac surgery or Purtscher retinopathy.
  - Other: Eale's disease, pseudoxanthoma elasticum, neoplasia (Leukemia, Hodgkin's disease), Sickle cell retinopathy, radiation retinopathy
- The hallmark of Proliferative Diabetic Retinopathy (PDR) is the occurrence of neovascularization over the changes of severe Non-Proliferative Diabetic Retinopathy (NPDR).

- ❖ Retinal detachment surgery consists of three components—sealing retinal tears, reducing the vitreous traction on the retina and flattening of retina. Retinal tears are sealed by laser photocoagulation, diathermy or cryo application. Scleral buckling or encirclage is a procedure to push the wall of sclera inwards to close the tear, reduce the traction and flatten the retina. Drainage of subretinal fluid helps to flatten the retina against the sclera.
- ❖ Causes of retinal tear/hole (rhegmatogenous retinal detachment).
  - Myopia
  - Previous intraocular surgery: Cataract extraction, aphakia or pseudoaphakia
  - Trauma
  - Retinal degeneration
- ❖ Causes of cherry red spot
  - gM2 gangliosidoses (Tay Sachs and Sandhoff)
  - GM1 gangliosidoses
  - Niemann - Pick's disease
  - Gaucher' s disease
  - Metachromatic leukodystrophy
  - Central retinal artery occlusion (CRAO)
  - Trauma (Berlin's edema/commotio retinae)
- ❖ Berlin's oedema, also called commotio retinae, occurs in blunt trauma to eye. It manifests as milky white cloudiness involving a considerable area of the posterior pole with a 'cherry-red' spot in the foveal region.
- ❖ Proliferative diabetic retinopathy is a cause of tractional retinal detachment
- ❖ Pars plana vitrectomy is the most common approach to vitrectomy done in tackling various posterior segment disorders.
- ❖ *Ophthalmic complications of Diabetes*: Accelerated senile cataract, neovascular glaucoma, retinopathy, reduced corneal sensitivity and oculomotor nerve palsies
- ❖ The globe is displaced to inferonasal side in lacrimal gland tumours.

CORNEA AND CONJUNCTIVA

Between 25 and 35°C, the hydration of the cornea is nearly constant.

The corneal endothelium regulates corneal hydration and shows considerable changes in its metabolism over the same temperature range. The following explanation is proposed: as the outwardly directed active "pump" in the endothelium decreases in lowered temperatures so the inwardly directed passive "leak" across the endothelium correspondingly decreases to maintain a constant corneal hydration.

37. Corneal hydration is maintained by: *(NEET 2020)*

a. Stroma
b. Aqueous humor
c. Endothelium
d. Epithelium

Ans. is 'c' Endothelium

VERNAL KERATOCONJUNCTIVITIS (VKC)

- ❖ VKC or spring catarrh is a recurrent, bilateral, and self-limiting inflammation of conjunctiva, having a periodic seasonal incidence.
- ❖ *Symptoms*: VKC is characterised by marked burning and itchy sensations which accentuates when patient comes in a warm humid atmosphere. Associated symptoms include mild photophobia in case of corneal involvement, lacrimation, stringy discharge and heaviness of eyelids.

Important signs of VKC

Conjunctival		
Palpebral	***Bulbar***	***Corneal***
Papillary hypertrophy into polygonal papilla	Gelatinous thickening around limbus	Punctate epithelial keratitis
		Ulcerative vernal keratitis: shallow transverse ulcer (Shield ulcer)
Cobble stone (Pavement stone) appearance	Horner-Trantas spots	Vernal corneal plaques
Giant papilla (Cauliflower excrescence)	Dusky red triangular congestion	Subepithelial scarring
		Pseudogerontoxon: characterized by a classical "Cupid's bow" outline.
Follicles are not seen in VKC		

38. Pseudogerontoxon is seen in:

a. Vernal keratopathy
b. Choroidal melanoma
c. Trachoma
d. Retinoblastoma

Ans. is 'a' Vernal keratopathy

ACANTHAMOEBA KERATITIS

- Acanthamoeba is a free-living genus of amoeba. In humans, acanthamoeba causes: (i) Keratitis; (ii) Granulomatous encephalitis, (iii) Fulminant meningoencephalitis
- Acanthamoeba keratitis is the most common keratitis caused by a protozoan especially in contact lens users.
- Patient presents with very severe pain (which is out of proportion to the degree of clinical signs), watering, photophobia, blurred vision and blepharospasm.
- On examination, initially it shows typical reticular pattern due to radial keratoneuritis (Radial perineuritis).
- *Advanced cases (Stromal involvement)*: Over a period of weeks stromal signs develop with central or paracentral ring shaped lesion with stromal infiltrate and an overlying epithelial defect, ultimately presenting as ring abscess

39. Pain is out of proportion to signs in which corneal ulcer?

a. Herpes simplex keratitis
b. Acanthamoeba keratitis
c. Fungal keratitis
d. Pneumococcal keratitis

Ans. is 'b' Acanthamoeba keratitis

FUNGAL KERATITIS

- *Fusarium and Aspergillus fumigatus* are the most common causes around the world, while *candida* is the most common cause in temperate regions.

Predisposing Factors

- Injury by vegetative materials or animal tail–most common
- Long term use of topical steroids or antibiotics
- Prior corneal transplantation
- Contact lens wear
- Diabetes mellitus

Clinical Features

- Symptoms are mild as compared to the signs
- Mild pain, watering and photophobia are seen, but ciliary and conjunctival congestion are marked.
- Characteristic features of corneal ulcer are—dry looking, grayish white with elevated rolled out margins and feathery finger like extensions into surrounding stroma under intact epithelium, with satellite nodules
- A sterile immune ring of Wesseley is seen where fungal antigen and host antibody meet.
- Hypopyon is seen, which is often large and unsterile (pseudohypopyon) as fungi can penetrate into anterior chamber without perforation.

Diagnosis

- Examination of wet KOH mount, calcoflour white for fungal hyphae and culture on Sabouraud's medium.

Treatment

- Natamycin and amphotericin B are the 1st line drugs.
- Imidazole and flucytosine are used in candida infection.

Cycloplegics as atropine or scopolamine are used to reduce ciliary spasm, uveal inflammation and prevent posterior synechiae formation.

- Anti-inflammatory and analgesics
  - Topical steroids enhance fungal replication and corneal invasion and are contraindicated therapy of a fungal corneal ulcer.

40. Which is not a feature of fungal corneal ulcer?

a. White dry corneal ulcer
b. Immune ring
c. More symptomatic than bacterial ulcer
d. Non-sterile hypopyon

Ans. is 'c' More symptomatic than bacterial ulcer

Presenting clinical features that are specific to fungal keratitis include an infiltrate with feathery margins, elevated edges, rough texture, gray-brown pigmentation, **satellite lesions** and endothelial plaque. The spread of infection occurs through the channel network of the cornea. This mode of spread fully explains the satellite lesions.

- Fine or coarse granular infiltrate within the epithelium and anterior stroma
- Gray-white color, dry, and rough corneal surface that may appear elevated

- Typical irregular feathery-edged infiltrate
- **White ring in the cornea and satellite lesions near the edge of the primary focus of the infection**
- In advanced cases, suppurative stromal keratitis associated with conjunctival hyperemia, anterior chamber inflammation, hypopyon, iritis, endothelial plaque, or possible corneal perforation.

41. Most characteristic feature of fungal corneal ulcer is: *(NEET 2020)*

a. Dendritic processes
b. White hypopyon
c. Satellite lesions
d. Watery discharge

Ans. is 'c' Satellite lesions

PTERYGIUM

- Pterygium is a non-cancerous (non-neoplastic) growth of conjunctiva.
- Characterized by a wing-shaped fold of conjunctiva upon the cornea from either side within the interpalpebral fissure.
- Pterygium is always situated in the palpebral aperture.
- Pathologically, Pterygium is a degenerative and hyperplastic condition of con- junctiva.
- The subconjunctival tissue undergoes elastotic degeneration and proliferates as vascularised granulation tissue under the epithelium, which ultimately encroaches the cornea

Clinical Features

- More common in people with excess outdoor exposure to sunlight (UV rays) dry heat, high wind and abundance of dust.
- Clinically, presents as a triangular fold of conjunctiva encroaching the cornea in the area of palpebral aperture, usually on the nasal side.
- *Stocker's line*: Iron deposition line at edge of pterygium on corneal epithelium
- Pterygium is an asymptomatic condition in the early stages, except for cosmetic intolerance
- Visual disturbance or corneal astigmatism may occur due to encroachment on papillary area

Treatment

- Asymptomatic pterygium which is not progressive is best left alone
- Surgical excision is the only satisfactory treatment

42. False statement about given condition of eye: *(NEET 2019)*

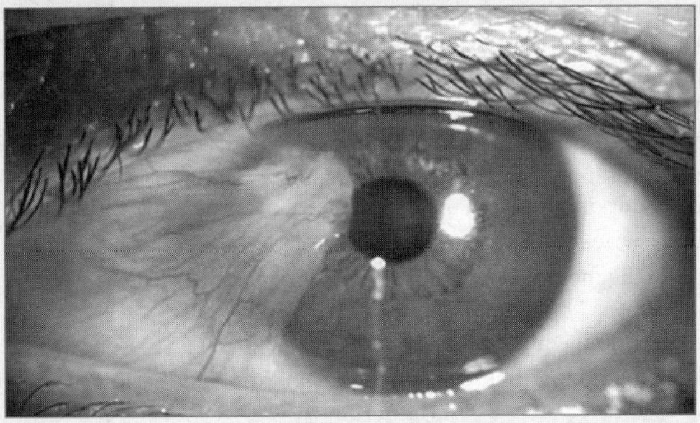

a. Arises from any part of conjunctiva
b. Can cause astigmatism
c. Surgery is the treatment of choice
d. UV exposure is risk factor

Ans. is 'a' Arises from any part of conjunctiva

Explanation: The clinical photograph shows a Pterygium

SCLEROMALACIA PERFORANS

- A specific type of non-inflammatory scleritis with progressive scleral thinning that typically affects elderly women with longstanding rheumatoid arthritis. Despite the nomenclature, perforation of the globe is extreme as integrity is maintained by a thin layer of fibrous tissue.

Ophthalmology

- *Symptoms*: Mild non-specific irritation; pain is absent and vision unaffected. Keratoconjunctivis sicca may be seen
- *Signs*: Necrotic scleral plaques near the limbus without vascular congestion, Coalescence and enlargement of necrotic areas and Slow progression of scleral thinning with exposure of underlying uvea
- *Treatment*: Immunosuppressives have been used. Underlying systemic disease should be treated aggressively. Protection from trauma is important. Surgical repair of scleral perforation (e.g. patch grafting) is mandatory to prevent phthisis bulbi.

43. All except one is true for Scleromalacia perforans:

a. It is noninflammatory scleritis
b. It affects only males
c. Perforation of the globe is extremely rare
d. Vision is unaffected

Ans. is 'b' It affects only males

Previously Asked Facts

- Most common malignant orbital tumor in children—Rhabdomyosarcoma
- Most common malignant orbital tumor in adult—Lymphoma
- Most common primary intraocular tumor in children—Retinoblastoma
- Most common primary intraocular tumor in adults—Uveal melanoma
- Microscopic features of a well differentiated Retinoblastoma include Flexner-Wintersteiner rosettes (specific for retinoblastoma), Homer-Wright rosettes, pseudo rosettes and fleurettes formation.
- Most common cause of unilateral proptosis in children is orbital cellulitis
- Most common cause of unilateral proptosis in adults is thyroid ophthalmopathy
- Most common cause of bilateral proptosis in children → Neuroblastoma (mc), Leukemia (Chloroma)
- Most common cause of bilateral proptosis in adults is thyroid ophthalmopathy
- Most serious cause of conjunctivitis that causes blindness in children is Trachoma
- Common Dyes used for Conjunctival Staining—Rose Bengal, Fluoroscein, Lissamine
- Goblets cells in conjunctiva are most dense nasally and least dense in upper temporal fornix. They are absent in palpebral mucocutaneous junction and the limbus.
- Placido disc is used for assessing Corneal sheen and surface.
- The processes involved in healing of corneal epithelial wounds is divided into three distinct components—cell migration, cell proliferation, and cell adhesion
- Mooren's ulcer is a rare disorder, typically seen in healthy adult men. Patients complain of redness, tearing, and photophobia. The pain is out of proportion to the inflammation . Treatment includes immunosuppressive drugs.
- Schwalbe's line is the anatomical line found on the interior surface of the eye's cornea, and delineates the outer limit of the corneal endothelium layer. Specifically, it represents the termination of Descemet's membrane.
- Iron deposition line at edge of pterygium on corneal epithelium is known as Stocker's line.
- Cornea contains three major glycosaminoglycans fractions namely: Keratan sulfate (50%), chondroitin sulfate (25%) and chondroitin (25%). GAGs play an important role in the maintenance of corneal hydration level and transparency.
- Mucin layer deficiency over cornea causes Keratoconjunctivitis sicca.
- Meibomianitis is inflammation of the meibomian glands. Treatment includes cleansing the lid edges, application of moist heat and local antibiotics.
- Most common site of basal cell carcinoma of the eye is Eyelid
- Ankyloblepharon is adhesion of margins of two eyelids. Symblepharon is adhesion of the lids to eyeball. Lagophthalmos is incomplete closure of the palpebral aperture when eyes are shut. Tylosis is thickening of lid margin.
- Vitreous is present in posterior segment of eye. It consists largely of water (99%), a network of collagen fibrils, large molecules of hyaluronic acid, peripheral cells (hyalocytes), and mucopolysaccharides, forming a gel-like material. Vitreous is attached anteriorly to the lens (Hyaloid capsular ligament of Weiger) and ciliary epithelium in the ora serrata. Posteriorly vitreous is attached to the edge of the optic disc and macula lutea (region) forming ring shaped structure around them.
- Causes of floaters:
  - Posterior vitreous detachment (PVD)
  - Retinal detachment
  - High myopia
  - Vitreous hemorrhage
  - Uveitis

CHAPTER 10 ENT

EAR

EAR EMBRYOLOGY

Pars superior: Semicircular canals and utricle takes place earlier than pars inferior (saccule and cochlea).

1. Saccule of inner ear develops from: *(NEET 2020)*

a. Pars inferior
b. Pars superior
c. Saccus posterior
d. Saccus superior

Ans. is 'a' Pars inferior

ANATOMY OF MIDDLE EAR

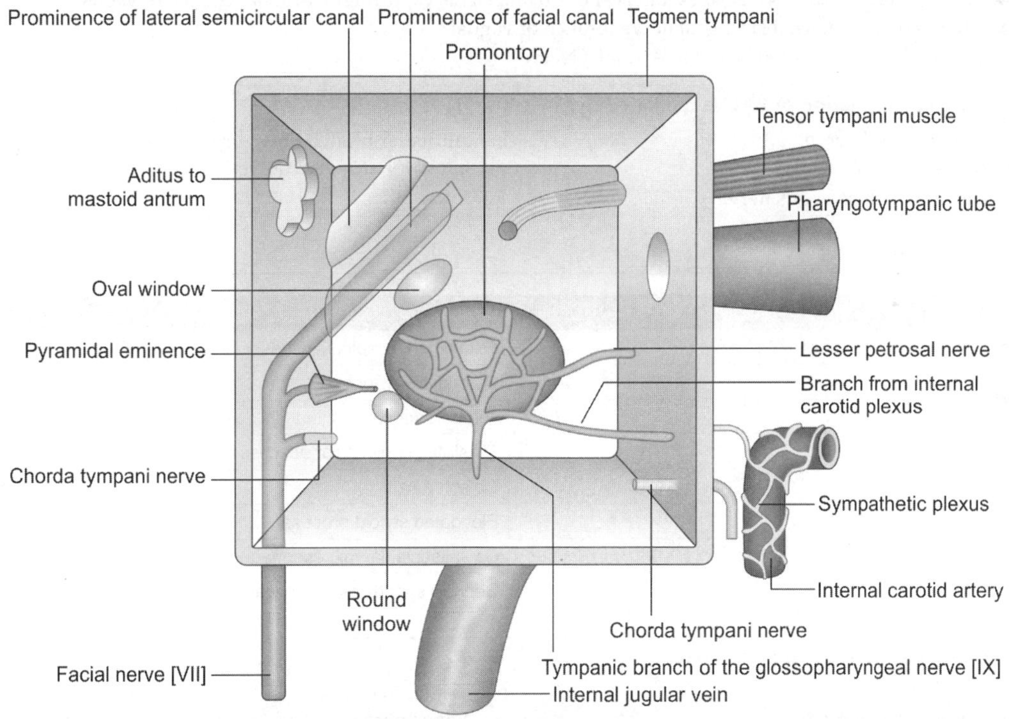

Tympanic cavity muscles				
Muscle	***Origin***	***Insertion***	***Nerve supply***	***Function***
Tensor tympani	Cartilaginous pharyngo-tympanic tube, greater wing of sphenoid, its own bony canal	Upper part of handle of malleus	Mandibular nerve (V3)	Tenses tympanic membrane to reduce the force of vibrations in response to loud noise
Stapedius	Pyramidal eminence	Neck of stapes	Branch of facial nerve	Contraction, usually in response to loud noises, pulls the stapes posteriorly and prevents excessive oscillation

2. Tensor tympani is attached at:

a. Malleus
b. Incus
c. Stapes
d. Tympanic membrane

Ans. is 'a' Malleus

Nerve supply of external ear	
Pinna	
Greater auricular nerve (C2,C3)	Medial surface; posterior part of lateral surface
Lesser occipital nerve (C2)	Upper part of medial surface
Auriculotemporal nerve (V3)	Tragus, crus of helix
Auricular branch of Vagus (X) and Facial (VII)	Concha
External auditory canal	
Auriculotemporal nerve (V3)	Anterior wall and roof
Auricular branch of vagus (X) and Facial (VII)	Posterior wall and floor
Tympanic membrane	
Auriculotemporal nerve (V3)	Anterior half of lateral surface
Auricular branch of Vagus (X) (Arnold's nerve)	Posterior half of lateral surface
Tympanic branch of CN IX (Jacobson's nerve)	Medial surface

Nerve supply of external acoustic meatus

- Anterior wall and roof by auriculotemporal nerve
- Posterior wall and floor by auricular branch of vagus nerve (Arnold N)
- Posterior wall of auditory canal also receives innervations by facial nerve through auricular branch of vagus
  - Cough reflex is due to internal laryngeal nerve [branch of vagus]
  - Cough's reflex during syringing is due to Arnold's Nerve

3. Cough reflex on stimulation of EAC is mediated by: *(NEET 2020)*

a. Auriculotemporal nerve
b. Auricular branch of vagus nerve
c. Sensory division of facial nerve
d. Glossopharyngeal nerve

Ans. is 'b' Auricular branch of vagus nerve

REFERRED OTALGIA

	Causes
Via CN V	Dental caries, apical abscess
	Ca oral cavity/tongue
	Temporomandibular joint dislocation, arthritis
Via CN IX	Tonsillitis, peritonsillar abscess
	Ca soft palate
	Elongated styloid process
Via CN X	Ca vallecula, larynx, esophagus
Via C2 and C3	Cervical spondylosis, cervical trauma

4. Pain referred to ear in tonsillitis is due to: *(NEET 2018)*

a. Facial nerve
b. Trigeminal nerve
c. Glossopharyngeal nerve
d. Vagus nerve

Ans. is 'c' Glossopharyngeal nerve

5. Pinna is not supplied by:

a. Facial nerve
b. Vagus nerve
c. Greater occipital nerve
d. Auriculotemporal nerve

Ans. is 'c' Greater occipital nerve

BRAINSTEM EVOKED RESPONSE AUDIOMETRY (BERA) OR AUDITORY BRAINSTEM RESPONSE (ABR)

- It is a non-invasive procedure which objectively helps to find the integrity of central auditory pathway through the VIII nerve, Pons and mid brain.
- It is the most reliable method of differentiating between cochlear and retrocochlear hearing losses. It is an objective test and can be done under sedation.
- *Waves of BERA*: The first, third and fifth waves are most stable and are used in measurements.

• Wave I	Distal part of eighth nerve
• Wave II	Proximal part of eighth cranial nerve
• Wave III	Cochlear nucleus
• Wave IV	Superior olivary complex
• Wave V	Lateral leminiscus
• Wave VI and VII	Inferior colliculus

❖ **Uses of BERA**

- As a screening procedure for infants.
- For identification of the site of lesion in retrocochlear pathologies and brainstem pathology, e.g. acoustic neuroma, multiple sclerosis, or pontine tumor.
- To monitor CN VIII intraoperatively in surgery of acoustic neuromas
- To determine the threshold of hearing in infants and in malingerers

6. Earliest age for doing BERA is:

a. In utero-before birth
b. At birth
c. 3 months
d. 6 months

Ans. is 'b' At birth

TUNING FORK TESTS

Rinne test: In this test air conduction of the ear is compared with its bone conduction. Rinne test is called positive when AC is longer or louder than BC. It is seen in normal persons or those having sensorineural deafness. A negative Rinne (BC > AC) is seen in conductive deafness. Remember that a negative Rinne for 256, 512 and 1024 Hz indicates a minimum air-bone gap of 15, 30, 45 dB, respectively.

Weber test: In this test, a vibrating tuning fork is placed in the middle of the forehead or the vertex and the patient is asked in which ear the sound is heard. Normally, it is heard equally in both ears. It is lateralized to the worse ear in conductive deafness and to the better ear in sensorineural deafness.

Schwabach test: It is done with the opposite ear masked, placing the stems of vibrating forks on the mastoid process first of the patient and then of the examiner. If heard longer by the patient it indicates that he or she has conductive hearing loss and if heard longer by the examiner it indicates that the patient has sensorineural hearing loss.

7. Negative Rinne test with 256 Hz tuning fork indicates a minimum air bone gap of:

a. 15–20 dB
b. 25–30 dB
c. 35–40 dB
d. 45–50 dB

Ans. is 'a' 15–20 dB

TYMPANOMETRY

Based on the principle that—stiffer tympanic membrane will reflect more sound energy than a compliant one.

Types of Tympanograms	
Type A	Normal tympanogram
Type As	Compliance is lower at or near ambient air pressure. Seen in fixation of ossicles; e.g otosclerosis or malleus fixation
Type A_D	High compliance at or near ambient pressure. Seen in ossicular discontinuity or thin and lax tympanic membrane
Type B	A flar or dome-shaped graph. No change in compliance with pressure changes. Seen in middle ear fluid or thick tympanic membrane
Type C	Maximum compliance occurs with negative pressure in excess of 100 mm H_2O. Seen in retracted tympanic membrane

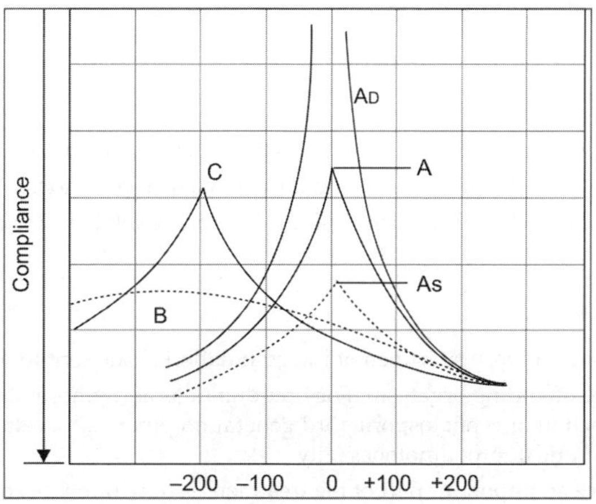

8. Serous Otitis media shows which type of tympanogram?

a. Type A
b. Type B
c. Type C
d. Type D

Ans. is 'b' Type B

FITZGERALD–HALLPIKE TEST (BITHERMAL CALORIC TEST)

The bithermal caloric test has proven to be highly sensitive to unilateral lesion of the peripheral vestibular system.

In this test, patient lies supine with head tilted 30° forward so that horizontal canal is vertical. Ears are irrigated for 40 s alternately with water at 30°C and at 44°C (i.e. 7° below and above normal body temperature) and eyes observed for appearance of nystagmus till its end point. Time taken from the start of irrigation to the end point of nystagmus is recorded and charted on a calorigram. If no nystagmus is elicited from any ear, test is repeated with water at 20°C for 4 min before labelling the labyrinth dead. A gap of 5 min should be allowed between two ears. Cold water induces nystagmus to opposite side and warm water to the same side (remember mnemonic COWS: cold–opposite, warm–same). Depending on response to the caloric test, we can find canal paresis or dead labyrinth, directional preponderance, i.e. nystagmus is more in one particular direction than in the other, or both canal paresis and directional preponderance.

9. Hallpike test is done for which of the following?

a. Eustachian tube
b. Semicircular canal
c. Cochlea
d. Endolymphatic duct

Ans. is 'b' Semicircular canal

MALIGNANT OTITIS EXTERNA

- Also called necrotizing external otitis, is a misnomer as it is not a neoplastic condition, rather it is an infectious condition.
- Inflammation and damage of the bones and cartilage at the base of skull in temporal bone as a result of spread of infection from outer ear.
- Often caused by difficult to treat bacteria such as Pseudomonas aeruginosa.

Predisposing Factors

- Elderly diabetics (most common predisposing factor)
- Immunodeficiency or Chemotherapy.

Clinical Features

- Severe pain, fever, itching in ear canal
- Granulation tissue in the external auditory canal, at the junction of bony and cartilaginous part.
- Drainage from the ear—yellow, yellow-green, foul smelling, persistent.

Complications

- Cranial nerve palsies: most commonly facial nerve is involved. Other cranial nerves can also be involved (glossopharyngeal, vagus, spinal accessory, hypoglossal, abducens, trigeminal)
- Jugular venous thrombosis/Cavernous sinus thrombosis
- Meningitis.

Imaging

- *CT scan:* defines the anatomical extent of the disease and remains the initial investigation of choice
- *MRI:* Excellent at delineating extent of soft tissue disease and intracranial complications.
- *Radioisotope scans (technetium 99/gallium 67):* A base line Gallium-67 scan is obtained for comparison followed by serial scans to monitor treatment response.

Treatment

- The external ear canal is cleansed and a biopsy specimen of the granulation tissue sent for culture.
- IV antibiotics is directed against the offending organism. For Pseudomonas aeruginosa, the most common pathogen, the regimen involves an anti-pseudomonal penicillin or cephalosporin (3rd generation piperacillin ceftazidime) with an aminoglycoside. Early cases can be managed with oral and otic fluoroquinolones only.
- Extensive surgical debridement once an important part of the treatment is now rarely needed

10. All of the following are true about malignant otitis externa *except*:

a. Occurs in patients with diabetes mellitus
b. Monitoring is done by gallium scan
c. Most common malignant tumor of the external ear
d. Surgical debridement is rarely needed

Ans. is 'c' Most common malignant tumor of the external ear

11. A 55-year-old uncontrolled diabetic patient presents with fever and severe pain in the right ear with active pus discharge since three days. On examination granulation tissue is evident in the external auditory canal. What is the most probable diagnosis?

a. Serous otitis media
b. Malignant otitis externa
c. Carcinoma of external auditory canal
d. Otitis media

Ans. is 'b' Malignant otitis externa

KERATOSIS OBTURANS

- Collection of pearly white mass of desquamated epithelial cells in deep meatus
- Causes absorption of bone leading to widening of meatus so much so that facial nerve may be exposed
- Common between 5 and 20 years of age
- May present with pain, hearing loss, tinnitus
- *Treatment:* Keratotic mass is removed by syringing or instrumentation. Keratolytic agents like 2% salicylic acid in alcohol can be used to prevent recurrence.

12. Identify the condition in the given image. *(NEET 2019)*

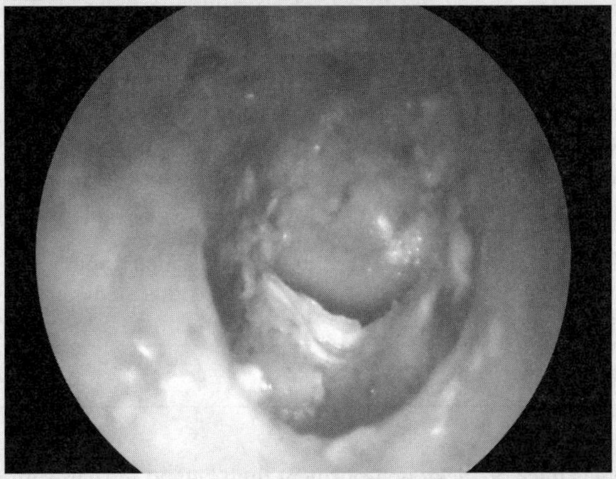

a. Acquired cholesteatoma
b. Congenital cholesteatoma
c. Ruptured tympanic membrane
d. Keratosis obturans

Ans. is 'd' keratosis obturans

Complications of Suppurative Otitis Media	
Intratemporal	***Intracranial***
Mastoiditis	Extradural abscess
Petrositis	Subdural abscess
Facial paralysis	Meningitis
Labyrinthitis	Brain abscess
	Lateral sinus thrombophlebitis
	Otitic hydrocephalus

- Most common complication of acute otitis media—Acute mastoiditis.
- Most common intracranial complication of acute otitis media—Meningitis

Gradenigo's syndrome: Classical presentation of Petrositis and consists of a triad of:

- External rectus palsy (VIth nerve/abducent nerve palsy) causing diplopia.
- Deep seated orbital or retroorbital pain (Vth nerve involvement).
- Persistent ear discharge due to ipsilateral acute or chronic otitis media

Abscesses in Relation to Mastoiditis

- *Postauricular abscess*: Commonest subperiosteal abscess associated with acute mastoiditis. It occurs lateral to the cortex of mastoid in MacEwen's triangle.
- *Bezold abscess*: Pus passes through mastoid tip and presents as upper neck swelling.
- *Zygomatic abscess*: Infection of zygomatic air cells.
- *Meatal (Luc's) abscess*: Pus breaks through the bony wall between the antrum and external osseous meatus
- *Citelli's abscess*: Abscess is formed behind the mastoid more towards occipital bone.
- Parapharyngeal and retropharyngeal abscess

Clinical Features of Lateral/Sigmoid Sinus Thrombophlebitis

- Hectic Picket-Fence type of fever with rigors
- Headache, Progressive anemia and emaciation.
- *Griesinger's sign*: Oedema over the posterior part of mastoid due to thrombosis of mastoid emissary veins.
- Papilloedema
- *Tobey-Ayer test*: Compression of vein on the thrombosed side produces no effect while compression of vein on healthy side produces rapid rise in CSF pressure which will be equal to bilateral compression of jugular veins.
- *Crowe-Beck test*: Pressure on jugular vein of healthy side produces engorgement of retinal veins. Pressure on affected side does not produce such change.

13. Gradenigo syndrome is characterized by all the following *except*:

a. Diplopia
b. Retro-orbital pain
c. Persistent ear discharge
d. Preauricular sinus

Ans. is 'd' Preauricular sinus

14. Citelli's abscess is:

a. Drained through external meatus
b. Formed over occipital bone
c. Presents as upper neck swelling
d. Retro-orbital abscess

Ans. is 'b' Formed over occipital bone

15. Tobey-Ayer test is done in:

a. Sigmoid sinus thrombosis
b. Sagittal sinus thrombosis
c. Uncal herniation
d. Serous otitis media

Ans. is 'a' Sigmoid sinus thrombosis

SEROUS OTITIS MEDIA (SOM)

- Secretory otitis media or 'Glue ear"
- Insidious condition in which there is thick or sticky non-purulent fluid behind the eardrum in the middle ear, but there is no ear infection. Fluid in the middle ear is sterile.
- SOM occurs most commonly in school going children and SOM is the commonest cause of childhood hearing loss.

Etiopathogenesis

- Eustachian Tube Dysfunction coupled with recurrent upper respiratory tract infection is the most important factor.
- Eustachian tube dysfunction may result from—respiratory tract infection, adenoid hypertrophy, rhinitis, tonsillitis, sinusitis, tumor of nasopharynx, unresolved otitis media or inadequate antibiotic therapy in ASOM.

Clinical Features

- Unlike children with ASOM, children with SOM do not appear sick.
- The only presenting symptom may be hearing loss with fullness in ear.
- Otoscopic findings of SOM:
  - Air bubbles on the surface of ear drum.
  - Fluid behind the eardrum.
  - Dullness of the eardrum when a light is used, with loss of light reflex.
  - Retracted eardrum with decreased mobility.

Treatment

- *Watchful waiting*: Active monitoring of the condition and hearing for about three months
- *Surgery*: Recommended in case of non-resolution of SOM.

- Myringotomy and aspiration of fluid: An incision is made in tympanic membrane and fluid as with suction.
- Grommet (ventilation tube): In case of recurrence following myringotomy, a grommet is inserted to provide continued aeration of middle ear. This is the most common surgical intervention for SOM. Most preferred site of grommet insertion is antero-inferior.
- Surgical treatment of causative factor: Adenoidectomy, tonsillectomy etc.

16. An 8-year-old child has history of adenoidectomy done one year back. He now complains of effusion in the middle ear. Which of the following is the most probable diagnosis?

a. Grisel syndrome
b. Velopharyngeal insufficiency
c. Recurrence
d. Rhinolalia clausa

Ans. is 'c' Recurrence

Explanation: Recurrence is due to regrowth of adenoid tissue left behind. It will lead to persistent symptoms of middle ear effusion.

17. All of the following are true about serous otitis media *except*:

a. Sterile effusion of the middle ear due to respiratory tract infection
b. Most common cause of childhood hearing loss
c. Loss of light reflex
d. Marked congestion of tympanic membrane

Ans. is 'd' Marked congestion of tympanic membrane

TUBERCULAR OTITIS MEDIA

Tuberculosis of the middle ear is most commonly seen in patients with previous history of tuberculosis in the lungs.

The most common features of tuberculous otitis media include **minimal discharge with pale granulation tissue in the middle ear, multiple perforations in tympanic membrane**, sometimes associated with facial nerve palsy, and white necrosis slough of middle ear mucosa. The patient develops rapid deterioration of hearing with more sensorineural component. They are more prone for developing profound hearing loss, if not treated timely. Because of variability in clinical presentations and lack of histopathological classical features most of the time, it is difficult to establish diagnosis. However, in case of strong clinical suspicion, even though first biopsy comes negative, one should follow-up the progression and response to routine antibiotic line of management. If recovery is not satisfactory, rapid deterioration of hearing and extensive involvement of the middle ear and mastoid cavity clinically and radiologically, it is always better to explore as emergency and resend the biopsy from antrum and middle ear and complete clearance of granulations should be done to prevent further hearing loss. **Antituberculosis treatment improves prognosis for most of the patients**. Surgical treatment should always be added to medical therapy in cases of complications and in cases of rapid deterioration of hearing. For complete cure, medical therapy should be given at least for 9 months according to INDEX-TB guidelines provided by government of India for extrapulmonary tuberculosis

18. All of the following are true for tubercular otitis media *except*: *(NEET 2020)*

a. Multiple TM perforations
b. Extremely painful condition
c. ATT is the treatment of choice
d. Pale granulation tissue is seen

Ans. is 'b' Extremely painful condition

FACIAL NERVE BRANCHES

1. *From intratemporal part*
   - Greater superficial petrosal nerve: It is the first branch and arises from geniculate ganglion (i.e., first genu). It joins the deep petrosal nerve to form Vidian nerve (nerve to pterygoid canal) and carries secretomotor fibres to the lacrimal gland, nasal gland, and minor salivary glands on palate and pharynx.
   - Nerve to stapedius: Arises at the level of second genu. It supplies the stapedius muscle and its damage can cause hyperacusis.
   - Chorda tympani: Arises from the middle of vertical segment. It carries secretomotor fibres to submandibular and sublingual glands and brings taste from anterior two-thirds of tongue.
   - Communicating branch: Joins the auricular branch of vagus.
2. *At its exit from stylomastoid foramen*
   - Posterior auricular nerve: It supplies muscles of pinna, occipital belly of occipitofrontalis.
   - Digastric nerve: Supplies posterior belly of digastric.
   - Stylohyoid nerve: Supplies the stylohyoid muscles.
3. *Terminal branches within Parotid gland*
   - Temporal branch
   - Zygomatic branch
   - Buccal branch
   - Mandibular branch
   - Cervical branch
   - These branched supply facial muscles

Symptoms of Facial Palsy

- *Loss of lacrimation*: Due to greater superficial petrosal nerve.
- *Loss of stapedial reflex*: Due to nerve to stapedius.
- *Lack of salivation*: Due to chorda tympani.
- *Loss of taste sensation from Anterior 2/3 of tongue*: Due to chorda tympani.
- *Paralysis of muscle of facial expression*: Due to terminal (peripheral) branches

Topodiagnosis of Facial Nerve Injury

- *Schirmer test*: It compares lacrimation of the two sides. A strip of filter paper is hooked in the lower fornix of each eye and the amount of wetting of strip measured. Decreased lacrimation indicates lesion proximal to the geniculate ganglion as the secretomotor fibres to lacrimal gland leave at the geniculate ganglion via greater superficial petrosal nerve.
- *Stapedial reflex*: Stapedial reflex is lost in lesions above the nerve to stapedius. It is tested by tympanometry.
- *Taste test*: It can be measured by a drop of salt or sugar solution placed on one side of the protruded tongue, or by electrogustometry. Impairment of taste indicates lesion above the chorda tympani.
- *Submandibular salivary flow test*: It also measures function of chorda tympani. Polythene tubes are passed into both Wharton ducts and drops of saliva counted during one minute period. Decreased salivation shows injury above the chorda.

19. Lesion at which point along the course of facial nerve would lead to loss of lacrimation and taste?

a. Distal to origin of chorda tympani
b. Between second genu and midportion of vertical segment
c. Distal to geniculate ganglion and proximal to second genu
d. Proximal to geniculate ganglion

Ans. is 'd' Proximal to geniculate ganglion

20. Topodiagnosis of facial nerve injury has all the tests *except*:

a. Schirmer test
b. Bing test
c. Taste test
d. Salivary flow test

Ans. is 'b' Bing test

FACIAL NERVE

Surgical landmarks of facial nerve for parotid Sx

1. *Cartilaginous pointer*: The nerve lies 1 cm deep and slightly anterior and inferior to the pointer. Cartilaginous pointer is a sharp triangular piece of cartilage of the pinna (tragus) and "points" to the nerve.
2. *Tympanomastoid suture*: Nerve lies 6–8 mm deep to this suture.
3. *Styloid process*: The nerve crosses lateral to styloid process.
4. *Posterior belly of digastric*: If posterior belly of digastric muscle is traced backwards along its upper border to its attachment to the digastric groove, nerve is found to lie between it and the styloid process.

21. Which of the following is not a surgical landmark for facial nerve during parotid surgery? *(NEET 2020)*

a. Tragus
b. Inferior belly of omohyoid
c. Posterior belly of digastrics
d. Retrograde dissection from terminal branches

Ans. is 'b' Inferior belly of omohyoid

MENIERE'S DISEASE

- Meniere's disease is also known as endolymphatic hydrops
- Disorder of the inner ear where the endolymphatic system is distended due to increased volume of endolymph

Cardinal Triad of symptoms: Episodic vertigo, Fluctuating hearing loss, Tinnitus

Tullio phenomenon: Vertigo is induced by loud noise due to distended saccule lying against the stapes footplate. Also seen when there are three functioning windows in the ear, e.g. fenestration of horizontal canal in the presence of mobile stapes.

Diplacusis: Condition in which the pitch of single tone is heard as two different pitches by the two ears. This causes distortion of sound.

- Patients with Meniere's disease cannot tolerate loud sounds due to recruitment phenomenon, they are thus poor candidates for hearing aids.

Investigations

- *Pure tone audiometry:* In early stages, lower frequencies are affected and the curve is of rising type. When higher frequencies are involved curve becomes flat or falling type.
- *Speech audiometry*: Discrimination score is usually 55–85% between the attacks but discrimination ability is much impaired during and immediately following an attack.
- *Special audiometry tests*: They indicate cochlear nature of disease and thus help to differentiate from retrocochlear lesions e.g. acoustic neuroma.
- *Electrocochleography*: It measures electrical potentials arising in the cochlea and CN VIII in response to auditory stimuli within fir milliseconds. The response is in the form of three phenomena: cochlear microphonics, summating potentials and the act potential of VIIIth nerve.
    - Electrocochleography is diagnostic of Meniere's disease. Ratio of Summating Potential (SP) to Action Potential (AP) is >30% in Meniere's disease.

Management

Medical: Medical management is the mainstay of treatment. Vestibular sedatives to relieve vertigo (Promethazine, Diazepam), Vasodilators: Carbogen, histamine drip, nicotinic acid (in chronic phase)

- **Intratympanic Gentamicin therapy:** Gentamicin is vestibulotoxic.

Surgical: Surgical treatment when medical management fails. Decompression of endolymphatic sac, shunt between endolymphatic sac and subarachnoid space, Sacculotomy (Fick's operation), Labyrinthectomy–done for refractory cases.

Others: Intermittent low pressure pulse therapy (Meniett device) using a myringotomy and a ventilation tube.

22. Triad of Meniere's disease includes all *except*:

a. Vertigo b. Hearing loss
c. Tinnitus d. Migraine

Ans. is 'd' Migraine

23. Electrocochleography helps in the diagnosis of:

a. ASOM b. Otosclerosis
c. Ossicular chain disruption d. Meniere's disease

Ans. is 'd' Meniere's disease

OTOSCLEROSIS

It is a primary disease of the bony labyrinth. In this, one or more foci of irregularly laid spongy bone replace part of normally dense enchondral layer of bony otic capsule.

Symptoms

1. *Hearing loss*: This is the presenting symptom and usually starts in twenties. It is painless and progressive with insidious onset. Often it is bilateral conductive type.
2. *Paracusis Willisii*: An otosclerotic patient hears better in noisy than in quiet surroundings. This is because a normal person will raise his voice in noisy surroundings.
3. *Tinnitus*: It is more commonly seen in cochlear otosclerosis and in active lesions.

Signs

1. A reddish hue may be seen on the promontory through the tympanic membrane (Schwartz sign). This is indicative of active focus with increased vascularity.
2. Tuning fork tests show negative Rinne (i.e. BC > AC) first for 256 Hz and then 512 Hz and still later, when stapes fixation is complete, for 1026 Hz. Weber test will be lateralized to the ear with greater conductive loss. Absolute bone conduction may be normal. It is decreased in cochlear otosclerosis with sensorineural loss.
3. *Gelle's test*: It is performed by placing a vibrating fork on the mastoid while changes in air pressure in the ear canal are brought about by Siegle's speculum. It is negative when ossicular chain is fixed or disconnected as in otosclerosis. It has been superseded by tympanometry.
   Pure tone audiometry shows loss of air conduction, more for lower frequencies.

Bone conduction is normal. In some cases, there is a dip in bone conduction curve. It is different at different frequencies but maximum at 2000 Hz and is called Carhart's notch (5 dB at 500 Hz, 10 dB at 1000 Hz, 15 dB at 2000 Hz and 5 dB at 4000 Hz). Carhart's notch disappears after successful stapedectomy.

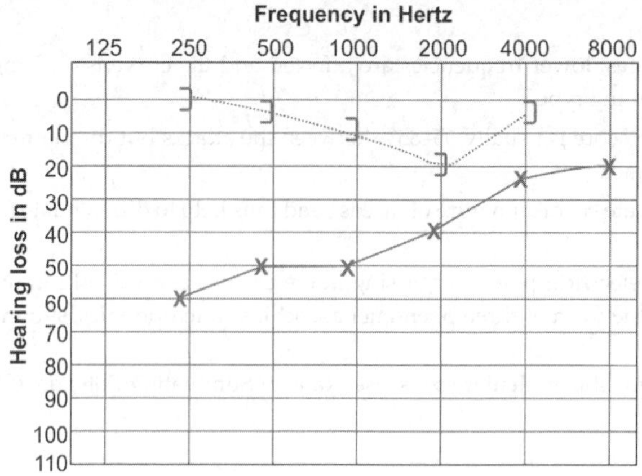

Cahart's notch

Treatment of Otosclerosis

Medical: Sodium fluoride has been tried to hasten the maturity of active focus and arrest further cochlear loss, but controversies exist and this treatment is not recommended generally.

Surgical: Stapedectomy/stapedotomy with a placement of prosthesis is the treatment of choice.

24. Paracusis willisii is seen in:

a. Tympanosclerosis b. Endolymphatic hydrops
c. Presbycusis d. Otosclerosis

Ans. is 'd' Otosclerosis

25. Pink reflex through intact tympanic membrane in active otosclerosis is known as:

a. Schwabach's sign b. Schwartz sign
c. Lyre's sign d. Chvostek's sign

Ans. is 'b' Schwartz sign

ACOUSTIC NEUROMA/VESTIBULAR SCHWANNOMA

- The commonest nerve of origin is the superior vestibular, followed by the inferior vestibular and rarely cochlear
- As it expands, it causes widening and erosion of the internal auditory canal and then appears in the cerebellopontine angle.

Clinical Features

- The commonest presenting symptoms are unilateral deafness or tinnitus. Hearing loss is retrocochlear sensorineural type. There is marked difficulty understanding speech, out of proportion to the pure tone hearing loss, a characteristic feature of acoustic neuroma.
- *Vth cranial nerve*: It is the earliest nerve to be involved after extension beyond the IAC. There is reduced corneal sensitivity and loss corneal reflex which is the earliest sign of acoustic neuroma.
- *VIIth nerve*: Sensory fibres of facial nerve are involved. There is hypoesthesia of posterior meatal wall (Hitzelberger's sign), loss of taste, and loss of lacrimation on Schirmer's test. Motor fibres are more resistant
- *IXth and Xth nerves*: Dysphagia and hoarseness due to palatal, pharyngeal and laryngeal paralysis.

Investigations

- Audiological tests show retrocochlear type of SNHL: SNHL is more marked in high frequencies on pure tone audiometry, Recruitment absent, Tone decay is significant, SISI score 0-20%. Rollover phenomenon is present, i.e. reduction in discrimination score when loudness is increased beyond a particular limit.
- Acoustic reflex show stapedial reflex decay.
- *Imaging*: Gadolinium enhanced MRI is the most sensitive and specific test to demonstrate acoustic neuroma.

26. Earliest reflex lost in acoustic neuroma is:

a. Pharyngeal reflex b. Laryngeal reflex
c. Stapedial reflex d. Corneal reflex

Ans. is 'd' Corneal reflex

27. All of the following are true about vestibular schwannomas *except*:

a. Commonly arise from superior vestibular nerve b. Leads to cochlear hearing loss
c. CT scan is the most sensitive investigation d. Hitzelberger's sign is seen due to involvement of VII nerve

Ans. is 'c' CT scan is the most sensitive investigation

ENT

EPLEY'S MANEUVER

- ❖ Used for treating Benign Paroxysmal Positional Vertigo (BPPV)
- ❖ *Principle*: The maneuver repositions otoconial debris from posterior semicircular canal back into utricle
- ❖ The doctor stands behind the patient and the assistant on the side
- ❖ The manoeuvre consists of five positions

Position 1. With the head turned 45°, the patient is made to lie down in head-hanging position (Dix-Hallpike manoeuvre). It will cause vertigo and nystagmus. Wait till vertigo and nystagmus subside.

Position 2. Head is now turned so that affected ear is facing up at a 90° rotation.

Position 3. The whole body and head are now rotated away from the affected ear to a lateral recumbent position in a 90°-rotation face-down position.

Position 4. Patient is now brought to a sitting position with head still turned to the unaffected side by 45°.

Position 5. The head is now turned forward and chin brought down 20°.

- ❖ Eighty per cent of the patients will be cured by a single manoeuvre. If the patient remains symptomatic, the manoeuvre can be repeated.

28. Name the manoeuvre shown in image. *(NEET 2019)*

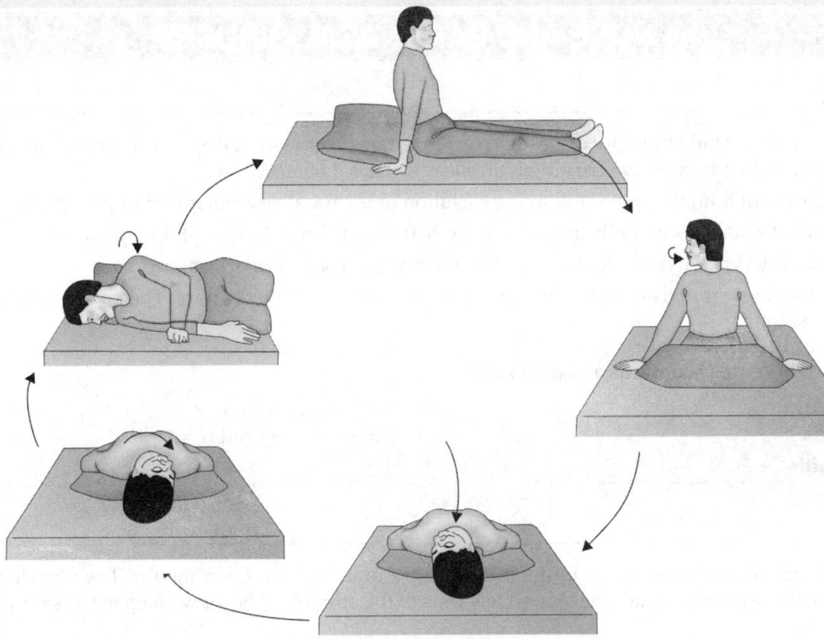

a. Epley b. Foster
c. Brandt-Daroff d. Semont

Ans. is 'a' Epley

Previously Asked Facts

- ❖ Angle made by tympani membrane with floor of the meatus is 55°
- ❖ Korner's septum is persistence of petrosquamous suture in the form of a bony plate. It is surgically important as it may cause difficulty in locating the antrum and the deeper cells and thus lead to incomplete removal of disease at mastoidectomy.
- ❖ The handle of malleus causes tenting which causes the reflection of light from the anteroinferior quadrant of tympanic membrane leading to cone of light.
- ❖ *Peripheral receptors in membranous labyrinth*: Macula (Otolith organs) in utricle and saccule; Cristae in semicircular canal.
- ❖ Auditory brainstem implant (ABI) is designed to stimulate the cochlear nuclear complex in the brainstem directly by placing the stimulator in the lateral recess of the fourth ventricle. Such an implant is needed when CN VIII has been severed in surgery of vestibular schwannoma.
- ❖ Deafness in a case of Paget's disease is due to VIII nerve compression
- ❖ *Tests for Eustachian tube patency*: Valsalva test, Politzer test, Toynbee test, Frenzel maneuver
- ❖ Cauliflower ear is seen in Perichondritis in boxers

- Ramsay Hunt syndrome is an acute lower motor neuron facial neuropathy associated with erythematous vesicular rash of the skin of the ear canal, auricle (also termed herpes zoster oticus), and/or mucous membrane of the oropharynx. It is due to Varicella Zoster Virus (VZV) infection of CN VII.
- Otitis externa is also known as Singapore ear, Swimmer's ear, Telephonist's ear.
- Pulsatile otorrhea (Lighthouse effect) is seen in Acute Suppurative Otitis Media.
- Chronic Suppurative Otitis Media (CSOM) presents with non-foul smelling mucopurulent discharge. Patient may report a paradoxical effect, i.e. hearing is better in the presence of discharge than when the ear is dry. This is due to round window shielding effect produced by discharge.
- Long process of incus is most commonly involved ossicle in attico-antral type of CSOM.
- SADE classification grades retraction of tympanic membrane.
- Mild retraction pocket is first treated with antibiotics followed by Tympanostomy and surgical excision in case of non-resolution.
- Posterior semicircular canal is most commonly involved in Benign Paroxysmal Positional Vertigo (BPPV)
- An aural polyp should never be avulsed as it may be arising from the stapes, facial nerve or horizontal canal and thus lead to facial paralysis or labyrinthitis.
- Most common malignancy of middle ear is squamous cell carcinoma.
- Most common benign tumor of the external auditory canal is Osteoma.

NOSE AND PARANASAL SINUSES

ATROPHIC RHINITIS

Atrophic Rhinitis: Atrophic chronic inflammatory disease characterized by progressive atrophy of the nasal mucosa and the underlying bone of the turbinates associated with excessive crusting which leads to nasal obstruction.

Sx- Young's operation: Closure of both the nostril following elevation of the nasal vestibular folds, opened after 6 months.

Modified Young's operation: Partial closure of the nostril leaving behind a 1–3 mm hole kept for a period of 2 years.

Allergic Rhinitis: IgE mediated Type I hypersensitive reaction of nasal mucosa to airborne allergens.

Vasomotor Rhinitis is a non-allergic rhinitis which occurs due to parasympathetic overactivity. The parasympathetic overactivity leads to congestion and vasodilatation.

29. Obliteration of nasal cavities is done as a treatment of: *(NEET 2020)*

a. Atrophic rhinitis
b. Vasomotor rhinitis
c. Allergic rhinitis
d. Acute viral rhinitis

Ans. is 'a' Atrophic rhinitis

X-RAYS FOR PNS

Occipitomental view (Water's view): X-ray taken in the nose-chin position with an open mouth. The film demonstrates mainly the maxillary sinuses, nasal cavity, septum, frontal sinuses and few cells of the ethmoid. The view taken in the standing position may show fluid level in the antrum.

Water's view with open mouth → PIERRE'S VIEW

Occipitofrontal view (Caldwell view): The patient's forehead and tip of the nose are kept in contact with the film. This view is particularly useful for fontal sinuses. A portion of the maxillary antrum and nasal cavity are also shown.

Sinuses best seen in water's view → Maxillary sinus and anterior ethmoid sinuses

Sinuses not seen in water's view → Posterior Ethmoidal > Sphenoid

Best view for frontal sinuses is CADLWELL'S VIEW/OCCIPITO FRONTAL VIEW

30. Occipitomental view with open mouth is known as: *(NEET 2020)*

a. Water's view
b. Caldwell's view
c. Pierre's view
d. Risse view

Ans. is 'c' Pierre's view

LATERAL NASAL WALL

- It has 3 bony projections called as turbinates or conchae. The inferior turbinate is a separate bone, while rest of the turbinates are a part of ethmoidal bone. Below and lateral to each turbinate is the corresponding meatus.

i. Inferior meatus
  - It is the largest meatus.
  - Nasolacrimal duct opens in the inferior meatus anteriorly. It is closed by a mucosal flap called Hasner's valve.

ii. Middle meatus
- The important structures in middle meatus are:
  - Hiatus semilunaris
  - Ethmoidal infundibulum: Frontal sinus, maxillary sinus and the anterior ethmoidal sinuses drain into it.
  - Uncinate process: It partly covers the opening of maxillary sinus.
  - Bulla ethmoidalis: Middle ethmoidal sinuses open on or above it.
  - Atrium is a shallow depression in front of the middle turbinate.
  - Agger nasi is an elevation just anterior to the attachment of middle turbinate. It represents the most anterior ethmoidal air cell and extends into lacrimal bone.

iii. Superior meatus
- Posterior ethmoidal sinuses open into it.

iv. Spheno-ethmoidal recess
- It lies above the superior turbinate and receives the opening of sphenoid sinus.
- Sometimes a fourth turbinate is also present just above superior turbinate. This fourth turbinate is known as supreme turbinate. Supreme turbinate is found in 30% of population.

31. Agger nasi is:

a. Mucosal flap covering the nasolacrimal duct
b. Opening of the sinuses
c. Depression in front of middle turbinate
d. Elevation anterior to middle turbinate

Ans. is 'd' Elevation anterior to middle turbinate

BLOOD SUPPLY OF NASAL SEPTUM

Little's Area and Kiesselbach's Plexus

- It is situated in the anterior inferior part of nasal septum, just above the vestibule. Four arteries—anterior ethmoidal, septal branch of superior labial, septal branch of sphenopalatine and the greater palatine, anastomose here to form a vascular plexus called "Kiesselbach's plexus." This area is exposed to the drying effect of inspiratory current and to finger nail trauma, and is the usual site for epistaxis in children and young adults.

Woodruff's Area

- It is situated under the posterior end of inferior turbinate.
- Sphenopalatine artery anastomoses with posterior pharyngeal artery.
- Posterior epistaxis occurs in this area.

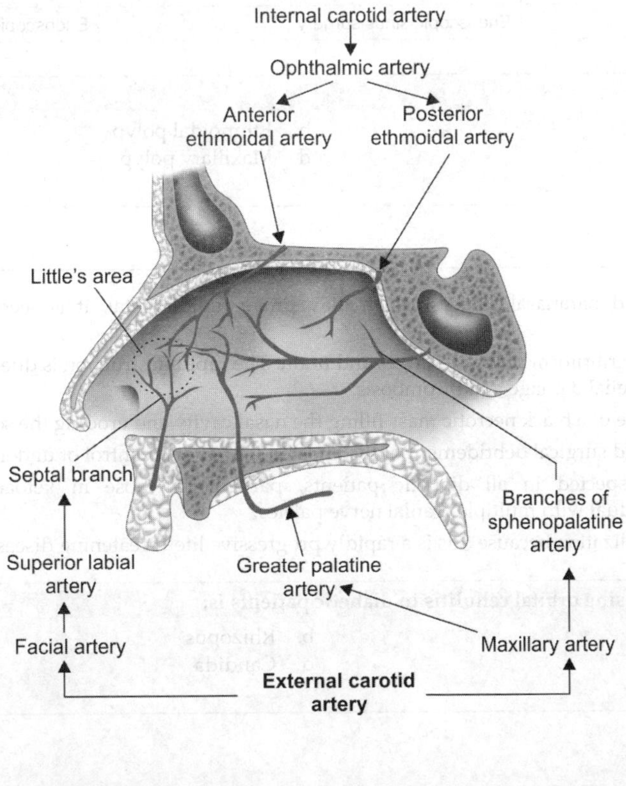

Surgical management of epistaxis: Done if bleeding persists after conservative measures and nasal packing

- Surgical treatment performed endoscopically includes ligation of the sphenopalatine or anterior ethmoidal artery.
- Angiographic embolization approximate to those of surgical treatment.
- For arterial ligation the choice of the specific vessel or vessels to be ligated depends on the location of the epistaxis.
  - External carotid artery: It is usually ligated just distal to the superior thyroid artery.
  - Internal maxillary artery: It is closer to bleeding site, therefore its ligation stops bleeding to a great extent.
  - Sphenopalatine artery at its exit from the sphenopalatine foramen.
  - Ethmoidal artery: If bleeding occurs high in the nasal vault, ligation of anterior ethmoidal artery, the posterior ethmoidal artery or both should be done.

32. Woodruff's plexus is located at:

a. Anterosuperior part of nose
b. Anteroinferior part of nose
c. Posteroinferior part of nose
d. Posterosuperior part of nose

Ans. is 'c' Posteroinferior part of nose

33. Epistaxis after ligating external carotid artery is due to which vessel?

a. Anterior ethmoidal artery
b. Superior labial artery
c. Sphenopalatine artery
d. Greater palatine artery

Ans. is 'a' Anterior ethmoidal artery

Explanation: Since external carotid artery is ligated, the bleeding comes from branches of internal carotid artery.

Differences between Antrochoanal and Ethmoidal Polyp

	Antrochoanal polyp (Killian's Polyp)	*Ethmoidal polyp*
Age	Children	Adults
Etiology	Infection	Allergy
Number	Solitary	Multiple
Laterality	Unilateral	Bilateral
Origin	Maxillary sinus near the ostium	Ethmoidal sinus, middle meatus
Growth	Grows backwards to choana	Grows anteriorly
Shape	Trilobed with antral, nasal and choanal parts. May fill nasopharynx	Small
Recurrence	Uncommon	Common
Treatment	Endoscopic sinus surgery	Endoscopic sinus surgery

34. Killian's Polyp is:

a. Antrochoanal polyp
b. Ethmoidal polyp
c. Frontal polyp
d. Maxillary polyp

Ans. is 'a' Antrochoanal polyp

MUCORMYCOSIS

- Fungal infection of nose and paranasal sinuses which may prove rapidly fatal. It is seen in uncontrolled diabetics or in immunocompromised.
- Infection can spread to orbit, cribriform plate, meninges and brain. The rapid destruction is due to affinity of the fungus to invade the arteries and cause endothelial damage and thrombosis.
- Typical finding is the presence of a black necrotic mass filling the nasal cavity and eroding the septum and hard palate.
- *Treatment*: Amphotericin B and surgical debridement of the affected tissues and control of underlying predisposing cause.
- Mucormycosis must be suspected in all diabetic patients, particularly those in ketoacidosis, and any debilitated or immunocompromised individual with multiple cranial nerve palsies.
- It requires immediate hospitalization because this is a rapidly progressive life-threatening disease.

35. Most common fungus causing orbital cellulitis in diabetic patients is:

a. Mucor
b. Rhizopus
c. Aspergillus
d. Candida

Ans. is 'a' Mucor

Previously Asked Facts

- PNS X-rays
  - Caldwell (occipito-frontal) view–Frontal sinus, superior orbital fissure
  - Towne's view–Inferior orbital fissure
  - Water's (Occipito-Mental) view–Maxillary sinus, orbital floor
  - Rheese view - Optic canal
- Shape of septal cartilage of nasal septum is Quadrilateral.
- Nasal vestibule is antero-inferior part of nasal cavity.
- Most prominent point of nasal tip is Pronasale.
- Most common sinus predisposed to malignancy is Maxillary sinus.
- Maxillay sinus is the first sinus to develop; Sphenoid sinus is the last sinus to develop
- Rhinolith can cause perforation of nasal septum by pressure necrosis.
- Most common ossicle affected due to trauma is Incus.
- Transverse fractures of petrous bone has the maximum chances of facial nerve injury
- Standard therapy for nasal fractures is to perform closed reduction or open reduction between 3 and 7 days, and up to 2 weeks. This is because soft tissue swelling can produce the misleading appearance of a deformity even in absence of fracture.
- Most common benign tumor of paranasal sinuses is Osteoma.
- Workers of furniture industry (wood workers) have propensity to develop adenocarcinoma of PNS; nickel industry workers develop squamous cell carcinoma
- Pott's Puffy tumor characterized by subperiosteal abscess associated with osteomyelitis of frontal bone.

PHARYNX

DIVISIONS OF PHARYNX

	Nasopharynx	*Oropharynx*	*Laryngopharynx*
A. Situation	Behind nose	Behind oral cavity	Behind larynx
B. Extent	Base of skull (body of sphenoid of soft palate)	Soft palate to upper border of epiglottis	Upper border of epiglottis to lower border of cricoid cartilage
C. Communication	Anteriorly with nose	1. Anteriorly with oral cavity 2. Above with nasopharynx 3. Below with laryngopharynx	Inferiorly with esophagus
D. Nerve supply	Pharyngeal branches of pterygo- palatine ganglion	IX and X nerves	IX and X nerves

36. Which of the following forms the lower border of hypopharynx?

a. Lower border of hyoid cartilage
b. Lower border of thyroid cartilage
c. Lower border of cricoid cartilage
d. First esophageal sphincter

Ans. is 'c' Lower border of cricoid cartilage

ADENOIDS

- Also known as nasopharyngeal tonsils.
- Situated at the junction of the roof and posterior wall of the nasopharynx.
- Unlike palatine tonsils, adenoids have no crypts and no capsule.
- Adenoid tissue is present at birth, shows physiological enlargement up to the age of 6 years, and then tends to atrophy at puberty and almost completely disappears by the age of 20.
- Adenoid hypertrophy leads to chronic nasal obstruction and mouth breathing leading to characteristic facial appearance called adenoid facies. Nose gives a pinched-in appearance due to disuse atrophy of alae nasi.
- Contraindications of adenoidectomy include—cleft palate or submucous palate, Hemorrhagic diathesis, Acute infection of upper respiratory tract.

37. All are true about adenoid *except*:

a. It is also known as nasopharyngeal tonsil
b. Capsulated
c. Atrophies at puberty
d. Adenoid hypertrophy leads to disuse atrophy of alae nasi

Ans. is 'b' Capsulated

PARAPHARYNGEAL SPACE

- It is the space on both sides of the pharynx, i.e. lateral to the pharynx
- It is also known as pharyngomaxillary space.
- It is pyramidal in shape with base at the base of skull and apex at the hyoid bone.

Relations

- *Medial*: Buccopharyngeal fascia covering the constrictor muscles
- *Posterior*: Prevertebral fascia covering prevertebral muscles and transverse processes of cervical vertebrae
- *Lateral*: Medial pterygoid muscle, mandible and deep surface of parotid gland

Divisions of Parapharyngeal Space

- Styloid process and the muscles attached to it divide the parapharyngeal space into anterior and posterior compartments.
- Anterior compartment is related to tonsillar fossa medially and medial pterygoid muscle laterally.
- Posterior compartment is related to posterior part of lateral pharyngeal wall medially and parotid gland laterally.
- Through the posterior compartment pass the carotid artery, jugular vein, IXth, Xth, XIth', XIIth cranial nerves and sympathetic trunk.

Clinical Features of Parapharyngeal Abscess

- Develops as a complication of tonsillitis or tonsillectomy and as a result of extraction of lower third molar tooth.
- Fever and marked trismus because of spasm in medial pterygoid muscle.
- The tonsil is pushed medially.
- Torticollis (due to spasm of prevertebral muscles), marked odynophagia and signs of toxemia.
- Further extension of disease may cause involvement of IX, X, XI, XII cranial nerve and sympathetic chain.

38. All of the following are true about parapharyngeal abscess *except*:

a. Mastoid process divides the space into anterior and posterior
b. Also known as pharyngomaxillary space infection
c. Tonsil is pushed medially
d. Occurs after tooth extraction

Ans. is 'a' Mastoid process divides the space into anterior and posterior

PERITONSILLAR ABSCESS (QUINSY)

Collection of pus between the fibrous capsule of the tonsil, and the superior constrictor muscle of the pharynx. Condition is generally unilateral. Tonsil is swollen, red, hot and congested. Uvula and soft palate are pushed to opposite side. Uvula Points towards Normal side as shown in the image below.
Organism involved are *Streptococcus*, Staph *aureus*, anaerobic organism, more often mixed growth is seen.

Parapharyngeal abscess (abscess of lateral pharyngeal space, pterygomaxillary space, pharyngomaxillary space: Swelling is on lateral wall of Pharynx pushing tonsils towards midline. Patient may also have a swelling in neck, posterior to SCM muscle. Patient may also present with Trimus.

Ludwig's angina is cellulitis of submandibular space.

39. A young boy presents with dysphagia, soft husky voice and drooling of saliva. Oral examination is shown below. What is the likely diagnosis? *(NEET 2020)*

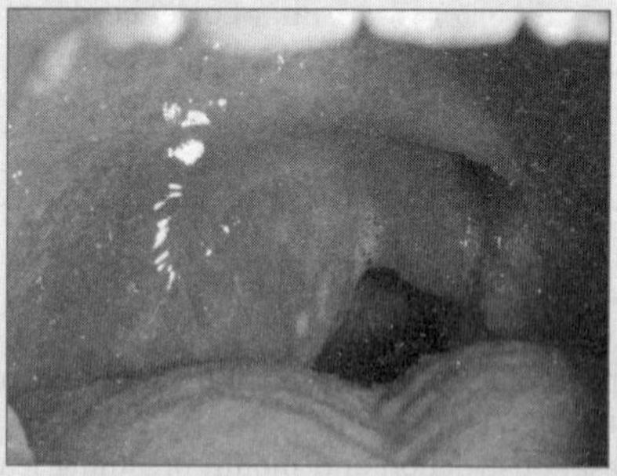

a. Ludwig angina
b. Peritonsillar abscess
c. Parapharyngeal abscess
d. Retropharyngeal abscess

Ans. is 'b' Peritonsillar abscess

BRANCHIAL ABNORMALITIES

Branchial Cyst

- Most commonly develops from vestigial remnants of 2nd branchial cleft
- Lined by squamous epithelium
- Contains thick, turbid fluid
- Cyst usually presents in the upper neck in early adulthood
- Found at the junction of upper third and middle third of Sternocleidomastoid at its anterior border
- Fluctuant swelling that may transilluminate and is often soft in its early stages

ENT

- USG helps in diagnosis
- Treatment: Complete excision

Branchial Fistula

- Represents a persistent 2nd branchial cleft
- External orifice situated in lower third of neck near the anterior border of sternocleidomastoid
- Internal orifice located on anterior aspect of posterior faucial pillar just behind the tonsil
- Requires complete excision

40. The most common site of branchial cyst is: *(NEET 2019)*

a. Posterior border of sternocleidomastoid
b. Anterior border of sternocleidomastoid
c. Digastric muscle
d. Omohyoid muscle

Ans. is 'b' Anterior border of sternocleidomastoid

Previously Asked Facts

- *Styalgia or Eagle syndrome*: Chronic throat pain along the anatomic course of thyrohyoid ligament. Elongated styloid process protrudes into the tonsillar fossa and puts pressure on the trigeminal, glossopharyngeal, vagus or facial nerves.
- Investigation of choice for diagnosing submandibular gland duct stones is Ultrasound as it permits assessment of the gland, duct system and calculus
- Lingual nerve is liable to get affected during submandibular gland excision.
- Most common tumor of oropharynx is Squamous cell carcinoma
- Trotter's triad occurs in nasopharyngeal carcinoma. It includes:
  - Conductive deafness (due to Eustachian tube blockage).
  - Temporo-parietal neuralgia (due to involvement of ipsilateral Vth cranial nerve).
  - Palatal paralysis (due to involvement of Xth cranial nerve)
- Four types of laser are generally used in ENT surgery:
  - Argon
  - KTP-532 (Potassium titanyl phosphate)
  - Nd: YAG (Neodymium-yttrium aluminium garnet)
  - CO_2: The carbon dioxide (CO_2) laser is the most common laser used for tracheal neoplasm.

LARYNX

LARYNGOTRACHEOBRONCHITIS (LTB)

The given X-ray shows Steeple Sign/ Pencil Tip Sign.

Acute laryngotracheobronchitis (CROUP): Narrowing of subglottic region is seen in chest X-ray of patients of laryngotracheobronchitis. Onset is gradual with prodrome of upper respiratory symptoms fever usually low grade, painful croupy cough (barking cough or seal barks cough) hoarseness and stridor.

Acute epiglottitis (supraglottic laryngitis): It is acute inflammatory condition of the supraglottic structures epiglottis, aryepiglottic fold and arytenoids. Child prefers sitting position with hyperextended neck (tripod sign) which relieves stridor. Drooling of saliva present as child has dysphagia, lateral soft tissue X-ray of neck shows: Swollen epiglottis (Thumb sign), absence of deep well-defined vallecula (vallecula sign).

41. The following sign is seen in: *(NEET 2020)*

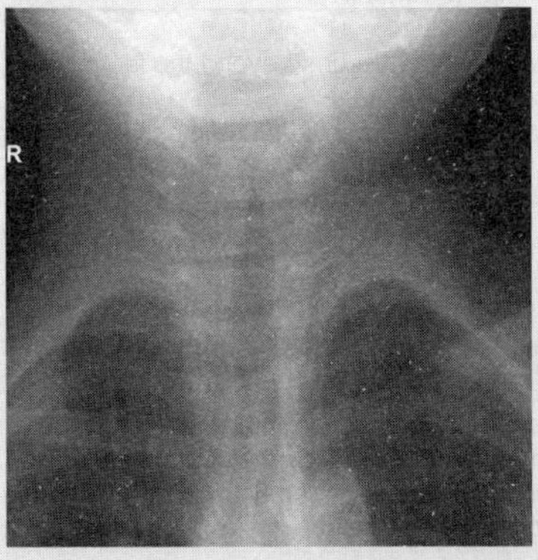

a. Acute epiglottitis
b. Adenoid hypertrophy
c. Laryngotracheobronchitis
d. Subglottic stenosis

Ans. is 'c' Laryngotracheobronchitis

ENT

RECURRENT LARYNGEAL NERVE PARALYSIS

- *Recurrent laryngeal nerve supplies*: All intrinsic muscles of the larynx except cricothyroid.
- So, paralysis of RLN causes paralysis of all intrinsic muscles including all adductors (except for cricothyroid) and all abductors. Though, there is paralysis of both adductors (except cricothyroid) and abductors, the manifestations are due to paralysis of abductors.
- Wagner and Grossman hypothesis states that cricothyroid muscle which receives innervation from superior laryngeal nerve, provide some adductor function, and keeps the cord in paramedian position.
- Most common overall cause of vocal cord paralysis is iatrogenic in origin following surgery, most commonly thyroidectomy.
- Most common cause of unilateral left vocal cord paralysis is bronchial carcinoma at the left hilum.

42. In recurrent laryngeal nerve palsy which muscle keeps vocal cord in median position?

a. Posterior cricoarytenoid
b. Cricothyroid
c. Vocalis
d. All of the above

Ans. is 'b' Cricothyroid

43. Bilateral recurrent laryngeal nerve is most commonly affected in:

a. Neck trauma
b. Bronchogenic carcinoma
c. Carcinoma esophagus
d. Post thyroid surgery

Ans. is 'd' Post thyroid surgery

CARCINOMA LARYNX

- Most common site for Ca larynx is Glottis
- Best prognosis—Ca Glottis
- Hoarseness of voice is earliest seen is Glottic cancer

TNM Classification of Cancer Larynx (American Joint Committee on Cancer, 2002)	
Supraglottis	
T_1	Tumour limited to one subsite of supraglottis with normal vocal cord mobility.
T_2	Tumour invades mucosa of more than one adjacent subsites of supraglottis or glottis or region outside the supraglottis (e.g., mucosa of base of tongue, vallecula, medial wall of pyriform sinus) without fixation of the larynx.
T_3	Tumour limited to larynx with vocal cord fixation and/or invades any of the following: postcricoid area, pre-epiglottic tissues, paraglottic space and/or minor thyroid cartilage invasion.
T_4a	Tumour invades through the thyroid cartilage and/or invades tissues beyond the larynx (e.g., trachea, soft tissues of neck including deep extrinisic muscle of tongue, strap muscles, thyroid or oesophagus).
T_4b	Tumour invades prevertebral space, encases carotid artery or invades mediastinal structures.
Glottis	
T_1	Tumour limited to vocal cord(s) (may involve anterior or posterior commissures) with normal mobility.
T_1a	Tumour limited to one vocal cord.
T_1b	Tumour involves both vocal cords.
T_2	Tumour extends to supraglottis and/or subglottis, and/or with impaired vocal cord mobility.
T_3	Tumour limited to the larynx with vocal cord fixation and/or invades paraglottic space and/or minor thyroid cartilage erosion.
T_4a	Tumour invades through thyroid cartilage and/or invades tissues beyond the larynx (e.g., trachea, soft tissues of neck including deep extrinsic muscles of the tongue, strap muscles, thyroid, or oesophagus).
T_4b	Tumour invades prevertebral space, encases carotid artery or invades mediastinal structures.
Subglottis	
T_1	Tumour limited to the subglottis.
T_2	Tumour extends to vocal cord(s) with normal or impaired mobility.
T_3	Tumour limited to larynx with vocal cord fixation.
T_4a	Tumour invades cricoid or thyroid cartilage and/or invades tissues beyond the larynx (e.g., trachea, soft tissues of neck including deep extrinsic muscle of tongue, strap muscles, thyroid or oesophagus).
T_4b	Tumour invades prevertebral space, encases carotid artery or invades mediastinal structures.
Regional lymph nodes (N)	
N_x	Regional lymph nodes cannot be assessed.
N_0	No regional lymph node metastasis.
N_1	Metastasis in a single ipsilateral lymph node, 3 cm or less in greatest dimension.
N_2	Metastasis in a single ipsilateral lymph node, more than 3 cm but not more than 6 cm in greatest dimension, or multiple ipsilateral lymph nodes, none more than 6 cm in greatest dimension, or bilateral or contralateral lymph nodes, none more than 6 cm in greatest dimension.
N_2a	Metastasis in a single ipsilateral lymph node more than 3 cm but not more than 6 cm in greatest dimension.
N_2b	Metastasis in multiple ipsilateral lymph nodes, none more than 6 cm in greatest dimension.
N_2c	Metastasis in bilateral or contralateral lymph nodes, none more than 6 cm in greatest dimension.
N_3	Metastasis in a lymph node more than 6 cm in greatest dimension.
Distant metastasis (M)	
M_x	Distant metastasis cannot be assessed.
M_0	No distant metastasis.
M_1	Distant metastasis.

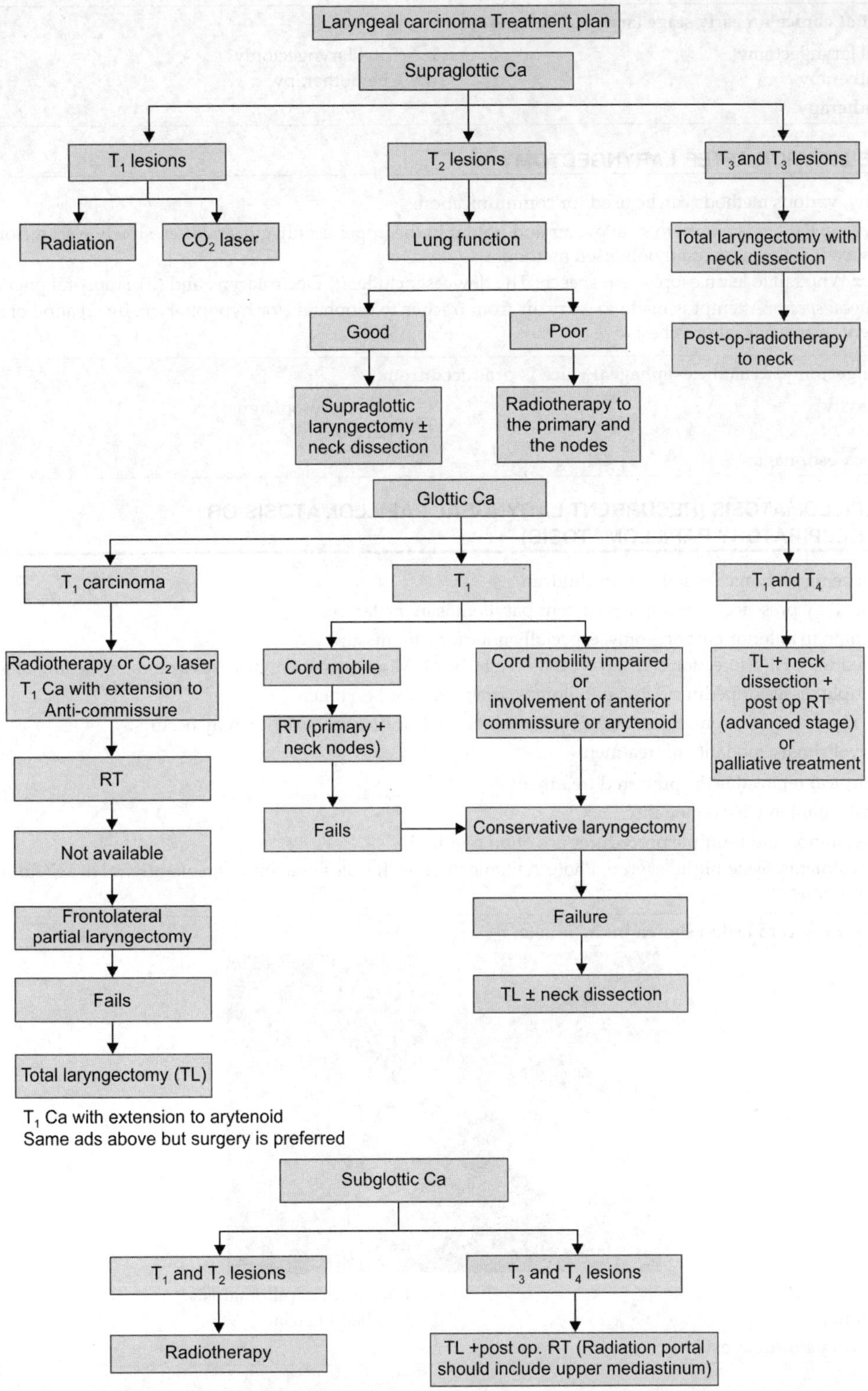

44. A patient presents with Ca larynx involving left false cord, left arytenoid and left aryepiglottic fold with bilateral mobile true cords. The treatment of choice in this patient is which of the following?

a. Vertical hemilaryngectomy
b. Horizontal partial hemilaryngectomy
c. Total laryngectomy
d. Radiotherapy following by chemotherapy

Ans. is 'b' Horizontal partial hemilaryngectomy

Explanation: For T2 stage voice conservative surgery should be done. Supraglottis is excised by partial horizontal laryngectomy.

45. Treatment of choice for early stage laryngeal carcinoma is:

a. Partial laryngectomy
b. Total laryngectomy
c. Radiotherapy
d. Chemotherapy

Ans. is 'c' Radiotherapy

VOICE REHABILITATION AFTER LARYNGECTOMY

After laryngectomy, various methods can be used for communication:

- *Oesophageal speech*: Patient is taught to swallow air and hold it in the upper esophagus and then slowly eject it from the esophagus into the pharynx. It is the most commonly used method.
- *Artifciai larynx*: Who fail to learn esophageal speech. The devices include: (i) Electrolarynx and (ii) Transoral pneumatic device
- *Tracheo-esophageal speech*: Attempt is made to carry air from trachea to esophagus or hypopharynx by creation of skin-lined fistula or by placement of an artificial prosthesis

46. After laryngectomy, dynamic esophageal voice is produced from:

a. Oral cavity
b. Pharynx- esophagus
c. Trachea
d. Pharynx

Ans. is 'b' Pharynx-esophagus

JUVENILE PAPILLOMATOSIS (RECURRENT LARYNGEAL PAPILLOMATOSIS OR RECURRENT RESPIRATORY PAPILLOMATOSIS)

- Most common benign laryngeal neoplasm in children
- It is characterized by presence of multiple recurrent papillomas in the larynx
- It is most common in anterior part of glottis, especially anterior commissure

Etiology: Associated with HPV infection (HPV-6 & HPV-11); HPV-11: More aggressive disease & more prone to malignant change.

Morphology: Multiple sessile or pedunculated papillomas, friable & bleed on touch

Clinical Features: Hoarse cry, Dyspnea, stridor & eventually complete airway obstruction may occur.

Treatment: Surgery: Primary modality of treatment

- Endoscopic surgical removal is the preferred treatment
- CO_2 laser: Most commonly used modality
- Recurrence is common and multiple procedures are often required

Nonsurgical treatments: Systemic interferon, Photodynamic therapy, Intralesional injection of antiviral drug (cidofovir), Interferon alpha-2a, 13-cis-retinoic acid

47. Identify the vocal cord lesion shown in the image. *(NEET 2019)*

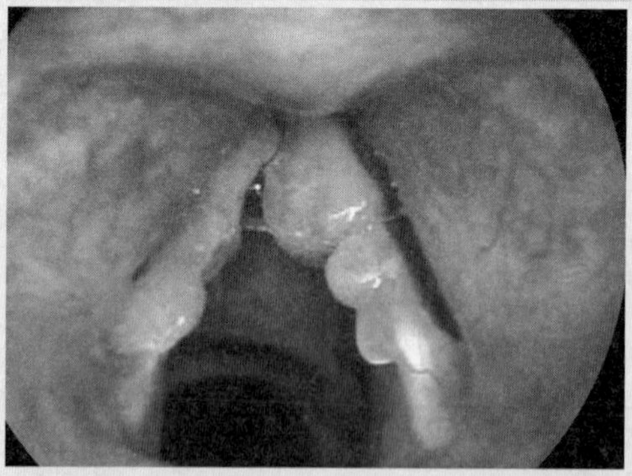

a. Reinke's edema
b. Laryngeal papillomatosis
c. Malignancy
d. Tracheomalacia

Ans. is 'b' Laryngeal papillomatosis

STRIDOR

- Stridor is noisy respiration produced by turbulent airflow through the narrowed air passages.
- **Inspiratory stridor** is often produced in obstructive lesions of supraglottis or pharynx, e.g. laryngomalacia or retropharyngeal abscess.
- **Expiratory stridor** is produced in lesions of thoracic trachea, primary and secondary bronchi, e.g. bronchial foreign body, and tracheal stenosis.
- **Biphasic stridor** is seen in lesions of glottis, subglottis and cervical trachea, e.g. laryngeal papillomas, vocal cord paralysis and subglottis stenosis

48. Inspiratory stridor is found in what kind of lesion? *(NEET 2019)*

a. Supraglottic
b. Subglottic
c. Tracheal
d. Bronchus

Ans. is 'a' Supraglottic

Previously Asked Facts

- Vocal nodules (Singer's nodules) are benign non-neoplastic growth on free edge of both the vocal cords at the junction of anterior 1/3 with posterior 2/3rd. The major cause is voice abuse. Hoarseness is the most common symptom. Usually treated conservatively by educating the patient in proper use of voice.
- Reinke's space is a potential subepithelial space between the glottic epithelium and the vocal ligament.
- Lining epithelium of vocal cord is Stratified squamous epithelium
- Most common site of distant metastasis from Ca larynx is Lung
- Most common site of metastasis for laryngeal Ca is cervical lymph nodes

SURGICAL PROCEDURES IN ENT

MEATOPLASTY

Meatoplasty: Operation in which crescent of conchal cartilage is excised to widen the meatus.
Myringoplasty is repair of a perforation of the tympanic membrane (the pars tensa).
Tympanoplasty is ossicular reconstruction with myringoplasty.
Otoplasty is reconstruction of Pinna

49. Surgical widening of cartilaginous part of EAC is known as: *(NEET 2020)*

a. Myringoplasty
b. Meatoplasty
c. Otoplasty
d. Tympanoplasty

Ans. is 'b' Meatoplasty

TRACHEOSTOMY

Tracheostomy is making an opening in the anterior wall of trachea and converting it into a stoma on the skin surface.

- Sites of Tracheostomy
  - ***High tracheostomy***: Performed above the level of thyroid isthmus
    - Indicated in carcinoma larynx when laryngectomy is anticipated.
    - Drawback: can cause perichondritis of the cricoid cartilage and subglottic stenosis, so it is better avoided.
  - ***Mid tracheostomy***: Performed at the level of thyroid isthmus. The opening is made at the level of II, III tracheal rings.
    - It is the preferred site for tracheostomy
  - ***Low tracheostomy***: Performed below the level of thyroid isthmus. Indicated in laryngeal papillomatosis to avoid implantation
    - Drawback: At this level trachea lies close to several large vessels which can get injured.

INDICATIONS OF TRACHEOSTOMY

Indications for tracheostomy
1. **Respiratory obstruction** a. Infections i. Acute laryngo-tracheo-bronchitis, acute epiglottitis, diphtheria ii. Ludwig's angina, peritonsillar, retropharyngeal or parapharyngeal abscess, tongue abscess b. Trauma i. External injury of larynx and trachea ii. Trauma due to endoscopies, especially in infants and children iii. Fractures of mandible or maxillofacial injuries c. Neoplasms d. Foreign body larynx e. Oedema larynx due to steam, irritant fumes or gases, allergy (angioneurotic or drug sensitivity), radiation f. Bilateral abductor paralysis g. Congenital anomalies – Laryngeal web, cysts, tracheo-oesophageal fistula – Bilateral choanal atresia

Contd...

ENT

Contd...

Indications for tracheostomy
2. **Retained secretions** a. Inability to cough i. Coma of any cause, e.g. head injuries, cerebrovascular accidents, narcotic overdose ii. Paralysis of respiratory muscles, e.g. spinal injuries, polio, Guillain-Barre syndrome, myasthenia gravis iii. Spasm of respiratory muscles, tetanus, eclampsia, strychnine poisoning b. Painful cough c. Aspiration of pharyngeal secretions 3. **Respiratory insufficiency** Chronic lung conditions, viz. emphysema, chronic bronchitis, bronchiectasis, atelectasis.

50. High tracheostomy is done in a patient with consideration of the following in future:

a. Diphtheria infection
b. Ca larynx
c. Papillomatosis
d. Vocal polyps

Ans. is 'b' Ca Larynx

51. Elective tracheostomy is done at what levels?

a. Above thyroid isthmus
b. At the level of thyroid isthmus
c. Below thyroid isthmus
d. Depends on the indication

Ans. is 'b' At the level of thyroid isthmus

MASTOIDECTOMY

Indications of Simple Cortical Mastoidectomy (Schwartz Operation)

- Acute coalescent mastoiditis
- Incompletely resolved acute otitis media with reservoir sign
- Masked mastoiditis
- As a initial step to perform: Endolymphatic sac surgery, Decompression of facial nerve

Indications of Radical Mastoidectomy

- When all cholesteatoma cannot be safely removed, e.g. that invading eustachian tube, round window niche, perilabyrinthine or hypotympanic cells
- As an approach to petrous apex
- Removal of glomus tumour
- Carcinoma middle ear

52. Simple mastoidectomy is done in which of the following indication?

a. Acute coalescent mastoiditis
b. Carcinoma of middle ear
c. Removal of glomus tumor
d. As an approach to petrous apex

Ans. is 'a' Acute coalescent mastoiditis

53. Radical mastoidectomy is done for:

a. Removal of glomus tumor
b. Acute coalescent mastoiditis
c. Masked mastoiditis
d. Cholesteatoma confined to attic and antrum

Ans. is 'a' Removal of glomus tumor

THYROPLASTY

Isshiki divided thyroplasty procedures into 4 categories:

- Type 1: Medial displacement of vocal cord (done by injection of gel foam/Teflon paste)
- Type 2: Lateral displacement of cord (done to improve the airway)
- Type 3: Shortening (relaxing) the cord, to lower the pitch (gender transformation from female to male)
- Type 4: Lengthening (tightening) the cord, to elevate the pitch (gender transformation from male to female), for example as a treatment of androphonia or puberphonia

54. Hoarseness/virilization of female voice secondary to exposure to androgens, can be surgically treated by:

a. Thyroplasty type 1
b. Thyroplasty type 2
c. Thyroplasty type 3
d. Thyroplasty type 4

Ans. is 'd' Thyroplasty type 4

CHAPTER 11 Preventive and Social Medicine

CONCEPTS OF HEALTH AND DISEASE

HEALTH

As defined by the World Health Organization (**WHO**), is "a state of complete physical, mental and social well-being and not merely the absence of disease or infirmity and an ability to lead a socially and economically productive life."

The well-being of an individual has two components:

- Objective component: Standard of living or level of living
- Subjective component: Quality of life

Standard of Living

- It depends on 'Per capita GDP'.

Human Development Index (HDI)

- HDI is a composite index combining indicators representing three dimensions.
  - *Longevity*: Life expectancy at birth
  - *Knowledge*: Mean years of schooling (gross enrolment ratio) and expected year of schooling and literacy rate
  - *Income*: GNI or GDP Per Capita
- *Range*: 0 to +1

Characteristics of Health Indicators (Health Index)

It should be:

- **Valid**, i.e. they should actually measure what they are supposed to measure
- **Reliable** and objective, i.e. the answers should be the same if measured by different people in similar circumstances
- Sensitive, i.e. they should be sensitive to changes in the situation concerned
- Specific, i.e. they should reflect changes only in the situation concerned
- **Feasible**, i.e. they should have the ability to obtain data needed
- Relevant, i.e. they should contribute to the understanding of the phenomenon of interest.

Disability Adjusted Life Years (DALYs)

- It is a measure of:
  - Burden of disease in a defined population
  - Effectiveness of interventions
- It expresses years lost to premature death and years lived with disability adjusted for the severity of the disability.
- DALYs can measure 'both mortality and disability together' (Sullivan's index is related to disability only).
- One DALY is one lost year of healthy life.

Physical Quality of Life Index

- Physical quality of life index consolidates three indicators:
  - Literacy rate
  - Infant mortality rate
  - Life expectancy at age 1 year (LE1)
- For each component, the performance of individual countries is placed on a **scale of 0 to 100**, where 0 represents an absolutely defined worst performance and 100 represents an absolutely defined best performance.
- The composite index is calculated by averaging the three indicators, giving equal weight to each of them
- The resulting PQLI thus also is scaled **0 to 100.**

1. Component of HDI are all *except*:

a. Life expectancy
b. Knowledge
c. Income
d. Social status

Ans. is 'd' Social status

2. Health index characteristics are all *except*:

a. Validity
b. Reliability
c. Affordability
d. Feasibility

Ans. is 'c' Affordability

3. DALY is defined as:

a. Years of life lost to disability
b. Years of life lived with disability
c. Years of life lost to disability and premature death
d. Years of life lived in hospital

Ans. is 'c' Years of life lost to disability and premature death

4. PQLI is:

a. Objective component of level of living
b. Subjective component of level of living
c. Objective component of quality of life
d. Subjective component of quality of life

Ans. is 'd' Subjective component of quality of life

Triage

- It is defined as categorization of the patients and treating them according to the available resource.
- When the quantity and severity of injuries overwhelm the operative capacity of health facilities, a different approach to medical treatment must be adopted.
- The usual principle of "first come, first treated", is not followed in mass emergencies
- Triage consists of rapidly classifying the injured and the likelihood of their survival with prompt medical intervention
- Higher priority is granted to victims whose immediate or long-term prognosis can be dramatically affected by simple intensive care
- Moribund patients who require a great deal of attention, with questionable benefit have the lowest priority
- Most common **triage classification** system used internationally is four color code system:
  1. ***Red***: High priority treatment or transfer
  2. ***Yellow***: Medium priority
  3. ***Green***: Ambulatory patients
  4. ***Black***: Dead or moribund patients.

5. Green color of triage is for which patient: *(NEET 2019)*

a. Low priority
b. Morbidity
c. Ambulatory
d. High priority

Ans. is 'c' Ambulatory

6. Triage is defined as:

a. Treating the most serious cases
b. Categorization of the patient and treating them according to the available resource
c. Cautery burns
d. Treating mentally ill patients

Ans. is 'b' Categorization of the patient and treating them according to the available resource

7. Highest priority is given to which color code in Triage:

a. Red color
b. Yellow color
c. Green color
d. Black color

Ans. is 'a' Red color

Evidence-based Medicine (EBM)

- Considered as 'Gold standard for clinical practice.'
- It is the conscientious, explicit, judicious and reasonable use of modern, best evidence in making decisions about the care of individual patient.
- It integrates clinical experience and patient values with the best available research information.
- It is a movement which aims to increase the use of high-quality clinical research in clinical decision making.
- It requires new skiffs of the clinician including efficient literature searching, and the application of formal rules of evidence in evaluating the clinical literature.
- The practice of evidence-based medicine is a process of lifelong, self-directed, problem-based learning in which caring for one's own patients creates the need for clinically important information about diagnosis, prognosis, therapy and other clinical and health care issues.

8. Evidence-based medicine refers to:

a. Clinical trials to prove adverse effects of drugs
b. Clinical trials to prove safety of drugs
c. Use of various research findings for taking decisions about best patients' care
d. All of the above

Ans. is 'c' Use of various research findings for taking decisions about best patients' care

EPIDEMIOLOGY

EPIDEMIOLOGICAL STUDIES

Types of epidemiological studies:

Types of epidemiological study	Unit of study
1. Observational studies	
a. Descriptive studies b. Analytical studies	
I. Cohort study II. Case control study III. Cross sectional study IV. Ecological study	Individual Individual Individual Population
2. Experimental studies	
a. Randomized controlled trial b. Field trial c. Community trial d. Clinical trial	Patients Healthy people Community Patients

- **Confounding factor** is defined as one which is associated with both the exposure and the disease and is distributed unequally in study and control groups. It is itself a risk factor for the disease.

Cohort Study

- Longitudinal studies (cohort studies) are used to study natural history of disease.
- *There are following types of cohort study:*

a. **Prospective cohort study**
   - Known as 'Concurrent cohort study'
   - Outcome has not yet occurred when the study has begun: Only exposure has occurred; we look for development of same disease in both exposed and non-exposed groups.

b. **Retrospective cohort study**
   - Known as 'Historical cohort study' or 'Non-concurrent cohort study'
   - Combines advantages of both Cohort study and Case control study
   - Both exposure as well as outcome have occurred when the study has begun: First we go back in time and take only exposure into consideration (cohorts identified from past hospital of college records), then look for development of same disease in both exposed and non-exposed groups
   - Sample size required is same as that of prospective cohort study
   - Usually used in occupational cancer studies.

c. **Combined prospective-retrospective cohort study**
   - Known as 'Mixed cohort study'
   - Combines designs of both prospective cohort study and retrospective cohort study
   - Both exposure as well as outcome has occurred when the study has begun: First we go back in time and take only exposure into consideration (cohorts identified from past hospital/college records), then look for development of same disease in both exposed and non-exposed groups; later cohort is followed prospectively into future for outcome. Examples: Court-Brown and Doll Study on effects of radiation therapy.

Cross-Sectional Study

- Cross-sectional study is the simplest form of an observational study.
- It is also known as prevalence study.
- It is based on a single examination of a cross-section of population at one point of time.

- Results of this examination can be projected on the whole population.
- Cross-sectional study tells about the distribution of a disease rather than its etiology.
- Cross-sectional studies can be thought of as providing a snapshot of the frequency and characteristic of a disease in a population at a particular point in time.
- Cross-sectional study is more useful for chronic disease.
- As population is studied at once, no follow-up is required.
- Cross-sectional study is an analytic type of observational study. It is also called as prevalence study.

Case Control Study

- Case control study is a common first approach to test causal hypothesis.
- Case is an individual who has developed the disease.
- Control- is an individual who has not developed the disease but is otherwise comparable to case (e.g. age, sex, occupation, social status, etc.)
- The case-control study has three distinct features:
  - Both exposure (risk factor) and outcome (disease) have occurred before the start of study
  - Study proceeds backwards from effect to cause—retrospective study
  - It uses a control or comparison group to support or refute an inference
- The focus is on a disease that has already developed.
- Association between risk factor and disease can be tested—risk factor can be identified.

Suspected risk factor	Cases (disease present)	Control (disease absent)
Present	A	B
Absent	C	D
	A + C	B + D

e.g. If the frequency of smoking, a/(a+c) is higher in cases than in control b/(b + d), an association is said to exist between smoking and lung cancer.

Cross Product Ratio

Risk in case control study is calculated by odds ratio (cross product ratio). Odds ratio is a measure of the strength of the association between risk factor and outcome.

	Disease	
	Yes	No
Exposed	a	b
Not exposed	c	d

Odds' ratio = ad/bc

Main difference between case control and cohort studies	
Case Control study	***Cohort study***
• Proceeds from "effect to cause" • Starts with the disease • Tests whether the suspected cause occurs more frequently in those with the disease than among those without the disease • Usually the first approach to the testing of a hypothesis, but also useful for exploratory studies	• Proceeds from "cause to effect" • Starts with people exposed to risk factor or suspected cause • Tests whether disease occurs more frequently in those exposed, than in those not similar exposed • Reserved for testing of precisely formulated hypothesis
• Involves fewer number of subjects • Yields relatively quick results • Suitable for the study of rare diseases • Generally, yields only estimate of OR (odds ratio) • Cannot yield information about diseases other than that selected for study • Relatively inexpensive	• Involves larger number of subjects • Long follow-up period often needed, involving delayed results • Inappropriate when the disease or exposure under investigation is rare • Yields incidence rates, RR as well as AR • Can yield information about more than one disease outcome • Expensive

ECOLOGICAL STUDY

An ecological study is an observational study defined by the level at which data are analyzed, namely at the population or group level, rather than individual level. Ecological studies are often used to measure prevalence and incidence of disease, particularly when disease is rare. They are inexpensive and easy to carry out, using routinely collected data, but they are prone to bias and confounding. Also, because they are area-level studies, care must be taken when extrapolating either to individuals within the area level of measurement, or to a higher population level.

9. A person wants to analyse the link of association between bronchial asthma and cigarette smoking. He collects the data of asthmatic patients from various government. Hospitals and number of cigarette packs sold by the vendors. What is the type of study method used? *(NEET 2020)*

a. Cross sectional study
b. Ecological study
c. Pesiological study
d. Experimental study

Ans. is 'b' Ecological study

10. Confounding factor is defined as: *(NEET 2019)*

a. Factor associated with both the exposure and the disease and is distributed unequally in study and control groups
b. Factor associated with exposure only and is distributed unequally in study and control groups
c. Factor associated with both the exposure and the disease and is distributed equally in study and control groups
d. Factor associated with the disease and is distributed equally in study and control groups

Ans. is 'a' Factor associated with both the exposure and the disease and is distributed unequally in study and control groups.

11. Which method is used to study the following timeline? *(NEET 2019)*

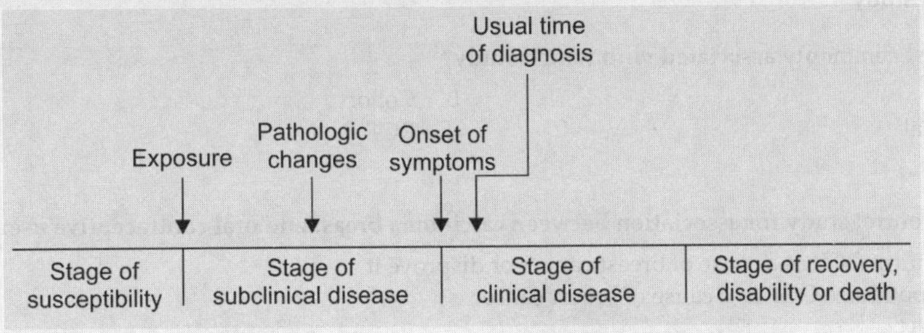

a. Cohort study
b. Cross-sectional study
c. Randomized control trials
d. Interventional studies

Ans. is 'a' Cohort Study

12. Cohort study is which type of study?

a. Descriptive observational
b. Analytic observational
c. Experimental
d. Controlled trial

Ans. is 'b' Analytic observational

13. Natural about cohort study:

a. Cross-sectional study
b. Ecological study
c. Longitudinal study
d. Community trial

Ans. is 'c.' Longitudinal study

14. True about cohort study:

a. Cheaper than case control study
b. Small subjects are required
c. More reliable than case control study for association of risk factor and disease
d. Proceeds from effect to cause

Ans. is 'c' More reliable than case control study for association of risk factor and disease

15. A cohort of nurses with control group is studied for use if IUD and abdominal pain as side effect, in case-control manner. This type of study is:

a. Current cohort study
b. Non-concurrent cohort study
c. Concurrent cohort study
d. Mixed cohort study

Ans. is 'b' Non-concurrent cohort study

16. Study that gives prevalence of delusion in elderly at a given point of time:

a. Control study
b. Cohort study
c. Cross-sectional study
d. Ecological study

Ans. is 'c' Cross-sectional study

17. Cross-sectional study is an example of all *except*:

a. Observational study
b. Incidence study
c. Prevalence study
d. Analytic study

Ans. is 'b' Incidence study

18. Residents of three villages participated in study to identify cholera carriers. All carriers were identified and compared. The type of study is:

a. Cohort
b. Cross-sectional
c. Case-control
d. Experimental

Ans. is 'b' Cross-sectional

19. Cross product ratio is determined by which study? *(NEET 2019)*

a. Case control
b. Cohort
c. Cross-sectional
d. RCT

Ans. is 'a' Case control

20. Retrospective study is also known as:

a. Case control study
b. Cross-sectional study
c. Cohort study
d. Experiment studies

Ans. is 'a' Case control study

21. Recall bias is most commonly associated with which study?

a. Case-control
b. Cohort
c. Cross-sectional
d. RCT

Ans. is 'a' Case-control

22. True about case control study for association between carcinoma breast and oral contraceptive use:

a. Study can confirm OCP as a cause of breast cancer or disprove it
b. Study can hypothesize OCP as a cause of breast cancer
c. Both are correct
d. None of the above correct

Ans. is 'a' Study can confirm OCP as a cause of breast cancer or disprove it

23. In a study there were 35 cases of lung carcinoma and 82 controls were there. On taking history, 33 cases had positive history of smoking and 55 individuals among controls had positive history of smoking. What is the odds ratio?

a. 8
b. 20
c. 50
d. 100

Ans. is 'a' 8

Explanation:

Odds ratio is cross product of entries in the table.

- Total cases 35
- Among these smokers = 33(a)
- Nonsmokers 35–33 = 2 (c)
- Controls
  - Total = 82
  - Smokers = 55 (b)
  - Nonsmokers = 82–55 = 27 (d)

	Lung cancer	
	Present (cases)	*Absent (controls)*
Smoking present Smoking absent	(a) 33 (c) 2	(b) 55 (d) 27
Total	35 (a + c)	82 (b + d)

Odds ratio = ad/bc = 33 × 27/55 × 2 = 8.1

Epidemiological Triad

- The occurrence and manifestations of any disease, whether communicable or non-communicable, are determined by the interaction of three factors, which together constitute epidemiological triad:
  - Agent
  - Host
  - Environment

Interaction of these three is required for causation of a disease.

- ❖ Advanced model of the triangle of Epidemiology
- ❖ This new model includes all facets of the communicable disease model.
- ❖ The term 'agent' is replaced by causative factors and this model shows the interaction of:
  - Causative factors
  - Group of population and their characteristic
  - Environment behavior, culture, physiological factors, ecological elements
  - Time

Epidemiological studies can be classified as observational studies and experimental studies with further subdivisions, which are as follows:

- ❖ Observational studies
- ❖ Descriptive studies
- ❖ Analytical studies
  - Ecological or correlational with populations as unit of study
  - Cross-sectional or prevalence with individuals as unit of study
  - Case-control or case reference with individuals as unit of study
  - Cohort or follow-up with individuals as unit of study.
- ❖ Experimental studies or intervention studies.

24. Triangle of epidemiology stands for: *(NEET 2018)*

a. Interaction of agent, host and environment
b. Interaction of agent, host, environment and time
c. Interaction and interdependence of agent, host, environment and time
d. None of the above

Ans. is 'c' Interaction and interdependence of agent, host, environment and time

25. Study unit of ecological study is: *(NEET 2018)*

a. Population b. Individual
c. Society d. Community

Ans. is 'a' Population

26. Epidemiological study with population as a unit of study:

a. Ecological study b. Cohort study
c. Case reference study d. Experimental study

Ans. is 'a' Ecological study

Strength of association in a cohort study is:

- ❖ Relative risk (RR)
- ❖ Attributable risk (AR)
- ❖ Population attributable risk (PAR)

Relative Risk (Risk Ratio)

- ❖ Relative risk is the ratio of the incidence of the disease (or death) among exposed and the incidence among non-exposed.
- ❖ *Relative risk (RR)* = Incidence among exposed/ Incidence among non-exposed
- ❖ RR = Iexposed/Inon-exposed
- ❖ RR is a direct measure of the strength of the association between the suspected cause and effect.
- ❖ A relative risk of one indicates no association.
- ❖ A relative risk greater than one indicates positive association between the exposure and the disease understudy.
- ❖ For example, a RR of 2 indicates that the incidence rate of disease is 2 times higher in exposed group as compared with unexposed - 100% increase in risk.
- ❖ A relative risk of less than one indicates negative association, i.e. exposure to a factor will decrease the incidence of disease (e.g. exposure to vit A decreases the incidence of skin cancer).

Attributable Risk (Risk Difference)

- ❖ Attributable risk is the difference in incidence rates of disease (or death) between an exposed group and non-exposed group.
- ❖ *Attributable risk (AR)* = (Incidence among exposed–Incidence among nonexposed)/ Incidence among exposed × 100
- ❖ AR = (Iexposed–Inon-exposed)/Iexposed × 100
- ❖ AR is also known as absolute risk or excess risk or risk difference.
- ❖ Attributable risk indicates to what extent the disease can be attributed by risk factor.
- ❖ For example, AR of 90% means 90% of disease (e.g. lung cancer) among exposed (e.g. smoker) is due to exposure to risk factor (smoking).
- ❖ This suggests the amount of disease that might be eliminated if the factor could be controlled or eliminated, i.e. AR of 90% indicates that there will be 90% reduction in incidence of disease (e.g. lung cancer) if risk factor (smoking) is eliminated.

Relative Risk vs Attributable Risk

- Relative risk is a direct measure of the strength of association between suspected cause and effect. For example, a relative risk of 2 means that the incidence rate is 2 times higher in the exposed group as compared with unexposed® i.e. a 100% increase in risk.
- On the other hand, attributable risk indicates the extent which is attributed by risk factor (exposure) to disease. For example, attributable risk of 90% means 90% of disease among exposed is due to exposure to risk factor.
- In simple words:
  - Relative risk indicates the increased percentage of risk of developing a disease, of person is exposed to risk factor.
  - Attributable risk indicates the percentage of disease which is attributed by risk factor among the exposed.
  - Relative risk is a better index than is attributable risk for assessing the etiological role of a factor in disease.
  - On the other hand, attributable risk gives a better idea than does relative risk of the impact of successful preventive or public health program might have in reducing the problem. That means attributable risk reflects the public health importance better than relative risk.

Population Attributable Risk (PAR)

- It is the incidence of disease (or death) in the total population minus the incidence of disease (or death) among those who are not exposed.
- *Population attributable risk (PAR)* = (Incidence among total–Incidence among nonexposed)/ Incidence among total × 100
- PAR = (Itotal–Inon-exposed)/Itot × 100
- The concept of population attributable risk is useful in that it provides an estimate of the amount by which disease could be reduced in that population, if the suspected factor is modified or eliminated.
- So, population attributable risk gives a better idea than does relative risk of the impact of successful preventive or public health program might have in reducing the problem.
- Population attributable risk is broader and better than attributable risk.

27. Risk among exposed by risk among us on-exposed is defined to be: *(NEET 2018)*

a. Relative risk b. Odds ratio
c. Attributable risk d. None of the above

Ans. is 'a' Relative risk

28. Incidence of disease in exposed divided by incidence among nonexposed is: *(NEET 2018)*

a. Attributable risk b. Population attributable risk
c. Odds ratio d. Risk ratio

Ans. is 'd' Risk ratio

29. Strength of association of outcome and risk factor is measured by: *(NEET 2018)*

a. Relative risk b. Attributable risk
c. Population attributable risk d. None of the above

Ans. is 'a' Relative risk

30. Important measure for National Health Policy: *(NEET 2018)*

a. Relative risk b. Odds ratio
c. Population attributable risk d. Attributable risk

Ans. is 'c' Population attributable risk

31. 100 individuals are diagnosed with lung cancer in a population of 100,000. Out of 100 patients, 80 were smokes and 20,000 were smokers in totals population. What is PAR? *(NEET 2018)*

a. 60 b. 75
c. 80 d. 90

Ans. is 'b' 75

Explanation:

- *Population attributable risk (PAR)* = (Incidence among total–Incidence among nonexposed)/ Incidence among total × 100
- PAR = (Itotal–Inon-exposed)/ Itot × 100
- Incidence in total population = 100 per 1 lac
- Number of exposed = 20,000 (All exposed)
- Number of non-exposed 80,000 (10,0000–20,000)
- Nonexposed having lung cancer = 20 (out of 100 patients 80 were smoker. Thus 20 are nonexposed).
- Incidence among nonexposed = 20 per 80,000 or 25 per 10,0000
- Thus, PAR = [(100–25)/100] × 100 = 75.

Attributable risk (AR) or risk difference is the difference between the incidence rates in exposed and non-exposed groups. This reflects the absolute risk of the exposure or the excess risk of the outcome (e.g. disease) in the exposed group compared with the non-exposed group. AR is sometimes referred to as attributable risk in the exposed because it is used to quantify risk in the exposed group that is attributable to the exposure.

Incidence is the rate of new (or newly diagnosed) cases of the disease. It is generally reported as the number of new cases occurring within a period of time (e.g., per month, per year).

Prevalence is the actual number of cases alive, with the disease either during a period of time (period prevalence) or at a particular date in time (point prevalence).

A risk ratio (RR), also called relative risk, compares the risk of a health event (disease, injury, risk factor, or death) among one group with the risk among another group. It does so by dividing the risk (incidence proportion, attack rate) in group 1 by the risk (incidence proportion, attack rate) in group 2.

32. Difference between the incidence of disease among exposed and nonexposed to a risk factor is termed as: *(NEET 2020)*

a. Incidence
b. Prevalence
c. Attributable risk
d. Risk ratio

Ans. is 'c' Attributable risk

33. If effective treatment for a disease is introduced in a community, what will be the effect on incidence (I) and prevalence (P)?

a. No change in P and I
b. Both P and I will decrease
c. P will decrease and I will increase
d. P will decrease and I will remain the same

Ans. is 'd' P will decrease and I will remain the same

Prevalence

- Prevalence refers specifically to all current cases (old and new) existing at a given point in time or over a period of time in a given population
  - Prevalence depends upon 2 factors:
    - Incidence
    - Duration of illness
  - Prevalence: Incidence x mean duration
- Prevalence is of two types: (i) Point prevalence, and (ii) Period prevalence

I. Point prevalence

- Point prevalence is defined as the number of all current cases (old and new) of a disease at one point of time, in relation to a defined population.
  Prevalence = No. of total (new + old) cases of a disease in a year × 100/Total population
- When the term prevalence rate is used, without any further qualification it is taken to mean "point prevalence"

II. Period prevalence

- It measures the frequency of all current cases (old and new) existing during a defined period of time (e.g. annual prevalence) expressed in relation to a defined population
- It includes cases arising before but extending into or through to the year as well as those cases arising during the year.

34. Point prevalence is defined as:

a. Number of few cases at a given point of time
b. Number of new cases in a given year
c. Number of total cases in a given year
d. Number of total cases at a given point of time

Ans. is 'd' Number of total cases at a given point of time

35. Relationship between incidence and prevalence:

a. Incidence = Prevalence × Duration
b. Prevalence = Incidence × Duration
c. Incidence = Prevalence + Duration
d. Prevalence = Incidence + Duration

Ans. is 'b' Prevalence = Incidence × Duration

36. Incidence of a disease is 4 per 1000 of population with duration of 2 years. Calculate the prevalence:

a. 8/1000
b. 4/1000
c. 2/1000
d. 6/1000

Ans. is 'a' 8/1000

37. Prevalence of leprosy in India:

a. 7 per 10,000 population
b. 0.7 per 10,000 population
c. 15 per 10,000 population
d. 1.5 per 10,000 population

Ans. is 'b' 0.7 per 10,000 population

Natural Experiments

Those in which exposure to the event or intervention of interest has not been manipulated by researcher. The individuals exposed to the experimental and control conditions are determined by nature or by other factors outside the control of the investigators.

- ❖ When a naturally occurring event or situation is exploited by a researcher help to answer a research question, it is called a natural experiment. There searcher has little or no control over the situation that is being observed. A good example of natural experiment is one by **James Lind** in 1747 on the prevention of scurvy among sailors. He compared the effects of different acidic substances, ranging from vinegar to cider, on groups of afflicted sailors, and found that the group who form vinegar to cider, on group so afflicted sailors, and found that the group who were given oranges and lemons had largely recovered from scurvy after 6 days.
- ❖ Other important example is John Snow's natural experiment on cholera linked with contaminated water.
- ❖ RCT is not natural experiment as researcher allocate the individuals in study and control group by randomization.
- ❖ Randomized controlled trials or clinical trials with patients as unit of study.

38. All are true about natural experiments, *except*:

a. Researcher has no control over the allocation of subjects
b. James Lind experiment is an example
c. Includes randomized controlled trials (RCTs)
d. All are correct

Ans. is 'c' Includes randomized controlled trials (RCTs)

39. In a study a patient does not know the nature of drug (whether a placebo or curative drug) he is taking. The researcher knows the drug type to be given to the individuals in study. Types of blinding in this study is:

a. Single
b. Double
c. Triple
d. Combined double/triple

Ans. is 'a' Single

40. Individual in a village population are arranged alphabetically and then every 8th person is selected for the study; the type of study is:

a. Simple random sampling
b. Stratified random sampling
c. Systemic random sampling
d. Cluster sampling

Ans. is 'c' Systemic random sampling

41. Definition of surveillance:

a. Analysis of routine measurements
b. Continuous scrutiny of factor
c. Systemic collection and analysis of data
d. All of the above

Ans. is 'Both b and c' Continuous scrutiny of factor and Systemic collection and analysis of data

42. The difference between descriptive and analytic studies:

a. Descriptive studies are used to test hypothesis
b. Analytic studies are used to formulate a hypothesis
c. Descriptive studies are first phase in epidemiology
d. Analytic studies observe distribution of disease

Ans. is 'c' Descriptive studies are first phase in epidemiology

43. In a population of 60,000; 20,000 are smokers and 40,000 are nonsmokers. 200 smokers and 40 nonsmokers developed lung cancer. What is the relative risk of smoking for causing lung carcinoma?

a. 5
b. 10
c. 15
d. 20

Ans. is 'b' 10

Explanation:

- ❖ Relative risk is the ratio of the incidence of the disease (or death) among exposed and the incidence among nonexposed.

RR = Incidence of disease among exposed/incidence of disease among nonexposed

Smoking	Developed lung cancer	Did not develop lung cancer	Total
Yes	200	19,800	20,000
No	40	39,960	40,000

Incidence of lung cancer among smoker = 200/20,000 = 10 per 1000 Incidence of lung cancer among nonsmokers = 40/40,000 = 1 per 1000
Relative risk = incidence among exposed/incidence among nonexposed = 10/1 = 10.

Selection bias may be of following types:

- ❖ Surveillance/detection bias:
  - It results from the use of a particular diagnostic technique or type of equipment
- ❖ Neyman survival bias (incidence-prevalence bias):
  - This type of bias is due to missing of fatal cases, mild cases or cases of shorter duration from the study

- ❖ Referral bias (volunteer bias):
  - Volunteer or referral bias occurs because people who volunteer to participate in a study (or who are referred to it) are often different than non-volunteers/non-referral
  - This bias usually favors the treatment group, as volunteers tend to be more motivated and concerned about their health.
- ❖ Response bias:
  - This type of bias occurs when those who respond to a survey differ in important ways from who do not respond.
- ❖ Berksonian bias:
  - Berksonian bias results from the greater probability of hospital admission for people with two or more disease than for people with one disease. So, it is also known as admission rate bias.

44. Berksonian bias is a type of:

a. Admission rate bias
b. Interviewer bias
c. Information bias
d. Recall bias

Ans. is 'a' Admission rate bias

Types of random sampling are:

- ❖ Simple random sampling
  - It is also known as "unrestricted random sampling". Each individual is chosen randomly and entirely by chance. There is no stratification in similar groups. Thus, each individual has the same probability of being chosen.
  - Methods of simple random sampling are:
    - Lottery method
    - Random number table
    - Computer technique.
  - It is suitable for small homogeneous population and is used in clinical trials. It provides the greatest number of possible samples.
- ❖ Systemic random sampling
  - In order to do systematic random sampling, the individuals in a population are arranged in a certain way (for example, alphabetically).
  - A random starting point is selected and then every nth (for example 10th or 15th) individual is selected for the sample.
  - That is, after arranging the individuals in certain pattern (e.g. alphabetically) a starting point is chosen at random, and choices thereafter at regular intervals.
- ❖ Stratified random sampling
  - When sub-populations vary considerably, it is advantageous to sample each subpopulation (stratum) independently.
  - Stratification is the process of grouping members of the population into relative homogeneous subgroups before sampling.
  - The strata should be mutually exclusive, every element in the population must be assigned to only one stratum. Then systematic random sampling method is applied within each stratum.
  - Stratified random sampling is particularly useful where one is interested in analyzing the data by a certain characteristic of the population, viz. Hindus, Muslims, Christians, age group, etc. —as we know these groups are not equally distributed in the population.
- ❖ Cluster sampling
  - Cluster sampling is a sampling technique used when natural groupings are evident in a statistical population. In this technique, the total population is divided into these groups (Or clusters) and a sample of groups is selected.
  - The characteristic feature is that selected groups act as samples (while in other types of random sampling individuals act as sample).
  - Cluster sampling is rapid, simple and economic (less expensive).
  - Sample size may vary according to study.
  - Cluster sampling is an example of two-stage sampling
  - There are chances of sampling error
  - Cluster sampling is used in India to evaluate immunization coverage. WHO used 30 × 7 technique (total 210 children) for cluster sampling in which there are 30 clusters, each containing 7 children who are 12–23 months old and are completely immunized for primary immunization (till measles vaccine at 9 month).
- ❖ Multistage random sampling
  - It is done in successive stages; each successive sampling unit is nested in the previous sampling unit Advantage: Introduces flexibility in sampling.
  - For example, in large country surveys, states are chosen, then districts, then villages, then every 10th person in village as final sampling unit.
- ❖ Multiphase random sampling
  - It is done in successive phase; part of information is obtained from whole sample and part from the sub-sample
  - For example, in a TB survey, Mantoux test done in first phase, then X-ray done in all Mantoux positive then sputum examined in all those with positive X-ray findings.

45. In a psychiatric hospital, all patients are arranged chronologically according to height [from lower to higher]. Then every 4th patient is taken into study. Type of sampling:

a. Simple random sampling
b. Stratified random sampling
c. Systemic random sampling
d. All of the above

Ans. is 'c' Systemic random sampling

46. Heart of controlled trial is:

a. Binding
b. Matching
c. Randomization
d. Stratification

Ans. is 'c' Randomization

47. True about standardization are all *except*:

a. Most commonly used for age differences
b. Direct standardization is used when population is large
c. Age specific rates are required in indirect standardization
d. All are correct

Ans. is 'c' Age specific rates are required in indirect standardization

48. Standardization is most important for:

a. Sex distribution
b. Age distribution
c. Disease distribution
d. None of the above

Ans. is 'b' Age distribution

49. Secondary attacks rate is defined as:

a. Number of total cases developing disease within maximum incubation period
b. Number of cases developing disease within incubation period following exposure to primary case
c. Number of cases developing disease after exposure to primary case in any period of time
d. Number of cases developing after exposure to secondary case

Ans. is 'b' Number of cases developing disease within incubation period following exposure to primary case

50. Stratified sampling is ideal for:

a. Small homogeneous population
b. Natural population group
c. Hidden population
d. When subpopulation very considerably

Ans. is 'd' When subpopulation very considerably

51. Sex ratio as per 2011 census:

a. 970
b. 940
c. 921
d. 915

Ans. is 'b' 940

52. Bed occupancy rate is an indicator of:

a. Morbidity
b. Mortality
c. Utilization
d. Health care delivery

Ans. is 'c' Utilization

Carrier

❖ Carrier is a person who harbors the pathogenic microorganism without suffering from any disease from it.

Classification

❖ *Healthy carriers*: These are the persons who harbor the microorganism bud had never suffered from any disease by it.
❖ *Convalescent carriers*: These are the persons who had been infected by that microorganism and are recovering from that infection. Even though they have no more symptoms of the disease, they continue to shed the microorganism into the environment.
❖ *Temporary carriers*: The carrier state lasts for less than 6 months.
❖ *Chronic carriers*: The carrier state extends beyond 6 months and may even last for years.
❖ *Contact carrier*: A person can become a contact carrier when he acquires the microorganism due to his contact with the patient.
❖ *Paradoxical carrier*: A person is a paradoxical carrier when he acquires the microorganism from another carrier.

53. Paradoxical carriers are: *(NEET 2019)*

a. A person who acquires the microorganism due to his contact with the patient
b. A person who acquires the microorganism another carrier
c. A person who is clinically recovered from an infectious disease but still capable of transmitting the infectious agent to others
d. None

Ans. is 'b' A person who acquires the microorganism another carrier

54. Carrier is defined as:

a. Person, animal or object from which infectious agent passes to host
b. Person, animal or object in which an infectious agent lives and multiplies
c. Infected person harboring infectious agent without clinical features and acts as source of infection
d. A person in which infectious agent lie dormant

Ans. is 'c' Infected person harboring infectious agent without clinical features and acts as source of infection

SCREENING OF DISEASE

Screening Test

- The criteria for screening are based on two considerations:
  - Disease to be screened
  - Screening test to be applied

a. **Disease to be screened**
   - The disease should be an important health problem with a recognizable latent or asymptomatic stage
   - There should be a test (screening test) which can detect the disease prior to clinical stage, with also availability of a diagnostic (confirmatory) test
   - There should be an effective treatment which should reduce morbidity and mortality if started early.

b. **Screening test to be applied**
   - The screening test to be applied should fulfill following criteria:

   1. **Acceptability**
      - The test should be acceptable to the people whom is aimed
   2. **Repeatability (reliability)**
      - The test must give consistent results when it is repeated more than once on the same individual under same condition, i.e. results of test must by precise(exact).
      - Thus, repeatability is also known as precision, reliability or reproducibility
   3. **Validity (accuracy)**
      - It refers to what extent the test accurately measures which is purports to measure
      - *Validity has two components*:
        - Sensitivity
        - Specificity
      - A test should have high sensitivity and specificity

      Accuracy = (Sensitivity) (Prevalence) / (Specificity) (1-Prevalence)

      Accuracy = True positive + true negative/True positive + false positive + true negative + false negative
   4. **Others**
      - *Other important criteria are:* Simplicity, rapidity, low cost (cost effectiveness), safety, and ease of administration.
      - There are two major statistical measures for the validity of a screening test:

55. Which of the following is an example of prospective screening? *(NEET 2020)*

a. Screening of immigrants
b. Screening of newborn
c. Screening of cervical cancer
d. Screening for blood sugar levels in pregnant females

Ans. is 'a' Screening of immigrants

Sensitivity

- It is the ability of a test to identify correctly all those who have the disease, i.e. true positive
- In other words, sensitivity measures the percentage of sick people who are identified as having disease
- For example, if a test is 90% sensitive, that means out of 100 diseased people, it will diagnose 90 (90% of diseased people will be diagnosed). Remaining 10% will be wrongly identified as not having the disease, i.e. false negative.

False negative rate = 1 – sensitivity

or

Sensitivity = 1 – false negative rate

Specificity

- It is the ability of a test to identify correctly those who do not have the disease, i.e. true negative
- In other words, specificity measures the percentage of well people who are identified as not having the disease
- For example, a 90% specificity means that 90% of non-diseased people will be identified as not having the disease. The remaining 10% will be wrongly classified as diseased, i.e. false positive.

False positive rate = 1 – specificity

or

Specificity = 1 – false positive rate

- True positive is directly related to sensitivity
- False negative is inversely related to sensitivity
- True negative is directly related to specificity
- False positive is inversely related to specificity

- If a test has high sensitivity—More true positive, less false negative, and also more false positive
- If a test has high specificity—More true negative, less false positive and also more false negative.

Evaluation of a Screening Test

Screening test result by diagnosis			
	Diagnosis		
Screening test results	*Diseased*	*Not diseased*	*Total*
Positive	a. (True-positive)	b. (False-negative)	a + b
Negative	c. (False-negative)	d. (True-positive)	c + b
Total	a + c	b + d	a + b + c + d

The following measures are used to evaluate a screening test:

- Sensitivity = a/(a + c) x 100
- Specificity = d/(b + d) x 100
- Predictive value of a positive test = a/(a + b) x 100
- Predictive value of a negative test = d/(c + d) x 100
- Percentage of false-negative = c/(a + c) x 100
- Percentage of true-positive = b/(b + d) x 100
- When a screening test is used to diagnose a disease, the test outcome can be positive (diseased) or negative (healthy), while the actual health status of the person may be different. In that setting:
  - *True positive*: Diseased people correctly diagnosed as diseased
  - *False positive*: Healthy people wrongly identified as diseased
  - *True negative*: Healthy people correctly identified as healthy
  - *False negative*: Diseased people wrongly identified as healthy.

Case Scenario

- If a population has more false positive cases:
  - Screening test is more sensitive
  - Positive predictive value of the test is low
  - Prevalence of disease is low.
- If a population has more false negative cases
  - Screening test is more specific
  - Negative predictive value of the test is low.

Positive predictive value is related to sensitivity specificity and prevalence.

PPV = TP/(TP + FP) × 100

- This relationship is represented by Baye's theorem:

$$\text{PPV} = \frac{\text{Sensitivity} \times \text{Prevalence}}{(\text{Sensitivity} \times \text{prevalence}) + (100 - \text{Spcificity})\ (100 - \text{prevalence})} \times 100$$

- Positive predictive value is the ability of a test to correctly diagnose the proportion of cases in which persons with a positive screening test result have the disease in question.
- Negative predictive value is the proportion of cases in which people with negative test result do not have the disease in question.
- Sensitivity is defined as the ability of the test to identify correctly all those who have the disease, i.e. true positive.
- Specificity is defined as the ability of the test to identify correctly those who do not have the disease, i.e. true negative.

Remember

Predictive accuracy (Predictive value) of screening test

- Predictive value reflects the diagnostic power of the test
- Predictive value depends upon sensitivity, specificity and prevalence
  - Positive predictive value (Post-test probability of a disease or precision rate)
- It is the probability a patient with positive test result has the disease in question, i.e. the proportion of patients with positive test results who are correctly diagnosed.

A high positive predictive value indicates that a person with a positive test has the disease for diagnostic power of a screening test to correctly identify the disease.

- It is the most important measure of a diagnostic method as it reflects the probability that a positive test reflects the underlying condition being tested for.
  - Negative predictive value

- ❖ It is the probability that a person with negative test results, is in fact healthy
- ❖ In other words, the percentage of healthy people among those who show negative test results
- ❖ A high negative predictive value means there is high probability that a negative test rules out the disease diagnostic power of a screening test to exclude the disease.

56. Diagnostic power of a test to correctly diagnose a disease is: *(NEET 2019)*

a. Negative predictive value b. Positive predictive value
c. Sensitivity d. Specificity

Ans. is 'b' Positive predictive value

57. Positive predictive value is:

a. Diagnostic power to identify all positive cases (true and false)
b. Diagnostic power to identify all negative cases (true andfalse)
c. Diagnostic power to exclude a disease
d. Diagnostic power to correctly identify a disease

Ans. is 'd' Diagnostic power to correctly identify a disease

58. True about sensitivity:

a. Directly related to false negative b. Sensitivity = 1–true positive
c. Ability to detect true positive d. All are correct

Ans. is 'c' Ability to detect true positive

59. Screening test was applied on a particular disease, out of 1000 population 90 were tested positive, it was compared with gold standard test which showed 100 were positive. What is the sensitivity of the new screening test:

a. 90/1000 b. 90/100
c. 100/100 d. 90–10/100

Ans. is 'b' 90/100

60. Ideal screening test should be:

a. Safe b. Reliable
c. Valid d. All of the above

Ans. is 'd' All of the above

61. More false positive cases in screening test make the test:

a. More specific b. More sensitive
c. Less sensitive d. More specific and more sensitive

Ans. is 'b' More sensitive

62. A screening test has sensitivity of 90% and specificity to 99%. The prevalence of disease under investigation is 5 per 1000 population. What is the PPV of the given screening test:

a. 10 b. 70
c. 33 d. 99

Ans. is 'c' 33

Explanation:

- ❖ One thing should be remembered that prevalence is in percentage (per 100 population) not per1000.
- ❖ So, in this question, prevalence 5 per 1000 = 0.5 per 100 or 0.5%

$$PPV = \frac{99 \times 0.5}{(99 \times 0.5) + (100 - 99)\,(100 - 0.5)} \times 100 = 33.2$$

63. A screening test is applied for screening of liver cancer in a population of 500. The test result is positive in 80 individuals and negative in remaining 420. Out of 80 positive individuals 60 confirmed to be diagnosed liver cancer by diagnostic test and 20 were ruled out. Out of negative 420 individuals 40 had liver cancer. The sensitivity of the test is:

a. 60% b. 80%
c. 90% d. 95%

Ans. is 'a' 60%

Explanation:

- ❖ Total positive = 80
- ❖ True positive = 60
- ❖ False positive = 20

- False negative = 40
- True negative = 380 (420 – 40)
- Sensitivity = True positive/True positive + false negative × 100 = 60/(60 + 40) × 100 + 60%
- Specific = True negative/true negative + false positive × 100 = 380/(380 + 20) × 100 = 95%

64. Specificity of a test refers to its ability to detect:

a. True positive b. True negative
c. False negative d. False positive

Ans. is 'b' True negative

65. A population of 50 children is having 10 immunized against chickenpox. 5 children developed chickenpox on 1st march 2017. Other 28 children developed chickenpox within next 2 week what is the SAR of chickenpox:

a. 60% b. 70%
c. 80% d. 90%

Ans. is 'c' 80%

Explanation:

- Primary cases in the question developing chickenpox on same day
- Immune children = 10
- Susceptible contacts Total children – (Primary cases + immunized children) = 50 – (5 + 10) = 35
- No. of susceptible developing disease = 28
- SAR No. of susceptible developing disease/Total number of susceptible × 100 = 28/35 × 100 = 80%

Lead Time

The lead time is the time period between diagnosis by early detection (i.e. earliest point of diagnosis by screening test) and diagnosis by standard diagnostic tests. Lead time is the advantage gained by screening.

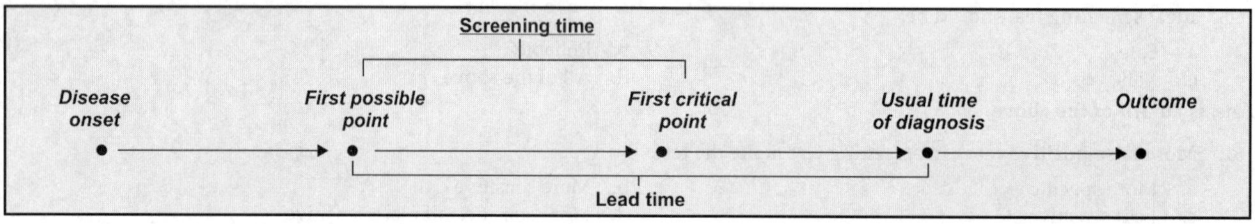

- *Generation time*: Period from receipt of infection to maximal infectivity
- *Serial interval*: Gap between onset of primary case and secondary case.
- *Primary case*: First case of communicable disease introduced into the population
- *Index case*: First case to come for attention of the investigator.

66. Lead time is defined as:

a. Time between diagnosis and treatment
b. Time between points where the diagnosis is made by screening test to usual diagnosis
c. Time between disease onset and outcome
d. Time between usual time of diagnosis and outcome

Ans. is 'b' Time between points where the diagnosis is made by screening test to usual diagnosis

67. Serial interval is:

a. Interval between primary and secondary case
b. Interval between first case and last case
c. Interval between primary case and all subsequent cases multiplied by secondary attack rate
d. Interval between incubation period and gestational period

Ans. is 'a' Interval between primary and secondary case

68. Time period between entry of organism to body to maximum infectivity is:

a. Lead time b. Median incubation period
c. Generation time d. Serial interval

Ans. is 'c' Generation time

Levels of prevention

Level	Phase of disease	Aim	Actions	Target
Primordial	Underlying economic, social, and environmental conditions leading to causation	Establish and maintain conditions that minimize hazards to health	Measures that inhibit the emergence of environmental, economic, social and behavioral conditions	Total population or Selected groups; achieved through public health policy and health promotion
Primary	Specific causal factors	Reduce the incidence of disease	Protection of health by personal and community efforts, such as enhancing nutritional status. Providing immunizations and eliminating environmental risks • Immunization (vaccination) • Chemoprophylaxis • Nutritional supplementation programs (e.g. vitamin A supplementation) • Chlorination of water • Using a mosquito net • Health education	Total population, selected groups and individuals at high-risk achieved through public health programs
Secondary	Early stage of disease	Reduce the prevalence of disease by shortening its duration	Measures available to individuals and communities for early detection and prompt intervention to control disease and minimize disability) e.g. through screening programs) • Screening test • Case finding programs • Early diagnosis and treatment	Individuals with established disease; achieved through early diagnosis and treatment
Tertiary	Late stage of disease (treatment, rehabilitation)	Reduce the number and/ or impact of complication	Measures aimed at softening the impact of long-term disease and disability; minimizing suffering; maximizing potential years of useful life. • Disability limitation • Resting the affected limb in neutral position in PRPP to prevent deformity • Rehabilitation • Establishing schools for blind • Provision of aids for crippled • Reconstructive surgery in leprosy • Muscle re-education and graded exercise in neurological disorder like polio • Changing profession for a more suitable one	Patients; achieved through rehabilitation

69. Vitamin A supplementation is which type of presentation?

a. Primordial
b. Primary
c. Secondary
d. Tertiary

Ans. is 'b' Primary

70. Target group is secondary prevention:

a. Total population
b. High risk group
c. Individuals with established disease
d. Patient with disability

Ans. is 'c' Individuals with established disease

COMMUNICABLE DISEASES

Time Distribution of Disease

- *Sporadic*: Disease occurring irregularly from time to time.
- *Endemic*: Disease occurring regularly in expected frequency.
- *Epidemic*: Disease occurring in excess of expected frequency.
- *Pandemic*: Epidemic affecting a large proportion of population over a wide geographic area.

71. Endemic disease is defined as a disease:

a. Occurrence regularly in expected frequency
b. Occurrence irregularly from time to time
c. Occurrence in excess of expected frequency
d. Occurrence in large population

Ans. is 'a' Occurrence regularly in expected frequency

Sources and Reservoirs

- Source is 'the person, animal, object or substance from which infectious agent passes to host', i.e. man acquires infection from source.
- Reservoir is 'any person, animal, insect, plant, soil or substance in which an infectious agent lives and multiplies'. Infectious agent is dependent on reservoir for survival. From reservoir it can be transmitted to susceptible host. Thus, a reservoir may act as a source of infection when a person acquires infection directly from a reservoir.

- Source and reservoir are same, Tetanus spores survive in soil (reservoir) and a person acquires infection directly from soil (source). So, soil acts as reservoir as well as source.
- Source and reservoir different–In typhoid, bacillus survives and multiplies inside human cases or carriers (act as reservoir), but immediate source of infection is feces or urine of patients, or contaminated food, water or milk (act as source).

Carrier in Cholera

There are following types of carrier in cholera:

- *Incubatory*: Shed vibrios only in the brief incubation period of 1–5 days
- *Convalescent*: Shed vibrios for 2–3weeks
- *Healthy or contact carrier*: Has had subclinical infection and shed vibrios for less than 10 days
- *Chronic carriers*: Can shed vibrios for months or years and may have persistent infection in gallbladder.

72. Healthy carrier is seen in:

a. Measles
b. Rubella
c. Meningococcal meningitis
d. Influenza

Ans. is 'c' Meningococcal meningitis

73. Infectivity of convalescent carrier of cholera lasts for:

a. 1–5 days
b. 1–2 weeks
c. 2–3 weeks
d. 4–5 weeks

Ans. is 'c' 2–3 weeks

Modes of Transmission

The route which an infectious agent is transmitted from a reservoir to another host is called the mode of transmission. Various direct and indirect modes of transmission are:

- *Direct modes of transmission*: Direct transmission refers to the transfer of an infectious agent from an infected host to a new host without the need for intermediates such as air, food, water or other animals. Direct modes of transmission can occur in two main ways:
    - *Person to person*: The infectious agent is spread by direct contact between people through touching, biting, kissing, sexual inter-course or direct projection of respiratory drop lets into another person's nose or mouth during coughing, sneezing or talking. A familiar example is the transmission of HIV from an infected person to others through sexual intercourse.
    - *Transplacental transmission*: This refers to the transmission of an infectious agent from a pregnant woman to her fetus through the placenta. An example is mother-to-child transmission (MTCT) of HIV.
- *Indirect modes of transmission*: Indirect transmission is when infectious agents are transmitted to new hosts through intermediates such as air, food, water, objects or substances in the environment, or other animals. Indirect transmission has three subtypes:
    - *Air-borne transmission*: The infectious agent may be transmitted in dried secretions from the respiratory tract, which can remain suspended in the air for some time. For example, the infectious agent causing tuberculosis can enter a new host through airborne transmission.
    - *Vehicle-borne transmission*: A vehicle is any non-living substance or object that can be contaminated by an infectious agent, which then transmits it to a new host. Contamination refers to the presence of an infectious agent in or on the vehicle.
    - *Vector-borne transmission*: A vector is an organism, usually an arthropod which transmits an infectious agent to a new host. Arthropods, which act as vectors, include houseflies, mosquitoes, lice and ticks.

74. Which of the following is not an example of direct transmission in communicable diseases: *(NEET 2018)*

a. Transplacental
b. Soil
c. Respiratory
d. STDs

Ans. is 'b' Soil

Kala-azar

- Kala-azar has re-emerged from near eradication. The annual estimate for the incidence and prevalence of kala-azar cases worldwide is 0.5 million and 2.5 million, respectively. Of these, 90% of the confirmed cases occur in India, Nepal, Bangladesh and Sudan.
- In India, it is a serious problem in Bihar, West Bengal and eastern Uttar Pradesh where there is under-reporting of kala-azar and post kala-azar dermal leishmaniasis is seen in women and children 0–9 years of age.
- Untreated cases of kala-azar are associated with up to 90% mortality, with treatment reduces to 15% and 3.4% even in specialized hospitals. It is also associated with up to 20% in subclinical infection.
- Spraying of DDT helped control kala-azar; however, there are reports of the vector *Phlebotomusargentipes* developing resistance. Also, lymphadenopathy, a major presenting feature in India raises the possibility of a new vector or a variant of the disease.
- The wide spread coexistence of malaria and kala-azar in Bihar may lead to a difficulty in diagnosis and in appropriate treatment. In addition, reports of the organism developing resistance to sodium antimony gluconate—the main drug for the treatment—would make its eradication difficult.

- ❖ Resistance to DDT has not been demonstrated in sand flies.
- ❖ A single application of DDT or lindane has been found effective in reducing sand flies.
- ❖ DDT residue may remain effective for a period of 1 to 2 years and lindane only for a period of 3 months.
- ❖ Clinical trials in India have reported encouraging results with amphotericin B (recommended as a third-line drug by the National Malaria Eradication Programme).
- ❖ Phase III Trials with a first-generation vaccine (killed Leishmania organism mixed with a low concentration of BCG as an adjuvant) have also yielded promising results. Preliminary studies using autoclaved Leishmania major mixed with BCG have been successful in preventing infection with *Leishmania donovani*.
- ❖ Until a safe and effective vaccine is developed, a combination of sand-fly control, detection and treatment of patients and prevention of drug resistance is the best approach for controlling kala-azar.

75. Prevalence of Kala-azar is not seen in: *(NEET 2018)*

a. UP b. Bihar
c. West Bengal d. Assam

Ans. is 'd' Assam

76. Insecticide of choice to prevent Kala-azar: *(NEET 2018)*

a. DDT b. HCH
c. Malathion d. Paris green

Ans. is 'a' DDT

Diagnosis of tuberculosis is made by following methods:

a. **Direct examination of specimen**
- These are rapid methods of diagnosis. These may be:
    - Smear microscopy (staining and microscopy)
        - It is the most rapid method for diagnosis. but sensitivity and specificity are low
        - At least 10,000 bacilli should be present per ml of sputum for demonstration indirect
        - Most commonly used method for staining is Ziehl-Neelsen acid fast staining. At least 10 are examined before giving a negative report.
        - Fluorescence microscopy using auramine-rhodamine stain is more sensitive and rapid method it is used when several smears are to be examined daily.
    - Detection and identification of mycobacteria directly from specimen
    - These are alternative for smear microscopy. These are also rapid methods for diagnosis (more rapid than microscopy)
    - *Important tests are*:
        - Genotypic methods (molecular methods): PCR, TMA (transcription mediated amplification), NAA (nucleic acid amplification), Gene Xpert MTB/RIF.
        - Phenotypic methods: FAST plaque TB.
    - Gene Xpert MTB/ RIF detects DNA sequence specific for M. tuberculosis and rifampicin resist by PCR. Results are obtained within 90 minutes.

b. **Culture of tubercular bacilli**
- Isolation of mycobacteria from clinical samples by culture is the most reliable method for diagnosis.
    - For culture ~10 100 bacilli per mL.
    - For microscopy ~10000 (10^4) bacilli per mL.
    - In genitourinary tuberculosis culture of three morning urine specimens yield a definitive diagnosis in 90% of cases.
    - M. tuberculosis can be cultivated by:

    a. On conventional media
    - Mycobacterial culture on conventional media is the gold standard for primary isolation
    - Various liquid and solid media are used
    - The solid medium most widely employed for routine culture of tubercular is Lowenstein—Jensen Medium (LJ medium)
    - The major disadvantage of isolation on conventional culture media is that it takes 4–8 weeks to produce visible colonies.

    b. Automated culture-method (Liquid-medium culture with automated growth detection)
    - These methods detect growth much faster than conventional culture methods
    - Methods are:
        - » Radiometric BACTEC 460 TB
        - » MGIT-960 (Mycobacterial growth indicator tube) OR BACTEC -MGIT 960 system
        - » MB/BacT system
        - » ESP II culture system
        - » Septi-chek AFB method

    c. Serological tests
    - These are TB STA T-PAK and Insta test TB. Other serological tests are:

Name of the assays	Antigen used
Myco Dot (Dot-blot)	Lipoarabinomannan (LAM)
Detect-TB (ELISA)	Recombinant protein peptide
PathozymeMyco (ELISA)	38 kDa (recombinant Ag) and LAM
Pathozyme TB (ELISA)	38 kDA (recombinant)
Antigen A60 (ELISA)	Antigen-60
ICT diagnostics (membrane based)	38 kDa (recombinant)

The following epidemiological-indices are used in tuberculosis problem measurement and program strategy:

- Prevalence of Infection
- Incidence of infection (Annual infection rate)
  - It is the best indicator for evaluation of TB problem and its trend
  - In India, annual infection rate/tuberculin conversion index is 1.7%
- Prevalence of disease or case rate
  - It is the best available practical index to estimate the number of infectious cases or case load in a community
- Incidence of new cases
  - It is the percentage of new TB cases (confirmed by bacteriological examination) per 1000 population occurring during one year
- Prevalence of suspected cases
  - This is based on X-ray examination of chest
- Prevalence of drug resistant cases
  - It is the prevalence of patient excreting tubercle bacilli resistant to anti-tubercular drugs.
- Mortality rate.

Directly Observed Treatment Short Course (DOTS)

In the Revised National Tuberculosis Control Programme (RNTCP), patients are provided short course chemotherapy as DOTS. All patients are provided short-course chemotherapy free of charge.

- During the intensive phase of treatment, a health worker watches as the patient swallows the drug in his presence (i.e. supervised drug intake).
- During continuation phase, the patient is issued medicine for one week in a multiblistercombipack of which the first dose is swallowed by the patient in the presence of health worker. The consumption of medicine in the continuation phase is also checked by return of empty multiblistercombipack when the patient comes to collect medicine for the next week.
- In this program, alternate day treatment is given.
- Under RNTCP, active case finding is no longer pursued. Case finding is passive. Patients presenting themselves with symptoms suspicious of tuberculosis are treated with DOTS therapy.
- DOTS agents are teachers, anganwadi workers, dais, ex-patients, social workers, etc.
  National tuberculosis programme (NTP) was started in 1962. The NTP was reviewed in 1992 by Government of India, WHO and World Bank. Based on the findings a 'Revised National Tuberculosis Control Programme (RNTCPY) was launched. The objectives and salient features are:
  - To achieve at least 85% cure rate
  - To detect at least 7096 cases (achieve a case detection rate of at least70%)
  - Involvement of NGOs.

77. For diagnosis of TB, sputum microscopy has:

a. High sensitivity and high specificity
b. High sensitivity and low specificity
c. Low sensitivity and high specificity
d. Low sensitivity and low specificity

Ans. is 'd' Low sensitivity and low specificity

78. Not a component of DOTS:

a. Free drug delivery
b. Alternate day treatment
c. Medicine given for 1 month
d. All are true

Ans. is 'c' Medicine given for 1 month

79. Best indicator for spread of TB in a community:

a. Annual infection rate
b. Prevalence of infection
c. Case rate
d. Incidence of new cases

Ans. is 'a' Annual infection rate

80. Objectives of RNTCP:

a. Detects at least 85% of cases
b. Achieve at least 85% cure rate
c. No help from NGO
d. Achieve at least 90% cases are treated

Ans. is 'b' Achieve at least 85% cure rate

81. Under RNTCP, sputum microscopy should detect how much cases?

a. At least 95% b. At least 85%
c. At least 80% d. At least 70%

Ans. is 'd' At least 70%

Influenza virus: An RNA virus, belongs to orthomyxovirus.

- There are three viral subtypes: (i) Type A (causes all pandemics and most epidemics); type B; and type C (not circulating currently).
- Currently the influenza viruses circulating in the world are: H1 N1 of type A (causes swine flu); $H_2 N_2$ of type A; $H_3 N_2$ of type A; $H_5 N_1$ of type A (causes bird flu or avian influenza); $H_7 N_9$ of type A (caused epidemic of avian influenza in China in 2013); and type B.
- Influenza shows cyclic trend with epidemic occurring every 2–3 years in case of influenza - A and every 4–7 years in case of influenza-B. Pandemics are caused by only influenza-A every 10–15 years.
- Influenza affects all ages and both sexes
- Source of infection of influenza is a clinical case or subclinical case
- Major reservoir of influenza virus exists in animal and birds
- Incubation period is 18–72 hours. Most of the infections are subclinical. Clinical cases present with cough, fever, myalgia and head-ache.

Complications include pneumonia, encephalitis, Reye's syndrome (with type-B virus); GB syndrome and gastric flu/GIT symptoms (with type-B virus).

82. Most common influenza virus causing disease:

a. Type A b. Type B
c. Type C d. Type D

Ans. is 'a' Type A

83. H1 N1 strain of influenza is responsible for:

a. Avian influenza b. Bird flu
c. Swine flu d. None of the above

Ans. is 'c' Swine flu

Arthropod-Borne Diseases and Their Vectors

Arthropods	Arthropod-borne diseases	
Mosquito:	• Anopheles	Malaria Filaria (not in India)
	• Culex	Japanese encephalitis, West Nile fever, Bancroftian filariasis, Viral arthritis
	• Aedes	Yellow fever, Dengue Dengue hemorrhagic fever, Chikungunya fever Rift valley fever, Filaria (not in India) Zika virus
	Mansonoides	Brugian filariasis
• Sandfly	Kala-azar, Oriental sore, Orya fever Sand fly fever	
• Tsetse fly	Sleeping sickness	
• Louse	Epidemic typhus, relapsing fever, trench fever, pediculosis, vagabond disease	
• Rat flea	Bubonic plague, endemic typhus, chiggerosis, *Hymenolepis diminuta*	
• Black fly	Onchocerciasis	
• Reduviid bug	Chagas disease	
• Hard tick	Tick typhus, viral encephalitis, viral hemorrhagic fever, KFD tularemia, tick paralysis, human babesiosis, Lyme's disease	
• Soft tick	Q fever, relapsing fever, KFD	
• Trombiculid mite	Scrub typhus, rickettsial pox	
• Itch mite	Scabies	
• Cyclops	Guinea worm disease, fish tape worm (*D. latum*)	
• Cockroaches	Enteric pathogens	
• Housefly	Typhoid and paratyphoid fever, diarrhea, cholera gastroenteritis, amebiasis, helminthic infestations, poliomyelitis, conjunctivitis, trachoma, anthrax, yaws, etc.	

84. Louse transmits:

a. Trench fever
b. Chagas disease
c. Sleeping sickness
d. Chikungunya fever

Ans. is 'a' Trench fever

85. Which of the following is not spread by Aedes mosquito?

a. Dengue fever
b. Chikungunya
c. Japanese encephalitis
d. Yellow fever

Ans. is 'c' Japanese encephalitis

86. Reduviid bug transmits:

a. Kala-azar
b. Relapsing fever
c. Trench fever
d. Chagas disease

Ans. is 'd' Chagas disease

87. Rat flea transmits all the following *except*:

a. Plague
b. Salmonellosis
c. Hymenolepis
d. Endemic typhus

Ans. is 'b' Salmonellosis

Japanese Encephalitis (JE)

- JE is caused by flavivirus, a group B arbovirus. It is a zoonotic disease infecting mainly animals and incidentally man.
- In south, epidemics have occurred in Karnataka, Andhra Pradesh, Tamil Nadu and Kerala. Now Gorakhpur district of UP contributes largest number of cases.
- Main vector of JE transmission is *Culex* mosquito (*Culex tritaeniorhynchus*), a zoophilic rural mosquito that breeds in rice paddy fields, shallow ditches and pools. Other important vector species are *Culex vishnui* and *Culex gelidus*.
- Pigs are amplifier host; i.e. infected pigs do not manifest overt symptoms but circulate the virus so that mosquito get infected and can transmit virus to man. Horses are the only domestic animals showing symptoms of JE. Man is an 'incidental dead-end host', there is no man-to-man transmission. 'Cattle and buffaloes' act as mosquito attractants, i.e. infected but are not the natural hosts. Herons (birds) are the reservoir hosts.

88. Amplifier host in Japanese encephalitis:

a. Horse
b. Pigs
c. Dogs
d. Monkey

Ans. is 'b' Pigs

Biological Transmission

Propagative

- Agent undergoes multiplication (increase in number), but there is no development (no change in the form), for example, plague bacilli in rat flea.

Cyclo-developmental

- Agent undergoes only development (change in form) but there is no multiplication (no change in number), for example, microfilaria in mosquito.

Cyclo-propagative

- There is both development (change in form) and multiplication (change in number), for example, malarial parasite (plasmodium) in mosquito.

Diagnosis of Filariasis

A. Detection of microfilariae (Mf)

- The most commonly used method for diagnosis of filariasis is detection of micro filariae in blood smear. The blood collection should be done at night because of nocturnal periodicity of microfilariae
- Thick film is most commonly used method for detection of microfilariae
- Concentration technique by membrane filter concentration (MFC) method is the most sensitive method which can detect low density of microfilariae in blood.

Other Methods

- Detection of circulating filarial antigen (only in *W. brancrofti*) in blood by ELISA or immuno-chromatographic card test
- Detection of adult worm in lymphatics
- Detection of filarial DNA in blood
- Serological tests detecting antibodies against Mf and adults

89. Cyclo-developmental mode of transmission is seen in:

a. Plague in rat flea
b. Malaria in mosquito
c. Microfilariae in mosquito
d. Scrub typhus in mite

Ans. is 'c' Microfilariae in mosquito

90. Diagnosis of filariasis is confirmed most commonly:

a. Clinical features
b. Detection of microfilariae
c. PCR
d. Serological test

Ans. is 'b' Detection of microfilariae

Malaria

- Malaria is a protozoal disease caused by infection with parasite of genus plasmodium and transmitted to man by certain species of infected female Anopheline Mosquito
- Definitive host—Mosquito (sexual lifecycle)
- Intermediate host—Man (A sexual cycle)
- Season—In India maximum prevalence is from July to November
- Reservoir—With possible exception of chimpanzees intropical Africa, which may carry the infection with *P. malariae*, no other animal reservoir is known to exist. Man harboring sexual forms (gametocytes) is the only reservoir
- Extrinsic incubation period (inmosquito)—10 to 20 days. It is the period of time required for the development of parasite from gametocyte to sporozoite stage (infective stage to man) in the body of mosquito.
- Vector for malaria is female anopheline mosquito. There are more than 55 species in India. Six primary vectors are:
  - *An. culfacies*: Main vector of rural malaria
  - *An. stephensi*: Main vector of urban malaria. It is the most important vector in India
  - *An. fluvitalis*: Main vector in hilly areas, forests and forests fringes, especially in the east
  - *An. minimum*: Vector in the foot hills of North-Eastern states
  - *An. dirus*: Vector in the forest of North-East
  - *An. epiroticus*: Restricted to Andaman and Nicobar Islands.

Diagnosis and Treatment of Malaria

All fever cases should be investigated for malaria either by microscopy or by rapid diagnostic test (RDT) for both vivax and falciparum, i.e. combo RDT (bivalent RDT).

Further treatment is as follows:

- *For Plasmodium vivax*: 3 days chloroquine plus 14 days primaquine.
- *For Plasmodium falciparum*: Treatment for falciparum malaria is Artemisinin combination therapy (ACT). It includes:
  - *ACT-AL for North-Eastern states*: Artemether with lumefantrine for 3 days plus single dose primaquine on 2nd day.
  - *ACT-SP for all other states*: Artesunate for 3 days plus sulfadoxine-pyrimethamine on day 1 plus single dose primaquine on day2.
- *Treatment of mixed infection*: Should be treated as falciparum malaria. But primaquine is given for total 14 days (not a single dose on day 2 as is given for falciparum infection).
- When microscopy results are not available within 24 hours or if RDT for only falciparum (monovalent RD) is used:

B. Patient at high risk area for Pf (TfR> 1% and Pf% > 30% in, last 3 years)
  - *P. falciparum* RDT positive—Treat as falciparum malaria (as above).
  - *P. falciparum* RDT negative—Send blood slide to laboratory, and give chloroquine for 3 days, arid await microscopy results:
  - +ve for vivax - Primaquine for 14 days.
  - +ve for falciparum—Treatment of falciparum malaria as above.

C. Patient not at high-risk area for Pf
  - Weight for slide results, give chloroquine for 3 days and treat definitely according to species of slide results.
  - When Microscopy results are not available within 24 hours and bivalent RDT (for both vivax and falciparum) is used:
    - Positive for *P. vivax*: Treat for vivax infection (see above)
    - Positive for *P. falciparum*: Treat for falciparum infection (see above)
    - Positive for mixed infection: Treat for mixed infection (see above).
  - Treatment of severe malaria: Severe manifestations (e.g. Unconsciousness, Convulsions, Coma, Metabolic acidosis, etc.) can develop in *P. falciparum* infection. Treatment is as follows:

- Start with parenteral artemisinin derivative (artesunate, artemether, arteether) orquinine.
- *Once patient can take oral therapy:*
- Patients receiving parenteral quinine should be treated with oral quinine along with doxycycline for 7 days. In pregnant women clindamycin is given instead of doxycycline.

Patients receiving artemisinin derivatives should get full course of oral ACT.

91. Anopheles species spreading malaria in urban area:

a. *Anopheles stephensi*
b. *Anopheles subpictus*
c. *Anopheles fluviatilis*
d. *Anopheles dirus*

Ans. is 'a' *Anopheles stephensi*

92. Maximum spread of malaria occurs in which month?

a. March–April
b. January–February
c. April–May
d. September–October

Ans. is 'd' September-October

93. Incubation period of *Plasmodium vivax* is:

a. 5–7 days
b. 7–10 days
c. 10–14 days
d. 5–30 days

Ans. is 'c' 10–14 days

94. Drug of choice for falciparum malaria in endemic area:

a. Artemisinin
b. Chloroquine
c. Mefloquine
d. Halofantrine

Ans. is 'a' Artemisinin

Incubation Periods of Important Infections

Disease	Causative organism	Incubation period
Poliomyelitis	Poliovirus	7–14 days
Hepatitis A	Enterovirus 72 (Picornavirus)	15–45 days
Hepatitis B	Hepadnavirus	45–180 days
Hepatitis C	Hepacivirus	30–120 days
Hepatitis D	Deltavirus	30–90 days
Hepatitis E	Calcivirus	21–45 days
Cholera	Vibrio cholerae	1–2 days
Typhoid fever	Salmonella typhi	10–14 days
Staphylococcal food poisoning	Staphylococcus aureus	1–6 hours
Ascariasis	Ascaris lumbricoides	2 months
Ancylostomiasis (Hookworm)	Ancylostoma duodenale	5 weeks–9 months
Guinae worm (Dracunculiasis)	Dracunculus medinensis	1 year

Incubation periods of important respiratory infections

Disease	*Causative organism*	*Incubation period*
Smallpox	Variola virus	7–14 days
Chickenpox	Human (alpha) herpes virus	14–16 days
Measles (Rubella)	RNA paramyxovirus	10–14 days
Rubella (German measles)	RNA Togavirus	14–21 days
Mumps	RNA Myxovirus	14–18 days
Influenza	Orthomyxovirus	18–72 hours
Diphtheria	Corynebacterium diphtheriae	2–6 days
Pertussis (Whooping cough)	Bordetella pertussis	7–14 days
Meningococcal meningitis	Neisseria meningitis	3–4 days
SARS	Corona virus	3–5 days
Tuberculosis	Mycobacterium tuberculosis	Weeks-years

- Incubation period is the time interval between invasion by an infectious agent and appearance of the first sign and symptom.
- 'Median incubation period' is the time required for 50% cases to occur following exposure.

95. Incubation period of chickenpox:

a. 1–2 days
b. 3–5 days
c. 7–14 days
d. 14–16 days

Ans. is 'd' 14–16 days

96. Incubation period of poliomyelitis:

a. 7–14 days
b. 1–3 days
c. 15–20 days
d. 35–40 days

Ans. is 'a' 7–14 days

97. Median incubation period is:

a. Maximum time from exposure to development of symptoms in all cases
b. Minimum time from exposure to development of symptoms in all cases
c. Time for exposure to development in 50% of cases
d. None of this above

Ans. is 'c' Time for exposure to development in 50% of cases

98. Varicella zoster virus infection is more likely to occur in which of the following month:

a. March
b. August
c. October
d. November

Ans. is 'a' March

Vaccine Derived Polio Virus (VDPV)

- VDPVs resemble WPVs biologically and differ from the majority of vaccine-related poliovirus (VRPV) isolates in that they have genetic properties consistent with prolonged replication or transmission, which is substantially longer than the normal period of vaccine virus replication of 4–6 weeks in OPV recipients.
- VDPVs are divided into three categories: (1) Circulating VDPV (cVDPV), which is transmitted from person to person; (2) immunodeficiency- associated VDPV (iVDPV), which is isolated from patients with primary immunodeficiency; and (3) Ambiguous VDPV (aVDPV), which are either clinical isolates from person with no immunodeficiency or sewage isolates whose source is unknown.
- Because of emergence of VDPV, OPV use will be discontinued worldwide once all WPV transmission has been interrupted, i.e. IPV will replace OPV.

"The main cause of vaccine derived poliovirus (VDPV) outbreaks is currently type 2 component of OPV". (Previously it was due to type-3 component of OPV).

99. VDPV is due to which type of poliovirus?

a. Type-1
b. Type-2
c. Type-3
d. Type-4

Ans. is 'b' Type-2

HIV Transmission

Transmission rate:

- During pregnancy: 5–10%
- During labour and delivery: 10–15%
- During breastfeeding: 5–20%
- Overall without breastfeeding: 15–25%
- Overall with breastfeeding to six months: 20–35%
- Overall with breastfeeding to 18–24 months: 30–45%

- Vaginal and emergency caesarean section deliveries, prematurity, and low CD4 cell count were most strongly associated with infant's infection status in univariate analysis.
- Children delivered vaginally or by emergency caesarean section were more likely to be infected than those delivered by elective caesarean section with a reduction in risk of 79% associated with the latter (P<0.001).
- Similarly, infants delivered before 37 weeks were more than twice as likely to be infected than infants who were not premature.
- Caesarean section before onset of labour and rupture of membranes approximately halves the risk of mother-to-child transmission.

100. Vertical transmission of HIV is highest with: *(NEET 2019)*

a. Elective caesarean section
b. High viral RNA load
c. Breastfeeding
d. Term delivery

Ans. is 'b' High viral RNA load

Treatment of Pneumonia in Children

Antibiotics of choice for treatment of acute respiratory infections in children aged 2 months–5 years
- No pneumonia (Cough or cold)—Noantibiotic
- Pneumonia (not severe)—Co-trimoxazole
- Severe pneumonia—Benzyl penicillin or ampicillin or chloramphenicol
- Very severe disease—Chloramphenicol

Antibiotics of choice for treatment of acute respiratory infections in infants younger than 2 months
- No pneumonia (Cough or cold)—No antibiotic
- All pneumonia (severe or not severe)—(Benzyl penicillin or ampicillin) plus gentamicin.

101. Antibiotic of choice for severe pneumonia in 1 year old child:

a. Co-trimoxazole
b. Ciprofloxacin
c. Benzyl penicillin
d. Tetracycline

Ans. is 'c' Benzyl penicillin

NON-COMMUNICABLE DISEASES

"There were 69.1 million cases of diabetes in India in 2015".
- "India had 69.2 million people living with diabetes (8.7%) as per the 2015 data" WHO website
- This is around 8.7% of adult population.

The decline in infectious diseases and a rise in chronic diseases, particularly cardiovascular disease (CVD), underlies the health trajectory of the 20th century. While much was known about CVD, particularly myocardial infarction and stroke, population data were problematic. Importantly, the peak and decline of the CVD epidemic in the 1960s and 1970s in some countries was not well recognized, leading to calls for more population-based disease surveillance. The WHO Multinational **Monitoring of trends and determinants in cardiovascular disease (MONICA)** Project was the most comprehensive approach to better understanding disease etiology, incidence and trends at the population level. For a period of ten years or more in each center, from the early 1980s to the mid 1990s, MONICA implemented CVD surveillance in 21 countries. It included mortality, morbidity, coronary care, and population-based risk factor surveillance. The study is characterized by well-described methods and high quality data. The findings show large differences between different centers in 21 countries and provide information for disease treatment and prevention. Many MONICA centers continued to actively collect data on populations within their countries. This experience provides a comprehensive approach for CVD patterns in the developed countries and the oncoming epidemic in the developing world.

102. MONICA project is aimed for: *(NEET 2020)*

a. Methods of new diagnostic tests for cardiovascular disease
b. Monitoring of trends and determinants of cardiovascular disease
c. Emerging risk factors for cardiovascular disease
d. Assessing the mortality rates due to cardiovascular disease

Ans. is 'b' Monitoring of trends and determinants of cardiovascular disease

Occupational Diseases

Disease	Cause
• Anthracosis	Coal dust
• Silicosis	Silica
• Siderosis	Iron
• Byssinosis	Cotton dust (textile industry)
• Farmer's lung	Hay or grain dust (micropolysporafaeni)
• Sequoias	Moldy red wood saw dust
• Suberosis	Moldy cork dust
• Detergent worker's lung	Enzyme additives
• Bagassosis	Sugarcane dust (thermoactinomyces sacchari)

103. Prevalence of diabetes in India in adult population:

a. 1–2%
b. 3–5%
c. 5–6%
d. 7–8.5%

Ans. is 'd' 7–8.5%

104. Anthracosis is caused by:

a. Silica
b. Iron
c. Coal dust
d. Cotton dust

Ans. is 'c' Coal dust

NATIONAL HEALTH PROGRAMS, POLICIES AND LEGISLATIONS IN INDIA

Nikshay

- *New Initiatives in RNTCP*: The RNTCP has completed the feasibility study of introducing Gene-Xpert in RNTCP in 18 Tuberculosis Units in 12 states. RNTCP is currently using CB-NAAT for the diagnosis of tuberculosis and MDR-TB in high-risk population like HIV positive and pediatric groups.
- *Nikshay*: TB surveillance using case-based web-based IT system. Central TB Division in collaboration with National Informatics Center has undertaken the initiative to develop a case-based web-based application named Nikshay. This software was launched in May 2012 and has following functional components:
  - Master management
  - User details
  - TB patient registration and details of diagnosis, DOT provider, HIV status, follow-up, contact tracing, outcomes
  - Details of solid and liquid culture and DST, LPA, CBNMT details
  - MDR-TB patient registration with details
  - Referral and transfer of patients
  - Private health facility registration and TB notification
  - Mobile application for TB notification
  - SMS alerts to patients on registration
  - SMS alerts to program officers
  - Automated periodic reports
    - Case finding
    - Sputum conversion
    - Treatment outcome.
- *TB notification*: In order to ensure proper diagnosis and management of TB cases, and to reduce TB transmission and the emergence and spread of MDR-TB, it is essential to have complete information of all TB cases. According to the Government of India notification dated 7th May 2012, it is now mandatory for all healthcare providers to notify every TB case to local authorities, i.e. District Health Officer/Chief Medical Officer of a district and Municipal Health Officer, every month in a given format. At present, 57,000 health facilities have been registered and 35,000 patients have been notified.
- *Ban on TB serology*: The serological tests are based on antibody response, which is highly variable in TB and may reflect remote infection rather than active disease. Currently available serological tests are having poor specificity and should not be used for the diagnosis of pulmonary or extrapulmonary TB. Their import, manufacturing, sale, distribution and use are banned by the Government of India.

105. New RNTCP software online TB monitoring is: *(NEET 2018)*

a. Nikshay b. Nirbhaya
c. e-DOT d. Nischay

Ans. is 'a' Nikshay

Children Rights in Constitution of India

The Indian constitution accords rights to children as citizens of the country, and in keeping with their special status the state has even enacted special laws. The government has the flexibility to undertake appropriate legislative and administrative measures to ensure children's rights; no court can make the government ensure them, as these are essentially directives. These directives have enabled the judiciary to give some landmark judgments promoting children's rights, leading to Constitutional Amendments as is in the case of the 86th Amendment to the Constitution that made Right to Education a fundamental right.

Constitutional guarantees that are meant specifically for children include

- Right to free and compulsory elementary education for all children in the 6–14 year age group (Article 21A)
- Right to be protected from any hazardous employment till the age of 14 years (Article 24)
- Right to be protected from being abused and forced by economic necessity to enter occupation sun suited to their age or strength (Article 39(e))
- Right to equal opportunities and facilities to develop in a healthy manner and in conditions of freedom and dignity and guaranteed protection of childhood and youth against exploitation and against moral and material abandonment (Article 39(f))
- Right to early childhood care and education to all children until they complete the age of six years (Article 45).

Besides, children also have rights as equal citizens of India, Just as any other adult male or female

- Right to equality (Article 14)
- Right against discrimination (Article 15)
- Right to personal liberty and due process of law (Article 21)

- Right to being protected from being trafficked and forced into bonded labor (Article 23)
- Right of minorities for protection of their interests (Article 29)
- Right of weaker sections of the people to be protected from social injustice and all forms of exploitation (Article 46)
- Right to nutrition and standard of living and improved public health (Article 47).
- *Employment of young persons*: The Factory Act prohibits employment of children below the age of 14 years and declares persons between the ages 15 and 18 to be adolescents. Adolescents should be duly certified by the 'certifying surgeons, regarding their fitness for work. Restrictions have been laid down on employment of women and children in certain dangerous occupations. Child who has not completed his fourteenth year of age has been restricted from employment in any factory. Adolescent employee is allowed to work only between 6 am and 7 pm.
- *Hours of work*: The Act has prescribed a maximum of 48 working hours per week, not exceeding 9 hours per day with rest for at least half hour after 5 hours of continuous work. For adolescents, the hours of work have been reduced from 5 to 4½ per day. The 1976 amendment makes a provision to increase the spread-over period of work (including rest intervals) of an employee in a factory upto 12 hours from the existing 101/2 hours. The total number of hours of work in a week including overtime shall not exceed 60.

106. Which of the following constitutional article is not related to children rights? *(NEET 2018)*

a. 46
b. 39
c. 45
d. 23

Ans. is 'a' 46

107. Which of the following statement regarding factory Act is correct? *(NEET 2018)*

a. Child age less than 14 years cannot be employed in dangerous work
b. Child age less than 18 years cannot be employed
c. Working hours should not be more than 40 hours per week for adults
d. Working hours are 8 hours per day for children

Ans. is 'a' Child age less than 14 years cannot be employed in dangerous work

Important Days of Public Health Importance

30th January	Anti-Leprosy day
4th February	World cancer day
2nd Wednesday of March	No Smoking day
8th March	International Women's day
15th March	World Disabled day
24th March	Anti-TB day
7th April	World Health day
8th May	World Red Cross day
31st May	No Tobacco day
5th June	World Environment day
1st July	Doctors day
11thJuly	World Population day
8th September	World Literacy day
28th September	World Rabies day
29th September	World heart day
1st October	International day for older persons
10th October	World Mental Health day
24th October	UN Day
10th November	Universal Immunization day
17th November	National epilepsy day
1st December	World AIDS day
3rd December	International Day of Disabled persons
10th December	Human Rights Day

- The day 16th October on which WTG Morton demonstrated the first surgical anesthesia to the world by using ether is called as "Etherday" and now popularly known as "World Anesthesia Day".

108. World Anesthesia day is celebrated on:

a. 11 September
b. 16 October
c. 30 April
d. 11 August

Ans. is 'b' 16 October

109. National epilepsy day:

a. 7th April
b. 31st May
c. 17th November
d. 1st July

Ans. is 'c' 17th November

110. World breastfeeding week is celebrated in:

a. 1st week of September
b. Last week of September
c. 1st week of March
d. 1st week of August

Ans. is 'd' 1st week of August

111. World heart day is celebrated on:

a. 29th September
b. 28th September
c. 8th September
d. 1st December

Ans. is 'a' 29th September

MEASUREMENT OF MALARIA

Measurements of Malaria in the Pre-eradication Era

- *Spleen rate*: Defined as the percentage of children between 2 and 10 years of age showing enlargement of spleen. Spleen rate is widely used for measuring the endemicity of malaria in a community.
- *Average enlarged spleen*: A refinement of spleen rate, denoting the average size of spleen.
- *Parasite rate*: Defined as on the percentage of children between the ages of 2 and 10 yrs showing malarial parasites in their blood films.
- *Parasite density index*: Average degree of parasitemia.
- *Infant parasite rate*: Percentage of infants showing malarial parasites in their blood films. It is the most sensitive index of recent transmission of malaria in a locality. If the infant parasite rate is zero for three consecutive years in a locality, it is regarded as absence of malaria transmission even though, the Anopheline vectors responsible for previous transmissions may remain.

Eradication Era

- Annual Parasite Incidence (API) (Confirmed cases during one year/population under surveillance) x 1000. It is the sophisticated measure of malaria incidence and burden of disease in a community.
- Annual Blood Examination Rate (ABER) = (No. of slides examined/population) x 100.
- ABER is an index of operational efficiency. In the modified plan of operation, the minimum prescribed is 10% of the population in a year.
- ABER or Annual Blood Examination Rate is not an epidemiological indicator but an indicator of operational efficiency of Malaria Control Programme.
- Annual falciparum index.
- *Slide positivity rate*: Slide positivity rate is the percentage of slides found positive for malarial parasite, irrespective of the type of species.
- *Slide falciparum rate*: It is the percentage of slides positive for *P. falciparum*.

112. Which is not an epidemiological indicator? *(NEET 2019)*

a. ABER
b. Annual parasite index
c. Annual falciparum incidence
d. None of the above

Ans. is 'a' ABER

113. Under National Vector Borne Disease Control Programme, operational efficiency of anti-malarial measures is assessed by:

a. Annual Parasite Incidence (API)
b. Annual Blood Examination Rate (ABER)
c. Infant parasite rate
d. Slide positivity rate

Ans. is 'b' Annual Blood Examination Rate (ABER)

114. Jai Vigyan National Mission is for:

a. Adolescent girl's health
b. Mother and child health (MCH)
c. Science and technology
d. Child labor prevention

Ans. is 'c' Science and technology

115. National health policy was adopted India in:

a. 1977
b. 1983
c. 1995
d. 2001

Ans. is 'b' 1983

Reproductive and Child Health Programme

The various activities of Reproductive and child Health Programme (RCH) are targeted at the district level.

"The RCH programme is based on a differential approach. Inputs in all the districts have not been kept uniform.

While the care component is the same for all districts, the weaker districts will get more support and sophisticated facilities are proposed for relatively advanced districts. On the basis of crude birth rate and female literacy rate–all the districts have been divided into three categories 'A, B, and C'. All the districts will be covered in a phased manner over a period of three years."

The Sub-Centre is the most peripheral and first contact point between the primary health care system and the community. Sub-Centres are assigned tasks relating to interpersonal communication in order to bring about behavioral change and provide services in relation to maternal and child health, family welfare, nutrition, immunization, diarrhea control and control of communicable diseases programmes.

The Sub-Centres are provided with basic drugs for minor ailments needed for taking care of essential health needs of men, women and children.

116. Last point where reproductive and child health programme are targeted is: *(NEET 2019)*

a. Sub-center
b. Anganwadi
c. District
d. Taluka

Ans. is 'c' District

117. Health center in remotest area for planning and management of schemes: *(NEET 2019)*

a. Anganwadi
b. Block center
c. Sub-center
d. PHC

Ans. is 'c' Sub-center

DEMOGRAPHY, FAMILY PLANNING AND CONTRACEPTION

Maternal Mortality Ratio (MMR)

- MMR = Total no. of female death due to complications of pregnancy child birth or with 42 days of delivery from puerperal causes within an area during a given year × 1000 (or 100,000)/Total no. of live birth in the same area and year
- Maternal death occurring after 42 days (7 weeks) of birth is not included in maternal mortality ratio
- It is called late maternal death—Death of women from direct or indirect obstetric causes more than 42 days but less than 1 year after termination of pregnancy.

Maternal Mortality Rate

- It is the number of maternal deaths in a given period per 1000 (or 100,000) women of reproductive age during same period
- Maternal mortality rate = Total no. of female death due to complication of pregnancy, childbirth or within 42 days of delivery/Total no, of women of reproductive age × 1000 (or 100,000)
- Denominator in maternal mortality ratio: 1000 live birth (or 100,000 live birth)
- Denominator in maternal mortality rate: 1000 (or 100,000) women of reproductive age.

118. Denominator in MMR:

a. 1000 live birth
b. 1000 women of reproductive age
c. Mid-year population
d. Mid-year women population

Ans. is 'a' 1000 live birth

119. 10 women got pregnant out of 100 women; mean interval was 2 years. Calculate Pearl index: *(NEET 2018)*

a. 5
b. 10
c. 2
d. 4

Ans. is 'a' 5

Explanation:

The Pearl index is defined as the number of 'failures per 100 woman-years of exposure (HWY). This rate is given by the formula: Failure rate per HWY = Total accidental pregnancies/total months of exposure × 1200

From question, Pearl index = 10/24 × 1200 = 500 or 5%.

Couple Protection Rate

- The National Health Policies approved by the Parliament in1983.
- It laid down the long-term demographic goal of NRR = 1 by the year 2000 which implies a 2-child family norm—through the attainment of a birth rate of 21 and a death rate of 9 per thousand population, and a couple protection rate of 60% by the year 2000.
- The Sixth and Seventh Five-Year Plans were accordingly set to achieve these goals. The National Health Policy also called for restructuring the healthcare delivery system to achieve HFA/2000AD, and family planning has been accorded a central place in the health development.
- Couple protection rate (CPR) is an indicator of the prevalence of contraceptive practice in the community. It is defined as the percent of eligible couples effectively protected against childbirth by one or the other approved methods of family planning, viz, sterilization, IUD condom or oral pills. Sterilization accounts for over 60% of effectively protected couples. Demographers are of the view that the demographic goal of NRR= 1 can be achieved only if the CPR exceeds 60%.

120. For Net NFR to be 1 couple protection rate should be: *(NEET 2018)*

a. 60% b. 100%
c. 40% d. 80%

Ans. is 'a' 60%

Child Death Rate

- CDR = (No. of deaths of children aged 1—4 years in a year /Mid year population of children aged 1—4 years) x 1000
- Under 5 proportional mortality rate = No. of deaths under 5 years of age/Total no. of death during same period x 100

Proportional Mortality Rate (Ratio)

- Proportional mortality rate measures the proportion of total death due to specific cause or proportion of deaths in a particular age group
- It is defined as "number of deaths due to a particular cause (or in specific age group) per 100 total deaths"
- It is the 'simplest measure of estimating the burden of disease' in the community
- It is a useful 'health Status indicator'; indicates magnitude of preventable mortality
- It is used when population data is not available
- It does not indicate the risk of members of population contracting or dying from the disease.

121. Which does not have live births as denominator?

a. Infant mortality rate b. Neonatal mortality rate
c. Child mortality rate d. Child death rate

Ans. is 'd' Child death rate

122. Denominator in proportional mortality rate:

a. Mid-year population b. Total number of deaths in a year
c. Total deaths due to specific cause d. Total number of cases

Ans. is 'b' Total number of deaths in a year

123. Denominator in under-5 proportional mortality rate:

a. Number of deaths under 5 years of age b. Mid-year under-5 population
c. Total deaths d. Mid-year population

Ans. is 'c' Total deaths

124. Dual record system is useful for estimation of:

a. Literacy b. Fertility
c. Population density d. Sex ratio

Ans. is 'b' Fertility

125. A community of 500,000 people had 100 deaths in a year. Out of those 100 deaths 10 individuals died due to pulmonary TB. What is the proportional mortality rate from TB:

a. 10% b. 50%
c. 75% d. None

Ans. is 'a' 10%

(**Solution:** Proportional mortality from TB = No. of deaths due to TB in a year/Total no. of deaths in that year x 100)

Preventive and Social Medicine

126. A village has a population of 100,000. 100 died due to TB, 5 due to electrocution, 25 due to RTA and 50 due to cardiovascular accident. What is the crude death rate?

a. 2 per 1000
b. 20 per 1000
c. 1 per 1000
d. 10 per 1000

Ans. is 'a' 2 per 1000

Explanation:

- Crude death rate = No. of death during the year/Mid-year population × 1000
- Total deaths in the question are 180 (100 + 5 + 25 + 50).
- Thus CFR = 180/100,000 × 1000 = 1.8 per 1000

Mid-year Population Estimation

- Mid-year population estimates refer to population of 1st July
- In some places it can be calculated by knowing the population on 1st Jan and 31st Dec. Mid-year population is Arithmetic mean of population on 1st January and the population on 31st December of a year.

Remember

- Denominator in crude death rate is mid-year population, which is estimated on first of July of a year.

127. Mid-year population is estimated on:

a. 1st March
b. 1st July
c. 1stApril
d. 15thAugust

Ans. is 'b' 1st July

128. Mid-year population is calculated by:

a. Mean of population at 1st April of one year and 31st March of next year
b. Mean of population at 1st Jan and 31st Dec of same year
c. Mean of population on 1st Feb of one year and 31st Jan of next year
d. None of the above

Ans. is 'b' Mean of population at 1st Jan and 31st Dec of same year

PREVENTIVE OBSTETRICS, PEDIATRICS AND GERIATRICS

Daily Iron Requirement

Groups	Iron to be absorbed per day in mg	Recommended daily intake in mg
Adult male	0.84	17
Adult female (menstruating)	1.65	21
Pregnant woman	2.80 (extra-1.15)	35 (extra 14 mg/day)
Lactating woman (0–6 months)	1.65	21
Infant (6–12 months)	0.7	5
Adolescent boys (13–15 years)	1.6	32
Adolescent girls (13–15 years)	1.36	27
Adolescent boys (16–18 years)	1.37	28
Adolescent girls (16–18 years)	1.30	26

129. Daily iron recommendation in menstruating adult female: *(NEET 2018)*

a. 17
b. 21
c. 35
d. 37

Ans. is 'b' 21

Daily Iodine Requirement

The daily requirement of iodine for adults is placed at 150 mcg. The recommendations of WHO of 250 mcg per day for iodine during pregnancy have also been adopted. This amount is normally supplied by the well-balanced diet and drinking water except in regions where food and water are deficient in iodine.

130. Iodine requirement in pregnant women in micrograms per mL is: *(NEET 2018)*

a. 200
b. 150
c. 100
d. 250

Ans. is 'd' 250

Treatment of Vitamin-A Deficiency in Children

- *Oral therapy*: The oral regimen of vitamin A is 200,000 IU on day of presentation, next day and 2-4 weeks later.
- Children less than 1 year of age or less than 8 kg should receive half the dose of the above dose. Repeat 2,00,000 IU every 6 months up to 6 years of age to prevent recurrence.
- *Parenteral therapy*: If the patient has severe disease, is unable to take oral feeds, or has malabsorption, the preferable dose is 100,000 IU of vitamin A given intramuscularly.
- Children with severe measles should also receive vitamin A as they are very likely to be benefited from such therapy both in terms of saving sight and reducing case fatality.

Prevention

- Prophylaxis consists of periodic administration of Vitamin A supplements. WHO recommended schedule, which is universally recommended is as follows:
  - Infants 6–12 months old and any older children weighing less than 8 kg–100,000 IU orally every 3–6 months
  - Children over 1 year and under 6 years of age–200,000 IU orally every 6 months
  - Infants less than 6 months old, who are not being breastfed–50,000 IU orally should be given before they attain the age of 6 months

131. A 2-year-old boy of weight 12 kg with vitamin A deficiency what is oral dose of vitamin A? *(NEET 2019)*

a. 50, 000 IU
b. 1 lakh IU
c. 1.5 lakh IU
d. 2 lakh IU

Ans. is 'd' 2 lakh IU

Breathing Rate in Children

As the children get older, their breathing rate slows down.
Therefore, the cut-off point has fast breathing will depend on the age of the child. Fast breathing is present when the respiratory rate is:

- Child less than 2 months of age—60 breaths per minute
- Child aged 2 months upto 12 months—50 breaths per minute
- Child aged 12 months upto 5 years—40 breaths per minute

132. According to IMNCI, in a baby of 6-month-old age criteria for fast breathing is more than___/min *(NEET 2019)*

a. 60
b. 50
c. 40
d. 30

Ans. is 'b' 50

Consanguinity

Consanguinity is a marriage between relatives and has various degrees. Closely related individuals have a higher chance of carrying the same alleles than those less closely related and therefore children from consanguineous marriages are more frequently homozygous for various alleles than those from non-consanguineous unions.

Generally speaking, frequency of congenital malformations among newborns of first cousin unions is about 2 times the frequency among the general population. In other words, instead of a rate of 2–3% of birth defects in the general population, the risk to first cousin couples is around 4–6%.

133. Risk of genetic diseases in consanguineous marriage between first cousins? *(NEET 2019)*

a. 1–2%
b. 4–8%
c. 8–10%
d. 12–14%

Ans. is 'b' 4–8%

NUTRITION AND HEALTH

Criteria for Indian reference Man and Woman		
	Indian reference man	*Indian reference woman*
Energy requirements		
Light work	2320 kcal/day	1900 kcal/day
Moderate work	2730 kcal/day	2230 kcal/day
Heavy work	3490 kcal/day	2850 kcal/day

134. A 70 kg farmer is consuming 56 grams proteins, 275 grams carbohydrate and 60 grams lipids. He is consuming:

a. Less calories
b. More calories
c. Adequate calories
d. Cannot be commented

Ans. is 'a' Less calories

135. Energy requirement for woman doing heavy work (in Kcal/d):

a. 1500 b. 1900
c. 2250 d. 2850

Ans. is 'd' 2850

Recommended Protein Allowances

Recommended Protein Allowances		
Group	*Particulars*	*g/kg/day*
Man (60 kg)	Sedentary work Moderate work Heavy work	1
Woman (55 kg)	Sedentary work Moderate work Heavy work	1
Infants	0-6 months	1.16
	6-12 months	1.69
Children	1-3 years	1.3
	4-6 years	1.12
	7-9 years	1.18
Adolescent Males	10-12 years	1.16
	13-15 years	1.14
	16-18 years	1.11
Adolescents Females	10-12 years	1.15
	13-15 years	1.11
	16-18 years	1.06
Adult male and female		1

136. Protein requirement in an adult male per day:

a. 1 g/kg/day b. 1.5 g/kg/day
c. 2 g/kg/day d. 5 g/kg/day

Ans. is 'a' 1 g/kg/day

There are two major forms of iron:

1. **Heme-iron**
   - It is better absorbed but is less important source of iron in Indian diet. It is mainly found in foods of animal origin, e.g. liver, meat, poultry and fish
   - Red meat is the richest source of iron.
2. **Non-heme iron**
   - It is poorly absorbed but is the important source of iron in Indian diet. It is mainly found in foods of vegetable origin, e.g. cereals, green leafy vegetables
   - Among dry fruits, cashew nut has maximum iron (9%) followed by almonds (7%), and pistachios (7%)
   - Iron of milk is low in all mammalian species
   - Jaggery is considered as poor man's iron source. It contains good amount of iron along with vitamin-A.

137. Poor man's iron source is:

a. Almond b. Grapes
c. Soya d. Jaggery

Ans. is 'd' Jaggery

Body Mass Index

Classification	BMI (kg/m²)	
	Global population (WHO international)	Indian population
Grade III severe under weight	<16	
Grade II (moderate) under weight	16.0–16.9	
Grade I (mild) under weight	17.0–18.49 (<18.5)	<18.5
Normal	18.5–24.99	18.5–22.99
Overweight (pre- obese)	25–29.99	23–24.99
Obesity	> 30	> 25
• Class I	30.00–34.99	
• Class II • Class III	35.00–39.99 > 40.00	

Indices for Obesity

- Body mass Index (Quetelets Index)
  - It is used internationally as reference standard for assessing the prevalence of obesity
  - It is dependent both on height and weight.

$$BMI = \text{Weight in kg}/(\text{Height in meters})^2$$

- Ponderal Index
  - It is dependent both on height and weight
  - It is defined as height (cm) divided by cube root of weight(kg).
- Broca Index = Ideal weight = Height (cm)–100
  It is the simplest Index.
- Corpulence Index = Actual weight/Desirable weight
  It is dependent only on weight (height independent). It should be < 1.2

138. To define obesity on the basis of BMI, it should be:

a. > 20　　b. >30
c. > 35　　d. >40

Ans. is 'b' >30

139. An adult male has weight 50 kg and height 150 cm. He is:

a. Underweight　　b. Normal
c. Pre-obese　　d. Obese

Ans. is 'b' Normal

140. Ponderal Index is:

a. Height–100　　b. Height/3 root weight
c. Weight/Height　　d. Weight/[height^2]

Ans. is 'b' Height/3 root weight

Gomez Classification

- It is based on weight retardation (not on height retardation)
- The child on the basis of his/her weight is compared with a 'normal' child of the same age
- The 'normal' reference child is the 50th centile of the Boston standards.

Weight for age (%) = (Weight of child / weight of normal child of same age) × 10	
90–110%	Normal nutritional status
75–89%	Mild malnutrition 1st degree
60–70%	Moderate malnutrition 2nd degree
Under 60%	Severe malnutrition 3rd degree

- Classification is easy to compute as weight is widely recorded parameter
- Classification has prognostic value for hospitalized patients (This is because the Cut off values were set during a study of risk of death based on weight for age at admission to a hospital unit).

141. Gomez classification is based on:

a. Weight retardation　　b. Height retardation
c. Mid-arm circumference　　d. Stunting

Ans. is 'a' Weight retardation

Dietary Fiber

- Constituents of dietary fiber:
  - Cellulose
  - Hemicellulose
  - Inulin
  - Pectins
  - Mucilages
  - Gums
  - Lignin
  - Algal polysaccharides

- Dietary fibre consists of unabsorbable cell wall and other constituents of vegetable food like cellulose, lignin, hemicellulose, gums, pectins, glycoproteins and other polysaccharides.
- Dietary fibre absorbs water in the intestine, swells, increase bulk of stood by increasing water content of faeces and soften it, decreases transit time by facilitating colonic transit.
- "The presence of fibre shortens the transit times and increases the stool bulk".

Dietary fibre is of two types:

1. *Soluble fibre*: It absorbs upto 15 times its weight in water as it moves through GIT, producing softer stools. Its good sources are oat, flaxseeds, peas, beans, apple, citrus fruits, carrots, barley and psyllium.
2. *Insoluble fibre*: It promotes movement of material through digestive system and increases stool bulk. Its good sources are wheat flour, wheat bran, nuts and vegetables.

142. All of the following are examples of Dietary fibre *except*: *(NEET 2019)*

a. Pectin b. Lignin
c. Cellulose d. Gums

Ans. is None (All options are dietary fibres)

SOCIAL SCIENCES AND HEALTH

Acculturation

- **Acculturation** is a process of social, psychological, and cultural change that stems from the balancing of two cultures while adapting to the prevailing culture of the society.
- Acculturation is a process in which an individual adopts, acquires and adjust to a new cultural environment. Individuals of a differing culture try to incorporate themselves into the new more prevalent culture by participating in aspects of the more prevalent culture, such as their traditions, but still hold onto their original cultural values and traditions.
- The effects of acculturation can be seen at multiple levels in both the devotee of the prevailing culture and those who are assimilating into the culture
- It is a Culture contact, when there is contact between two peoples with different types of culture. There is diffusion of culture in both ways.

143. Acculturation is defined as:

a. Loss of culture sense b. Isolation of two culture
c. Fading away of culture d. Cultural contact

Ans. is 'd' Cultural contact

ENVIRONMENT AND HEALTH

Yellow Fever Vaccination for Travelers

- Measures designed to restrict the spread of yellow fever are specified in the "International health regulation" of WHO.
- These are implemented by the Govt. of India through stringent aerial and maritime traffic regulations. Broadly these comprise:

I. Travelers

- All travelers (including infants) exposed to yellow fever or passing through endemic zones of yellow fever must possess a valid international certificate of vaccination against yellow fever before they are allowed to enter yellow fever receptive areas like India.
- The validity of the certificate begins 10 days after the date of vaccination and extends up to 10 years.
- Revaccination performed before the end of the validity of certificate renders the certificate valid for a further period of 10 years starting on the day of revaccination.
- If no such certificate of vaccination is available, the traveler is placed on quarantine for 6 days from the date of leaving an infected area.

II. Mosquitoes

- The aircraft and ships arriving from endemic areas are subjected to aerosol spraying with prescribed insecticides.
- Airports and Seaports are kept free from the breeding of insect vectors over an area extending at least 400 meters around their perimeters.
- The "*Aedes aegypti* index" is kept below 1.
- Aedes do not fly over long distances; usually less than 100 metres (110 yards).

Anopheles	3–5 km
Culex	11 km
Aedes	100 m

144. To control yellow fever Airports should be kept mosquito free around their perimeters for up to:

a. 400 m
b. 200 m
c. 500 m
d. 100 m

Ans. is 'a' 400 m

145. Range of flight of Aedes mosquito is:

a. 1 km
b. Less than 100 m
c. 400 m
d. 10 km

Ans. is 'b' Less than 100 m

Chlorination

- Chlorination is one of the greatest advances of water purification. It is a supplement not a substitute to sand filtration. Chlorine kills pathogenic bacteria, but it has no effect on spores and certain viruses (e.g. polio, viral hepatitis) except in high doses. Apart from its germicidal effect, chlorine has several important secondary properties of value in water treatment: It oxidizes iron, manganese and hydrogen sulfide; it destroys some taste and odor producing constituents; it controls algae and slime organisms; and aids coagulation.
- *Action of chlorine*: When chlorine is added to water, there is a formation of hydrochloric and hypochlorous acids. The hydrochloric acid is neutralized by the alkalinity of the water. The hypochlorous acid ionizes to form hydrogen ions and hypochlorite ions.
- The disinfecting action of chlorine is mainly due to the hypochlorous acid, and to a small extent due to the hypochlorite ions. The hypochlorous acid is the most effective form of chlorine for water disinfection. It is more effective (70–80 times) than the hypochlorite ion. Chlorine acts best as a disinfectant when the pH of water is around 7 because of the predominance of hypochlorous acid. When the pH value exceeds 8.5 it is unreliable as a disinfectant because about 90% of the hypochlorous acid gets ionized to hypochlorite ions. It is fortunate that most waters have a pH value between 6–7.5.
- *Principles of chlorination*: The mere addition or chlorine to water is not chlorination. There are certain rules which should be obeyed in order to ensure proper chlorination:
  - First of all, the water to be chlorinated should be clear and free from turbidity. Turbidity impedes efficient chlorination.
  - Secondly, the 'chlorine demand' of the water should be estimated. 'The chlorine demand of water is the difference between the amount of chlorine added to the water and the amount of residual chlorine remaining at the end of a specific period of contact (usually 60 minutes) at a given temperature and pH of the water'. In otherwords, it is the amount of chlorine that is needed to destroy bacteria and to oxidize all the organic matter and ammoniacal substances present in the water. The point at which the chlorine demand of the water is met is called the 'breakpoint'. If further chlorine is added beyond the breakpoint, free chlorine (HOCI and OCI) begins to appear in the water.
  - Thirdly the contact period. The presence of free residual chlorine for a contact period of at least 1 hour is essential to kill bacteria and viruses. It should be noted however, that chlorine has no effect on spores, protozoan cysts and helminthic ova, except in higher doses.
  - The minimum recommended concentration of free chlorine is 0.5 mg/L for one hour. The free residual chlorine provides a margin of safety against subsequent microbial contamination such as may occur during storage and distribution.
  - The sum of the chlorine demand of the specific water plus the free residual chlorine of 0.5mg/L constitutes the correct dose of chlorineto be applied.

Water type	Recommended	
	Residual chlorine level	*Contact period*
Drinking water	>0.5 mg per litre (ppm)	1 hour
Water bodies, post disaster	>0.7 mg per litre (ppm)	1 hour
Swimming pool sanitation	>1.0 mg per litre (ppm)	1 hour

Remember

Instrument	Utility
Horrock' Apparatus	Chlorine demand estimation
Chlorinator/Chloronome	Mixing or regulating dose of chlorine
Chloroscope	Measuring residual level of chlorine

146. Chlorine disinfection of water is due to which ions?

a. Hypochlorous acid
b. Hypochlorite ions
c. Hydrogen ions
d. Hydrochloric acid

Ans. is 'a' Hypochlorous acid

147. Disinfective action of chlorine is mainly due to:

a. Hypochlorous acid
b. Hypochlorous ion
c. Hypochlorite ion
d. None

Ans. is 'a' Hypochlorous acid

148. Residual chlorine in drinking water should be:

a. 0.5 mg/L
b. 0.7 mg/L
c. 1 mg/L
d. 2 mg/L

Ans. is 'a' 0.5 mg/L

149. Horrock's apparatus is used for:

a. Wind velocity
b. Chlorine demand
c. Water contamination
d. Coliform count

Ans. is 'b' Chlorine demand

Hardness of Water

Hardness may be defined as the soap destroying power of water. The consumer considers water is hard if large amounts of soap are required to produce lather. The hardness in water is caused mainly by four dissolved compounds. These are:

1. Calcium bicarbonate
2. Magnesium bicarbonate
3. Calcium sulfate
4. Magnesium sulfate

The presence of any one of these compounds produces hardness. There are others which are of less importance. Chlorides and nitrates of calcium and magnesium can also cause hardness but they occur generally in small amounts. Iron, manganese and aluminium compounds also cause hardness, but as they generally are present in such small amounts, it is customary not to consider them in connection with hardness.

Hardness is classified as carbonate and non-carbonate. The carbonate hardness which was formerly designated as 'temporary' hardness is due to the presence of calcium and magnesium bicarbonates. The non-carbonate hardness formerly designated as 'permanent' hardness is due to calcium and magnesium sulfates, chlorides and nitrates.

Hardness in water is expressed in terms of 'milliequivalents per litre (mEq/L)'. One mEq/L of hardness producing ion is equal to 50 mg $CaCO_3$ (50 ppm) in 1litre of water. The terms soft and hard water are used when the levels of hardness are as given in the table. Drinking water should be moderately hard. Softening of water is recommended when the hardness exceeds 3 mEq/L (150 mg per liter).

Classification of hardness in water

Classification	*Level of hardness (mEq/litre)*
Soft water	Less than 1 (<50 mg/L)
Moderately hard	1–3 (50–150 mg/L)
Hard water	3–6 (150–300 mg/L)
Very hard water	Over 6 (>300 mg/L)

150. Hardness of water is not due to: *(NEET 2018)*

a. Calcium carbonate
b. Calcium sulfate
c. Calcium bicarbonate
d. Magnesium bicarbonate

Ans. is 'a' Calcium carbonate

Air Pollutants

Primary Pollutants

- These are substances directly emitted from a process, e.g. from factories.
- SO, NO, ammonia, chlorofluorocarbons (OECs), particulate material (smoke and dust), Volatile organic compounds VOCs (methane, benzene, toluene, xylene), and toxic metals (lead, cadmium).

Secondary Pollutants

- They form in air when primary pollutants react
- Examples are ground level ozone and peroxyacetyl nitrate
- Ground level ozone is formed by reaction of nitrogen oxides and volatile organic compounds, e.g. methane.

151. Not a primary air pollutant:

a. SO_2
b. CO_2
c. Ozone
d. VOCs

Ans. is 'c' Ozone

Monitoring of Air Pollution

The best **indicators** of air pollution are **sulphur dioxide., smoke** and **suspended particles**. These are monitored on a daily basis over several sites. The results are then collected by a central agency.

- *Sulphur dioxide:* This gas is a major contaminant in many urban and industrial areas. Its concentration is estimated in all air pollution surveys.
- *Smoke* or *soiling Index:* A known volume of air is filtered through a white filter paper under specified conditions and the stain is measured by photoelectric meter. Smoke concentration is estimated and expressed as micrograms/cubic metre of air as an average age level over a period of time.
- *Grit* and *dust measurement:* Deposit gauges collect grit, dust and other solids. These are analyzed monthly.
- *Coefficient of haze:* A factor used, particularly in the USA in assessing the amount of smoke or other aerosol in air.
- *Air pollution Index:* It is an arbitrary index which takes into account one or more pollutants as a measure of the severity of pollution.

152. Indicators used for routine assessment of air pollution are: *(NEET 2020)*

a. CO, SO_2, H_2S
b. SO_2, smoke, lead
c. CO, H_2S, lead
d. SO_2, smoke, suspended particles

Ans. is 'd' SO_2, smoke, suspended particles

Explanation: Direct line from Park's Textbook of PSM.

153. Which is an indoor air pollutant?

a. Benzene
b. Ozone
c. Asbestos
d. All of the above

Ans. is 'd' All of the above

Sound Intensity

Whisper	30 dB
Normal conversation	60 dB
Shout	90 dB
Discomfort of ear	120 dB
Pain in ear	130 dB

154. Sound intensity of whispering:

a. 30 dB
b. 60dB
c. 90 dB
d. 120dB

Ans. is 'a' 30 dB

155. Household insecticide used for malaria:

a. Malathion
b. Pyrethrum
c. Paris green
d. Permethrin

Ans. is 'a' Malathion

Indian Factories Act

- The first Indian Factories Act dates as far back as 1881.
- The Act was revised and amended several times, the latest being the Factories (Amendment) Act, 1987
- The standards laid down by the factories Act:

Health, Safety and Welfare

- Following standards are recommended:
  - A minimum of 500 Cu ft of space for each worker (not taking into account space more than 14 feet above the group level).
  - For factories installed before the 1948 Act, a minimum of 350 Cuft of space per worker.
  - A Safety Officer in every factory where in 1000 or workers are employed
  - A Welfare Officer in every factory where in 500 or more workers are employed.
  - A canteen where in more than 250 or more workers are employed.
  - Creches where in more than 30 women workers are employed.

Employment of Young Persons

- *Standards are*:
  - Children less than 14 years have been restricted from employment in factories.
  - Adolescents (15–18 years) need to be duly certified by certifying surgeons regarding their fitness for work.
  - Adolescent employee is allowed to work only between 6 AM to 7 PM.

Standards of Work

- A maximum of 48 hours per week, not exceeding 9 hours per day with rest for at least l hour after 5 hours of continuous work.
- For adolescent - 4/2 hours per day
- The total number of hours of work in a week including overtime shall not exceed 60.

Leave with Wages

- Leave with wages after 12 months continuous service:
  - One day for every 20 days of work in adult
  - One day for every 15 days of work in children
- The leave can be accumulated up to 30 days in case of adults and 40 days in case of children.

156. Minimum floor space recommended for worker according to Factories Act:

a. 1000 Cu ft b. 500 Cu ft
c. 200 Cu ft d. 100 Cu ft

Ans. is 'b' 500 Cu ft

Under the Factories Act, no adult worker shall be required or allowed to work in a factory for more than nine hours in any day or No adult worker shall be required or allowed to work in a factory for more than forty-eight hours in any week.

Under special circumstances these can be increased yet:

- The total number of hours of work in any day shall not exceed ten
- The spread over, inclusive of intervals for rest, shall not exceed twelve hours in any one day
- **The total number of hours of work in a week, including overtime, shall not exceed sixty**
- The total number of hours of overtime shall not exceed fifty for any one quarter.

157. Maximum hours of work in a week under Factories Act including overtime is: *(NEET 2020)*

a. 48 hrs b. 60 hrs
c. 72 hrs d. 84 hrs

Ans. is 'b' 60 hrs

ESI ACT

Sickness Benefit under ESI scheme represents periodical cash payments made to an insured person (IP) during the period of certified sickness occurring in a benefit period when IP requires medical treatment and attendance with abstention from work on medical grounds. **Sickness benefit is 70% of the average daily wages and is payable for 91 days during 2 consecutive benefit periods.**

Extended Sickness Benefit (ESB)

Insured persons suffering from long term diseases were experiencing great hardship on expiry of 91 days Sickness benefit. Often they, though not fit for duty, pressed for a Final certificate. Hence, a provision for paying **Sickness Benefit for an extended period (Extended Sickness Benefit) of up to 2 years in a ESB period of 3 years**

Following are eligible for ESB (NO NEED TO REMEMBER ALL, just have a glance but remember TB)

- **Infectious Diseases**
  - Tuberculosis
  - Leprosy
  - Chronic Empyema
  - AIDS
- **Neoplasms**
  - Malignant Diseases
- **Endocrine, Nutritional and Metabolic Disorders**
  - Diabetes Mellitus-with proliferative retinopathy/diabetic foot/nephropathy.
- **Disorders of Nervous System**
  - Monoplegia
  - Hemiplegia
  - Paraplegia
  - Hemiparesis
  - Intracranial Space Occupying Lesion
  - Spinal Cord Compression
  - Parkinson's disease
  - Myasthenia Gravis/Neuromuscular Dystrophies

- ❖ **Disease of Eye**
  - Immature Cataract with vision 6/60 or less
  - Detachment of Retina
  - Glaucoma
- ❖ **Diseases of Cardiovascular System**
  - Coronary Artery Disease: (a) Unstable Angina (b) Myocardial infraction with ejection less than 45%
  - Congestive Heart Failure: Left, Right
  - Cardiac Valvular Diseases with failure/complications
  - Cardiomyopathies
  - Heart disease with surgical intervention alongwith complications
- ❖ **Chest Diseases**
  - Bronchiectasis
  - Interstitial Lung Disease
  - Chronic Obstructive Lung Diseases (COPD) with congestive heart failure (Cor Pulmonale)
- ❖ **Diseases of the Digestive System**
  - Cirrhosis of liver with ascities/chronic active hepatitis
- ❖ **Orthopaedic Diseases**
  - Dislocation of vertebra/prolapse of intervertebral disc
  - Non union or delayed union of fracture
  - Post Traumatic Surgical amputation of lower extremity
  - Compound fracture with chronic osteomyelitis
- ❖ **Psychoses**
  - Sub-group under this head are listed for clarification (a) Schizophrenia, (b) Endogenous depression, (c) Manic Depressive Psychosis (MDP) and (d) Dementia
- ❖ **Others**
  - More than 20% burns with infection/complication
  - Chronic Renal Failure
  - Reynaud's disease/Burger's disease.

158. 7. Sickness benefit that a TB patient receives under ESI Act is for: *(NEET 2020)*

a. 1 year
b. 2 years
c. 90 days
d. 6 months

Ans. is 'b' 2 years

Instruments and their Use

Instruments	Measure
Sling psychrometer	Humidity
Assmann psychrometer	Humidity
Dry and wet bulb hygrometer	Humidity
Kata thermometer	Cooling power and air velocity
Globe thermometer	Radiant temperature
Anemometer	Air velocity
Wind vine	Wind (air) direction
Sound level meter	Intensity of sound
Bond frequency analyzer	Characteristic (pitch) of sound

159. Kata Thermometer is used to measure:

a. Maximum temperature
b. Minimum temperature
c. Radiant heat
d. Cooling power of air

Ans. is 'd' Cooling power of air

160. Sling psychrometer is used to measure:

a. Cooling power
b. Air velocity
c. Wind direction
d. Humidity

Ans. is 'd' Humidity

161. For trench type of sanitary filling the amount of land required for 2-meter-deep trench for 10000 population is: *(NEET 2019)*

a. 1 acre
b. 2 acres
c. 3 acres
d. 4 acres

Ans. is 'a' 1 acre

Solution: General WHO Guidelines for Shallow Trenches is 3–5 metre for 100 People. So, about 300–500 Meter of Shallow Trenches for 10,000 People. Also, there should be a perimeter of 30 m around the trench. Now 1 Acre = 4046 Sq Meter [200 m × 200 m].

BIOMEDICAL WASTE MANAGEMENT

CATEGORIES OF BIOMEDICAL WASTES (BMW)

Schedule: Categories of biomedical wastes (BMW)		
Waste category n.	***Waste category type***	***Treatment and disposal options***
Category 1	Human anatomical waste: Human tissues, organs, body parts	Incineration/deep burial
Category 2	Animal waste: Animal tissues, organs, body parts carcasses, bleeding parts, fluid, blood and experimental animals used in research, waste generated by veterinary hospital, animal house	Incineration/deep burial
Category 3	Microbiology and biotechnology waste: waste from laboratory culture, stocks or specimens of microorganisms live or attenuated vaccines. Human and animal cell culture used/research and infectious agents from research and industrial laboratories, waste from production of biologicals, toxins, dishes and devices used for transfer of cultures	Local autoclaving/microwaving incineration
Category 4	Waste sharps: Needles, syringes, scalpels, blades, glass, etc. that may cause puncture and cuts. This includes both used and unused sharps	Disinfection (chemical treatment/autoclaving/ microwaving and mutilation/shredding)
Category 5	Discarded medicines and cytotoxic drugs: wastes comprising of outdated, contaminated and discarded medicines	Incineration/autoclaving/microwaving
Category 6	Soiled waste: Items contaminated with blood, and body fluids, including cotton, dressings, soiled plaster casts, lines, bedding, other material contaminated with blood	Incineration/autoclaving/microwaving
Category 7	Solid waste: Waste generated from disposable items other than the waste sharps such as tubing, catheters, intravenous sets, etc.	Disinfection by chemical treatment/autoclaving/ microwaving and mutilation/shredding
Category 8	Liquid waste: Waste generated from laboratory and washing, cleaning, housekeeping and disinfecting activities	Disinfection by chemical treatment and discharge into drain
Category 9	Incineration ash: Ash from incineration of any biomedical waste	Disposal in municipal landfill
Category 10	Chemical waste: chemicals used in the production of disinfection, insecticides, etc.	Chemical treatment and discharges into drains for liquids and secured landfill for solids

Advantages and Disadvantages of Treatment and Disposal for BMW

Treatment/disposal	Advantages	Disadvantages
Incineration	• High efficiency of disinfection • Suitable for infectious and hazardous waste	• Cytotoxic may be partially destructed • High capital and O and M costs
Kiln	Suitable for infectious and hazardous waste.	High capital and OandM costs.
Disinfection by chemical	• Disinfection is effective under suitable operational parameters • Few disinfectants are inexpensive • Significant waste volume reduction	• Qualified manpower for O and M is required • Hazardous chemicals require safety measures • Unsuitable for selected chemicals and contagious wastes
Single chamber incineration	• Good disinfection efficiency • Reduced weight and volume of waste. • Residues can be disposed inland fills • Trained manpower may not be required • Low capital and O and M costs	• Substantial emissions to atmosphere • Removal of air pollutants is important • Inefficient in destruction of thermally resistant wastes
Thermal treatment	• Significant waste volume reduction • Low capital and O and M costs	• Qualified manpower for O and M is required • Not suitable for BMW.
Drum incinerator	• Significant reduction of weight/volume of waste • Low capital and O and M costs	• Selected chemicals do not get destructed • Substantial emissions to atmosphere (flow gas smoke, and odor)
Encapsulation	• Low capital and O and M costs • Suitable for other hazardous wastes	• Not suitable for BMW
Burial	• Low capital and O and M cost	• Suitable where site access is restricted and precautionary measures are followed.
Irradiation	Good disinfection efficiency Significant waste volume reduction	High capital and OandM cost Possibility of OandM problems

Category	Type of waste (Older cat no.)	Bag/Container	Treatment and disposal options
Yellow	(a) Human anatomical waste (1) (b) Animal anatomical (2)	Yellow non-chlorinated plastic bags	Incineration/Plasma pyrolysis/Deep burial
	(c) Soiled waste (6)		Incineration/Plasma pyrolysis/Deep burial OR Autoclaving/Microwaving/Hydroclaving THEN Shredding/Mutilation
	(d Expired/ Discarded Medicines (5) (e) Chemical waste	Yellow non-chlorinated plastic bags or containers	Incineration/Encapsulation/Plasma pyrolysis
	(f) Chemical liquid waste (8)	Separate collection system leading to effluent treatment system	Pretreatment THEN Drain
	(g) Discarded linen, mattresses, beddings contaminated with blood or body fluid	Non-chlorinated yellow plastic bags or suitable packing material	Non-chlorinated chemical disinfection THEN Incineration/Plasma pyrolysis/Energy recovery OR shredding mutilation
	(h) Microbiology, Biotechnology Clinical laboratory waste (3)	Autoclave safe plastic bags or containers	Pre-treat with non-chlorinated chemicals THEN Incineration
Red		Red non-chlorinated plastic bags or containers	Autoclaving/Microwaving/Hydroclaving THEN Shredding/Mutilation THEN Energy recovery/Plastics to diesel or fuel oil/road making
White (Translucent)		Puncture proof, Leak proof, Tamper proof containers	Autoclaving / Dry heat THEN Shredding/ Mutilation/Encapsulation THEN Iron foundries/ Sanitary landfill/Waste sharp pit
Blue	(a) Glassware (4) (b) Metallic body implants	Cardboard boxes with blue colored making	Sodium hypochlorite/Autoclaving/Microwaving/ Hydroclaving THEN Recycling

162. Cytotoxic and expired drugs are disposed by: *(NEET 2018)*

a. Incineration
b. Deep burial
c. Chemical treatment
d. Autoclaving

Ans. is 'a' Incineration

163. Advantage of single chamber incinerator: *(NEET 2018)*

a. Low pollutant emissions
b. Effective for thermally resistant articles
c. Good efficiency
d. All of the above

Ans. is 'c' Good efficiency

164. Human anatomical waste should be disposed in: *(NEET 2018)*

a. Yellow bag
b. Red bag
c. Blue bag
d. Black bag

Ans. is 'a' Yellow bag

165. Category 4 biochemical waste includes: *(NEET 2018)*

a. Human anatomical waste
b. Animal waste
c. Cytotoxic drug
d. Waste sharps

Ans. is 'd' Waste sharps

DISASTER MANAGEMENT

DISEASES COMMON IN POST-DISASTER PHASE

- Gastroenteritis (MC)
- Acute respiratory tract infections (Pneumonia)
- Leptospirosis

- Rickettsiosis
- Rabies
- Equine encephalitis

166. Most common epidemic after disaster is:

a. Gastroenteritis
b. Respiratory infection
c. Wound infection
d. Leptospirosis

Ans. is 'a' Gastroenteritis

HEALTH EDUCATION AND COMMUNICATION

HEALTH EDUCATION VS PROPAGANDA

Education	Propaganda or publicity
• Knowledge and skills actively acquired	Knowledge instilled in the mind of people
• Makes people think for themselves	Prevents or discourages thinking by ready-made slogans
• Disciplines primitive desires	Arouses and stimulates primitive desires
• Develops reflective behavior; Trains people to use judgment before acting	Develops reflexive behavior; aims at making impulsive actions
• Appeals to reason	Appeals to emotion
• Develops individuality personality and self-expression	Develops a standard pattern at attitudes and behaviors according to the mold used
• Knowledge acquired through self-reliant activity	Knowledge is spoon-fed and passively received
• The process is behavior centered—aims at developingfavorable attitudes, habits and skills	The process is information-centered, no change of attitude or behavior designed

Types of Communication

1. **One-way communication (Didactic method)**
   - One-way communication is one in which information is always transferred in only one pre-assigned direction, i.e. from communicator to the audience.
   - *Example*: Lectures, demonstration, mass media communication (TV radio, internet).
2. **Two-way communication (Socratic method)**
   - It is method of communication in which both the communicator and the audience take part and the information is transferred in both directions.
   - *Examples*: Group discussion, Panel discussion, **symposium**, workshop, conferences.
3. **Verbal communication**
   - Communication by words of mouth.
4. **Nonverbal communication**
   - Communication without words, by whole range of bodily movements, postures, gestures, facial expressions (e.g. smiling, frown).
5. **Formal and informal education**
   - *Follows lines of authority*: Formal communication.
   - From channels that fall outside the formal communication—informal (grape-vine) communication.
6. **Visual communication, charts, graphs, tables etc.**
7. **Telecommunication and internet**
   - Telecommunication is the process of communication over distance using electromagnetic instruments designed for the purpose, e.g. Radio, TV and internet

167. Propaganda is defined as:

a. Knowledge by active learning
b. Knowledge forced into the mind
c. Facilitates learning
d. Develops reflective behavior

Ans. is 'b' Knowledge forced into the mind

168. Which of the following is Socratic method of communication?

a. Lectures
b. Group discussion
c. Demonstration
d. Mass media

Ans. is 'b' Group discussion

169. Two-way communication is:

a. Symposium
b. Lectures
c. Demonstration
d. All of the above

Ans. is 'a' Symposium

HEALTH CARE IN INDIA, HEALTH PLANNING AND MANAGEMENT

Designated microscopy center (DMC): The most peripheral laboratory under the RNTCP network is the DMC which Serves a population of around 100,000 (50,000 in tribal and hilly areas).

- Currently all the districts in the country are implementing EQA. For quality improvement purposes, the NRL on-site evaluation (OSE) recommendations to IRLs and districts are discussed in the RNTCP laboratory committee meetings, quarterly at CTD.
- Quality improvement workshops for the state level TB officer sand laboratory managers are conducted at NRL5 based on the observations of the NRL-OSE5. These workshops focus on issues such as human resources, training, AMC for binocular microscopes, quality specifications for ZN stains, RBRC blinding and coding issues, biomedical waste disposal, infection control measures, etc.

The quality assurance activities include:

- On-site evaluation
- Panel testing
- Random blinded rechecking

170. Most peripheral unit of microscopic center of TB is: *(NEET 2018)*

a. District microscopy center
b. TB unit
c. PHC
d. Peripheral microscopy unit

Ans. is 'd' Peripheral microscopy unit

Mukhya Sevika

- "Anganwadi workers are supervised by an anganwadi supervisor or anganwadi supervisor worker, also called Mukhya Sevika"
- The Anganwadi system is mainly managed by the Anganwadi worker (AWW). She is a health worker chosen from the community and given 4 months training in health, nutrition and childcare. She is in-charge of an Anganwadi which covers a population of 1000. About 20–25 Anganwadi workers are supervised by a Supervisor called Mukhya-sevika. 4 Mukhyasevikas are headed by a Child Development Projects Officer.
- Integrated health service (which is a part of primary health care) is provided at village health unit, subcentre and PHC. Amongst these, PHC is the highest level.
- Infrastructure of primary healthcare
- At present, in India, the health infrastructure is based on a 3 tier system of services provided at three levels:
  - *Primary health care*: Provided at village health unit, sub-center and PHC
  - *Secondary health care*: At CHC, District hospital
  - *Tertiary health care*: At teaching hospitals, super specialty hospital, Regional hospitals.

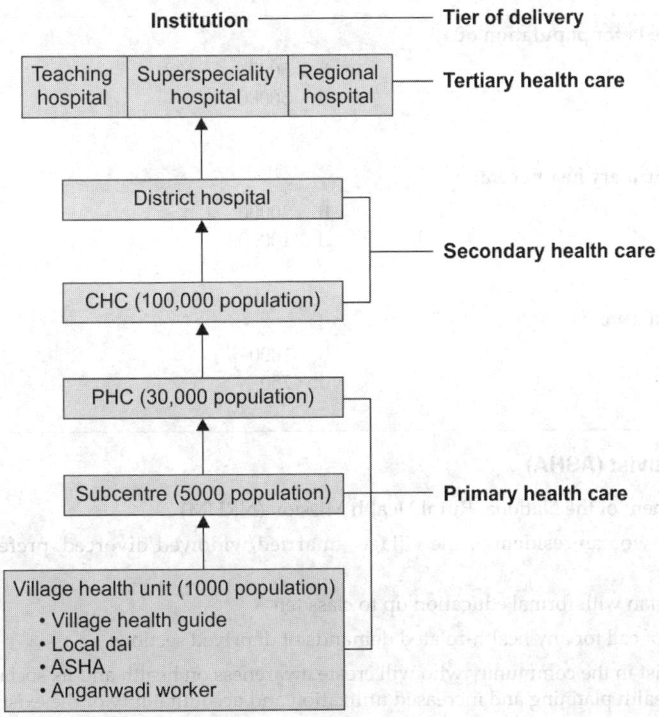

Preventive and Social Medicine

- ❖ Integrated health service means integration of all aspects of health, i.e. preventive, promotive, and curative aspects.
- ❖ The concept of PHC is to provide integrated health service in the rural population.

171. Who looks after the work of Anganwadi worker?

a. Auxiliary nurse midwife
b. Mukhyasevika
c. Village health guide
d. ASHA

Ans. is 'b' Mukhyasevika

172. Highest level of integration in health service is:

a. PHC
b. Subcentre
c. CHC
d. District hospital

Ans. is 'a' PHC

Population Norms in India

Centre/health personnel	*Population covered*
One doctor	3500
One nurse	5000
One subcentre - One female health worker (auxiliary nurse midwife; ANM) One male health worker (multipurpose worker)	5000 in plains, 3000 in hilly/tribal/backward areas
One PHC - One health assistant male One health assistant female (lady health visitor; LHV)	30,000 in plains, 80,000 in hilly/tribal areas
One CHC	1,20,000 in plains, 80,000 in hilly/tribal areas
One ASHA	1000 village
One trained dai	1000 village
One village health guide	1000 village
One anganwadi worker	400–800 in plains, 300–800 in hilly/tribal areas
One pharmacist	100,000
One lab technician	10,000

173. One village health guide is for population of:

a. 1000
b. 5000
c. 10000
d. 50000

Ans. is 'a' 1000

174. Population covered by primary health center:

a. 5000
b. 30000
c. 50000
d. 100000

Ans. is 'b' 30000

175. One ASHA caters a population is:

a. 500
b. 1000
c. 10000
d. 750

Ans. is 'b' 1000

Accredited Social Health Activist (ASHA)

- ❖ ASHA is the central component of the National Rural Health Mission (NRHM)
- ❖ ASHA must primarily be a woman resident of the village—married/widowed/divorced, preferably in the age group of 25 to 45 years.
- ❖ She should be a literate woman with formal education up to class ten
- ❖ ASHA will be the first port of call for any health-related demands of deprived sections
- ❖ ASHA will be a health activist in the community who will create awareness on health and its social determinants and mobilize the community towards local health planning and increased utilization and accountability of the existing health services.

- She will counsel women on birth preparedness, importance of safe delivery, breastfeeding and complementary feeding, immunization, contraception and prevention of common infections including Reproductive Tract Infection/Sexually Transmitted Infection (RTIs/STIs) and care of the young child
- She will arrange escort/accompany pregnant women and children requiring treatment
- Admission to the nearest pre-identified health facility
- ASHA will provide primary medical care for minor ailments such as diarrhea, fevers, and first aid form in or injuries. She will be a provider of Directly Observed Treatment Short-course (DOTS) under Revised National Tuberculosis Control Program
- She will also act as a depot holder for essential provisions being made available to every habitation like Oral Rehydration Therapy (ORS), Iron Folic Acid Tablet (IFA), chloroquine, Disposable Delivery Kits (DDK), Oral Pills and Condoms, etc. A Drug Kit will be provided to each ASHA.
- The general norm will be 'One ASHA per 1000 population. In tribal, hilly, desert areas the norm could be relaxed to one ASHA per habitation, dependent on workload etc.

176. Role of ASHA in DOTS:

a. Referring the TB cases to government hospital
b. Helping in diagnosis
c. Providing DOTS
d. Giving BCG vaccine

Ans. is 'c' Providing DOTS

177. Village health nutrition day is observed:

a. Every week
b. Every month
c. Every 6 month
d. Every year

Ans. is 'b' Every month

Principles of Primary Health Care

- Equitable distribution
  - It means, health services must be shared equally by all people irrespective of their ability to pay and all people (urban or rural, rich or poor) have access to health services
  - Community participation
  - The local community is involved in planning and implementation of health services
  - Primary health care is thus described as—Health by the people, placing people's health in people hands
  - Village health guides and trained dais are perfect examples of community participation. They belong to the community they serve
- Inter-sectoral coordination
  - The primary health care is not provided by health sector alone
  - It involves all other related sectors of national and community development, in particular agriculture, animal husbandry, food, industry, education, housing, public works (e.g. an adequate supply of safe water and basic sanitation), communication and other sectors
- Appropriate technology
  - Appropriate technology is defined as 'technology that is scientifically sound, adaptable to local needs, and acceptable to those who apply it and those for whom it is used, and that can be maintained by the people themselves in keeping with the principles of self-reliance with the resources the community and country can afford.

178. Standpipe in rural areas is an example of which principle of primary health care?

a. Equitable distribution
b. Community participation
c. Intersectoral coordination
d. Appropriate technology

Ans. is 'c' Intersectoral coordination

Community Health Centre

- First referral unit is community health centre (CHC).
- Each community health centre covers a population of 80000 to 1.20 Lakh. It has 30 beds and specialist in Surgery, Medicine, Obstetrics and Gynecology, and Pediatrics with X-ray and laboratory facilities. For strengthening preventive and promotive aspects of health care, new nonmedical (not medical) post called community health officer (CHO) has been created at each CHC. The CHO is selected with a minimum of 7 years experience in rural health programs.
- Staff at CHC consists of 30–31 workers:
  - 4 specialist medical officers (Surgeon, Physician, Obstetrician/Gynecologist, Pediatrician-1 each)
  - 23–24 staff [Nurse-midwife (9), Dresser (1), Pharmacist (1), Radiographer (1), Lab technician (1), Ophthalmic Assistant (1), Ward boy (2), Sweepers (3), Chowkidar (1), OPD attendant (1), OT attendant (1), Statistical assistant (1), Registration clerk(1)].
  - *Proposed 3 new staff*: Anesthetist, Eye surgeon, Public health program manager (1 each).

	Subcentre	PHC	CHC
Level of care	Primary	Primary	Secondary
Population norm Plains Hilly/tribal areas	 5000 3000	 30,000 20,000	 1,20,000 80,000
Staff	3	15	30
Maintenance	Central Govt.	State Govt.	State Govt.
Rural area covered	21 sq. km	140 sq. km.	770 sq. km.
Redial distance covered	2.6	6.6	15.6
Average no. of villages covered	4	29	158

179. Not criteria of first referral unit:

a. Covers a population of 1 lac
b. Provide secondary care
c. Has 30 beds
d. Community health officer is medical graduate or post graduate

Ans. is 'd' Community health officer is medical graduate or post graduate

180. Not true about first referral unit in urban areas:

a. 30–50 beds
b. Covers 2.5 lakh population
c. Salary is given by state government
d. Setting up cost is given by state government

Ans. is 'd' Setting up cost is given by state government

HEALTH MANAGEMENT

- Management techniques were initially developed for organizations' managers for ensuring efficient functioning of these organizations
- These were found useful in health sector too, some more than others
- Management techniques are based on:
  - Organizational behavior and
  - Quantitative methods

  The quality and performance of health services are difficult to quantify. Management Techniques Useful in Health Sector

Those based on organizational behavior (behavioral sciences)

1. Organizational design
2. Personnel management
3. Communication
4. Information systems
5. Management by objectives

Those based on quantitative methods

1. Cost benefit analysis
2. Cost effective analysis
3. Cost accounting
4. Input–output analysis
5. Model
6. System analysis
7. Network analysis- PERT and CPM
8. Planning programming budgeting system
9. Work sampling
10. Decision taking

Management by Objectives

- Short term objectives are set for each unit and subunit comprising the organization
- Each unit then chalks out its own plan of action for achieving these objectives in the allotted time
- Efficient achievement of the objectives by the units and subunits contributes to achievement of the broad objective of the organization
- Objectives are JOINTLY set i.e. in consultation with the top management and the employees
- The objectives should be feasible and clear
- Top management should provide support to the subunits for achieving the objectives MBO- Advantages
- Measurement of performance of each unit is automatically set—the % age of the objective achieved
- Offers motivation to the workers and sets accountability.

181. Which of the following management techniques is based upon behavioural sciences? *(NEET 2020)*

a. Systematic analysis
b. Network analysis
c. Decision making
d. Management by objectives

Ans. is 'd' Management by objectives

COST BENEFIT ANALYSIS

Cost Benefit Analysis

- Compares costs and benefits of an intervention.
- **Standardizes all costs and benefits in monetary terms.**
- Can include non-health benefits.
- Used primarily in regulatory policy analyses.
- Increasingly applied to public health.
- *Benefit*: Cost analysis is used to decide whether to implement one specific intervention or program, which can be determined if net benefits are greater than zero. It can also be used when choosing between competing options. In this case, you would choose the intervention with the highest return on investment or highest net benefit.

182. When the economic benefits of a program are compared to the cost of the program, it is known as: *(NEET 2020)*

a. Cost benefit analysis
b. Cost effective analysis
c. Cost accounting
d. Input output analysis

Ans. is 'a' Cost benefit analysis

INTERNATIONAL HEALTH

DISEASES NOTIFIABLE TO WHO

- At the international level, the following diseases are notifiable to WHO in Geneva under International health regulation:
  - Cholera
  - Plague
  - Yellow fever
  - These are notifiable diseases as well as under surveillance
- Few other diseases are also subjected to international surveillance:
  - Louse-borne typhus fever
  - Relapsing fever
  - Polio
  - Influenza
  - Malaria
  - Rabies
  - Salmonellosis

183. Disease under international surveillance by WHO:

a. Measles
b. Relapsing fever
c. Typhoid
d. Rubella

Ans. is 'b' Relapsing fever

Headquarters

Health agencies	Headquarters
WHO (World Health Organization)	Geneva, Switzerland
UNICEF (United Nations Children Fund)	New York, USA
UNDP (United Nations Development Programme)	New York, USA
FAO (Food and Agricultural Organization)	Rome, Italy
ILO (International Labour Organization)	Geneva, Switzerland
UNESCO	Paris

184. Headquarter of UNICEF:

a. Geneva, Switzerland
b. New York, USA
c. Rome, Italy
d. Paris

Ans. is 'b' New York, USA

Red Cross

- The International Committee of the Red Cross (ICRC) is a private humanitarian institution founded in 1863 Geneva, Switzerland, by Henry Dunant and Gustave Moynier. Its 25-member committee has a unique authority under international humanitarian law to protect the life and dignity of the victims of international and internal armed conflicts. The ICRC was awarded the Nobel Peace Prize on three occasions (in 1917, 1944 and 1963).

185. International red cross was founded by:

a. Henry Dunant
b. Claude Bernard
c. Samuel Hahnemann
d. Gregor Mendel

Ans. is 'a' Henry Dunant

Declarations

Year	Declaration	Key topic
1948	The declaration of Geneva	Humanitarian goals of medicine
1964	The declaration of Helsinki	Human experimentation and clinical trials
1968	The declaration of Sydney	Determination and the recovery of organs
1970	The declaration of Oslo	Therapeutic abortion
1975	The declaration of Tokyo	Torture and other cruel and degrading treatment or punishment
1981	The declaration of Lisbon	Rights of the patient
1983	The declaration of Venice	Terminal illness
1987	The declaration of euthanasia	Euthanasia
1989	The declaration of Hong Kong	The abuse of the elderly
1991	The declaration of Malta	Hunger strikers
1997	The declaration of Hamburg	Support for medical doctors who refuse to condone or participate in torture
1998	The declaration of Ottawa	Child health
2000	The declaration of Edinburgh	Prison conditions and the spread of TB and other communicable diseases
2002	The declaration of Washington	Biological weapons
2002	The declaration of patient safety	Patient safety
2008	The declaration of Seoul	Professional autonomy and clinical independence
2009	The declaration of Delhi	Health and climate change
2011	The declaration of Montevidoe	Disaster preparedness and medical response
2011	Declaration of end-of life medical care	End of life care

186. Declaration of Oslo deals with:

a. Human experimentation
b. Therapeutic abortion
c. Euthanasia
d. Hunger strikers

Ans. is 'b' Therapeutic abortion

187. Declaration of Lisbon is related to:

a. Human experimentation
b. Right of patient
c. Hunger strikers
d. Patient safety

Ans. is 'b' Right of patient

Small Pox Eradication

- Eradication implies termination of all transmission of infection by extermination of infectious agent
- It is an absolute process, i.e. all or none phenomenon
- It literally means "tearing out by roots"
- Eradication is a "global term" used only cessation of infection from the whole world
- It is the only infectious disease which has been eradicated globally. The world's Last case occurred in Somalia on 26 October 1977. The WHO declared on 8 may 1980 that smallpox had been eradicated.

- ❖ In April 1977, India was declared smallpox free. The last indigenous case in India occurred on 17 may 1975 in Bihar and India's last known case of smallpox was an importation from Bangladesh, which occurred on 24 May 1975.
- ❖ Other diseases which are candidates for global eradication—Polio, measles, dracunculiasis, diphtheria.

188. Only disease which is eradicated worldwide:

a. Smallpox b. Polio
c. Diphtheria d. Measles

Ans. is 'a' Smallpox

189. The last case of small pox was reported in the world:

a. 1977 b. 1978
c. 1979 d. 1982

Ans. is 'a' 1977

WHO Vision 2020

The diseases identified for global elimination include:

1. Cataract blindness
2. Trachoma blindness and transmission
3. Onchocerciasis
4. Avoidable causes of childhood blindness
5. Refractive errors and low vision

   Above 5 diseases were for global vision 2020. Indian vision 2020 includes following seven diseases.

   - Cataract blindness
   - Glaucoma
   - Trachoma blindness and transmission
   - Diabetic retinopathy
   - Childhood blindness
   - Corneal blindness
   - Refractive errors and low vision.

Note

- ❖ Corneal ulcer (corneal blindness) and diabetic retinopathy are included in India Vision-2020 **not** in WHO vision 2020.

190. WHO Vision 2020 initiative includes:

a. Corneal ulcer b. Trachoma blindness
c. Diabetic retinopathy d. Vernal keratoconjunctivitis

Ans. is 'b' Trachoma blindness

SUSTAINABLE DEVELOPMENT GOAL

Maternal mortality reduction remains a priority under "Goal 3: Ensure healthy lives and promote well-being for all at all ages" in the new **Sustainable Development Goals** (SDGs) agenda through 2030.

Global Target

By 2030, reduce the global maternal mortality ratio (MMR) to fewer than 70 maternal deaths per 100,000 live births.

National Targets

- ❖ By 2030, countries should reduce their MMRs by at least two-thirds from their 2010 baseline; countries with the highest maternal mortality burdens will need to achieve even greater reduction.
- ❖ By 2030, no country should have an MMR greater than 140 maternal deaths per 100,000 live births, a number twice the global target.

191. SDG 3.1 goal for MMR to be achieved by 2030 is: *(NEET 2020)*

a. <70 b. <100
c. <140 d. <50

Ans. is 'a' <70

BIOSTATISTICS

P VALUE

According to convention, if P is less than or equal to 0.05, it is regarded as 'statistically significant'. The smaller the P value, the greater the statistical significance or probability that the association is not due to chance alone. However, statistical association (P value) does not imply causation. Statement of P value is thus an inadequate, although common end-point of case-control studies.

- A small p-value (typically 0.05) indicates strong evidence against the null hypothesis. So, you reject the null hypothesis
- A large p-value (> 0.05) indicates weak evidence against the null hypothesis, so you fail to reject the null hypothesis
- P-values very close to the cutoff (0.05) are considered to be marginal (could go either way). Always report the p-value so that readers can draw their own conclusions.

192. In a study, the remission rate of the new drug was found to be equal to the remission rate of a drug already in use. P value = 0.4. Which of the following is true? *(NEET 2018)*

a. Insufficient data to compare the two drugs
b. Both drugs are ineffective
c. Both drugs are effective
d. Power of study is 60%

Ans. is 'c' Both drugs are effective

Standard Normal Curve

- It is also known as Bell curve or Gaussian distribution
- The shape of the curve is like a bell—bell shaped curve
- The data are distributed symmetrically on either side of a central value
- Normal distribution curve looks symmetrical in the dispersion with the largest frequencies in the middle score and tapering down of frequencies towards the highest as well as the lowest score—No tail
- Normal distribution curve is based on mean and standard deviation
- Mean median and mode all coincide—No skew
- Mean = median = mode = 0
- Total area of curve is 1
- Its standard deviation is 1
- Variance is 1

193. Area under standard normal distribution curve:

a. 0.5
b. 1
c. 1.5
d. 2.0

Ans. is 'b' 1

194. True about Bell's curve is:

a. It skewed to the left
b. Has mean = 1.0
c. Has standard deviation = 0.0
d. Has variance = 1.0

Ans. is 'd' Has variance = 1.0

Type of Curves

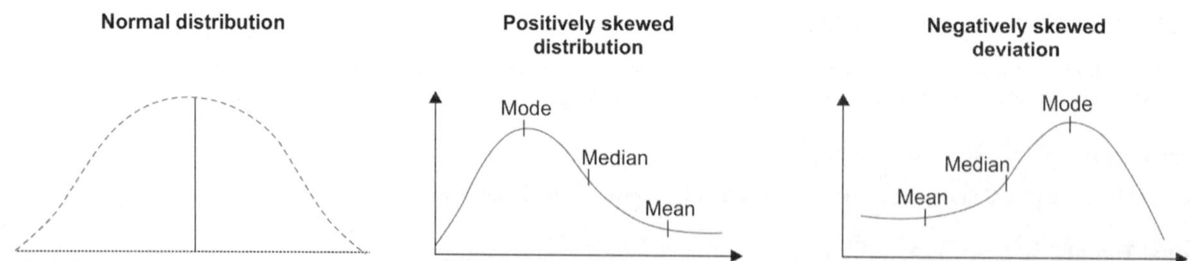

Normal distribution:
- No tail
- Bell shaped curve: Gaussian distribution
- **Mean = Median = Mode**

Positively skewed distribution:
- Tail is towards right side
- Large no. of low scores, small no of high scores
- **Mean > Median > Mode**

Negatively skewed deviation:
- Tail is towards left side
- Large no of high scores, small no of low scores
- **Mean < Median < Mode**

- Sidedness of the skewed distribution is towards the side of tail. For example, right sided skewed deviation means the tail is towards the right
- Facts to remember the relation between mean, media and mode (see above figure):
  - Mean is right of the median under right skew, and left of the median under left skew
  - Mode is left of the median under right skew, and right of the median under left skew.

Remember:

Relationship b/w the measures of central tendency

- In a symmetrical curve Mean = Median = Mode
- In a Positive (Right) skewed curve Mean > Median > Mode
- In a Negative (left) skewed curve Mean < Median < Mode

195. In positive skewed deviation, what is true?

a. Mode < Median < Mean
b. Mode > Median > Mean
c. Median > Mean > Mode
d. Mode > Mean > Median

Ans. is 'a' Mode < Median < Mean

196. Mean < Median < Mode is seen in which type of curve?

a. Negative skewed
b. Positively skewed
c. Normal distribution
d. No correlation

Ans. is 'a' Negative skewed

- The commonly used statistical average (measures of central tendency) are: (i) Arithmetic mean, (ii) Median and (iii) Mode.

Arithmetic Mean

- It is the most commonly used statistical average. It is obtained by sum of all the values divided by total number of values.
- The major disadvantage of mean is that it may be unduly influenced by abnormal high or low values in the distribution.

Median

- It is the middle most value in a distribution arranged in ascending or descending order. If there are two values in the middle, instead of one, the median is worked out by taking the average of two middle values.
- The main advantage of median is that it is not affected by abnormal high or low values (unlike mean). Therefore, median is used in skewed distribution (distribution which is skewed/deviated due to small number of very high or low values).

Mode

- It is the most frequently occurring value in a distribution. If there are two most frequent values, there are two modes and the distribution is called 'bimodal distribution'. In bimodal distribution the mode is the average of two modes.
- For bimodal distribution

$$\text{Mode} = (3 \times \text{median}) - (2 \times \text{mean})$$

- Mode is the central tendency which is least affected by extreme values or skewness (But median is the preferred central tendency in skewed distribution).

197. In set of date with highly variable values (very high and low), the best measure of central tendency is:

a. Mean
b. Median
c. Mode
d. SD

Ans. is 'b' Median

198. Most commonly used measure of central tendency:

a. Mean
b. Median
c. Mode
d. None

Ans. is 'a' Mean

199. Not a measure of central tendency:

a. Mean
b. SD
c. Mode
d. Median

Ans. is 'b' SD

200. Bimodal distribution is represented by:

a. Mode = 3 median – 2 mean
b. Mode = 3 median + mean
c. Mode = 2 median + 2 mean
d. Mode = 3 mode – 3 median

Ans. is 'a' Mode = 3 median – 2 mean

Chi-square Tests

- It is a non-parametric test to measure the association between two or more qualitative variables, i.e. when observations are in proportions, percentage or fractions. It tests the significance of difference between two proportions. As with all non-parametric tests, it is used for non- Normal (non-Gaussian) distribution.

- The chi square test has an added advantage, it can be applied to find association or relationship between two discrete attributes when there are more than two class or groups as happens in multinomial samples.
- Studies often collect data on categorial (qualitative) variables that can be summarized as a series of counts. These counts are commonly arranged in a tubular format known as a contingency table. For example, a study designed to determine whether or not there is association between cigarette smoking and asthma attack might collect data that could be assembled into a 2–2 table—table containing two columns and two rows.
- The chi-square test can be used to evaluate whether there is an association between the rows and columns in a contingency table i.e. between two variables (smoking and asthma attack).
- The chi-square test assumes that no association occurs between two events in question unless proved otherwise—Null hypothesis. The chi-square test is designed to test the null hypothesis which says that there is no association between two variables (the rows and columns of a contingency table).
- Chi-square test only tells about the presence or absence of association, but it does not measure the strength of association.

Degree of Freedom

- Degree of freedom is the number of observations in the final calculation that are free to vary. The number of degrees of freedom of contingency table is the product of one less the number of rows(r) and one less the number of column(c).

$$DOF = (C-1)\ (r-1)$$

- Chi-Square test offers a method of testing the significance of difference between the proportions.
- Its advantage lies in the fact that it can also be used when more than two groups are to be compared.
- By using this test, we can find out if the difference between two proportions or ratios has occurred by chance. The steps involved are:
  1. Testing the null hypothesis.
  2. Applying chi-square test.
  3. Calculating the degree of freedom.
  4. Comparing with probability tables.

201. True about chi-square test:

a. Parametric test
b. Used for Gaussian distribution
c. Measure the strength of association
d. Used when there are more than 2 group

Ans. is 'd' Used when there are more than 2 group

202. The significance of difference between proportions can also be tested by: *(NEET 2019)*

a. t' test
b. Chi square test
c. ANOVA
d. Correlation and regression

Ans. is 'b' Chi square test

Paired T-Test

- It is used to compare the values of means from two related samples; for example, in a before and after scenario.
- The difference between the means of the samples is unlikely to be equal to zero (due to sampling variation) and the hypothesis test is designed to answer the question "Is the observed difference sufficiently large enough to indicate that the alternative hypothesis is true".

203. Paired T-test is defined as: *(NEET 2019)*

a. Test used to assess quantitative observations before and after an intervention
b. Test that is used when the observation is in the form of proportions (for qualitative data)
c. Test applied when separate observations are made on individuals of two separate groups, and these need to be compared
d. None

Ans. is 'a' Test used to assess quantitative observations before and after an intervention

Correlation

A correlation expresses the strength and direction of the association between two variables (continuous quantitative variables). But correlation does not tell about causation or about the risk of disease.

Coefficient of correlation (Correlation coefficient 'r') measures the degree or strength of correlation between two variables. Value of r varies from –1 to +1.

The strength of the relationship is indicated by the size of the correlation coefficient, whereas its direction is indicated by the sign (+ or –). Both –1.0 and +1.0 implies a perfect linear relationship.

Regression

- Correlation quantifies the strength of association between two variables, but it cannot predict one-unit change of one variable will cause how much change of the other variable
- If two variables are highly correlated, it then becomes possible to predict the value of the dependent variable from the value of the independent variable by using regression technique
- Regression analysis is the mathematical modeling to describe the effect that one or more independent variables have on a dependent variable
- While correlation indicates the degree (strength) of association between two variables, regression does quantification of this relationship i.e. regression indicates the nature of the relationship algebraically.
- For example, height to weight is an association:
  - Strength of this association will be determined by correlation ®strong positive/negative or weak positive/negative
  - Quantification is done by regression—by regression we might predicts the weight by measuring height.

REGRESSION COEFFICIENT

Regression **coefficients are *estimates* of the unknown *population parameters* and describe the relationship between a *predictor variable* and the *response*.** In linear regression, coefficients are the values that multiply the predictor values. Suppose you have the following regression equation: y = 3X + 5. In this equation, + 3 is the coefficient, X is the predictor, and + 5 is the constant.

The sign of each coefficient indicates the direction of the relationship between a predictor variable and the response variable.

- A positive sign indicates that as the predictor variable increases, the response variable also increases.
- A negative sign indicates that as the predictor variable increases, the response variable decreases.

The coefficient value represents the **mean** change in the response given a one unit change in the predictor. For example, if a coefficient is +3, the mean response value increases by 3 for every one unit change in the predictor.

204. If value of one variable is known and another variable is calculated from it, it is known as: *(NEET 2020)*

a. Regression coefficient
b. Coefficient of variance
c. Correlation coefficient
d. Multivariate analysis

Ans. is 'a' Regression coefficient

Scatter Diagram (Dot Diagram)

- A scatter diagram is a tool for analyzing relationships between two variables
- One variable plotted on the horizontal axis and the other is plotted on the vertical axis
- The pattern of their intersecting points can graphically show relationship patterns
- While the diagram shows relationships, it does not by itself prove that one variable causes the other, i.e. scatter diagram only show relationship between cause and effect (change in one will change other), but cannot prove the variable as a cause of the other
- Correction and regression are plotted on scatter diagram—also known as correlation diagram

Line Diagram (Line chart/Line Graph)

- It is used to show the trend of events with passage of time and show the frequency of a particular event or variable vary overtime.
- Line diagrams are used to show the trend of events with passage of time.
- It is used to show the trend of events with passage of time and shows how the frequency of a particular event or variable vary over time.

205. All of the followings how relationship between two variables, *except*:

a. Correlation coefficient
b. Regression
c. Scatter diagram
d. Line diagram

Ans. is 'd' Line diagram

206. Best representative of incidence of disease in different timeline: *(NEET 2019)*

a. Histogram
b. Line diagram
c. Scattered diagram
d. Bar diagram

Ans. is 'b' Line diagram

Division of Distributions

- Distributions can be divided into multiple equal parts by various measures of location. For example, a Quartile divides the distribution into four equal parts (25% each).

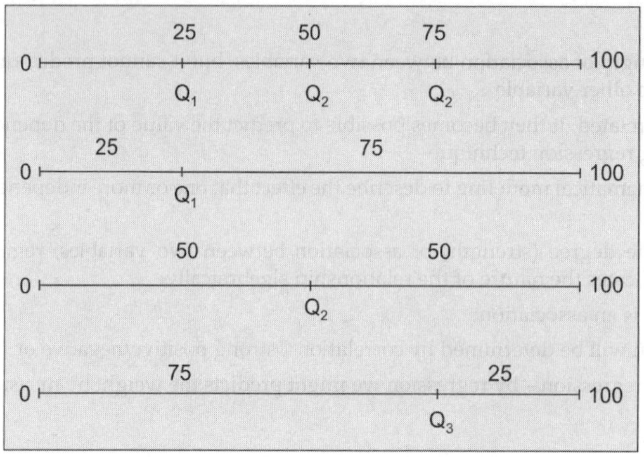

- So, in Quartile the number of intercepts required are three: Q (first/lowest quartile), Q (second quartile) and Q (third/highest quartile).
- Similarly, tertile divides the distribution into three equal parts (33.33% each) by two intercepts.

	Divides distribution into	No. of intercepts
Tertile	3 equal parts	2
Quartile	4 equal parts	3
Pentik (Quintile)	5 equal parts	4
Hextite	6 equal parts	5
Heptile	7 equal parts	6
Octile	8 equal parts	7
Decile	10 equal parts	9
Centile (Percentile)	100 equal parts	99

207. Percentile divides the data into how many equal parts?

a. Two
b. Four
c. Fifty
d. Hundred

Ans. is 'd' Hundred

Bar Charts

- Bar charts is a chart with rectangular bars with length proportional to the values that they represent
- Bar charts are used for comparing two or more values that were taken overtime or on different conditions.
- It is for visual comparison of magnitude of different frequencies in qualitative data.

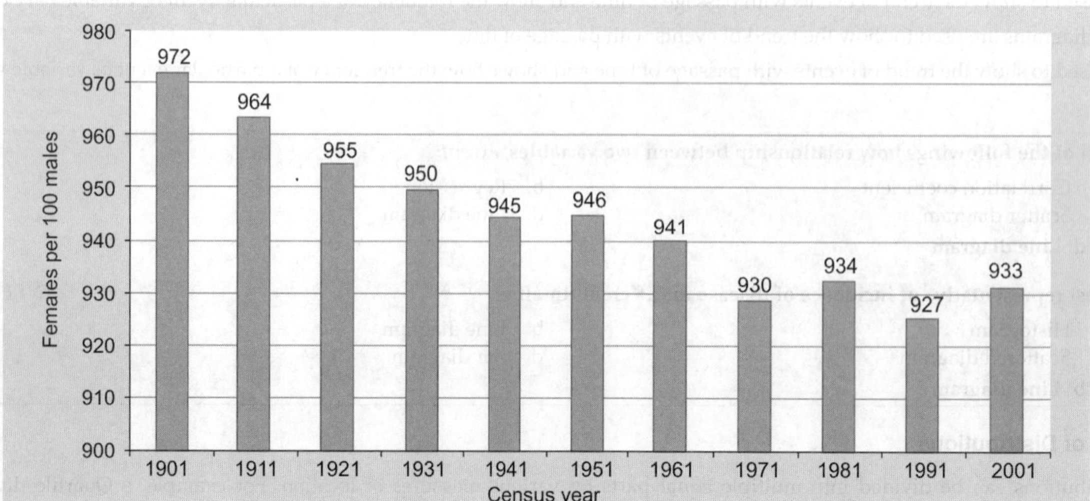

Preventive and Social Medicine

Histogram

- ❖ It is graphic display of tabulated frequencies shown as bar.
- ❖ "Histogram is presentation of a frequency distribution by means of bars whose width represent class and whose areas are proportional to corresponding frequencies."
- ❖ In other words, Histogram shows the numbers of cases per unit interval so that the height of each bar is equal to the proportion of total people in the survey who fall in the category. The area under curve represents the total number of cases.
- ❖ The categories (bars) are usually specified as non-overlapping intervals of some variable.
- ❖ Categories (bars) must be adjacent.
- ❖ Intervals are generally of the same size.
- ❖ For example, the data set of blood cholesterol level of a group (mg/dL)—3, 11, 12, 19, 22, 23, 24, 25, 27, 29, 35, 36, 37, 45, 49.
- ❖ Information in this data set can be divided into interval and frequencies.

Interval	Width	Quantity (frequencies)
0–10	10	1
10–20	10	3
20–30	10	6
30–40	10	4
40–50	10	2

- ❖ *Histogram will be:*

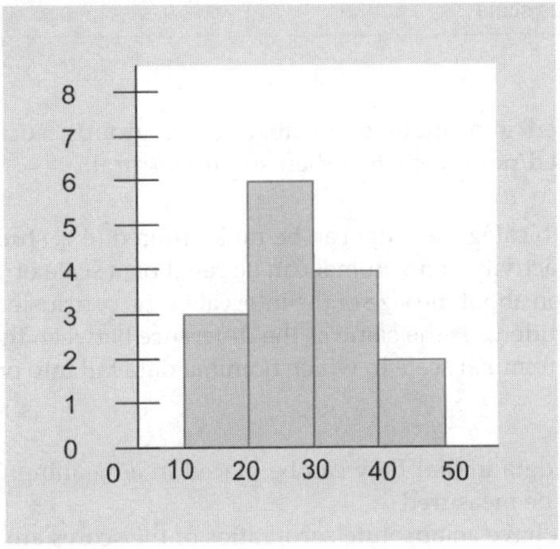

208. True about Bar chart:

a. Width of bar is proportional to representative values
b. Used for quantitative data
c. Same as histogram
d. Rectangular bars are used to represent data

Ans. is 'd' Rectangular bars are used to represent data

- ❖ Continuous (quantitative) data is represented by histogram:

Data	Scale	Graph/diagram
Quantitative	Interval scale Ratio scale	Histogram Frequency polygon Cumulative frequency curve Line Chart graph
Quantitative	Normal scale Ordinal scale	Bar diagram Pie chart Pictogram Map diagram or spot map

209. Continuous data is represented by:

a. Bar diagram
b. Pie chart
c. Histogram
d. Pictogram

Ans. is 'c' Histogram

Data	Method
Frequency of occurrence (comparisons of magnitude)	Bar chart Pie chart
Trends over time	Line graph
Distribution (not related to time)	Histogram Frequency polygon
Association (Looking for correlation between two variables)	Scatter diagram

210. Scatter diagram represents:

a. Frequency of occurrence b. Trend overtime
c. Correlation/Association d. None of the above

Ans. is 'c' Correlation/Association

Statistical Scales

❖ There are following type of statistical scales to measure statistical data:

For qualitative data (categorical scale)	For quantitative data (metric scale)
• Nominal scale • Ordinal scale • Dichotomous scale	• Interval scale • Ratio scale

a. **Categorical scale**

1. **Nominal scale**
   - Nominal scale data are divided into qualitative categories or groups, such as male/female, black/white, died/cured, attacked/not attacked, vaccinated/not vaccinate, urban/suburban/rural.
2. **Ordinal Scale**
   - Here the data can be placed into categories that can be rank ordered (e.g. students maybe ranked 1st/2nd/3rd/4th in their class or into grades A/B/C, the activity of an animal can be rated on a scale of 1 to 6, hardness scale for water etc.)
   - However, there is no information about the size of the interval i.e. no conclusion can be drawn about whether the difference between the first and second students is the same as the difference between the second and third
   - Dichotomous Scale is a type of nominal scale in which nominal data fall into only two groups e.g. black/white, died/cured, failed/passed.

b. **Metric scale interval scale**

- Interval scale data are like ordinal data in that they can be placed in a meaningful order; in addition, they have meaningful intervals between items, which can be measured
- However, interval scale data do not have an absolute zero, ratios of the scores are not meaningful i.e. 80°C temperature is not twice as hot as 40 °C because 0 °C does not indicate a complete absence of heat.

Ratio Scale

❖ A ratio scale has the same properties as an interval scale, however, because it has an absolute zero, meaningful ratio doesexist.
❖ Ratio of one value to other is meaningful. For example, pulse rate of 120 beats/minute is twice as fast as a pulse rate of 60 beats per minute, and 300°k is twice as hot as 150°k.
❖ If data on anemia are placed into categories that are ordered mild, moderate, sever—ordinal scale should be used.

211. Anemia is classified into mild, moderate and severe on which scale?

a. Interval b. Nominal
c. Ordinal d. Ratio

Ans. is 'c' Ordinal

Parametric Test Vs Non-parametric Test

	Parametric test	Non-parametric test
Data	Quantitative, e.g. weight, BP etc.	Qualitative, e g. gender, Blood group etc.
Observation form	Mean, standard deviation, range, variance	Proportions, percentage, fractions
Scales	Interval or ratio	Nominal or ordinal.
Examples	Student 't-test' • Paired t test • Unpaired test Z test ANOVA (f test/F ratio)	Chi square test Fisher exact test Sign test Wilcoxon Rank sum test (Mann Whitney U test) Wilcoxon signed rank test

212. Not a parametric test:

a. Z-test
b. ANOVA
c. Student 't-test'
d. Chi-square test

Ans. is 'd' Chi-square test

213. In a normal curve what is the area that comes under 1 standard deviation? *(NEET 2019)*

a. 50%
b. 68%
c. 95%
d. 100%

Ans. is 'b' 68%

Solution

1 SD includes → 68% of values
2 SD includes → 95% of values
3 SD includes → 99.7% of values

The empirical rule states that for a HYPERLINK "https://www.statisticshowto.datasciencecentral.com/probability-and-statistics/normal-distributions/"normal distribution, nearly all of the data will fall within three HYPERLINK "https://www.statisticshowto.datasciencecentral.com/probability-and-statistics/standard-deviation/"standard deviations of the HYPERLINK "https://www.statisticshowto.datasciencecentral.com/mean/"mean. The empirical rule can be broken down into three parts:

1. 68% of data falls within the first standard deviation from the mean.
2. 95% fall within two standard deviations.
3. 99.7% fall within three standard deviations.

The rule is also called the HYPERLINK "https://www.statisticshowto.datasciencecentral.com/empirical-rule-2/"68-95-99 7 Rule or the **Three Sigma Rule.** HYPERLINK "https://www.statisticshowto.datasciencecentral.com/wp-content/uploads/2013/09/standard-normal-distribution.jpg" *Standard normal distribution showing standard deviations. Image credit: University of Virginia.* When applying the Empirical Rule to a data set the following conditions are true:

- Approximately 68% of the data falls within one standard deviation of the mean (or between the mean–one times the standard deviation, and the mean + 1 times the standard deviation). In mathematical notation, this is represented as: $\mu \pm 1\sigma$
- Approximately 95% of the data falls within two standard deviations of the mean (or between the mean–2 times the standard deviation, and the mean + 2 times the standard deviation). The mathematical notation for this is: $\mu \pm 2\sigma$
- Approximately 99.7% of the data falls within three standard deviations of the mean (or between the mean–three times the standard deviation and the mean + three times the standard deviation). The following notation is used to represent this fact: $\mu \pm 3\sigma$
- In this question, applying the empirical rule, 68% population lies between 200 ± 20, i.e. 180-220

214. In a normal distribution, if mean is 200 and SD is 20, 68% population lies within what range? *(NEET 2020)*

a. 180–220
b. 160–240
c. 190–210
d. 140–260

Ans. is 'a' 180–220

215. A survey was made to assess malnutrition among children. 100 children from rural area and 100 from urban area were taken. 30 from rural area and 20 from urban area were found to be malnourished. which test can be used to find out if this difference is significant? *(NEET 2020)*

a. Chi square test
b. Paired T-test
c. Student T-test
d. ANOVA test

Ans. is 'a' Chi square test

Explanation: In this case, we intend to measure the proportion of malnutrition between rural (30/100 = 30%) and urban (20/100 = 20%) populations. So the best method applicable will be Chi square test.

- Other 3 tests given in options are used for comparing quantitative data.
- Paired T-test—for paired data (before and after an intervention)
- Student T-test—for comparing quantitative data of 2 populations
- ANOVA test—for comparing quantitative data of >2 populations

VACCINES AND VACCINATION

Mission Indradhanush

The Government of India has launched Mission Indradhanush on 25th December 2014 to cover children who are either unvaccinated or partially vaccinated against seven vaccine preventable diseases, i.e. diphtheria, whooping cough, tetanus, polio, tuberculosis, measles and hepatitis B. The goal is to vaccinate all under-fives by the year 2020. Under the program, four special vaccination campaigns will be conducted between January and June 2015. Intensive planning and monitoring experience of pulse polio immunization program will be used. 201 high focus districts will be covered in the first phase. Of these 82 districts are from Uttar Pradesh, Bihar, Madhya Pradesh and Rajasthan. These 201 districts have nearly 50% of all unvaccinated children of the country. The drive will be through a 'catch-up' campaign mode. The mission will be technically supported by WHO, UNICEF, Rotary International and other donor partners.

216. Which one of the following is not included in the mission Indradhanush scheme of vaccine? *(NEET 2018)*

a. TB
b. Diphtheria
c. Polio
d. Japanese encephalitis

Ans. is 'd' Japanese encephalitis

The ultimate goal of Mission Indradhanush is to ensure **full immunization with all available vaccines for children up to two years of age and pregnant women.** The Government has identified 201 high focus districts across 28 states in the country that have the highest number of partially immunized and unimmunized children.

Earlier the increase in full immunization coverage was 1% per year which has increased to 6.7% per year through the first two phases of Mission Indradhanush. Four phases of Mission Indradhanush have been conducted till August 2017 and more than 2.53 crore children and 68 lakh pregnant women have been vaccinated.

217. Mission INDRADHANUSH is meant for: *(NEET 2020)*

a. Mother and child health
b. Immunization
c. Cleanliness in ESI hospitals
d. Family planning

Ans. is 'b' Immunization

Rabies Vaccination

Type of prophylaxis	Schedule
Post-exposure	
• Intramuscular	
– Routine	Day 0, 3, 7, 14, 28, 90 (all one site)
– Abbreviated multi site (2-1-1)	Day 0 (2 sites), 7 (one site), 21 (one site)
• Intradermal	
– 2 sites	Day 0, 3, 7, 28 (all two sites each)
– 8 sites	Day 0 (8 sites), 7 (4 sites), 28 (one site), 90 (one site)
Pre-exposure	Day 0, 7 and 21 or 28
Post-exposure in previously immunized	
• 1 site 2 days intradermal	Day 0, 3
• Intramuscular	Day 0
• Single visit 4-site intradermal	Day 0 (4 sites)

218. Post-exposure prophylaxis abbreviated multisite intramuscular schedule for rabies vaccination:

a. 0, 3, 7, 14, 28, 90
b. 0, 7, 21
c. 0, 7, 28, 90
d. 0, 3, 7, 28

Ans. is 'b' 0, 7, 21

Vaccines

Varicella vaccine is live attenuated vaccine and is recommended for children between 12–18 months of age

Live 'attenuated' vaccines	Killed 'inactivated' vaccines
BCG Pertussis	IPV (Salk—Inactivated polio vaccine)
OPV (Sabin—Oral polio vaccine)	Rabies vaccine
Measles vaccine	Cholera vaccine
Mumps vaccine	Meningococcal vaccine
Rubella vaccine	Hepatitis B vaccine
Chickenpox vaccine	Typhim Vi vaccine
Yellow fever vaccine	
Typhoral	

219. Chicken pox vaccine is:

a. Live vaccine
b. Killed vaccine
c. Conjugated vaccine
d. Toxoid

Ans. is 'a' Live vaccine

Malaria Vaccine

Circumsporozoite protein (CSP) is a secreted protein of the sporozoite stage of the malaria parasite (*Plasmodium* sp) and the antigenic target of RTS, Sapre-erythrocyte malaria vaccine currently undergoing clinical trials. The amino-acid sequence of CSP consists of an immuno dominant central repeat region flanked by conserved motifs at the N-and C-termini that are implicated in protein processing as the parasite travels from the mosquito to the mammalian vector.

- ❖ The structure and function of CSP is highly conserved across the various strains of malaria that infect humans, non-human primates and rodents. It can first be detected in large quantities as sporozoites are forming within oocysts residing the midgut walls of infected mosquitoes. Upon egression from mature oocysts, sporozoites begin migrating to the salivary glands, and CSP is known to be an important mediator of this process. Additionally, CSP is involved in hepatocyte binding in the mammalian host. Here the N-terminus and central repeat region initially facilitate parasite binding. Once the hepatocyte surface proteolytic cleavage at region 1 of the N-terminus exposes the adhesive domain of the C-terminus, thereby priming the parasites for invasion of the liver.

220. Specific content in malaria vaccine is:

a. Gametocytic protein
b. Polysaccharide sheath
c. Sporozoite protein
d. Lipoprotein envelope

Ans. is 'c' Sporozoite protein

Oral Polio Vaccine

Bivalent oral polio vaccine (BOPV) contains suspension of type 1 and type 3 attenuated Polio viruses (Sabin strains), prepared in primary monkey kidney cell.

- ❖ Trivalent OPV contains type 1, 2 and 3 attenuated polioviruses. It contains:
  - Over 300,000 TCID 50 of type 1 poliovirus
  - Over 100,000 TCID 50 of type 2 poliovirus
  - Over 300,000 TCID 50 of type 3 poliovirus

"Polio Sabin (oral) vaccine is a magnesium chloride stabilized preparation of live attenuated polio viruses of sabin strains type 1, 2, and 3".

Additional Component in Vaccines (Excipients)

1. **Adjuvant:** It is added to a vaccine to enhance immune response. Commonly used adjuvants are aluminium salts (aluminium hydroxide, aluminium phosphate or potassium aluminium sulfate).
2. **Antibiotics:** Antibiotics are used during manufacturing phase to prevent bacterial contamination of tissue culture cells in which viruses are grown. For example, MMR vaccine and IPV contain neomycin (<25 g per dose).
3. **Preservatives:** These are chemicals (e.g. thimerosal, formaldehyde) used in killed or subacute vaccines in order to inactivate viruses, detoxify bacterial toxins, and to prevent serious secondary infections.
4. **Stabilizers:** These are used to confirm product quality or stability. Examples are potassium or sodium salts, lactose, human serum albumin, gelatin and bovine serum albumin.

221. Role of magnesium (Mg) in OPV:

a. Adjuvant
b. Preservative
c. Stabilizer
d. Anti-infective

Ans. is 'c' Stabilizer

222. Bivalent oral polio vaccine contains which strains of polio virus?

a. 1 and 2
b. 2 and 3
c. 1 and 3
d. 3 and 4

Ans. is 'c' 1 and 3

Rotavirus Vaccines

- ❖ The Rotavirus vaccines are live—attenuated vaccines given orally.
- ❖ Two new vaccines are now in use:
  - RVS oral pentavalent vaccine (Rotateq) contains five reassortant rotaviruses developed from 5 human strains on bovine rotavirus background [These five strains are G1, G2, G3, G4 and G9]
  - RV1 monovalent vaccine (Rotarix) contains one live attenuated rotavirus strain [the strain is G1P(8)]
- ❖ The administration of Rotarix (2 doses) and Rota Teq (3 doses) needs to be completed by 32 weeks of age to minimize any potential risk of intussusceptions.

223. Rotavirus vaccine is:

a. Live oral
b. Killed intramuscular
c. Killed subcutaneous
d. Live subcutaneous

Ans. is 'a' Live oral

DPT Vaccine

Total three doses are given in primary immunization with an interval of 4 weeks between three doses. First booster is given at 16–24 months with second booster at 5–6 years.

Dose	Age
DPT 1	6 weeks of age
DPT 2	10 weeks of age
DPT 3	14 weeks of age
DPT Booster	16–24 months of age
DPT Booster	5 years of age

❖ Important infections in which immunity is transferred from mother to child (congenital passive immunity): Chicken pox, mumps, measles, rubella, polio, diphtheria. Maternal passive immunity is not transferred in pertussis (whooping cough), Hepatitis B and TB.

224. Passive immunity from mother to child is transferred in:

a. Hepatitis B
b. Diphtheria
c. TB
d. Pertussis

Ans. is 'b' Diphtheria

225. Minimum accepted interval between two doses of DPT vaccine:

a. 2 weeks
b. 4 weeks
c. 6 weeks
d. 8 weeks

Ans. is 'b' 4 weeks

Anti-typhoid Vaccines

Two safe and effective vaccines are licensed and available:

1. **The Vi polysaccharide vaccine (TYPHIM Vi Vaccine)**
   - It contains purified Vi capsular polysaccharide from Type 2 strain
   - It is given as single dose by subcutaneous or intramuscular route
   - It confers protection 7 days after the injection
   - To maintain protection, re-vaccination is recommended every 3 years
   - It is given in individuals 2 years of age (not given < 2 years of age)
   - The vaccine can be co-administered with other vaccines relevant for international travelers
   - The vaccine has no serious systemic or local side effects. There is no major contraindication, except for hypersensitivity.
2. **The Ty 21a Oral vaccine (TYPHORAL Vaccine)**
   - It is an orally administered live attenuated vaccine
   - It contains > 10 viable organisms of live attenuated Ty 21a strain which lacks enzyme UDP-galactose 4-epimerase (Gal E mutant)
   - Vaccine is administered on 1, 3 and 5th day, i.e. a 3-dose regimen
   - Vaccine confers the protection 7 days after the last dose
   - The recommendation is to repeat this (3 doses) every 3 years for people living in endemic areas and every year for individuals travelling from non-endemic to endemic countries.

226. Schedule of typhoid oral vaccine is:

a. Day 1, 2, 3
b. Day 2, 3, 5
c. Day 1, 3, 5
d. Day 2, 4, 6

Ans. is 'c' Day 1, 3, 5

227. Which of the following is live attenuated bacterial vaccine?

a. OPV
b. Measles
c. Typhoid
d. Mumps

Ans. is 'c' Typhoid

Vaccine which must be stored in the cold part but never allowed to freeze.

❖ Typhoid
❖ DPT
❖ TT

- Hepatitis B
- DT
- BCG
- Diluents

228. Which vaccine is not stored in freezer?

a. OPV
b. Measles
c. DPT
d. Rubella

Ans. is 'c' DPT

Pertussis Vaccine

- Mainstay of prevention is active ammunition by vaccine. There are two types of vaccines
  1. **Whole cell vaccine (killed)**
     - Three injections at intervals of 4–6 weeks are given before the age of 6 months, followed by booster at the end of the first year of life
     - Usually administered with diphtheria and tetanus toxoid as triple vaccine (DPT)
     - It can cause neurological complication with a risk of 1:170000.
  2. **Acellular vaccine**
     - It contains PT, FHA, agglutinogen 5 (1, 2, 3), pertactin and fimbrial –2 and 3 antigens
     - It causes less neurological complications
     - Efficacy of both vaccines is about 90%.

229. True about pertussis vaccine *except:*

a. Neurological complications are more with whole cell vaccine
b. Efficacy is 85–90%
c. Administered as triple vaccine
d. It is live attenuated vaccine

Ans. is 'd' It is live attenuated vaccine

Measles Vaccine

- Measles vaccine is live attenuated, lyophilized (Freeze dried) vaccine.
- Strains of virus used to prepare vaccine are Edmonston-Zagreb strain (most common), Schwartz strain and Moraten strain.
- It is given subcutaneously in to middle one-third of anterolateral aspect of thigh.
- It is given at the age of 9 months (age can be lowered to 6 months in epidemics and malnutrition) and is repeated at 16–24 months of age.
- Diluent used for measles vaccine reconstitution is distilled water or sterile water
- Reconstituted vaccine should be used within 1 hour.
- Usual temperature for cold chain storage is +2 to +8°C.
- Three vaccines have potential of reducing death from pneumonia:
  - Measles vaccine
  - RIB vaccine (*Haemophilus influenzae* type B)
  - Pneumococcal vaccine
- These vaccines work to reduce the incidence of bacterial pneumonia

230. Which vaccine is used to prevent death from pneumonia in children?

a. Measles vaccine
b. Rubella vaccine
c. Chickenpox vaccine
d. Influenza viral vaccine

Ans. is 'a' Measles vaccine

231. After reconstitution, measles vaccine should be used within:

a. 5 minutes
b. 1 hour
c. 5 hours
d. 1 day

Ans. is 'b' 1 hour

Meningococcal Vaccine

- Vaccines are available for group A, C, Y and W-125. There is no group B vaccine available at present. Vaccines are prepared from capsular polysaccharide
- Bivalent (A, C), trivalent (A, C, W135), and tetravalent (A, C, W135, Y) vaccines are available
- The vaccines contain 50 µg of each of the individual polysaccharide.
- Monovalent Men A conjugate vaccine should be given as a single dose to individuals 1–29 years of age
- For monovalent Men C conjugate vaccine, one single intramuscular dose is recommended for children aged > 12 months, teenagers and adults

- Children 2–11 months of age require 2 dose administration at an interval of at least 2 months and a booster about 1 year thereafter
- Quadrivalent vaccines are administered as a single dose to individuals aged 2 years.

232. Meningococcal vaccine contains:

a. 50 mcg of polysaccharide of each strain
b. 100 mcg of polysaccharide of each strain
c. 1000 mcg of polysaccharide of each strain
d. 5000 mcg of polysaccharide of each strain

Ans. is 'a' 50 mcg of polysaccharide of each strain

233. How many doses of monovalent meningococcal 'C' vaccine is given in infants?

a. One
b. Two
c. Three
d. Four

Ans. is 'b' Two

MENINGOCOCCAL VACCINE

The methods for the prevention of meningococcal infection include antimicrobial chemoprophylaxis following identification of an index case, use of droplet precautions, vaccination prior to exposure, and avoidance of risk factors

Antimicrobial chemoprophylaxis: Antimicrobial chemoprophylaxis was first used successfully to abort the spread of meningococcal infection in the 1930s. The reported attack rate for close contacts of patients with sporadic meningococcal disease is approximately 4 in 1000 persons exposed (0.4 percent), which is 500 to 800 times higher than the general population.

Chemoprophylaxis is indicated in close contacts of patients with meningococcal infection and should be given as early as possible following the exposure.

Close contacts may include individuals exposed in the following ways:

1. Household members, roommates, intimate contacts, contacts at a childcare center, young adults exposed in dormitories, military recruits exposed in training centers
2. Travelers who had direct contact with respiratory secretions from an index patient or who were seated directly next to an index patient on a prolonged flight (i. e., one lasting ≥8 hours)
3. Individuals who have been exposed to oral secretions (i. e., intimate kissing, mouth-to-mouth resuscitation, endotracheal intubation, or endotracheal tube management)

Regimens for antimicrobial prophylaxis have been defined by the CDC and include **rifampin, ciprofloxacin, and ceftriaxone**

234. A 12-year-old-girl is exposed to a case of meningococcal meningitis in school. What should she prophylactically receive? *(NEET 2020)*

a. Polysaccharide conjugate vaccine single dose
b. Two doses of polyvalent vaccine 4 weeks apart
c. No vaccination
d. Empirical ceftriaxone

Ans. is 'b' Two doses of polyvalent vaccine 4 weeks apart

Diphtheria Anti-toxin (DAT)

- DAT manufactured by Instituto Butantan is a sterile, clear transparent serum solution supplied in 10 mL ampoules containing 10,000 IU each.
- DAT must be stored in the refrigerator at 2–8°C (36–46°F).
- DO NOT FREEZE. Once an ampoule is opened, the DAT serum solution should be used immediately.

235. Dose of diphtheria anti-toxin is: *(NEET 2019)*

a. 1000 to 5000 IU
b. 10000 to 100000 IU
c. 1000 to 2000 IU
d. None

Ans. is 'b' 10000 to 100000 IU

Live vaccines are contraindicated in pregnancy.

- Important ones are:
  - Measles
  - Mumps
  - Poliomyelitis
  - Rubella
  - Yellowfever
  - Varicella (Chicken pox)
  - BCG

236. Which vaccine is contraindicated in pregnancy? *(NEET 2019)*

a. Chicken pox
b. Rabies
c. Tetanus toxoid
d. Hepatitis B

Ans. is 'a' Chicken pox

CHAPTER 12 Medicine

CARDIOLOGY

CONGESTIVE HEART FAILURE (CHF)

Heart failure (HF) is a complex clinical syndrome that can result from any structural or functional cardiac disorder that impairs the ability of the ventricle to fill with or eject blood. It is characterized by specific symptoms, such as dyspnea and fatigue, and signs, such as those related to fluid retention. There are many ways to assess cardiac function. However, there is no diagnostic test for HF, since it is largely a clinical diagnosis that is based upon a careful history and physical examination.

Modified Framingham Clinical Criteria for the Diagnosis of Heart Failure

Major
• Paroxysmal nocturnal dyspnea Orthopnea
• Elevated jugular venous pressure Pulmonary rales
• Third heart sound Cardiomegaly on chest X-ray
• Pulmonary edema on chest X-ray
• Weight loss ≥ 4.5 kg in five days in response to treatment of presumed heart failures*
Minor
• Bilateral leg edema Nocturnal cough
• Dyspnea on ordinary exertion Hepatomegaly
• Pleural effusion
• Tachycardia (heart rate ≥ 120 beats/min)
• Weight loss ≥ 4.5 kg in five days
Diagnosis
The diagnosis of heart failure requires that **two major or one major and two minor criteria** cannot be attributed to another medical condition.

*This criterion was noted in the text of the source paper.

1. An elderly male came to OPD with bilateral basal crepitations, dyspnea, pedal edema, distended jugular veins and positive hepatojugular reflex. What is the likely diagnosis? *(NEET 2020)*

a. Congestive heart failure
b. Left ventricular hypertrophy
c. Dilated cardiomyopathy
d. Acute pericarditis

Ans. is 'a' Congestive heart failure

TYPES OF PULSES

Pulsus alternans: Large and small volume pulses alternating with each other with normal rhythm. Difference of 10–40 mm Hg in systolic pressure between beats.

❖ Seen typically in left heart failure, in which the ventricles beats strongly, then weakly, alternating with each other.

Pulsus bigeminus: A pulse wave with normal beat followed by premature beat and compensatory pause, thereby producing irregular rhythm.

❖ Formed as a result of an ectopic beat following each regular beat.
❖ Seen in digitalis toxicity.

Anacrotic pulse: Low amplitude pulse with slow rise and slow fall.

❖ Seen in aortic stenosis.

Dicrotic pulse: Two palpable waveforms one in systole and the other in diastole.

❖ Seen in cases with low stroke volume with decreased peripheral resistance.
❖ Seen in LVF, dilated cardiomyopathy, cardiac tamponade.

Collapsing or water hammer pulse: Large volume pulse with rapid upstroke and rapid downstroke.

❖ Rapid upstroke is because of increased stroke volume
❖ Rapid downstroke is due to decrease in peripheral resistance and diastolic leak back into left ventricles
❖ Best felt in radial artery with patient's arm elevated
❖ Seen in aortic regurgitation, patent ductus arteriosus and hyperdynamic states. Various hyperdynamic states are: thyrotoxicosis, beri-beri, anemia, AV fistula, pregnancy, etc.

Pulsus bisferiens: Single pulse wave with two peaks, both occurring in systole.

- ❖ Due to ejection of rapid jet blood through aortic valve
- ❖ Best felt in brachial artery and femoral artery
- ❖ Seen in AR + AS, severe AR, hypertrophic obstructive cardiomyopathy.

Pulsus parvus et tardus: Small volume pulse like anacrotic pulse but anacrotic wave is not felt.

- ❖ Usually seen if left ventricular stroke volume or systemic arterial pressure is reduced.
- ❖ Seen in severe hypotension (shock), severe AS, severe PS.

Pulsus paradoxus: Exaggerated decrease in strength of arterial pulse during inspiration.

- ❖ Radial pulse gets smaller in volume with inspiration and larger in volume with expiration
- ❖ Seen in cardiac tamponade, SVC obstruction, COPD, acute severe asthma, constrictive pericarditis, pulmonary embolism, hypovolemic shock.

Pulsus paradoxus is measured by noting the difference between the systolic pressure at which the Korotkoff sounds are first heard (during expiration). While examining the patient for pulsus paradoxus, patient is required to breathe normally since deep breathing can give false positive results. Korotkoff sounds are heard with each heartbeat, independent of the respiratory phase. Between these two pressures, the Korotkoff sounds are heard only intermittently and during expiration. The cuff pressure must be decreased slowly to appreciate the finding. It can be difficult to measure pulsus paradoxus in patients with tachycardia, atrial fibrillation, or tachypnea. A pulsus paradoxus may be palpable at the brachial artery or femoral artery level when the pressure difference exceeds 15 mm Hg. This inspiratory fall in systolic pressure is an exaggerated consequence of interventricular dependence.

The water hammer or Corrigan (or hyperkinetic) pulse is characterized by an abrupt, very rapid upstroke of the peripheral pulse (percussion wave), followed by rapid collapse. It is best appreciated by raising the arm abruptly and feeling for the characteristics in the radial pulse.

The water hammer pulse probably results from very rapid ejection of a large left ventricular stroke volume into a low resistance arterial system. Thus, it occurs most commonly in chronic, hemodynamically significant aortic regurgitation. A bounding arterial pulse with widened pulse pressure is not diagnostic of aortic regurgitation; it can occur in many conditions associated with increased stroke volume such as patent ductus arteriosus, large arteriovenous fistulas, hyperkinetic states, thyrotoxicosis anemia, and extreme bradycardia. The typical pulse characteristics of chronic aortic regurgitation may not occur in acute aortic regurgitation.

2. Water hammer pulse is seen in: *(NEET 2020)*

a. AR b. MS
c. AS d. MR

Ans. is 'a' AR

3. Water hammer pulse is seen in:

a. Aortic regurgitation b. Anemia
c. Pregnancy d. All of the above

Ans. is 'd' All of the above

4. Pulsus bisferiens, which of the following is not true?

a. It is seen in aortic regurgitation b. It is better felt in peripheral arteries
c. It has one peak in systole and one in diastole d. It has two peaks

Ans. is 'c' It has one peak in systole and one in diastole

MURMURS

Type of murmur	Examples
Diastolic Murmurs	
Early	Aortic regurgitation, pulmonary regurgitation, Graham-Steell murmur
Mid	Mitral stenosis, Austin-Flint murmur
Late	Rheumatic carditis (Carey-Coombs murmur)
Systolic Murmurs	
Ejection mid-systolic	Aortic stenosis, pulmonary stenosis
Holosystolic	Mitral regurgitation, aortic regurgitation
Late	Mitral valve prolapse

Named diastolic murmurs		Seen in
Early diastolic	Graham Steell	Pulmonary regurgitation
Late diastolic	Carey-Coombs	Rheumatic carditis
Mid diastolic	Austin-Flint	Severe aortic regurgitation

Bedside maneuver	Effect
Inspiration (↑ venous return to RA)	↑ intensity of right heart sounds
Handgrip (↑ afterload)	↑ intensity of MR, AR, VSD ↓ HOCM and AS murmurs MVP–later onset of click/murmur
Valsalva (phase II), Standing up (↓ preload)	↓ intensity of most murmurs (including AS) ↑ intensity of HOCM MVP–earlier onset of click/murmur
Rapid squatting (↑ venous return, ↑ preload, ↑ afterload)	↓ intensity of HOCM ↑ intensity of MR, AR, VSD MVP–later onset of click/murmur

5. Which murmur increases on standing? *(NEET 2019)*

a. HOCM
b. MR
c. MS
d. VSD

Ans. is 'a' HOCM

6. Carey-Coombs murmur is seen in:

a. Acute rheumatic fever
b. Infective endocarditis
c. Systemic lupus erythematosus
d. Patent ductus arteriosus

Ans. is 'a' Acute rheumatic fever

ELECTROCARDIOGRAPHY (ECG)

Rhythm Abnormalities on ECG

Junctional Rhythm

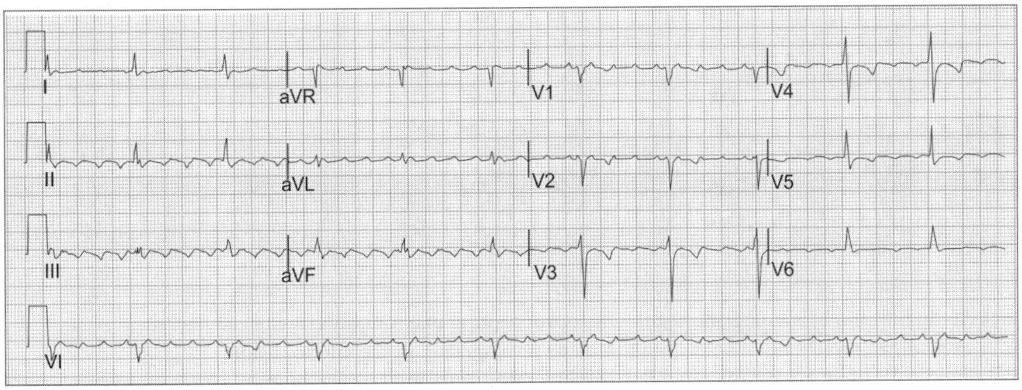

- The QRS complex is narrow, with a rate typically between 40 and 60 bpm.
- P waves are absent, retrograde, very slow, or unrelated to the QRS complex

Ventricular Rhythm

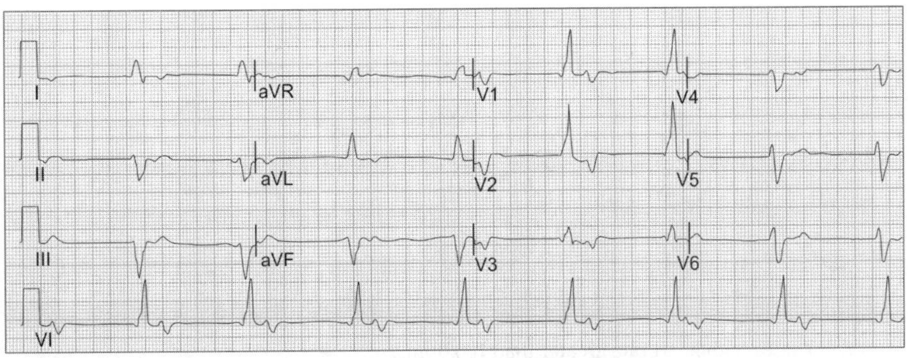

- The QRS complex is wider than 120 ms, with a rate typically between 20 and 40 bpm.
- The T wave is discordant relative to the QRS.

Atrial Fibrillation

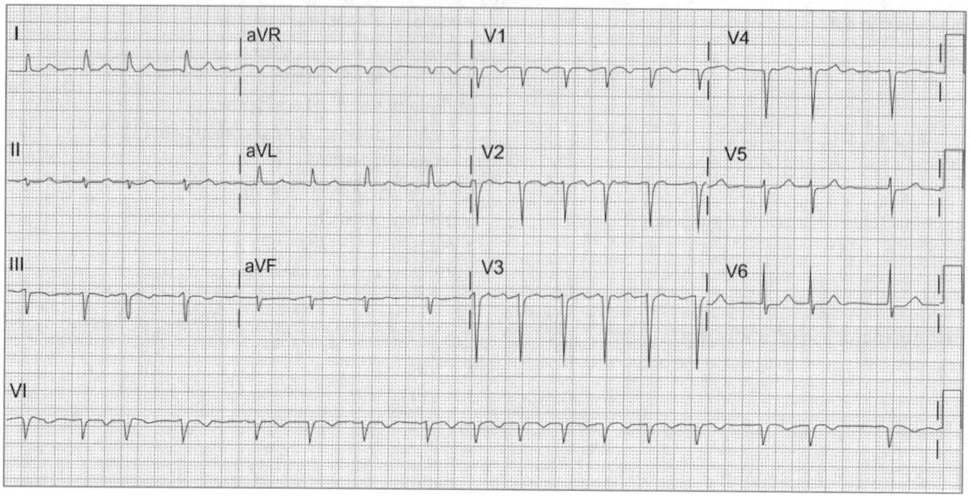

- ❖ Electrical activity in the atria is chaotic. The ECG baseline, representing the ongoing chaotic atrial activity, is unorganized. The resulting "rumbling" baseline may have large or indiscernibly small amplitude.
- ❖ The AV node has a refractory period, and therefore does not conduct every signal it receives from the atria. Thus, ventricles depolarize variably creating varying R-R intervals and an "irregularly irregular" pattern.

Atrial Flutter

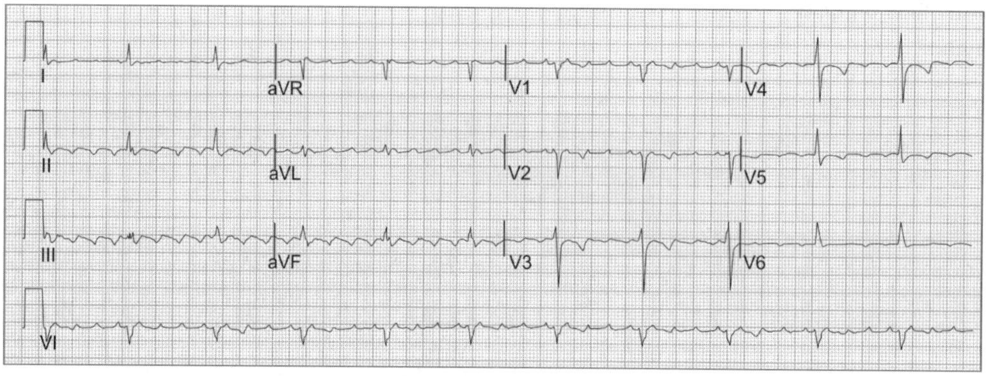

- ❖ Electrical activity in the atria is ongoing and regular, self-propagating in a roughly circular movement.
- ❖ Flutter waves appear in a rapid sine wave or "sawtooth" pattern, usually in the inferior leads.
- ❖ Atrial activity in lead V1 often appears as rapid P waves at a rate approximating 300 bpm.

Multifocal Atrial Tachycardia

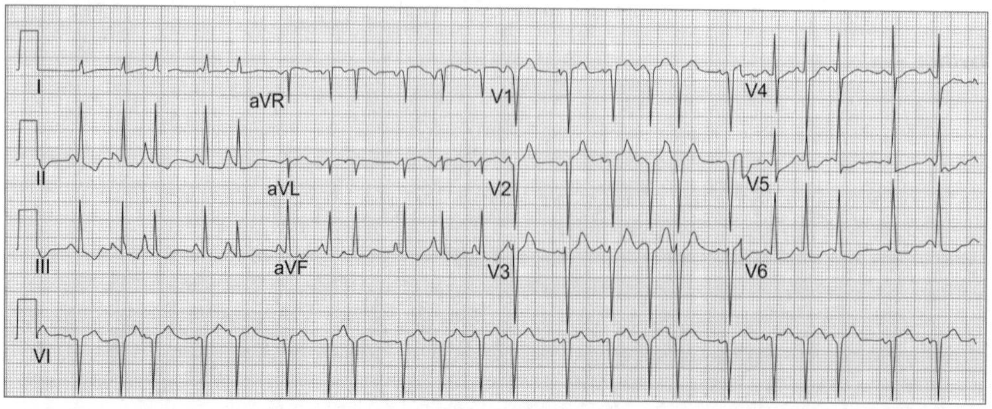

- ❖ Multiple P-wave morphologies with heart rate greater than 100 bpm
- ❖ A chaotic R-R interval
- ❖ Varying PR intervals.

Ventricular Tachycardia

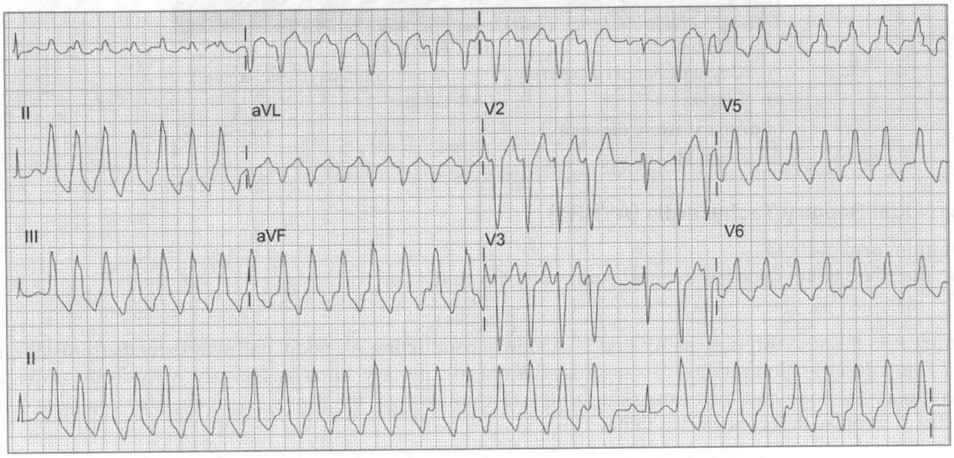

- Tachycardia (usually >120 bpm) with a wide QRS complex.
- AV dissociation is present; P waves may appear periodically in the T wave or baseline.
- "Capture" beats may occur if atrial depolarization occurs prior to the intrinsic firing of the ventricle.
- "Fusion" beats may occur if atrial depolarization passes through the AV node at the same time as the intrinsic ventricle depolarization, producing a QRS that appears to be different or narrower than the other VT QRS complexes.

Ventricular Flutter

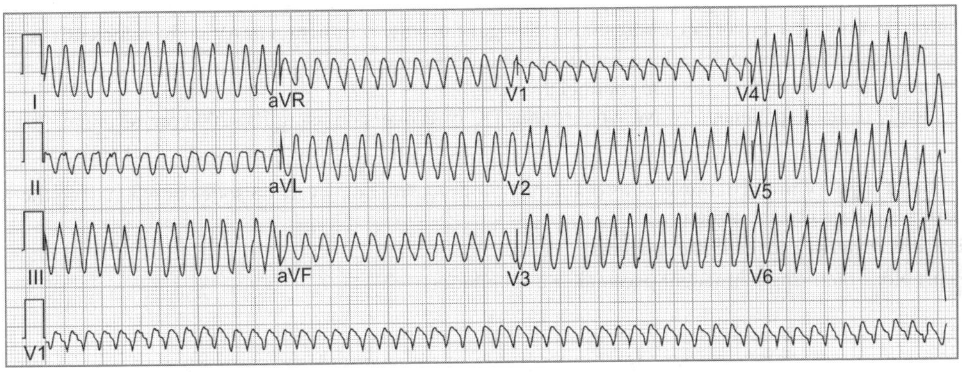

- Tachycardia with a wide monomorphic QRS complex.
- Ventricular rate may be very rapid (300 bpm).
- Sine wave appearance with regular large oscillations.

Atrioventricular (AV) Block

AV block is classified into 3 categories based on the severity of conduction block:

- First degree AV block presents as a prolonged PR interval with 1:1 conduction, i.e. all P waves are conducted into the ventricles.
- Second degree AV blocks is further divided into 2 categories:
  - Mobitz I: progressive prolongation of PR interval over successive beats followed by an absent QRS complex. (Wenckebach phenomenon)
  - Mobitz II: PR interval remains constant, but the P waves get conducted into the ventricles only intermittently.
- Third degree AV block or complete AV block—Atrioventricular dissociation occurs as a result of complete failure of atrial impulses to get conducted into the ventricles. There is no relationship between P wave and QRS complex. However, the P-P interval and R-R interval remains constant.

Etiologies of atrioventricular block	
Autonomic	
• Carotid sinus hypersensitivity	• Vasovagal
Metabolic/endocrine	
• Hyperkalemia • Hypermagnesemia	• Hypothyroidism • Adrenal insufficiency
Drug-related	

Contd...

Medicine

Contd…

Etiologies of atrioventricular block	
• Beta blockers • Calcium channel blockers • Digitalis	• Adenosine • Antiarrhythmics (class I and III) • Lithium
Coronary artery disease	
• Acute MI	

Atrioventricular Nodal Reentry Tachycardia (AVNRT)

- ❖ It is most common form of PSVT
- ❖ Individuals in their 2nd to 4th decades are most commonly affected.

Mechanism:

- ❖ Electrical reentry into the atria through the AV node—A slowly conducting AV nodal pathway extends from compact AV node near the bundle of His, inferiorly along tricuspid annulus, adjacent to coronary sinus os. Reentry wave-front propagates up this slow pathway to compact AV node and then exits through the fast pathway at the top of AV node. This creates a continuously active source of electrical impulse, triggering arrhythmia.

Clinical Features:

- ❖ It is usually well tolerated and not associated with structural heart diseases
- ❖ Angina, pulmonary edema, hypotension, or syncope may be seen in the elderly.

ECG Findings:

- ❖ Long PR interval, narrow QRS complex tachycardia
- ❖ P-wave is buried inside QRS complex.

Immediate Treatment:

- ❖ Vagal stimulation (Valsalva maneuver or carotid sinus massage) can slow conduction in AV node sufficiently to terminate AVNRT
- ❖ If physical maneuvers do not terminate tachyarrhythmia, 1st-line treatment: Adenosine
- ❖ *2nd-line treatment*: IV beta blockade or calcium channel therapy
- ❖ In hemodynamically unstable patients, R-wave synchronous DC cardioversion using 100–200 J can terminate the tachyarrhythmia.

Catheter Ablation:

- ❖ Catheter ablation of slow AV nodal pathway is recommended for recurrent or severe episodes or when drug therapy is ineffective, not tolerated, or not desired by the patient
- ❖ Catheter ablation is curative in over 95% of patients
- ❖ *Major risk*: Heart block requiring permanent pacemaker implantation

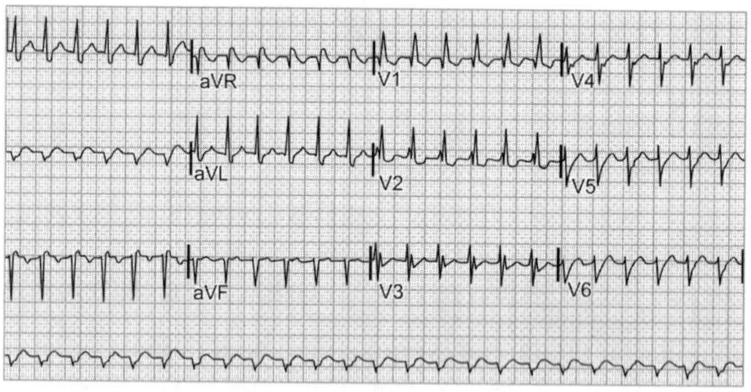

- ❖ **p-mitrale**–Notched / Bifid p-wave seen in Left Atrial Enlargement
- ❖ **p-pulmonale**–Tall peaked p-wave seen in Right Atrial Enlargement
- ❖ Similar picture seen in hypokalemia–**'Pseudo p-pulmonale'**

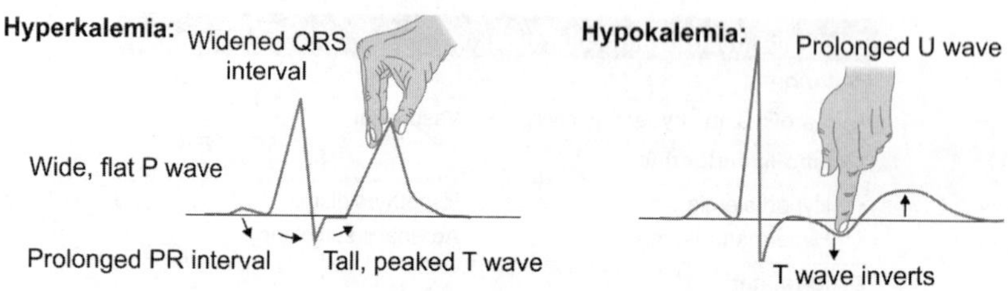

"Pull and push effects" of potassium on T wave of ECG

- **Hypercalcemia**: Bradycardia, AV block, short QT interval
- **Hypocalcemia**: Prolongation of QT interval.

J wave: Also known as Osborn wave, camel-hump sign, late delta wave, hypothermic wave, K wave, H wave or current of injury — is an abnormal ECG finding.

J waves are positive deflections occurring at the junction between the QRS complex and the ST segment, where the S point, also known as the J point, has a myocardial infarction-like elevation.

Causes: They are usually observed in people suffering from hypothermia with a temperature of less than 32°C (90°F), though they may also occur in people with hypercalcemia, brain injury, vasospastic angina or ventricular fibrillation and could also be a normal variant.

Wolff-Parkinson-White Syndrome

- Most common type of ventricular pre-excitation syndrome.
- Abnormal fast accessory conduction pathway from atria to ventricles (Bundle of Kent) bypasses the rate-slowing AV node → ventricles begin to partially depolarize earlier → characteristic delta wave with widened QRS complex and shortened PR interval on ECG.
- May result in reentry circuit → supraventricular tachycardia.

Conditions associated with prolonged QT syndrome
Congenital
• Romanoward syndrome → normal hearing
• Jervell and Lange-Nielsen syndrome → sensorineural hearing loss
Acquired
• Antiarrhythmic drugs–IA, IC, III
• TCAs
• Antibiotics (macrolides, cotrimoxazole)
• Terfenadine (when combined with macrolides or antifungal)
Metabolic
• Hypokalemia
• Hypocalcemia
• Hypomagnesemia
T/T acquired prolonged QT syndrome
• DC shock (unstable patient)
• Magnesium sulphate IV

ECG Findings in Pulmonary Embolism

- Sinus tachycardia—most common abnormality.
- S1Q3T3 sign: An S wave in lead I, Q wave in lead III, and an inverted T wave in lead III. This finding is relatively specific but insensitive.
- T-wave inversion in leads V1 to V4.

7. Osborn J wave is seen in: *(NEET 2019)*

a. Hypothermia b. Hyperkalemia
c. Hypocalcemia d. Hypokalemia

Ans. is 'a' Hypothermia

8. Which of these statements is true for Bundle of Kent? *(NEET 2019)*

a. An abnormal pathway between the two atria
b. It is a muscular or nodal pathway between atria and ventricle in WPW
c. It is slower than AV nodal pathway
d. None

Ans. is 'b' It is a muscular or nodal pathway between atria and ventricle in WPW

9. Which of the following causes AV block?

a. Hypothyroidism b. Hyperthyroidism
c. Pheochromocytoma d. Carcinoid

Ans. is 'a' Hypothryroidism

10. Which of the following is the most common abnormality in ECG manifestation of pulmonary embolism?

a. T wave inversion in V1 to V4 b. Sinus tachycardia
c. U wave d. S1Q2T3 pattern

Ans. is 'b' Sinus tachycardia

11. Identify the condition in ECG: *(NEET 2019)*

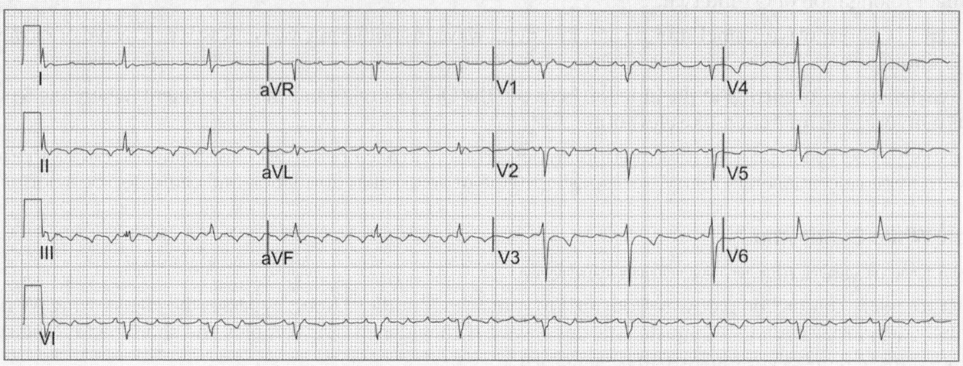

a. Atrial fibrillation
b. Ventricular tachycardia
c. Atrial flutter
d. Cardiomyopathy

Ans. is 'c' Atrial flutter

12. Identify the ECG: *(NEET 2019)*

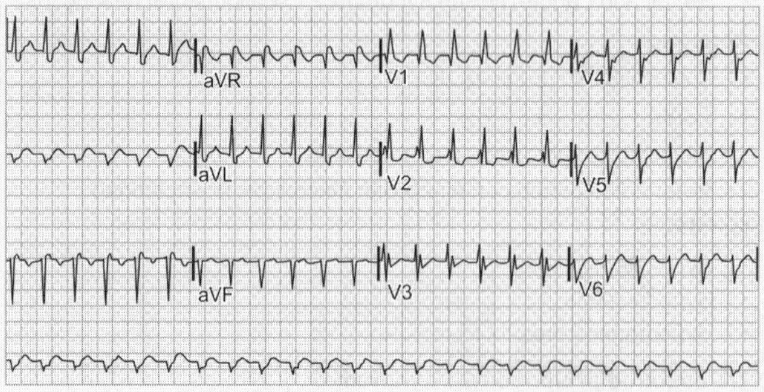

a. VT
b. PSVT
c. AT
d. VF

Ans. is 'b' PSVT

MITRAL STENOSIS

- **Major causes**
  - Rheumatic fever–Leading cause
  - Congenital (cor triatriatum)
  - Severe mitral annular calcification
  - SLE, RA
  - Myxoma
  - Infective endocarditis.
- **X-ray findings of MS**
  - Left atrial enlargement is responsible for X-ray findings
  - Earliest sign–Splaying of carina
  - Straightening of left heart border
  - 'Double Density'– Retrocardiac shadow of enlarged left atrium
  - Posterior displacement of esophagus on barium swallow—Left atrium is the most posterior chamber of heart.
- **Auscultation findings**
  - S1 is usually accentuated in the early stages of the disease and slightly delayed. The pulmonic component of the second heart sound (P2) also is often accentuated with elevated PA pressures, and the two components of the second heart sound (S2) are closely split.
  - The opening snap (OS) of the mitral valve is most readily audible in expiration at, or just medial to, the cardiac apex. This sound generally follows the sound of aortic valve closure (A2) by 0.05–0.12 s. The time interval between A2 and OS varies inversely with the severity of the MS.
  - The OS is followed by a low-pitched, rumbling, diastolic murmur, heard best at the apex with the patient in the left lateral recumbent position. In general, the duration of this murmur correlates with the severity of the stenosis in patients with preserved CO.

- **Management**
  - Percutaneous balloon mitral valvotomy (PMBV)—splitting of fused commissures. Contraindications include moderate or severe MR, left atrial thrombus, commissural calcification and thickened fibrotic leaflets with decreased mobility. If no C/I, PMBV is indicated in symptomatic (NYHA II-IV) patient with severe MS (<1.5 cm^2 or < 1 cm^2/m^2 BSA).
  - Mitral valve replacement (MVR)—Indicated in NYHA III-IV patients with severe MS or MS + severe MR or in presence of contraindications for PMBV.

13. Which of the following is not a cause of mitral stenosis?

a. Cor triatriatum
b. Atrial myxoma
c. Systemic lupus erythematosus
d. Cryoglobulinemia

Ans. is 'd' Cryoglobulinemia

14. In mitral stenosis "the double shadow' on X-ray chest PA view is due to enlargement of:

a. Right atrial enlargement
b. Right ventricular enlargement
c. Left atrial enlargement
d. Left ventricular enlargement

Ans. is 'c' Left atrial enlargement

15. Which heart chamber enlargement can be seen on barium swallow in mitral stenosis? *(NEET 2019)*

a. Left atrium
b. Right atrium
c. Left ventricle
d. Right ventricle

Ans. is 'a' Left atrium

16. Contraindication for percutaneous balloon mitral valvotomy include the following *except*:

a Presence of pulmonary hypertension
b. Left atrial thrombus
c Severe mitral regurgitation
d Commissural calcification

Ans. is 'a' Presence of pulmonary hypertension

ISCHEMIC HEART DISEASE

Stable Angina Pectoris

- The typical patient with angina is a man >50 years or a woman >60 years of age who complains of episodes of chest discomfort, usually described as heaviness, pressure, squeezing, smothering, or choking and only rarely as frank pain.
- When the patient is asked to localize the sensation, he or she typically places a hand over the sternum, sometimes with a clenched fist, to indicate a squeezing, central, substernal discomfort (Levine's sign).
- Angina is usually crescendo-decrescendo in nature, typically lasts 2 to 5 min, and can radiate to either shoulder and to both arms (especially the ulnar surfaces of the forearm and hand).
- It also can arise in or radiate to the back, interscapular region, root of the neck, jaw, teeth, and epigastrium. Angina is rarely localized below the umbilicus or above the mandible.

Prinzmetal's Variant Angina

- Severe ischemic pain that occurs at rest but not usually with exertion and is associated with transient ST segment elevation.
- This syndrome is due to focal spasm of an epicardial coronary artery, leading to severe myocardial ischemia.
- Patients with Prinzmetal's variant angina (PVA) are generally younger and have fewer coronary risk factors with the exception of cigarette smoking.
- Focal spasm is most common in the right coronary artery, and it may occur at one or more sites simultaneously.
- Nitrates and calcium channel blockers are the main agents used to treat acute episodes and to a recurrent episodes of PVA.
- Aspirin may actually increase the severity of ischemic episodes.

ECG localization of MI

Infarct location	*Leads with ST elevation*
Anteroseptal (LAD)	V1, V2
Anteroapical (distal LAD)	V3, V4
Anterolateral (LAD or LCX)	V5, V6
Lateral (LCX)	I, aVL
Inferior (RCA)	II, III, aVF; Reciprocal changes in I, aVL
Posterior (PDA)	V7-V9; ST depression in V1-V3

Complications of MI

- *Cardiac arrhythmia*: Occurs within the first few days after MI. Important cause within first 24 hours post-MI.
- Postinfarction fibrinous pericarditis: 1–3 days, friction rub present.
- *Papillary muscle rupture*: 2–7 days; posteromedial papillary muscle rupture ↑ risk due to single blood supply from PDA. Can result in severe mitral regurgitation.
- *Ventricular pseudoaneurysm formation*: 3–14 days; free wall rupture contained by adherent pericardium or scar tissue; ↓ cardiac output, risk of arrhythmia, embolus from mural thrombus.
- *Ventricular free wall rupture*: 5–14 days; free wall rupture → cardiac tamponade. May lead to sudden death.
- *True ventricular aneurysm*: 2 weeks to several months; outward bulge with contraction (dyskinesia). Approximately 80% of left ventricular aneurysms are located in anterior and/or apical walls, most commonly with LAD occlusion. Only 10–15% involve inferior wall; lateral aneurysms are rare.
- *Dressler syndrome*: Several weeks; Autoimmune phenomenon resulting in fibrinous pericarditis.
- LV failure.

17. Infarcts involving which portion of myocardium cause aneurysm as a post-MI complication? *(NEET 2019)*

a. Subendocardial
b. Anterior transmural
c. Posterior transmural
d. Inferior wall

Ans. is 'b' Anterior transmural

18. Which of the following is not true about Prinzmetal's angina?

a. Severe ischemic pain at rest with ST segment elevation
b. Focal spasms are common in right coronary artery
c. Nitrates and calcium channel blockers are the mainstay of management
d. Aspirin treatment decreases the episodes of angina

Ans. is 'd' Aspirin treatment decreases the episodes of angina

19. Reciprocal changes in ECG in patients with inferior wall myocardial infarction are seen in which lead?

a. I
b. II
c. III
d. IV

Ans. is 'a' I

DILATED CARDIOMYOPATHY

- Most common cardiomyopathy (90% of cases).
- *Often idiopathic or familial.*
- *Other etiologies include*: Chronic alcoholism, Coxsackie B viral myocarditis, chronic cocaine use, Chagas disease, Doxorubicin toxicity, hemochromatosis, sarcoidosis, peripartum cardiomyopathy.
- Leads to systolic dysfunction.
- *Findings*: Heart failure, S3, systolic regurgitant murmur, dilated heart on echocardiogram.
- *Treatment*: Sodium restriction, ACE inhibitors, Beta-blockers, diuretics.

20. Alcohol causes which type of cardiomyopathy?

a. Hypertrophic cardiomyopathy
b. Dilated cardiomyopathy
c. Pericarditis
d. Myocarditis

Ans. is 'b' Dilated cardiomyopathy

INFECTIVE ENDOCARDITIS

Criteria for the Clinical Diagnosis of Infective Endocarditis

Major Criteria

1. Positive blood culture for IE
    - Typical microorganism for infective endocarditis from two separate blood cultures:
        - *Viridans streptococci, Streptococcus gallolyticus*, HACEK group, *Staphylococcus aureus*, or
        - Community-acquired enterococci in the absence of a primary focus, or
    - Persistently positive blood culture, defined as recovery of a microorganism consistent with infective endocarditis from:
        - Blood cultures drawn >12 h apart; or
        - All of 3 or a majority of ≥ 4 separate blood cultures, with first and last drawn at least 1 h apart
    - Single positive blood culture for *Coxiella burnetii* or phase I IgG antibody titer of >1:800.

Medicine

2. Evidence of endocardial involvement
   - Positive echocardiogram:
     - Oscillating intracardiac mass on valve or supporting structures or in the path of regurgitant jets or in implanted material
     - Abscess, or
     - New partial dehiscence of prosthetic valve, or
   - New valvular regurgitation (increase or change in preexisting murmur not sufficient).

Minor Criteria

1. *Predisposition*: Predisposing heart condition or injection drug use
2. *Fever*: ≥38.0°C (≥100.4°F)
3. *Vascular phenomena*: Major arterial emboli, septic pulmonary infarcts, mycotic aneurysm, intracranial hemorrhage, conjunctival hemorrhages, Janeway lesions
4. *Immunologic phenomena*: Glomerulonephritis, Osler's nodes, Roth's spots, rheumatoid factor
5. *Microbiologic evidence*: Positive blood culture but not meeting major criterion as noted previously or serologic evidence of active infection with organism consistent with infective endocarditis
   - Definite endocarditis is defined by documentation of two major criteria, of one major criterion and three minor criteria, or of five minor criteria.

21. Essential major blood culture criteria for infective endocarditis: *(NEET 2019)*

a. Single positive culture of HACEK
b. Single positive culture of coxiella
c. Single positive culture of Corynebacterium
d. Both A and B

Ans. is 'a' Single positive culture of HACEK

PERICARDITIS

Causes of hemorrhagic pericarditis
• Tuberculosis
• Malignant involvement of pericardial sac
• Bleeding diathesis
• Cardiac surgery
• Post-myocardial infarction
• Dissecting aneurysm of aorta
• Uremic pericarditis

Acute Pericarditis ECG Manifestations

- The electrocardiogram (EGG) in acute pericarditis without massive effusion usually displays changes secondary to acute subepicardial inflammation.
- It typically evolves through four stages:
  1. In stage 1, there is widespread elevation of the ST segments, often with upward concavity, involving two three standard limb leads and V2 to V6, with reciprocal depressions only in aVR. Usually there are significant changes in QRS complexes.
  2. In stage 2, after several days, the ST segments return to normal, and only then, or even later, do the T waves become inverted (stage 3).
  3. Ultimately, weeks or months after the onset of acute pericarditis, the EGG returns to normal in stage 4.
  4. Sequential ECGs are useful in distinguishing acute pericarditis from MI. In the latter, elevated ST segments return to normal within hours.

22. Following ECG manifestations are seen in acute pericarditis *except*:

a. ST segment elevation with upward concavity in V2–V6
b. ST depression in aVR
c. T wave inversion
d. Prolongation of QRS complexes

Ans. is 'd' Prolongation of QRS complexes

23. Hemorrhagic pericarditis can be caused by:

a. Tuberculosis
b. After cardiac surgery
c. Metastatic disease
d. All the above

Ans. is 'd' All the above

IMPLANTABLE CARDIOVERTER DEFIBRILLATOR (ICD)

Terminate arrhythmia by a shock applied to a lead in right ventricle

Indications: Secondary prophylaxis (survivors of cardiac arrest) and Primary prophylaxis

Class I indications (the benefit greatly outweighs the risk and treatment should be administered)

- Structural heart disease, sustained VT
- Idiopathic VT, inducible VT or VF at electrophysiologic study (EPS)
- **Post-MI**, Left ventricular ejection fraction (LVEF) ≤35% or inducible VT.

Class IIa indications (the benefit outweighs the risk and it is reasonable to administer the treatment)

- Hypertrophic cardiomyopathy with 1 or more major risk factors
- **Arrhythmogenic right ventricular dysplasia** with risk factors for sudden cardiac death (SCD)
- **Long QT syndrome**, syncope or VT while receiving beta-blockers
- **Brugada syndrome**, syncope or VT
- Catecholaminergic polymorphic VT, syncope or VT while receiving beta-blockers
- Cardiac sarcoidosis.

24. Implantable cardioverter defibrillator is useful in: *(NEET 2018)*

a. Brugada syndrome
b. Arrhythmogenic RV dysplasia
c. Post MI with structural damage
d. All of the above

Ans. is 'd' All of the above

PERMANENT CARDIAC PACEMAKER

Indications

- SA node dysfunction with symptomatic bradycardia
- Second or third degree AV block with symptomatic bradycardia
- Chronic bifascicular and trifascicular block
- Post-MI with second or third-degree AV block, bundle branch block or advanced infranodal AV block
- Hypersensitive carotid sinus syndrome and neurocardiogenic syncope.

25. Permanent cardiac pacing is helpful in: *(NEET 2018)*

a. Brugada syndrome
b. Post-myocardial infarction AV block
c. Ventricular fibrillation
d. Transient AV block

Ans. is 'b' Post-myocardial infarction AV block

Previously Asked Facts

- Drug of choice for rheumatic chorea: Sodium Valproate > Haloperidol
- On auscultation, Mitral Valve Prolapse (MVP) shows mid-late systolic click and late systolic murmur at cardiac apex
- Signs of wide pulse pressure in aortic regurgitation

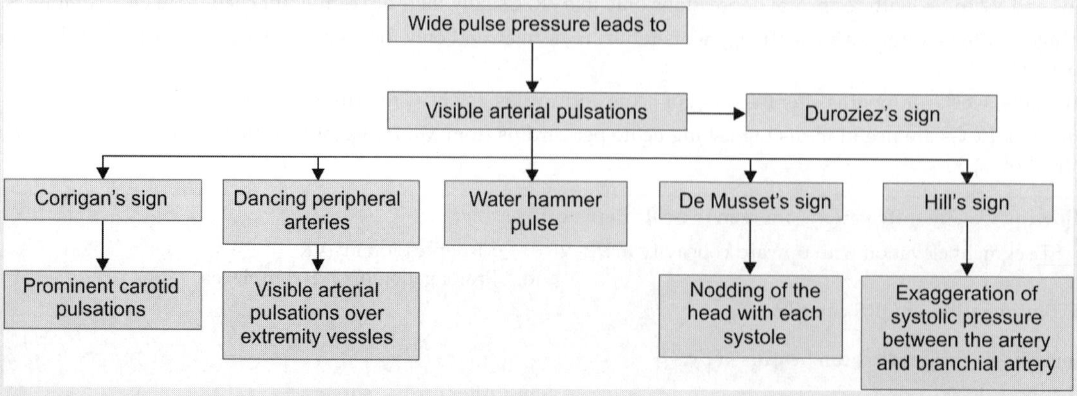

- In aortic stenosis, there is a pressure gradient between left ventricle and aorta. More severe the stenosis, higher the gradient between LV and aorta.

HEMATOLOGY

ANEMIAS

Treatment of Iron Deficiency Anemia

Oral iron therapy: Indicated in asymptomatic patients with established IDA.

- Dose: 200 mg elemental iron per day.
- It should be taken on an empty stomach because food inhibits absorption.
- The anemia should be corrected so as to have extra stores of 0.5–1 g of iron in the body. Oral iron must be given for 6–12 months to achieve this.
- *Side effects*: Abdominal pain, nausea, vomiting, or constipation.

Parenteral iron therapy: Indicated in patients who are unable to tolerate oral iron, or who are non-compliant with oral iron.

- Total dose administered would contain the iron required to correct hemoglobin deficit and provide at least 500 mg of iron stores
- Iron required is calculated by the formula: 23 × Body weight (kg) × (15-patient's hemoglobin g/dL) + 500 or 1000 mg (for stores).
- Test dose is given before iron dextran, since anaphylaxis may occur.
- Iron sucrose is given as infusion diluted in 5% dextrose or normal saline.

Red cell transfusion: Reserved for individuals with symptoms of anemia, cardiovascular instability, continued and excessive blood loss requiring immediate intervention.

Sickle Cell Anemia Symptoms

- *Vaso-occlusion symptoms*: Strokes, acute chest syndrome (associated with fever, hypoxia and pulmonary infarcts, most common cause of death in adults with sickle cell anemia), hand and feet swelling (ischemic dactylitis), aseptic necrosis of femoral or humeral head, splenic infarcts as well as autosplenectomy leads to increased susceptibility to encapsulated bacteria (most common cause of death from bacterial infections in children with sickle cell).
- *Sequestration symptoms*: Acute pooling of RBCs in spleen, usually post-infection; presents with acute splenomegaly and septic shock-like state.
- *Hemolytic symptoms*: Pallor from chronic hemolytic anemia, mostly intravascular hemolysis. Massive erythroid hyperplasia due to expansion of hematopoiesis into skull (crewcut), facial bone (chipmunk face) and extramedullary hematopoiesis.
- *Aplastic symptoms*: ↑ risk of Parvovirus B19 infection.

Clinical and hematological features of β-thalassemia

Syndrome	*T-major* *Homozygous*	*T- Intermedia* *Double heterozygotes*	*T-minor* *Heterozygotes*
Clinical features			
• Severity of disease	++++	++	±
• Growth and development	Impaired	–	–
• Splenomegaly	++++	++	–
• Skeletal changes	+++	±	–
• Thalassemia facies	+++	+	–
Hematological findings			
• Hb (g/dL)	<7 (severe)	7–10 (moderate)	>10
• Red cell count	$<4 \times 10^{12}$/L	$<5 \times 10^{12}$/L	$>55 \times 10^{12}$/L
• Microcytosis	+++	++	+
• Hypochromia	+++	++	+
• Basophilic stippling	++	+	+
• Anisopoikilocytosis	+++	++	±
• Target cells	+++	++	+
• Nucleated red cells	++	Occasional	–
• HbF	30–90%	(20–100%)	0–5%
• HbA2	<3.5%	<3.5%	3.6–8%
• BM iron	++++	++	±
• Iron overload			
– Myocardium	+	–	–
– Endocrine involvement	+	–	–
• Life expectancy	20–28 years	Normal	Normal

COOMB'S TEST

Direct Coomb's Test

- It detects antibodies of complement bound to RBC surface antigens in vivo.
- It is used in the diagnosis of immune-mediated hemolytic anemia (e.g. SLE), hemolytic disease of the newborn, drug-induced hemolysis, mismatch transfusion reaction.

Indirect Coomb's Test

- This test detects circulating antibodies in the serum.
- It is used in the detection of very low concentrations of antibodies in a patient's plasma/serum prior to a blood transfusion and in pregnant women for diagnosing Rh isoimmunization.
- It can also be used in compatibility testing, RBC phenotyping.

26. Ischemic dactylitis is seen in:

a. Hemophilia b. Thalassemia
c. Sickle cell anemia d. Hereditary spherocytes

Ans. is 'b' Thalassemia

27. All but one is true for beta thalassemia major:

a. Growth and development is impaired b. Red cell count < 4×10^{12}/L
c. Levels of HbA2<3.5% d. Bone marrow iron is depleted

Ans. is 'd' Bone marrow iron is depleted

28. Coomb's positive hemolytic anemia is associated with:

a. TTP b. SLE
c. PAN d. HUS

Ans. is 'b' SLE

HEMOPHILIA

- 2nd most common inherited coagulation disorder (after von Willebrand disease)
- X-linked recessive hereditary disorder
- Males affected.

Types

- Hemophilia A (classic hemophilia: 80%): defective or deficient coagulation factor VIII.
- Hemophilia B (Christmas disease: 10–15%): defective or deficiency of coagulation factor IX.

Clinical Features

Hemarthrosis:

- Most common presentation.
- Physically, economically and psychologically debilitating manifestation.
- Most common: Knee, but there are others as elbows, wrists and ankles (toddlers).

Chronic involvement with joint deformity 'hemophilic arthropathy.

Hemorrhage:

- Prolonged bleed from umbilical cord, tooth extraction.
- Gum bleeds while brushing teeth.
- Gastrointestinal and genitourinary bleeds.
- Intracranial bleeds—presents with unusual headache.

Hematomas:

- Subcutaneous and muscular hematomas.
- *Muscle hematomas*: 1. Calf, 2. thigh, 3. buttocks, 4. forearms.
- *Psoas hematoma*: If right sided may mimic acute appendicitis.

29. Characteristic features of hemophilia:

a. Hematemesis b. Hemarthrosis
c. Hemoptysis d. Bleeding varices

Ans. is 'b' Hemathrosis

Medicine

IMMUNE THROMBOCYTOPENIA

Immune thrombocytopenia			
Clinical presentation	• Antecedent viral infection • Asymptomatic petechiae and ecchymosis most common • Mucocutaneous bleeding (e.g., epistaxis, hematuria, gastrointestinal bleeding)		
Laboratory findings	• Isolated thrombocytopenia <100,000/μL • Peripheral smear with megakaryocytes and no other abnormalities		→ Normal Hct and leukocyte count
Treatment	Children	• Skin manifestations only: Observe • Bleeding • IVIg OR • Glucocortcoids	→ Usually spontaneous recovery withing 6 months–hence, treat only if bleeding +ve regardless of platelet count
	Adults	• Platelets ≥30,000/μL without bleeding: Observe • Platelets <30,000/μL OR bleeding: • IVIg OR • Glucocortcoids	

- ❖ Last resort is Splenectomy.
- ❖ ITP is termed secondary if it is associated with an underlying disorder; autoimmune disorders, particularly systemic lupus erythematosus (SLE), and infections, such as HIV and hepatitis C, are common causes.

30. Which of the following is not a cause of secondary idiopathic thrombocytopenic purpura?

a. Systemic lupus erythematosus b. Hepatitis C infection
c. Rheumatoid arthritis d. HIV infection

Ans. is 'c' Rheumatoid arthritis

MULTIPLE MYELOMA

Both criteria must be met for diagnosis:

- ❖ Clonal bone marrow plasma cells or biopsy-proven bony or extramedullary plasmacytoma.
- ❖ Any one or more of the following myeloma defining events:
  - Evidence of end organ damage that can be attributed to the underlying plasma cell proliferative disorder, specifically:
    - *Hypercalcemia*: Serum calcium >0.25 mmol/L (>1 mg/dL) higher than the upper limit of normal or >2.75 mmol/L (>11 mg/dL)
    - *Renal insufficiency*: Creatinine >2 mg/dL
    - *Anemia*: Hemoglobin value of >2 g/dL below the lower limit or normal, or a hemoglobin value <10 g/dL.
    - *Bone lesions*: One or more osteolytic lesions on skeletal radiography, computed tomography (CT), or positron emission tomography- CT (PET-CT)
  - Clonal bone marrow plasma cell percentage ≥ 60%.
  - Involved:Uninvolved serum free light chain (FLC) ratio ≥ 100 (involved free light chain level must be ≥ 100 mg/L)
  - > 1 focal lesions on magnetic resonance imaging (MRI) studies (at least 5 mm in size).

Diagnosis

Immunoelectrophoresis in Multiple Myeloma

- ❖ The monoclonal antibody must be present at a concentration of at least 5 g/L (0.5 g/dL) to be accurately quantitated by this method.
- ❖ Confirmation that such an M component is truly monoclonal and the type of immunoglobulin is determined by immunoelectrophoresis that reveals a single heavy and/or light chain type.
- ❖ Hence, immunoelectrophoresis and electrophoresis provide qualitative and quantitative assessment of the M component, respectively.
- ❖ The serum M component in multiple myeloma will be IgG in 53% of patients. IgA in 25% and lgD in 1%; 20% of patients will have only light chains in serum and urine.

Imaging

- ❖ The skull demonstrates the typical punched out' lesions characteristic of multiple myeloma.
- ❖ The lesion represents a purely osteolytic lesion with little or no osteoblastic activity.

Bone lesions are most common in vertebral column. Other locations are ribs, skull, pelvis, femur and clavicle

Medicine

Treatment of M myeloma	
Autologous SCT	***No SCT***
• CSF (colony stimulating factor) → stem cell split into plasma → collect cells (stem) • Then give lenalidomide + dexamethasone +bortezomib • Bortezomib can be replaced by ixazomib or carfilzomib • Thalidomide can be used as a cheaper alternative of lenalidomide	Melphalan → MP → Prednisolone Melphalan → MPT → Prednisolone + thalidomide > 70 years

Management of relapsed/refractory multiple myeloma is:

❖ Relapsed myeloma can be treated with novel agents including lenalidomide and/or bortezomib. These agents target not only the tumor cell but also the tumor cell-bone marrow interaction and the bone marrow milieu. These agents in combination with dexamethasone can achieve up to 60% partial responses and 10–15% complete responses in patients with relapsed disease.
❖ The combination of bortezomib and liposomal doxorubicin is active in relapsed myeloma.
❖ Thalidomide, if not used as initial therapy, can achieve responses in refractory cases.
❖ High-dose melphalan and stem cell transplant, if not used earlier, also have activity in patients with refractory disease.

31. A 55-year-old male having bone pains for the last 2 years with X-ray of skull shown below. Most probable diagnosis is:

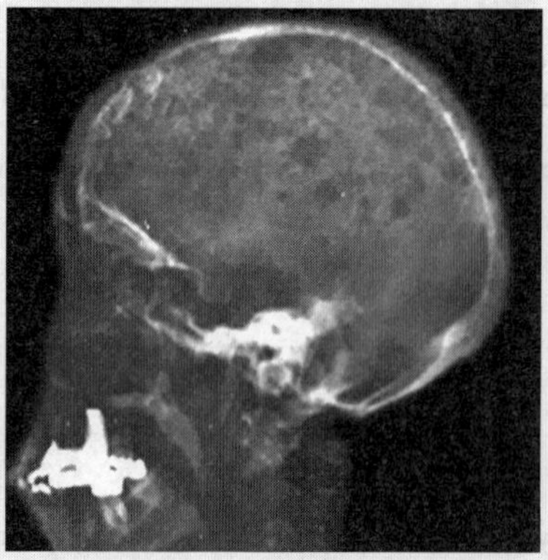

a. Multiple myeloma
b. Paget's disease
c. Hyperparathyroidism
d. Eosinophilic granuloma

Ans. is 'a' Multiple myeloma

32. M protein on immunoelectrophoresis in multiple myeloma patients in most commonly formed by:

a. IgM
b. IgG
c. IgA
d. IgD

Ans. is 'b' IgG

33. Drugs used in management relapsed multiple myeloma is:

a. Bortezomib
b. Lenalidomide
c. Doxorubicin
d. All of the above

Ans. is 'd'All of the above

Previously Asked Facts

❖ Z track injection technique is used for deep intramuscular injection of iron dextran and other irritating solutions (antipsychotics; etc.) to prevent leakage.
❖ Plummer-Vinson syndrome is characterized by dysphagia, iron deficiency anemia, glossitis and esophageal webs. Female preponderance is seen.
❖ Sickle cell disease is caused by a point mutation in sixth codon of β-globin chain that leads to replacement of glutamate residue with valine residue.
❖ Fanconi anemia is caused by a DNA repair defect and is characterized by skin hyperpigmentation of trunk, neck and intertriginous areas, short stature, upper limb bony abnormalities and hypogonadism.
❖ Various definitions of Massive blood transfusion (MBT)
  • Replacement of one entire blood volume within 24 hours
  • Transfusion of 10 or more units of Packed RBCs within 24 hours
  • Transfusion of 4 or more units of Packed RBCs within 1 hour when on-going need is foreseeable
  • Replacement of 50% of total blood volume within 3 hours.

RHEUMATOLOGY

CHARACTERISTIC JOINT INVOLVEMENT IN HANDS IN VARIOUS ARTHRITIS

Joint involved	Arthritis
Distal interphalangeal joint	Osteoarthritis, psoriasis
Proximal interphalangeal joint	Osteoarthritis, rheumatoid arthritis
Metacarpophalangeal joint	Rheumatoid arthritis, hemochromatosis
1st Carpometacarpal joint	Osteoarthritis
Wrist	Rheumatoid arthritis
Joint spared	**Arthritis**
Wrist, metacarpophalangeal joint	Osteoarthritis
Distal interphalangeal joint	Rheumatoid arthritis

In patients with interphalangeal joint osteoarthritis, pain and inflammatory signs subside over years and only swellings (nodes) remain:

Bouchard's Nodes–PIP

Heberden's Nodes–DIP

34. PIP, DIP joints involved with wrist sparing points to the diagnosis of:

a. Osteoarthritis
b. Rheumatoid arthritis
c. Psoriatic arthritis
d. CPPD

Ans. is 'a' Osteoarthritis

35. Heberden's nodes are the clinical manifestations seen in:

a. Osteoarthritis
b. Rheumatoid arthritis
c. Ankylosing spondylitis
d. Reactive arthritis

Ans. is 'a' Osteoarthritis

GOUT

Hyperuricemia is the strongest risk factor for gout. Other risk factors–male sex, obesity, hypertension

Causes of hyperuricemia	
Diminished renal excretion of uric acid	Renal failure Drugs–Thiazides Lead nephropathy Lactic acidosis Alcohol Von-Gierke's disease
Overproduction of uric acid	Myeloproliferative diseases Lesch-Nyhan syndrome (HGPRT mutation) Trauma/surgery (tissue breakdown)
Increased intake	Red meat, seafood

Chronic lead poisoning (occupational exposure or illicitly distilled beverages) may cause proximal tubule dysfunction in kidney. This causes diminished urate excretion–leading to hyperuricemia and thus predisposition for gout. This condition is called Saturnine Gout.

Diagnosis

Arthrocentesis–Confirmatory

- Elevated WBC counts: 20,000–50,000/μL
- 'Negatively Birefringement' gout crystals: Monosodium urate crystals are confirmatory.

Serum Uric Acid Levels

- Normal or Low levels during an acute attack: Limited value for diagnosis
- 24-hour-urine excretion of uric acid: Assessment of risk for stones.

36. Saturnine gout is seen with:

a. Lead
b. Arsenic
c. Mercury
d. Cadmium

Ans. is 'a' Lead

37. Which of the following is not true for the investigations used for diagnosis of gout?

a. Aspirate of joint fluid for microscopy to identify the needle shaped crystals is confirmatory
b. Serum levels of uric acid are diagnostic of acute gout
c. 24 hour urine for uric acid levels is used for assessing the risk of uric acid stones
d. Synovial fluid leukocyte counts are elevated during the acute attack

Ans. is 'b' Serum levels of uric acid are diagnostic of acute gout

AUTOIMMUNE DISEASES

Autoantibodies in autoimmune diseases			
Disease	***Autoantibody***	***% Positive***	***Association***
SLE	dsDNA	50	Nephritis; Specific for SLE
	U1-RNP		
	Smith Antigen	30	Specific for SLE
	Ro (SS-A)/La (SS-B)	40	Congenital heart block, Neonatal lupus
	Anti-phospholipid	30	Antiphospholipid syndrome
	Anti-nuclear antibodies (ANAs)	98	Very sensitive (Good screening test); Not specific
Systemic sclerosis	DNA topoisomerase I	50	Diffuse skin disease, lung disease; specific for SS
	Centromeric proteins		Limited skin disease, pulmonary HTN
	RNA polymerase III		Renal crisis
Sjogren syndrome	Ro/SS-A La/SS-B	80	
Rheumatoid arthritis	Cyclic citrullinated protein (CCP)	70	Specific for RA
	Rheumatoid factor	70	Not specific for RA
Autoimmune myositis	Jo1 Mi-2 nuclear antigen		

Systemic Lupus Erythematosus

Systemic lupus international collaborating clinic criteria for classification of systemic lupus erythematosus

Clinical manifestations	Immunologic manifestations
Skin • Acute, subacute cutaneous LE (photosensitive, malar, maculopapular, bullous) • Chronic cutaneous LE (discoid lupus, panniculitis, lichen planus-like, hypertrophic verrucous, chillblains) Oral or nasal ulcers Nonscarring Alopecia Synovitis involving ≥2 joints Serositis (pleurisy, pericarditis) Renal • Prot/Cr ≥ 0.5 • RBC casts • Biopsy[a] Neurologic • Seizures, psychosis, mononeuritis, myelitis, peripheral or cranial neuropathies, acute confusional state Hemolytic anemia Leukopenia (<4000/μL) or Lymphopenia (<1000/μL) Thrombocytopenia (<100,000/μL)	ANA > reference negative value Anti-dsDNA >reference, if by ELISA 2x reference Anti-Sm Antiphospholipid (any of lupus anticoagulant, false-positive RPR, anti-cardiolipin, anti-β glycoprotein I Low serum complement (C3, C4 or CH50) Positive direct Coombs test in absence of hemolytic anemia

[a] Renal biopsy read as systemic lupus qualifies for classification as SLE if any lupus autoantibodies are present, even if total criteria are fewer than 4.

Interpretation: Presence of any four criteria (must have at least 1 in each category) qualifies patient to be classified as having SLE with 93% specificity and 92% sensitivity

Shrinking Lung Syndrome

- Diaphragmatic dysfunction leading to reduced lung volumes
- Restrictive disease on PFT with absence of parenchymal lung abnormalities
- Typical feature of SLE.

Scleroderma

Two clinical forms

- ❖ Diffuse (Diffuse skin thickening and visceral involvement)
- ❖ Limited (CREST–Calcinosis, Raynaud's phenomenon, Esophageal dysmotility, Sclerodactyly, Telangiectasias).

Pulmonary disease in scleroderma

- ❖ Interstitial Lung Disease–Non-specific Interstitial Pneumonia (NSIP) pattern is most common; Velcro crackles at lung bases on auscultation
- ❖ Pulmonary Arterial Hypertension–Can progress to right heart failure.

38. A female of 26-years, presents with oral ulcers, photosensitivity and malar rash sparing the nasolabial folds. What is the diagnosis? *(NEET 2019)*

a. Stuge-Weber syndrome
b. SLE
c. Dermatitis
d. psoriasis

Ans. is 'b' SLE

39. Shrinking lung syndrome is seen most commonly in:

a. SLE
b. Scleroderma
c. Rheumatoid arthritis
d. Ankylosing spondilitis

Ans. is 'a' SLE

40. Which of the following is used as screening for systemic lupus erythematosus?

a. Antinuclear antibody
b. Anti Smith antibody
c. Anti-RNP antibody
d. Anti-phospholipid antibody

Ans. is 'a' Antinuclear antibody

41. Presence of Velcro crackles at the lung base on auscultation is a sign of:

a. Scleroderma
b. Systemic lupus
c. Wegener's granulomatosus
d. Polyarteritis nodosa

Ans. is 'a' Scleroderma

SCLERODERMA

These symptoms and chest X-ray findings are suggestive of systemic sclerosis related interstitial lung disease.

Interstitial lung disease (ILD) is one of the major types of lung involvement in systemic sclerosis (SSc). SSc-associated ILD consists of various histopathologic subtypes, most commonly nonspecific interstitial pneumonitis and usual interstitial pneumonitis. Affected patients have a worse prognosis than patients with SSc who are free of pulmonary involvement.

The diagnosis of SSc-associated ILD is generally based on the presence of the characteristic **high resolution computed tomography (HRCT)** features of ILD in a patient with known SSc and exclusion of other etiologies of pulmonary parenchymal disease, such as heart failure, drug-induced lung toxicity, recurrent aspiration, or pulmonary vascular disease.

42. A 30-year-old lady with systemic sclerosis for the past so many year, with chest X-ray showing bilateral basal reticular opacities, with 4 months progressive exertional breathlessness and pedal edema ,what should be the most appropriate next investigation for thus patient? *(NEET 2020)*

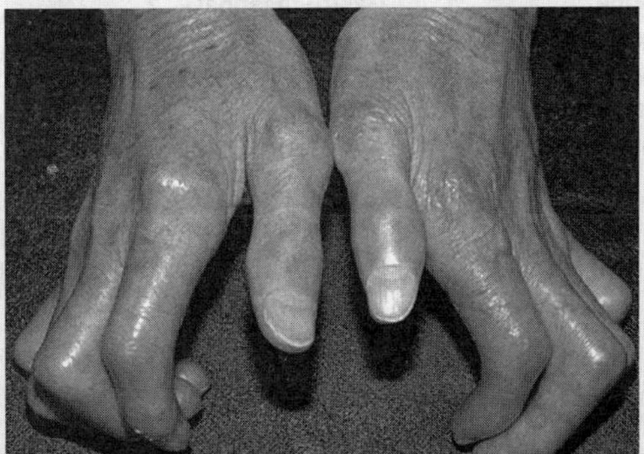

a. Echo to look for cor pulmonale
b. HRCT
c. Pulmonary function test
d. CECT

Ans. is 'b' HRCT

BISPHOSPHONATES

- Pyrophosphate analogs; Inhibit Osteoclasts
- *Oral drugs*: Alendronate, Risedronate
- *IV drugs*: Pamidronate, Ibandronate, Zoledronate
- Uses
  - Osteoporosis (postmenopausal, idiopathic, steroid-induced)
  - Paget's Disease
  - Hypercalcemia of malignancy
  - Osteolytic bone metastases
- Adverse effects
  - GERD, esophageal ulcers–Oral drugs
  - Flu-like symptoms–IV drugs
  - Atypical femur fractures, Jaw osteonecrosis–Serious rare adverse effects.

Oral bisphosphonates (Alendronate) are to be taken with water on empty stomach; patient should remain upright for 30 minutes (to prevent esophagitis).

Zoledronate is drug of choice for metastatic bone disease and hypercalcemia as it is more effective and faster acting than pamidronate.

Management of Hypercalcemia

No treatment is required for mild, asymptomatic hypercalcemia.

Management of symptomatic hypercalcemia includes the following:

- IV fluids are the 1st line of treatment: 4—6 L of IV saline is given over the first 24 h. Loop diuretics can be given concomitantly.
- In diseases involving increased calcium mobilization from bone, drugs inhibiting bone resorption are given.
- Bisphosphonates including zoledronate, pamidronate and ibandronate are used for treatment of hypercalcemia of malignancy.
- Gallium nitrate: inhibits bone resorption, but is nephrotoxic.
- Dialysis may be needed in some cases.

43. Drug of choice for management of hypercalcemia with metastatic bone diseaseis:

a. Alendronate
b. Risedronate
c. Pamidronate
d. Zoledronate

Ans. is 'd' Zoledronate

NEPHROLOGY

SYSTEMIC MANIFESTATIONS IN CHRONIC KIDNEY DISEASE AND UREMIA

Fluid and Electrolytes	**Cardiopulmonary**
Dehydration Edema Hyperkalemia Metabolic acidosis	Hypertension Congestive heart failure Pulmonary edema Uremic pericarditis
Calcium and Bone Hyperphosphatemia Hypocalcemia Secondary hyperparathyroidism Renal osteodystrophy	**Gastrointestinal** Bleeding Esophagitis, gastritis Peptic ulcer
Hematological Anemia Bleeding diasthesis	**Dermatological** Pruritus Uremic frost–Crystallized urea deposits on skin
Neurological Peripheral neuropathy Encephalopathy	

44. Which of the following are the clinical abnormalities of uremia?

a. Hyperphosphatemia
b. Uremic frost
c. Peptic ulcer
d. All of the above

Ans. is 'd' All of the above

GLOMERULAR DISEASES

- Breakdown of components of filtration barrier.

Spectrum

- Nephrotic Syndrome
  - Massive proteinuria: >3.5 g/day
  - Hypoalbuminemia: Plasma albumin < 3 g/dL
  - Generalized edema
  - Hyperlipidemia and lipiduria
- Nephritic Syndrome
  - Dysmorphic RBCs: Hematuria
  - Mild proteinuria: <3.5 g/day
  - Renal failure.

Immunological Abnormalities in Nephrotic Syndrome

- Decreased IgG antibody level
- Increased IgE and IgM antibody levels
- Increased beta-microglobulin level
- Decreased production of IL-2.

Major causes	
Nephritic syndrome	***Nephrotic syndrome***
Post-streptococcal	Focal segmental glomerulosclerosis (FSGS)
Berger's (IgA) nephropathy	Minimal change disease
Rapidly proliferative glomerulonephritis (RPGN)	Membranous nephropathy
Alport syndrome	DM, amyloidosis
Membranoproliferative glomerulonephritis	Membranoproliferative glomerulonephritis

IgA Nephropathy

- Episodic hematuria immediately following an upper respiratory tract or diarrheal illness
- Diffuse mesangial deposits of IgA immune complexes
  - IgA deposited in mesangium is typically polymeric and of IgA1 subclass
- Leads to end stage renal disease in 50% patients
- Poor prognostic factors
  - Hypertension or proteinuria
  - Older age of onset
  - Persistent proteinuria for 6 months or longer
- Henoch-Schonlein purpura: IgA nephropathy + extrarenal involvement.

45. Which of the following is not true about IgA nephropathy?

a. Characterized by episodic hematuria and deposition of IgA in mesangium
b. Nephrotic syndrome commonly develops
c. Persistent proteinuria for 6 months or longer points towards bad clinical outcomes
d. Majority of the IgA deposited is polymeric form of IgA1 subclass

Ans. is 'b' Nephrotic syndrome commonly develops

46. Patient with nephrotic syndrome has decreased amount of with which antibody?

a. IgG b. IgE
c. IgM d. IgA

Ans. is 'a' IgG

ACUTE KIDNEY INJURY (AKI)

Definition

- Rise of serum creatinine > 0.3 mg/dL within 48 hours or > 50% higher than baseline in 1 week
- Urine output <0.5 mL/kg/hr for longer than 6 hours.

RIFLE Criteria for AKI

Stage	GFR criteria	Urine output criteria
Risk	Increase SCr × 1.5 or Decrease in GFR > 25%	<0.5 mL/kg/h × 6 h
Injury	Increase SCr × 2 or Decrease in GFR > 50%	<0.5 mL/kg/h × 12 h
Failure	Increase SCr × 3 or Decrease in GFR 75% or Increase in SCr >0.5 mg/dL (if baseline SCr > 4 mg/dL)	<0.3 mL/kg/h × 24 h or anuria × 12 h
Loss of kidney function	Need for RRT × 4 weeks	
End-stage kidney disease	Need for RRT × 3 months	

Types of AKI

- Pre-renal (Insufficient blood flow to kidney)—Dehydration, shock, heart failure
- Renal/Intrinsic (Renal dysfunction)—Acute tubular necrosis, glomerulonephritis
- Post-renal (Obstruction to urine flow)—Renal stones, BPH, tumors

The differences between prerenal and renal AKI are summarized below:

Clinical and laboratory variables in the differential diagnosis between prerenal and renal AKI		
	Prerenal	*Renal*
History	GI, urinary, skin volume loss, blood loss or third spacing	Drugs or toxin exposure, hemodynamic change
Clinical presentation	Hypotension or volume depletion	No specific symptoms or signs
Laboratory studies		
BUN/Scr	>20	<20
Sediment	Normal to few casts	"Muddy brown" casts
U_{osm} (mmol/kg)	>500	<350
Proteinuria	None to trace	Mild to moderate
U_{Na} (mmol/L)	<20	>40
Fe_{Na} (%)	<1	>1
FE_{Urea} (%)	<35	>35
$U_{Cr/SCr}$	<20	>40
Novel biomarkers	None	KIM-1. cystatin C, NGAL, CYR61, others

Fe_{Na} = Sodium clearance/creatinine clearance (Fractional Excretion of Na)

- *Oliguria*: 24-hours urine output < 400 mL
- *Anuria*: Complete absence of urine formation (<100 mL in 24 hours)
- *Polyuria*: Urine output > 3L/day

Salt-Wasting Nephropathy

- Clinical state rather than a specific disease.
- Associated with chronic kidney disease due to tubulointerstitial disease or glomerulonephritis.
- Example of toxic nephropathy causing salt losing nephropathy is analgesic abuse.

47. RIFLE criteria is used for diagnosis of:

a. Acute kidney injury
b. Acute splenic injury
c. Acute liver injury
d. Acute bowel injury

Ans. is 'a' Acute kidney injury

48. Laboratory findings differentiating prerenal azotemia from oliguria acute renal failure include the following *except*:

a. > 2% fractional excretion of Na
b. Urine osmolality > 500 mOsmol/L H_2O
c. Urine/plasma creatinine ratio > 40
d. None of the above

Ans. is 'a' > 2% fractional excretion of Na

49. Oliguria is defined as:

a. 24 hour urine output < 200 mL
b. 24 hour urine output < 300 mL
c. 24 hour urine output < 400 mL
d. 24 hour urine output < 500 mL

Ans. is 'c' 24 hour urine output < 400 mL

Medicine

VASCULITIS

Classification

Vessel	Disease	Associated features
Large	Temporal arteritis Takayasu's arteritis	Elderly female, headache Asian female, pulseless
Medium	Kawasaki disease Buerger's disease Polyarteritis nodosa	Asian child, red rash, Strawberry tongue Smoker's hands Hepatitis B
Small	Henoch-Schonlein purpura Churg-Strauss Wegener's granulomatosis Microscopic polyangiitis	Child, URI, melena Asthma, eosinophils, p-ANCA Sinus, kidneys, lungs, c-ANCA Kidneys, lungs, p-ANCA

Kawasaki Disease

- Also known as Mucocutaneous Lymph Node Syndrome
- Medium vessel vasculitis
- Asian children; 80% are less than 4 years
- Classic involvement—skin (red rash), lips, tongue ('Strawberry tongue')
- Conjunctival erythema, desquamative rash on palms and soles, Cervical lymphadenopathy
- Feared complication—Coronary artery aneurysms–rupture may cause myocardial infarction
- 20% patients develop cardiovascular sequelae (ranging from asymptomatic coronary arteritis to giant aneurysms)
- *Treatment*: Intravenous Immunoglobulin and Aspirin (to reduce risk of symptomatic coronary artery disease).

Henoch-Schonlein Purpura (HSP)

- Most common childhood systemic vasculitis
- Often follows upper respiratory tract infection
- Symptoms
  - Skin: Palpable purpura on buttocks/legs
  - GIT: Colicky abdominal pain, melena
  - Renal: Nephritis
  - Joints: Polyarthralgias in absence of frank arthritis

Churg-Strauss Syndrome

- Also known as Allergic Angiitis and Granulomatosis
- Asthma, allergic rhinitis and sinusitis
- Neuropathy (Mononeuritis multiplex)
- Palpable purpura
- Renal involvement is less common and less severe than Wegener's and Microscopic Polyangiitis
- Eosinophilia, p-ANCA +ve.

Cryoglobulinemic Vasculitis

- Cryoglobulins are cold-precipitable monoclonal or polyclonal immunoglobulins
- Underlying disorders associated with cryoglobulinemia
  - Hepatitis C virus infection: Vast majority
  - Multiple myeloma, Lymphoproliferative diseases, Liver diseases
- Common clinical manifestations of cryoglobulinemic vasculitis—Cutaneous vasculitis, peripheral neuropathy, arthritis, glomerulonephritis (most commonly Membranoproliferative glomerulonephritis)
- *Diagnosis*: Circulating cryoprecipitates, Rheumatoid Factor +ve, Hypocomplementemia
- Hepatitis C antibodies and HCV RNA should be tested for evidence of HCV infection
- *Treatment*: Antiviral therapy in patients with HCV infection.

50. A 50-year-old male patient presenting with cutaneous vasculitis, proteinuria and cryoglobulinemia and glomerulonephritis. What test should be most appropriate for diagnosis?

a. ANCA b. HBsAG
c. Anti-HCV antibody d. MIF

Ans. is 'c' Anti-HCV antibody

51. Triad of skin lesions, mononeuritis multiplex, eosinophils are seen in:

a. Alport's syndrome
b. Churg-Strauss syndrome
c. Cryoglobulinemia
d. Wegener's granulomatosis

Ans. is 'b' Churg-Strauss syndrome

52. A 5-year-old female presents with palpable purpura over the buttocks, arthralgias, abdominal pain with diarrhea with passage of blood per rectum. Patient also has presence of proteinuria. What is the most probable diagnosis?

a. Henoch-Schonlein purpura
b. Nephrotic syndrome
c. Nephritic syndrome
d. Thalassemia

Ans. is 'a' Henoch-Schonlein purpura

53. Which of the following is not true about Kawasaki disease?

a. It is also called mucocutaneous lymph node syndrome
b. 80% of the patients are 4 years old or older
c. It can result in acute myocardial infarctions
d. 20% of the untreated patients develop cardiovascular sequel

Ans. is 'b' 80% of the patients are 4 years old or older

INHERITED CYSTIC KIDNEY DISEASES

Inherited cystic kidney diseases

Diseases	*Inheritance*	*Renal involvement*	*Extra-renal involvement*	*Gene*
Autosomal dominant polycystic kidney disease	AD	Cortical and medullary cysts	Liver, pancreatic cysts, cerebral aneurysms	PKD1 (16p; Polycystin-1); PKD2 (4p; Polycystin-2)
Autosomal recessive polycystic kidney disease	AR	Distal and collecting duct cysts	Hepatic fibrosis	PKHD1 (6p; Fibrocystin)
Nephronophthisis	AR	Small fibrotic kidneys; medullary cysts	Growth retardation, anemia, retinal atrophy	NPHP (Nephrocystin)
Medullary cystic kidney	AD	Small fibrotic kidneys; medullary cysts	In adults, gout	UMOD, MUC1
Tuberous sclerosis	AD	Renal cysts, angiomyolipomas, RCC	Facial angiofibromas, cortical tubers	TSC1 (9p; Hamartin); TSC2 (16p; Tuberin)
Von Hippel-Lindau disease	AD	Renal cysts, RCC	Cerebellar hemangioblastomas, retinal hemangioblastomas, pheochromocytomas	VHL (3p; VHL tumor suppressor protein)

Von Hippel-Lindau Disease

- Autosomal Dominant
- Mutation in VHL gene on Chromosome 3; codes for VHL tumor suppressor protein
- Multiple hemangioblastomas—Cerebellum, spinal cord, retina
- Renal cysts, bilateral renal cell carcinoma—Clear cell RCC
- Pheochromocytomas
- Screening protocol
    - Annual USG Abdomen (for RCC)
    - Baseline MRI Brain at 20 years of age; annual neurological examination (for Hemangioblastomas)
    - Annual urinary VMA level (for Pheochromocytoma)
    - Annual ophthalmoscopy (for retinal hemangioblastomas).

54. True about VHL syndrome is:

a. It is an autosomal recessive condition
b. Central nervous system is not involved
c. Regular screening for clear cell carcinoma of kidneys is essential
d. VHL is a growth promoter gene

Ans. is 'c' Regular screening for clear cell carcinoma of kidneys is essential

55. Synthesis of which protein is affected in patients with autosomal recessive polycystic kidney disease?

a. Polycystin 1
b. Fibrocystin
c. Hamartin
d. Nephrocystin III

Ans. is 'b' Fibrocystin

DIAGNOSTIC MODALITIES FOR RENAL ARTERY STENOSIS

Modality	Role	Comments
Duplex sonography	Shows renal arteries and measures flow velocities for severity assessement	Velocities > 200 cm/s predict hemodynamically important lesions (>60% vessel occlusion)
CT / MR angiography	Shows renal arteries	Concern for Gadolinium toxicity
Captopril renography (^{99m}Tc MAG3)	Captopril mediated fall in filtration pressure amplifies differences in renal perfusion	Normal study exciudes renal artery stenosis
Intra-arterial angiography	Shows location and severity of vascular lesion	Considered 'Gold Standard' for RAS; simultaneous intervention possible

56. Hemodynamically important lesions of renal artery stenosis are predicted by renal artery velocities more than_______on Doppler ultrasound.

a. 150 cm/s
b. 125 cm/s
c. 150 cm/s
d. 200 cm/s

Ans. is 'd' 200 cm/s

URINARY CASTS

Urinary casts are formed only in Distal Convoluted Tubule and Collecting Duct.
Casts are formed by solidification of materials in tubules of nephrons.

Casts	Associations
Hyaline casts	MC type of casts; can be normal Consist of Tamm-Horsfall protein Seen with exercise, dehydration, fever, diuretics
Granular casts	Textured appearance ranging from fine to coarse in character Result from breakdown of cellular casts 'Muddy-Brown' heme-granular casts are seen in acute tubular necrosis
Broad casts	Form in dilated chronically damaged collecting ducts due to stasis Also known as Renal Failure casts; seen in Advanced kidney disease
Waxy casts	Cylinders of smooth highly refractive material Seen in Advanced kidney disease
RBC casts	Glomerulonephritis
WBC casts	UTI (Pyelonephritis), Tubulointerstitial nephritis
Renal tubular epithelial cell casts	Tubular injury, like acute tubular necrosis

57. Broad casts seen in cases of:

a. Advanced renal failure
b. Hypotension
c. Severe hydronephrosis
d. Renal papillary necrosis

Ans. is 'a' Advanced renal failure

URINARY TRACT INFECTIONS: TERMINOLOGIES

- **Asymptomatic bacteriuria**: Bacteria in urinary tract in absence of symptoms
- **Urinary Tract Infection (UTI)**: Symptomatic disease
- **Uncomplicated UTI**: Acute cystitis/pyelonephritis in nonpregnant women without anatomic abnormalities or instrumentation of urinary tract
- **Complicated UTI**: All scenarios that do not conform to description for uncomplicated UTI. Examples:
  - UTI in males
  - Anatomical abnormalities like obstruction, calculi or colovesical fistula
  - Pregnant women
  - Non-resolution within 2 weeks of adequate therapy
  - Recurrent episodes despite adequate treatment (resistant organisms).

58. Definition of complicated urinary tract infection is, the infection which fails to resolve or recur within_______weeks of standard therapy.

a. 1 week
b. 2 weeks
c. 3 weeks
d. 4 weeks

Ans. is 'b' 2 weeks

INHERITED CHANNELOPATHIES

Bartter Syndrome

- Autosomal recessive disorder
- Abnormal solute transfer in thick ascending limb
- Similar to effects of loop diuretics
- 4 types
  - Type 1–Na-K-2Cl pump mutation
  - Type 2–Potassium channel ROMK mutation
  - Type 3–Chloride channel CIC-Kb mutation
  - Type 4–Barttin mutation; associated deafness
- May present in neonatal period or early childhood
- Salt-wasting, hypercalciuria with stones
- Growth and mental retardation.

Gitelman Syndrome

- Autosomal recessive disorder
- Mutation in Na-Cl co-transporter in Distal Convoluted Tubule (DCT)
- Similar to effect of Thiazides

Bartter	Gitelman
Less common	More common
Defect in thick ascending limb	Defect in distal tubule
Hypokalemic metabolic alkalosis, salt-wasting	Hypokalemic metabolic alkalosis, salt-wasting
Similar to loop diuretics	Similar to thiazides
Severe clinical course; early childhood	Milder clinical course; later age of onset
Hypercalciuria (stones or nephrocalcinosis)	Hypocalciuria
Mild hypomagnesemia	Severe hypomagnesemia
Mild or absent neuromuscular symptoms	Prominent neuromuscular symptoms (muscle spasms, weakness)

Liddle's Syndrome

- Autosomal dominant disorder
- Gain of function mutation in Epithelial sodium channels (principal cells in collecting ducts)
- Similar to effects like aldosterone
- Hypertension (early onset)
- Hypokalemic metabolic alkalosis (weakness, fatigue, myalgias).

Fanconi Syndrome

- Loss of proximal tubule functions
- Impaired reabsorption of solutes (Bicarbonate, glucose, amino acids, phosphate)
- Presentation
  - Polyuria, polydipsia—diuresis from glucose (normal blood glucose in contrast with diabetes)
  - Non-anion gap acidosis (loss of bicarbonate)—Type II Renal Tubular Acidosis
  - Hypokalemia
  - Hypophosphatemia
  - Amino acids in urine
- Causes
  - Inherited: Cystinosis
  - Acquired: Lead poisoning, multiple myeloma, drugs (Cisplatin, Ifosfamide, Tenofovir, Valproate).

59. Which type of Bartter's syndrome is associated with mutations in barttin? *(NEET 2016)*

a. Type 1 b. Type 2
c. Type 3 d. Type 4

Ans. is 'd' Type 4

60. Gitelman's syndrome resembles the effects of which of the following drugs? *(NEET 2016)*

a. Thiazide b. Furosemide
c. Spironolactone d. Amiloride

Ans. is 'a' Thiazide

61. In Bartter syndrome, defect is present in which part of kidney? *(NEET 2018)*

a. Proximal tubule
b. Descending limb of loop of Henle
c. Ascending limb of loop of Henle
d. Collecting duct

Ans. is 'c' Ascending limb of loop of Henle

62. A young child with mental retardation, hypokalemia and metabolic alkalosis suggests the diagnosis of: *(NEET 2018)*

a. Gitelman syndrome
b. Bartter syndrome
c. Liddle syndrome
d. Fanconi syndrome

Ans. is 'b' Bartter syndrome

63. Child with alkalosis, hypertension and hypokalemia. What can be the cause? *(NEET 2018)*

a. Bartter's syndrome
b. Gitelman syndrome
c. Liddle syndrome
d. Fanconi syndrome

Ans. is 'c' Liddle syndrome

DIABETES INSIPIDUS

Nephrogenic diabetes insipidus (DI) refers to a decrease in urinary concentrating ability that results from resistance to the action of antidiuretic hormone (ADH). This problem can reflect resistance at the ADH site of action in the collecting tubules, or interference with the countercurrent mechanism due, for example, to medullary injury or to decreased sodium chloride reabsorption in the medullary aspect of the thick ascending limb of the loop of Henle

- Patients with moderate to severe nephrogenic or central DI typically present with polyuria, nocturia, and polydipsia. The first manifestation of a mild to moderate loss of concentrating ability is often nocturia.
- The most common causes of nephrogenic DI in children are genetic mutations; in adults, nephrogenic DI is most often due to drugs, hypercalcemia, and hypokalemia.
- Mutations in the vasopressin V2 receptor (V2R) gene, which is X-linked, and the aquaporin-2 gene, which is autosomal, are the two most frequent causes of hereditary nephrogenic DI.

64. Impaired function of aquaporins result in: *(NEET 2020)*

a. Liddle syndrome
b. Barter syndrome
c. Cystic fibrosis
d. Nephrogenic DI

Ans. is 'd' Nephrogenic DI

NEUROLOGY

MULTIPLE SCLEROSIS

The characteristic neuropathologic feature of MS is the presence of focal demyelinated plaques within the central nervous system, accompanied by variable degrees of inflammation and gliosis, with partial preservation of axons. These lesions tend to be located in the optic nerves, spinal cord, brainstem, cerebellum, and the juxtacortical and periventricular white matter . In addition, demyelinated lesions can also be found in the corpus callosum and cortical gray matter. **This demyelination leads to slow conduction of motor and sensory pathways.**

Axonal injury can be a prominent pathologic feature of the MS plaque, though not in the acute phase.

65. In multiple sclerosis, slow conduction of motor and sensory pathways is due to: *(NEET 2020)*

a. Defect in node of Ranvier
b. Loss of myelin sheath
c. Leaking of sodium channels
d. Axonal damage

Ans. is 'b' Loss of myelin sheath

REFLEXES

Reflexes	Afferent nerve	Center	Efferent nerve
Superficial Reflexes			
Corneal	Cranial V	Pons	Cranial VII
Pharyngeal and uvular	Cranial IX	Medulla	Cranial X
Upper abdominal	T7, 8, 9, 10	T7, 8, 9, 10	T7, 8, 9, 10

Contd...

Contd...

Reflexes	Afferent nerve	Center	Efferent nerve
Lower abdominal	T10, 11, 12	T10, 11, 12	T10, 11, 12
Cremasteric	Femoral	L1	Genitofemoral
Plantar	**Tibial**	**S1, 2**	**Tibial**
Anal	Pudendal	S4, 5	Pudendal
Deep Reflexes			
Jaw	Cranial V	Pons	Cranial V
Biceps	Musculocutaneous	C5, 6	Musculocutaneous
Triceps	Radial	C6, 7	Radial
Periosteoradial	Radial	C6, 7, 8	Radial
Wrist (flexion)	Median	C6, 7, 8	Median
Wrist (extension)	Radial	C7, 8	Radial
Patellar	Femoral	L2, 3, 4	Femoral
Achilles	Tibial	**S1**	Tibial
Visceral Reflexes			
Light	Cranial II	Midbrain	Cranial III
Accommodation	Cranial II	Occipital cortex	Cranial III
Carotid sinus	Cranial IX	Medulla	Cranial X
Bulbocavemosus	Pudendal	S2, 3, 4	Pelvic autonomic
Bladder and rectal	Pudendal	S2, 3, 4	Pudendal and autonomies

Bulbocavernosus Reflex

- Dependent on an intact S1 and S2 spinal reflex.
- If the bulbocavernosus reflex is preserved in the presence of complete perineal sensory loss and flaccid paralysis of the lower extremities, it indicates that the period of spinal shock has passed and that the neurologic deficit is due to a lesion above the S1 segment.
- Absence of the bulbocavernosus reflex may indicate either the presence of spinal shock or a spinal cord lesion including the S1 and S2 segments.
- Spinal shock usually resolves within 24 hours and is accompanied by return of the bulbocavernosus reflex if the S1 and S2 segments are not directly involved in the spinal cord lesion.

Plantar Response

- Three responses possible:
  - Flexor: The toes curve down and inwards, and the foot everts; this is the normal response. **Its main root value (myotome) is S1.**
  - Indifferent: There is no response.
  - Extensor: The hallux dorsiflexes, and the other toes fan out; this is Babinski's sign, which indicates upper motor neuron lesion.

66. First reflex response to reappear after spinal shock is:

a. Cremasteric reflex
b. Bulbocavernosus reflex
c. Ankle reflex
d. Superficial abdominal reflex

Ans. is 'b' Bulbocavernosus reflex

67. Ankle reflex is mediated by: *(NEET 2016)*

a. L2
b. L4
c. S1
d. None

Ans. is 'c' S1

68. What is the root value of normal plantar response? *(NEET 2016)*

a. L4
b. L5
c. S1
d. S4

Ans. is 'c' S1

Medicine

APHASIA

	Comprehension	Repetition of spoken language	Naming	Fluency
Wernicke's	Impaired	Impaired	Impaired	Preserved or increased
Broca's	Preserved (except grammar)	Impaired	Impaired	Decreased
Global	Impaired	Impaired	Impaired	Decreased
Conduction	Preserved	Impaired	Impaired	Preserved
Nonfluent (motor) transcortical	Preserved	Preserved	Impaired	Impaired
Fluent (sensory) transcortical	Impaired	Preserved	Impaired	Preserved
Isolation	Impaired	Echolalia	Impaired	No purposeful speech
Anomic	Preserved	Preserved	Impaired	Preserved except for word-finding pauses
Pure word deafness	Impaired only for spoken language	Impaired	Preserved	Preserved
Pure alexia	Impaired only for reading	Preserved	Preserved	Preserved

Aphasia	Area affected in left (dominant) hemisphere
Broca's aphasia	Inferior frontal gyrus
Wernicke's aphasia	Superior temporal gyrus
Conduction aphasia	Arcuate fasciculus
Global aphasia	Arcuate fasciculus, Broca and Wernicke areas Stroke in entire left MCA distribution Associated right hemiplegia and visual loss
Pure word deafness	Superior temporal gyrus; left MCA infarct

69. Right hand dominant patient presents with normal comprehension but speaks with short utterances of a few words at a time, comprised mostly of nouns. What is the most probable location of the lesion?

a. Left inferior frontal gyrus
b. Right inferior frontal gyrus
c. Left superior temporal gyrus
d. Right superior temporal gyrus

Ans. is 'a' Left inferior frontal gyrus

70. Pure word deafness is associated with:

a. Middle cerebral artery stroke
b. Posterior cerebral artery stroke
c. Vertebral artery aneurysm
d. Basilar artery aneurysm

Ans. is 'a' Middle cerebral artery stroke

71. Global aphasia is seen due to:

a. Strokes involving entire middle cerebral artery distribution in left hemisphere
b. Strokes involving entire middle cerebral artery distribution in right hemisphere
c. Strokes involving entire posterior cerebral artery distribution in left hemisphere
d. Strokes involving entire posterior cerebral artery distribution in right hemisphere

Ans. is 'a' Strokes involving entire middle cerebral artery distribution in left hemisphere

Acute Ischemic Stroke Syndromes According to Vascular Territory

Artery involved	Syndrome
Anterior cerebral artery	Motor and/or sensory deficit (leg > face, arm) Grasp, sucking reflexes Abulia, paratonic rigidity, gait apraxia
Middle cerebral artery	Dominant hemisphere: aphasia, motor and sensory deficit (face, arm > leg > foot), may be complete hemiplegia if internal capsule involved, homonymous hemianopia Non-dominant hemisphere: neglect, anosognosia, motor and sensory deficit (face, arm > leg > foot), homonymous hemianopia
Posterior cerebral artery	Homonymous hemianopia; alexia without agraphia (dominant hemisphere); visual hallucinations, visual perseverations (calcarine cortex); sensory loss, choreoathetosis, spontaneous pain (thalamus); III nerve palsy, paresis of vertical eye movement, motor deficit (cerebral peduncle, midbrain)
Penetrating vessels	Pure motor hemiparesis (classic lacunar syndromes) Pure sensory deficit Pure sensory-motor deficit Hemiparesis, homolateral ataxia Dysarthria/clumsy hand

Contd...

Contd...

Artery involved	Syndrome
Vertebrobasilar	Cranial nerve palsies Crossed sensory deficits Diplopia, dizziness, nausea, vomiting, dysarthria, dysphagia, hiccup Limb and gait ataxia Motor deficit Coma Bilateral signs suggest basilar artery disease
Internal carotid artery	Progressive or stuttering onset of MCA syndrome, occasionally ACA syndrome as well if insufficient collateral flow

72. A 60-year-old man, known case of hypertension and past MI operated by CABG. He was prescribed warfarin but he was not compliant to treatment. One day he developed sudden onset of paralysis and inability to speak. Which of the following is not true regarding his management? *(NEET 2020)*

a. Monitoring of PT-INR is required
b. EEG is one of the first lines of management
c. Brain imaging is not required if EEG is normal
d. 2D echo is recommended in this patient.

Ans. is 'c' Brain imaging is not required if EEG is normal

UPPER AND LOWER MOTOR NEURON PARALYSIS

Sign	UMN lesion	LMN lesion
Weakness	+	+
Atrophy	–	+
Fasciculations	–	+
Reflexes	Increased	Decreased
Tone	Increased	Decreased
Babinski sign	+	–
Spastic paresis	+	–
Flaccid paralysis	–	+
Clasp knife rigidity	+	–
EMG	Normal	Denervation potentials (Fibrillations, fasciculations, positive sharp waves)
Nerve conduction studies	Normal	Abnormal

73. Which of the following is not a feature of upper motor neuron lesion?

a. Positive Babinski sign
b. Normal nerve conduction study
c. Positive sharp waves on EMG
d. Hyperactive tendon reflexes

Ans. is 'c' Positive sharp waves on EMG

FRONTAL LOBE LESIONS

Key areas in Frontal Lobe

- Motor cortex
- *Frontal eye fields*: Conjugate eye movements to contralateral side
- *Broca's Speech area*: Lesion in dominant hemisphere causes expressive aphasia
- *Pre-frontal cortex*: Anterior 2/3 of frontal lobe
  - Lesions cause Disinhibition, Disorientation, Indifference, Euphoria, Irritability and re-emergence of primitive reflexes—Frontal Lobe Syndrome.

74. Frontal lobe syndrome consists of:

a. Euphoria
b. Indifference
c. Irritability
d. All of the above

Ans. is 'd' All of the above

AGNOSIA

Inability to recognize objects by a particular sensory modality even though the sensory modality itself is intact.

- *Astereognosis*: Inability to identify objects by feeling them; lesion in non-dominant parietal lobe.
- *Unilateral neglect/inattention*: Lesions in inferior parietal lobule in non-dominant hemisphere.

- **Prosopagnosia–Inability to recognize faces; Lesion in occipito-temporal network for face and object recognition.** Prosopagnosia occurs most often in association with bilateral occipito-temporal lesions involving the inferior and mesial visual association cortices in the lingual and fusiform gyri causing a visual field defect, most often a left superior quadrantanopia or hemianopia.
- Visual agnosia–Failure to identify an object by sight.
- Anosmia–Absence of the ability to smell.
- Alexia–Loss of the ability to read.
- Apraxia–Inability to perform purposive movement although there is no sensory or motor impairment.

75. Prosopagnosia is defined as: *(NEET 2018)*

a. Inability to read
b. Inability to identify faces
c. Inability to write
d. Inability to speak

Ans. is 'b' Inability to identify faces

76. Prospagnosia is caused by lesion of: *(NEET 2016)*

a. Parietal lobe
b. Frontal lobe
c. Occipito-temporal
d. Parieto-occipital

Ans. is 'c' Occipito-temporal

BRAINSTEM SYNDROMES

Midbrain

Benedikt Syndrome	Weber's Syndrome
CNIII–Occulomtor palsy	CNIII–Occulomotor palsy
Medial lemniscus–Contralateral loss of proprioception/vibration	Corticospinal tract–Contralateral hemiparesis
Red nucleus–Tremors, Ataxia	Corticobulbar tract–Pseudobulbar palsy (UMN cranial nerve motor weakness; Exaggerated gag reflex, Spastic dysarthria, No tongue wasting)

Medulla

Medial medullary syndrome	Lateral medullary syndrome (Wallenberg syndrome)
Corticospinal tract–Contralateral hemiparesis	Vestibular nuclei–Nystagmus, vertigo
Medial lemniscus–Contralateral loss of proprioception/vibration	Sympathetic tract–Horner's syndrome
CNXII–Flaccid paralysis of tongue	Spinothalamic tract–Contralateral pain/temp loss
	Spinal V nucleus–Ipsilateral face pain/temp loss
	Nucleus ambiguus (IX, X)–Hoarseness, dysphagia
Anterior spinal artery stroke	Posterior Inferior Cerebellar Artery stroke

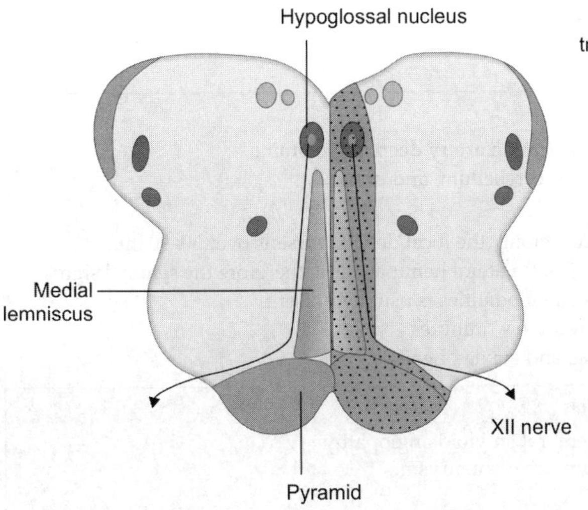

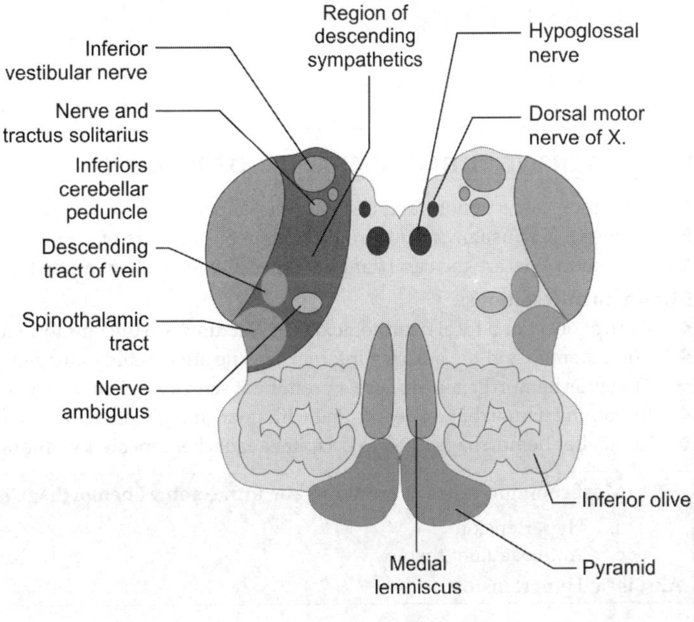

Horner's Syndrome

- Compression/disruption along sympathetic pathway from Hypothalamus to T1 vertebral level
- *Miosis*: Small/constricted pupil; Unequal pupils
- *Ptosis*: Drooping eyelid
- *Anhydrosis*: No sweat.

77. Weber's syndrome includes all *except*:

a. Cranial 3rd nerve palsy
b. Contralateral hemiparesis
c. Dorsal midbrain involvement
d. Anterior cerebellar peduncle

Ans. is 'd' Anterior cerebellar peduncle

78. Embolism of PICA causes:

a. Horner syndrome
b. Wallenberg syndrome
c. Weber syndrome
d. Medial medullary syndrome

Ans. is 'b' Wallenberg syndrome

Acute Ischemic Stroke Syndromes According to Vascular Territory

Artery involved	Syndrome
Anterior cerebral artery	Motor and/ or sensory deficit (leg > face, arm) Grasp, sucking reflexes Abulia, paratonic rigidity, gait apraxia
Middle cerebral artery	Dominant hemisphere: aphasia, motor and sensory deficit (face, arm > leg > foot), may be complete hemiplegia if internal capsule involved, homonymous hemianopia Non-dominant hemisphere: neglect, anosognosia, motor and sensory deficit (face, arm > leg > foot), homonymous hemianopia
Posterior cerebral artery	Homonymous hemianopia; alexia without agraphia (dominant hemisphere); visual hallucinations, visual perseverations (calcarine cortex); sensory loss, choreoathetosis, spontaneous pain (thalamus); III nerve palsy, paresis of vertical eye movement, motor deficit (cerebral peduncle, midbrain)
Penetrating vessels	• Pure motor hemiparesis (classic lacunar syndromes) • Pure sensory deficit • Pure sensory-motor deficit • Hemiparesis, homolateral ataxia • Dysarthria/ clumsy hand
Vertebrobasilar	• Cranial nerve palsies • Crossed sensory deficits • Diplopia, dizziness, nausea, vomiting, dysarthria, dysphagia, hiccup • Limb and gait ataxia • Motor deficit • Coma • Bilateral signs suggest basilar artery disease
Internal carotid artery	Progressive or stuttering onset of MCA syndrome, occasionally ACA syndrome as w ell if insufficient collateral flow

79. A person presents with cortical blindness and nystagmus, ataxia and dysdiadochokinesia. Which artery is likely to be involved? *(NEET 2020)*

a. ACA
b. MCA
c. PCA
d. ICA

Ans. is 'c' PCA

HYPERTENSIVE INTRACEREBRAL HEMORRHAGE

Most common cause of nontraumatic intracerebral hemorrhage.

Hypertensive ICH usually results from spontaneous rupture of a small penetrating artery deep in the brain.

Most common sites are the basal ganglia (especially the putamen), thalamus, cerebellum, and pons.

Clinical manifestations:

- Abrupt onset of a focal neurologic deficit. Seizures are uncommon. Commonly the focal deficit worsens over 30–90 min.
- The putamen and the adjacent internal capsule are usually damaged. Contralateral hemiparesis is therefore the sentinel sign.
- Thalamic hemorrhages produce a prominent sensory deficit involving all modalities is usually present.
- In pontine hemorrhages, deep coma with quadriplegia often occurs over a few minutes.
- Cerebellar hemorrhages lead to occipital headache, repeated vomiting, and ataxia of gait.

80. Most common cause of nontraumatic intracerebral hemorrhage is:

a. Hypertension
b. Cerebral amyloid angiopathy
c. Anticoagulant therapy
d. Rupture of aneurysm

Ans. is 'a' Hypertension

DIFFUSE AXONAL INJURY

- Loss of consciousness (Poor GCS), initial imaging often minimally abnormal
- Small petechial hemorrhages at GM-WM junction
- CT—less sensitive
- Susceptibility—Weighted Imaging (SWI)–More sensitive for hemorrhages
- IOC for DAI—MRI (Hyperintensities on FLAIR, Blooming on SWI).

81. IOC for diffuse axonal injury is:

a. Radiograph	b. CT Scan
c. MRI	d. PET Scan

Ans. is 'c' MRI

ALZHEIMER'S DISEASE

Most common cause of dementia.

Characterized by loss of Ach activity in cortex.

Pathology

- Cortical atrophy in frontal, temporal and parietal lobes
- Medial temporal lobe structures (Hippocampus, entorhinal cortex and amygdale) are involved early in the course
- Extracellular Beta Amyloid plaques and Neurofibrillary tangles (Tau protein) in neurons.

Risk Factors

- Major risk factor is Age
- *Down's Syndrome*: APP gene on Chromosome 21
- *Familial form*: Presenilin 1 and 2 gene mutations
- *Others*: Family history, African-American race, Type II Diabetes.

Clinical Manifestations

- Cognitive changes may not follow any characteristic pattern, but usually the disease begins with memory impairment progressing to language and visuospatial deficits.
- *Early stages*: Amnestic state.
- *Middle stages*: Impaired language (Dysnomia), Visuospatial deficits (Apraxias).
- *Late stages*: Delusions, Depression, Personality changes.

Vascular Dementia

- Second most common cause of dementia
- Multi-infarct dementia
- *Risk factors*: Similar to CVA, i.e. HTN, hypercholesterolemia, smoking
- Multiple gray and white mater infarcts over course of months-years
- *Binswanger's Disease*: Preferential involvement of subcortical white mater.

82. Risk factors for Alzheimer's disease include:

a. Klinefelter syndrome	b. Down syndrome
c. Low BP	d. None

Ans. is 'b' Down syndrome

83. Which lobe is affected in the early course of Alzheimer's disease ?

a. Frontal lobe	b. Parietal lobe
c. Medial temporal lobe	d. Lateral temporal lobe

Ans. is 'c' Medial temporal lobe

84. Vascular dementia develops secondary to infarcts in:

a. Gray mater	b. White mater
c. Both a and b	d. Neither a nor b

Ans. is 'c' Both a and b

MOVEMENT DISORDERS

Disorder	Presentation	Characteristic lesion	Associations
Chorea	Sudden, jerky purposeless movements	Basal Ganglia (Striatum; mainly caudate)	Huntington's disease, Sydenham chorea in rheumatic fever
Dystonia	Sudden, involuntary muscle contractions		Blepharospasm, torticollis
Athetosis	Slow snake-like writhing movements	Basal Ganglia	Huntington's disease
Hemiballismus	Sudden wild flailing of one arm	Contralateral subthalamic nucleus	E.g. Lacunar stroke
Myoclonus	Sudden, brief uncontrolled muscle contraction		Jerks, hiccups
Essential tremor	High frequency tremor with sustained posture (e.g. outstretched arms)		Treatment–Non-selective Beta-blockers (e.g.–Propranolol)
Intention tremor	Slow zigzag motion when extending towards a target	Cerebellum	
Resting tremor	Uncontrolled movement most noticeable in hands	Substantia nigra (Parkinson disease)	'Pill-rolling tremor' of Parkinson disease.
Fine tremors	High frequency, low amplitude tremors felt in hands		Catecholamine excess (anxiety, hypoglycemia, smoking); Drugs (Lithium, Valproate); Toxins (Caffeine, Mercury)

Parkinson's Disease

- Degenerative disease of substantia nigra; Deletion of dopamine in SN Pars Compacta.
- *Pathology*: Lewy Bodies in SN (alpha-synuclein inclusions in neurons)
- Mean age on onset–60 years
- Cardinal motor features
  - Rest tremor (Pill-Rolling tremor)
  - Bradykinesia
  - Rigidity
  - Postural instability

Huntington's Disease

- Autosomal Dominant Disease
- Degeneration in Striatum; atrophy of frontal/temporal lobes
- Mutation in HTT gene
- CAG repeats in gene (Normal–10–35; 36–120 in HD)
- Onset of symptoms—25–45 years; death after 10–20 years
- Rapid, semi-purposeful involuntary choreiform movements
- Dementia in late stage.

Wilson's Disease

- Autosomal recessive disorder of copper metabolism
- Mutation of ATP7B gene
  - *Lack of copper excretion in bile*: Copper accumulates in liver
  - *Lack of ceruloplasmin secretion into plasma*: Low ceruloplasmin level; Increased free serum copper; Low total serum copper (despite copper overload).
- Mean age of onset: 12–23 years
  - *Liver*: Cirrhosis, high risk of HCC
  - *CNS*: Dyskinesia, dysarthria, tremors, dementia
  - *Hemolysis*: Coombs' negative hemolytic anemia
  - *Kayser-Fleischer Rings*: Corneal copper deposits in Descemet's membrane at corneo-scleral junction; seen in 50% cases with liver disease and 90% cases with CNS disease.
- Diagnosis
  - *Low ceruloplasmin levels*: Diagnostic hallmark
  - High urinary copper excretion (24 hour test)
  - Kayser-Fleischer rings (Slit lamp exam)
  - *Liver biopsy*: Gold standard
- Treatment: Penicillamine (Binds copper).

Ataxia-Telangiectasia

- Autosomal recessive
- *Cause*: DNA hypersensitivity to ionizing radiation; defective repair of double-strand breaks in DNA

❖ Clinical features
- Ataxia (Cerebellar atrophy)—1st year of life
- Oculomotor apraxia
- Telangiectasias (dilated capillaries) over ear, nose, face—5–8 years
- Recurrent sinus/respiratory infections
- Diabetes in adolescence or later; Delayed puberty
- Increased risk of cancer.

85. Chorea occur due to damage of: *(NEET 2016)*

a. Subthalamus
b. Globus pallidus
c. Sybstantia nigra
d. Striatum

Ans. is 'd' Striatum

86. A child presents with neurological symptoms and has following feature; what test is to be done next?

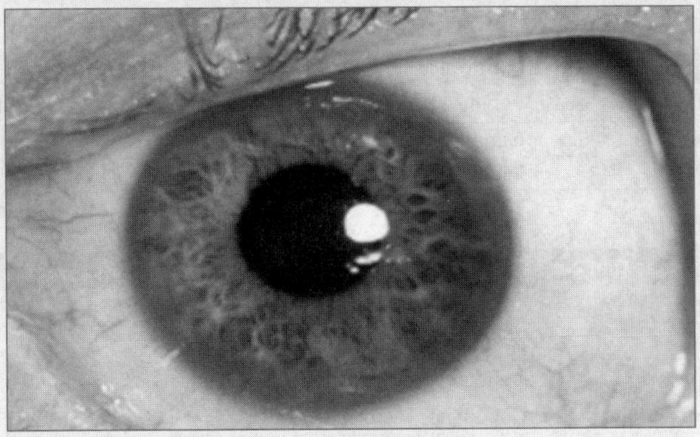

a. Serum ceruloplasmin
b. Keryotyping
c. Serum copper
d. PCR

Ans. is 'a' Serum ceruloplasmin

87. True about ataxia telangiectasia are all *except*:

a. Autosomal dominant
b. Occurs in adults
c. Poor coordination and telangiectasia present
d. Oculomotor apraxia

Ans. is 'a' Autosomal dominant

88. Huntington's disease is commonly seen in age group between:

a. 15–35 years
b. 25–45 years
c. 35–55 years
d. 45–65 years

Ans. is 'b' 25–45 years

89. Violent abnormal flinging movements which are irregular and affecting one side are called as:

a. Chorea
b. Athetosis
c. Dystonia
d. Hemiballismus

Ans. is 'd' Hemiballismus

90. Which of the following disease are not caused by misfolding of proteins?

a. Familial hypercholesterolemia
b. Alpha 1 antitrypsin deficiency
c. Alzheimer disease
d. Parkinson's disease

Ans. is 'd' Parkinson's disease

Explanation: Diseases caused by misfolding of proteins
❖ Cystic fibrosis - CFTR
❖ Familial hypercholesterolemia–LDL receptor
❖ *Tay-Sachs disease*: Hexosaminidase B
❖ Alpha-1-antitrypsin deficiency–Alpha-1-antitrypsin
❖ Creutzfeldt-Jacob disease–Prions
❖ *Alzheimer disease*: Amyloid-Beta peptide.

SEIZURES

Transient signs/symptoms due to abnormal excessive synchronous neuronal activity in brain

Classification of seizures

1. **Focal onset (Partial)**: Intact (Simple partial) or impaired (Complex partial) consciousness
   - Important features of focal motor seizures
     - *Jacksonian March*: Motor movements begin in restricted region (e.g. fingers) and gradually progress (over seconds to minutes) to involve larger portion of extremity
     - *Todd's paralysis*: Localized paresis for minutes to hours in involved region
     - *Epilepsia partialis continua*: Seizure continuing for hours or days refractory to medical therapy.
2. **Generalized**: Entire brain
   - Absence (Petit mal)
   - Tonic-clonic (Grand mal)
   - Atonic (Drop seizure)
   - Myoclonic.

Causes of Seizures

Neonates	Children	Adults	Elderly
Perinatal hypoxia	Febrile seizures	Trauma	Stroke
Intracranial hemorrhage	Genetic	Tumor	Tumor
CNS infection	Infection	Drugs	Drugs
Metabolic	Tumor	Infections	Metabolic

Drugs and Substances that cause seizures	
Alkylating agents	Busulfan, Chlorambucil
Antimicrobials	Beta-lactams, Quinolones, Isoniazid
Anesthetics	Meperidine, Tramadol, Local anesthetics
Immunomodulatory drugs	Cyclosporine, Tacrolimus
Psychotropics	Antidepressants (e.g. Bupropion), Antipsychotics (e.g. Clozapine), Lithium
Drug withdrawal	Alcohol, Barbiturates, Benzodiazepines
Drugs of abuse	Amphetamine, Cocaine, Phencyclidine

Features	Seizure	Syncope
Immediate precipitating factor	None	Emotional stress, Valsalva, orthostatic hypotension
Premonitory symptoms	None or aura (e.g. odd odor)	Tiredness, nausea, diaphoresis, tunneling of vision
Posture at onset	Variable	Erect
Transition to unconsciousness	Immediate	Gradual (over seconds)
Duration of unconsciousness	Minutes	Seconds
Duration of tonic/clonic movements	30–60 s	Never >15 s
Facial appearance	Cyanosis, frothing at mouth	Pallor
Disorientation after event	Minutes to hours	<5 min
Aching of muscles after event	Often	Sometimes
Biting of tongue	Sometimes	Rarely
Incontinence	Sometimes	Sometimes
Headache	Sometimes	Rarely

(Harrison's 20th Edition Pg–3060)

91. Todd's paralysis is experience following episode of:

a. Focal seizure
b. Generalized seizure
c. After correction of hyponatremia
d. After correction of hypokalemia

Ans. is 'a' Focal seizure

92. Features which differentiate seizures from syncope include the following *except*:

a. No immediate precipitating factors like stress, Valsalva, orthostatic hypotension
b. Immediate transition to unconsciousness
c. Presence of cyanosis and frothing of mouth
d. Presence of premonitory symptoms like diaphoresis and tunneling of vision

Ans. is 'd' Presence of premonitory symptoms like diaphoresis and tunneling of vision

WERNICKE'S ENCEPHALOPATHY

- Seen in alcoholic patients with chronic thiamine (B1) deficiency
- Acute encephalopathy; Reversible with thiamine
- Pathogenesis
  - Thiamine is a cofactor of enzymes like transketolase, pyruvate dehydrogenase and alpha-ketoglutarate dehydrogenase
  - Glutamate accumulates due to reduced alpha-ketoglutarate dehydrogenase activity and causes cell damage
  - Often precipitated by glucose infusion without thiamine (thiamine is utilized as a cofactor for glucose metabolism)
- Characteristic clinical triad–Ophthalmoplegia, Ataxia and Confusion
- Atrophy of mammillary bodies.

Korsakoff Psychosis

- Chronic neurological condition; usually a consequence of Wernicke's
- Non-reversible condition
- Amnestic state with impaired recent memory, confabulation and personality changes.

93. Wernicke's encephalopathy develops secondary to accumulation of which substrate?

a. Glutamate b. Aspartate
c. Lactate d. Acetate

Ans. is 'a' Glutamate

SPINAL CORD SYNDROMES

Structure of Spinal Cord

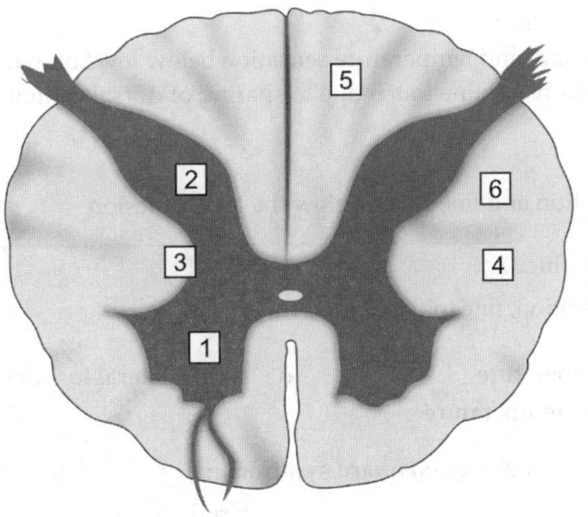

1. *Anterior horn*: Motor nerves
2. *Posterior horn*: Sensory nerves (pain/temp)
3. *Lateral horn*: Autonomic nerves
4. *Spinothalamic tract*: Pain/Temperature
5. *Medial lemniscus*: Vibration/Propriception
6. *Corticospinal tract*: Motor.

Brown-Sequard Syndrome

Loss of half of spinal cord

Causes–Trauma, Tumor, Infarction

Findings

1. Ipsilateral loss of all sensation at level of lesion
   Ipsilateral Lower Motor Neuron signs at level of lesion (If level above T1–Horner's syndrome)
2. Ipsilateral Upper Motor Neuron signs below level of lesion (corticospinal tract damage)
   Ipsilateral loss of proprioception, vibration and light touch below level of lesion (dorsal column damage)
3. Contralateral loss of pain, temperature and crude touch below level of lesion (spinothalamic tract damage).

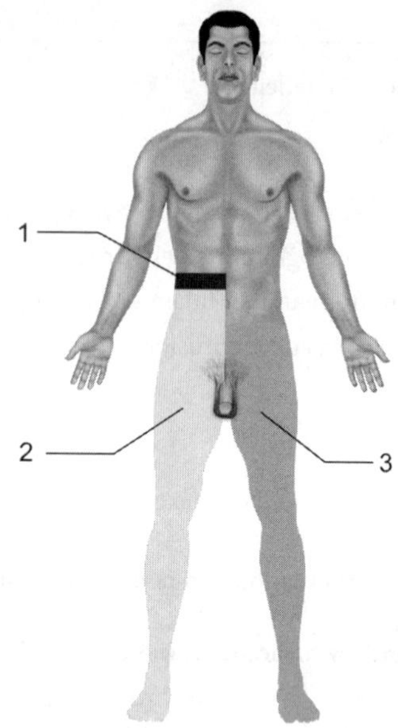

Central Cord Syndrome

- Bilateral sensory and motor deficits with upper extremity weakness greater than lower extremity (Dissociative motor weakness)
- Sacral sparing.

Anterior Cord Syndrome

- Ischemia in territory of anterior spinal artery
- Complete loss of motor function and pain and temperature sensation below level of injury
- Preservation of vibration, proprioception and fine touch due to sparing of dorsal column.

Posterior Cord Syndrome

- Bilateral loss of vibration, proprioception and fine touch below the level of lesion.

94. True about Brown-Sequard syndrome: *(NEET 2018)*

a. Contralateral loss of proprioception, fine touch and vibration
b. Contralateral paralysis
c. Ipsilateral loss of pain and temperature
d. Contralateral loss of pain and temperature

Ans. is 'd' Contralateral loss of pain and temperature

95. Type of sensation lost on same side in Brown-Sequard syndrome: *(NEET 2019)*

a. Pain
b. Crude touch
c. Proprioception
d. Temperature

Ans. is 'c' Proprioception

ROMBERG TEST

Investigate the cause of loss of motor coordination (ataxia).
Differentiate Sensory (loss of proprioception due to dorsal column damage) vs Cerebellar (cerebellum dysfunction) ataxia.
Test and interpretation

- Patient is asked to stand, keep feet together and close eyes
- Positive test—Patient loses balance
- Patients with sensory ataxia compensate for loss of proprioception through vision; if Romberg test positive–Sensory ataxia
- Cerebellar ataxia occurs even with eyes open.

96. Which of the following clinical test when positive suggests presence of sensory ataxia?

a. Romberg test
b. Adson test
c. Stinchfield test
d. Crossed SLR test

Ans. is 'a' Romberg test

NEUROCUTANEOUS SYNDROMES

Neurofibromatosis

Autosomal dominant familial cancer syndromes.

Neurofibromatosis–1 (von Recklinghausen Disease)

- Mutation of NF-1 gene on Chromosome 17; encodes for neurofibromin
- Diagnostic criteria (at least 2 required)
  - Six or more café-au-lait spots
  - Two or more neurofibromas
  - Freckles in axilla or groin
  - Optic glioma
  - Two or more Lisch nodules
  - Bone lesions
  - 1st degree relative with NF-1.

Neurofibromatosis-2

- Less common than NF-1; mutation of NF-2 gene on Chromosome 22
- Bilateral vestibular schwannomas
- Meningiomas.

Tuberous Sclerosis

- Autosomal Dominant
- Mutation in TSC1 (Hamartin) or TSC2 (Tuberin) genes
- *Hallmark*: Hamatomas in multiple organ systems
- Epilepsy, Mental retardation, Adenoma Sebaceum—VOGT's TRIAD.

Tuberous Sclerosis		
Cutaneous	***Neurological***	***Other benign neoplasms***
Adenoma Sebaceum: Facial angiofibromas	Epilepsy, Mental retardation	Cardiac Rhabdomyoma
Ash-leaf spots: Hypopigmented macules	Cortical tubers: Distorted cortex	Renal Angiomyolipomas: MC renal manifestation
Shagreen patches: Leathery thickening over lower back	Subependymal nodules: Calcified on CT	
Ungual fibromas: Fibromas beneath nailbeds	Subependymal Giant Cell Astrocytomas (SEGAs): at Interventricular foramen	

97. Criteria of NF1 include all *except*:

a. Lisch nodule
b. Optic gliomas
c. Bilateral schwannomas
d. Cafe au lait spots

Ans. is 'c' Bilateral schwannomas

98. Tuberous sclerosis is caused by mutations in the following proteins:

a. Hamartin
b. Neurofibromin
c. Merlin
d. Ankyrin

Ans. is 'a' Hamartin

99. Features of tuberous sclerosis are all *except*:

a. Ash leaf macules
b. Adenoma sebaceum
c. Angiomyolipoma of kidney
d. Erythema migrans

Ans. is 'd' Erythema migrans

100. The gene for Neurofibromatosis type II is located on which chromosome?

a. 11
b. 14
c. 17
d. 22

Ans. is 'd' 22

MYASTHENIA GRAVIS

Autoimmune disease, Antibodies block nicotinic Ach receptors.

Despite the muscle weakness, deep tendon reflexes are preserved.

Muscle bulk is also normal and there are no fasciculations as there is involvement of neuromuscular junction rather than LMN.

Diagnosis

History

- Diplopia, ptosis, bulbar symptoms
- Worse with repeated activity.

Laboratory Testing

- *Anti-AChR radioimmunoassay*: 85% positive in generalized MG; 50% in ocular MG; definite diagnosis if positive; negative result does not exclude MG; 40% of AChR antibody—negative patients with generalized MG have anti-MuSK antibodies.
- *Repetitive nerve stimulation*: Decrement of >15% at 3 Hz: highly probable.
- *Single-fiber electromyography*: Blocking and jitter, with normal fiber density; confirmatory, but not specific.
- Edrophonium chloride 2 mg + 8 mg IV; highly probable diagnosis if unequivocally positive.

Most specific test to diagnose myasthenia gravis—Anti-AchR antibody test.

Most sensitive test to diagnose myasthenia gravis—Single fiber electromyography.

Drugs that may exacerbate myasthenia gravis	
Antibiotics	Aminoglycosides (streptomycin, tobramycin); Quinolones (levofloxacin); Macrolides (erythromycin, azithromycin, tobramycin)
Nondepolarizing muscle relaxants	Curare, pancuronium, vecuronium, atracurium
Beta-blockers	Propranolol, atenolol, metoprolol
Botulinum toxin	
Quinine derivatives	Quinidine, chloroquine, mefloquine
Magnesium	
Penicillamine	

Lambert-Eaton Myasthenic Syndrome

- Also a disorder of NMJ
- Paraneoplastic syndrome asscociated with small cell ca of lung
- IgG autoantibodies against pre-synaptic calcium channels—Prevent Ach release

	Myasthenia gravis	Lambert-Eaton myasthenic syndrome
Cause	Post-synaptic Ach receptor Ab	Pre-synaptic Calcium channel Ab
Muscle use	Worsens	Improves
Eye symptoms	Classic	Less common
Proximal muscles	Rare	Common
Deep Tendon Reflexes	Intact	Absent
Autonomic symptoms (dry mouth, impotence)	Absent	Common
Tensilon test	Symptom reversal	Mild improvement
Repetitive nerve stimulation	Decremental response	Incremental response

101. About myasthenia gravis pathogenesis, true is:

a. Antibody against Ach receptor
b. Antibody against Ca receptor
c. Ach is not secreted
d. Blockage of nerve conduction through myoneural junction

Ans. is 'a' Antibody against Ach receptor

102. Decremental response on EMG is seen in:

a. Myasthenia gravis
b. Lambert-Eaton syndrome
c. Duchenne muscular dystrophy
d. UMN lesion

Ans. is 'a' Myasthenia gravis

103. Lambert-Eaton syndrome true is:

a. It is a paraneoplastic syndrome associated with squamous cell carcinoma of lung
b. IgM antibodies against ligand gated calcium channels
c. There is increase in release of presynaptic acetylcholine
d. With continuous stimulation there is marked increase in amplitude of action potentials

Ans. is 'd' With continuous stimulation there is marked increase in amplitude of action potentials

MISCELLANEOUS TOPICS

Frey's Syndrome

- Rare disorder resulting from damage to Auriculotemporal nerve often from surgery
- *Symptoms*: Excessive sweating and flushing of the cheek in response to food—'gustatory sweating'
- *Cause*: Auriculotemporal nerve carries postganglionic parasympathetic fibers from cranial nerve IX to parotid gland and sympathetic fibers to sweat glands. Following injury, there is aberrant reinnervation of these postganglionic parasympathetic fibers to nearby denervated sweat glands and cutaneous blood vessels. This results in sweating and flushing of skin in response to parasympathetic activation during salivation and mastication.

Myotonic Dystrophy

- Autosomal dominant inherited muscular dystrophy
- Distal muscle weakness more than proximal weakness
- Two overlapping subtypes—DM1 and DM2
  - DM1: Trinucleotide explansion in Gene DMPK on chromosome 19
  - DM2: DNA expansion mutation in Gene CMBP.

Charcot-Marie-Tooth Disease

- Most common type of hereditary neuropathy
- Multiple subtypes
- Progressive muscle weakness and atrophy that begins in first two decades of life
- Often atrophy of muscles below knee
- Present with foot deformities like pes cavus, scoliosis
- Motor symptoms predominate over sensory symptoms.

Peripheral Nerve Damage

Seddon's classification: In order of increasing severity

- *Neuropraxia*: Only focal demyelination, axon intact; continuity maintained; excellent recovery
- *Axonotmesis*: Axon and myelin sheath damaged, peri and epineurium intact; continuity maintained; prognosis depends on extent of injury
- *Neurotmesis*: Axon, myelin sheath, peri and epineurium damages; continuity lost; bad prognosis

Morphology after Injury

- *Distal to the lesion*: 'Wallerian Degeneration'—Axon degenerates, myelin sheath involutes into spherical structures (Myelin ovoids)
- *Proximal to the lesion*: 'Axonal Reaction'—Central Chromatolysis (Nissl granules break up), nucleus moves to periphery
- *Regeneration*: Starts at site of injury with formation of a growth cone and outgrowth of branches from proximal stump
  - If there is a wide gap between the stumps, regeneration does not occur without surgical repair
  - Failure of outgrowing axons to find their distal target produces a Neuroma—whorled proliferation of axons and Schwann cells that is painful
  - Axonotmesis produces Neuroma in continuity (nerve is not completey transected)
  - Neurotmesis produces Neuroma not in continuity (nerve is completely transected).

Alien Limb Syndrome/Alien Hand Syndrome

- Interesting situation in which a person loses control of his or her hand, which starts to act independently
- Complex goal-directed activity of one limb has been described
- Patient has a feeling that the limb is foreign or that it has a will of its own
- This rare syndrome has been reported after surgery on corpus callosum, brain tumor removal, aneurysm, stroke and degenerative brain conditions like Alzheimer's disease and Creutzfeldt-Jakob disease.

Lumbar Puncture

Positioning:

- Patient in lateral position, with thighs, knees, neck and back flexed in such a way that the knees touch the abdomen. This position widens the intervertebral space.
- Performed at or below the L3–L4 interspace (at the level of a line drawn between posterior superior iliac crests)

Technique:

- Local disinfection.
- 3–5 mL of local anesthetic (1% lidocaine), is injected into subcutaneous tissue.

- LP needle (usually 20–22 G) is inserted in midline, midway between two spinous processes and slowly advanced, with slight angulation directed upwards.
- Bevel of needle should be maintained in a horizontal position, parallel to direction of dural fibers and with flat portion of bevel pointed upward; this minimizes injury to fibers as dura is penetrated.
- In most adults, needle is advanced 4–5 cm before the subarachnoid space is reached; a sudden loss of resistance is felt when the ligamentum flavum is punctured.
- A manometer is attached to needle and opening pressure measured. Upper limit of normal opening pressure with the patient supine is 180 mm Hg in adults but may be as high as 200–250 mm Hg in obese adults.
- CSF is allowed to drip into collection tubes; it should not be withdrawn with a syringe.

During lumbar puncture, the needle passes through the following anatomic structures before it enters the subarachnoid space:

- Skin
- Subcutaneous tissue
- Supraspinous ligament
- Interspinous ligament
- Ligamentum flavum
- Dura mater
- Arachnoid mater.

Absolute Contraindications

- Sepsis at site of injection
- Coagulopathy including low platelet count of < 20,000/mcL
- Features of raised ICP.

Post-dural Puncture Headache (PDPH)

- Occurs due to CSF leak. Typical location is bifrontal or occipital.
- Worse on sitting or upright posture—hallmark of PDPH.
- Onset usually 12–72 hours following procedure; lasts for 7–10 days.
- Increased incidence in young patients, females, pregnancy, large bore needle and multiple punctures.
- Small bore needle can prevent PDPH.
- **Treatment**:
  - Conservative treatment with recumbent position, NSAIDs, oral/IV fluids and Sumatriptan.
  - *Epidural blood patch*: If conservative treatment fails; involves injecting 15–20 mL autologous blood into epidural space.

Other complications of lumbar puncture

- Cerebral herniation (in case of raised ICP), low back pain, infection and bleeding complications.

Varicella Zoster

- Reactivation of Varicella Zoster Virus (primary infection is chickenpox)
- Virus lies dormant in dorsal root ganglia
- Reactivated lesions follow sensory dermatome (most commonly thoracic dermatome); do not cross midline
- Pre-eruptive phase (sensory symptoms) followed by vesicular eruptive phase
- *Risk factors*: Elderly, immunocompromised, inflammatory bowel disease
- *Pathology*: Affected ganglia show neuronal death with axonal degeneration; intranuclear inclusions are not found in peripheral nervous system
- *Rare complications*: Ophthalmic zoster (blindness), encephalitis

Obstructive Sleep Apnea

- Multiple episodes of apnea (cessation of breathing) during sleep
- Recurrent soft-tissue collapse in pharynx; strongest risk factor is obesity
- Polysomnography (sleep study)
  - EEG, eye movements, O_2 level, Heart rate, Respiratory rate
  - Number of apnea episodes recorded
  - **Apnea-Hypopnea Index (AHI)**: Number of apnea events per hour of sleep
  - Indicates severity of OSA
  - *AHI values*: Normal < 5; Mild OSA 5–15; Moderate 15–30; Severe >30.

104. Following are the features of neuropathy associated with varicella-zoster infection *except*:

a. Persistent infection in neurons of sensory ganglia
b. With reactivation virus transported along nerves to skin
c. Shingles are distributed along motor dermatomes
d. Intranuclear inclusions are not found in peripheral nervous system

Ans. is 'c' Shingles are distributed along motor dermatomes

105. Frey's syndrome develops secondary to aberrant innervation of the skin over parotid by which cranial nerve?

a. IX
b. X
c. XI
d. XII

Ans. is 'a' IX

106. Following is not used in the management of post dural headache:

a. Propped up position
b. Sumatriptan
c. Hydration
d. Epidural blood patch

Ans. is 'a' Propped up position

PULMONOLOGY

LUNG CANCER

TNM 8th–Primary tumor characteristics	
T_X T_0 T_{is}	Tumor in sputum/bronchial washings but not be assessed in imaging or bronchoscopy No evidence of tumor Carcinoma in situ
T_1 $T_{1a(mi)}$ T_{1a} T_{1b} T_{1c}	$\leq$ 3 cm surrounded by lung/visceral pleura, not involving main bronchus Minimally invasive carcinoma $\leq$ 1 cm 1 to $\leq$ 2 cm 2 to $\leq$ 3 cm
T_2 T_{2a} T_{2b}	3 to $\leq$ 5 cm or Involvement of main bronchus without carina, regardless of distance from carina or invasion visceral pleural *or* atelectasis or postobstructive pneumonitis extending to hilum >3 to $\leq$ 4 cm >4 to $\leq$ 5 cm
T_3	>5 to $\leq$ 7cm in greatest dimension *or* tumor of any size that involves chest wall, pericardium, phrenic nerve or satellite nodules in the same lobe
T_4	> 7 cm in greatest dimension *or* Any tumor with invasion of mediastinum, **diaphragm**, heart, great vessels, recurrent laryngeal nerve, carina, trachea, oesophagus, spine *or* Separate tumor in different lobe of ipsilateral lung
N_1 N_2 N_3	Ipsilateral peribronchial and/or hilar nodes and intrapulmonary nodes Ipsilateral mediastinal and/or subcarinal nodes Contralateral mediastinal or hilar; ipsilateral/contralateral scalene/supraclavicular
M_1 M_{1a} M_{1b} M_{1c}	Distant metastasis Tumor in contralateral lung or pleural/pericardial nodule/malignant effusion Single extrathoracic metastasis, including single non-regional lymph node Multiple extrathoracic metastases in one or more organs

107. What is the T stage of a 2.5 cm lung carcinoma, which is not involving the pleura. *(NEET 2020)*

a. T_{1a}
b. T_2
c. T_{1b}
d. T_{1c}

Ans. is 'd' T_{1c}

Medicine

HAI

Hospital-acquired (or nosocomial) pneumonia (HAP) is a pneumonia that occurs 48 hours or more after admission and did not appear to be incubating at the time of admission.

Ventilator-associated pneumonia (VAP) is a type of pneumonia that develops ≥48 hours after endotracheal intubation.

108. Onset of symptoms after ___ hrs of hospital admission in a previously asymptomatic patient is termed as HAI: *(NEET 2020)*

a. 24 hrs
b. 48 hrs
c. 72 hrs
d. 90 hrs

Ans. is 'b' 48 hrs

CRACKLES

Brief, discontinuous, popping sounds heard on chest auscultation. They can be further classified into:

Coarse crackles	Fine crackles
It occurs in both phases of respiration	Heard during mid to late inspiration
No predilection for any particular area of lung	Usually starts in basal part of lungs
It can be altered by coughing, but not by body position changes	It can be altered by body position change, but remains unaltered by coughing
It can be transmitted to mouth	It is not transmitted to mouth
It is produced by gas passing through airways which undergo intermittent opening and closing	It is produced by sudden inspiratory opening of small airways which were held closed during the previous expiration

Classification based on the respiratory phase in which it is heard:

- *Early inspiratory crackles (inspiratory squeaks)*: Small airway disease (bronchiolitis)
- *Mid-inspiratory crackles*: Pulmonary edema, Pulmonary fibrosis (fine)
- *Late inspiratory crackles*: Bronchial secretions in COPD, Pneumonia, lung abscess, Tubercular lung cavities
- Crackles throughout inspiration and expiration—Bronchiectasis (coarse).

109. Inspiratory squeaks are the physical examination finding of:

a. Bronchiolitis
b. Pulmonary hypertension
c. Pneumonia
d. Pulmonary edema

Ans. is 'a' Bronchiolitis

PULMONARY FUNCTION TESTS (PFTs)

- The **FEV1/FVC ratio**, also called Tiffeneau-Pinelli index, is used in the diagnosis of obstructive and restrictive lung disease.
- It represents the proportion of a person's vital capacity that they are able to expire in the first second of forced expiration to the full vital capacity.
- Normal values are approximately 80%.
- It is usually decreased in obstructive lung disease and normal or increased in restrictive lung disease (as the FEV1 and FVC are equally reduced).

Pulmonary function measurement	Obstructive pulmonary disease	Restrictive pulmonary disease
FVC	Decrease/Normal	Decrease
FEV1	Decrease	Decrease/Normal
FEV1/FVC	Decrease	Normal/Increase

Obstructive lung diseases	Restrictive lung diseases
Emphysema	Neuromuscular disorders–Polio, ALS
Chronic bronchitis	Scoliosis
Bronchiectasis	ARDS
Asthma	Interstitial lung disease

110. FEVI/FVC decreased in all of the following *except*:

a. Asthma
b. COPD
c. Bronchiectasis
d. ARDS

Ans. is 'd' ARDS

CHRONIC BRONCHITIS

Chronic cough and productive sputum for at least 3 months over two consecutive years in the absence of any other identifiable cause.

- ❖ Strongly associated with smoking
- ❖ Appearance—Blue Bloater (cyanosis with air trapping)–Vs Pink Puffer in Emphysema (hyperventilation maintains O_2 level initially)
- ❖ Can lead to pulmonary hypertension and right heart failure (cor pulmonale).

GOLD (Global initiative for COPD) criteria for COPD severity			
Stage	***Severity***	***Spirometry***	***Treatment***
I	Mild	FEV1 >80%, Normal FEV1/FVC	Short-acting bronchodilator as needed
II	Moderate	FEV1 50–79%	Add long-acting bronchodilator
III	Severe	FEV1 30–49%	Add inhaled corticosteroid
IV	Very severe	FEV1 <30%	Oxygen/surgery

COPD EXACERBATION

Rapid overview: Initial emergency management of severe COPD exacerbations

Clinical Features

Features of COPD exacerbation: Diffuse wheezing, distant breath sounds, barrel-shaped chest, tachypnea, tachycardia, smoking >20 pack years

Features of severe respiratory insufficiency: Use of accessory muscles; brief, fragmented speech; inability to lie supine; profound diaphoresis; agitation; asynchrony between chest and abdominal motion with respiration; failure to improve with initial emergency treatment

Features of impending respiratory arrest: Inability to maintain respiratory effort cyanosis hemodynamic instability, and depressed mental status

Features of cor pulmonale: Jugular venous distension, prominent left parasternal heave, peripheral edema COPD exacerbations are most often precipitated by infection (viral or bacterial)

Severe respiratory distress in a patient with known or presumed COPD can be due to an exacerbation of COPD or a comorbid process, such as a cute coronary syndrome, decompensated heart failure pulmonary embolism, pneumonia, pneumothorax:, sepsis.

Management

Assess patient's airway, breathing, and circulation; secure as necessary.

Provide supplemental oxygen to target a pulse oxygen saturation of 88 to 92% or PaO_2 of 60 to 70 mm Hg (7.98 to 9.31 kPa); Venturi mask can be useful for titrating FiO_2; high FiO_2 usually not needed and can contribute to hypercapnia (high FiO_2 requirement should prompt consideration of alternative diagnosis [e. g., PE])

Determine patient preferences regarding intubation based on direct questioning or advance directive whenever possible Provide combination of aggressive bronchodilator therapy and ventilatory support (NIV or invasive ventilation)

Noninvasive ventilation (NIV): Appropriate for the majority of patients with severe exacerbations of COPD unless immediate intubation is needed or NIV is otherwise contraindicated

Contraindications to NIV include: Severely impaired consciousness, inability to clear secretions or protect airway, high aspiration risk.

Initial settings for bilevel NIV: 8 cm H_2O inspiratory pressure (may increase up to 15 cm H_2O if needed to aid ventilation); 3 cm H_2Oexpiratory pressure.

Administer bronchodilators via nebulizer or MDI: Nebulizer usually requires interruption of NIV; MD is can be delivered in line using adaptor (see dosing below)

Obtain ABG after two hours of NIV and compare with baseline: Worsening or unimproved gas exchange and pH <7.25 are indications for invasive ventilation

Tracheal intubation and mechanical ventilation: Indicated for patients with acute respiratory failure, hemodynamic instability (e.g., heart rate < 50/minute uncontrolled arrhythmia) and those in whom NIV is contraindicated or who fail to improve with NIV and aggressive pharmacotherapy.

Rapid sequence induction (e.g. etomidate, ketamine, or propofol)

Intubate with #8 endotracheal tube (8 mm internal diameter) or larger, if possible

Initial ventilator settings aim to maintain adequate oxygenation and ventilation while minimizing elevated airway pressures: SIMV, tidal volume 6 to 8 mL/kg, respiratory rate 10 to 12/minute, inspiratory flow rate 60 to 80 L/min (increase if needed to enable longer expiratory phase), PEEP 5 cm H_2O. May need to tolerate elevated $PaCO_2$ to avoid barotrauma (i. e., permissive hypercapnia). In patients with chronic hypercapnia, aim for $PaCO_2$ close to baseline.

Administer inhaled bronchodilator therapy: Usually via MDI, with in-line adaptor (see dosing below)

Diagnostic Testing

- ❖ Assess oxygen saturation with continuous pulse oximetry
- ❖ Obtain ABG in all patients with severe COPD exacerbation
- ❖ $ETCO_2$ monitoring (capnography) has only moderate correlation with arterial $PaCO_2$ in COPD exacerbations

- Do not assess peak expiratory flow or spirometry in acute severe COPD exacerbations as results are not accurate
- Obtain portable chest radiograph: Look for signs of pneumonia, acute heart failure, pneumothorax.
- Obtain complete blood count, electrolytes (Na+, K^+, Cl^-, HCO_3^-), BUN, and creatinine; also obtain cardiac troponin, BNP, or NT-pro BNP, if diagnosis uncertain Test for influenza infection during influenza season*
- Obtain ECG: Look for arrhythmia, ischemia, cor pulmonale

Pharmacotherapy

- **Inhaled beta agonist:** Albuterol 2.5 mg diluted to 3 mL via nebulizer or 4 to 8 inhalations from MDI every hour or more frequently if needed
- **Inhaled anticholinergic agent:** Ipratropium 500 micrograms via nebulizer or 4 to 8 inhalations from NIDI every four hours
- Intravenous glucocorticoid (e.g., methylprednisolone 60 mg to 125 mg IV, repeat every 6 to 12 hours)
- **Antibiotic therapy*:** Appropriate for majority of severe COPD exacerbations; select antibiotic based on likelihood of particular pathogens (e.g., *Pseudomonas*¶ risk factors, prior sputum cultures, local patterns of resistance)
  - **No *Pseudomonas*¶ risk factor(s):** Ceftriaxone 1 to 2 grams IV, **OR** cefotaxime 1 to 2 grams IV, **OR** levofloxacin 500 mg IV or orally, **OR** moxifloxacin 400 mg IV or orally
  - ***Pseudomonas*¶ risk factor(s):** Levofloxacin 750 mg IV or orally, OR piperacillin-tazobactam 4.5 grams IV, OR cefepime 2 grams IV, OR ceftazidime 2 grams IV
- **Antiviral therapy (influenza suspected)*:** Oseltamivir 75 mg orally every 12 hours **OR** peramivir 600 mg IV once (for patients unable to take oral medication)

Monitoring

- Perform continual monitoring of oxygen saturation, blood pressure, heart rate, respiratory rate
- Close monitoring of respiratory status
- Continuous ECG monitoring
- Monitor blood glucose

Disposition

Criteria for ICU admission include:

- Patients, with high-risk comorbidities (pneumonia, cardiac arrhythmia, heart failure, diabetes mellitus, renal failure, liver failure) Continued need for NIV or invasive ventilation
- Hemodynamic instability
- Need for frequent nebulizer treatments or monitoring

COPD: chronic obstructive pulmonary disease; PaO_2: arterial tension of oxygen; FiO_2: fraction of inspired oxygen; PE: pulmonary embolism; NIV: noninvasive ventilation; MDI: metered dose inhaler; ABG: arterial blood gas; SIMV: synchronized intermittent mechanical ventilation; PEEP: positive end-expiratory pressure; $PaCO_2$: arterial tension of carbon dioxide; $ETCO_2$: end-tidal carbon dioxide; BUN: blood urea nitrogen; BNP: brain natriuretic peptide; NT-ProBNP: N-terminal pro-BNP; ECG: electrocardiogram; IV: intravenous; ICU: intensive care unit.

*When influenza is suspected, therapy should not be delayed while awaiting results of testing. Doses shown are for patients with normal renal function. Some agents require dose adjustment for renal impairment; refer to separate Up To Date algorithms of antibiotic treatment of exacerbations of COPD.

¶***Pseudomonas* infection risk factors:** Frequent administration of antibiotics (four or more courses over the past year); recent hospitalization (two or more days duration in the past 90 days); isolation of *Pseudomonas* during a previous hospitalization; severe underlying COPD (FEV1 <50 percent predicted).

There has been increasing recognition that mechanical ventilation can cause acute parenchymal lung injury (ventilator-induced lung injury, or VILI) in addition to the more widely recognized forms of barotrauma. In patients with acute asthma, chronic obstructive pulmonary disease, or acute lung injury, however, accepting abnormal blood-gas tensions, particularly an elevated $PaCO_2$ (permissive hypercapnia), to improve survival and reduce complications is frequently necessary. Extensive experience has shown that ventilated patients usually tolerate moderate hypercapnia and frequently some degree of hypoxemia in the absence of shock, anemia, severe cardiac disease, or other contraindications.

111. A known case of COPD with acute exacerbation of COPD, on examination patient conscious and alert, pulse-110/min, on examination bilateral wheeze. Which of the following is not true? *(NEET 2020)*

a. IV Steroids
b. Inhalation with salbutamol
c. Permissible hypercapea allowed
d. Noninvasive ventilation not indicated

Ans. is 'd' Noninvasive ventilation not indicated

ASTHMA

Signs of impending respiratory failure in asthma:

- Drowsiness
- Diaphoresis
- Bradycardia
- Hypotension

- ❖ Peak expiratory flow rate < 33%
- ❖ Pulsus paradoxus
- ❖ Hypercapnia
- ❖ Silent chest.

Treatment of Asthma

- ❖ *Beta 2–agonists*: Albuterol (short acting), Salmeterol, Formoterol (long acting)
- ❖ *Muscarinic antagonists*: Ipratropium (short acting), Tiotropium (long acting)
- ❖ *Steroids*: Inhaled (Beclomethasone, Fluticasone), Oral (Prednisone), IV (Methylprednisolone).

Special Asthma Drugs

- ❖ Leukotriene Antagonists (Montelukast, Zafirlukast): Block cys-LT1 receptors
  - Used as add-on therapy in patients not controlled by low dose inhaled glucocorticoids
  - Aspirin-sensitive asthma
- ❖ 5-Lipoxygenase inhibitors: Zileuton
- ❖ Theophylline: Narrow therapeutic index
- ❖ Omalizumab: Anti-IgE
- ❖ Cromolyn: Inhibits mast cell degranulation.

BRONCHIECTASIS

Causes

- ❖ Obstruction (tumor, foreign body)
- ❖ Infections
- ❖ Genetic causes (CF, Kartagener's syndrome)
- ❖ Aspiration
- ❖ Allergic bronchopulmonary aspergillosis (ABPA)

Symptoms

- ❖ *Recurrent infections*: Common cause of death before era of antibiotics
- ❖ Cough, excessive foul smelling sputum
- ❖ Hemoptysis
- ❖ *Right heart failure (Cor Pulmonale)*: Common cause of death in patients with chronic bronchitis.

Investigation of choice in Lung diseases

Disease	*Investigation of choice*
Interstitial lung disease	HRCT chest
Bronchiectasis	HRCT chest
Pulmonary embolism	CT pulmonary angiography
Solitary pulmonary nodule	CECT chest
Pulmonary malignancy	CECT chest
Superior sulcus/Pancoast tumor	MRI

112. Imaging modality for confirming the diagnosis of bronchiectasis is?

a. Chest CT scan
b. MRI chest
c. X-ray chest
d. Bronchoscopy

Ans. is 'a' Chest CT scan

113. Life-threatening features of asthma are the following *except*:

a. Drowsy or confused patient
b. Presence of pulsus paradoxus
c. Silent chest
d. Tachycardia

Ans. is 'd' Tachycardia

114. Leukotriene inhibitors are used in asthma for:

a. Monotherapy for acute attack
b. Add-on therapy in patients not controlled by low dose inhaled glucocorticoids
c. Status asthmaticus
d. None of the above

Ans. is 'b' Add-on therapy in patients not controlled by low dose inhaled glucocorticoids

ALLERGIC BRONCHOPULMONARY ASPERGILLOSIS (ABPA)

Hypersensitivity reaction to aspergillus.

Predisposing conditions: Bronchial asthma, Cystic fibrosis.

Symptoms: Chronic cough, wheeze, recurrent pneumonias/sinus infections.

Diagnostic criteria

- Elevated serum IgE levels (>1000 IU/mL)
- Eosinophil count >1000 cells/microliter in peripheral blood (peripheral eosinophilia)
- Chest radiographic opacities
- Central bronchiectasis on HRCT chest
- Immediate type I reaction to *A. fumigatus antigen*.

115. Which of the following is not seen in ABPA?

a. Wheeze, cough, fever
b. Peripheral eosinophilia
c. Skin rash
d. Recurrent pneumonia

Ans. is 'c' Skin rash

Empirical antibiotic treatment of community-acquired pneumonia	
Outpatient	
• Previously healthy; No antibiotics in past 3 months	• Macrolide (clarithromycin, azithromycin) or • Doxycycline
• Comorbities; Antibiotics in past 3 months	• Fluoroquinolone (moxifloxacin, levofloxacin) or • Beta-lactam (amoxicillin, cefuroxime) plus Macrolide
Inpatient, Non-ICU	• Fluoroquinolone (moxifloxacin, levofloxacin) or • Beta-lactam plus Macrolide
Inpatients, ICU	• Beta-lactam (ceftriaxone, cefotaxime) plus either azithromycin or fluoroquinolone
Special concerns	
• Pseudomonas	Antipseudomonal Beta-lactam (Piperacillin/Tazobactam, cefepime, imipenem) plus cipro/levofloxacin or aminoglycoside
• MRSA	Add linezolid or vancomycin plus clindamycin

116. What is the following therapy for management of suspected case of pneumonia who requires outpatient management and does not have any other comorbidities and has not received any antibiotic treatment in the past 3 months?

a. Oral clarithromycin
b. Oral ciprofloxacin
c. Oral amoxicillin
d. Oral linezolid

Ans. is 'a' Oral clarithromycin

ACUTE RESPIRATORY DISTRESS SYNDROME (ARDS)

- Clinical syndrome of severe dyspnea of rapid onset, hypoxemia and diffuse pulmonary infiltrates leading to respiratory failure
- Triggered by various lung injuries

Direct lung injury	Indirect lung injury
Pneumonia	Sepsis
Aspiration of gastric contents	Pancreatitis
Pulmonary contusion	Flail chest, Head trauma
Drowning	Postcardiopulmonary bypass
Toxic inhalation	Multiple transfusions

Diagnostic criteria for ARDS			
Severity: Oxygenation	***Onset***	***Chest radiograph***	***Normal LA pressure***
Mild: 200 mm Hg < $PaO_2/FiO_2 \le 300$ mm Hg *Moderate*: 100 mm Hg < $PaO_2/FiO_2 \le 200$ mm Hg *Severe*: $PaO_2/FiO_2 \le 100$ mm Hg	Acute: Within 1 week of a clinical insult or new or worsening respiratory symptoms	Bilateral opacities consistent with pulmonary edema	PCWP < 18 mm Hg or no clinical evidence of increased LA pressure

Lung Compliance

- Measure of volume change for given pressure
- *Compliant lung*: Small pressure change for large volume change
- *Non-compliant lung*: Large pressure change for small volume change.

	Lung conditions
Decreased compliance	Pneumonia, Pulmonary edema, Pulmonary fibrosis
Increased compliance	Emphysema, Aging

117. All are seen in ARDS *except*:

a. PCWP more than 18 mm of Hg
b. Severe hypoxemia
c. Decreased pulmonary compliance
d. Pulmonary infiltrates

Ans. is 'a' PCWP more than 18 mm of Hg

COMPLICATIONS OF TB

Acute complications: Pneumothorax, Pleural effusion/empyema, Collapse, Tubulointerstitial nephritis.

Chronic complications: Bronchiectasis, Cor Pulmonale, Pulmonary fibrosis, Aspergilloma, Reactivation.

Brock syndrome: Right middle lobe collapse secondary to hilar node involvement; acute complication of pulmonary TB.

118. Brock syndrome is due to which lobe of lung?

a. Right middle lobe
b. Right lower lobe
c. Left upper lobe
d. Left lower lobe

Ans. is 'a' Right middle lobe

MANAGEMENT OF PULMONARY EDEMA

Reduction of preload	
Loop diuretics (Furosemide, Torasemide)	Drug of choice Effective in most forms of pulmonary edema
Nitrates	Venodilators, coronary vasodilation DOC for acute cardiogenic pulmonary edema
Morphine	Transient venodilator
Others	ACE Inhibitors, Nesiritide (Recombinant BNP)
Support of oxygen and ventilation	
Oxygen therapy	Goal is O_2 saturation ≥ 92%
Positive pressure ventilation	PPV by face / nasal mask / endotracheal intubation

119. Drug of choice for management of acute pulmonary edema is:

a. Furosemide
b. Hydrochorthiazide
c. Spironolactone
d. Triamterene

Ans. is 'a' Furosemide

INFECTIOUS DISEASES

HUMAN IMMUNODEFICIENCY VIRUS (HIV)

Enveloped RNA retrovirus (uses reverse transcriptase: RNA to dsDNA)

Genome

- Diploid genome (carries two copies of +ve stranded RNA)
- 3 structural genes
  - *env*
    - gp120–attachment to host CD4 + T cell; rapid mutation (antigenic variation)
    - gp41–fusion and entry into T-cells
  - *gag*: Capsid (p24) and matrix (p17) proteins
  - *pol*: Reverse transcriptase, Integrase, Protease enzymes.

Symptoms

- Initial infection asymptomatic 10–60%
- Acute HIV syndrome—2–4 weeks after exposure
  - Fever, myalgias, sore throat, cervical adenopathy, maculopapular rash.

Medicine

- Severe immunosuppression (AIDS)
  - Average time of 10 years from exposure
  - *Diagnosis*: CD4 ≤ 200 cells/mm³ or AIDS-defining illness
  - Opportunistic infections present.

Diagnosis

- Combination antigen/antibody immunoassays
  - Detect p24 Antigen capsid protein and IgG antibodies to HIV
  - Very high sensitivity/specificity
  - *Presumptive diagnosis*: If positive, HIV 1–2 antibody differentiation assay or nucleic acid tests for confirmation
  - Western blot tests no longer recommended for confirmatory testing.
- Viral load tests
  - High viral load associated with poor prognosis
  - Therapy monitoring; HIV genotyping to determine appropriate therapy
  - Used for diagnosis of perinatal HIV (as maternal antibodies persist for months).
- Window period
  - Time between exposure to HIV infection and the point when diagnostic immunoassays give accurate result
  - Patient can be infectious but still test HIV negative
  - Length of window period–22 days for western blot, 16 days for p24 antigen and 12 days for nucleic acid tests.

AIDS-defining illnesses

CD4 < 500/mm³	
HHV-8	Kaposi sarcoma
HPV	Squamous cell carcinoma (cervix, anus)
CD4 < 200/mm³	
Histoplasma capsulatum	Disseminated infection
HIV	Dementia
JC virus (reactivation)	Progressive Multifocal Leukoencephalopathy
Pneumocystis jiroveci	Pneumocystic pneumonia
CD4 < 100/mm³	
Aspergillus fumigatus	Invasive aspergillosis
Candida albicans	Esophagitis, bronchi, trachea, lungs
CMV	Retinitis, esophagitis, colitis, pneumonitis
Cryptococcus neoformans	Meningitis
Cryptosporidium/Isospora	Watery diarrhea
EBV	CNS lymphoma, Non-Hodgkin lymphoma
Mycobacterium avium-intracelluare	Disseminated infection
Toxoplasma	Brain abscesses

Others

- Reactivation of past infections (TB, HSV, shingles)
- Disseminated bacterial and fungal (coccidiodomycosis)
- Wasting syndrome attributed to HIV.

Prophylaxis for Opportunistic Infections

CD4 < 200/mm³	
Trimethoprim-Sulfamethoxazole	Pneumocystis pneumonia
CD < 100/mm³	
Trimethoprim-Sulfamethoxazole	Pneumocystis pneumonia and Toxoplasmosis
Itraconazole	Histoplasmosis (endemic areas)
CD < 50/mm³	
Azithromycin	Mycobacterium avium complex

Anti-HIV Drugs

NRTI (Nucleoside reverse transcriptase inhibitors)		
Didanosine Emtricitabine Lamivudine Stavudine Zidovudine	Competitively inhibit reverse transcriptase	Bone marrow suppression (Zidovudine), peripheral neuropathy, pancreatitis (Didanosine), lactic acidosis
NNRTI (Non-nucleoside reverse transcriptase inhibitors)		
Efavirenz Nevirapine	Inhibit reverse transcriptase (bind at different site than NRTIs)	Skin rash, hepatotoxicity
Protease Inhibitors		
Indinavir Rotinavir Lopinavir	Inhibits HIV protease, blocks production of structural proteins and enzymes	Hyperglycemia, renal stones (Indinavir), lipodystrophy
Integrase inhibitors		
Raltegravir	Inhibits HIV genome integration into host DNA	
Fusion inhibitors		
Enfuvirtide	Binds gp41	
Maraviroc	Binds CCR5 on T-cells/macrophages	

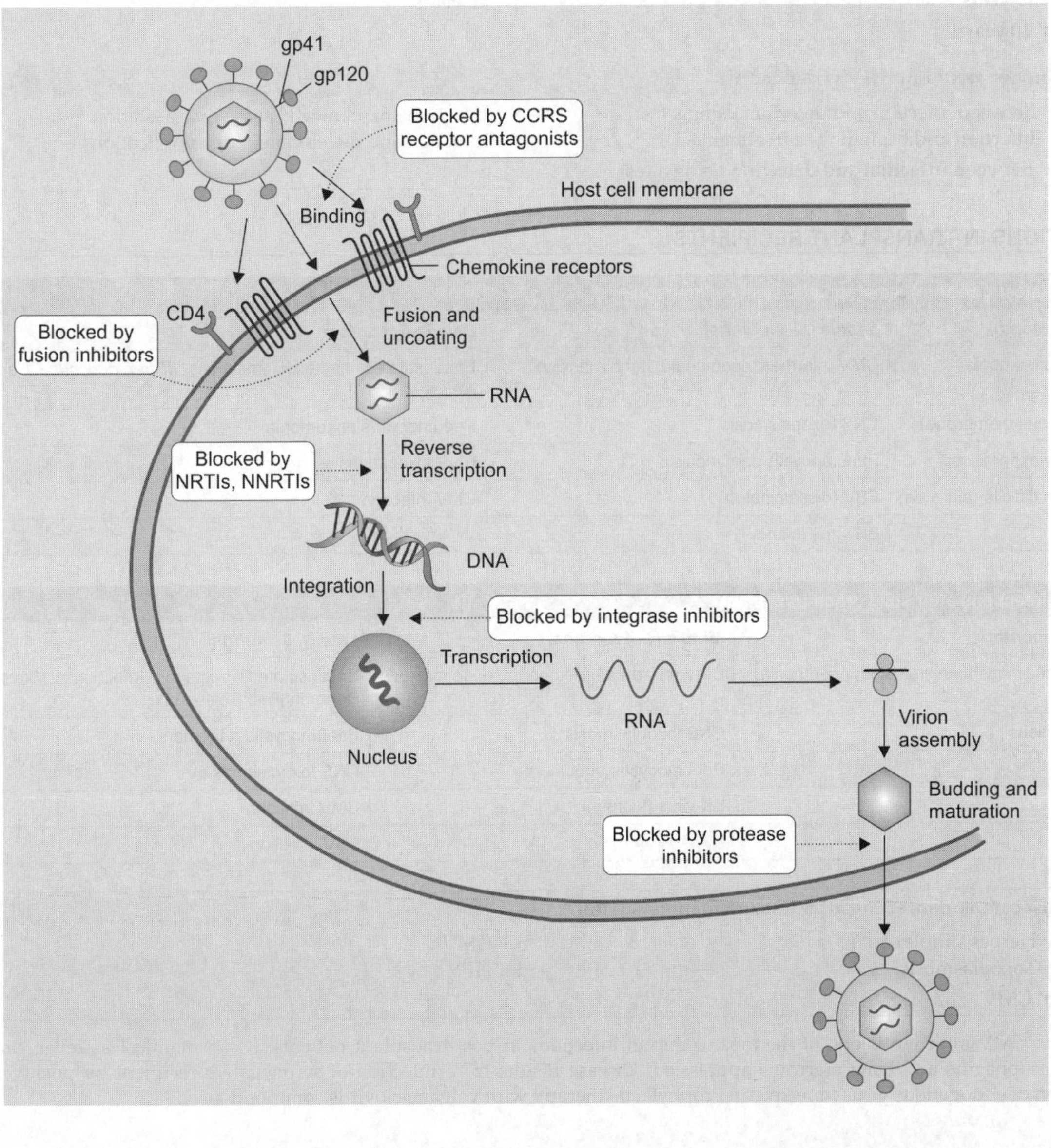

Anti-HBV Drugs in HIV Patients

- Lamivudine, emtricitabine, adefovir/tenofovir/entecavir and telbivudine alone or in combination
- These drugs also have activity against HIV—must not be used alone in HIV patients to avoid emergence of HIV resistance

Seven approved drugs for treatment of chronic hepatitis B

- *Injectables*: Interferon-alpha and pegylated interferon
- *Oral agents*: Lamivudine, adefovir, entecavir, telbivudine, tenofovir.

120. Which is not related to HIV? *(NEET 2019)*

a. Primary CNS lymphoma
b. Tertiary syphilis
c. Esophageal candidiasis
d. Cryptosporidiasis

Ans. is 'b' Tertiary syphilis

121. Antiviral drug used in both HIV and HBV infection is: *(NEET 2018)*

a. Abacavir
b. Emtricitabine
c. Stavudine
d. Enfuvirtide

Ans. is 'b' Emtricitabine

122. Mean time interval from HIV to AIDS manifestation is: *(NEET 2018)*

a. 7.5 years
b. 10 years
c. 15 years
d. 12 years

Ans. is 'b' 10 years

123. Window period for HIV is defined as: *(NEET 2018)*

a. Between infection and detection using a test
b. Infection and clinical disease manifestation
c. Infection and beginning of treatment
d. Infection and development of complications

Ans. is 'a' Between infection and detection using a test

INFECTIONS IN TRANSPLANT RECIPIENTS

Common infections after hematopoietic stem cell transplant		
Early (<1 month)	***Middle (1–4 months)***	***Late (> 6 months)***
Bacterial pneumonia	CMV (diarrhea, pneumonia, bone marrow)	Encapsulated bacterial infections (*Streptococcus*, *Haemophilus*, *Neisseria*)
HSV (mucous membrane)	CNS toxoplasmosis	Pneumocystis pneumonia
Pulmonary aspergillosis	Pneumocystis pneumonia	CNS toxoplasmosis
Costridium difficile (diarrhea)	EBV (disseminated)	CMV infection
	BK virus (kidney)	

Common infections after solid organ transplant		
Early (<1 month)	***Middle (1–4 months)***	***Late (> 6 months)***
Bacterial infections (disseminated, pneumonia)	CMV (diarrhea, pneumonia, bone marrow)	Encapsulated bacterial infections (Streptococcus, Haemophilus, Neisseria)
Graft infections	CNS toxoplasmosis	Pneumocystis pneumonia
	Pneumocystis pneumonia	CNS toxoplasmosis
	BK virus (kidney)	CMV infection
		EBV infection

124. Most common infection after transplantation is with: *(NEET 2018)*

a. Herpes simplex
b. CMV
c. Toxoplasmosis
d. HPV

Ans. is 'b' CMV

Explanation: CMV infection is one of the most common infections in post-transplant patients. It can manifest as fever, diarrhea, GI bleeding, esophagitis and bone marrow suppression. Disease results from infection of seronegative recipient by positive donor or reactivation of endogenous virus in recipient. Prophylactic therapy with valganciclovir is commonly used.

Drug of choice for prophylaxis	
Rheumatic fever	Benzathine penicillin
Tuberculosis	Isoniazid (alone or with Rifampicin)
Meningococcal meningitis	Rifampicin/ciprofloxacin
Gonorrhea/Syphilis	Procaine penicillin
Influenza	Oseltamivir
Surgical prophylaxis	Cefazolin
Diphtheria	Penicillin/Erythromycin
HSV	Acyclovir
Haemophilus influenza	Rifampicin
Pneumocystis	Cotrimoxazole
Toxoplasmosis	Cotrimoxazole
Recurrent cystitis	Nitrofurantoin/cotrimoxazole
Dental procedure in patients with cardiac disease (risk of endocarditis)	Amoxicillin/ampicillin
Recurrent Staph aureus skin infections	Mupirocin
Recurrent spontaneous bacterial peritonitis in cirrhotic patients	Fluoroquinolone
Recurrent pneumococcal meningitis with CSF leak or humoral immunodeficiency	Penicillin
High risk neutropenia (< 100/mm^3)	Levofloxacin/ciprofloxacin

125. For prophylaxis of meningococcal meningitis, drug used is: *(NEET 2018)*

a. Rifampicin
b. Tetracycline
c. Ceftriaxone
d. Azithromycin

Ans. is 'a' Rifampicin

GASTROENTEROLOGY

CELIAC DISEASE

The patient characeristics point to a diagnosis of celiac disease (the exact question might have had more clues)

The diagnostic approach is based on the risk for celiac disease and whether the patient is on a gluten-containing diet. All testing for celiac disease should ideally be performed while patients are on a gluten-containing diet.

Individuals with low celiac disease probability: The probability of celiac disease is low in individuals with one or more of the following clinical scenarios:

- Absence of suggestive signs or symptoms of malabsorption such as significant chronic diarrhea/steatorrhea or weight loss
- Absence of family history of celiac disease
- Chinese, Japanese, or Sub-Saharan African descent

Individuals at low risk for celiac disease should undergo serologic testing. Patients with positive serologic testing, should undergo an upper endoscopy with small bowel biopsy to diagnose celiac disease. The serum tissue transglutaminase (tTG)-IgA and endomysial (EMA)-IgA antibody tests have similar sensitivities. A negative result for either test in individuals at low-risk for celiac disease has a high negative predictive value and obviates the need for small bowel biopsy.

Individuals with high celiac disease probability: Both serologic testing and small bowel biopsy (regardless of celiac specific serology results) should be performed in individuals with a high probability of celiac disease **(Serology is always performed first)**

Individuals with a high celiac disease probability include:

- Individuals whose clinical presentation is highly suggestive for celiac disease such as chronic diarrhea/steatorrhea with weight loss
- Individuals with both risk factors that place them at moderate to high risk of celiac disease and consistent gastrointestinal or extraintestinal symptoms/signs of celiac disease.

Risk factors that place an individual at moderate to high risk for celiac disease include:

- First and second degree relative with confirmed celiac disease
- Type 1 diabetes
- Autoimmune thyroiditis
- Down and Turner syndromes
- Pulmonary hemosiderosis (moderate risk)

Serologic evaluation: Tissue transglutaminase (tTG)-IgA antibody is the single preferred test for detection of celiac disease in adults.

Histologic features: Histologic features of celiac disease in the small intestine range from a mild alteration characterized only by increased intraepithelial lymphocytes, to a severely atrophic mucosa with complete loss of villi, enhanced epithelial apoptosis, and crypt hyperplasia.

126. A 21-year-old female type 1 diabetic is unable to gain weight and average 6 episode of loose stool.Next investigation to diagnosis.? *(NEET 2020)*

a. Anti tissue transglutaminase antibody
b. Duodenal biopsy
c. ANCA antibodies
d. Schillings test

Ans. is 'a' Anti tissue transglutaminase antibody

ESOPHAGITIS

Reflux Esophagitis

- Inflammation of epithelial layer secondary to gastroesophageal reflux disease (GERD)
- Mucosal erythema and edema
- *Histology*: Basal zone hyperplasia, Eosinophils and neutrophils present
- *Feline esophagus*: Transient transverse bands seen in mid and lower esophagus on barium swallow (associated with GERD).

Infectious Esophagitis

- Seen in immunosuppressed patients
- In AIDS patients, infectious esophagitis (Candida, HSV, CMV) are seen at CD4 counts < 200/mm^3
- Most useful investigation—Endoscopy with biopsy
- Candida
    - Characteristic white plaques with friability
    - Pseudohyphae on biopsy
- Herpetic esophagitis (HSV-1)
    - Small, punched-out ulcerations
    - *Biopsy*: Ground glass nuclei, eosinophilic Cowdry's type A inclusion bodies and giant cells
- CMV esophagitis
    - Linear, serpiginous ulcers
    - Large nuclear or cytoplasmic inclusion bodies.

Eosinophilic Esophagitis

- Immune-mediated esophageal dysfunction
- Diagnosis of exclusion (must exclude other causes of esophagitis)
- *Ringed esophagus*: Permanent concentric ring-like strictures of the esophagus on barium swallow
- *Endoscopy*: Esophageal edema, multiple esophageal rings, longitudinal furrows
- *Biopsy*: Eosinophil-predominant inflammation.

127. Punched out ulcers in esophagus is seen in: *(NEET 2019)*

a. Herpes
b. CMV
c. Pill-esophagitis
d. Candida

Ans. is 'a' Herpes

128. Feline esophagus is seen in: *(NEET 2018)*

a. Eosinophilic esophagitis
b. Herpetic esophagitis
c. Reflux esophagitis
d. Radiation-induced esophagitis

Ans. is 'c' Reflux esophagitis

PEPTIC ULCER DISEASE

Location of PUD: Proximal duodenum (90%) > Pyloric antrum along lesser curvature (10%). Less commonly in prepyloric region and proximal stomach

Risk Factors

- *Helicobacter pylori*
- NSAIDs
- Smoking.

	Gastric ulcer	Duodenal ulcer
Pain	Greater with meals–weight loss	Decreases with meals–weight gain
H. pylori infection	70%	90%
Mechanism	Less mucosal protection against gastric acid	Less mucosal protection or More gastric acid secretion
Other causes	NSAIDs	Zollinger-Ellison syndrome
Risk of carcinoma	Higher	Benign
	Biopsy margins to rule out malignancy	Hypertrophy of Brunner glands

Ulcer Complications

- *Hemorrhage*: Most common complication
  - Ruptured gastric ulcer on lesser curvature—Left gastric artery bleed
  - Ruptured ulcer on posterior wall of duodenum—Gastroduodenal artery bleed
- Perforation
  - More common with anterior wall duodenal ulcers
  - Cause pneumoperitoneum
- Obstruction–Pyloric channel or duodenal ulcer.

129. Most common site of peptic ulcer is: *(NEET 2018)*

a. Upper part of lesser curvature
b. Lower part of lesser curvature
c. Pyloric antrum
d. Incisura angularis

Ans. is 'c' Pyloric antrum

UPPER GASTROINTESTINAL BLEEDING

Bleeding proximal to ligament of Treitz.

Presents with hematemesis, melena (black, tarry stool) [Vs hematochezia (bright red blood per rectum) in lower GI bleed]

Sources of upper GI bleed (in order of decreasing incidence)
Peptic ulcers (~ 50%)
Mallory-Weiss tears
Esophageal varices
Erosions in esophagus, stomach, duodenum
Neoplasms
Vascular ectasias (Hereditary hemorrhagic telangiectasias)

Evaluation and Management of UGI Bleed

- Risk assessment tools may be used for risk stratification
  - Rockall Scoring system–uses both clinical and endoscopic findings
  - Glasgow-Blatchford score–uses clinical and blood lab parameters
- Manage shock (if present)
- Upper GI endoscopy–performed within 24 hours
- Peptic ulcer
  - PPI infusion (IV pantoprazole) given
  - Endoscopic cauterization in case of active bleeding or visible vessel
  - Angiographic embolization of bleeding gastroduodenal/left gastric artery
  - Surgical ligation
- Esophageal varices
  - IV vasoactive drug (Octreotide)
  - Endoscopic ligation/banding
- Mallory-Weiss tears
  - Endoscopic cautery if active bleeding.

130. True about upper GI bleeding is: *(NEET 2018)*

a. Most common cause is variceal bleeding
b. It is bleeding up to ampulla of Vater
c. Most common management is endoscopic banding
d. Rockall scoring is used for risk stratification

Ans. is 'd' Rockall scoring is used for risk stratification

HELICOBACTER PYLORI

Gram negative rod; urease +ve.
Causes acute and chronic gastritis; Most common cause of chronic gastritis.
Mostly occurs in antrum of stomach.
Associated with MALT lymphoma and gastric adenocarcinoma.

Diagnosis

- Endoscopic biopsy
  - Stained with Silver stain
  - Rapid urease test +ve
- Urea breath test
  - Patient swallows C-13 labeled urea
  - Detection of isotope-labeled carbon dioxide in exhaled breath
  - Indicates urea was split (i.e. urease present)
- Stool antigen test.

Treatment

- Triple therapy for 7–10 days
  - Proton pump inhibitor
  - Clarithromycin
  - Amoxicillin/Metronidazole
- Testing often repeated to confirm eradication

131. Urea breath test is used for diagnosis of:

a. H. pylori
b. Campylobacter jejuni
c. E. coli
d. Lactobacillus

Ans. is 'a' H. pylori

INFLAMMATORY BOWEL DISEASE

Feature	Crohn disease	Ulcerative colitis
Macroscopic findings		
Bowel region	Ileum ± colon; rectal sparing	Colon only; starts in rectum
Distribution	Skip lesions; Cobblestone mucosa	Diffuse
Stricture	Early	Late/rare
Wall appearance	Thickened	Thin
Dilatation	No	Yes (Loss of haustra; lead pipe colon)
Microscopic findings		
Inflammation	Transmural, Creeping fat Aphthous ulcers–Earliest lesion	Limited to mucosa
Pseudopolyps	No to slight	Marked
Crypt abscesses	Yes	Yes
Ulcers/fissures	Deep, linear	Superficial
Lymphoid reaction	Marked	Mild
Fibrosis/Strictures	Marked	Mild
Non-caseating granulomas	Yes (50%)	No
Clinical findings		
Fistulae/sinuses	Yes	No
Fat/vitamin malabsorption	Yes	No
Malignant potential	Yes (only when colon involved)	Yes
Response to surgery	Poor	Good
Extra-intestinal manifestations	Erythema nodosum, Migratory polyarthritis, Uveitis Renal/Gallstones Ankylosing spondylitis Anti-Saccharomyces cerevisiae antibodies +ve	Pyoderma gangrenosum, Uveitis Primary Sclerosing Cholangitis Ankylosing spondylitis p-ANCA +ve
Smoking	Worsens outcome	Improves outcome

Ulcerative colitis: Disease presentation			
	Mild	*Moderate*	*Severe*
Bowel movements	<4 per day	4–6 per day	>6 per day
Blood in stool	Small	Moderate	Severe
Tachycardia	None	<90	>90
Sedimentation rate	<30 mm		>30 mm
Endoscopic appearance	Erythema, decreased vascular pattern, fine granularity	Marked erythema, absent vascular markings, coarse granularity	Spontaneous bleeding, ulcerations

Treatment

- *5-ASA (Mesalazine), Sulfasalazine:* Ulcerative colitis
- *Glucocorticoids*: Moderate/severe UC; Moderate/severe CD
- *Antibiotics (Metronidazole)*: Fistulizing CD
- *Azathioprine, 6-Mercaptopurine*: Concomitant with biological therapy
- *Methotrexate*: Concomitant with biological therapy
- *Cyclosporine*: Glucocorticoid-resistant severe UC
- *Tacrolimus*: Glucocorticoid-resistant UC/CD
- *Biologic Therapies*
  - Anti-TNF (Infliximab, Adalimumab, Certolizumab)–Moderate/severe CD/UC; Fistulizing CD
  - Anti-Integrins (Natalizumab, Vedolizumab, Ustekinumab)–Moderate/severe CD/UC.

132. Which of the following is used in steroid-resistant ulcerative colitis? *(NEET 2018)*

a. Cyclosporine b. Tacrolimus
c. Azathioprine d. None

Ans. is 'a' Cyclosporine > b' Tacrolimus

Explanation: Large clinical trials have proven efficacy of Cyclosporine although both Cyclosporine and Tacrolimus have indication for steroid-resistant UC.

133. Which of the following is not a feature of severe ulcerative colitis? *(NEET 2018)*

a. 4–6 bowel movements per day b. Pulse rate of 96 per minute
c. Spontaneous bleeding seen on endoscopy d. ESR 50 mm

Ans. is 'a' 4–6 bowel movements per day

134. Earliest feature of Crohn's disease is: *(NEET 2018)*

a. Aphthous ulcers b. Fissures
c. Perforation d. Granuloma

Ans. is 'a' Aphthous ulcers

VITAMIN K

Only fat soluble vitamin that acts as a coenzyme.

Function

- Activates clotting factors in liver
- Vitamin K dependent factors—II, VII, IX, X, Protein C, S
- Post-translational modification by vitamin K by carboxylation of glutamate residues (forming gamma-carboxyglutamate).

Sources

- Green leafy vegetables (K1 form or Phylloquinone)
- Synthesized by GI bacteria (K2 form or Menaquinone).

Causes of Vitamin K Deficiency

- Antibiotic therapy (eliminate normal intestinal flora)
- Warfarin (Vitamin K antagonists)
- Newborn babies (sterile GI tract at birth and insufficient Vitamin K in breast milk)
- Dietary deficiency rare because GI bacteria produce sufficient quantities.

Presentation

- Results in bleeding (coagulopathy)
- Deficiency of Vitamin K dependent factors
- Elevated PT/INR (due to short half-life of factor VII in Extrinsic pathway)
- Elevation in PTT is less sensitive
- Newborn infants with inadequate vitamin K stores may suffer from Hemorrhagic Disease of Newborn–so, babies given IM vitamin K at birth.

135. True about Vitamin K is: *(NEET 2018)*

a. Is a water soluble vitamin
b. Helps in synthesis of factor VIII
c. Prolonged antibiotic therapy for bacterial infection can cause vitamin K deficiency
d. Vitamin K deficiency leads to thrombosis

Ans. is 'c' Prolonged antibiotic therapy for bacterial infection can cause vitamin K deficiency

Serum-to-Ascites Albumin Gradient (SAAG)

- The serum-to-ascites albumin gradient (SAAG) identifies the presence of portal hypertension.
- The SAAG is calculated by subtracting the ascitic fluid albumin value from the serum albumin value.
- The presence of a gradient 1.1 g/dL (11 g/L) predicts that the patient has portal hypertension.
- A gradient <1.1 g/dL (g/dL) indicates that the patient does not have portal hypertension.
- The SAAG will be elevated with any disorder leading to portal hypertension and is not specific to ascites due to cirrhosis.

Classification of ascites by the serum-to-ascites albumin gradient	
High albumin gradient (SAAG ≥ 1.1 g/dL)	***Low albumin gradient (SAAG < 1.1 g/dL)***
• Cirrhosis • Alcoholic hepatitis • Heart failure • Massive hepatic metastases • Heart failure/constrictive pericarditis • Budd-Chiari syndrome • Portal vein thrombosis • Idiopathic portal fibrosis	• Peritoneal carcinomatosis • Peritoneal tuberculosis • Pancreatitis • Serositis • Nephrotic syndrome

136. Ascitic fluid SAAG<1.1; what is the disease associated with it?

a. Hepatic failure
b. Idiopathic portal fibrosis
c. Constrictive pericarditis
d. Peritoneal carcinomatosis

Ans. is 'd' Peritoneal carcinomatosis

LIVER CIRRHOSIS SCORING SYSTEMS

Modified Child-Pugh Classification

- Predictor of survival and likelihood of major complications of cirrhosis
- Score ranges from 5 to 15
  - 5–6—Child-Pugh Class A cirrhosis
  - 7–9—Child-Pugh Class B cirrhosis
  - 10–15—Child-Pugh Class C cirrhosis (worst prognosis)

Child-Pugh classification of cirrhosis			
Factor	***Points towards total score***		
	1	**2**	**3**
Serum bilirubin (mg/dL)	<2.0	2.0–3.0	>3.0
Serum albumin (g/dL)	>3.5	3.0–3.5	<3.0
Prothrombin time (INR)	<1.7	1.7–2.3	>2.3
Ascites	None	Easily controlled	Poorly controlled
Hepatic encephalopathy	None	Minimal	Advanced

Model for End-Stage Liver Disease (MELD) Score

- Scoring system for prioritization of patients awaiting liver transplantation
- Factors included
  - Serum bilirubin
  - Serum creatinine
  - Prothrombin time (INR)
  - Modified MELD - Serum sodium concentration is also included
- MELD is a more objective means of assessing disease severity than Child-Pugh score

Pediatric End-Stage Live Disease (PELD) Score

- Used to establish priority listing in children (<12 years)

137. MELD score includes: *(NEET 2019)*

a. Serum creatinine
b. Transaminase
c. Albumin
d. Alkaline phosphatase

Ans. is 'a' Serum creatinine

HEPATITIS

138. A 42-year-old patient presented with yellow coloured urine and clay coloured stools. His ALT= 100 IU/L, ALP = 1500 IU/L, increased GGT and serum haptoglobin levels. What is the likely diagnosis? *(NEET 2020)*

a. Hemolytic jaundice
b. Alcoholic hepatitis
c. Obstructive jaundice
d. Acute pancreatitis

Ans. is 'b' Alcoholic hepatitis

Explanation:

- Yellow urine + clay coloured stools are suggestive of conjugated hyperbilirubinemias
- Haemolytic jaundice is classically unconjugated so can be ruled out. Also serum haptoglobin levels are low in haemolytic jaundice
- Acute pancreatitis does not present with jaundice initially. It is an acute presentation with vomiting and abdominal pain. Diagnostic tests would be elevated serum amylase and lipase levels. Hence it is ruled out here
- Now our differentials are hepatitis vs. Obstructive jaundice:
- GGT is a classical marker of liver pathology. Elevated haptoglobin suggest inflammatory lesions (as it is an acute phase reactant). ALT and ALP both can be elevated in hepatic cause of jaundice. It can cause both unconjugated as well as conjugated hyperbilirubinemias. Hence the most probable answer here.

ENDOCRINOLOGY

PHEOCHROMOCYTOMA

An Addisonian crisis results from an acute lack of glucocorticoids or mineralocorticoids. This condition most often occurs in a patient with known adrenal insufficiency, either primary or secondary.

The salient feature of patients in acute adrenal crisis is circulatory collapse. They might have symptoms like nausea, vomiting, fever and lower chest/ abdominal pain along with the low blood pressure. They may appear cyanotic due to shock. Sometimes the patients are confused, delirious, or lethargic. Patients may have hyperpyrexia, with temperatures reaching 105°F or higher, and may be comatose. In acute adrenal hemorrhage, the patient can deteriorate with sudden collapse, abdominal or flank pain, and nausea with or without hyperpyrexia. Bilateral adrenalectomy for any reason can lead to addisonian crisis.

The surgical removal of a unilateral cortisol-producing adrenal adenoma in a patient with Cushing syndrome can cause an acute adrenal crisis from secondary adrenocortical insufficiency.

This is due to the atrophy of the normal adrenal cortex from lack of the stimulant effect of pituitary ACTH.

139. A patient who undervent bilateral adrenalectomy for pheochromocytoma presented with hypotension. The blood volume was normal. What is the diagnosis? *(NEET 2020)*

a. Cushing disease
b. Cardiogenic shock
c. Sepsis
d. Addisonian crisis

Ans. is 'd' Addisonian crisis

CONGENITAL ADRENAL HYPERPLASIA (CAH)

Autosomal recessive disorder caused by deficiency of enzymes in synthesis of steroid hormones in adrenal cortex.

Deficient enzymes can be

- 21-α hydroxylase–Most common cause
- 11-β hydroxylase
- 17-α hydroxylase
- 3-β hydroxysteroid dehydrogenase

Pathophysiology

- In all these enzyme deficiencies, there is reduced cortisol synthesis with loss of feedback inhibition on ACTH—Excessive ACTH causes hyperplasia of adrenals; hence the name Congenital adrenal hyperplasia
- Common precursor Pregnenolone (derived from cholesterol) is used for excessive production of mineralocorticoids (Aldosterone) and/or androgens according to the pathway not affected by deficient enzyme.

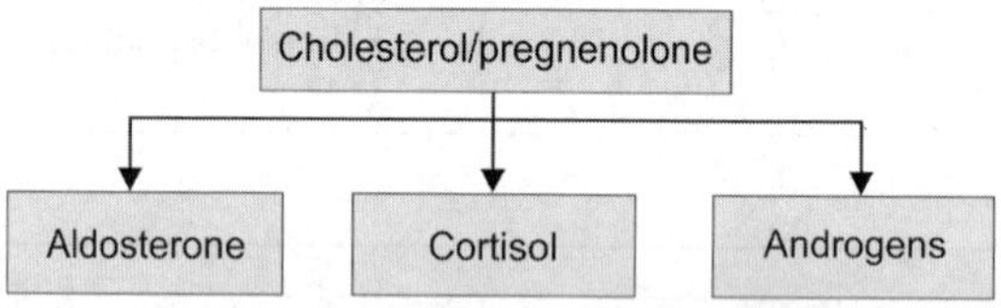

Presentations

1. *21-α hydroxylase*
   - Low cortisol–Hypoglycemia, hyperpigmentation (due to excess ACTH)
   - Low aldosterone–Hyponatremia, hypotension, hyperkalemia
   - Excess androgens–in girls (XX)–Female pseudohermaphroditism (ambiguous genitalia); in boys (XY)–Precocious puberty.
2. *11-β hydroxylase*
   - Low cortisol symptoms
   - Excess androgens symptoms
   - High mineralocorticoid activity due to excess 11-deoxycorticosterone (intermediate for aldosterone)–Hypertension, hypernatremia, hypokalemia.
3. *17-α hydroxylase*
   - Low cortisol symptoms
   - Excess mineralocorticoids
   - Low androgens–Male pseudohermaphroditism (feminization of male genitalia); female development normal.
4. *3-β hydroxysteroid dehydrogenase*
   - Low cortisol and mineralocorticoids
   - Excess androgens.

140. Most common outcome of congenital adrenal hyperplasia: *(NEET 2018)*

a. Male pseudohermaphroditism
b. Female pseudohermaphroditism
c. True hermaphroditism
d. Precocious puberty

Ans. is 'b' Female pseudohermaphroditism

BODY MASS INDEX (BMI)

Most widely used index to define obesity.
Also called Quetelet's index.
Calculated as body weight (in kg) divided by height squared (in meters).

Classification	BMI (kg/m²)	
	Global population	*Indian population*
Underweight	<18.5	<18.5
Normal	18.5–24.99	18.5–22.99
Overweight (Pre-obese)	25–29.99	23–44.99
Obesity	≥30	≥25

Lethal BMI—Lowest BMI compatible with life is 13 in males and 11 in females.

141. Lethal BMI for adult males is: *(NEET 2018)*

a. 11
b. 13
c. 15
d. 17

Ans. is 'b' 13

METABOLIC SYNDROME

ATP III criteria define metabolic syndrome as the presence of any **three** of the following five traits:

1. Abdominal obesity, defined as a waist circumference ≥102 cm (40 in) in men and ≥88 cm (35 in) in women
2. Serum triglycerides ≥ 150 mg/dL (1.7 mmol/L) or drug treatment for elevated triglycerides
3. Serum high-density lipoprotein (HDL) cholesterol <40 mg/dL (1 mmol/L) in men and <50 mg/dL (1.3 mmol/L) in women or drug treatment for low HDL cholesterol
4. Blood pressure ≥ 130/85 mm Hg or drug treatment for elevated blood pressure
5. Fasting plasma glucose (FPG) ≥ 100 mg/dL (5.6 mmol/L) or drug treatment for elevated blood glucose.

142. As per NECP-ATP-III, which is not included in metabolic syndrome? *(NEET 2020)*

a. Hypertriglyceridemia
b. Hypertension
c. Central obesity
d. High LDL

Ans. is 'd' High LDL

CYSTINURIA

- Autosomal recessive disorder
- Defective reabsorption of Cystine and dibasic amino acids (Ornithine, Lysine, Arginine) in proximal renal tubule and small intestine
- Thus, four amino acids excreted in urine
  - Cystine
  - Ornithine
  - Lysine
  - Arginine
- Presents with recurrent cystine renal stones.

143. In cystinuria, none of the following amino acid is reabsorbed, *except*: *(NEET 2018)*

a. Lysine
b. Arginine
c. Citrulline
d. Ornithine

Ans. is 'c' Citrulline

CARCINOID SYNDROME

- Carcinoid tumors are Neuroendocrine tumors
- Produce a variety of polypeptides, prostaglandins and biogenic amines
- *Most important are*: Serotonin, histamine, kallikrein and prostaglandins
- *Various locations*: GI tract, lungs, pancreas.

Carcinoid Syndrome: Symptoms secondary to high serotonin levels in systemic circulation.

Pathophysiology: Altered tryptophan metabolism

- Normally only 1% of tryptophan is metabolized into serotonin
- Upto 70% tryptophan is converted into serotonin in carcinoid syndrome patients
- Results in tryptophan deficiency–symptoms of niacin deficiency (tryptophan is a source of niacin)–Pellagra-like symptoms
- Serotonin is metabolized to **5-Hydroxyindoleacetic acid (5-HIAA)–Raised urinary levels**
- More common with midgut carcinoids (as compared to foregut and hindgut carcinoids)
- No carcinoid syndrome in absence of liver metastases (liver and lungs inactivate serotonin).

Symptoms

- Diarrhea (serotonin stimulates GI motility)
- *Carcinoid heart disease*: Fibrous deposits in tricuspid/pulmonary valves (Left heart disease rare due to inactivation of serotonin by lungs)
- *Flushing*: Not due to serotonin; other mediators like histamine and kallikreins.

Treatment

- Octreotide–Somatostatin analog
- Surgical excision of tumor.

144. Increases 5-hydroxyindoleacetic acid (5-HIAA) in urine is seen in: *(NEET 2018)*

a. Cushing's syndrome
b. Pheochromocytoma
c. Acromegaly
d. Carcinoid syndrome

Ans. is 'd' Carcinoid syndrome

MYXEDEMA COMA

It is the end stage of untreated or inadequately treated hypothyroidism. The clinical picture is often that of an elderly obese female, presenting in midwinter with increased lethargy, somnolence, and confusion. Myxedema coma is most frequently associated with discontinuation of thyroid hormone therapy. It presents less frequently as the first manifestation of hypothyroidism. It may be precipitated by an illness such as a cerebrovascular accident, myocardial infarction, or an infection such as a urinary tract infection or pneumonia. Other precipitating factors include gastrointestinal hemorrhage; acute trauma; excessive hydration; or administration of a sedative, narcotic, or potent diuretic drug.

Diagnosis

The physical findings are not specific. The patient may be semicomatose or comatose with dry, coarse skin, hoarse voice, thin scalp and eyebrow hair, possibly a scar on the neck, and slow reflex relaxation time. There is marked hypothermia, with body temperature sometimes falling to as low as 24°C (75°F), particularly in the winter months. It is important to be alert to the presence of complicating factors such as pneumonia, urinary tract infection, ileus, anemia, hypoglycemia, or seizures. Often there are pericardial, pleural, or peritoneal effusions. Hypoventilation leads to hypoxia and hypercapnea. The key laboratory tests are a low free thyroxine (FT4) and elevated thyroid-stimulating hormone (TSH). It is essential to check blood gases, electrolytes, creatinine, and an electrocardiogram in evaluating pulmonary, renal, cardiac, and central nervous system status. Myxedema may cause prolongation of the Q-T interval leading to torsade de pointes.

Management

1. Admit to ICU for ventilatory support and for intravenous medications.
2. Parenteral thyroxine: Give a loading dose of 300–400 μg IV, then 50–100 μg IV daily. (May also give liothyronine sodium, 10 μg IV every 8 h for the first 48 h if necessary. Nasogastric route can also be used.)
3. *Electrolytes*: Water restriction for hyponatremia. Avoid fluid overload.
4. *Limit sedation*: Appropriate reduction in drug dosage.
5. *Glucocorticoids*: Controversial but necessary in hypopituitarism or polyglandular failure. Dosage: Hydrocortisone sodium phosphate or sodium succinate, 50–100 mg every 6 h initially and tapered downward over 1 wk. (If initial serum cortisol was >30 μg/dL, corticosteroids are unnecessary.)
6. *Hypothermia*: Do not externally rewarm.

145. Which of the following is not a feature of myxedema coma?

a. Reduced level of consciousness and seizures with other features of hypothyroidism is seen
b. Hypoventilation leading to hypoxia and hypercapnea play a major role
c. Levothyroxine can be given via intravenous and nasogastric route
d. Levothyronine should not be used in the management

Ans. is 'd' Levothyroxine should not be used in the management

GLUCOSE TOLERANCE TEST

Oral glucose tolerance testing

Time	*75- g glucose*		*Interpretation*
Fasting	<110 mg/dL	<6.1 mmol/L	Normal
	110–125 mg/dL	6.1–7.0 mmol/L	Impaired fasting glucose
	126 mg/dL	>7.0 mmol/L	Diabetes
1 hour	180 mg/dL	10.0 mmol/L	Normal
2 hours	<140 mg/dL	<7.8 mmol/L	Normal
	140–200 mg/dL	7.8–11.1 mmol/L	Impaired glucose tolerance
	>200 mg/dL	>11.1 mmol/L	Diabetes

146. Patient presents with fasting plasma glucose level of 124 mg/dL and 2 hour post-prandial levels of 180 mg/dL. Which of the following is the patient diagnosis?

a. Normal glucose tolerance
b. Impaired glucose tolerance or prediabetes
c. Diabetes mellitus
d. Diabetic ketoacidosis

Ans. is 'b' Impaired glucose tolerance or prediabetes

Multiple endocrine neoplasia (MEN) syndromes			
	Men 1 (Werner syndrome)	*Men 2A (Sipple syndrome)*	*Men 2B*
Pituitary	Adenomas, hyperplasia	–	–
Parathyroid	Hyperplasia, adenomas	Hyperplasia or adenoma	–
Pancreatic islets	Hyperplasia adenomas carcinomas	–	–
Adrenal	Cortical hyperplasia	Pheochromocytoma	Pheochromocytoma
Thyroid	–	C-cell hyperplasia, medullary carcinoma	C-cell hyperplasia medullary carcinoma
Extraendocrine changes	Foregut carcinoid subcutaneous or visceral dermal angiofibroma orcollagenoma	Cutaneous lichen, Amyloidosis Hirschsprung disease	Mucosal and gastrointestinal neuroma, ganglio-neuromas, marfanoid habitus
Mutant gene locus	MEN1	RET	RET

147. Which of the following are the extraintestinal manifestations of Sipple syndrome?

a. Cutaneous lichen
b. Amyloidosis
c. Hirschsprung disease
d. All the above

Ans. is 'd' All the above

TREATMENT OF HYPERKALEMIA

It is divided into three stages:

1. Immediate antagonism of the cardiac effects of hyperkalemia- Intravenous calcium serves to protect the heart, whereas other measures are taken to correct hyperkalemia. Calcium raises the action potential threshold and reduces excitability, without changing the resting membrane potential. By restoring the difference between resting and threshold potentials, calcium reverses the depolarization blockade due to hyperkalemia. The recommended dose is 10 mL of 10% calcium gluconate (3–4 mL of calcium chloride), infused intravenously over 2–3 min with cardiac monitoring.
2. Rapid reduction in plasma K^+ concentration by redistribution into cells- Insulin lowers plasma K^+ concentration by shifting K^+ into cells. The recommended dose is 10 units of intravenous regular insulin followed immediately by 50 mL of 50% dextrose (D50W, 25 g of glucose total).

   β2-agonists, most commonly albuterol, are effective but underused agents for the acute management of hyperkalemia. The recommended dose for inhaled albuterol is 10–20 mg of nebulized albuterol in 4 mL of normal saline, inhaled over 10 min.

   Intravenous bicarbonate has no role in the acute treatment of hyperkalemia, but may slowly attenuate hyperkalemia with sustained administration over several hours.
3. *Removal of potassium*: This is typically accomplished using cation exchange resins, diuretics, and/or dialysis. The cation exchange resin sodium polystyrene sulfonate (SPS) exchanges Na^+ for K^+ in the gastrointestinal tract and increases the fecal excretion of K^+; alternative calcium-based resins, when available, may be more appropriate in patients with an increased ECFV. Whenever possible, alternative therapies for the acute management of hyperkalemia (i.e., aggressive redistributive therapy, isotonic bicarbonate infusion, diuretics, and/or hemodialysis) should be used instead of SPS.

148. Which of the following is not true about treatment of severe hyperkalemia?

a. Calcium gluconate causes transcellular shift of potassium
b. Calcium gluconate onset of action is within 5 mins of administration
c. Calcium gluconate is the fastest acting agent
d. Most effective and rapid way of lowering potassium is by hemodialysis

Ans. is 'a' Calcium gluconate causes transcellular shift of potassium

EMERGENCY MEDICINE

PNEUMOPERITONEUM

Pneumoperitoneum describes gas within the peritoneal cavity.

Causes

1. Perforated hollow viscus (Most common)
   a. Peptic ulcer disease, ischemic bowel, bowel obstruction, necrotizing enterocolitis, appendicitis, diverticulitis, malignancy, inflammatory bowel disease.
   b. Mechanical perforation: trauma, colonoscopy, foreign bodies, iatrogenic.
2. Postoperative free intraperitoneal gas.
3. Peritoneal dialysis.
4. Vaginal "aspiration": cunnilingus, douching, sudden squatting,
6. Mechanical ventilation.
7. Pneumomediastinum, Pneumothorax.

Radiographic Features

An erect chest X-ray—most sensitive plain radiograph for the detecton of free intraperitoneal gas and shows subdiaphragmatic free gas.

a. Bowel related signs.
   - Double wall sign (Rigler's or bas-relief sign): Air on either side of intestinal wall
   - Telltale triangle sign.

b. Peritoneal ligament related signs
   - Football sign: large oval radiolucency due to massive pneumoperitoneum.
   - Silver sign: visualization of falciform ligament
   - Lateral umbilical ligament sign (also known as inverted V sign)
   - Urachus sign

c. Right upper quadrant signs.
   - Lucent liver sign.
   - Hepatic edge sign.
   - Fissure for ligamentum teres sign.
   - Morison's pouch sign (doge cap sign).
   - Cupola sign.

Management

- In presence of peritoneal signs/shock–Exploratory laparotomy
- Broad-spectrum antibiotics (signs of sepsis)
- Benign causes usually do not require any treatment

149. A patient came in the emergency with severe abdominal pain, pulse 112/min and systolic BP 80 mm Hg. Chest X-ray is shown. What will be the next appropriate step? *(NEET 2019)*

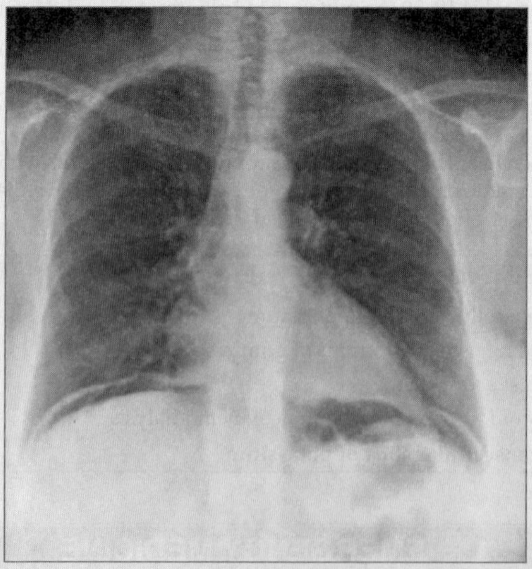

a. Exploratory laparotomy
b. Saline wash of stomach
c. Intercostal tube drainage
d. None

Ans. is 'a' Exploratory laparotomy

Medicine

MANAGEMENT OF ACUTE PANCREATITIS

- Aggressive fluid resuscitation with **isotonic crystalloid solution** (Ringer's Lactate and Normal saline)–to maintain BP and renal perfusion
- Nil per oral with nasogastric decompression to give rest to pancreas. However, enteral nutrition should be commenced after initial fluid resuscitation and within first 24 hours of admission
- *Analgesics*: NSAID (Metamizole) for mild pain; Opioid (Buprenorphine) for severe pain
  - Morphine is avoided due to its propensity to cause sphincter of Oddi spasm
- Prophylactic antibiotics are not recommended. Cephalosporins are preffered in established infection
- Therapeutic ERCP is not recommended, unless presence of concomitant cholangitis
- *Laparoscopic cholecystectomy*: In case of gallstone pancreatitis (except severe cases and old patients)
- Operative treatment in cases of
  - Phlegmon of pancreas
  - *Infected collection*: Percutaneous drainage done
  - Perforation
  - Hemorrhage/ischemia.

150. In a case of acute pancreatitis with shock, initial management is: *(NEET 2018)*

a. Central line and isotonic crystalloid solution
b. Wide bore peripheral line and hypertonic colloid solution
c. Urgent laparotomy
d. ERCP

Ans. is 'a' Central line and isotonic crystalloid solution

CHAPTER 13 Surgery

BREAST

FIBROADENOMA

Fibroadenoma is the **most common benign growth** in the breast and usually occurs in **women of a reproductive age**. They are proliferations of **stromal and epithelial tissue** of the duct lobules.

On examination, they are **highly mobile** lesions (historically termed a "breast mouse") that are **well-defined and rubbery** on palpation, with most less than 5 cm in diameter. They can be **multiple** and **bilateral**.

Phyllodes Tumours

Phyllodes tumours* are **rare fibroepithelial tumours**. Phyllodes tumours are commonly larger, occur in an **older age group**, and are comprised of **both epithelial and stromal tissue**. They often grow rapidly.

They are difficult to clinically and microscopically differentiate from fibroadenomas, however around one third of Phyllodes tumours have **malignant potential** and 10% of benign tumours will recur after excision. Consequently, most Phyllodes tumours should be **widely excised** (or mastectomy if the lesion is large).

Breast Abscess

A breast abscess is a collection of pus within the breast lined with granulation tissue, most commonly developing from acute mastitis.

They present with tender fluctuant and erythematous masses, with a puncutum potentially present. Associated systemic symptoms include fever and lethargy. A suspected abscess can be confirmed via an ultrasound scan if there is any doubt regarding the diagnosis.

The initial phase is often fully reversible with prompt empirical antibiotics and US-guided needle therapeutic aspiration. More advanced abscesses may require incision and drainage under a local anaesthetic.

Breast Cancer

Patients can present **symptomatically** or **asymptomatically via screening**.

Clinical features may include **breast lump(s)**, **asymmetry**, or **swelling** (all or part of breast), **abnormal nipple discharge**, **nipple retraction**, **skin changes** (dimpling/Peau d' Orange, or Paget's-like changes), **mastalgia**, or with a **palpable lump in the axilla**.

1. A 30-year-old female presented with asymptomatic lump in the upper outer quadrant of right breast. On examination, the size of breast was normal, the lump was nontender and freely mobile. What is the diagnosis? *(NEET 2020)*

a. Phyllodes tumor
b. Breast abscess
c. Fibroadenoma
d. CA breast

Ans. is 'c' Fibroadenoma

VAN NUYS PROGNOSTIC INDEX FOR DCIS

VNPI scoring system	1	2	3
Tumor size (diameter in mm)	Less or equal to 15	16–40	Greater or equal to 41
Margin width (in mm)	More than or equal to 10	1–9	< 1
Pathologic Classification	Non-high grade, (nuclear grades 1 and 2) no necrosis	Non-high grade, (nuclear grades 1 and 2) with necrosis	High grade (nuclear grade 3) with or without necrosis
Age (years)	>60	40–60	<40

	Treatment recommendation
Low score (4–6)	Wide Local Excision (WLE)
Intermediate (7–9)	WLE + Radiotherapy
High (10–12)	Mastectomy

2. Van Nuys classification of DCIS includes all *except*:

a. Grade
b. Size
c. Microinvasion
d. Receptors

Ans. is 'd' Receptors

BREAST CARCINOMA STAGING (AJCC, 8TH EDITION)

Primary Tumor (T)

TX	Primary tumor cannot be assessed
T0	No evidence of primary tumor
Tis	Carcinoma in situ
T1	Tumor ≤ 20 mm in greatest dimension
T1mi	Tumor ≤ 1 mm in greatest dimension
T1a	Tumor > 1 mm but ≤ 5 mm in greatest dimension (round any measurement >1.0-1.9 mm to 2 mm)
T1b	Tumor > 5 mm but ≤ 10 mm in greatest dimension
T1c	Tumor > 10 mm but ≤ 20 mm in greatest dimension
T2	Tumor > 20 mm but ≤ 50 mm in greatest dimension
T3	Tumor > 50 mm in greatest dimension
T4	Tumor of any size with direct extension to the chest wall and/or to the skin (ulceration or skin nodules), not including invasion of dermis alone
T4a	Extension to chest wall, not including only pectoralis muscle adherence/invasion
T4b	Ulceration and/or ipsilateral satellite nodules and/or edema (including peau d'orange) of the skin, which do not meet the criteria for inflammatory carcinoma
T4c	Both T4a and T4b
T4d	Inflammatory carcinoma

Lymph Nodes (N)

cNx	Regional lymph nodes cannot be assessed (e.g, previously removed)
cN0	No regional lymph node metastasis (on imaging or clinical examination)
cN1	Metastasis to movable ipsilateral level I, II axillary lymph node(s)
cN1mi	Micrometastases (approximately 200 cells, larger than 0.2 mm, but none larger than 2.0 mm)
cN2	Metastases in ipsilateral level I, II axillary lymph nodes that are clinically fixed or matted; *or* in ipsilateral internal mammary nodes in the absence of clinically evident axillary lymph node metastases
cN2a	Metastases in ipsilateral level I, II axillary lymph nodes fixed to one another (matted) or to other structures
cN2b	Metastases only in ipsilateral internal mammary nodes and in the absence of axillary lymph node metastases
cN3	Metastases in ipsilateral infraclavicular (level III axillary) lymph node(s), with or without level I, II axillary node involvement, *or* in ipsilateral internal mammary lymph node(s) with level I, II axillary lymph node metastasis; *or* metastases in ipsilateral supraclavicular lymph node(s), with or without axillary or internal mammary lymph node involvement
cN3a	Metastasis in ipsilateral infraclavicular lymph node(s)
cN3b	Metastasis in ipsilateral internal mammary lymph node(s) and axillary lymph node(s)
cN3c	Metastasis in ipsilateral supraclavicular lymph node(s)

Distant Metastases (M)

M0	No clinical or radiographic evidence of distant metastasis
cM0 (i+)	No clinical or radiographic evidence of distant metastases in the presence of tumor cells or deposits no larger than 0.2 mm detected microscopically or by molecular techniques in circulating blood, bone marrow, or other nonregional nodal tissue in a patient without symptoms or signs of metastases
cM1	Distant metastases detected by clinical and radiographic means

AJCC Anatomic Stage Groups

When T is...	And N is...	And M is ...	Then the stage group is ...
Tis	N0	M0	**0**
T1	N0	M0	**IA**
T0	N1 mi	M0	**IB**
T1	N1 mi	M0	**IB**
T0	N1	M0	**IIA**

Contd...

Surgery

Contd...

When T is...	And N is...	And M is ...	Then the stage group is ...
T1	N1	M0	IIA
T2	N0	M0	IIA
T2	N1	M0	IIB
T3	N0	M0	IIB
T0	N2	M0	IIIA
T1	N2	M0	IIIA
T2	N2	M0	IIIA
T3	N1	M0	IIIA
T3	N2	M0	IIIA
T4	N0	M0	IIIIB
T4	N1	M0	IIIIB
T4	N2	M0	IIIB
Any T	N3	M0	IIIC
Any T	Any N	M1	IV

3. A 52-year-old female patient present with 4 cm diameter diagnosed breast cancer lesion with ipsilateral axillary and contralateral supraclavicular lymphadenopathy. As per AJCC system, patient belongs to which stage of breast cancer?

a. IIIa
b. IIIb
c. IIIc
d. IV

Ans. is 'd' IV

Explanation: Metastasis to contralateral supraclavicular lymph node is classified as distant metastasis. Metastasis to ipsilateral supraclavicular lymph nodes is classified as N3C.

TREATMENT OF BREAST CANCER

Surgery

Breast conservation surgery or wide local excision is preferred over mastectomy in early breast cancers, as long as adequate negative resection margins can be achieved.

Adjuvant Chemotherapy

- Indicated in all patients of Invasive ductal carcinoma.
- Chemotherapy may be avoided in some selected patients with favorable tumors <1 cm in size and based on recurrence genetic signatures like Oncotype DX, MammaPrint etc.

Adjuvant Radiotherapy

For most women treated with breast-conserving surgery, whole breast radiation therapy (WBRT) is recommended. There are a few possible exceptions to this approach, e.g. women ≥65 years old with node-negative, hormone receptor-positive primary tumors up to 3 cm for whom endocrine therapy is planned, RT may reasonably be excluded.

Adjuvant Hormonal Therapy

5 years of Tamoxifen/Aromatase inhibitors (if post-menopausal) is indicated in patient with ER/PR positive tumors.

Management of Axillary Lymph Nodes in Ca Breast

- Sentinel lymph node biopsy is considered the standard for evaluation of the axillary lymph nodes for metastasis in women who have clinically negative lymph nodes (the sentinel lymph node is the first regional lymph node to receive tumor cells that metastasize along the lymphatic pathway from the primary breast cancer).
- Axillary lymph node dissection (ALND) is performed for clinically palpable axillary lymph nodes or metastatic disease detected in sentinel lymph node biopsy
- Sentinel lymph node biopsy is done using the dual tracer method, combining blue dye with either radioactive colloid or fluorescent dye. Radioactive Tc 99m sulphur colloid is injected below the nipple areola complex in the morning on the day of the surgery. Further, methylene blue dye is injected into peritumoral and subareolar regions just before the surgical incision is given. If fluorescent dye is used, it is injected below the nipple areola complex just before the incision is given. Sentinel nodes are identified intraoperatively by their blue color, fluorescence, or high radioactivity detected on gamma probe.

Poor Prognostic Factors in Ca Breast: Advanced Tumor staging, High histologic Grade, Negative for Estrogen receptor [ER] and Progesterone receptor [PR], Positive for Human Epidermal Growth Factor Receptor-2 [Her-2-neu], Presence of breast cancer cells in circulation or bone marrow, High Ki-67 index, Scirrhous histological type of breast cancer.

Breast Reconstruction

- ❖ The easiest type of reconstruction is using a silicone gel implant under the pectoralis major muscle.
- ❖ Commonly used **flaps in breast reconstruct on** include:
  - **TRAM flap: Transverse rectus abdominis muscle**
  - LD FLAP: Latissimus dorsi flap
  - DIEP: Deep inferior epigastric perforator flap
  - SEIA: Superficial inferior epigastric artery perforator flap
- ❖ If a patient is likely to need postoperative radiotherapy then a delayed reconstruction using a flap often gives a better result. Radiotherapy onto a prosthesis often leads to a high incidence of capsular contracture and unacceptable results.
- ❖ Nipple reconstruction is a relatively simple procedure that can be performed under a local anesthetic.

4. Best prognosis for carcinoma breast is seen with which of the following?

a. <1 cm size, nodes –ve, ER/PR +ve, her 2/neu –ve
b. <1 cm size, nodes –ve, ER/PR –ve, her 2/neu +ve
c. <2 cm size, nodes –ve, ER/PR +ve, her 2/neu –ve
d. <2 cm size, nodes –ve, ER/PR –ve, her 2/neu +ve

Ans. is 'a' <1 cm size, nodes –ve, ER/PR +ve, her 2/neu –ve

5. Among the following the primary indication of sentinel lymph node biopsy:

a. Metastasis
b. Breast lump with palpable axillary lymph node
c. Breast lump without palpable axillary lymph node
d. None

Ans. is 'c' Breast lump without palpable axillary lymph node

6. Which of the following is true about breast reconstruction surgery?

a. Easiest reconstruction is done using silicon gel implant
b. TRAM flap gives better cosmetic results then LD flap
c. Radiotherapy in postoperative does not influence the outcome after breast reconstruction
d. Nipple reconstruction cannot be performed under local anesthesia

Ans. is 'a' Easiest reconstruction is done using silicon gel implant

The serratus anterior muscle takes origin from the lateral scapula. Only a portion of the muscle is used for flap reconstruction: the lower three slips of muscle arise at the very inferior scapula and have an independent blood and nerve supply, making them a good source of a medium to small sized muscle for free flap coverage. The vascular anatomy of the serratus is related to the latissimus and axillary vessels, familiar territory for the reconstructive surgeon. **The subscapular artery, a branch of the third part of the axillary artery, descends inferiorly to supply the serratus artery**. Before branching into the serratus it gives off a circumflex scapular branch and the thoracodorsal artery.

Free transverse rectus abdominis myocutaneous flaps: The free TRAM flap gets its blood supply from below, from the **deep inferior epigastric vessels.** This requires the division and microsurgical reanastomosis of these vessels.

The latissimus muscle blood supply is via the **subscapular artery, a branch of the axillary artery**. The subscapular sends off a circumflex scapular branch posteriorly and then distributes a serratus branch before it enters the substance of the muscle on its undersurface. On the subscapular system a 5 to 15 centimeter pedicle can be obtained

7. What is the anatomical basis of the flap of anterior abdominal wall used for reconstruction after breast surgery? *(NEET 2020)*

a. Serratus anterior flap based on superior epigastric artery
b. Transverses abdominis flap based on deep inferior epigastric artery
c. Transversus abdominis flap based on superficial epigastric artery
d. Latissimus dorsi flap based inferior epigastric artery

Ans. is 'b' Transverses abdominis flap based on deep inferior epigastric artery

THYROID AND PARATHYROID

RETROSTERNAL GOITER

Radiologic testing: Substernal goiters are often seen on chest radiograph as a mass that causes tracheal narrowing or deviation or as superior mediastinal widening. Past radiographs, if available, permit an estimate of the rate of growth of the goiter, and neck radiographs may show narrowing of the airway. However, the extent of the goiter and its effect upon surrounding structures should be assessed by CT or MRI. CT is very useful for evaluating the extent of both large cervical goiters and substernal goiters.

Asymptomatic substernal goiter: The main treatment options for patients with asymptomatic substernal goiter are surgery or observation with monitoring. The choice of therapy depends upon the extent of substernal extension and patient characteristics.

Surgery is advised for most patients with asymptomatic substernal goiters that extend below the level of the brachiocephalic vein, if they are good surgical candidates

The majority of obstructive and substernal goiters can be excised through a standard cervical incision, while partial or complete sternotomy or even thoracotomy may be required in patients with previous cervical thyroidectomy, very large substernal goiters, or invasive cancer. In a major study only 6.5 percent required sternotomy

The vast majority of **retrosternal goiter** are secondary, which originate from the downward extension of the gland along the planes of the cervical and mediastinal fascia. The **blood supply** arises principally from the inferior thyroid arteries and most of the venous return is through the inferior thyroid veins.

8. Which of the following statements is true regarding retrosternal goitres? *(NEET 2020)*

a. Operated only if patient is symptomatic
b. Almost always operated by a midline sternotomy
c. Majority of the goitres derive their blood supply from mediastinal vessels
d. CT/MRI has to be done routinely in all patients

Ans. is 'd' CT/MRI has to be done routinely in all patients

MEDULLARY CARCINOMA OF THYROID

- Are neuroendocrine neoplasms derived from the calcitonin secreting parafollicular cells (C cells) of thyroid
- Account for approximately 5% of thyroid neoplasms
- Most MTCs (75–80%) arise sporadically. The remainder (20–25%) occurs in the setting of MEN syndromes 2A or 2B or as familial tumors without an associated MEN syndrome.
- Bilaterality, young age of presentation and multicentricity is common in familial cases.
- The familial cases are also associated with C-cell hyperplasia, which is considered premalignant lesion of MTC.
- RET proto-oncogenes play an important role in the development of both familial and sporadic MTCs.
- Associated with palpable cervical lymphadenopathy (early spread to lymphatics is common)
- Tumor cells secrete calcitonin, the measurement of which plays an important role in the diagnosis and postoperative follow-up of patients. In some instances the tumor cells elaborate other polypeptide hormones, such as serotonin, ACTH, and vasoactive intestinal peptide (VIP).
- Diarrhea is a feature in 30% of cases due to 5-hydroxytryptamine or prostaglandins produced by the tumor cells.
- Distal blood-borne metastasis to the liver, bone (frequently osteoblastic), and lung occur late in the disease
- Diagnosis is established by:
  - FNAC-presence of amyloid stroma is diagnostic
  - Raised serum calcitonin and CEA levels (Calcitonin is a more sensitive tumor marker, but CEA is a predictor of prognosis)
- All new patients with MTC should be screened for:
  - RET point mutations
  - Pheochromocytoma (24 hr urinary levels of VMA, catecholamine and metanephrine)
  - Hyperparathyroidism (serum calcium)
- MTC tumors do not take up radioiodine and are not hormone dependent.

9. Medullary carcinoma of thyroid, which of the following is not correct?

a. They secrete calcitonin
b. 20–25% are familial
c. Associated diarrhea can be seen in 30% of the patients
d. Medullary carcinomas of thyroid take up iodine

Ans. is 'd' Medullary carcinomas of thyroid take up iodine

10. Which of the following is not true about medullary thyroid carcinoma?

a. Are a type of neuroendocrine tumors
b. Associated with MEN 2A and 2B syndrome
c. Form about 25% of the thyroid malignancies
d. Tumor cells may secrete serotonin, ACTH and VIP

Ans. is 'c' Form about 25% of the thyroid malignancies

MANAGEMENT OF PAPILLARY CARCINOMA

Total thyroidectomy is reserved for risk of specific indications (namely those in which there is a preoperative diagnosis of high-risk cancer, bilateral disease or when there is a clear indication for postoperative radioiodine therapy).

'Small' cancers confined to one lobe can be managed by lobectomy and TSH suppression (arbitrary limits of between 1 and 4 cm). According to the radical approach routine total thyroidectomy, is done.

Total thyroidectomy facilitates the use of radioiodine for postoperative scanning to detect and subsequently ablate metastases. If metastases take up radioiodine they may be detected by scanning and treated with large doses of radioiodine.

Radioactive iodine is indicated in patients with unresectable disease, local recurrence or metastatic disease, high-risk patients and in those with a rising serum thyroglobulin level. But radioiodine is contraindicated in pregnant and lactating women.

11. Radio iodine preferred in treatment in:

a. Young patients
b. Pregnancy
c. Recent onset of toxic goiter
d. Post surgery for papillary thyroid cancer

Ans. is 'd' Post surgery for papillary thyroid cancer

HASHIMOTO'S THYROIDITIS

- ❖ Most common cause of hypothyroidism in areas of the world where iodine levels are sufficient
- ❖ Lymphocytes infiltrate thyroid gland (Struma lymphomatosa); Autoimmune disorder (T-cell attack thyroid; B cell activation); Associated with HLA-DR5
- ❖ Antibodies produced- Anti-TPO, Anti-thyroglobulin
- ❖ Histology: Massive lymphocytic infiltrate (germinal centers) with Hurthle cells (enlarged eosinophilic follicular cells)
- ❖ Primarily occurs in women, most prevalent between 45 and 65 years of age
- ❖ Enlarged non-tender thyroid gland
- ❖ Gradual loss of thyroid function → hypothyroid symptoms
- ❖ Treatment: thyroid hormone replacement
- ❖ Increased risk of non Hodgkin B cell lymphoma
- ❖ Increased risk for developing other immune diseases, both endocrine (type 1 diabetes, autoimmune adrenalitis) and nonendocrine (systemic lupus erythematosus, myasthenia gravis, and Sjögren syndrome).

12. Which of the following is not true regarding Hashimoto thyroiditis?

a. It is the most common cause of hypothyroidism where iodine levels are sufficient
b. It is more common in women
c. Patients have increased risk of development of systemic lupus erythematosus
d. It is most prevalent in 65 to 85 years age group

Ans. is 'd' It is most prevalent in 65 to 85 years age group

THYROGLOSSAL CYST

- ❖ Thyroglossal cyst is the only midline neck swelling mass/lump which moves with both deglutition and swallowing.
- ❖ A fibrous cyst that forms from a persistent thyroglossal duct.
- ❖ Thyroglossal cysts are the most common cause of midline neck masses.
- ❖ They can occur anywhere along the path of the thyroglossal duct, from the base of the tongue to the suprastemal notch.
- ❖ Most often present with a palpable asymptomatic midline neck mass above the level of the hyoid bone (suprahyoid location). Some patients may have neck or throat pain, or dysphagia.
- ❖ The mass on the neck moves during swallowing or on protrusion of the tongue because of its attachment to the tongue (foramen of cecum) via the tract of thyroid descent.
- ❖ *Differential diagnosis*: Other swellings which move with swallowing—Thyroid, ectopic thyroid, subhyoid bursitis, enlarged lymph nodes fixed to trachea, dermoid cysts and laryngocele.
- ❖ Treatment involves the "Sistrunk operation" which consists of en bloc cystectomy and excision of the central hyoid bone to minimize recurrence.

13. Most common site of thyroglossal cyst is:

a. Subhyoid
b. Suprahyoid
c. Floor of mouth
d. Beneath foramen cecum

Ans. is 'b' Suprahyoid

PARATHYROID SURGERY: AUTOTRANSPLANTATION

- ❖ Whenever multiple parathyroids are resected, it is preferable to cryopreserve tissue, so that it may be autotransplanted should the patient becomes hypoparathyroid.
- ❖ Each parathyroid gland is sliced into 1–3 mm slices and three or four grafts are implanted into separated muscle pockets in the anterior forearm (non-dominant) muscles (in **brachioradialis** muscle), then the muscle is closed with nonabsorbable sutures.

14. Parathyroid gland is implanted in which muscle? *(NEET 2019)*

a. Flexor digitorum
b. Extensor carpi radialis
c. Biceps
d. Brachioradialis

Ans. is 'd' Brachioradialis

MIAMI CRITERIA

With the development of imaging and localization studies, focused parathyroidectomy with use of intraoperative parathormone monitoring (IPM) is the mainstay of treatment for primary hyperparathyroidism at many health care centers both nationally and internationally. Focused parathyroidectomy guided by IPM allows for surgical excision of the offending parathyroid gland through smaller incisions. **The Miami criterion is a protocol that uses a "> 50% parathormone (PTH) drop" from either the greatest pre-**

Surgery

incision or pre-excision measurement of PTH in a blood sample taken 10 min following resection of hyperfunctioning glands. Following removal of the hyperfunctioning parathyroid gland, a > 50% PTH drop at 10 min indicates completion of parathyroidectomy, and predicts operative success at 6 mo. IPM using the Miami criterion has demonstrated equal curative rates of > 97%, which is comparable to the traditional bilateral neck exploration. The focused approach, however, is associated with shorter recovery times, improved cosmesis, and lower risk of postoperative hypocalcemia.

15. As per Miami criteria for parathyroidectomy, successful removal of lesion is confirmed by: *(NEET 2020)*

a. 50% reduction in PTH within 10 mins of gland removal
b. 50% reduction in PTH within 5 mins of gland removal
c. 25% reduction in PTH within 10 mins of gland removal
d. 25% reduction in PTH within 5 mins of gland removal

Ans. is 'a' 50% reduction in PTH within 10 mins of gland removal

GASTROINTESTINAL SURGERY

CA ESOPHAGUS

There is a rapid change in the caliber of the lumen of the esophagus in the mid-esophagus. There is a segment with irregular margins and apparent destruction of the normal smooth mucosal pattern. The findings are most suggestive of a carcinoma of the esophagus. Most carcinomas of the esophagus are of the squamous cell variety. They frequently spread longitudinally along the esophageal wall in part because of the lack of a serosal lining to the esophagus.

16. What is the diagnosis based on the barium studies shown below? *(NEET 2020)*

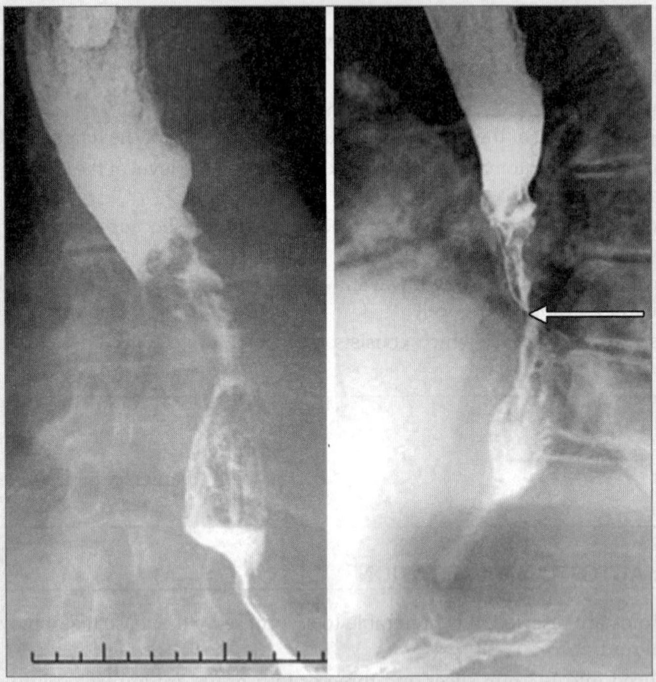

a. Achalasia cardia
b. Schatzki ring
c. Cancer esophagus
d. Hiatus hernia

Ans. is 'c' Cancer esophagus

DIVERTICULITIS

While most patients with freely perforated diverticulitis require surgery, the choice of techniques largely depends upon the extent of peritoneal contamination as assessed by the **Hinchey classification system**:

- Stage I – Pericolic or mesenteric abscess
- Stage II – Walled-off pelvic abscess
- Stage III – Generalized purulent peritonitis
- Stage IV – Generalized fecal peritonitis

17. A patient presents with vomiting, abdominal guarding and tenderness in surgical emergency. Emergency laparotomy revealed purulent peritonitis following a perforated diverticulitis. What is the grade of this complicated colonic diverticulitis? *(NEET 2020)*

a. Grade 1 b. Grade 2
c. Grade 3 d. Grade 4

Ans. is 'c' Grade 3

CA ANAL CANAL

Testicular tumor: Retroperitoneal nodes are the first landing site of metastatic disease with tumors originating from the right testicle often spreading to the inter-aortocaval lymph nodes while tumors originating in the left testicle will spread to the para-aortic lymph nodes.

Prostate and sigmoid colon malignancy spreads to pelvic lymph nodes.

Anal canal malignancy: Tumors originating above the dentate line, similar to rectal cancers, drain to the mesorectal and internal iliac nodes. In contrast, tumors arising below the dentate line may also spread to the superficial inguinal and external iliac (deep inguinal) nodes.

18. A patient presents with mass in inguinal region which is hard, indurated and nontender. On examination, most probably they were lymph nodes. What is the likely source of primary in this patient? *(NEET 2020)*

a. Testis b. Prostate
c. Sigmoid colon d. Anal canal

Ans. is 'd' Anal canal

SMALL INTESTINE RESECTION

Absorption of vitamin B12

- Vitamin B12 in foods is protein-bound, and this is dissociated in the acid milieu of the stomach with the help of pepsin.
- Additional vitamin B12-binding proteins known as R-binders or haptocorrins (HC) are secreted in the saliva and bind to the vitamin B12 in the stomach.
- Gastric parietal cells produce intrinsic factor. Pancreatic proteases secreted into the higher pH duodenum cleave off the R-binders, allowing the vitamin B12 to bind intrinsic factor.
- The vitamin B12-intrinsic factor complex is taken up by mucosal receptors in the ileum.

Small intestinal inflammation or surgery: A number of disorders of the small intestine have the potential to interfere with vitamin B12 absorption and may lead to clinically important vitamin B12 deficiency, especially if intake is low and/or if stores are borderline.

These disorders include small intestinal bacterial overgrowth, inflammatory bowel disease (IBD), radiation enteritis, celiac disease (especially if the patient is nonadherent to a gluten-free diet), lymphoma, tuberculous ileitis, amyloidosis, or ileal resection for any reason (e.g., IBD, bowel ischemia, urinary diversion)

19. Following a blunt trauma to abdomen, emergency resection of entire ileum and a part of distal jejunum was done. What is likely to occur as a sequelae? *(NEET 2020)*

a. Atrophic gastritis b. B12 deficiency
c. Folate deficiency d. Constipation

Ans. is 'b' B12 deficiency

PARALYTIC ILEUS

An Addisonian crisis results from an acute lack of glucocorticoids or mineralocorticoids. This condition most often occurs in a patient with known adrenal insufficiency, either primary or secondary.

The salient feature of patients in acute adrenal crisis is circulatory collapse. They might have symptoms like nausea, vomiting, fever and lower chest/ abdominal pain along with the low blood pressure. They may appear cyanotic due to shock. Sometimes the patients are confused, delirious, or lethargic. Patients may have hyperpyrexia, with temperatures reaching 105°F or higher, and may be comatose. In acute adrenal hemorrhage, the patient can deteriorate with sudden collapse, abdominal or flank pain, and nausea with or without hyperpyrexia. Bilateral adrenalectomy for any reason can lead to addisonian crisis.

The surgical removal of a unilateral cortisol-producing adrenal adenoma in a patient with Cushing syndrome can cause an acute adrenal crisis from secondary adrenocortical insufficiency.

This is due to the atrophy of the normal adrenal cortex from lack of the stimulant effect of pituitary ACTH.

20. A pregnant female underwent LSCS for delivery and had meconium stained liquor. After 3–4 days of operation, she developed complain of pain and constipation. Her BP and HR were normal. What is the likely diagnosis? *(NEET 2020)*

a. Bowel stricture b. Paralytic ileus
c. Bowel injury d. Meconium peritonitis

Ans. is 'b' Paralytic ileus

21. A patient who undervent bilateral adrenalectomy for pheochromocytoma presented with hypotension. The blood volume was normal. What is the diagnosis? *(NEET 2020)*

a. Cushing disease
b. Cardiogenic shock
c. Sepsis
d. Addisonian crisis

Ans. is 'd' Addisonian crisis

INTUSSUSCEPTION

Intussusception occurs when one segment of bowel is pulled into itself or a neighboring loop of the bowel by peristalsis.

While the classic triad of intermittent abdominal pain, vomiting, and right upper quadrant mass, plus occult or gross blood on rectal examination has great positive predictive value for intussusception in children, these findings are seen in less than 20% of intussusception cases.

A contrast enema remains the gold standard, demonstrating the intussusception as an occluding mass prolapsing into the lumen, giving the "coiled spring" appearance (barium in the lumen of the intussusceptum and in the intraluminal space). The main absolute contraindication for an enema is a perforation, which needs to be treated surgically.

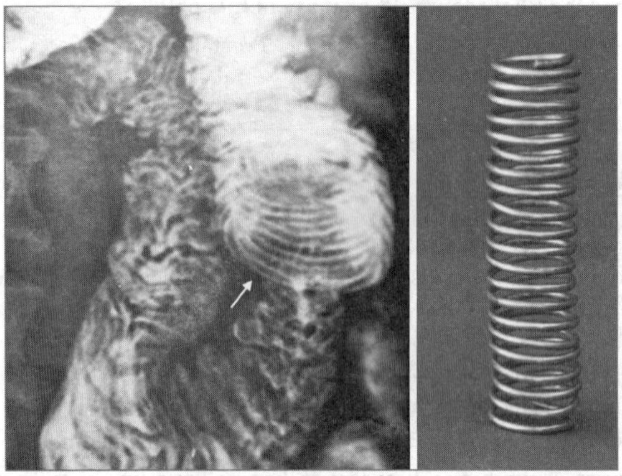

22. A patient presented with acute onset of abdominal pain, occult blood in stool and palpable lump on examination. X-ray is shown below. What is the diagnosis? *(NEET 2020)*

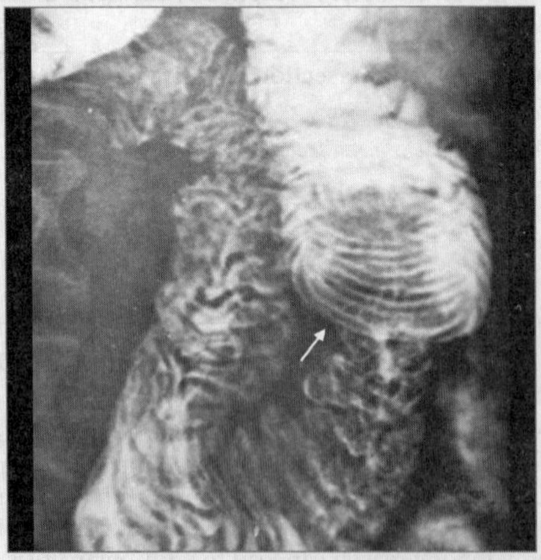

a. Diverticulitis
b. Sigmoid volvulus
c. Intussusception
d. Ogilvie's disease

Ans. is 'c' Intussusception

ESOPHAGEAL DIVERTICULA

Esophageal diverticula are of two types: pulsion and traction

- In pulsion diverticulum increased intraluminal pressures (secondary to abnormal esophageal motility push the mucosa and submucosa through a muscular defect in the wall of the esophagus creating a pulsion diverticulum. It is a false diverticulum (not containing all the layers of the esophageal wall)

- In traction diverticulum extraluminal forces (like inflamed and scarred peribronchial and mediastinal lymph nodes) pull the full thickness of the esophagus out, creating a true diverticulum.

Zenker's Diverticulum

- Mucosal outpouching occurring through Killian's triangle between the upper oblique fibers (also known as thyropharyngeus muscle) and lower horizontal fibers (also known as cricopharyngeus muscle) of the inferior constrictor muscle.
- Underlying pathology is neuromuscular incoordination due to different nerves supply of the two parts of the inferior constrictor muscle—the thyropharyngeus supplied by the pharyngeal plexus and the cricopharyngeus by recurrent laryngeal nerve.
- Zenker's diverticulum is a pulsion diverticulum (false diverticulum)
- The diverticula arises posteriorly in the midline of neck. The mouth of the diverticula is in the midline but the sac projects laterally (usually left laterally)
- Most patients are over 50.
- Dysphagia is the most common symptom. Undigested food is regurgitated into the mouth, gurgling noises after eating, halitosis (bad mouth odor) and a sour metallic taste in the mouth are common symptoms.
- Barium swallow is diagnostic.
- Cervical webs are seen associated in 50% of patients with Zenker's diverticula and can cause dysphagia postoperatively if not treated.
- Treatment
  - Excision of pouch and cricopharyngeal myotomy through cervical approach
  - Dohlman's procedure: The partition wall between the esophagus and the pouch is divided by diathermy through an endoscope. This is done in poor risk debilitated patients
  - Endoscopic laser treatment similar to Dohlman's procedure.

23. Which of the following is false about Zenker's diverticulum?

a. Most patients are above 50 years of age
b. It is the most common esophageal diverticulum
c. Mucosal outpouching through the Killian's triangle
d. Cervical webs can be associated with Zenker's diverticulum in 80% of the patients

Ans. is 'd' Cervical webs can be associated with Zenker's diverticulum in 80% of the patients

24. Dohlman's procedure is used for: *(NEET 2019)*

a. Zenker's diverticulum
b. Carcinoma esophagus
c. Carcinoma larynx
d. Nasal carcinoma

Ans. is 'a' Zenker's diverticulum

Zenker's diverticulum: Patient present with intermittent dysphagia, regurgitation of food and foul smelling breath later on progressive dysphagia progressive.

Laryngocele is an air-filled cystic swelling due to dilatation of saccule.

It is a diverticulum of mucous membrane which starts from the anterior part of ventricular cavity and extends upward between vestibular folds and lamina of thyroid cartilage and abnormally enlarges to forms the air containing sac—Laryngocele.

25. An elderly male presents with halitosis and aspiration of food at night. On examination, there is a gurgling sound on neck palpation. Barium studies is as below. What is the diagnosis? *(NEET 2020)*

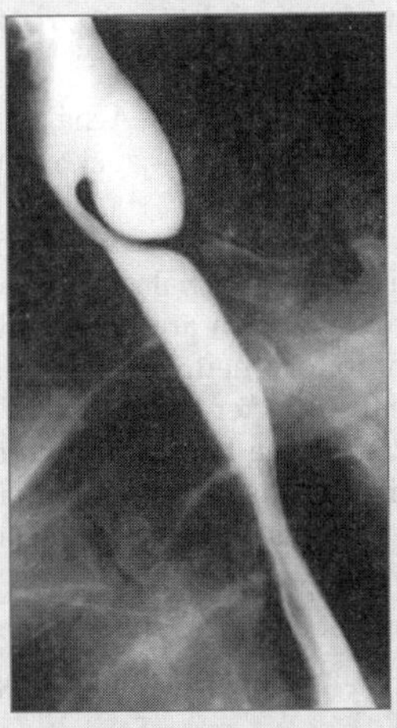

a. Pharyngeal pouch
b. Plummer Vinson syndrome
c. Dysphagia lusoria
d. Laryngocele

Ans. is 'a' Pharyngeal pouch

ACHALASIA CARDIA

- Failure of LES to relax due to loss of myenteric (Auerbach) plexus due to loss of postganglionic inhibitory neurons (which contain NO and VIP)
- Common in females between 20 and 40 years age group
- Progressive dysphagia, which is more for liquid than to solid food
- Barium swallow is diagnostic; shows:
  - Pencil like smooth narrowing of lower esophagus—Bird beak appearance
  - Dilatation of proximal esophagus
  - Absence of fundic gas bubble
  - Sigmoid esophagus or megaesophagus
- Manometry
  - The most confirmatory investigation
  - Incomplete lower esophageal sphincter relaxation (<75% relaxation)
  - Elevated LES pressure
  - Loss of primary peristaltic waves in the esophageal body
  - Increased intraesophageal baseline pressure relative to gastric baseline
- The most common surgical procedure for achalasia is laparoscopic Heller myotomy, usually performed in conjunction with an antireflux procedure (partial fundoplication).

26. Heller's operation is done for:

a. Achalasia cardia
b. Zenker's diverticulum
c. Esophageal spasm
d. Esophageal perforation

Ans. is 'a' Achalasia cardia

27. All of the following is true about achalasia cardia *except*:

a. Lower esophageal sphincter does not relax normally
b. Males are affected more than the females
c. Absence of gastric air bubble is a sign seen on X-ray
d. Manometry is the most confirmatory investigation

Ans. is 'b' Males are affected more than the females

ACHALASIA CLASSIFICATION

Esophageal pressure topography (EPT) criteria for achalasia subtypes:

- Type I: Median IRP >upper limit of normal, 100 percent failed peristalsis, minimal pressurization within the esophagus.
- Type II: Median IRP >upper limit of normal, no normal peristalsis, panesophageal pressurization with ≥20 percent of swallows.
- Type III: Median IRP >upper limit of normal, no normal peristalsis, preserved fragments of nonpropagating distal peristalsis or premature (spastic) contractions with DCI >450 mmHg·s·cm with ≥20 percent of swallows. The published upper limit of normal for the IRP is 15 mmHg

28. A patient presented with dysphagia to both solid and liquids. Manometry revealed IRP > 15 with panesophageal pressurization and >20% premature spastic contractions but no peristalsis and DCI >450 mm Hg. What is the diagnosis? *(NEET 2020)*

a. Achalasia type 1
b. Achalasia type 2
c. Achalasia type 3
d. Jackhammer esophagus

Ans. is 'c' Achalasia type 3

Histologic examination of the esophagus in patients with achalasia reveals decreased numbers of neurons (ganglion cells) in the myenteric plexuses, and the ganglion cells that remain often are surrounded by lymphocytes. This inflammatory degeneration preferentially involves the nitric oxide-producing, inhibitory neurons that affect the relaxation of esophageal smooth muscle; the cholinergic neurons that contribute to lower esophageal sphincter (LES) tone by causing smooth muscle contraction may be relatively spared. **Loss of inhibitory innervation in the LES causes the basal sphincter pressure to rise, and renders the sphincter muscle incapable of normal relaxation. Loss of peristalsis in the distal esophagus** and a failure of LES relaxation with swallowing both impair esophageal emptying; however, most of the symptoms and signs of achalasia are due primarily to the defect in LES relaxation (esophagogastric junction outflow obstruction).

Barium esophagram: Findings on barium esophagram that are suggestive of achalasia include:

- *Dilation of the esophagus*: In patients with late- or end-stage achalasia the esophagus may appear significantly dilated (megaesophagus), angulated, and tortuous, giving it a sigmoid shape.
- Narrow EGJ with "bird-beak" appearance caused by the persistently contracted LES
- Aperistalsis
- Delayed emptying of barium.

29. Which of the following is true about achalasia cardia? *(NEET 2020)*

a. Decreased esophageal peristalsis
b. Decreased LES tone
c. Decreased levels of NO and VIP
d. Decreased diameter of lower esophagus

Ans. is 'a' Decreased esophageal peristalsis

PEPTIC ULCER DISEASE

Vagotomy

Vagotomy is an essential component of surgical management of peptic ulcer disease. With the availability of excellent acid secretion control with H_2-receptor antagonists and proton pump inhibitors, the need for surgical management of this condition has greatly decreased.

The basic types of vagotomy are as follows:

- Truncal vagotomy (TV)
- Selective vagotomy (SV)
- Highly selective vagotomy (HSV)

Indications

- *Elective:* Failure of medical treatment (with the availability of effective acid suppression with H2RAs and PPIs; however, this indication has virtually become nonexistent)
- *Semielective:* Pyloric stenosis (obstruction) due to PUD
- *Emergency:* Upper gastrointestinal (GI) bleeding due to PUD or stress gastric ulcers (erosive gastric mucosal disease) or perforated PUD that is causing peritonitis.

Highly Selective Vagotomy

- In highly selective vagotomy (also known as parietal cell vagotomy or proximal gastric vagotomy) the vagal innervation to the antrum and pylorus (nerves of Latarjet) are preserved, only the vagal supply to the proximal two-thirds of stomach (where essentially all the parietal cells are located) is cut. This preserves gastric motility.
- *Advantages:* Technical simplicity and preservation of entire gastric reservoir capacity, Lowest mortality and side effects.
- *Disadvantage:* Recurrence rates are higher than less selective vagotomy.

Management of Peptic Ulcer Perforation

- Nasogastric tube, intravenous crystalloid, intravenous broad-spectrum antibiotics.
- Surgery is mostly indicated, although occasionally nonsurgical treatment can be used in stable patients without peritonitis. Surgery whether laparoscopy or laparotomy involves two components:
  I. Thorough peritoneal toilet to remove all the fluid and food debris. Drain is not indicated
  II. Management of perforation—The most frequently performed operation for a perforated duodenal ulcer is simple closure with an omental onlay reinforcement or patch. Postoperative *H. pylori* eradication (antibiotics + antisecretory agents) regimen is given.

Acute gastric ulcer associated with CNS injury—**Cushing ulcer** (↑ intracranial pressure stimulates vagal gastric H+ secretion)

Acute gastric ulcer associated with severe burns—**Curling ulcer** (greatly reduced plasma volume results in sloughing of gastric mucosa)

30. Surgery for perforated duodenal ulcer:

a. Vagotomy
b. Pyeloplasty
c. Omental patch repair
d. Roux-en- Y gastrectomy

Ans. is 'c' Omental patch repair

31. Not true about highly selective vagotomy:

a. It is also known parietal cell vagotomy
b. Nerves of Latarjet are sacrificed
c. Recurrence rates are higher than vagotomy
d. Entire gastric reservoir capacity is preserved

Ans. is 'b' Nerves of Latarjet are sacrificed

32. Cushing ulcer is seen in case of: *(NEET 2019)*

a. Burns
b. Head injury
c. Cell necrosis
d. Stress

Ans. is 'b' Head injury

MANAGEMENT OF SWALLOWED BATTERIES

- Immediate chest X-rays to make sure the battery is not stuck in the esophagus.
- Most swallowed batteries that pass through the esophagus will pass in the stool without complication.
- However, if a battery gets stuck in the esophagus, it can cause esophagitis and subsequent perforation.
- Radiographic studies of the entire digestive system may be taken.
- Disk batteries have a characteristic double- density (two-layer) shadow on X-rays. Laterally, their edges are rounded, and they contain a step-off junction at the positive and negative terminal. This can help distinguish them from coins and buttons.
- If a battery is located in the esophagus (food pipe), immediate removal is necessary.

33. A child swallowed a watch battery containing alkaline content. What next?

a. Immediate X-ray
b. Remove surgically immediately
c. CT abdomen
d. Laxatives

Ans. is 'a' Immediate X-ray

CORROSIVE INJURY OF ESOPHAGUS

- The type of agent, its concentration and the volume ingested largely determine the extent of damage.
- In general, alkalis are relatively odorless and tasteless, making them more likely to be ingested in large volume.
- Alkalis cause liquefaction, saponification of fats, dehydration and thrombosis of blood vessels that usually leads to fibrous scarring.
- Acids cause coagulative necrosis with eschar formation, and this coagulant may limit penetration to deeper layers of the esophageal wall
- Acids also cause more gastric damage than alkalis because of the induction of intense pylorospasm with pooling in the antrum
- Symptoms and signs are unreliable in predicting the severity of injury
- The key to management is early endoscopy to inspect the whole of the esophagus and stomach
- Deep ulcers and the recognition of a gray or black eschar signify the most severe lesions with the greatest risk of perforation.
- Regular endoscopic examinations are the best way to assess stricture development.
- Other than the need for emergency surgery for bleeding or perforation, elective esophageal resection should be deferred for at least 3 months until the fibrotic phase is established.

34. In corrosive injury of esophagus correct statement is all *except*:

a. Alkalis are usually ingested in larger volumes
b. Alkalis cause more gastric damage than acids
c. Alkalis form fibrous scar
d. Acids form eschar

Ans. is 'b' Alkalis cause more gastric damage than acids

ESOPHAGEAL PERFORATION

Effort rupture of the esophagus, or Boerhaave syndrome, is a spontaneous perforation of the esophagus that results from a sudden increase in intraesophageal pressure combined with negative intrathoracic pressure. Spontaneous rupture of the esophagus can be caused by straining or vomiting and, much less frequently, childbirth, seizure, prolonged coughing or laughing, or weightlifting.

- Boerhaave syndrome can occur in patients with a normal underlying esophagus. However, a subset of patients with Boerhaave syndrome have an underlying esophageal malignancy, pill esophagitis, eosinophilic esophagitis, Barrett's or infectious ulcers. The esophageal perforation usually involves the left posterolateral aspect of the distal esophagus. Rupture of the esophagus results in contamination of the mediastinal cavity with gastric contents and inflammation, and subsequently bacterial infection and mediastinal necrosis. If untreated, sepsis and organ failure result.
- Patients with Boerhaave syndrome often present with excruciating retrosternal chest pain. Patients may present with neck, chest, or back pain, hoarseness, dysphagia, odynophagia, dyspnea, subcutaneous emphysema, and symptoms of an acute abdomen. Within hours of the perforation, patients can develop odynophagia, dyspnea, and sepsis and shock
- *Thoracic and cervical radiography*: Findings suggestive of an esophageal perforation on chest radiograph include mediastinal or free peritoneal air or subcutaneous emphysema, pleural effusions, mediastinal widening, hydrothorax, hydropneumothorax, or subdiaphragmatic air. **While thoracic and cervical radiography can be supportive of the diagnosis, the diagnosis is established by contrast esophagram or computed tomography scan.**

35. A middle-aged man complains of upper abdominal pain after a heavy meal. There is tenderness in the upper abdomen and on X-ray, widening of the mediastinum is seen with pneumo-mediastinum. What is the diagnosis? *(NEET 2020)*

a. Spontaneous perforation of the esophagus
b. Perforated peptic ulcer
c. Foreign body causing perforation in esophagus
d. Rupture of emphysematous bulla

Ans. is 'a' Spontaneous perforation of the esophagus

GASTROINTESTINAL STROMAL TUMORS (GISTs)

- Gastrointestinal stromal tumors (GISTs) commonly occur in the stomach and duodenum
- Universally associated with a mutation in the tyrosine kinase c-kit oncogene.
- These tumors are sensitive to the tyrosine kinase inhibitor imatinib, and an 80% objective response rate can be observed.
- The biological behavior of these tumors is unpredictable but size and mitotic index are the best predictors of metastasis.
- Peritoneal and liver metastases are most common; metastatic lymphadenopathy is extremely rare.
- Obvious tumors are considerably less common than gastric cancer
- As the biological behavior is difficult to predict, the best guide to treatment is to consider the size of the tumor.
- If easily resectable, surgery is the primary mode of treatment. Smaller tumors can be treated by wedge excision. Larger tumors may require a gastrectomy or duodenectomy but lymphadenectomy is not required.
- Larger tumors are treated for 3–6 months with imatinib before surgery as this will usually radically reduce their size and vascularity

36. Which of the following is not true about gastrointestinal stromal tumor [GIST]?

a. It rarely occurs in duodenum
b. It is universally associated with mutation in tyrosine kinase c kit oncogene
c. Size and mitotic index are best predictors of metastases
d. It is sensitive to imatinib

Ans. is 'a' It rarely occurs in duodenum

GALLSTONES

Increased cholesterol and/or bilirubin, ↑ bile salts, and gallbladder stasis all cause stones.

There are two types of stones:

1. Cholesterol stones (radiolucent with 10–20% opaque due to calcifications)- 80% of stones. Associated with obesity, Crohn disease, advanced age, estrogen therapy, multiparity, rapid weight loss, Native American origin.
2. Pigment stones (black = radiopaque, Ca^2 + bilirubinate, hemolysis; brown = radiolucent, infection). Associated with Crohn disease, chronic hemolysis, alcoholic cirrhosis, advanced age, biliary infections, total parenteral nutrition (TPN).
   Risk factors (4 Fs): Female, Fat, Fertile (multiparity), Forty
   Most common complication is cholecystitis; can also cause acute pancreatitis, ascending cholangitis.
   Diagnose with ultrasound. Treat with elective cholecystectomy if symptomatic.

Indications of Cholecystectomy in Asymptomatic Gallstones

- Large stone, >3 cm in diameter
- Multiple small stones (more chances of passing into CBD and causing obstruction)
- Stone associated with polyp
- Calcified gallbladder (Porcelain gallbladder)
- Congenitally anomalous gallbladder
- Gallstones with diabetes (because emphysematous cholecystitis is common in diabetics with gallstones)
- Immunocompromised / transplant patients (because complication rate is high)
- Few authorities are now also recommending routine cholecystectomy in all young patient with silent stones.

Management of Suspected or Proven CBD Stones Associated with Gallbladder Stones

For gallstones—laparoscopic cholecystectomy is the procedure of choice

For CBD stones two things can be done:

1. If the surgeon is experienced in laparoscopic techniques of CBD stone removal then both cholecystectomy and transduodenal choledocholithotomy is done in the same sitting
   - CBD stones are first confirmed by an intraoperative cholangiogram then the stones are removed laparoscopically via the cystic duct or by choledochotomy.
2. If the surgeon is not experienced with laparoscopic methods of CBD stone removal, preoperative endoscopic sphincterotomy with stone removal and later laparoscopic cholecystectomy is done.

37. Asymptomatic gallstone > 3 cm what is the treatment?

a. Laparoscopic cholecystectomy
b. Cholecystectomy
c. Dissolution therapy
d. ERCP

Ans. is 'a' Laparoscopic cholecystectomy

38. Most common type of gallstone is: *(NEET 2019)*

a. Black pigment stones
b. Cholesterol stones
c. Pigment stones
d. Calcium bilirubinate stones

Ans. is 'b' Cholesterol stones

PRIMARY SCLEROSING CHOLANGITIS

Primary sclerosing cholangitis (PSC) is an uncommon inflammatory condition, which affects the biliary tree resulting in multiple strictures, liver damage, and eventually cirrhosis.

PSC is strongly associated with inflammatory bowel disease (IBD) (in 70% cases), especially ulcerative colitis, and thus shares similar demographics: young to middle-aged males (~4th decade) are most frequently affected.

The average age of diagnosis is 54 years (range 6–93) with increased occurrence in men (63%). A large number of asymptomatic individuals are identified upon investigation of persistently deranged liver function tests. Symptomatic individuals commonly present non-specifically with fatigue. More specific symptoms include pruritus, jaundice or GI bleeding.

ERCP has traditionally been the gold standard for the depiction of the biliary tree, and also offers the ability to perform cholangioplasty, if necessary. In practice, however, MRCP is used before ERCP since it is noninvasive, can visualize the liver, and it avoids the 10% risk of hospitalization from ERCP in PSC patients.

The characteristic findings on direct imaging of the biliary tree are:

- ❖ Multiple segmental strictures
  - Typically short segment
  - Intervening segments are of normal caliber or slightly dilated (beading)
- ❖ Biliary dilatation: may be present in ~85% of cases
  - General: ~35%
  - Segmental: ~50%
- ❖ Biliary diverticula
- ❖ Mural irregularities
- ❖ Distortion of the biliary tree due to associated cirrhosis

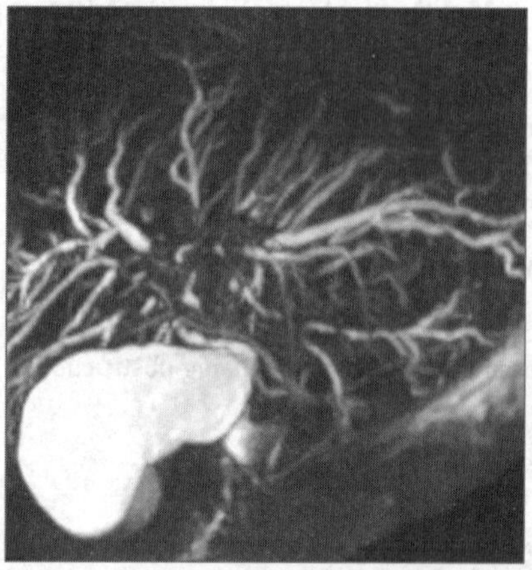

Typical gross central stricturing of the ducts with proximal dilatation. 3D MRCP nicely shows gross stricturing centrally involving the right and left hepatic ducts with segmental and subsegmental involvement.

39. A man presents with deep jaundice, fever and chills. MRCP is shown below. What is the diagnosis? *(NEET 2020)*

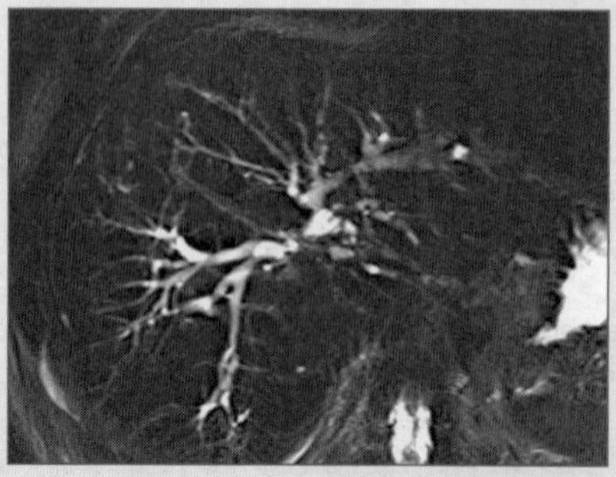

a. Primary sclerosing cholangitis
b. Primary biliary cirrhosis
c. Caroli's disease
d. Oriental cholangiohepatits

Ans. is 'a' Primary sclerosing cholangitis

COMMON BILE DUCT (CBD) STONES

Risk assessment: In a 2010 guideline, the American Society for Gastrointestinal Endoscopy (ASGE) proposed the following approach to stratify patients based on their probability of having choledocholithiasis. Patients were stratified using the following predictors:

- **"Very strong" predictors (Just remember these)**
  - **The presence of a common bile duct stone on transabdominal ultrasound**
  - **Clinical acute cholangitis**
  - **A serum bilirubin greater than 4 mg/dL**
- "Strong" predictors
  - A dilated common bile duct on ultrasound (more than 6 mm in a patient with a gallbladder in situ)
  - A serum bilirubin of 1.8 to 4 mg/dL
- "Moderate" predictors
  - Abnormal liver biochemical test other than bilirubin
  - Age older than 55 years
  - Clinical gallstone pancreatitis

Using the above predictors, patients are stratified as:

- High risk
  - At least one very strong predictor **and/or**
  - Both strong predictors
- Intermediate risk
  - One strong predictor **and/or**
  - At least one moderate predictor
- Low risk
  - No predictors

Patients at **high risk** for having common bile duct stones and with intact gallbladder **generally proceed to endoscopic retrograde cholangiopancreatography (ERCP) with stone removal, followed by elective cholecystectomy**, or they undergo cholecystectomy with intraoperative cholangiography, followed by intraoperative or postoperative ERCP; where available, laparoscopic common duct exploration can be performed. Pre-cholecystectomy ERCP with postponed cholecystectomy is appropriate in patients with **acute cholangitis**, in those with ongoing evidence of biliary obstruction and acute pancreatitis, and in patients who are poor surgical candidates.

Patients at **intermediate risk** either undergo **preoperative endoscopic ultrasound or magnetic resonance cholangiopancreatography**, or they proceed to laparoscopic cholecystectomy with intraoperative cholangiography or ultrasonography. Subsequent management choices are as above. **(EUS and MRCP have largely replaced ERCP for the diagnosis of choledocholithiasis in patients at intermediate risk for choledocholithiasis).**

Patients at **low risk can proceed directly to cholecystectomy** without additional testing, provided gallstones or sludge were seen on preoperative imaging.

40. A patient presents with fever, jaundice and upper abdominal pain. USG revealed a stone in common bile duct with dilated bile duct and biliary radicles. What is the next appropriate step in management? *(NEET 2020)*

a. Cholecystectomy
b. MRCP/ERCP
c. CECT abdo.
d. Percutaneous drainage

Ans. is 'b' MRCP/ERCP

ACUTE PANCREATITIS

Radiological IOC-CECT (shows prognosis also)

Revised Atlanta Classification (2012)

Acute pancreatitis		
Types	*Acute interstitial edematous*	*Acute necrotizing*
Fluid collections <4 weeks	Acute peripancreatitic fluid collection, Ill-defined Homogenous	Aute necrotic collection, Ill-defined Heterogenous
Fluid collections <4 weeks	Pseudocyst, Thickwall, Homogenous	Walled-off necrosis, Thick-wall, Heterogenous

Blood Tests in Acute Pancreatitis

- Sernun amylase is the most widely used laboratory test because of its simplicity. However, it lacks the specificity to pancreas and may be raised in a number of conditions causing high false positive reactions. Serum amylase level usually return to normal after 48 to 72 hours of acute episode, further limiting its usefulness.
- Serum Lipase is now the single best enzyme to measure for the diagnosis of acute pancreatitis. Its level remains elevated for much longer duration of time (7 to 14 days).

41. Pancreatic pseudocyst is developed in how much duration following an attack of acute pancreatitis?

a. Less than 1 week
b. Less than 2 weeks
c. 3 or more weeks
d. 4 or more weeks

Ans. is 'd' 4 or more weeks

42. Case of acute pancreatitis diagnostic test:

a. Secretin stimulation test
b. Serum lipase
c. Impaired glucose tolerance
d. S. amylase

Ans. is 'b' Serum lipase

GASTRINOMA TRIANGLE

- Also known as Passaros triangle.
- Anatomical area in the abdomen where majority (90%) of gastrinomas are thought to arise
- Boundaries – Triangle is formed by joining the three points
  - Superiorly – confluence of the cystic and common bile ducts
  - Inferiorly – Junction of second and third parts of duodenum
  - Medially – Junction of neck and body of pancreas

43. Identify the triangle in the given image. *(NEET 2019)*

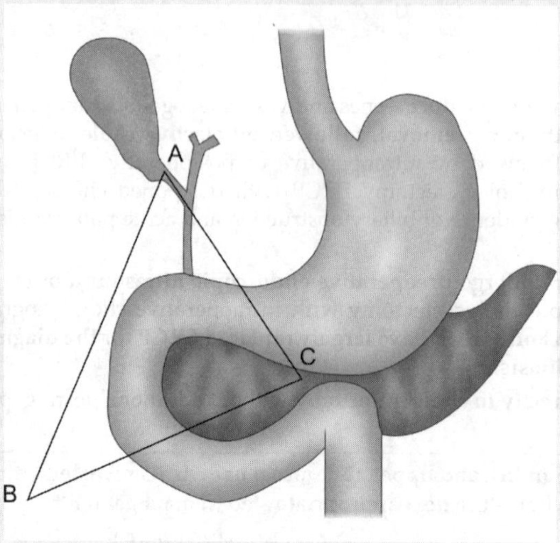

a. Koch's triangle
b. Hesselbach's triangle
c. Gastrinoma triangle
d. Sherren's triangle

Ans. is 'c' Gastrinoma triangle

BUDD-CHIARI SYNDROME

- Venous drainage of the liver is occluded by hepatic venous thrombosis or obstruction from a venous web.
- Commonly affects young females
- Liver becomes acutely congested, with the development of impaired liver function and, subsequently, portal hypertension, ascites and esophageal varices
- In an acute thrombosis, the patient may rapidly progress to fulminant liver failure but, in the majority of cases abdominal discomfort and ascites are the main presenting features
- An underlying myeloproliferative disorder or procoagulant state is commonly found, such as anti-thrombin 3, protein C or protein S deficiency.
- The diagnosis is commonly suspected in a patient presenting with ascites, in whom a CT scan shows a large congested liver (early stage) or a small cirrhotic liver (late stage) in which there is gross enlargement of segment I (the caudate lobe). This feature results from preservation and hypertrophy of the segment with direct venous drainage to the IVC in the face of atrophy of the rest of the liver due to venous obstruction.
- IVC compression or occlusion from the segment I hypertrophy is also a common feature, as is thrombosis of the portal vein.

44. A young female who is a known case of myeloproliferative disorder presents with a 3 day history of progressive abdominal discomfort and ascites. Which of the following is the possible diagnosis?

a. Budd-Chiari syndrome
b. Hepatitis A
c. Perforation peritonitis
d. Acute pancreatitis

Ans. is 'a' Budd-Chiari syndrome

FISTULA IN-ANO

- Track, lined by granulation tissue, that connects internally in the anal canal or rectum and superficially on the skin around the anus
- Usually results from an anorectal abscess (cryptoglandular abscess). Other causes are Crohn's disease, malignancy, radiation, tuberculosis
- 2 types—high and low, according to whether their internal openings is below or above the anorectal ring
- A low level can be treated by fistulotomy (opening the tract) without causing damage to the sphincter.
- High level fistulas can be treated only by 'staged' operation as there is risk of incontinence.

Goodsall's Rule

- Is used to determine the location of internal opening of perianal fistula
- It states that Fistulas with external opening anterior to horizontal imaginary line drawn across the mid point of anus, connect to the internal opening by short straight tract
- Fistulas with external opening posterior to the horizontal line—run a curvilinear course and open internally into the posterior midline
- Exceptions to this rule often occur if an anterior external opening is greater than 3 cm from the anal margin. Such fistulas track to the posterior midline. Also, when there is an anterior and also a posterior opening of the same fistula, the rule of posterior opening applies.

45. Exception to Goodsall's rule is considered when the anterior external opening is more situated more than ________ cm from anal margin:

a. 2
b. 3
c. 4
d. 5

Ans. is 'b' 3

46. Treatment of choice for low fistula in ano is:

a. Fistulotomy
b. Intravenous antibiotics
c. Staged surgical resection
d. None of the above

Ans. is 'a' Fistulotomy

Previously Asked Facts

- Peau d'orange is due to cutaneous lymphatic edema due to obstruction of subdermal lymphatics, where the infiltrated skin is tethered by sweat ducts, it cannot swell, leading to an appearance like orange skin.
- Lymphangiosarcoma is a rare complication of lymphedema with an onset many years after the original treatment. It takes the form of multiple subcutaneous nodules in the upper limb and must be distinguished from recurrent carcinoma of the breast.
- Discrete breast lump without tenderness in an 18-year-old female is most likely a fibroadenoma.
- Hadfields operation is performed for Duct ectasia.
- Microdochotomy is treatment for Duct papilloma.
- Most common type of carcinoma breast in males is infiltrating ductal carcinoma.
- Zuska disease is an eponym for Squamous metaplasia of lactiferous ducts in breast.
- FNAC cannot distinguish between a benign thyroid follicular adenoma and thyroid follicular carcinoma, as this distinction is dependent not on cytology but on histological criteria, which include capsular and vascular invasion.
- Sistrunk operation is used for treatment of Thyroglossal cyst.
- Anaplastic carcinoma is highly aggressive and uniformly lethal of all the thyroid cancers
- Most common cause of chronic pancreatitis is Alcoholism
- Pringles maneuver is used to stop bleeding from Liver.
- 10% of gallstones are radio-opaque. 90% of renal stones are radio-opaque.
- T2 gallbladder cancers discovered incidentally during or after simple cholecystectomy should be treated by segment resection 4b and 5, dissection of N1-2 lymph nodes and excision of the port sites. If T2 gallbladder cancer is discovered postoperatively re-resection should be performed as soon as possible.
- The activities of three enzymes—alkaline phosphatase, 5′ -nucleotidase, and γ-glutamyl transpeptidase (GGT)—are usually elevated in cholestasis.

- The standard resection for a tumor of the pancreatic head or the ampulla is a pylorus-preserving Pancreatico-duodenectomy (PPPD) – Modified Kaush-Whipple Operation.
- Initial imaging technique for diagnosis of primary sclerosing cholangitis is Magnetic Resonance Cholangio-pancreatography (MRCP).
- Rapid measurement of urinary trypsinogen-2 level is useful in the emergency department as a screening test for acute pancreatitis. A negative test rules out acute pancreatitis with high degree of probability.
- For most patients with chronic pancreatitis, abdominal pain is the presenting symptom.
- Boas' sign - Right Shoulder Tip Pain in Cholecystitis via nerve roots C3-C5.
- The surgical treatment of choice for duodenal obstruction due to duodenal stenosis or atresia or annular pancreas is a duodenoduodenostomy.
- Specific signs in abdominal examination
  - Courvoisier sign - Palpable gallbladder and jaundice seen in Carcinoma of the head of the pancreas
  - Cullen sign - Periumbilical bruising seen in hemorrbagic pancreatitis > ectopic pregnancy
  - Grey Turner sign - Bruising of flank seen in Hemorrhagic appendicitis
  - Rovsing sign - Pain on extension of the hip joint (due to psoas irritation) seen in retrocecal appendicitis
  - Murphy sign - Right upper quadrant tenderness exacerbated by inspiration seen in acute cholecystitis
- Among peptic ulcers, Anterior duodenal ulcers are most likely to perforate.
- Boerhaave's syndrome is spontaneous perforation of the esophagus, occurring usually due to severe barotrauma when a person vomits against a closed glottis. Most common location of perforation is in the left posterolateral aspect 3–5 cm above the gastroesophageal junction.
- Nigro protocol includes combined radiation and chemotherapy with 5FU and mitomycin C. It is commonly used in management of anal canal carcinoma.
- Most common site for colorectal cancer is Rectum.
- Dysphagia more for solids than liquids implies mechanical obstruction (Ca, stricture, webs). Dyspahgia equal for solids and liquids from the very onset suggest motor disorders (Achalasia)
- 24 hour pH recording is the gold standard for diagnosis of GERD.
- Total Nissen's fundoplication is used for the surgical management of GERD, tends to be associated with short-term dysphagia but is the most durable repair in terms of long-term reflux control. Partial fundoplication, whether performed posteriorly (Toupet) or anteriorly (Dor, Watson), has fewer short- term side effects at the expense of a slightly higher long-term failure rate.
- Meckel's diverticulum is present in 2% of the population; it is situated on the anti-mesenteric border of the small intestine, 2 inch in length, 2 feet proximal to ileocecal valve, Half of those who are symptomatic are less than 2 years of age. It represents the patent intestinal end of the vitellointestinal duct. It is a true diverticulum and ectopic gastric mucosa is present in 50% cases.
- Cleft lip occurs due to by failure of fusion of the medial nasal process and the maxillary prominence.
- Kernahan's striped 'Y' classification - is used to classify cleft lip and cleft palate. The incisive foramen is taken as reference point.
- Internal hemorrhoids typically cause bright red bleeding per rectum but are painless. External hemorrhoids cause severe pain when thrombosed.
- Uphill esophageal varices are seen most commonly in the setting of cirrhosis and portal hypertension and result from reversal of venous flow from the coronary vein into the distal esophageal venous plexus. Downhill esophageal varices are produced by the obstruction of the superior vena cava, which results in collateral drainage from the head, neck and upper extremity venous systems into the veins surrounding the mid and upper thoracic esophagus.
- Coins are the most commonly impacted foreign bodies in children in esophagus and oropharynx followed by the food products.
- Amebic liver abscess is the most common extraintestinal manifestation of amebiasis.
- Critical diameter of cecum when perforation is considered eminent in pseudo-obstruction is > 9 cm.
- Typhoid intestinal perforation is usually occurs 2nd – 3rd week of typhoid fever.
- Most common small intestinal tumor is adenocarcinoma. The risk of developing small bowel carcinoma correlates positively with the colorectal cancer.

Surgery

UROLOGY

RENAL CELL CARCINOMA (RCC)

47. Management of RCC less than 4 cm size: *(NEET 2020)*

a. Partial nephrectomy
b. Radical nephrectomy
c. Radical nephrectomy with radiotherapy
d. Radical nephrectomy with chemotherapy

Ans. is 'a' Partial nephrectomy

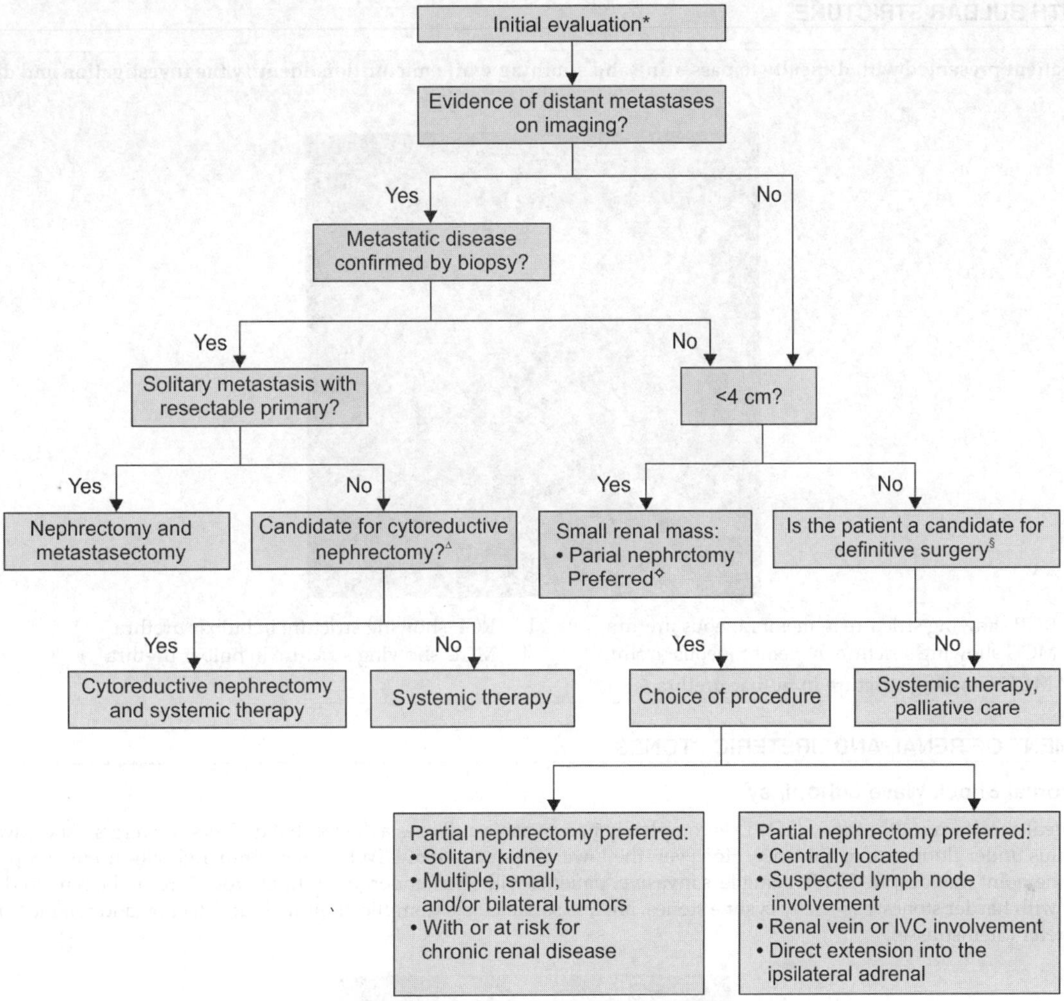

URETHRAL INJURY

The most relevant clinical and diagnostic imaging findings are summarized as follows:

- **Bladder injury:** Gross hematuria, suprapubic tenderness, and/or difficulty voiding are the main signs associated with bladder injury. Other clinical presentations include peritonitis related to intraperitoneal leakage of urine. Retrograde cystography demonstrating extravasation of contrast from the bladder confirms the diagnosis
- **Urethral injury:** Clinical features associated with a urethral injury include **blood at the meatus, difficulty voiding, scrotal/perineal ecchymosis, scrotal hematoma, pelvic fracture, and/or a high-riding prostate in men**. **Retrograde urethrography** demonstrating extravasation of contrast from the urethra confirms the diagnosis
- **Straddle injury:** Straddle injuries are caused by direct trauma to the perineum and **compress the bulbar urethra against the pubic bone.** Straddle injury is the most common cause of anterior urethral injury. The clinical manifestations of these injuries can present acutely if there are accompanying clinical symptoms (i.e., hematuria, **hematoma**) or in a delayed fashion following obstructive voiding secondary to a urethral stricture.
- **Urethra:** The male urethra is divided into the anterior (bulbous and pendulous) and posterior (prostatic and membranous) urethra. Traditionally, this division was described at the level of the urogenital diaphragm. **An injury below the urogenital diaphragm is more likely to cause a large perineal swelling.**

48. A man is brought to the emergency after he fell into a man hole and injured his perineum. He feels the urge to micturate but is unable to pass urine and there is blood at the tip of the meatus with extensive swelling of the perineal region. What is the location of the injury? *(NEET 2020)*

a. Bulbar urethra
b. Prostatic urethra
c. Bladder
d. Membranous urethra

Ans. is 'a' Bulbar urethra

MCU WITH BULBAR STRICTURE

49. A patient presented with difficulty to pass urine and straining while micturition. Identify the investigation and diagnosis? *(NEET 2020)*

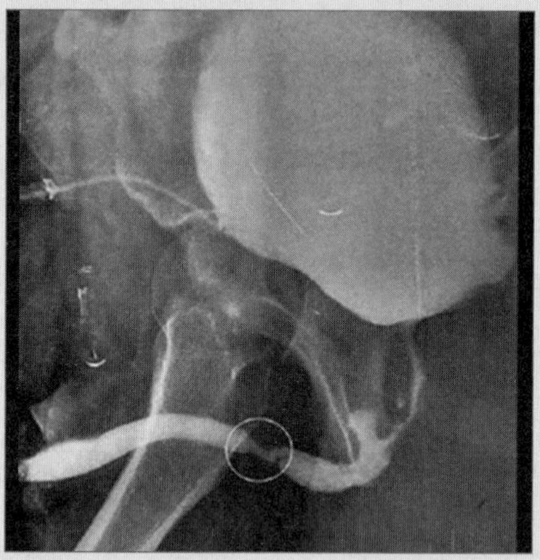

a. RGP showing stricture in membraneous urethra
b. RGP showing stricture in bulbar urethra
c. MCU showing stricture in membraneous urethra
d. MCU showing stricture in bulbar urethra

Ans. is 'd' MCU showing stricture in bulbar urethra

TREATMENT OF RENAL AND URETERIC STONES

Extracorporeal Shock Wave Lithotripsy

Extracorporeal shock wave lithotripsy (ESWL) is completely noninvasive and uses a device that delivers convergent shockwave energy to the calculus under fluoroscopic guidance. However, the lower efficacy rate of ESWL, when compared with ureteroscopy or PCNL, highlights the point that despite ESWL being less invasive, patients will often undergo multiple procedures to be rendered stone free. The results with harder stones, especially cystine stones, are less satisfactory. Complications include infection and retained fragmented stones in ureter (Steinstrasse).

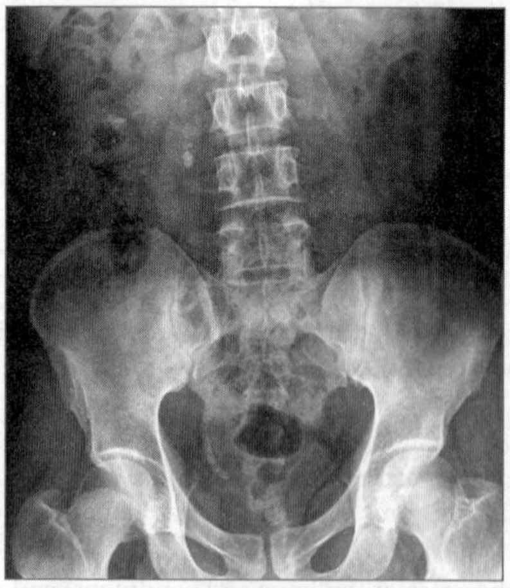

Steinstrasse formation in right distal ureter after ESWL

Ureteroscopic Stone Extraction

Ureteroscopic stone extraction is highly efficacious for lower ureteral calculi. The use of small-caliber ureteroscopes and the advent of balloon dilation or ureteral access sheaths have increased stone-free rates dramatically.

Percutaneous Nephrolithotomy

Percutaneous removal of renal and proximal ureteral calculi is the treatment of choice for large (>2.5 cm) calculi; those resistant to SWL; select lower pole calyceal stones with a narrow, long infundibulum and an acute infundibulopelvic angle; and instances with evidence of obstruction; the method can rapidly establish a stone-free status.

Surgery

Ureterolithotomy

Long-standing ureteral calculi—those inaccessible with endoscopy and those resistant to SWL—can be extracted with an ureterolithotomy. Again, a preoperative radiograph documents stone location and directs an appropriate incision. The proximal ureter may be approached with a dorsal lumbotomy.

50. Plan KUB shows complication of which procedure?

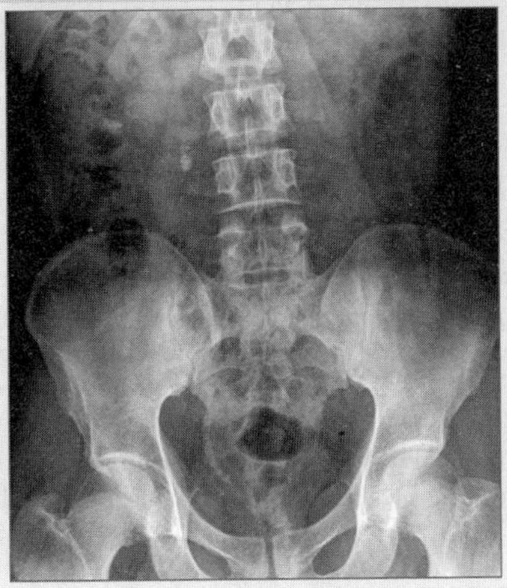

a. ESWL for renal stone
b. ESWL for bladder stones
c. ESWL for renal TB
d. Stent for benign prostatic hyperplasia

Ans. is 'a' ESWL for renal stone

URETERIC COLIC

- There is a pattern of severe exacerbation on a background of continuing pain
- Radiates to the groin, penis, scrotum or labium as the stone progresses down the ureter
- The severity of pain is not related to the size of the stone
- The pain is almost invariably associated with hematuria
- There may be few physical signs
- Sharp stabbing pain of ureteric colic is carried by Slow Type A fibres. Continuous dull pain is carried by Fast Type C fibres.

51. A 40-year-old male complains of loin pain for 1 month. Patient's complaint of pain has severely increased over last 2 hours and pain now radiates from loin and to groin and anterior thigh and patient is writhing in bed for comfort. What is the most probable etiology?

a. Bladder calculus
b. Ureteric calculus
c. Vesicoureteric reflux
d. Hydronephrosis

Ans. is 'b' Ureteric calculus

UNDESCENDED TESTIS

- The testis is arrested in some part of its path to the scrotum
- Approx 70–77% of cryptorchid testes will spontaneously descend, usually by 3 months of age
- More common in preterm, small for gestational age, LBW and twin neonates
- More common on right side
- Secondary sexual characteristics are normal
- ↓ inhibin B, ↑ FSH, ↑ LH; testosterone ↓ in bilateral cryptorchidism, normal in unilateral.
- Complications of incomplete descent.
  - Torsion of testis
  - Epididymo-orchitis
  - An associated indirect inguinal hernia is frequent
  - Atrophy
  - Pain: A testis situated in the inguinal canal is often liable to trauma and give rise to pain in the groin
  - Sterility: If the condition is bilateral
  - Malignancy: Risk is 40 times more than a normally placed testis. Surgery for undescended testes does not decrease the chances of development of testicular carcinoma
- An ectopic testis is one which has passed through the external inguinal ring in the normal pathway and then is misdirected to an abnormal location (MC site – superficial inguinal ring). The main hazard is liability to injury.

52. Which of the following is not true about undescended testes?
a. Surgery for undescended testes does not decrease the chances of development of testicular carcinoma
b. Approximately 70% of the cryptorchid testis descend by 3 months of age
c. Risk of developing testicular malignancy is about 20 times more
d. Patients have normal secondary sexual characteristics

Ans. is 'c' Risk of developing testicular malignancy is about 20 times more

HYDROCELE

- An abnormal collection of serous fluid in a part of the processus vaginalis, usually the tunica.
- Hydrocele fluid contains albumin and fibrinogen.
- About 5% of inguinal hernias are associated with a vaginal hydrocele on the same side.
- Hydroceles are typically translucent and it is possible to 'get above the swelling' on scrotal examination.
- In congenital hydrocele, the processus vaginalis is patent and connects with the peritoneal cavity. The communication is usually too small to allow herniation of intra-abdominal contents. Pressure on the hydrocele does not always empty it but the hydrocele fluid may drain into the peritoneal cavity when the child is lying down; thus, the hydrocele is often intermittent; thus a scrotal swelling nonreducible but disappears when the child wakes up from sleep is most likely a congenital hydrocele.
- Encysted hydrocele of the cord is a smooth oval swelling near the spermatic cord, which is liable to be mistaken for an inguinal hernia. The swelling moves downwards and becomes less mobile if the testis is pulled gently downwards.
- Hydrocele of the canal of Nuck is a similar condition in females. The cyst lies in relation to the round ligament and is always at least partially within the inguinal canal.

53. Scrotal swelling nonreducible but disappears when the child wakes up from sleep is most likely to be:
a. Congenital hydrocele
b. Varicocele
c. Indirect inguinal hernia
d. None of the above

Ans. is 'a' Congenital hydrocele

54. Which of the following is not true about hydrocele?
a. Abnormal collection of serous fluid in tunica vaginalis
b. It is not possible to get above the swelling on examination of the scrotum
c. Vaginal hydrocele is associated with 5% of the inguinal hernia
d. In congenital hydrocele processus vaginalis is patent and connects to the peritoneal cavity

Ans. is 'b' It is not possible to get above the swelling on examination of the scrotum

ANATOMY OF PROSTATE

Anatomical Division

- Prostate has 5 lobes
- Anterior lobe: Is a small isthmus connecting the two lateral lobes in front of the urethra,
- Posterior lobe: It connects the two lateral lobes behind the urethra. It lies behind the median lobe and the ejaculatory ducts. Carcinomas are most common in this lobe.
- Median lobe: Lies behind the upper part of the urethra, in front of the ejaculatory ducts just below the neck of the bladder. The mucous membrane just behind the internal urethral orifice presents a slight elevation, the uvula vesicae of urinary bladder, caused by the median lobe of prostate. Benign hyperplasia of prostate arises in this lobe.
- Lateral lobes: Lie one on each side of the urethra.

Zonal or Surgical Division of Prostate

- Prostate has 3 distinct zones
- The peripheral zone (PZ)—accounts for 70% of volume of young adult prostate
- The central zone (CZ)—accounts for 25%
- The transition zone (TZ)—accounts for 5%
- Carcinoma of prostate arises most commonly in → the peripheral zone
- Benign prostatic hyperplasia originates in → the transition zone

55. Uvula vesicae is produced by which lobe of prostate? *(NEET 2019)*
a. Anterior lobe
b. Posterior lobe
c. Lateral lobe
d. Median lobe

Ans. is 'd' Median lobe

Previously Asked Facts

- Most common organism causing acute bacterial prostatitis – *E. coli*
- Commonest site of urethral opening in hypospadias is Just proximal to glans. Surgical correction of distal hypospadias is frequently undertaken before 2 years of age, often as a single stage operation.
- Radiolucent stones – Uric Acid and Xanthine.
- Content of Staghorn calculus is Ammonium magnesium Phosphate (Struvite stone)
- Radical nephrectomy involves en bloc removal of Gerota's fascia and its contents, including the kidney, the ipsilateral adrenal gland, and adjacent hilar lymph nodes.
- Carcinomas are most common in Posterior lobe. Benign Prostatic Hyperplasia arises in Median lobe.
- Carcinoma of prostate arises most commonly in Peripheral zone. Benign prostatic hyperplasia originates in Transition zone.
- Normal serum level of Prostate Specific Antigen (PSA) is <4 ng/ml.
- Elongated and constricted posterior urethra on MCU in a patient with obstructive uropathy – s/o Benign Prostatic Hyperplasia (Figure below)

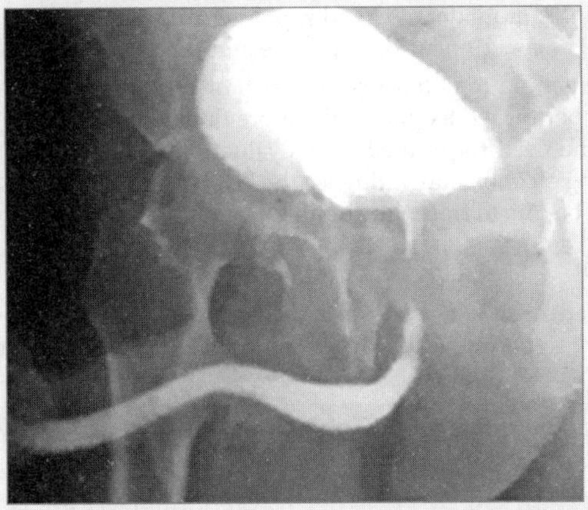

- Delayed postoperative hemorrhage is an uncommon but life-threatening complication of TURP.
- Phimosis is a condition in which the foreskin of the penis cannot be pulled back past the glans. The physiological adhesions between the foreskin and the glans penis may persist until 6 years of age or more, giving the false impression that the prepuce will not retract.
- The common metabolic complication associated with ureterosigmoidostomy is Hyperchloremic hypokalemic metabolic acidosis.
- Hunner's ulcers on cystoscopy are seen in interstitial cystitis.
- Palpable plaque with curved penis pointing to the side of plaque is a feature of Peyronie's disease.
- Bag of worms appearance in scrotum is seen in Varicoceles.
- In renal transplant, the transplant kidney is placed in the iliac fossa in the retroperitoneal position leaving the native kidneys in situ.
- CT KUB is the gold standard for imaging ureteric stones.
- Schistosoma hematobium infection of urinary bladder is a risk factor for both Transitional Cell Carcinoma and Squamous Cell Carcinoma.

TRAUMA

PRIMARY SURVEY IN TRAUMA

Primary Survey

The first and key part of the assessment of patients presenting with trauma is called the primary survey. During this time, life-threatening injuries are identified and simultaneously resuscitation is begun. A simple mnemonic, ABCDE, is used as a mnemonic for the order in which problems should be addressed.

Airway Maintenance with Cervical Spine Protection

The first stage of the primary survey is to assess the airway. If the patient is able to talk, the airway is likely to be clear. If the patient is unconscious, he/she may not be able to maintain his/her own airway. The airway can be opened using a chin lift or jaw thrust. Airway adjuncts may be required. If the airway is blocked (e.g., by blood or vomit), the fluid must be cleaned out of the patient's mouth by the help of suctioning instruments. In case of obstruction, pass an endotracheal tube.

Breathing and Ventilation

The chest must be examined by inspection, palpation, percussion and auscultation. Subcutaneous emphysema and tracheal deviation must be identified if present. The aim is to identify and manage six life-threatening thoracic conditions as Airway Obstruction, Tension Pneumothorax, Massive Haemothorax, Open Pneumothorax, Flail chest segment with Pulmonary Contusion and Cardiac Tamponade. Flail chest, tracheal deviation, penetrating injuries and bruising can be recognized by inspection. Subcutaneous emphysema can be recognized by palpation. Tension Pneumothorax and Haemothorax can be recognized by percussion and auscultation.

Circulation with Bleeding Control

Hemorrhage is the predominant cause of preventable post-injury deaths. Hypovolemic shock (low BP) is caused by significant blood loss. Two large-bore intravenous lines are established and crystalloid solution may be given. If the person does not respond to this, type-specific blood, or O-negative if this is not available, should be given. External bleeding is controlled by direct pressure. Occult blood loss may be into the chest, abdomen, pelvis or from the long bones

Disability/Neurologic Assessment

During the primary survey a basic neurological assessment is made, known by the mnemonic AVPU (alert, verbal stimuli response, painful stimuli response, or unresponsive). A more detailed and rapid neurological evaluation is performed at the end of the primary survey. This establishes the patient's level of consciousness, pupil size and reaction, lateralizing signs, and spinal cord injury level.

The Glasgow Coma Scale is a quick method to determine the level of consciousness, and is predictive of patient outcome. If not done in the primary survey, it should be performed as part of the more detailed neurologic examination in the secondary survey. An altered level of consciousness indicates the need for immediate reevaluation of the patient's oxygenation, ventilation, and perfusion status. Hypoglycemia and drugs, including alcohol, may influence the level of consciousness. If these are excluded, changes in the level of consciousness should be considered to be due to traumatic brain injury until proven otherwise.

Exposure and Environmental Control

The patient should be completely undressed, usually by cutting off the garments. It is imperative to cover the patient with warm blankets to prevent hypothermia in the emergency department. Intravenous fluids should be warmed and a warm environment maintained. Patient privacy should be maintained.

56. Which of the following is not done in primary survey of a trauma patient? *(NEET 2020)*

a. Airway assessment
b. Measuring BP
c. Exposure to look for injuries
d. Performing a CT

Ans. is 'd' Performing a CT

FOCUSSED ASSESSMENT WITH SONOGRAPHY FOR TRAUMA (FAST)

- Initial investigation for abdominal trauma
- FAST +ve – detects fluid in abdomen suggestive of hemoperitoneum
- Source of bleeding is not localized on FAST.
- IOC for abdominal trauma is CECT – To look for specific organ injury
- 4 views in FAST – Hemoperitoneum, Pericardial effusion, Hemothorax
  - Right upper quadrant
  - Left upper quadrant
  - Suprapubic view
  - Subxiphoid view of heart
- E-FAST – Extended FAST
  - + Pneumothorax
  - B/l Parasagittal chest view for pneumothorax

57. USG FAST does not involve scanning of which region from the following?

a. Pericardial
b. Pleural
c. Pelvic
d. Hepatic

Ans. is 'b' Pleural

Pericardial tamponade: Any patient with a penetrating wound to the chest, back, neck, or abdomen can develop pericardial tamponade. If the rate of bleeding is slow or the pericardium periodically decompresses by emptying blood into the pleural space, patients may initially appear stable. Some patients may complain of shortness of breath. Beck's triad (hypotension, jugular venous distension (JVD), muffled heart sounds) can be difficult to detect and may not be present. In hypovolemic patients, JVD may be absent. Ultimately, tamponade physiology causes diminished cardiac output, leading to a decrease in systolic blood pressure and a narrowing of the pulse pressure. Diagnosis should be determined rapidly by ultrasound, if immediately available.

Hemothorax: Patients with injuries to the great vessels rarely survive to reach the hospital. Survivors with a significant hemothorax have often sustained injuries to the lung parenchyma, or possibly intercostal blood vessels. Depending upon the size of the hemothorax, breath sounds are diminished and signs of shock may be present. Hemothorax often occurs concomitantly with pneumothorax and other injuries.

58. Patient with stab injury to the right lower chest presented with low pulses and BP improved after giving IV fluids. Chest X-ray showed clear lung fields. Next appropriate step in the management? *(NEET 2020)*

a. Chest tube insertion
b. CECT abdomen
c. CECT chest
d. E-FAST

Ans. is 'd' E-FAST

THORACOSCORE

Parameters of thoracoscore for predicting in-hospital mortality for patients requiring thoracic surgery.
Age (<55, 55-65, >65 years)
Sex
ASA classification (≤ 2, ≥ 3)
Performance status according to Zubrod scale (≤ 2, ≥ 3)
Severity of dyspnea according to Medical Research Council Scale (≤ 2, ≥ 3)
Priority of surgery (elective, urgent/emergency)
Extent of resection (pneumonectomy, other)
Diagnosis (malignant, benign)
Comorbidity score

(ASA: american Society of Anesthesiologists).

59. Which one of the following is not a component of THORACOSCORE? *(NEET 2020)*

a. Performance status
b. Complication of surgery
c. ASA grading
d. Priority of surgery

Ans. is 'b' Complication of surgery

CHEST TRAUMA

Traumatic Pneumothorax

- Traumatic pneumothoraxes can result from both penetrating and nonpenetrating chest trauma.
- Traumatic pneumothoraxes should be treated with tube thoracostomy unless they are very small, i.e, insertion of intercostal chest drainage tube in the 5th Intercostal space.
- If a hemopneumothorax is present, one chest tube should be placed in the superior part of the hemithorax to evacuate the air and another should be placed in the inferior part of the hemithorax to remove the blood.
- Iatrogenic pneumothorax is a type of traumatic pneumothorax that is becoming more common.
- The leading causes are transthoracic needle aspiration, thoracentesis, and the insertion of central intravenous catheters.
- Most can be managed with supplemental oxygen or aspiration, but if these measures are unsuccessful, a tube thoracostomy should be performed.

Tension Pneumothorax

- It develops when air flows into the thoracic cavity through a one-way valve mechanism, resulting in collapse of the affected lung.

Clinical Features:

- It is essentially a clinical diagnosis.
- Patient presents with sudden onset dyspnea and distended neck veins.
- Mediastinal shift to the opposite side with tracheal deviation, hyperresonance and absent breath sounds over the affected hemithorax.

Treatment:

- Treatment consists of immediate decompression by rapid insertion of a large-bore needle into 2nd intercostal space in the mid-clavicular line of the affected hemithorax.
- This is immediately followed by insertion of a chest tube through the 5th intercostal space in anterior axillary line.

Indications for Thoracotomy in Blunt Chest Trauma

- Initial drainage of blood > 1000 mL, especially if fresh
- Continued brisk bleeding > (100 mL/15 minutes) from intercostal drain
- Continued bleeding of > 200 mL/hour for > 3 hours
- Rupture of bronchus, aorta, esophagus or diaphragm
- Cardiac tamponade (if needle aspiration unsuccess).

Flail Chest

- Flail chest is a life-threatening medical condition that occurs when a segment of the rib cage breaks and becomes detached from the rest of the chest wall.
- Three of more ribs should be broken at two or more places
- The flail segment moves in the opposite direction to the rest of the chest wall.
- This so-called "paradoxical breathing" is painful and increases the work involved in breathing
- Treatment consists of oxygen administration, adequate analgesia (including opiates) and physiotherapy.

60. What is the first line of management in a case of tension pneumothorax?

a. Needle in 2nd intercostal space
b. Needle in 5th intercostal space
c. Chest drain in 2nd intercostal space
d. Chest drain in 5th intercostal space

Ans. is 'a' Needle in 2nd intercostal space

61. Indications of thoracotomy in blunt chest trauma include all *except*:

a. Initial drainage of > 500 mL of fresh blood
b. Rupture of bronchus
c. Continued bleeding of >200 mL/hour for ≥3 hours
d. Unsuccessful attempt at drainage of cardiac tamponade

Ans. is 'a' Initial drainage of > 500 mL of fresh blood

62. About Flail chest, which of the following is not true?

a. It can be life threatening
b. Three of more ribs should be broken at two or more places
c. The flail segment moves opposite to the chest wall
d. Work of breathing in not increased

Ans. is 'd' Work of breathing in not increased

The situation here refers to a case of tension pneumothorax with patient having respiratory distress, hypotension and decreased/absent breath sounds.

Patients with a tension pneumothorax may manifest tachypnea, chest pain, hypoxia, unilateral diminished or absent breath sounds, subcutaneous air, or unilateral hyper-resonance to percussion, depending on the extent of the pneumothorax. Suspected tension pneumothorax is treated with immediate tube thoracostomy or needle decompression using a large angiocatheter.

Needles as long as 7 to 8 cm may be necessary to decompress a pneumothorax, depending upon the size of the patient. Acceptable sites for needle insertion include the second or third intercostal space in the midclavicular line or the fifth intercostal space in the anterior or mid-axillary line.

63. A 20-year-old boy is brought to the emergency following a RTA with respiratory distress and hypotension. He has subcutaneous emphysema and no air entry on the right side. What is the next best step in the management? *(NEET 2020)*

a. Start IV fluids after insertion of wide bore IV line
b. Needle decompression in the 5th intercostal space
c. Shift to ICU and intubate
d. Positive pressure ventilation

Ans. is 'b' Needle decompression in the 5th intercostal space

NEUROTRAUMA

Skull Base Fractures

Clinical signs can often be used to diagnose basilar skull fractures and include the following:

- Retroauricular or mastoid ecchymosis (i.e., Battle sign) typically appears one to three days after the fracture is sustained

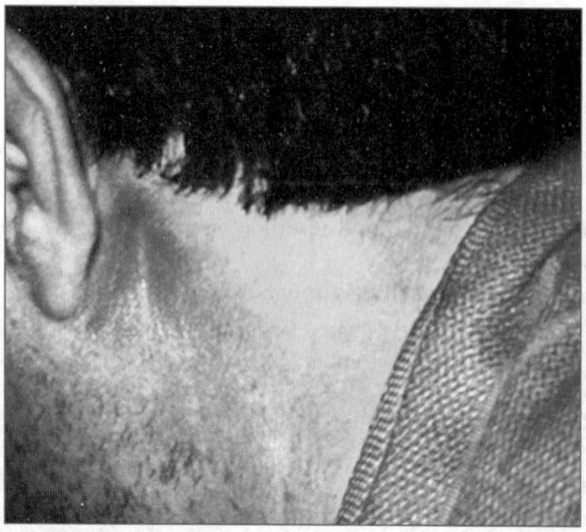

Surgery

❖ "Raccoon eyes" is a common term for periorbital ecchymosis, which suggests a basilar skull fracture or anterior or middle fossa facial trauma like Battle sign, raccoon eyes are typically **NOT** present during the examination immediately following the injury but appear one to three days later.

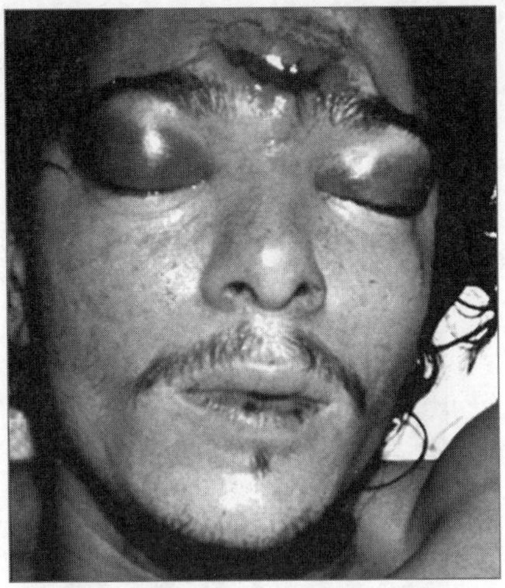

❖ Clear rhinorrhea or otorrhea is found in up to 20% of temporal bone fractures. Such leaks may be detected within hours or up to several days after trauma.

❖ Hemotympanum is blood behind the tympanic membrane. It is a common finding in basilar skull fractures that involve the petrous ridge of the temporal bone and generally appears within hours of injury

64. A person sustained injury to skull base and presented with the following sign. What is it? *(NEET 2020)*

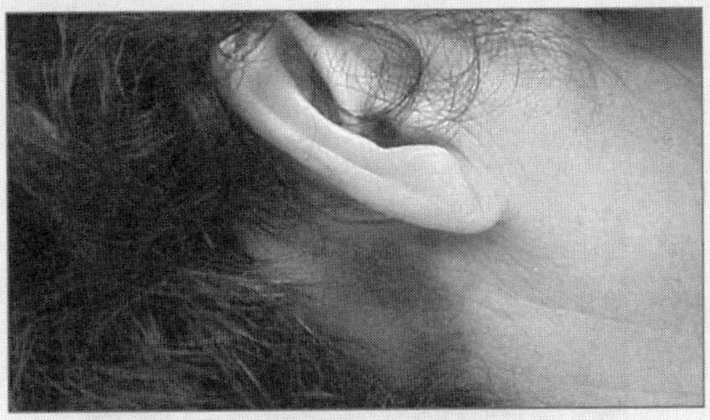

a. Battle sign
b. Bezold sign
c. Raccoon sign
d. Grisinger sign

Ans. is 'a' Battle sign

Classification of CNS Injuries

A. *Extra-axial injuries*

❖ **Extra Dural Hematoma (EDH)** – Blood between skull and dura

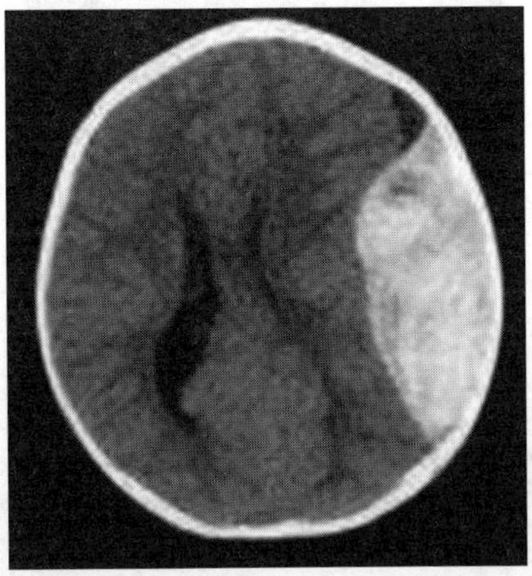

- Less common, young adults, lucid internal in approx. 50%
- Arterial (90%), Venous (10%), Associated skull fracture (90%)

- Lucid interval classically seen
- Hyperdense biconvex (Lens-Shaped) collection
- Does not cross suture line
    - Need for Surgical Intervention-
        - Thickness > 15 mm
        - Volume > 30 mL
        - Midline shift > 5 mm
        - Swirl sign on NCCT—Hypodense areas within hyperdense hematoma, represents active bleeding.

❖ **Subdural Hematoma (SDH)**

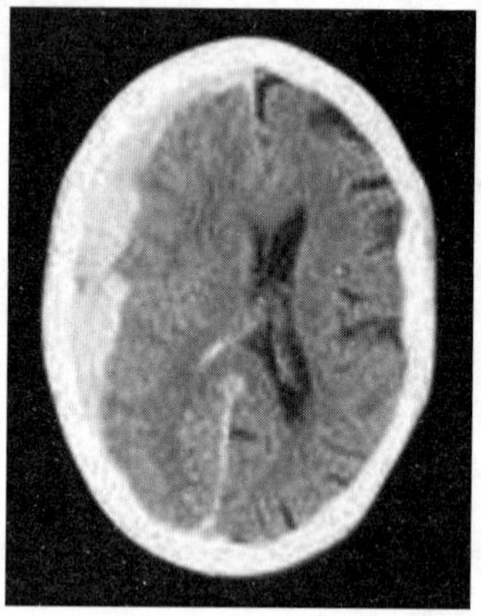

- Blood between dura and arachnoid
- Tear of bridging cortical veins
- Seen with trivial trauma in elderly
- 'Crescentic' collection of blood
- SDH cross sutures; SDH does not cross dual attachments

❖ **Traumatic subarachnoid Hemorrhage (SAH)**

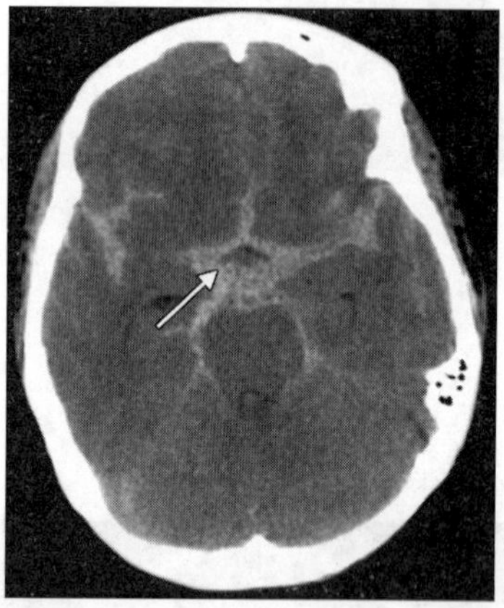

- It is the most common traumatic extra-axial injury
- Adjacent to cortical contusions
- Blood is seen more commonly in superficial sulci than basilar cisterns

B. *Intra-Axial Injuries*

❖ Cerebral contusions: Parenchymal hematoma

❖ Diffuse Axonal Injury (DAI)

- Loss of consciousness; initial imaging often minimally abnormal
- Small petechial hemorrhages at gray-white matter junction

65. Investigation of choice for SDH is:

a. NCCT b. USG

c. Doppler US d. X-ray pelvis

Ans. is 'a' NCCT

GLASGOW COMA SCALE (GCS)

Eye opening		Verbal response		Best motor response	
Spontaneous	4	Oriented	5	Obeys commands	6
To loud voice	3	Confused disoriented	4	Localizes pain	5
To pain	2	Inappropriate words	3	Flexion (withdrawal) to pain	4
No response	1	Incomprehensible sounds	2	Abnormal flexion posturing	3
		No response	1	Extension posturing	2
				No response	1

- Maximum score-15, minimum score-3
- Best predictor of outcome: Motor response
- GCS is a predictor of mortality following head trauma. Endotracheal intubation is indicated if GCS is < 8.

66. Glasgow Coma Scale of patient presenting after injury, confused, eye opening on painful stimulus, flexion withdrawal on left side and localizing to pain on right side?

a. 8 b. 9
c. 10 d. 11

Ans. is 'd' 11

STAGES OF HYPOVOLEMIC SHOCK

Initial Stage

- Decrease in Mean Arterial Pressure (MAP) of 5–10 mm Hg from baseline
- Increased sympathetic stimulation (mild vasoconstriction and tachycardia)

Compensated Reversible Stage (Non-progressive Stage)

- Decrease in MAP of 10–15 mm Hg from baseline
- Kidney and hormonal compensatory mechanisms are activated
- Continued sympathetic stimulation (moderate vasoconstriction, tachycardia)
- Renin, aldosterone and ADH secretion
- **Afferent arteriole constriction – Decreased renal blood flow – Decreased GFR and urine output**
- Mild acidosis and hyperkalemia

Decompensated Reversible Stage (Progressive Stage)

- Decrease in MAP > 20 mm Hg from baseline
- Anoxia of non-vital organs
- Hypoxia of vital organs
- Anaerobic metabolism metabolites (Acidosis, hyperkalemia)

Refractory Stage

- Severe tissue hypoxia with ischemia
- Build up of toxic metabolites
- Multiple Organ Dysfunction Syndrome (MODS)

Classification of Hemorrhagic Shock

Class of hemorrhagic stock				
	I	*II*	*III*	*IV*
Blood loss (mL)	Up to 750	750–1500	1500–2000	>2000
Blood loss (% blood volume)	Up to 15	15–30	30–40	>40
Pulse rate (per minute)	Normal	Normal	Decreased	Decreased
Pulse pressure (mm Hg)	Normal or increased	Decreased	Decreased	Decreased
Respiratory rate (per minute)	14–20	20–30	30–40	>35
Urine output (mL/hour)	>30	20–30	5–15	Negligible
Central nervous system/mental status	Slightly anxious	Mildly anxious	Anxious confused	Confused, lethargic

67. Which of the following is seen in kidney in hypovolemic shock? *(NEET 2018)*

a. Increased GFR
b. Increased renal blood flow
c. Afferent arteriole constriction
d. Increased urine output

Ans. is 'c' Afferent arteriole constriction

68. Following road traffic accident patient suffers polytrauma and is evaluated in the emergency section of the hospital. His pulse rate is 116, respiratory rate is 24, blood pressure of 122/78 mm of Hg and patient is mildly anxious. What is the approximate blood loss patient has following trauma?

a. <750 mL
b. 750–1500 mL
c. 1500–2000 mL
d. >2000 mL

Ans. is 'b' 750–1500 mL

DAMAGE CONTROL SURGERY (DCS)

- DCS centers on coordinating staged operative interventions with periods of aggressive resuscitation to salvage trauma patients sustaining major injuries.
- Damage control includes an abbreviated laparotomy, temporary packing, and closure of the abdomen in an effort to blunt the physiologic response to prolonged shock and massive hemorrhage.
- These patients are often at limits of their physiological reserve when they present to operating room and persistent operative stress results in exacerbation of their underlying hypothermia coagulopathy and acidosis, initiating a vicious cycle that culminates in death.
- In these situations, abrupt termination of the procedure after control of surgical hemorrhage and contamination, followed by ICU resuscitation and staged reconstruction, can be life saving.

Phase of Damage Control Surgery

Phase I (initial exploration)—Consists of an initial operative exploration to attain rapid control of active hemorrhage and contamination

Phase II (secondary resuscitation)—Following completion of initial exploration, critically ill patients is transferred to ICU.

Phase III (definitive operation)—It consists of planned re-exploration and definitive repair of injuries

69. Control of active hemorrhage and contamination is a part of which stage of damage control surgery?

a. I
b. II
c. III
d. IV

Ans. is 'b' II

VASCULAR SURGERY

INTERMITTENT CLAUDICATION

Intermittent: Pain within a defined group of muscles that is induced by exercise and relieved with rest defines classic intermittent claudication (derived from the Latin word for limp). It is a symptom of peripheral vascular disease.

Classic symptoms of claudication manifest as exertional leg pain that begins after a certain walking distance, causes the patient to stop walking, and resolves within 10 minutes of rest, allowing the patient to resume walking again, typically for the same distance after which the pain recurs. Claudication can present unilaterally or bilaterally, as buttock and hip, thigh, calf, or foot pain, singly or in combination. The usual relationships between pain location and corresponding anatomic site of PAD are as follows:

- *Buttock and hip claudication*: Patients with aortoiliac disease may complain of buttock, hip, and, in some cases, thigh claudication. The pain is often described as aching in nature and may be associated with weakness of the hip or thigh with walking. Pulses in one or both groins are diminished. Bilateral aortoiliac PAD that is severe enough to cause lower extremity symptoms almost always causes erectile dysfunction in men. Leriche syndrome is the triad of claudication, absent or diminished femoral pulses, and erectile dysfunction.
- *Thigh claudication*: Atherosclerotic occlusion of the common femoral artery may induce claudication in the thigh, calf, or both. Patients with disease isolated to the superficial femoral or popliteal arteries have normal groin pulses but decreased pulses distally.
- *Calf claudication*: **Calf claudication is the most common complaint**. It is usually described as escalating pain that is consistently reproduced with exercise and relieved with rest. Pain in the upper two-thirds of the calf is usually due to superficial femoral artery stenosis, whereas pain in the lower third of the calf is due to popliteal disease.
- *Foot claudication*: Claudication of the foot is usually accompanied by occlusive disease of the tibial and peroneal vessels. Isolated foot claudication is uncommon with PAD.

70. True statement about intermittent claudication: *(NEET 2020)*

a. Maximum at rest
b. Most common site is the calf
c. Claudication distance can vary from day to day in the same person
d. Relieved after getting out of bed and walking

Ans. is 'b' Most common site is the calf

AORTO-ILIAC OBSTRUCTION

Buttock and hip claudication: Patients with aortoiliac disease may complain of buttock, hip, and, in some cases, thigh claudication. The pain is often described as aching in nature and may be associated with weakness of the hip or thigh with walking. Pulses in one or both groins are diminished. Bilateral aortoiliac PAD that is severe enough to cause lower extremity symptoms almost always causes erectile dysfunction in men. Leriche syndrome is the triad of claudication, absent or diminished femoral pulses, and erectile dysfunction.

71. A 30-year-old man presents with cramping gluteal pain and pain in the leg after walking 500 meter. Which is the vessel involved? *(NEET 2020)*

a. Arterial disease with aorto-iliac involvement
b. Arterial disease with femoral artery involvement
c. Femoral venous insufficiency
d. Sciatic nerve compression

Ans. is 'a' Arterial disease with aorto-iliac involvement

DEEP VENOUS THROMBOSIS (DVT)

Acute unilateral or asymmetric edema: It is essential to consider the diagnosis of deep venous thrombosis (DVT) in patients with acute unilateral or asymmetric leg edema. In addition to edema, patients with a DVT can have calf tenderness, pain or firmness along the course of a vein, or unilateral warmth or erythema. A larger calf circumference in the affected leg is the most useful finding, whereas Homans' sign (calf pain upon passive dorsiflexion of the foot) is **not** a reliable sign of DVT. The findings of DVT may be subtle; patients may present with only unilateral or asymmetric edema.

72. A middle-aged pregnant female, with history of HTN, DM and cardiac bypass from coastal region of india, presented with nontender swelling in left lower limb. Which of the following investigations should be performed? *(NEET 2020)*

a. Venous Doppler
b. CT pelvis
c. 2D echo
d. Midnight blood samples for microscopy

Ans. is 'a' Venous Doppler

LYMPHEDEMA

Chronic unilateral or asymmetric edema: The most common cause of chronic unilateral or asymmetric edema is lower extremity chronic venous disease. Less common causes include primary or secondary lymphedema, a pelvic neoplasm compromising venous return, and complex regional pain syndrome.

- *Chronic venous disease*: There may be an antecedent history of thrombophlebitis in the affected leg. If the edema is longstanding, it often leads to characteristic pigmentary changes and skin ulceration
- *Lymphedema*: Patients with lymphedema may have a history of an ipsilateral inguinal or pelvic lymph node dissection, or of radiation therapy. The edema is initially pitting, but becomes non-pitting as cutaneous fibrosis occurs.
- *Complex regional pain syndrome*: Complex regional pain syndrome usually occurs four to six weeks after limb trauma, and is characterized by pain, edema, and alteration in skin color and temperature.
- A neoplasm should be suspected when CUS is suggestive of pelvic outflow obstruction, particularly in patients with a history of cancer or concerning symptoms such as unexplained weight loss. If a neoplasm is suspected, imaging of the pelvis should be obtained.

The presence of lymphedema is usually suggested by the following findings:

- The edema is typically localized and characterized by slowly progressive ipsilateral (unilateral) swelling of an upper extremity following axillary node dissection or lower extremity following inguinal node dissection
- *A history of cancer treatment or trauma*: Cancer treatments include surgery, lymph node dissection or removal (e.g., axillary, inguinal lymph nodes), and radiation therapy.
- The absence of a cause of generalized edema (e.g., heart failure, nephrotic syndrome)
- The presence of cutaneous and subcutaneous thickening, which is seen in severe lymphedema
- Nonpitting edema is suggestive of lymphedema; however, the presence of pitting does **not** exclude lymphedema, since, as noted above, pitting is present in early stages of lymphedema.

73. A patient presents with unilateral long standing progressive swelling of left lower limb which is more in proximal part compared to distal. There is nonpitting edema. What is the diagnosis? *(NEET 2020)*

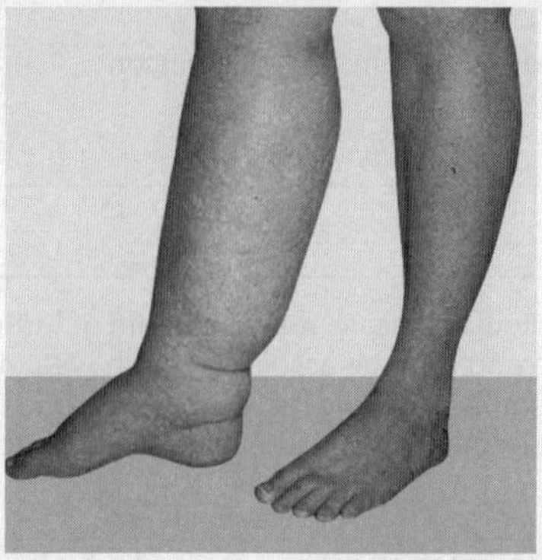

a. Arterial insufficiency
b. Venous insufficiency
c. Lymphedema
d. Congestive heart failure

Ans. is 'c' Lymphedema

WELL'S CRITERIA

Well's criteria and modified Well's criteria: Clinical assessment for pulmonary embolism	
• Clinical symptoms of DVT (leg swelling, pain with palpation)	3.0
• Other diagnosis less likely than pulmonary embolism	3.0
• Heart rate >100	1.5
• Immobilization (≥ 3 days) or surgery in the previous four weeks	1.5
• Previous DVT/PE	1.5
• Hemoptysis	1.0
• Malignancy	1.0
Probability	Score
Traditional clinical probability assessment (Well's criteria)	
High	>6.0
Moderate	2.0 to 6.0
Low	<2.0
Simplified clinical probability assessment (Modified Well's criteria)	
PE likely	>4.0
PE unlikely	≤4.0

74. A patient presented with dyspnea, palpitation and tachyacardia with HR 120 bpm. She has a unilateral tender leg swelling and she is a known case of ovarian malignancy. What is the risk of pulmonary embolism in this patient? *(NEET 2020)*

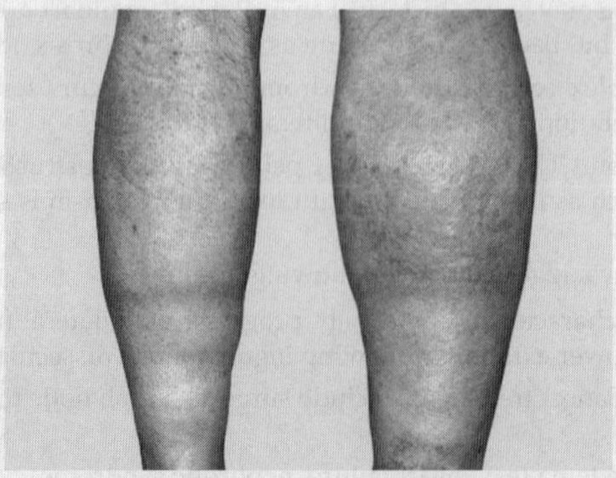

a. High
b. Moderate
c. Low
d. Cannot be assessed

Ans. is 'a' High

MANAGEMENT OF ABDOMINAL AORTIC ANEURYSM

Conservative/Medical Treatment

- It is done in low-risk abdominal aortic aneurysm (age below 70 years; active physically without cardiac, respiratory, renal impairment and noninflammatory aneurysm); if aneurysm size is < 5 cm; if growth rate is < 0.5 cm/year)
- It includes risk factor modifications; cessation of smoking; control of blood pressure, cholesterol.
- Periodic size measurement of an aneurysm using ultrasound once in 6 months to find out growth rate is essential during conservative treatment

Surgical Treatment: Indications for surgery are:

- Asymptomatic aneurysm more than 5.5 cm
- Growth rate more than 0.5 cm/year
- Painful, tender aneurysm
- Thrombosed aneurysm, aneurysm with distal emboli.

75. Asymptomatic aortic aneurysm is to be operated when diameter is more than:

a. 55 mm
b. 75 mm
c. 50 mm
d. 60 mm

Ans. is 'a' 55 mm

Elective abdominal aortic aneurysm (AAA) repair is the most effective management to prevent rupture. However, elective aortic surgery is associated with risks, and thus, elective AAA repair is not recommended until the risk of rupture exceeds the risks associated with repair (anesthetic risk, technique-related risks). For asymptomatic patients, randomized trials comparing observation with open or endovascular AAA repair have found that the risk of AAA rupture generally does not exceed the risk associated with elective AAA repair until aneurysm diameter exceeds 5.5 cm. We agree with guidelines from the Society for Vascular Surgery that recommend observation for asymptomatic AAA <5.5 cm in diameter based upon these trials.

Although repair may not be warranted in patients with AAA diameter < 5.5 cm, these patients remain at risk for aneurysm expansion. As such, management consists of ongoing clinical evaluation and AAA surveillance, and risk modification.

76. Male patient with hypertension presents to the hospital with abdominal pain and is incidentally detected with an abdominal aortic aneurysm. What is the appropriate management of this patient? *(NEET 2020)*

a. Immediate surgery
b. USG monitoring till size of the aneurysm reaches 70 mm
c. Elective surgery after size reaches 55 mm
d. Conservative management

Ans. is 'c' Elective surgery after size reaches 55 mm

GRAFTS IN VASCULAR SURGERY

- Autologous saphenous vein achieves superior patency rates than prosthetic materials, especially in femorodistal bypass.
- In situ and reversed vein graft bypasses perform equally well and the choice of technique should be based upon anatomical considerations that are specific to individual patients.
- The patency of PTFE grafts may be improved by interposition of a vein cuff at the distal anastomosis
- Patency rates associated with pre-cuffed PTFE grafts are comparable to that obtained from standard PTFE grafts with an interposed vein cuff.
- Doppler ultrasound assessment is the method of choice for quality assurance on completion of the operative procedure.
- In the absence of specific contraindications, aspirin should be prescribed for all patients with peripheral vascular disease whether or not they are treated by an operative intervention. Clopidogrel may be prescribed in those with sensitivity to aspirin and those at particularly high risk of graft failure or other adverse cardiovascular event
- Controversy remains regarding routine postoperative duplex surveillance of autologous vein grafts. Present evidence does not support routine surveillance of prosthetic bypass grafts.

77. Which of the following is not true about use of graft in vascular surgery?

a. Autologous saphenous vein achieves superior patency rates to prosthetic materials especially in femorodistal bypass
b. The patency of the PTFE grafts may be improved by interposition of a vein cuff a proximal anastomosis
c. Doppler ultrasound assessment is the method of choice for quality assurance on completion of operative procedure
d. In the absence of specific contraindications aspirin should be prescribed for all the patients of peripheral vascular disease

Ans. is 'b' The patency of the PTFE grafts may be improved by interposition of a vein cuff a proximal anastomosis

VENOUS LEG ULCERS

- Venous disease is responsible for between 60% and 70% of all ulcers in the lower leg.
- Venous ulcers occur secondary to superficial venous incompetence or deep venous thrombosis.
- The venous ulcer of the leg characteristically develops in the skin of the gaiter region, the area between the muscles of the calf and the ankle. This is the region where many of the Cockett perforators join the posterior tibial vein to the surface vein, known as the posterior arch vein. The majority of ulcers develop on the medial side of the calf.
- Venous ulcers rarely extend on to the foot or into the upper calf and, if there is ulceration at these sites, other diagnoses should be seriously considered
- Almost all venous ulcers have surrounding lipodermatosclerosis—thickening, pigmentation, inflammation and induration of the calf skin.

Management of Venous Leg Ulcers

- When the diagnosis of a 'probable venous ulcer' has been made, patients are initially treated by a compression bandaging regimen. A low-compression regimen is desirable for mixed venous/arterial ulcers.
- The alternative to these bandaging regimens is to apply a bland absorbent leak-proof dressing beneath a graduated elastic compression stocking
- These compression regimens are ideally applied by trained staff on a weekly basis until the ulcer is starting to heal and the amount of exudate is reduced.
- Antibiotics do not speed ulcer healing and all other specific ulcer-healing drugs are of dubious validity.
- A number of biological dressings have been developed, including fetal keratinocytes and collagen meshes, which have been shown to improve healing.
- Failure to heal an ulcer may indicate another cause (e.g. malignancy, rheumatoid arthritis or arterial ischemia).

78. Characteristic site for development of venous leg ulcers is:

a. Skin of gaiter region
b. Behind lateral malleolus
c. Shin of tibia
d. Medial aspect of knee

Ans. is 'a' Skin of gaiter region

79. Which of the following is true about the management of venous ulcer of lower limb?

a. Initial treatment is debridement and surgery
b. Compression dressings should ideally be applied on twice weekly basis
c. Antibiotics dressings do not have potential to improve healing
d. Biological dressings do not have potential to improve healing

Ans. is 'c' Antibiotics dressings do not have potential to improve healing

BURNS

Burn depth classification

Depth	Histology	Appearance	Sensation	Healing
First degree	Epidemis only	Erythema, blanches with pressure	Intact, mild to moderate pain	3–6 days without scarring
Second degree • Superficial	Epidemis and superficial dermis, skin appendages intact	Erythema, blisters, moist elastic; blanches with pressure	Intact, severe pain	1–3 weeks, scarring unusual
• Deep	Epidermis and most dermis, most skin appendages destroyed	White appearing with erythematous areas, dry, waxy, less elastic, reduced blanching to pressure	Decreased; may be less painful	>3 weeks, often with scarring and contracture
Third degree	Epidermis and all of dermis; destruction of all skin appendages	White charred, tan, thrombosed vessels; dry and leathery; does not blanch	Anesthetic, not painful (although surrounding areas of second-degree burns are painful	Does not heal, severe scarring and contractures

Adult body		Child body	
Part	***BSA***	***Part***	***BSA***
Arm	9%	Arm	9%
Head and neck	9%	Head and neck	18%
Leg	18%	Leg	14%
Anterior trunk	18%	Anterior trunk	18%
Posterior trunk	18%	Posterior trunk	18%
Perineum	1%		

Fluid Resuscitation in Burns

Parkland formula

Volume of Ringer's lactate = 4 mL × %BSA × weight (kg)

1/2 → First 8 hours

1/2 → Next 16 hours

There are three types of fluids used. The most common is Ringer's lactate

Others: Human albumin solution or fresh-frozen plasma, and hypertonic saline.

Only **area covered by second-degree burns or greater is taken into consideration**, as first-degree burn does not cause hemodynamically significant fluid shift to warrant fluid replacement.

The thermal injury leads to a massive fluid shift from intravascular compartment to the extravascular compartment (interstitial + intracellular) leading to edema formation; maximum in first 24 hours.

Management of Burns

Degree of burn	Management
First	Topical soothing agents, leaves wound open
Superficial second (partial thickness)	Needs daily dressing
Deep second	Excision and grafting
Third full thickness	Escharotomy and serial excision with grafting

❖ Most common immediate cause of death in burn patients is Multi-organ failure.

80. Dermoepidermal burn is what degree of burn?

a. I
b. II
c. III
d. IV

Ans. is 'b' II

81. Which of the following is not true about resuscitation in burns patient?

a. Ringer's lactate is the preferred crystalloid solution
b. Fluid shift from intravascular to extravascular compartment in the burns patient is maximum in the first 24 hours
c. Quantity of crystalloid needed is calculated using the Parkland formula - 6 mL/kg body weight per % of the total body surface area burnt
d. Target means arterial pressure in resuscitation is 60 mm Hg

Ans. is 'c' Quantity of crystalloid needed is calculated using the parkland formula - 6 mL/kg body weight per % of the total body surface area burnt

82. A 50-kg-man having 40% second degree burns. How much fluid will be needed in first 8 hours?

a. 8 liters
b. 4 liters
c. 2 liters
d. 6 liters

Ans. is 'b' 4 litres

Previously Asked Facts

- Duret hemorrhage is secondary midline hemorrhage resulting from rapid asymmetrical herniation of brainstem downwards; involves midbrain and pons, never the medulla.
- Most common cause of sub-arachnoid hemorrhage is trauma.
- Most common abdominal organ involved in penetrating trauma is small intestine. Most commonly injured abdominal organ in blunt trauma is Spleen.
- Compartment syndrome is confirmed when intracompartmental pressure is more than 40 mm Hg.
- Best graft for femoropopliteal bypass is Reverse saphenous vein graft. Saphenous vein is reversed to nullify the action of valves so as to allow easy flow of blood.
- Allen's test detects adequacy of the blood supply to the hand from the radial and ulnar arteries and the arcade between them.
- Glomus tumor arises from modified smooth muscle cells.
- Cardinal rule for dressing of pressure ulcer is to keep ulcer tissue moist and surrounding intact tissue dry.
- The treatment of air embolism is to put the patient in a head-down (Trendelenburg) position to encourage the air to enter the veins in the lower part of the body. The patient should also be placed on the left side to help the air to float to the ventricular apex, away from the ostium of the pulmonary artery.
- The most commonly used myocutaneous pedicle graft for pelvis surgeries contains muscle segments from Rectus abdominis muscle.
- Full thickness skin graft (Wolfes graft)—it includes all epidermis and dermis; Partial thickness skin graft (Thiersch graft)—it includes all epidermis and part of dermis.

MISCELLANEOUS

NECK SWELLINGS

83. Middle-aged man with a swelling over the neck since childhood. Neck swelling has a bag of worm appearance and palpable thrill and audible bruit. Diagnosis? *(NEET 2020)*

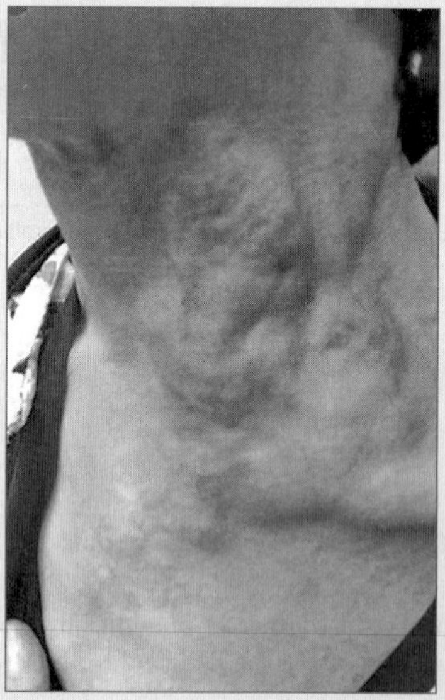

a. Cricoid aneurysm
b. Toxic nodular goiter
c. Varicocele
d. Neurofibroma

Ans. is 'a' Cricoid aneurysm

Explanation: Neurofibromas do have a bag of worms appearance and childhood presentation—but site is face and less likely to be neck. Also bruit and thrill are uncommon findings in NF palpable thrill, bruit and bag of worms appearance are suggestive of vascular pathology. So our differentials are narrowed to cricoid aneurysm and varicocele. Neck varix are unlikely to present since childhood and are relatively rare finding (varicocele technically is a scrotal pathology—but lets consider here in broad sense as varix). Cricoids (or crisoid) aneurysm can present as AVM since childhood with progressive growth. Hence the most probable diagnosis here. (Note—controversial)

MALIGNANT MELANOMA

Superficial spreading melanoma	Nodular melanoma	Lentigo maligna melanoma	Acral lentiginous melanoma
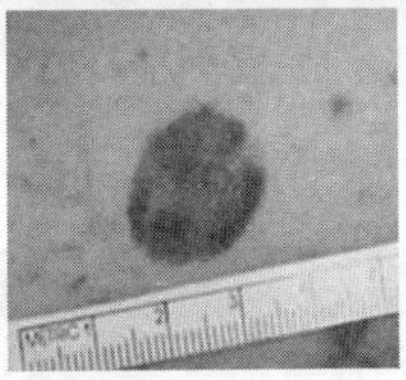	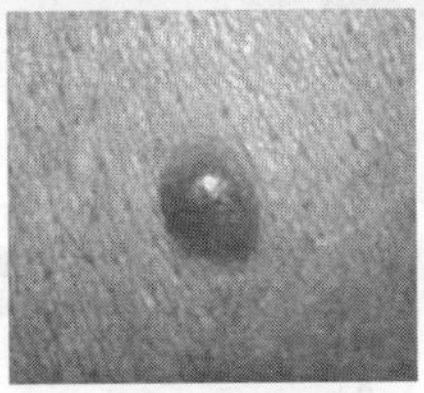	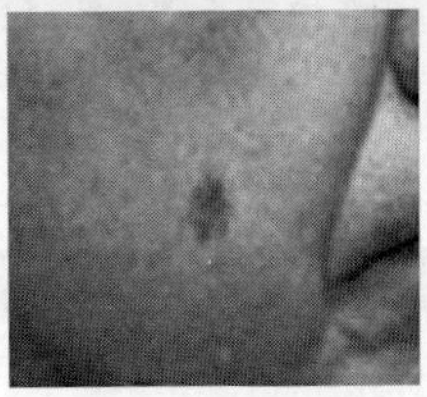	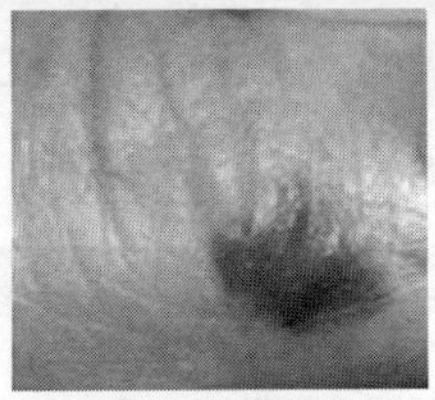
• Most Common • Flat and irregular in shape and color • Shades of black and brown	• Usually starts as a raised area • Dark black/blue or bluish/red • Some are not colored	• Usually occurs in older skin types • Commonly on face, neck, arms, etc • Abnormal skin areas usually large, flat, and tan with areas of brown	• Least common • Usually found on palms, soles, and even under fingernails

Superficial spreading melanoma: Superficial spreading melanoma is the most common histologic subtype, accounting for approximately 70% of all melanomas.

Lentigomaligna melanoma most commonly arises in chronically **sun-damaged areas** of the skin in older individuals and begins as a tan or brown macule. The lesion gradually enlarges over years and may develop darker, asymmetric foci of pigmentation, color variegation, and raised areas that signify vertical growth within the precursor in situ melanoma, which is termed "lentigomaligna".

84. A farmer presented with a black mole on the cheek. It increased in size, more than 6 mm with sharply defined borders with central pigmentation, what could be the diagnosis? *(NEET 2020)*

a. Superficial spreading melanoma
b. Lentigomaligna
c. Acral melanoma
d. Nodular melanoma

Ans. is 'b' Lentigomaligna

FROSTBITE

Rewarming: Rewarming is most effectively accomplished by immersing the affected area in water heated to 37 to 39°C (98.6 to 102.2°F), ideally in a whirlpool so a steady temperature can be maintained. Gentle active motion of the extremity while rewarming may help. Care should also be taken to avoid trauma to the injured area against the container walls during treatment. Higher temperatures do not warm the injured area appreciably faster and cause the warming process to be much more painful. Dry heat is difficult to regulate and is not recommended.

Thawing is usually complete when the tissue is red or purple and soft to the touch. This usually takes 15 to 30 minutes. Rewarming of frostbitten tissue may be painful. Appropriate analgesia, generally opioids, should be administered.

85. What is the temperature of water bath used for rewarming of a frostbite injury? *(NEET 2020)*

a. 37 degrees
b. 32 degrees
c. 42 degrees
d. 46 degrees

Ans. is 'c' 42 degrees

TYPE OF NECK DISSECTION

Classical Radical Neck Dissection (Crile)

- Involves resection of the cervical lymphatics and lymph nodes (level I to level V) and those structures closely associated: the internal jugular vein, the accessory nerve, the submandibular gland, sternocleidomastoid muscle, tail of the parotid and omohyoid muscle. These structures are all removed en bloc and in continuity with the primary disease if possible.
- The main disability that follows the operation is weakness and drooping of the shoulder due to paralysis of the trapezius muscle as a consequence of excision of the accessory nerve.
- Structures spared are: Carotid artery, Brachial plexus, phrenic nerve, vagus nerve, cervical sympathetic chain, marginal mandibular branch of facial, lingual and hypoglossal nerve.

Modified Radical Neck Dissection

- One or more of the three following structures are preserved: the accessory nerve, the sternocleidomastoid muscle or the internal jugular vein. Otherwise, all major lymph node groups and lymphatics are excised; i.e. level I to level V nodes.

Selective Neck Dissection

- One or more of the major lymph node groups is preserved along with the sternocleidomastoid muscle, accessory nerve and internal jugular vein.

86. Modified radical neck dissection includes which level of cervical lymph nodes?

a. I–III
b. I–IV
c. I–V
d. I–VII

Ans. is 'c' I-V

ASEPSIS SCORE

ASEPSIS wound score	Proportion of wound affected					
Wound characteristic	0	<20	20–39	40–59	60–79	>80
Serous exudate	0	1	2	3	4	5
Erythema	0	1	2	3	4	5
Purulent exudate	0	2	4	6	8	10
Separation of deep tissues	0	2	4	6	8	10
Points are scored for daily wound inspection.						
Criterion	**Points**					
Additional treatment: Antibiotics	10					
Drainage of pus under local anaesthesia	5					
Debridement of wound (general anaesthesia)	10					
Serous discharge*	daily 0–5					
Erythema*	daily 0–5					
Purulent exudate*	daily 0–10					
Separation of deep tissues*	daily 0–10					
Isolation of bacteria	10					
Stay as inpatient prolonged over 14 day	5					
*Given score only on five of seven days. Highest weekly score used Category of infection: Total score 0–10 = satisfactory healing; 11–20 = disturbance of healing: 20–30 = minor wound infection; 31–40 = moderate wound infection: >40 = severe wound infection.						

87. All of the following are part of ASEPSIS score *except*: *(NEET 2020)*

a. Serous discharge
b. Induration
c. Erythema
d. Isolation of bacteria

Ans. is 'b' Induration

CLASSIFICATION OF SURGICAL WOUNDS

Clean Wounds (Class I)

- Include those in which no infection is present; only skin microflora potentially contaminates the wound. No hollow visçus is entered. No inflammation
- Examples: Hernia repair, breast biopsy.

Clean/contaminated Wounds (Class II)

- Include those in which a hollow viscus such as the respiratory, alimentary or genitourinary tracts with indigenous bacterial flora is opened, but under controlled circumstances without significant spillage of contents. No inflammation.
- Examples: Cholecystectomy, elective GI surgery.

Contaminated Wounds (Class III)

- Include open accidental wounds encountered early after injury, those with extensive introduction of bacteria into a normally sterile area of the body due to major breaks in sterile technique (e.g. open cardiac massage); uncontrolled spillage of viscus contents such as from the intestine. Inflammation is apparent
- Examples: Penetrating abdominal trauma, large tissue injury.

Dirty Wounds (Class IV)

- Include traumatic wounds in which a significant delay in treatment has occurred and in which necrotic tissue is present; includes wounds in which pus is present. Includes those wounds created to access a perforated viscus accompanied by a high degree of contamination. Severe inflammation is seen.
- Examples: Perforated diverticulitis, necrotizing fasciitis.

88. Elective surgery in which a hollow viscus is opened, what is the class of surgical wound?

a. I
b. II
c. III
d. IV

Ans. is 'b' II

BARIATRIC SURGERY

- Procedures include:
  - Vertical banded gastroplasty
  - Adjustable gastric banding
  - Roux-en Y gastric bypass
  - Biliopancreatic diversion
  - Duodenal switch
- Indications for bariatric surgery
  - BMI > 40
  - BMI > 35 with serious comorbid conditions
  - Acceptable operative candidate
  - Motivated to adhere to the postoperative lifestyle changes
  - Well informed regarding risks of surgery
  - Able to participate in long-term follow-up
  - No substance abuse issues
  - No (or under control) significant psychiatric conditions

89. Indication for bariatric surgery:

a. BMI ≥40
b. BMI ≥35
c. In drug addicts
d. All of the above

Ans. is 'a' BMI ≥40

TRANSPLANTATION TERMINOLOGY

- *Autograft*: Tissue transplanted from one part of the body to another in the same individual. Also called an autotransplant
- *Isograft*: Is a graft of tissue between two individuals who are genetically identical (i.e. monozygotic twins). Transplant rejection between two such individuals virtually never occurs.
- *Allograft*: An organ or tissue transplanted from one individual to another.

90. Renal transplantation, in which mother acts as a donor of one kidney to her son is an example of: *(NEET 2019)*

a. Autograft
b. Heterograft
c. Allograft
d. Xenograft

Ans. is 'c' Allograft

LIVER TRANSPLANT

Common Indications

- Cirrhosis with end stage liver disease and decompensation
- Hepatocellular carcinoma / Hepatoblastoma in children
- Alcoholic Liver Disease
- *Hepatitis*: Autoimmune, chronic hepatitis B and C
- *Cholestatic diseases*: Primary biliary cirrhosis, Primary sclerosing cholangitis, Biliary atresia
- *Metabolic diseases*: Hemochromatosis, Wilson disease
- *Fulminant hepatic failure*: Viral/toxin/drug induced
- *Others*: Hepatic venous outflow tract obstruction, Polycystic liver disease

  Most common indication for liver transplant in children is—Biliary atresia

91. Most common indication for liver transplant in children is: *(NEET 2019)*

a. Biliary atresia
b. Cirrhosis
c. Hepatitis
d. Drug reactions

Ans. is 'a' Biliary atresia

KING'S COLLEGE CRITERIA

King's College criteria for liver transplantation in acute liver failure

Paracetamol	Non-paracetamol
pH < 7.3* or	Prothrombin time greater than 100 s (INR > 16.5) (irrespective of grade of encephalopathy) or any three of the following
Arterial lactate > 3.5 mmoL at 4 h or Arterial lactate > 3.0 mmoL/L at 12 h* or	1. Age less than 11 years or greater than 40 years 2. Aetiology of non-A/non-B hepatitis, halothane hepatitis, or idiosyncratic drug reactions
PT >100 s (INR > **6.5)**	3. Duration of jaundice of more than 7 days before onset of encephalopathy
Serum creatinine > 300 mmoL/1 (3. 4 mg/dL)	4. Prothrombin time greater than 50 s (INR >3.5)
Grade 3 or 4 encephalopathy	5. Serum bilirubin level greater than 17 mg/dL (300 μmol/L)

Adapted (with permission) from O'Grady, et al and Bernal, et al.
*After fluid resuscitation. INR, international normalised ratio.

92. A 5-year-old-child with acute liver failure due to Wilson disease. Which one of the following criteria are not included in the King's college criteria? *(NEET 2020)*

a. Age <10 years
b. INR >6.5
c. Bilirubin >17 mg/dL
d. Jaundice <7 days before development of encephalopathy

Ans. is 'd' Jaundice <7 days before development of encephalopathy

CTP SCORING

Child-Pugh Classification of Severity of Cirrhosis

	Points assigned		
Parameter	1	2	3
Ascites	Absent	Slight	Moderate
Bilirubin	< 2 mg/dL (< 34.2 micromol/L)	2 to 3 mg/dL (34.2 to 51.3 micromol/L)	> 3 mg/dL (> 51.3 micromol/L)
Albumin	> 3.5 g/dL (35 g/L)	2.8 to 3.5 g/dL (28 to 35 g/L)	< 2.8 g/dL (<28 g/L)
Prothrombin time			
Seconds over control	< 4	4 to 6	> 6
INR	< 1.7	1.7 to 2.3	> 2.3
Encephalopathy	None	Grade 1 to 2	Grade 3 to 4

Modified child-Pugh classification of the severity of liver disease according to the degree of ascites, the serum concentrations of bilirubin and albumin, the prothrombin time, and the degree of encephalopathy. A total Child-Turcotte-Pugh score of 5 to 6 is considered Child-Pugh class A (well-compensated disease); 7 to 9 is class B (significant functional compromise); and 10 to 15 is class C (decompensated disease). These classes correlate with one-and two-year patient survival: class A: 100 and 85%; class B: 80 and 60%; and class C: 45 and 35%.

93. A patient presented with encephalopathy grade 1-2, mild ascites, S.bilirubin 2.5 mg%, S.albumin<2.8 gm% and INR of 2.3. What is the Child-Turcotte-Pugh class of this patient? *(NEET 2020)*

a. CTP A
b. CTP B
c. CTP C
d. CTP D

Ans. is 'c' CTP C

VENTRAL WALL DEFECTS

❖ Developmental defects due to failure of rostral fold closure (e.g., sternal defects [ectopia cordis)), lateral fold closure (e.g., omphalocele, gastroschisis), or caudal fold closure (e.g., bladder exstrophy)

	Gastroschisis	Omphalocele
Etiology	Extrusion of abdominal contents through abdominal folds (typically right of umbilicus)	Failure of lateral walls to migrate at umbilical ring - persistent mid line herniation of abdominal contents into umbilical cord
Covering	Not covered by peritoneum or amnion	Surrounded by peritoneum (light gray shiny sac)
Associations	Not associated with chromosome abnormalities	Associated with congenital anomalies (e.g., trisomies 13 and 18, Beckwith-Wiedemann syndrome) and other structural abnormalities (e.g., cardiac, GU, neural tube)

Congenital Umbilical Hernia: Failure of umbilical ring to close after physiologic herniation of the intestines. Small defects usually close spontaneously.

94. Omphalocele is caused by: *(NEET 2019)*

a. Duplication of intestinal loops
b. Abnormal rotation of intestinal loops
c. Failure of gut to return to the body cavity after its physiological herniation
d. Reversed rotation of intestinal loops

Ans. is 'c' Failure of gut to return to the body cavity after its physiological herniation

Previously Asked Facts

- Transsphenoidal surgical resection is the preferred primary treatment for both microadenomas and macroadenomas. Transsphenoidal surgery + craniotomy is done for large tumors with suprasellar extension.
- Hyperventilation is used as a treatment in patients with raised intracranial pressure.
- Presence of Beta 2 - transferrin is the most definitive test for detection of CSF rhinorrhea.
- Hyponatremia is the most common electrolyte abnormality seen after head injury. Other Electrolyte disorders including hypernatremia, hypokalemia, hyperkalemia, hypophosphatemia and hypomagnesemia are also seen.
- Most common site for berry aneurysm in circle of Willis is seen at bifurcation between Anterior communicating artery and anterior cerebral artery.
- Salivary gland stone is most common in submandibular gland.
- Most of the sebaceous cysts are found on the hairy parts of the body. There are no sebaceous glands on the palms of the hands and soles of the feet, thus sebaceous cysts are not found here.
- Treatment of choice of cystic hygroma is: Complete surgical excision > Injection sclerotherapy
- Pleomorphic adenoma is the most common benign tumor of the salivary glands. It is the most common tumor of the parotid, submandibular and sublingual glands. Most common tumor of minor salivary glands are Adenoid cystic Ca and mucoepidermoid Ca.
- Common symptom of zygoma fracture is numbness on the cheek due to damage to the infraorbital nerve.
- LAHSAL code is used to represent congenital malformation of Lip, Alveolus and Hard palate.
- Killian's incision is used for submucous resection of nasal septum.
- For melanoma <1 mm deep, wide local excision with a 1 cm margin is sufficient. For deeper lesions, a 2 cm margin is recommended.
- The diagnosis of carcinoid syndrome relies on measurement of urinary or plasma serotonin or its metabolites in the urine. The measurement of 5-HIAA is used most frequently. Serum chromogranin A levels are not specific for carcinoid tumors. Plasma neuron specific enolase levels are also used as a marker of carcinoid tumors but are less sensitive than chromogranin A.
- Embolic materials commonly used for trans-arterial tumor embolization: Gelatin sponge particles, Microspheres, Autologous blood clots, Polyvinyl alcohol, N- butylcyanoacrylate (glue), Absolute ethanol.
- Most common site for penile carcinoma is Glans.
- Gleason score is used for Prostate carcinoma.
- Best investigation for carcinoma head of pancreas is FNAC by endoscopic ultrasound.
- Drug of choice for palliative treatment of pancreatic carcinoma is Gemcitabine.
- CT is the imaging modality of choice for evaluating liver metastases.
- Management plan for locally advanced (local bone invasion) tongue carcinomas includes subtotal glossectomy + selective neck dissection + mandibulectomy. Selective neck dissection is advisable for all oral tongue cancers as these patients have early lymph node involvement.
- Colonoscopy with biopsy of suspect lesions is the gold standard test for establishing the diagnosis of Ca colon.
- Slip sign is seen in Lipomas. When the edge of the swelling is pressed a finger the edge along with the swelling slips away from the palpating finger.
- Prostate, breast, and lung primaries account for 80% of all bone metastases.
- For noncolorectal, nonneuroendocrine tumors, metastases from genitourinary primaries have the best prognosis following hepatic metastasectomy.
- Hoarseness of voice in lung carcinoma is due to invasion of Recurrent laryngeal nerve.
- In patients with SVC syndrome secondary to non-small-cell carcinoma of the lung, radiotherapy is the primary treatment. Small cell carcinoma of lung presenting as SVC syndrome - Combination of chemotherapy and radiotherapy is used.
- Most common presentation of cholangiocarcinoma is Jaundice.
- For Ca maxilla, Combination of Surgery and radiotherapy is used for Squamous cell carcinoma. For adenocarcinoma, radiotherapy is ineffective, so only surgery is done.
- Weber-Fergusons incision is used for tumors of maxillary alveolus
- Burst abdomen usually occurs on 6th – 8th postoperative day

- Primary hemorrhage is hemorrhage occurring immediately as a result of an injury (or surgery). Reactionary hemorrhage is delayed hemorrhage (within 24 hours) and is usually caused by dislodgement of clot by resuscitation, normalization of blood pressure and vasodilatation, from technical failure such as slippage of a ligature. Secondary hemorrhage is caused by sloughing of the wall of a vessel. It usually occurs 7–14 days after injury and is precipitated by factors such as infection, pressure necrosis (such as from a drain) or malignancy.
- For reimplantation digits are stored in plastic bags with ice.
- Laparoscopic procedure patient develops shoulder pain due to subdiaphragmatic migration of gas.
- Carbon dioxide and N2O are preferred gases for creating pneumoperitoneum during laparoscopy.
- For parenteral nutrition, a peripheral venous catheter is preferred for short-term parenteral nutrition (less than 14 days). Tunneling subclavian line is recommended for long-term use (more than 30 days).
- Most common type of hiatal hernia is Sliding hernia.

SURGICAL INSTRUMENTS

SUTURES

	Types	Raw material	Tensile strength	Absorption rate
Silk	Braided or twisted multifilament coated (with max or silicone) or uncoated	Natural protein raw silk from silkworm	Loses 20% when wet; 80-100 % lost by 6 months	Fibrous encapsulation in body at 2–3 weeks absorbed slowly over 1–2 years
Catgut	Plain	Collagen derived from submucosa of healthy sheep or cattle	Lost within 7–10 days	Phagocytosis and enzymatic and degradation within 7–10 days
Catgut	Chromic	Tanned with chromium salts to improve handling and resist degradation in tissue°	Lost within 21–28 days	Phagocytosis and enzymatic degradation within 90 days
Polyglactin (Vicryl)	Braided multilfilament	Copolymer of lactide and glycolide in a ratio of 90:10, coated with polyglactin and calcium stearate	Approx., 60% remains at 2 weeks:. 30% remains at 3 weeks	Hydrolysis minimal until 5-6 weeks; Çomplete absorption 60–90 days
Polyglyconate	Monofilament dyed or undyed	Copolymer of glycolic acid andtrimethylene carbonate	Approx., 70% remains at 2 weeks; 55% remains at 3 weeks	Hydrolysis minimal until 8-9 weeks; Complete absorption 180 days
Polyglycarpone	Monofilament	Copolymer of glycolite and caprolactone	21 days maximum	Complete absorption 90–120 days
Polyglycolic acid (dexon)	Braided multifilament dyed or undyed coated or uncoated	Polymer of polyglycolic acid	Approx., 40% remains at 1 week; 20% remains at 3 weeks	Hydrolysis minimal at 2 weeks; significant at 4 weeks; Complete absorption 60–90 days
Polydioxane (PDS)	Monofilament dyed or undyed	Polyester polymer	Approx., 70% remains at 2 weeks; 50% remains at 4 weeks; 14% remains at 8 weeks	Hydrolysis minimal at 90 days; Complete absorption 180 days

- Non-absorbable sutures : Silk, Polypropylene (Prolene), Nylon

95. Which of the following statement is true about suture material in the image?

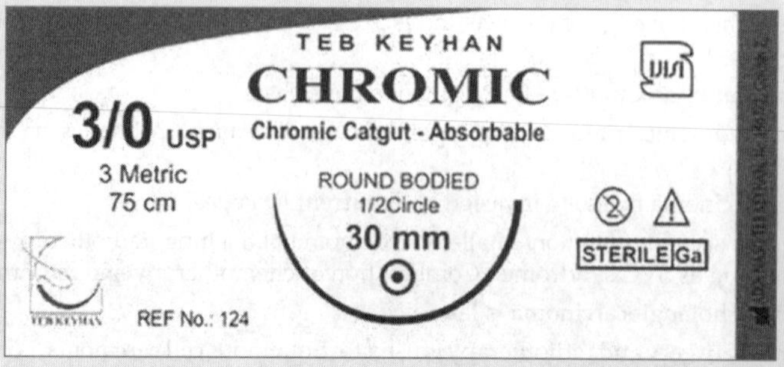

a. Made of rabbit submucosa
b Made of cat submucosa
c. Not degraded
d. Degraded by enzymatic degradation

Ans. is 'd' Degraded by enzymatic degradation

Morris Retractor: Used to retract abdominal wall

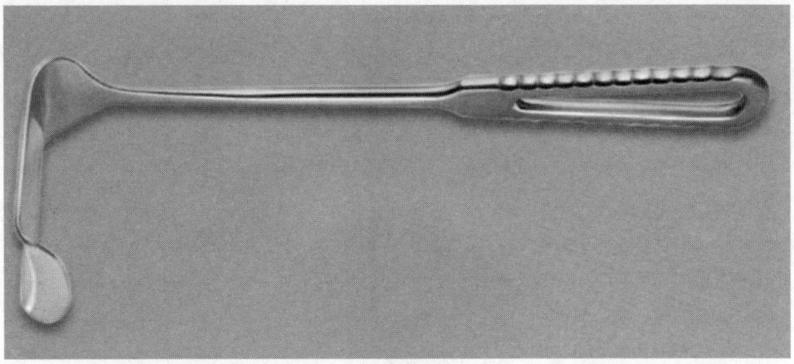

Langenbeck Retractor: Used in hernioplasty, thyroidectomy

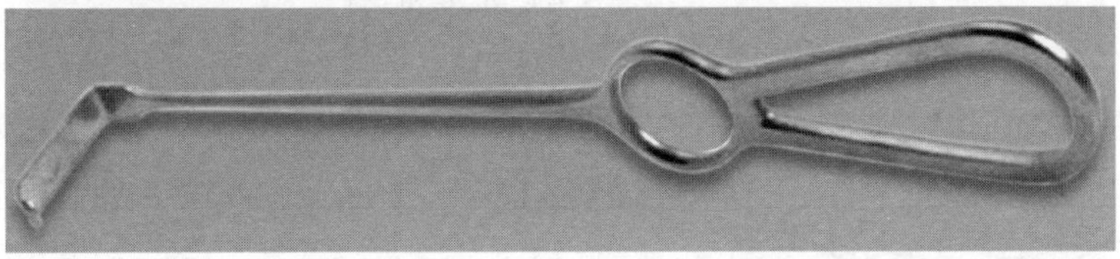

96. Identify the retractor? *(NEET 2018)*

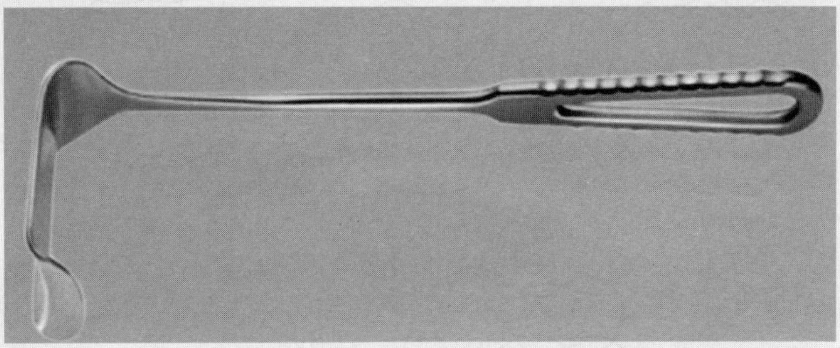

a. Morris retractor
b. Langenbeck retractor
c. Richardson retractor
d Deaver retractor

Ans. is 'a' Morris retractor

Scalpels: Common blades 10,11,15

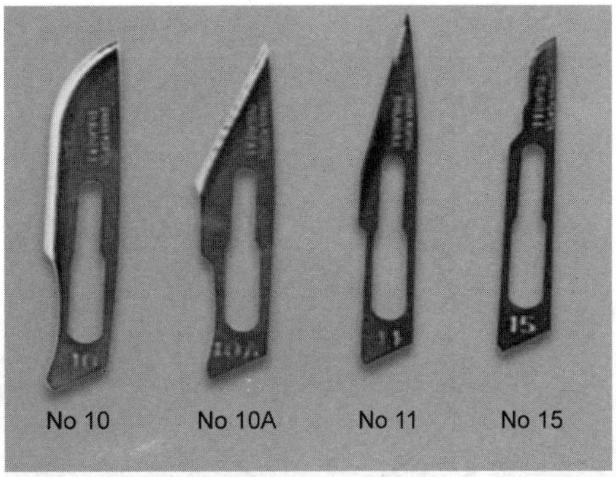

Blade No. 10: one of the more traditional blade shapes, this is generally used for making small incisions in skin and muscles.

Blade No. 11: this design is ideal for stab incisions. Used in procedures such as creating incisions for chest drains, opening coronary arteries, opening the aorta and removing calcifications in the aortic or mitral valves.

Blade No. 15: the most popular blade shape, ideal for making short and precise incisions. Utilised in a variety of surgical procedures including excision of a skin lesion or recurrent sebaceous cyst and for opening coronary arteries.

97. Identify the instrument. *(NEET 2019)*

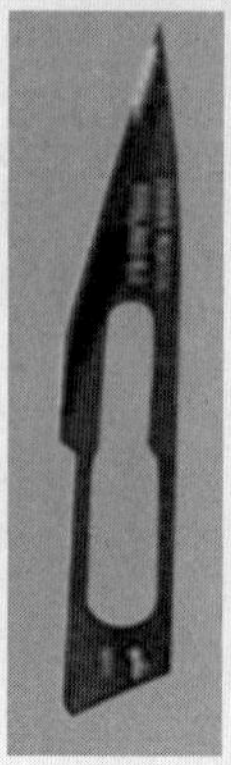

a. Blade No 10
b. Blade No 11
c. Blade No 12
d. Blade No 15

Ans. is 'b' Blade No 11

SURGICAL KNOTS

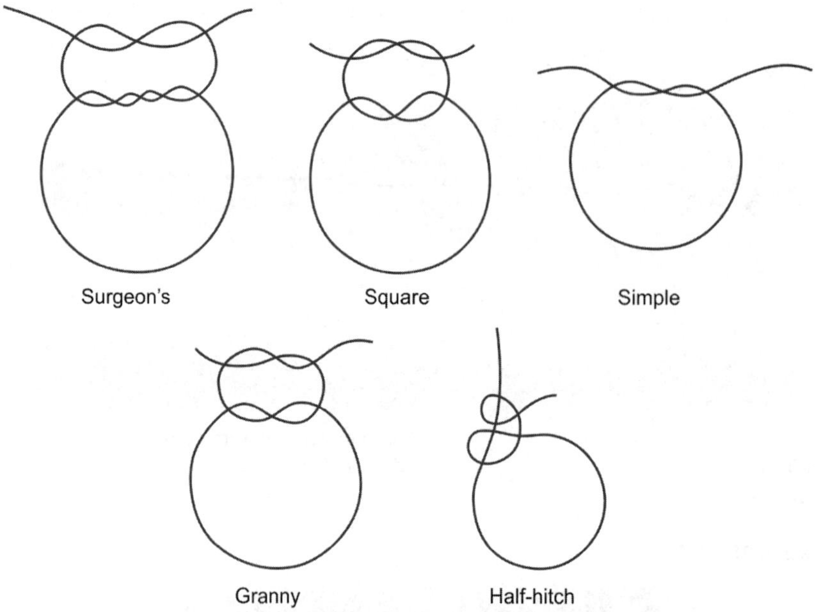

98. Identify the type of knot. *(NEET 2019)*

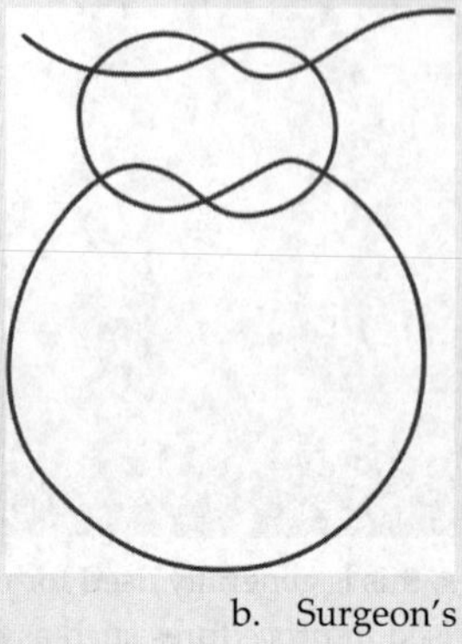

a. Granny knot
b. Surgeon's knot
c. Reef knot
d. None

Ans. is 'a' Granny knot

CHAPTER 14

Obstetrics and Gynecology

ANATOMY OF THE FEMALE GENITAL TRACT

EMBRYOLOGY-WOLFFIAN DUCT DERIVATIVES

During normal embryonic development, the **Wolffian** or paired **mesonephric ducts** form the reproductive organs in males and degenerate in females. **Remnants** of the **Wolffian duct** system in females may be retained within the leaves of the broad ligament.

1. Remnants of Wolffian ducts in a female are located in? *(NEET 2020)*

a. Pouch of douglas
b. Uterosacral ligament
c. Broad ligament
d. Round ligament

Ans. is 'c' Broad ligament

Lymphatic Drainage of Pelvic Organs

Organ	Lymphatic drainage
Uterus (fundus)	Para-aortic/lateral aortic (along, ovarian lymphatics superior lumbar)
Uterus (cornu)	Superficial inguinal nodes along with round ligament
Uterus (body)	Internal iliac >External iliac
Cervix	Internal iliac lymph nodes Hypogastric lymph nodes Obturator lymph nodes Presacral/paracervical lymph nodes External iliac lymph nodes
Fallopian tube	
Lateral part	Along with ovarian lymphatic drains into lateral aortic LN
Medial part	Along with cornua drains into superficial inguinal LN
Ovaries	Para-aortic
Vagina	
Upper1/3rd	Same as cervix
Middle 1/3rd	Internal iliac
Lower 1/3rd	Superficial inguinal LN
Vulva	
Labia majora (anterior ½)	Superficial inguinal
Labia majora (posterior ½)	Superficial inguinal, deep inguinal and external iliac
Labia minora and prepuce of clitoris	Superficial inguinal
Glans of clitoris	Deep inguinal and external iliac
Bartholin's gland	Superficial inguinal and anorectal

Delancey's Three Levels of Pelvic (Uterus, Vagina) Support

Level 1: The uterosacral-cardinal ligament complex provides attachment of the uterus and vaginal vault to the sacrum. Uterine prolapse occurs when this ligament complex breaks or is attenuated.

Level 2: The fascia overlying the levator ani muscles and the arcus tendineus fascia pelvis provide support to the middle part of the vagina.

Level 3: The perineal body and the urogenital diaphragm provide support to the lower part of the vagina

2. Lymphatic drainage of glans of clitoris is to this lymph nodes:

a. Obturator
b. Surficial inguinal
c. Deep inguinal
d. All of the above

Ans. is 'c' Deep inguinal

3. Level 1 support of uterus and vagina is:

a. Levator ani
b. Perineal body
c. Uterosacral ligaments
d. All of the above

Ans. is 'c' Uterosacral ligaments

PELVIS AND FETAL SKULL

Diameter of Fetal Skull

Diameter	Definition	Attitude of the head	Presentation
Suboccipitobregmatic 9.5 cm	Extends from the nape of the neck to the center of the bregma	Complete flexion	Vertex
Suboccipitofrontal: 10 cm (4")	Extends from the nape of the neck to the anterior end of the anterior fontanelle or center of the sinciput	Incomplete flexion	Vertex
Occipitofrontal 11.5 cm (41/2")	Extends from the occipital eminence to the root of the nose (Glabella)	Marked deflexion	Vertex
Mentovertical 14 cm (51/2")	Extends from the mid-point of the chin to the highest point on the sagittal suture	Partial extension	Brow
Submentovertical 11.5 cm (41/2")	Extends from junction of floor of the mouth and neck to the highest point on the sagittal suture	Incomplete extension	Face
Submentobregmatic 9.5 cm (33/4")	Extends from junction of floor of the mouth and neck to the centre of the bregma	Complete extension	Face

Some Important Points

- Normal female pelvis is–Gynaecoid pelvis
- Male type pelvis is–Android pelvis
- M/c type of pelvis–Gynaecoid pelvis
- Least common type pelvis–Platypelloid pelvis
- The only pelvis with AP diameter more than transverse diameter–Anthropoid pelvis
- Direct occipito–Posterior position is m/c in Anthropoid pelvis
- Persistant occipito–Posterior position is most common in Android pelvis
- Broad flat pelvis–Platypelloid pelvis
- Face to pubis delivery is most common in anthropoid pelvis
- The pelvic inlet usually is considered to be contracted if its shortest anteroposterior diameter is less than 10 cm or if the greatest transverse diameter is less than 12 cm.

Caput succedaneum is a neonatal condition involving a serous, subcutaneous, extra-periosteal fluid with poorly defined margins caused by the pressure of the presenting part of the scalp against the dilating (tourniquet effect of the cervix) during delivery.

- Caput succedaneum presents as a scalp swelling that extends across the midline and over suture lines associated with head moulding.
- Caput succedaneum does not usually cause complications and usually reason: within 24–48 hours.

4. Presenting diameter of full flexed head: *(NEET 2019)*

a. Suboccipito-bregmatic diameter
b. Suboccipito-frontal diameter
c. Occipito-frontal diameter
d. Occipito-posterior position

Ans. is 'a' Suboccipito-bregmatic diameter

5. After delivery, caput succedenum disappears:

a. Within 24–48 hours
b. 3–5 days
c. 5–7 days
d. 7–10 days

Ans. is 'a' Within 24–48 hours

BASICS OF REPRODUCTION

Semen Analysis

	WHO 1992	WHO 1999	WHO 2010
Parameters		**Normal values**	
Volume	2 mL	≥ 2 mL	≥1.5 mL
pH	—	—	7.2–7.8
Viscosity	—	—	< 3
Sperm concentration	20 million/mL	> 20 million/mL	15 million/mL
Total sperm count	—	≥ 40 million/ejaculate	39 million/ejaculate
Motility:			
Progressive motility	>50%	> 25%	> 32%
Total motility	—	> 50%	> 40%
Morphology:			
Normal forms	> 15%	> 14%	4%

Contd...

Contd...

Parameters	WHO 1992	WHO 1999	WHO 2010
		Normal values	
Viability/Living	—	≥ 75%	58%
Leucocyte	< 1 million/mL	—	< 1 million/mL
Round cells	—	—	< 5 million/mL
Sperm agglutination	< 10%	—	< 10%

Terminologies Related to Semen Analysis

- **Normospermia:** All parameters of semen analysis are normal
- **Oligospermia/oligozoospermia:** Decreased sperm number < 20 million/mL
- **Asthenospermia/asthenozoospermia:** Decreased sperm motility
- **Azoospermia:** No sperm in semen
- **Aspermia:** No ejaculate (ejaculation failure)
- **Teratozoospermia:** Increased abnormal forms of sperm
- **Oligoasthenoteratozoospermia:** All sperm viable abnormal
- **Necrozoospermia:** All sperm non-viable or non-motile
- **Leucocytospermia:** Increased white cells in semen

Method of Detecting Ovulation

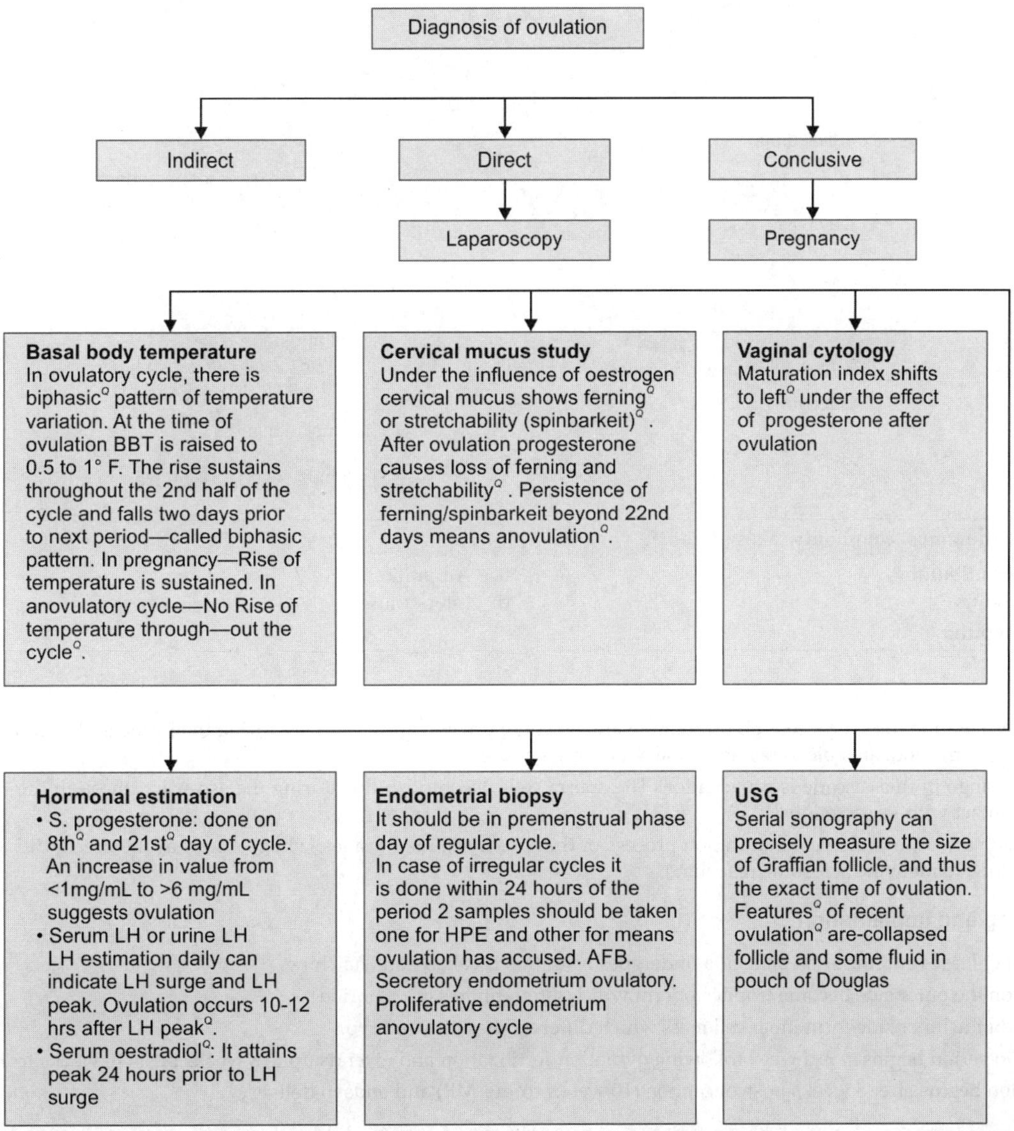

Indirect method	Direct method	Conclusive
• Serial vaginal cytology	Laparoscopy	Pregnancy
• Serial cervical mucus study		
• Premenstrual endometrial biopsy		
• Observing daily basal body temperature (BBT)		
• Estimation of blood progesterone levels (or urinary pregnanediol levels) in the postovulatory or immediate premenstrual phase		

Fertilization

- ❖ The uterine tubes, also known as oviducts or fallopian tubes, are the female structures that transport the ova from the ovary to the uterus each month.
- ❖ In the presence of sperm and fertilization, the uterine tubes transport fertilized egg to the uterus for implantation.
- ❖ The infundibulum gives rise to the fimbriae, finger like projections that are responsible for picking up the egg released by the ovary.
- ❖ Fertilization takes place in the ampullary part of the fallopian tube.
- ❖ **Human fertilization** is the union of a human egg and sperm, usually occurring in the ampulla of the fallopian tube. The result of this union is the production of a zygote cell, or fertilized egg.

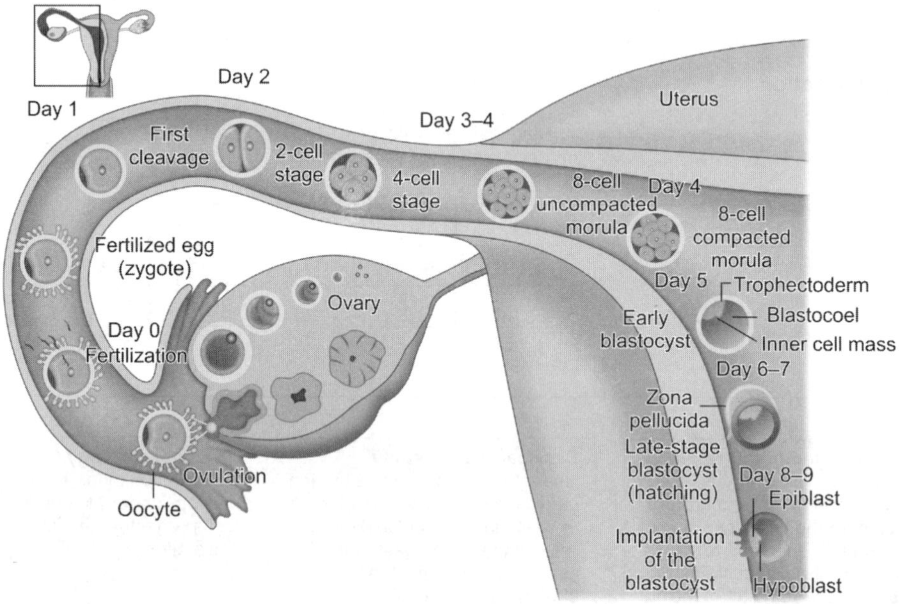

6. Fertilization most commonly takes place at? *(NEET 2020)*

a. Infundibulum
b. Ampulla
c. Isthmus
d. Interstitium

Ans. is 'b' Ampulla

Capacitation

- ❖ After the ejaculation the sperm cells go through several essential physiological changes during their time in the female genital tract before they, at the end, are able to penetrate the oocyte membrane.
- ❖ The first change in this cascade is capacitation. The sperm cells accomplish this during the ascension through the female genital tract (in contact with its secretions).
- ❖ It has to do with a physiological maturation process of the sperm cell membranes, which is seen as the precondition for the next step to follow, namely the acrosome reaction.

Zona Hatching and Implantation

- ❖ Blastocyst enlarges and the zona pellucida undergoes lysis, this is called zona hatching.
- ❖ The cells on the outer side become trophectoderm which differentiates into chorion
- ❖ The cells on the inner side form inner cell mass which differentiates into embryo.
- ❖ Embryonic period begins at 3rd week following ovulation/fertilization and extends up to 8 weeks post (10 weeks from LMP)
- ❖ Fatal period begins after 8 weeks postconception (10 weeks from LMP) and ends in delivery.

- The morula after spending about 3 days in the tube enters the uterine cavity via the narrow ostium (1 mm) on the fourth day in the 12–16 cell stage.
- Implantation occurs in the endometrium on the anterior or posterior wall of the body near the fundus on the sixth day following fertilization (corresponding to the 20th day of the menstrual cycle).
- The deeper penetration of the human blastocyst is called interstitial implantation, which happens by approximately the 13th day after fertilization.

Haematopoiesis

- Embryonic and fetal haematopoiesis occurs in three phases:
  1. Megaloblastic
  2. Hepatic
  3. Myeloid.
- **Sites and stages of fatal erythropoiesis**: Primitive erythropoiesis begins in the yolk sac at 2 to 3 weeks conception.
- By the end of the first trimester, the liver has become the main erythroid organ.
- The liver is primary source of red blood cells during the second trimester, and the bone marrow is the primary source of blood cells during the last trimester.

Basic Steps of IVF

- Ovarian stimulation with gonadotropins and follicular monitoring
- Oocyte retrieval (ovum pickup) done through TVS-guided needle
- Fertilization: 50,000 sperms are put on each oocyte retrieved
- Embryos kept in incubator for 48–72 h
- ET done on day 2 or day 3 (48–72 h) after oocyte retrieval
- Typically, embryos are transferred at the cleavage stage (Day 2 or 3 after oocyte retrieval)
- Day three embryos are called cleavage stage embryos and have approximately 4–8 cells.

Preimplantation Genetic Diagnosis (PGD)

- Preimplantation genetic diagnosis (PGD) is a reproductive technology used with an IVF cycle.
- PGD can be used for diagnosis of a genetic disease in early embryos prior to implantation and pregnancy.
- In addition, this technology can be utilized in the field of assisted reproduction for aneuploidy screening and diagnosis of unbalanced inheritance of chromosome abnormalities, such as translocations or inversions.
- PGD is considered in a similar fashion to prenatal diagnosis. When used to screen for a specific genetic disease, its main advantage is that it avoids selective pregnancy termination as the method makes it highly likely that the baby will be free of the disease under consideration.
- PGD thus is an adjunct to assisted reproductive technology, and requires in vitro fertilization (IVF) to obtain oocytes or embryos for evaluation.

7. Aspermia means:

a. Absence of sperms in semen
b. Absence of semen
c. 100% immobile sperms
d. None of the above

Ans. is 'b' Absence of semen

8. Endometrial biopsy to detect ovulation is done on which day of the menstrual cycle:

a. Day 8–9
b. Day 13–15
c. Day 21–23
d. Day 3–5

Ans. is 'c' Day 21–23

9. Fertilization occurs in:

a. Uterine cavity
b. Ampulla of fallopian tube
c. Infundibulum of fallopian tube
d. Isthmus of tube

Ans. is 'b' Ampulla of fallopian tube

10. Sperm capacitation takes place in:

a. Testes
b. Epididymis
c. Female genital tract
d. All of the above

Ans. is 'c' Female genital tract

11. In IVF, embryos are transferred back to uterine cavity at________ cells stage:

a. 2
b. 2–4s
c. 4–8
d. 8–1

Ans. is 'c' 4–8

REPRODUCTIVE PHYSIOLOGY AND HORMONES IN FEMALES

ANTI-MULLERIAN HORMONE (AMH)/MULLERIAN INHIBITING SUBSTANCE (MIS)

- Mullerian inhibiting substance (MIS)/Anti-Mullerian hormone (AMH) is the gonadal hormone that causes regression of the Mullerian ducts, during male embryogenesis.
- It is secreted at approximately 7 weeks gestation, when sertoli cell differentiation occurs.
- AMH exerts an inhibitory effect on oocyte meiosis, helps to control the descent of the testes, and inhibits surfactant accumulation in the lungs.
- AMH in males is secreted by Sertoli cells.
- Testosterone is secreted from Leydig cells.
- It is a peptide secreted by the granulosa cell in the ovary after puberty in females.
- Helps in follicular development and oocyte maturation
- It reflects the number of growing follicles
- The serum levels of MIS in women with normal cycles declines with age and becomes undetectable by the time of menopause.
- As the ovarian primordial follicle count decreases, the serum MIS concentration also decreases, making this hormone an ideal candidate for the early detection of ovarian reserve depletion.
- AMH test can be done on any day of a woman's cycle
- Since AMH is produced only in small ovarian follicles, blood levels of this substance have been used to measure the size of the pool of growing follicles in women
- Estimation of serum AMH used in:
  - Ovarian reserve in an infertile woman
  - Women with secondary amenorrhea
  - In IVF- predict the outcome after assisted reproductive techniques.
  - Woman with a smoking history
  - Poor response to gonadotropins
  - Age >35 years
  - Family history of early menopause
  - If there is history of ovarian surgery chemotherapy or irradiation

Values

- Normal value: 2-6.8 ng/mL
- *Poor ovarian reserve: < 1 ng/mL*
- PCOD and hyperstimulation syndrome: >10 ng/mL.

12. In low ovarian reserve, anti-Mullerian hormone level will be: *(NEET 2019)*

a. <1 b. 1-4
c. >7 d. >10

Ans. is 'a' <1

Superfecundation: It is the fertilization of two different ova released in the same cycle, by separate acts of coitus within a short period of time.

Superfetation is the fertilization of two ova released in different menstrual cycles. The nidation and development of one fetus over another fetus is theoretically possible until the decidual space is obliterated by 12 weeks of pregnancy.

Dysfunctional Uterine Bleeding (DUB) is a state of abnormal uterine bleeding without any clinically detect organic, systemic and iatrogenic cause.

Ormeloxifene

- A third generation benzopyran SERM which blocks the cytosol receptors by its competitive binding and selectively acts on estrogen receptors as agonist and antagonist in different reproductive tissues.
- It has anti-estrogenic action on endometrium and breast and estrogenic action on bones, vagina, liver, cardiovascular and central nervous system.
- It offers the additional advantage of relief of premenstrual syndrome in premenopausal women. However, it is not suitable for women desiring pregnancy in view of its contraceptive property.

Oestrous Cycle

- The oestrous cycle comprises of the recurring physiologic changes that are induced by reproductive hormone in most mammalian placental females.

- ❖ Humans undergo a menstrual cycle instead.
- ❖ Oestrous cycles starts puberty in sexually mature females and are interrupted by anoestrous phases or pregnancies. Typically cycles continue until death.
- ❖ Animals that have oestrous cycles reabsorb the endometrium if conception does not occur during that.
- ❖ Animals that have menstrual cycles shed the endometrium through menstruation instead.
- ❖ *Another different sexual activity*: In species with oestrous cycles, females are generally only sexually active during the oestrus phase their cycle.
- ❖ This is also referred to as being "in heat." In contrast, females of species with menstrual cycles can sexually active at any time in their cycle, even when they are not about to ovulate

Human Placenta Lactogen (hPL)

- ❖ Was named so, because of its potent lactogenic and growth hormone like bioactivity, as well as immunochemical resemblance to human growth hormone.
- ❖ It is detected as early as 2nd or 3rd week after fertilization.
- ❖ Maternal plasma concentrations are linked to placental mass and they rise steadily till 34–36 weeks of gestation.
- ❖ The half-life in maternal plasma is between 10 and 30 minutes
- ❖ The functions of hPL are:
  - It decreases maternal insulin sensitivity and ensures nutrient flow to the fetus
  - It promotes maternal lipolysis with the release of free fatty acids. This provides an energy source for maternal metabolism and foetal nutrition
  - It favours protein synthesis and provides a readily available amino acid source to the fetus
  - Potent angiogenic hormone, and may serve a function in foetal vasculature formation.

13. What is meant by superfecundation: *(NEET 2018)*

a. Fertilization of two or more ova in one intercourse
b. Fertilization of two of more ova in different intercourses in same menstrual cycle
c. Fertilization of ova and then it is division
d. Fertilization of second ovum first being implanted

Ans. is 'b' Fertilization of two of more ova in different intercourses in same menstrual cycle

14. SERM used in DUB is:

a. Clomiphene b. Raloxifene
c. Ormeloxifene d. Mifepristone

Ans. is 'c' Ormeloxifene

15. Ovarian cycle can be correlated with all *except*:

a. Endometrial sampling b. Vaginal cytology
c. Blood hormonal levels d. Estrous cycle

Ans. is 'd' Estrous cycle

16. HPL has activity similar to which hormone:

a. Oxytocin b. Growth hormone
c. Insulin d. All of the above

Ans. is 'b' Growth hormone

EFFECTS OF ESTROGEN

In girls, FSH stimulates the growth of ovarian follicles and, in conjunction with LH, stimulates production of estradiol by the ovaries). Early in puberty, estradiol stimulates breast development and growth of the skeleton, leading to pubertal growth acceleration. Later in puberty, the interplay between pituitary secretion of FSH and LH, and secretion of estradiol by ovarian follicles leads to ovulation and menstrual cycles. Estradiol also induces maturation of the skeleton, eventually resulting in fusion of the growth plates and cessation of linear growth.Estrogen stimulation of the vaginal mucosa causes a physiologic leukorrhea, which is a thin, white, non-foul-smelling vaginal discharge that typically begins 6 to 12 months before menarche.

Adrenarche begins when the zona reticularis of the adrenal gland begins to synthesize the adrenal androgens dehydroepiandrosterone (DHEA) and androstenedione. Though less potent than testosterone, these induce androgenic changes including growth of pubic and axillary hair, maturation of the apocrine sweat glands (leading to adult-type body odor), and development of acne

17. All of the following occur under the effect of estrogen *except*: *(NEET 2020)*

a. Cervical mucus b. Menstruation
c. Hair growth d. Breast development

Ans. is 'c' Hair growth

MENOPAUSE AND HRT

MENOPAUSE

- Menopause is defined as the time of cessation of ovarian function, which leads to permanent cessation of menses.
- It takes 12 months of cessation of menses to call as menopause.

Clinical Features of Menopause

Early features of menopause	Late features (due to chronic oestrogen deficiency)
Hot flushes	Arthritis
Sweating	Osteoporosis and fracture
Headache	Backache
Psychological	Cardiovascular accidents such as ischaemic heart disease, myocardial infarction, atherosclerosis
Dyspareunia, decreased libido	Hypertension
Pseudocyesis	Stroke
Irritability	Skin changes
Depression, insomnia, tiredness	Alzheimer's disease
Lack of concentration, loss of memory	Ano-colonic cancer
Urinary stress incontinence, dyspareunia	Tooth decay
	Prolapse genital tract
	Stress incontinence of urine and faecal incontinence
	Cataract, glaucoma and macular degeneration

Indication of HRT

a. **Short term**
   1. Hot flushes
   2. Vasomotor symptoms
   3. Dyspareunia
   4. Libido
   5. Urethral syndrome

b. **Long term**
   1. Osteoporosis
   2. Cardiovascular
   3. Alzheimer's disease

Risks of HRT

1. Endometrial cancer
2. Breast cancer
3. Ovarian cancer
4. Thromboembolism
5. Lipid profile dysfunction
6. Gall stones
7. Liver dysfunction

Gonadotropin Releasing Hormone

- Schally and Guillemin were the first to discover a decapeptide called gonadotropin-releasing hormone (GnRH) in 1971.
- GnRH is secreted by the median eminence and the arcuate nucleus, which modulates the neural control of follicle-stimulating hormone (FSH) and luteinizing hormone (LH) by the anterior pituitary gland.
- GnRH has a half-life of 2–4 min and is therefore difficult to assay.
- Its level is assessed through the LH level.
- It is released in a pulsatile manner into the portal vessels and reaches the anterior pituitary gland.
- The pulsatility and amplitude of its release vary with the various phases of the menstrual cycle.
- In the preovulatory phase (follicular phase), it pulses once in every 60 min, but it slows down to once in 3 h in the luteal phase, with increased amplitude of each pulse
- GnRH exhibits different actions depending on the manner in which it is released.
- Its continuous release causes suppression of gonadotropins and thereby the ovarian functions through the process of 'down-regulation' or desensitization of pituitary hormones.

❖ This mode of administration is now employed in therapy using synthetic analogues of GnRH in regulating ovulation in in-vitro fertilization and suppressing menstruation in precocious puberty, in reducing the size of the uterine fibroids and in causing shrinkage of endometriosis

Natural GnRH	Synthetic GnRH
Secreted in a pulsatile manner at different times of menstrual cycle.	Initially, there is a supra-physiological release of FSH and LH from pituitary (flare) followed by decrease in the synthesis and release of both FSH and LH
Initially secreted only at night	When given in pulsatile manner they stimulate gonadotropin secretion

GnRH agonist	*GnRH antagonist*
Leuproprolin	Centrorelix
Buserelin	Ganirelix
Nafarelin	
Goserelin	
Triptorelin	

Hormone Replacement in Turner Syndrome

❖ Growth hormone (GH) therapy has become the standard of care for girls with TS and should be considered as soon as decreased linear growth velocity is apparent.

❖ Final adult height is maximized if GH therapy is begun at a young age; and is positively associated with the duration of treatment.

❖ Recent studies have suggested that treatment initiated prior to 4 years of age significantly improved height outcome.

❖ Most girls with TS require hormone replacement therapy for breast development, uterine growth, and bone health.

❖ The consensus is to initiate hormone replacement therapy at a time that coincides with normal female pubertal development.

❖ Initial hormone replacement involves low dose estrogen monotherapy. Progestogen replacement is generally added 1–2 years after starting estrogen or upon breakthrough bleeding.

18. Menopause is defined as: *(NEET 2018)*

a. Presence of hot flushes
b. Cessation of menses for 1 year
c. Cessation of menses for 6 months
d. Cessation of menses for 2 years

Ans. is 'b' Cessation of menses for 1 year

19. Hormonal replacement therapy is indicated in menopausal women for: *(NEET 2018)*

a. Hot flushes
b. Ca breast
c. Endometriosis
d. Uterine bleeding

Ans. is 'a' Hot flushes

20. Symptoms of menopause are all *except*: *(NEET 2018)*

a. Hot flushes
b. Night sweats
c. Decrease libido
d. Intermittent hypotension

Ans. is 'd' Intermittent hypotension

21. All of the following are GnRH agonist *except*:

a. Ganirelix
b. Nafarelin
c. Goserelin
d. Triptorelin

Ans. is 'a' Ganirelix

22. Patient with 45XO, what HRT to be given:

a. Growth hormone + E + P
b. Estrogen
c. No HRT needed
d. HRT only after 45 years

Ans. is 'a' Growth hormone + E + P

Atrophic Vaginitis

❖ Occurs as a result of deterioration of the vaginal tissue.

❖ It's a common condition in postmenopausal women because as estrogen levels drop, the tissue that lines the vagina becomes thinner and more easily damaged.

- Women with atrophic vaginitis may also experience vaginal itching, burning, frequent urination, or vaginal discharge.
- Women can treat this condition topically with estrogen creams, tablets (Vagifem), or an estrogen-releasing ring placed in the vagina (Estring).
- Oral estrogen, available with a doctor's prescription, will also restore vaginal tissue.
- Vaginal lubricants offer an alternative for women wary of using estrogen.
- Moisturizers such as Replens, Astroglide, and Lubrin can reduce symptoms and make sexual intercourse more comfortable.

23. Vulvar atrophy and itching are treated by: *(NEET 2019)*

a. Estrogen ointment b. Antihistamines
c. Tamoxifen d. None

Ans. is 'a' Estrogen ointment

PLACENTA AND AMNIOTIC FLUID

PLACENTA

- At term, the "typical" placenta→ **Weight**: 470 g, **Shape:** Round to oval, **Size:** 22-cm diameter, and has a central thickness of 2.5 cm.
- It is composed of a placental disc, extraplacental membranes, and three-vessel umbilical cord.
- The maternal surface is the basal plate, which is divided by clefts into portions—termed cotyledons.
- The foetal surface is the chorionic plate, into which the umbilical cord inserts, typically in the centre.
- Large foetal vessels that originate from the cord vessels then spread and branch across the chorionic plate before entering stem villi of the placenta parenchyma.

Abnormal Placentation

Placenta accreta: is any placental implantation in which there is abnormally firm adherence to the uterine wall as a consequence of partial or total absence of the decidua basalis and imperfect development of the fibrinoid layer (Nitabuch layer), placental villi are attached to the myometrium in placenta accrete.

- When placental villi invade the myometrium **Placenta increta,** or penetrate through the myometrium in **Placenta Percreta**.
- The incidence of placenta accreta, increta, and percreta has increased, most likely because of the increased caesarean delivery rate.
- Abnormal placental adherence is found when decidual formation is defective.
- Associated conditions include implantation in the lower uterine segment over a previous surgical scar or after uterine curettage.

The Umbilical Cord

- The umbilical cord forms the connecting link between the foetus and the placenta through which the foetal blood flows to and from the placenta.
- It extends from the foetal umbilicus to the foetal surface of the placenta.
- Most umbilical cords are 40–70 cm long
- *The cord has three vessels*: 1 vein and 2 arteries. The right vein disappears (the left is left).
- The O_2 supply to the foetus is at the rate of 5–8 mL/kg/mm and this is achieved with cord blood flow of 165–330 mL/mm.

Placenta Previa

Clinical Features

1. Painless bleeding
2. Relaxed uterus
3. Floating head

Types

Type—I (Low-lying): The major part of the placenta is attached to the upper segment and only the lower margin encroaches onto the lower segment but not up to the os.

Type—II (Marginal): The placenta reaches the margin of the internal os but does not cover it.

Type—III (Incomplete or partial central): The placenta covers the internal os partially (covers the internal os when closed but does not entirely do so when fully dilated).

Type—IV (Central or total): The placenta completely covers the internal os even after it is fully dilated.

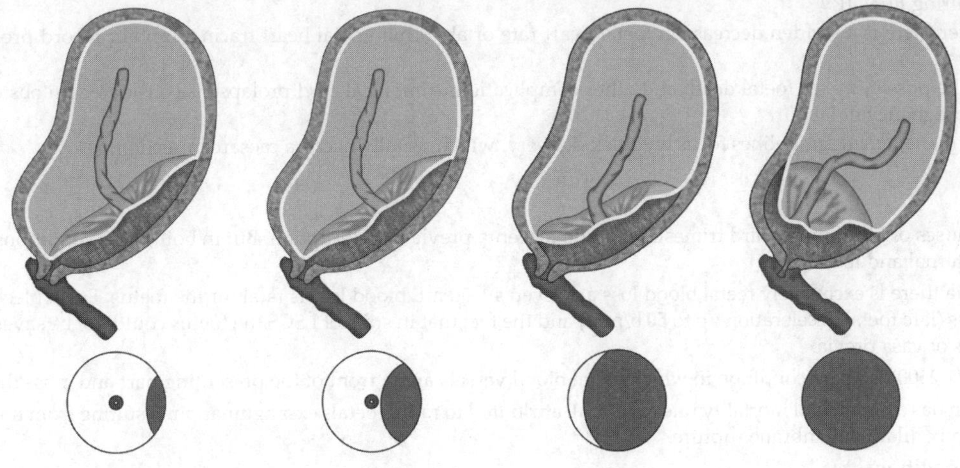

Conservative Management in Placenta Previa

McAfee and Johnson Regimen

- This consists of complete bed rest, tocolysis, and close observation of patient.
- Steroids are generally given to enhance lung maturity.
- To undertake this regimen (to wait and watch) all the three criteria should be fulfilled:
  - Mother should be hemodynamically stable
  - There should be no foetal distress
  - Pregnancy less than 36 weeks of gestation.
- If any one of the criteria is not met then the patient should be delivered by LSCS.
- If the same patient presented at 37 weeks, the answer would be LSCS.
- If there was foetal distress, the answer would be LSCS, and if there was maternal hemodynamic instability, the answer would be blood and IV fluids, followed by emergency LSCS
- The placenta serves as the interface between mother and foetus allowing for the exchange of physiologically important substances including oxygen, carbon dioxide, waste products of metabolism, drugs, etc.
- Foetal blood travels from the foetal heart to the placenta by way of two umbilical arteries and returns (nutrient enriched and waste free) to the foetus by means of a single umbilical vein.
- Uterine blood flow is one critical determinant of the proper functioning of the placenta and thus the health of the foetus.
- Uterine blood flow is not autoregulated and as a result the flow is proportional to uterine perfusion pressure (arterial pressure minus uterine venous pressure).
- Flow is also inversely related to uterine vascular resistance
- Uteroplacental blood flow increases progressively during pregnancy and ranges from 500–800 mL/mm at term.

Amniotic Fluid

- pH of amniotic fluid is 7.0–7.5
- The volume of amniotic fluid at term is 800 mL
- An osmolarity of 250 mOsmol/L of amniotic fluid is suggestive of fetal lung maturity
- Fetal urine is the major component of amniotic fluid.

Cord prolapse: It defined as the descent of the umbilical cord through the cervix alongside (occult) or past the presenting part (overt) in the vagina or outside the vulva in the presence of ruptured membranes.

Risk Factors for Cord Prolapse

- Long cord
- Polyhydramnios
- Malpresentations and Abnormal lie (transverse, breech, and oblique and compound presentation)
- Multiple pregnancies
- Floating (unengaged) head
- Prematurity
- Contracted pelvis

- Iatrogenic during ECV, IPV
    - Whenever there is a sudden decrease in foetal heart rate or abnormal foetal heart tracing, umbilical cord prolapse should be considered.
    - Due to the possibility for foetal death and other complications, umbilical cord prolapse is considered an obstetric emergency during pregnancy or labour.
    - Current management guidelines focus on quick delivery, which usually needs a caesarean section.

Vasa Previa

- Two main causes of bleeding in third trimester include placenta previa and abruption. But in both these conditions, the blood loss is mixed maternal and foetal.
- In vasa previa there is exclusively foetal blood loss and even 40–50 mL blood loss is fatal for the foetus. Fresh bleeding and severe foetal distress (late foetal deceleration up to 50 b/min) and the fact that in spite of LSCS the foetus could not be saved point towards the diagnosis of vasa previa.
- Vasa previa (1:2500) is a rare condition in which foetal blood vessels are in front of the presenting part and cross the cervix.
- The condition has a high foetal mortality rate (50–95%), attributed to rapid foetals exsanguination, resulting from the vessels tearing when the cervix dilates, membrane rupture.
- **Associated conditions**
    - Velamentous cord insertion
    - IVP pregnancies
    - Bibbed placenta
    - Multiple pregnancies
    - Succenturiate-lobed placenta
    - Maternal history of DandC or uterine surgery
    - Low-lying placenta or placenta previa

Management

- When vasa previa is detected prior to labour, the baby has a much greater chance of surviving.
- Vasa previa can be detected during pregnancy with use of USG and in combination with colour Doppler.
- Women with the above risk factors undergo colour Doppler test to rule out vasa previa.
- When it is diagnosed, elective LSCS (37–38 weeks) should be done before labour begins.

24. The major contribution of the amniotic fluid after 20 weeks of gestation: *(NEET 2019)*

a. Ultrafiltrate and maternal plasma
b. Fetal urine
c. Fetal lung fluid
d. Fetal skin

Ans. is 'b' Fetal urine

25. Identify the type of placenta praevia as shown in the picture below: *(NEET 2019)*

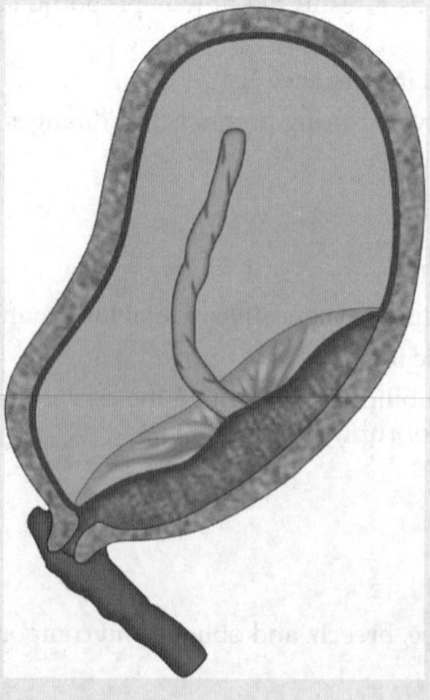

a. I.
b. II.
c. III.
d. IV.

Ans. is 'b' II.

26. G3P2L2 with previous 2 LSCS with anterior placenta previa has got a very high risk of which complications: *(NEET 2018)*

a. Placenta accreta
b. Vasa previa
c. Abruption
d. None of the above

Ans. is 'a' Placenta accreta

27. A primigravida with 36 weeks of pregnancy is in labor with 3 cm dilatation and minimal uterine contraction. On rupture of membranes, fresh bleeding is noted with late fetal deceleration up to 50 beats/min. The patient was taken for LSCS but fetus could not be saved. No abruptio or placenta previa was seen. The likely diagnosis is: *(NEET 2018)*

a. Placenta previa
b. Revealed abruptio
c. Circumvallate placenta
d. Vasa previa

Ans. is 'd' Vasa previa

28. A lady with 35 weeks of pregnancy is admitted in view of first episode of painless about of bleeding yesterday. On examination Hb 10 g% BP 120/70 mm Hg. Uterus relaxed and cephalic floating FHS regular. Next line of management is: *(NEET 2018)*

a. Caesarean section
b. Induction of labor
c. Wait and watch
d. Blood transfusion

Ans. is 'c' Wait and watch

29. Cord prolapse is least likely with:

a. Transverse lie
b. Fooling breech
c. Oligohydramnios
d. Floating head

Ans. is 'c' Oligohydramnios

OLIGOAMNIOS

First trimester: The etiology of first trimester oligohydramnios is often unclear. Reduced amniotic fluid prior to 10 weeks of gestation is rare because gestational sac fluid is primarily derived from the fetal surface of the placenta, transamniotic flow from the maternal compartment, and secretions from the surface of the body of the embryo.

Second trimester: By the beginning of the second trimester, fetal urine begins to enter the amniotic sac and the fetus begins to swallow amniotic fluid. Therefore, disorders related to the fetal renal/urinary system begin to play a prominent role in the etiology of oligohydramnios. These anomalies include intrinsic renal disorders (cystic renal disease) and obstructive lesions of the lower urinary tract (posterior urethral valves, urethral atresia, prune belly syndrome). Maternal and placental factors, as well as rupture of the fetal membranes, are also common causes of oligohydramnios in the second trimester. But fetal renal anomaly is the most common cause.

Third trimester: Oligohydramnios first diagnosed in the third trimester is often associated with PPROM or with uteroplacental insufficiency due to conditions such as preeclampsia or other maternal vascular diseases. Oligohydramnios frequently accompanies fetal growth restriction related to uteroplacental insufficiency. Fetal anomalies and abruptio placentae also play a role at this gestational age. Amniotic fluid volume normally decreases postterm, so oligohydramnios may develop in these pregnancies.

30. A woman with 18 weeks of gestation presented to opd. On examination, the uterus size corresponded to 16 weeks. On USG, oligohydramnios was found. Which of the following can be suspected? *(NEET 2020)*

a. Renal agenesis
b. Fetal anemia
c. Fetal cardiac anomalies
d. Neural tube defects

Ans. is 'a' Renal agenesis

MATERNAL ADAPTATIONS TO PREGNANCY

RENAL CHANGES IN PREGNANCY

Increased	Decreased
Renal blood flow	S. creatinine
GFR	S. BUN
Creatinine	Plasma osmolality
Aminoaciduria	S. uric acid
Serum aldosterone	S. $Na^+/K^+/Cl^-$
Glycosuria	

S. ADH (antidiuretic hormone) remains unchanged in pregnancy

Obstetrics and Gynecology

CVS Changes in Pregnancy

- Due to elevation of diaphragm because of gravid uterus, the heart is pushed upwards and outwards with slight rotation to the left.
- The apex beat is shifted to the 4th intercostal space about 2.5 cm outside the midclavicular line.
- Systolic murmur can be heard in pulmonary or apical area.
- Mammary murmur: Continuous hissing murmur in tricuspid area in left 2nd and 3rd intercostal space (due to increase in blood flow through internal mammary vessels).
- S3 and rarely S4 may be auscultated.
- *2D echo*: Increase in left ventricular end diastolic diameter.
- Increase in left and right atrial diameters.
- *EGG*: Left axis deviation.

Parameters that increase in pregnancy	Parameters that decrease in pregnancy
Cardiac output	Peripheral vascular resistances (as progesterone has a smooth muscle relaxant effect)
Stroke volume	Diastolic BP and systolic BP (Decrease in diastolic BP > systolic BP)
HR	Mean arterial BP Systolic BP+(Distolic BP × 2) 3

Cardiac Output (CO)

- Cardiac output increases by 40% during Pregnancy
- The cardiac output begins to rise from 5th week of gestation and reaches its peak at 30–32 weeks and then remains static to full term
- So the maximum risk of a heart disease patient to have cardiac failure during pregnancy is at 32 weeks
- CO increases by 50% during each uterine contraction in labour
- There is 80% increase in CO immediately postpartum (as the uterus contracts, blood from uterus is pushed back into the maternal system, also known as autotransfusion)
- Therefore, the risk of cardiac failure is maximum in the immediate postpartum period (followed by intrapartum). To avoid this, diuretics should be given after placental delivery to heart disease patients.
- CO returns to prelabour value by one hour following delivery and to prepregnant levels by another four weeks.

Respiratory Rate

- The respiratory rate is essentially unchanged, but tidal volume and resting minute ventilation increase significantly as pregnancy advances.
- The functional residual capacity and the residual volume are decreased as a consequence of the elevated diaphragm.
- The respiratory rate is essentially unchanged, but tidal volume and resting minute ventilation increase significantly as pregnancy advances.
- The functional residual capacity and the residual volume are decreased as a consequence of the elevated diaphragm.

Physiological Respiratory Changes During Pregnancy

Increases	Decreases	Unaffected
Tidal volume	Functional residual capacity	Respiratory rate
Minute ventilation	Expiratory reverse volume	Vital capacity
Inspiratory capacity	Residual volume	Inspiratory reserve volume
Minute O_2 uptake	Total lung capacity	
O_2 demand of causes (20%)	PCO_2 (∴ mild respiratory alkalosis)	

31. Which of the following is false as physiological change in pregnancy: *(NEET 2019)*

a. Increase cardiac output
b. Increase total protein
c. Increase residual volume
d. Increase GFR

Ans. is 'c' Increase residual volume

32. During pregnancy, true statement about CVS is:

a. Cardiac output decreases
b. Right axis deviation
c. Increase in left ventricular end diastolic diameter
d. All of the above

Ans. is 'c' Increase in left ventricular end diastolic diameter

PCOD, HIRSUTISM AND GALACTORRHOEA

POLYCYSTIC OVARIAN DISEASE (PCOD)

- It is a heterogeneous syndrome complex
- Characterized by chronic anovulation and hyperandrogenism
- Frequently associated with insulin resistance, resulting in menstrual irregularity, infertility and hirsutism

Diagnosis

Rotterdam 2003 criteria for diagnosis of PCOS/PCOD—at least two out of three should be present

1. Oligo/anovulation
2. Hyperandrogenism: biochemical or clinical
3. On USG: Twelve or more than 12 follicles 2–9 mm in size present within one or both ovaries on USG and/or ovarian volume >10 mL.

USG Features of Polycystic Ovarian Syndrome (PCOS)

- Greater than 12 follicles measuring between 2–9 mm in diameter, located peripherally, resulting in a pearl necklace appearance
- Increased echogenicity of ovarian stroma and/or ovarian volume greater than 10 mL

Management

Principles of Management Include

Irregular periods/amenorrhea = regularization of menses with OC pills/cyclical progesterone

Hirsutism/acne = suppression of androgens

Infertility = ovulation induction

Insulin sensitizers are also used to tackle insulin resistance

MC used drug metformin; Metformin will help the patient to lose weight and will either cause spontaneous ovulation or increase the success of ovulation induction drugs

Newer insulin sensitizer myo-inositol is now available.

It is better tolerated than metformin.

Danazol has no role in PCOS.

The Ferriman-Gallwey Score: Method used for evaluating and quantifying hirsutism in women.

33. Pearl necklace appearance is characteristic of:

a. Ectopic pregnancy b. PCOS
c. Endometriosis d. PID

Ans. is 'b' PCOS

34. What is not used in PCOS:

a. OC pills b. Cyclical progesterone
c. Myoinositol d. Danazol

Ans. is 'd' Danazol

35. Which of the following is used in quantifying hirsutism:

a. Bishop score b. Rotterdam criteria
c. Ferriman-Gallwey score d. All of the above

Ans. is 'c' Ferriman-Gallwey score

OVARIAN HYPERSTIMULATION SYNDROME (OHSS)

Ovarian hyperstimulation syndrome (OHSS) is a complication of ovarian stimulation treatment (ovarian induction therapy) for *in vitro* fertilisation. Rarely, it may also occur as a spontaneous event in pregnancy.

The clinical syndrome consists of ovarian enlargement with extra-vascular accumulation of exudates leading to varying degrees of:

- Weight gain
- Increase in abdominal circumference
- Ascites
- Pleural effusions
- Intravascular volume depletion with hemoconcentration
- Oliguria

Ultrasound

- Typically shows bilateral symmetric enlargement of ovaries (often >12 cm in size)
- Multiple cysts of varying sizes, giving the classic **spoke-wheel appearance**
- Associated ascites and pleural +/- pericardial effusion (which is due to capillary leak) may also be present

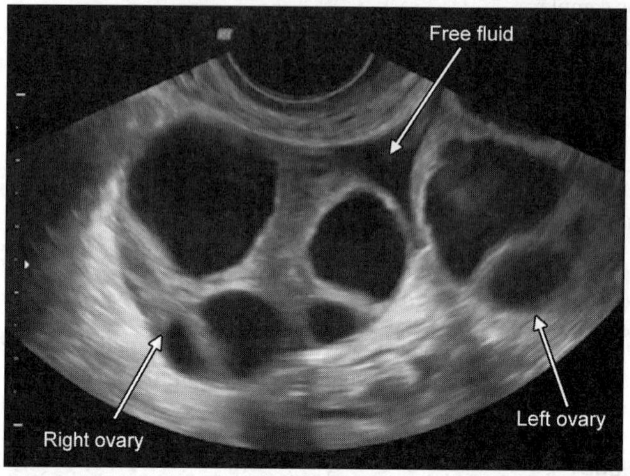

36. A woman on treatment for infertility received multiple injections of HMG. She complained of frequent menstrual bleeding and abdominal pain. USG is shown below. What is the diagnosis? *(NEET 2020)*

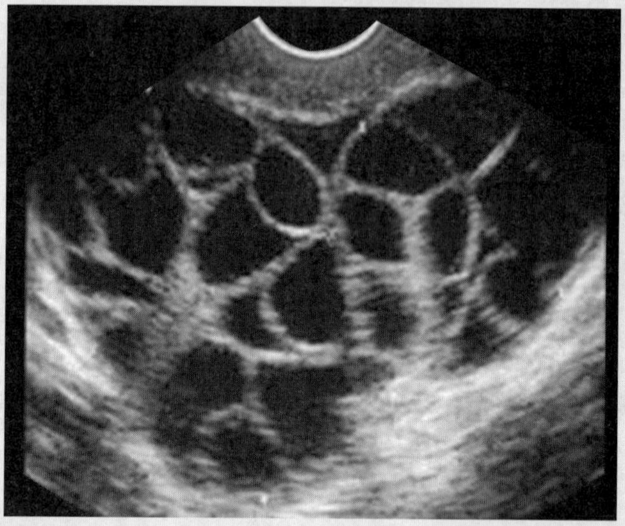

a. Polycystic ovarian syndrome
b. Complete mole
c. Ovarian hyperstimulation syndrome
d. CA ovary

Ans. is 'c' Ovarian hyperstimulation syndrome

CONGENITAL MALFORMATIONS

MULLERIAN ANOMALIES

WHO classification of Mullerian anomalies

- Class I = Mullerian agenesis (MRKH)
- Class II = Unicornuate uterus (10%)
- Class III = Didelphys uterus (complete duplication: two uteri, two cervices, and longitudinal vaginal septum (8%)
- Class IV = Bicornuate uterus (26%)
- Class V = Septate uterus (35%)

- Class VI = Arcuate uterus (18%)
- Class VII = DES-related abnormalities/T-shaped uterus

Mullerian agenesis (Mayer-Rokitansky-Kuster-Hauser syndrome): It presents as amenorrhea with absence of a vagina

- The karyotype is 46 XX.
- There is normal development of breasts, sexual hair, ovaries, external genitalia.
- There are associated urinary tract (33%) and skeletal (12%) anomalies.

Testicular feminization, or **congenital androgen insensitivity syndrome**, is an X-linked recessive disorder karyotype of 46 XY.

- The patient presents with an absent uterus and blind vaginal canal
- However, in patients the amount of sexual hair is significantly decreased/absent.

Gonadal dysgenesis present with lack of secondary sexual characteristics.

Klinefelter syndromes: have karyotype of 47 XXY and a male phenotype

Primary Amenorrhea

- In absence of secondary sexual characters, no menses till the age of 13 years.
- In presence of secondary sexual characters, no menses till the age of 15 years.
- MC cause of primary amenorrhea is ovarian dysgenesis/Turner syndrome.
- Mullerian agenesis (Mayer-Rokitansky-Küstner-Hauser or MRKH syndrome) is the second MC cause.
- Androgen insensitivity syndrome or testicular feminizing syndrome (AIS/TFS) is the third MC of primary amenorrhea.

Gartner's cyst (retention cyst in remnants of Wolffian duct):

- Situated anteriorly or anterolaterally in vagina and of variable size
- Rugosities of the overlying vaginal mucosa are lost
- Gartner's duct cyst is a cystic swelling at junction of lower one-third and upper two-thirds of anterior vaginal wall
- Vaginal mucosa over it becomes tense and shiny
- Not reducible
- No impulse on coughing

37. The most common Mullerian anomaly is:

a. Mullerian agenesis (MRKH)
b. Unicornuate uterus
c. Bicornuate uterus
d. Septate uterus

Ans. is 'd' Septate uterus

38. A 19-year-old patient presents to your office with primary amenorrhea. She has normal breast and pubic hair development. But the uterus and vagina are absent. Diagnostic possibility includes:

a. Testicular feminization syndrome
b. Gonadal dysgenesis
c. Mullerian agenesis
d. Klinefelter syndrome

Ans. is 'c' Mullerian agenesis

39. MC cause of primary Amenorrhea is:

a. Constitutional/idiopathic
b. MRKH syndrome
c. Ovarian dysgenesis
d. None of the above

Ans. is 'c' Ovarian dysgenesis

For women with septate uterus who are candidates for surgical repair, hysteroscopic(transcervical) metroplasty is the procedure of choice. Ideally, over 90 percent of the septum is removed during the procedure. A two-dimensional (2D) or three-dimensional (3D) ultrasound or a hysterosalpingogram should be performed two months after surgery to assess success; further repairs of the septum are indicated if more than 1 cm of septum remains. Attempts at pregnancy may begin two months postoperatively if the procedure is deemed adequate.

- For women with a bicornuate who are candidates for surgical repair, uterine reunification via laparotomy (Strassman procedure) is the procedure of choice, although evidence of efficacy are sparse. We do not prescribe exogenous estrogen postoperatively for women with normal ovarian function, but some authors routinely prescribe high-dose estrogen. We perform a hysterosalpingogram at approximately two months postoperatively to evaluate and document the resulting cavity. Women who conceive should delivery by cesarean as the transfundal incision places them at increased risk of uterine rupture.
- For women with a unicornuate uterus and an obstructed painful rudimentary horn, laparoscopic resection of the obstructed horn is the procedure of choice. These patients commonly have renal and ureteral anomalies and endometriosis, which increase the risk of organ injury during surgery. Intraoperative canalization of the single cervix and injection of blue dye will confirm which uterus communicates with the cervix. Most patients experience immediate improvement in pain. Endometriosis, if present, often resolves postoperatively.

40. A female presents with recurrent abortions. USG reveals a septate uterus. What is the best management for her? *(NEET 2020)*

a. Strassman metroplasty
b. Tompkins metroplasty
c. Johns metroplasty
d. Transcervical resection of septum

Ans. is 'd' Transcervical resection of septum

DIAGNOSIS OF PREGNANCY AND ANTENATAL CARE

SIGN AND SYMPTOMS OF PREGNANCY

Presumptive symptoms and signs	Probable sign	Positive or absolute sign
Amenorrhea	Abdominal enlargement	Palpation of foetal parts and or perception of active foetal movement by examiner at about 20 week
Frequency of micturition	Braxton hicks contraction	Auscultation of foetal heart sounds
Morning sickness	External ballottement	Ultrasound evidence of embryo/ foetus
Fatigue	Outlining of the foetus	Radiological evidence of foetus 16 weeks or beyond
Breast changes	Changes in the size, shape and consistency of the uterus	
Skin changes	Jacquemier's sign (softening of cervix)	
Quickening	Osiander's sign	
	Internal ballottement and immunological test	

Signs of Pregnancy

Name	Description
Jacquemier's or chadwick sign	Dusky hue of the vestibule and anterior vaginal wall due to local vascular congestion
Osiander sign	Increase pulsation felt through the lateral fornices
Goodell's sign	Softening of the cervix
Piskacek's sign	There is asymmetrical enlargement of the uterus if there is lateral implantation
Hegar's sign	On bimanual examination, the abdominal and vaginal fingers appose each other
Palmer's sign	Regular and rhythmic contractions during bimanual examination

Screening for Fetal Abnormalities

	Amniocentesis	CVS	Percutaneous umbilical blood sampling (PUBS)/ cordocentesis	Percutaneous skin biopsy
When to perform	Between 14–20 weeks of pregnancy	After 10 weeks of gestation (11–12 weeks)	After 16 weeks gestation	between 17–20 weeks of gestation
Procedure	under USG guidance 22-gauge needle is passed into the amniotic cavity and 10–20 mL of amniotic fluid that contains cells from amnion, foetal skin, lungs, and urinary tract epithelium are collected.	Under USG guidance a catheter is passed through the cervix or through the abdominal wall into the uterus, and a sample of chorionic villi surrounding the sac is obtained	Under USG guidance a needle is inserted into umbilical vein	done under USG guidance
To detect	Foetal karyotype	• Chromosome analysis is carried out to determine the foetal karyotype. • DNA can be extracted from the cells for molecular analysis. DNA analysis of CVS specimens is helpful for early diagnosis of hemoglobinopathies.	This technique apart from karyotyping is also useful for evaluating fetal metabolism and hematologic abnormalities	skin disorders, which can be diagnosed are anhidrotic ectodermal dysplasia, epidermolysis bullosa dystrophica, hypohidrotic ectodermal dysplasia, oculocutaneous albinism, and genetic forms of ichthyosis

Pseudocyesis/phantom/spurious Pregnancy

- ❖ Medical term for a false pregnancy. Woman has a strong belief that there is pregnancy, in absence of actual pregnancy.
- ❖ Pseudocyesis can cause many of the signs and symptoms of pregnancy, and often resembles the condition in every way except for the presence of a foetus.
- ❖ It is a psychological disorder in a patient with intense desire to have baby.

Determination of gestational age:

	Transvaginal ultrasonography (TVS)	Transabdominal ultrasonography (TAS)
Gestational sac	4 weeks + 5 days	5 weeks + 5 days
Yolk sac	5 weeks	6 weeks
Foetal pole	6 weeks	7 weeks
Foetal cardiac activity	6 weeks	weeks

- Gestational age at first trimester calculated by foetal crown rump length (CRL)
- In second trimester by Biparietal diameter and head circumference

Findings Diagnostic of Pregnancy Failure

1. Crown-rump length (CRL) of 7 mm and no heartbeat on a transvaginal scan
2. Mean sac diameter (MSD) of 25 mm and no embryo on a transvaginal scan
3. Absence of embryo with heartbeat 2 weeks after a scan that showed a gestational sac without a yolk sac
4. Absence of embryo with heartbeat 11 days after a scan that showed a gestational sac with a yolk sac.

Double decidual sac sign (DDSS) is a useful feature on early pregnancy ultrasound to confirm an early intrauterine pregnancy (IUP) when the yolk sac or embryo is still not visualized.

- The "Double Decidual Sign", first described by Nyberg and co-workers consists of two echogenic rings surrounding the hypoechoic gestational sac.
- The inner ring represents the chorion, embryonic disc and decidua capsularis.
- The outer ring represents the decidua parietalis.

Nuchal Translucency

Nuchal translucency is the normal fluid-filled subcutaneous space identified at the back of the fetal neck during the late first trimester and early second trimester (11.3-13.6 weeks).

- Nuchal translucency upto 3 mm- Normal
- NT > 3 mm- Marker for Down syndrome (Best way to measuring NT -Transvaginal sonography)
- *Note*: Increased nuchal translucency is not a fetal abnormality, but rather a marker or soft sign that confers increased risk of fetal abnormality.

Causes of Increased Nuchal Translucency

1. Down syndrome (Trisomy 21)
2. Trisomy 18
3. Trisomy 13
4. Turner syndrome
5. Klinefelter syndrome
6. Triploidy
7. Congenital heart disease

Foetal Pancreas

Begins to develop	4th week of gestation
Pancreatic alpha and beta cells have begun to emerge	9th week
Pancreas starts producing insulin, glucagon, somatostatin, and pancreatic polypeptide	8th -10th weeks of gestation
α-cells >β cells	During early stages of foetal development
Alpha cells reach their peak	Middle stage of gestation
Beta cells continue to increase in number	From the middle stage until term

Teratogenic Effects of Some Drugs

Drugs	Adverse effect on foetus
Phenytoin	Foetal hydantoin syndrome (craniofacial defects, limb defects, MR)
Valproic acids	Spina bifida (1-2% lumbosacral type)
Warfarin	Nasal hypoplasia, stippled vertebral and femoral epiphysis, agenesis of corpus callosum, dandy walker malformation, midline cerebellar atrophy, micro-ophthalmia, optic atrophy blindness, conradi syndrome
ACE inhibitors	Oligohydramnios, renal anomaly, neonatal renal failure, pulmonary hypoplasia, growth restriction, death
Isotretinoin	Craniofacial defects, cleft palate, cardiac defects, hydrocephalus, thymic defects

Human Chorionic Gonadotropin (hCG)

- Glycoprotein, with biological activity very similar to luteinizing hormone (LH), both act via the plasma membrane LH-hCG receptor.
- It is secreted by syncytiotrophoblasts.
- This hormone is structurally related to three other glycoprotein hormones: FH, FSH, and TSH.
- The amino acid sequence of the α-subunits of all four glycoproteins is identical.
- hCG is detectable in plasma of pregnant women as early as day 22 of menstrual cycle by RRA (radioreceptor assay) or day 25th of menstrual cycle by RIA (radioimmunoassay).
- hCG enters maternal blood at the time of blastocyst implantation.
- Blood levels increase rapidly, with maximal levels being attained at about 8–10 weeks of gestation.
- From 10 to 12 weeks the level begins to decline.
- Plasma levels are maintained at this lower level for the rest of pregnancy.
- It completely disappears from circulation 2 weeks postpartum.
- The best-known biological function of the hCG is the rescue and maintenance of function of the corpus luteum, that is, continued progesterone production.

Classic Congenital Toxoplasmosis

- Characterized by the tetrad 1. Chorioretinitis 2. Hydrocephalus 3. Intracranial calcification 4. convulsion.
- Maternal-foetal transmission occurs between 1 and 4 months following placental colonization by tachyzoites.
- There are 2 goals of drug therapy for toxoplasmosis, depending on whether or not foetal infection has occurred.
- If maternal infection has occurred but the foetus is not infected, Spiramycin is used for foetal prophylaxis (to prevent spread of organisms across the placenta from mother to foetus).
- Spiramycin is a macrolide antibiotic that is concentrated in but does not readily cross the placenta, and therefore is not reliable for treatment of foetal infection.
- Use is aimed at preventing vertical transmission of the parasite to the foetus, and it is indicated only before foetal infection.

Abdominal Pregnancy

- Although women with abdominal pregnancy usually report an increase in gastrointestinal symptoms, these are rarely severe enough to lead to investigation.
- Foetal death rates are reported to be above 90% with abdominal pregnancies.
- It is almost impossible and dangerous to salvage the foetus.
- Infections of the gestational products can occur especially when the placenta adheres to the intestines.
- This can lead to abscess formation and the possibility of rupture
- Although leaving the placenta in the abdomen following surgical delivery predisposes to risks of postoperative infections, the risk is much less severe than the haemorrhage associated with attempts at removal of placenta at the time of primary surgery
- If the placenta cannot easily be removed, recommendations are to leave it in place at the time of the first surgery
- Methotrexate should be given postoperatively to take care of the placenta in situ.

Vagitus uterinus: Crying of the foetus while still within the uterus, possible when the membranes have been ruptured and air has entered the uterine cavity. Very rare condition.

- The fetal mortality following vagitus uterinus is small, and in practically all cases is attributable to mechanical injury to the child in the efforts of delivery.
- The phenomenon is of interest from a medicolegal standpoint, because it proves that, under certain conditions, a child may be born dead, with lungs inflated

41. Nuchal translucency in USG can be detected at ______ weeks of gestation. *(NEET 2019)*

a. 11–13 weeks
b. 18–20 weeks
c. 8–10 weeks
d. 20–22 weeks

Ans. is 'a' 11–13 weeks

42. Double decidua sign is seen during: *(NEET 2019)*

a. 1st trimester
b. 2nd early trimester
c. 2nd late trimester
d. 3rd trimester

Ans. is 'a' 1st trimester

43. Most conclusive clinical sign of pregnancy is: *(NEET 2018)*

a. Uterine enlargement
b. Cervical softening
c. Amenorrhea
d. Fetal heart sound auscultation

Ans. is 'd' Fetal heart sound auscultation

44. Amniocentesis for fetal karyotyping is generally done at: *(NEET 2018)*

a. 8–10 weeks
b. 10–12 weeks
c. 14–18 weeks
d. 19–22 weeks

Ans. is 'c' 14–18 weeks

45. Fetal karyotyping can be done by all, *except*: *(NEET 2018)*

a. Cordocentesis
b. Amniocentesis
c. CVS
d. Foetal skin biopsy

Ans. is 'd' Foetal skin biopsy

46. True about Pseudocyesis is: *(NEET 2018)*

a. Belief there is no pregnancy in presence of actual pregnancy
b. Examination reveals pregnancy
c. Psychological disorder in a patient with intense desire to have baby
d. All of the above

Ans. is 'c' Psychological disorder in a patient with intense desire to have baby

47. Fetal heart starts beating at: *(NEET 2018)*

a. 10–12 days
b. 10–12 weeks
c. 3–5 weeks
d. 3–5 months

Ans. is 'c' 3–5 weeks

48. Poor prognosis in first trimester USG is:

a. No fetal pole at 5 weeks
b. No cardiac activity at 5 weeks
c. No gestational sac at 4 weeks
d. No cardiac activity at 8 weeks of gestation

Ans. is 'd' No cardiac activity at 8 weeks of gestation

49. Goodell's sign is:

a. Dusky hue of the vestibule
b. Softening of the cervix
c. Increased pulsations felt through the lateral fornices
d. Regular and rhythmic contractions during bimanual examination

Ans. is 'b' Softening of the cervix

50. In foetus, insulin production begins at __________ weeks of gestation:

a. 4–6
b. 8–12
c. 14–18
d. 24–28

Ans. is 'b' 8–12

51. In early pregnancy, doubling time of beta HCG is:

a. 24 hours
b. 48 hours
c. 96 hours
d. 2 weeks

Ans. is 'b' 48 hours

52. Folic acid required in first trimester of normal pregnancy:

a. 100 μg
b. 400 μg
c. 4 mg
d. 0.1 mg

Ans. is 'b' 400 μg

53. Drug of choice for preventing Fetal Toxoplasmosis infection during pregnancy is:

a. Pyrimethamine
b. Sulfadiazine
c. Spiramycin
d. Pyrimethamine + sulfadiazine

Ans. is 'c' Spiramycin

54. Which of the following statements concerning abdominal pregnancy is correct:

a. Gastrointestinal symptoms are quite often very severe
b. Foetal survival is approximately 80%
c. Aggressive attempt should be made to remove the placenta at the time of initial surgery
d. Placenta can be left in situ at the time of surgery

Ans. is 'd' Placenta can be left in situ at the time of surgery

- **Gravidity** is defined as the number of times that a woman has been pregnant.
- **Parity** is defined as the number of times that she has given birth to a fetus with a gestational age of 24 weeks or more, regardless of whether the child was born alive or was stillborn.
- Multiple pregnancies present a problem: a multiple gestation counts as a single event and a multiple birth should be interpreted as a single parous event.

55. An antenatal woman presents with 36 weeks of gestation. Previously she had a twin delivery. What is her GRAVIDA and PARA status? *(NEET 2020)*

a. G2P1
b. G2P2
c. G3P1
d. G1P1

Ans. is 'a' G2P1

NORMAL LABOUR

The position and relative frequency of the vertex at the onset of labour:

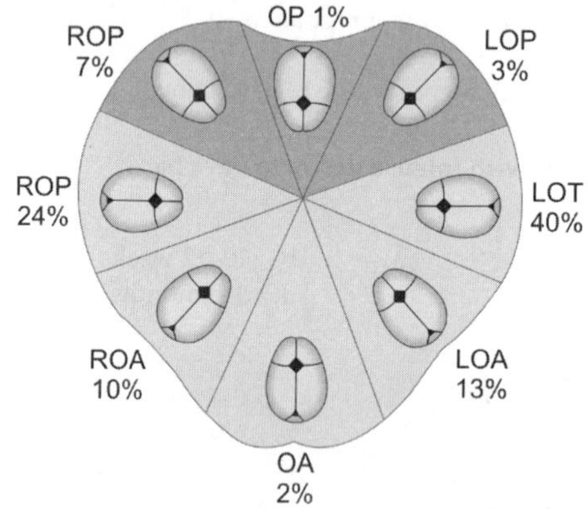

Stage	Definition
First	From the onset of true labour to full dilation of cervix. Average duration: 12 hours in primigravida and 6 hours in multigravida
Second	From full dilation of cervix to birth of the baby. Average duration: 2 hours in primigravida and 30 mins in multigravida
Third	From birth of the baby to delivery of the placenta. Duration- 15 minutes
Fourth	1 hour observation period following delivery of the placenta

56. Least common position in vertex is:

a. LOA
b. LOP
c. ROA
d. ROP

Ans. is 'b' LOP

57. Average duration of first stage of labour in primigravida is:

a. 6 hours
b. 12 hours
c. 16 hours
d. 18 hours

Ans. is 'b' 12 hours

SEXUALITY AND INTERSEXUALITY

PRECOCIOUS PUBERTY

Definition: Development of secondary sexual characters before the age of 8 years

Puberty before the age of 8 years in girls or 9 years in boys is considered precocious puberty.

Types: Two Varieties

1. Central/GnRH dependent (80%) and: Results from excessive GnRH, gonadotropins and target sex hormone elaborated by premature activation of hypothalamic pituitary-gonadal (HPG) axis.
2. Pseudo/peripheral/GnRH independent: Due to increased sex steroid secretion from either the adrenal gland or the gonads. It is independent of HPG axis activation
   - Most common cause of precocious puberty is constitutional/idiopathic.

Precocious menstruation is defined as onset of menses before 10 years

Causes of Precocious Puberty

Central precocious puberty	Peripheral precocious puberty isosexual blastoma	Heterosexual precocity
• **Idiopathic:** Sporadic or familial • **Central nervous system abnormalities**: – **Congenital anomalies of CNS:** hypothalamic hamartoma, hydrocephalus, porencephaly, arachnoid cysts. – **Acquired lesion of CNS:** inflammation, granuloma, trauma, surgery, radiation, chemotherapy – **Tumour of CNS:** pineal tumour, optic glioma, ependymoma, craniopharyngioma – **Hypothyroidism**	• **Ovary causes:** McCune Albright syndrome, granulosa theca cell tumour, gonadoblastoma • **Adrenal causes:** feminizing adrenal neoplasia • Exogenous oestrogen administration **Boys:** – **Testis:** Leyding cell tumour, Adrenal rest tumour, testotoxicosis – **Adrenal:** CAH (21 or 11 β hydroxylase deficiency), virilizing tumour – hCG secreting tumours hepatoma, choriocarcinoma, teratoma, dysgerminoma – Exogenous testosterone	**Girls:** Virilization in girls due to virilizing CAH, ovarian or adrenal neoplasia, polycystic ovarian disease **Boys:** Feminization due to oestrogen producing adrenal tumour, exogenous oestrogen, marijuana smoking.

58. MC cause of precocious puberty is:

a. Constitutional
b. McCune Albright syndrome
c. PCOS
d. Kalman syndrome

Ans. is 'a' Constitutional

59. Precocious puberty in girls is defined as development of secondary sexual characters before the age of:

a. 8 years
b. 9 years
c. 10 years
d. 6 years

Ans. is 'a' 8 years

Defective conversion of 17-hydroxyprogesterone (17OHP) to 11-deoxycortisol accounts for more than 95 percent of cases of congenital adrenal hyperplasia (CAH). This conversion is mediated by 21-hydroxylase due to mutations in the *CYP21A2* gene. Based upon neonatal screening studies that detect classic CAH, 21-hydroxylase deficiency (21OHD) is one of the more common inherited disorders.

The clinical spectrum of disease ranges from the most severe to mild forms, depending on the degree of 21-hydroxylase deficiency (21OHD). Three main clinical phenotypes have been described: classic salt-losing, classic non-salt-losing (simple virilizing), and nonclassic (late-onset):

- Females with the classic form (salt-losing and non-salt-losing) present with genital atypia.
- Males with the salt-losing form who are not identified by neonatal screening present with failure to thrive, dehydration, hyponatremia, and hyperkalemia typically at 7 to 14 days of life.
- Males with the classic non-salt-losing form who are not identified by neonatal screening typically present at two to four years of age with early virilization (pubic hair, growth spurt, adult body odor).
- Nonclassic or late-onset 21OHD may present as early pubarche or sexual precocity in school-age children, hirsutism and menstrual irregularity in young women, or there may be no symptoms

60. A young girl was brought by her parents as she had ambiguous genitalia, ammenorhea and clitoromegaly. She was diagnosed as a case of CAH. What is the most common enzyme defect in it? *(NEET 2020)*

a. 21 hydroxylase deficiency
b. 3 beta hydroxysteroid dehydrogenase deficiency
c. 11 hydroxylase deficiency
d. 17 hydroxylase deficiency

Ans. is 'a' 21 hydroxylase deficiency

INDUCTION OF LABOUR AND TRIAL OF LABOUR

TYPES OF BREECH

Complete: Full flexed attitude, thighs are flexed at the hips and legs are flexed at the knees, so the presenting part comprises of the buttocks, external genitalia and two feet. It is usually ***seen in multipara***.

Incomplete

- **Frank breech:** Thighs are flexed at the hips and legs are extended at the knees. The presenting part consists of external genitalia and buttocks. It is commonly seen in primigravida (70%) due to tight abdominal wall, good uterine tone and early engagement. Common in primigravida.
- **Footling presentation**: Both the thighs and the legs are partially extended bringing the legs at the pelvic brim.
- **Knee presentation**: Thighs are extended but the knees are flexed, bringing the knees to the pelvic brim.

Shoulder Dystocia

The term shoulder dystocia is defined to describe a wide range of additional obstetric manoeuvres to deliver the foetus after the head has been born and gentle traction has failed to deliver the shoulder.

Shoulder dystocia occurs when either the anterior or the posterior (rare) foetal shoulder impacts on the maternal symphysis or on the sacral promontory respectively.

Overall incidence varies between 0.2% and 1%.

Risk Factors

1. Previous shoulder dystocia
2. Macrosomia (> 4.5 kg)
3. Diabetes
4. Obesity (BMI>30kg/m^2)
5. Induced labour
6. Prolonged first stage or second stage of labour
7. Secondary arrest of labour
8. Post maturity
9. Multiparity
10. Anencephaly
11. Mid-pelvic instrumental delivery (more following ventouse than forceps)
12. Foetal ascites

Management

The following manoeuvres are commonly employed. There is no evidence that any method is superior to another in releasing the impacted shoulder or reducing the chance of injury. Head and neck should be grasped and taken posteriorly while suprapubic pressure is applied by an assistant slightly toward the side of foetal chest. This will reduce the bis-acromial diameter and rotate the anterior shoulder toward the oblique diameter.

Wood's Manoeuvre

- General anaesthesia is administered. The posterior shoulder is rotated to anterior position (1800) by a corkscrew movement.
- This is done by inserting two fingers in the posterior vagina.
- Simultaneous suprapubic pressure is applied.
- This pushes the bis-acromial diameter from the anteroposterior diameter to an oblique diameter. This helps easy entry of the bis-acromial diameter into the pelvic inlet.

Extraction of the Posterior Arm

- The operator's hand is introduced into the vagina along the foetal posterior humerus in the sacral hollow.
- The arm is then swept across the chest and thereafter delivered by gentle traction.
- This procedure may cause either fracture clavicle or humerus or both.

All Fours Position

- Changing the mother on to all fours may increase the pelvic dimensions and allow the foetal position to shift.
- Downward traction on the posterior shoulder helps to free the impacted shoulder.
- This may be done for a mobile and slim woman in a community setting.

McRoberts manoeuvre: to be done in cases of shoulder dystocia.

- Performed by flexing the mother's thighs toward her shoulders while she is lying on her back.
- No specific degree of elevation or flexion of the patient's legs has been defined for the McRoberts manoeuvre.
- Recent obstetric textbooks simply state that McRoberts is performed by "hyper flexing" or "sharply flexing" the maternal legs the abdomen.
- Care should be taken to avoid prolonged or overly aggressive application of the McRoberts manoeuvre, as the fibrocartilaginous articular surfaces of the symphysis pubis and surrounding ligaments may be unduly stretch.
- In addition, when the maternal thighs are markedly flexed and abducted, pressure from the overlying inguinal ligament may lead to femoral nerve injury.

Other techniques: May be used when all the above manoeuvres have failed

1. Deliberate fracture of the clavicle by linger pressure (fracture heals rapidly) or cleidotomy:

   One or both clavicles may be cut with scissors to reduce the shoulder girth.

   This is applicable to a living anencephalic baby as a first choice or in a dead foetus.
2. Zavanelli manoeuvre (pushing the foetus back to the uterus and delivering by caesarean section) or symphysiotomy is done rarely.

Various uses of prostaglandins in obstetrics
• Medical method of first trimester MTP (mifepristone followed by misoprostol)
• Second trimester MTP (PGE1 and PGF2 α, PGE1 preferred)
• Management of atonic postpartum haemorrhage (mainly PGF2 α and PGE1, PGE2 can also be used)
• Induction of labour (PGE2 and PGE1; PGE2 preferred as more safe, NEVER PGF2α)
• Augmentation of labour (PGE2 and PGE1)
• Medical management of tubal ectopic pregnancy

ACTIVE MANAGEMENT OF THE THIRD STAGE OF LABOUR (AMTSL)

- Current evidence indicates AMTSL (administration of uterotonic drugs, controlled cord traction, and fundal massage after delivery of the placenta) can reduce the incidence of postpartum haemorrhage by up to 60%.
- WHO recommends oxytocin as the drug of choice for AMTSL Administer a uterotonic drug at the delivery of the anterior shoulder or afterwards, within one minute of the baby's birth.
- Before performing AMTSL, gently palpate the woman's abdomen to rule out the presence of another baby.
- At this point, do not massage the uterus. If there is not another baby, begin the procedure by giving the woman 10 lU of oxytocin TM in the upper thigh.
- Clamp and cut the cord following strict hygienic techniques after cord pulsations have ceased or approximately 2–3 minutes after birth of the baby, whichever comes first.
- Perform controlled cord traction
- Massage the uterus immediately after delivery of the placenta and membranes until it is firm. Examine the foetal and maternal sides of the placenta and membranes to ensure they are complete. Perform a comprehensive examination of the woman and new-born one and six hours after childbirth. During the first two hours after the delivery of the placenta, monitor the woman at least every 15 minutes (more often if needed) to; — Palpate the uterus to check for firmness—Massage the uterus until firm. (Ask the woman to call for help if bleeding increases or her uterus gets soft.) — Check for excessive vaginal bleeding.

AMTSL Decreases

- Incidence of PPH
- Length of third stage of labour
- Percentage of third stages of labour lasting longer than 30 minutes
- Need for blood transfusion
- Need for uterotonic drugs to manage PPH.

61. Female with 41 weeks gestation confirmed by radiological investigation, very sure of her LMP, no uterine contractions, no effacement and no dilatation. What should not be done: *(NEET 2019)*

a. Intracervical foley's
b. PGE1 tab
c. PGE2 gel
d. PGF2 alpha

Ans. is 'd' PGF2 alpha

62. Which type of breech is seen more commonly in primigravidas: *(NEET 2018)*

a. Complete breech
b. Frank breech
c. Footling breech
d. Knee presentation

Ans. is 'b' Frank breech

63. In shoulder dystocia, next step in management is: *(NEET 2018)*

a. Immediate C-section
b. Flex hips on abdomen
c. O_2 ventilation is least effective
d. Rotate the shoulders 90° manually

Ans. is 'b' Flex hips on abdomen

64. Nerve injured in McRoberts manoeuvre is: *(NEET 2018)*

a. Lumbosacral trunk
b. Obturator nerve
c. Femoral nerve
d. Pudendal nerve

Ans. is 'c' Femoral nerve

65. All are components of active management of the third stage of labour *except*:

a. Uterotonic agent within 1 minute of birth
b. Massage of uterus before control cord traction
c. Control cord traction
d. None of the above

Ans. is 'b' Massage of uterus before control cord traction

INFECTIONS OF THE GENITAL TRACT

	Bacterial vaginosis	Candidiasis	Trichomonas vaginitis
Organism	Alteration of vaginal flora; *Lactobacilli* decreases whereas coccobacilli and *Gardnerella* increases	*Candida albicans* > *Candida galbrata*> *Candida tropicalis*	*Trichomonas vaginalis* (flagellated protozoa)
pH of discharge	> 4.5	< 4.5	5–6
m/c presenting feature	Foul smelling dirty white discharge No itching	Intense pruritis Curdy white discharge (or cotton cheese like discharge)	***Profuse frothy greenish yellow discharge*** Urinary symptoms Dysuria Dyspareunia
Sign	—	—	Strawberry vagina or angry looking vagina
IOC	**Saline microscopy** **'Clue cells'** i.e. vaginal epithelial cells to which bacteria are adhered seen	**Saline microscopy** Pseudohyphae seen	**Saline microscopy** typical motile flagellated trichomonas seen or motility
Gold standard investigation	**Gram stain** on gram staining **Nugent scoring** is done – the Nugent score is calculated by assessing the presence of lactobacillus (gram +ve rods- scored as 0 to 4), *Gardenella vaginalis* (scored 0 to 4) and *Mobiluncus* (gram variable rods scored as 0-2) A score of $\geq$ 7 is consistent with bacterial vaginosis	Culture on Sabouraud's medium or Nickerson medium	Culture on- Feinberg-whittington media or diamond media
Amine test/whiff test: 10% KOH added to discharge	*Positive*: on adding 10% KOH to discharge, fishy odour or amine like odour obtained.	Negative	May be positive or negative
T/t = non-pregnant females	Metronidazole (500 mg BD × 7 days or clindamycin	Fluconazole/miconazole orally as well as apply topically (150 mg, single dose)	Metronidazole (2 gm single dose oral)
Pregnancy = DOC		Metronidazole (250 mg TDS × 7 days) to be avoided in first trimester	Metronidazole (250 mg TDS × 7 days)
t/t of male partner	Not needed	Treatment needed if husband is symptomatic	Always done as trichomonas vaginalis is an STD

Fitz-High-Curtis Syndrome

Five percent to 10% of women with acute PID develop symptoms of perihepatic inflammation, the Fitz High-Curtis syndrome.

Aetiology

- Fitz-High-Curtis syndrome develops from transperitoneal or vascular dissemination of the gonococcal or chlamydia organism to produce the perihepatic inflammation.
- Other organisms, including anaerobic streptococci and coxsackievirus, have also been associated with this syndrome

Clinical Features

1. Persistent right upper quadrant pain
2. Pleuritic pain
3. Tenderness in the right upper quadrant when the liver is palpated.
4. The pain may radiate to the shoulder or into the back.
5. Liver transaminase levels may be elevated.

The condition is often mistakenly diagnosed as pneumonia or acute cholecystitis. When laparoscopy is performed, the liver capsule will appear inflamed, with classic violin string adhesions in the parietal beneath the diaphragm.

Differential Diagnosis of Acute Pelvic Pain

A. Women of reproductive age	B. Pregnant women
i. **Gastrointestinal:** Appendicitis; bowel obstruction; diverticulitis; gastritis; inguinal hernia; irritable bowel syndrome; mesenteric venous thrombosis; perirectal abscess ii. **Gynaecologic:** Adenomyosis; degenerating uterine fibroid; ectopic pregnancy; endometriosis; mittelschmerz; ovarian torsion; pelvic inflammatory disease; ruptured ovarian cyst; tubo-ovarian abscess iii. **Urinary:** Cystitis; pyelonephritis; ureterolithiasis iv. **Other:** Dissecting aortic aneurysm; lead poisoning; malingering; narcotic seeking; porphyria; sickle cell crisis; somatization disorder	1. Corpus luteum hematoma 2. Ectopic pregnancy 3. Endometritis (postpartum) 4. Ovarian torsion 5. Ovarian vein thrombosis (postpartum) 6. Placental abruption

Pelvic Inflammatory Disease (PID)

Clinical syndrome resulting from ascending infection from the lower genital tract to involve the endometrium, Fallopian tubes and/or adjacent pelvic structures.

Aetiology

Usually polymicrobial

Causative Organism

1. *Chlamydia trachomatis*
2. *Neisseria gonorrhoea*
3. *CMV*
4. Endogenous aerobic and anaerobic bacteria
5. Genital mycoplasma species

Sequelae of PID

- Increased rate of ectopic pregnancy
- Chronic and acute pelvic pain
- Infertility

Investigation

1. Laparoscopic appearance of Fallopian tube inflammation is "gold standard" for diagnosis:
   - The minimum criteria to diagnose PID laparoscopically include visible hyperaemia of the tubal surface, tubal wall oedema and the presence of exudate on the tubal surfaces and fimbriae.
   - It also helps to take samples for culture directly from fallopian tube, which is most preferred
   - Fluid in pouch of Douglas (POD) may also be aspirated for culture
2. Triad of lower abdominal pain + cervical motion tenderness + bilateral adnexal tenderness (minimal criterion for clinical diagnosis of PID)

Presumptive Treatment for PID

Should be initiated in sexually active young women and other women at risk for STDs if they are experiencing pelvic or lower abdominal pain, if no cause for the illness other than PID can be identified, and if one or more of the following minimum clinical criteria are present on pelvic examination—Cervical motion tenderness or Uterine tenderness or Adnexal tenderness.
Cervicitis is not included in PID

Tuberculosis-HSG Findings

- Lead pipe tubes
- Tobacco pouch appearance
- Beaded tubes
- Hydrosalpinx
- Cornual blocks
- Intravasation of the dye
- Golf club tube
- Sperm head tube
- Honeycomb appearance of uterus (Asher man syndrome)
- Pseudounicornuate appearance of uterus (due to intrauterine adhesions only on one side)

STI Syndromes in Women

Syndromes	Causes
Vaginal discharge syndrome	Gonorrhoea, Chlamydia, trichomoniasis, herpes simplex, candidiasis, bacterial vaginosis, cervicitis
Lower abdominal pain syndrome	Gonorrhoea, Chlamydia, Mycoplasma, Gardenerella, anaerobic bacteria (Bacteroides, Peptococci)
Genital ulcer syndrome	Syphilis, Chancroid, Genital herpes, Genital warts, Molluscum contagiosum, scabies

STI Syndromes in Men

Syndromes	Causes
Urethral discharge syndrome	Gonorrhoea, Chlamydia, trichomoniasis
Genital ulcer syndrome	Syphilis, Chancroid, Genital herpes
Inguinal bubo syndrome	Lymphogranuloma venerum, Chancroid
Painful scrotal swelling	Gonorrhoea, Chlamydia
Genital skin conditions	Genital warts, Molluscum contagiosum, scabies

Usually treatment given during syndromic management is ceftriaxone (for gonorrhoea), doxycycline or azithromycin (for chlamydia), metronidazole (for bacterial vaginosis and T. vaginalis), and fluconazole/clotrimazole (for candida).

66. Green frothy vaginal discharge is produced by: *(NEET 2019)*

a. Herpes simplex
b. Candida albicans
c. Trichomonas vaginalis
d. Normal vaginal flora

Ans. is 'c' Trichomonas vaginalis

67. Nugent score includes all *except*:

a. *Lactobacillus*
b. *Gardnerella*
c. *Mobiluncus*
d. *Gonococcus*

Ans. is 'd' *Gonococcus*

68. Violin string adhesion [violent string sign] is seen in:

a. PCOS
b. Endometriosis
c. Fitz-High-Curtis syndrome
d. Ruptured ectopic pregnancy

Ans. is 'c' Fitz-High-Curtis syndrome

69. Acute pelvic pain could be due to:

a. Ectopic pregnancy
b. PID
c. Corpus luteum hematoma
d. All of the above

Ans. is 'd' All of the above

70. Triad for clinical diagnosis PID includes all *except*:

a. Fever
b. Lower abdominal pain
c. Cervical motion tenderness
d. Bilateral adnexal tenderness

Ans. is 'a' Fever

71. During laparoscopy, the preferred site for obtaining cultures in a patient with acute pelvic inflammatory disease is:

a. Endocervix
b. Pouch of Douglas
c. Endometrium
d. Fallopian tubes

Ans. is 'd' Fallopian tubes

72. HSG finding suggestive of genital Koch:

a. Beaded tubes
b. Honeycomb uterus
c. Golf club tube
d. All of the above

Ans. is 'd' All of the above

GENITAL TB

The study shown here is a hysterosalpingogram. **Hysterosalpingogram (HSG)** is a fluoroscopic examination of the uterus and the Fallopian tubes, most commonly used in the investigation of infertility or recurrent spontaneous abortions.

Hydrosalpinx is a descriptive term and refers to a fluid-filled dilatation of the fallopian tube. If the fluid is infected, i.e. pus, then it is a pyosalpinx, if bloody, then hematosalpinx.

Hysterosalpingogram in hydrosalpinx will classically show a dilated fallopian tube, filling with contrast and with absence of free spillage

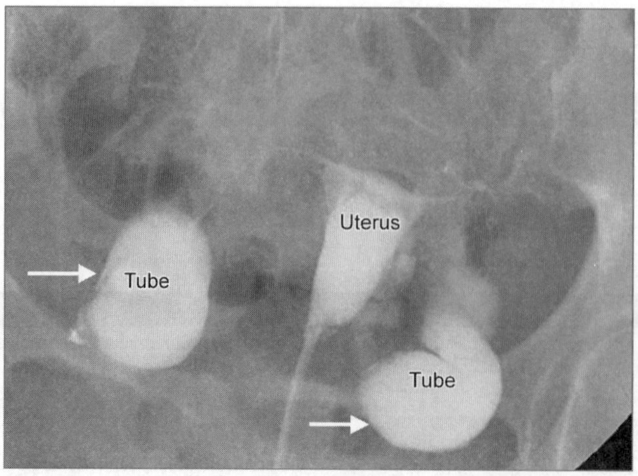

73. A young female suffering from infertility due to genital TB has the following HSG findings. What is the diagnosis?

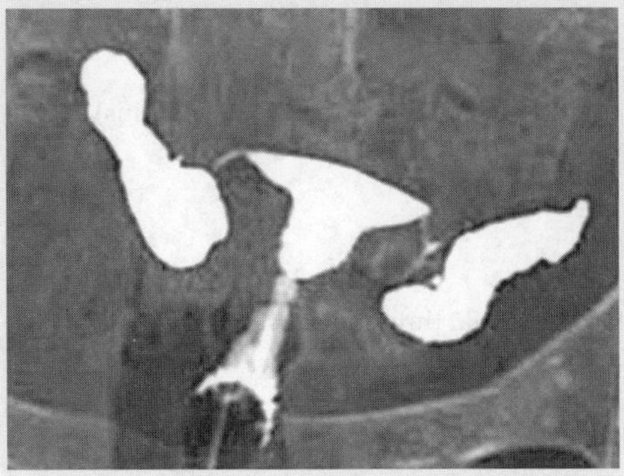

a. Bilateral hydrosalpinx
b. Ectopic pregnancy
c. Bilateral hydroureter
d. Bilateral endometriosis

Ans. is 'a' Bilateral hydrosalpinx

TO MASS

TOA is typically (but not exclusively) considered a complication of pelvic inflammatory disease (PID), and the classic presentation is the same as for PID, including acute lower abdominal pain, fever, chills, and vaginal discharge. Most women will not be overtly septic-appearing if their TOA is intact.

However, the presentation of some women with TOA differs from the classic scenario. Fever is not present in all patients, and some patients report only low-grade nocturnal fevers or chills. Also, not all women present in an acute fashion. As many as 40 percent of patients were afebrile upon presentation, 25 percent complained of chronic rather than acute abdominal pain, and 23 percent had normal white blood cell counts. Infrequently, women with TOA (often not associated with PID) present with seemingly unrelated symptoms, such as diffuse persistent upper abdominal pain or a change in bowel habits.

74. A 16 years old girl presented with low grade fever, weight loss, BMI of 19, left sided abdominal mass, mild ascites and amenorrhea for 6 months. What is the likely diagnosis? *(NEET 2020)*

a. Pelvic TB with tubo-ovarian mass
b. Ovarian malignancy
c. Ectopic pregnancy
d. Endometriosis

Ans. is 'a' Pelvic TB with tubo-ovarian mass

PUERPERIUM AND ITS ABNORMALITIES

NEUROLOGIC INJURY DURING CHILDBIRTH

- Neurologic injury during childbirth has long been recognized as a potential complication, with the **lateral femoral cutaneous nerve** as the most common obstetric-related nerve injury.
- Peroneal nerve injury is less commonly encountered and typically unilateral; the incidence of bilateral peroneal neuropathy following childbirth is extremely rare.
- Factors associated with lower extremity nerve injury in this study were nulliparous women and a prolonged second stage of labour.
- Most cases of bilateral peroneal neuropathy associated with childbirth occur in developed countries from prolonged mechanical external knee compression and forceful knee flexion.
- Additionally, nerve injury can result from an extended period of low pressure as well as a short interval of high pressure.
- Although the vast majority of neurologic injuries associated with childbirth are intrinsic obstetric palsies, neuraxial anaesthesia is a risk factor for an obstetric-related neurologic injury.
- Regional anaesthesia, in particular, increases the risk for developing a peroneal neuropathy as it blocks sensation to the lower extremities and, therefore, recognition of an impending nerve injury such as pain or altered sensation.

DURAL SINUS THROMBOSIS

- **The various aetiologies for dural sinus thrombosis are:**
  1. Thrombophilia (factor V Leiden mutation, prothrombin gene mutation 20210
  2. Deficiencies of antithrombin
  3. Protein C and protein S

4. APLA syndrome, hyper-homocysteinemia)
5. Pregnancy
6. Postpartum state
7. Hormonal contraceptive or replacement therapy
8. Infection (localized infections such as otitis, mastoiditis, sinusitis, meningitis)
9. Chronic inflammatory diseases
10. Vasculitis
11. Inflammatory bowel disease
12. Cancer
13. Hematologic disorders (polycythaemia, essential thrombocytosis, PNH)
14. Trauma
15. Nephrotic syndrome
16. Dehydration

Clinical Feature of Superior Sagittal Sinus

1. Headache is the most common presenting feature (75%).
2. Seizures occur in 10–37% patients.

Investigation

On non-contrast CT scan: The classic finding is the delta sign, which is a dense triangle due to hyperdense thrombus within the superior sagittal sinus (SSS).

On contrast-enhanced CT scan: The reverse delta sign (empty triangle) can be observed in the SSS from enhancement of the dural leaves surrounding the comparatively less dense thrombosed sinus.

- The presence of both these signs (delta and reverse delta) increases the likelihood of the diagnosis.

Other CT scan findings: Infarction in a nonarterial distribution in the white matter and/or cortical white matter junction, often associated with haemorrhage.

- Indirect CT signs include focal cerebral cortical ischemia with gyri enhancement, small ventricles due to compression by cerebral oedema, and intense tentorial enhancement.
- Absence of proteinuria, rule out eclampsia and besides postpartum.

75. Obstetric nerve palsy associated in Puerperium causes: *(NEET 2018)*

a. Median nerve
b. Facial nerve
c. Wrist drop
d. Foot drop

Ans. is 'd' Foot drop

76. A 32 years old female with mild hypertension. Two days after normal delivery, she develop seizures, headache. No proteinuria was there. On imaging she was found to have parasagittal infarction and hematoma 3 × 2 cm. the most probable cause is:

a. Eclampsia
b. Superior sagittal sinus thrombosis
c. Pituitary apoplexy
d. Subarachnoid haemorrhage

Ans. is 'b' Superior sagittal sinus thrombosis

ABORTION AND MTP, ALPA

CAUSES OF RECURRENT SPONTANEOUS ABORTION

- Hypothyroidism
- Uterine abnormalities can lead to impaired vascularization due to a distorted uterine cavity. In all, 12–15% women with recurrent abortions have a uterine malformation (e.g. septate uterus/T-shaped uterus).
- **Pathological causes**: fibroids and intra-uterine synechiae (Asherman syndrome) may also lead to recurrent spontaneous abortion, Hysteroscopy is a very useful tool in both diagnosis and correction of these factors.
- Anticardiolipin antibodies and lupus anticoagulant are antiphospholipid antibodies. They cause thrombosis spontaneous abortion, and foetal wastage. A total of 10–15% of women with recurrent abortions have then antibodies.
    - The recommended treatment for women with recurrent pregnancy loss associated with antiphospholipid syndrome includes combined Aspirin and Heparin therapy.
    - TORCH infection gives lifelong immunity so, TORCH infection can cause an abortion but not recurrent abortions.

MEDICAL METHOD FOR FIRST TRIMESTER MTP

It is now officially allowed in India up to 9 weeks (63 days) of gestation

Method: combination of RU486 followed by PGE1

Mifepristone: also known as RU-486, is an antiprogesterone compound

- It acts preferentially on target cells of the endometrium and decidua, counteracting the effect of progesterone, which is essential for establishment and maintenance of pregnancy.
- It affects the pituitary gonadotropic cells, producing a remarkable decrease of LH secretion, leading to luteolysis.
- It causes softening and ripening of the cervix and produces increased contractibility of the myometrium.
- It causes a marked increase in sensitivity of the uterus to exogenous PGs.

Misoprostol (PGE1): It acts by:

a. Enhancing uterine contraction and thus helping expulsion of the products of contraception and
b. Causing cervical ripening or priming.
   - It is used orally as tablets and vaginally as a suppository.
   - Success rate of this combination is 96%.

Dosage regimens: Recommended by World Health Organization are as follows: 200 mg mifepristone followed after 36–48 hours by: 800 g vaginal misoprostol or 400 g oral misoprostol

A registered medical practitioner shall have one or more of the following experience or training in gynaecology and obstetrics, namely:

1. In the case of a medical practitioner, who was registered in a State Medical Register immediately before the commencement of the Act, experience in the practice of gynaecology and obstetrics for a period of not less than three years.
2. In the case of a medical practitioner, who is registered in a State Medical Register:
   - If he has completed six months of house residency in gynaecology and obstetrics; or
   - If he has assisted a registered medical practitioner in the performance of 25 cases of MTP of which at least 5 have been performed independently, in a hospital or maintained or a training institute approved for this purpose by the government.
     - This training would enable the registered medical practitioner (RMP) to do only 1st trimester MTP (up to 12 weeks of gestation)
     - For terminations up to twenty weeks the experience or training as prescribed under sub rules shall apply.
     - In case of a medical practitioner who has been registered in a State Medical Register and who has graduate degree or diploma in gynaecology and obstetrics, the experience or training gained during such degree or diploma.

Abortus

The National Centre for Health Statistics defines an "abortus" as foetus or embryo removed or expelled from the uterus during the first half of gestation—20 weeks or less, or in the absence of accurate dating criteria, born weighing < 500 g."

77. Patient with recurrent abortion diagnosed to have antiphospholipid syndrome. What will be the treatment: *(NEET 2019)*

a. Aspirin only
b. Aspirin + Low molecular weight Heparin
c. Aspirin + Low molecular weight Heparin + Prednisolone
d. No Treatment

Ans. is 'b' Aspirin + Low molecular weight Heparin

78. In a case of recurrent spontaneous abortion the following investigation is unwanted:

a. Hysteroscopy
b. Testing for antiphospholipid antibodies
c. Testing for TORCH infections
d. Thyroid function tests

Ans. is 'c' Testing for TORCH infections

79. RMP can perform MTP in first trimester if he has assisted in ________ MTPs:

a. 5
b. 15
c. 25
d. 50

Ans. is 'c' 25

80. Mifepristone and misoprostol for MTP is allowed till:

a. 6 weeks
b. 7 weeks
c. 9 weeks
d. 12 weeks

Ans. is 'c' 9 weeks

INFERTILITY

Infertility: It is defined as an inability to conceive in spite of 1 year of regular unprotected intercourse

Primary never conceived

Secondary = conceived in the past (irrespective of outcome of that pregnancy)

Causes of Infertility

Male factor	Female factor	Both	Unexplained
30–40%	35–50%	20%	10%

SEMEN ANALYSIS

Semen analysis is the first and the most important investigation for evaluation of male factor

The ideal specimen for examination is after 3–5 days of abstinence. More prolonged period does not yield better results.

Methods of Semen Collection Include

- **Masturbation**, directing the sample into a sterile container. This is the most common way to collect a semen sample.
- **Sexual intercourse** in a special type of condom known as a collection condom. Collection condoms are made from silicone or polyurethane, as latex is somewhat harmful to sperm. Such samples are inferior to the ones collected by masturbation in clean cup.
- **Coitus interruptus (withdrawal):** With this technique, the man removes his penis from his partner near the end of intercourse and ejaculates into a wide-necked cup or bottle. Sample sent to laboratory as soon as possible so that examination is performed within 2 hours.
- Two other alternatives for men with an ejaculation due to spinal cord injury.
  1. Penile vibratory stimulation
  2. Electroejaculation

Motility

- The tail of the sperm—the flagellum—confers motility upon the sperm, and has a central skeleton constructed of 11 microtubules collectively termed the axoneme.
- Back and forth movement of the tail results from a rhythmical longitudinal sliding motion between the anterior and posterior tubules that make up the axoneme.
- The energy for this process is supplied by ATP produced by mitochondria.
- The velocity of a sperm in fluid medium is usually 1–4 mm/min.
- This allows the sperm to move towards an ovum in order to fertilize it.

Note: Following ejaculation, the semen forms a gel which provides protection for the sperm from the acidic environment of the vagina. The gel is liquefied within 20–30 minutes by enzymes from the prostate gland. This liquefaction is important to free the sperm so transportation may occur.

Causes of Male Infertility

- M/c cause of male infertility is Idiopathic
- M/c surgically correctable cause of male infertility is varicocele

Pretesticular	Testicular	Post-testicular
Hypogonadotropic hypogonadism	Varicocele, orchitis, trauma, torsion	Obstruction (infection)
Idiopathic	Heat/irradiation/chemotherapy	Kartagener syndrome/ young syndrome
Kallmann syndrome (deficient GnRH secretion associated with anosmia)	Bilateral cryptorchidism	Congenital bilateral absent vas deferens (associated with cystic fibrosis) Inguinal hernia repair (accidental damage to deferens)
Erectile dysfunction/ ejaculatory failure	Klinefelter syndrome, microdeletion Yq 11 idiopathic	Post-vasectomy

Site of pathology: Estimated by serum FSH level

- *A very high FSH*: Testicular cause
- *A very low FSH*: Pretesticular (hypothalamic/pituitary) cause
- *A normal FSH*: Post-testicular cause (as semen production is normal in post-testicular pathology).

Intracytoplasmic Sperm Injection

Indications

1. Severe oligo-astheno-teratospermia
2. Azoospermia
3. Repeated fertilization failure in IVF
   - The steps are identical to IVF (oocyte retrieval and embryo transfer), but for fertilization, one sperm mechanically injected into one oocyte.
   - Success rate of intracytoplasmic sperm injection (ICSI) per cycle is 30–35%.
   - If testes is producing sperm, then fertility is possible and Azoospermia patient can father of a child
   - Sperm retrieval techniques in case of azoospermia before doing ICSI:

PESA = percutaneous epididymal sperm aspiration
MESA = microscopic epididymal sperm aspiration
TESA = testicular sperm aspiration
TESE = testicular sperm extraction (testicular biopsy)

Test for Tubal Patency

1. **HSG (Hysterosalpingography)** – First line, but while pushing the dye, there can be cornual spasm. So HSG cannot differentiate between cornual blocks (pathological) and cornual spasm
2. **Laparoscopy (with chromopertubation with methylene blue dye):** Best investigation for tubal patency, as tubal patency can be confirmed under vision, and any pathology can simultaneously be corrected with operative laparoscopy (If on laparoscopy there is a presence of cornual block, cornual catheterization should be done simultaneously to remove the blocks)
   - IVF is the option in inoperable cases/severely damaged tubes or if surgery fails to remove the blocks.

Reasons for Infertility in Endometriosis

- Tubal adhesions/blocks or anatomy between the tube and ovary is distorted (main reason)
- Defective ovulation
- Impaired implantation
- ↑Sperm phagocytes
- Dyspareunia decreases coital frequency

Management of Endometriosis

- **Medical management** (aim is to induce amenorrhea in the patient)
  - **Pseudo pregnancy regimen**: OC pills DMPA POP, and Mirena
  - **Pseudo menopause regimen**: Danazol (Hardly ever used today because of androgenic side effects)
  - Medical castration: GnRH analogues (most common drug used for medical management)
- **Surgical Management**
  - **Patients with infertility**: Laparoscopic ovarian cystectomy, adhesiolysis, and electrocoagulation of endometriosis implants.
  - **If the family is complete and the patient has severe pain or menstrual complaints:** Hysterectomy with bilateral salpingo-oophorectomy.
  - Generally combined approach is adopted where laparoscopic surgery is followed by GnRH.

81. Causes of male infertility: *(NEET 2018)*

a. Idiopathic
b. Varicocele
c. q 11 microdeletion
d. All of the above

Ans. is 'd' All of the above

82. Abstinence period before semen analysis is: *(NEET 2018)*

a. 1–2 days
b. 3–5 days
c. 5–7 days
d. 7–9 days

Ans. is 'b' 3–5 days

83. Azoospermic patient can be a father of a child, by which of the following: *(NEET 2018)*

a. IUI
b. ZIFT
c. ICSI
d. No possible and counsel regarding adoption

Ans. is 'c' ICSI

84. Azoospermia with normal FSH would indicate: *(NEET 2018)*

a. Hypothalamic failure
b. Testicular failure
c. Obstruction of vas deferens
d. All of the above

Ans. is 'c' Obstruction of vas deferens

85. An infertile woman has bilateral tubal block at cornua diagnosed on hysterosalpingography. Next treatment of choice is:

a. IVF
b. Laparoscopy and hysteroscopy
c. Tuboplasty
d. Hydrotubation

Ans. is 'b' Laparoscopy and hysteroscopy

86. Treatment of choice in patient with infertility and endometriosis:

a. IUI
b. Surgery
c. Danazol
d. Ovulation induction

Ans. is 'b' Surgery

CONTRACEPTION

BARRIER CONTRACEPTIVES

All of the above options are types of Barrier contraceptives.

Barrier methods of birth control act as barriers to keep the man's ***sperm*** from reaching the woman's ***egg***. Some barrier methods also protect against ***sexually transmitted infections (STIs)***.

How effective are barrier methods of birth control in preventing pregnancy?

Barrier methods are not as effective at preventing pregnancy as other birth control methods, such as the birth control implant, injection, or ***intrauterine device (IUD)***. Out of 100 women per year, 18–28 women will become pregnant when using barrier methods. They work best when they are used correctly every time you have sex. Even one act of sex without using a barrier method can result in pregnancy. If barrier method breaks or becomes dislodged during sex, or if couple forget or are unable to use it, they may consider ***emergency contraception***.

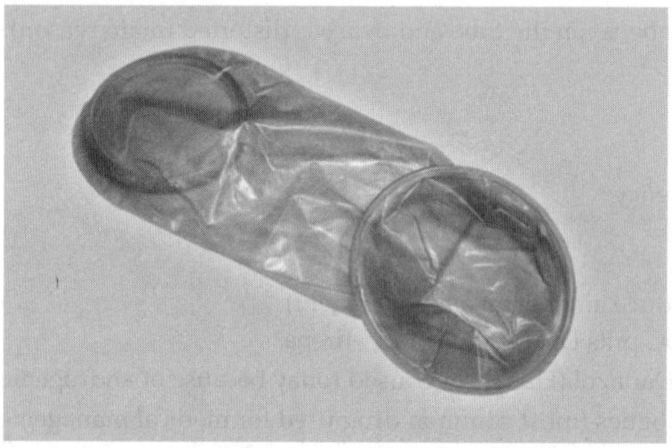

Female condom

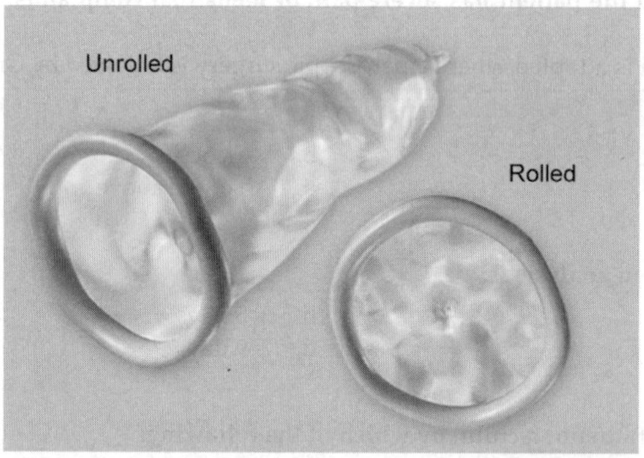

Male condom

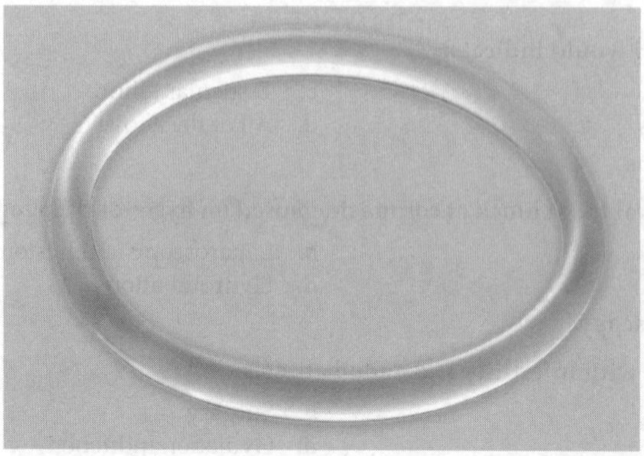

Vaginal ring

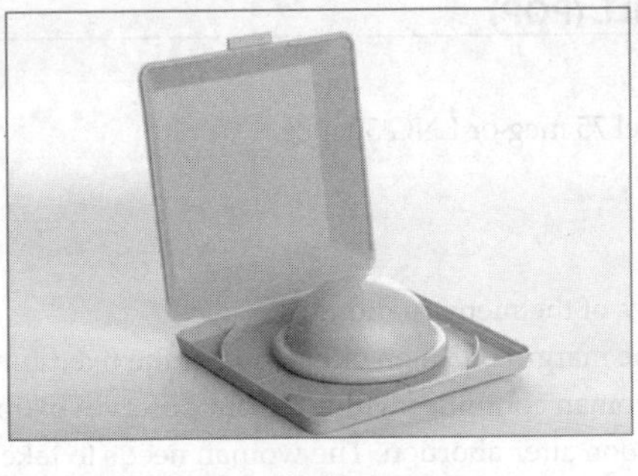

Diaphragm

87. Identify the contraceptive device? *(NEET 2020)*

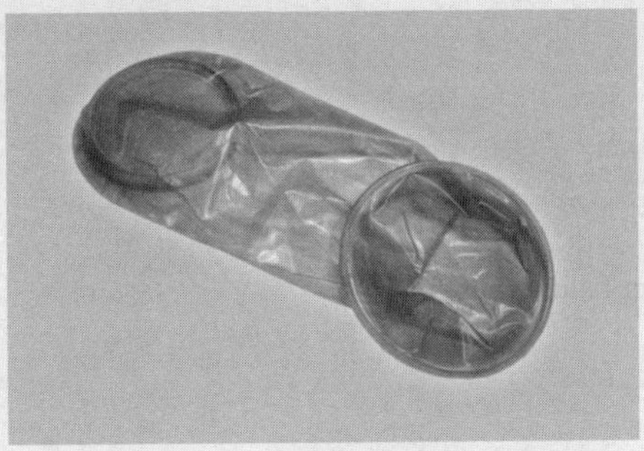

a. Male condom
b. Female condom
c. Vaginal ring
d. Diaphragm

Ans. is 'b' Female condom

TUBAL LIGATION

Falope ring technique for laparoscopic tubal ligation

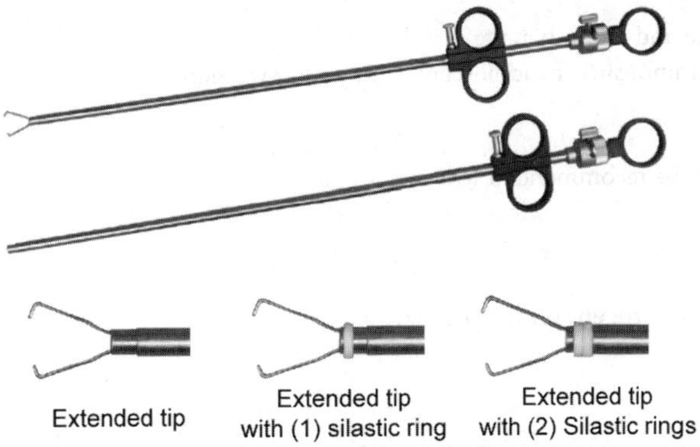

88. The following instrument is used for: *(NEET 2020)*

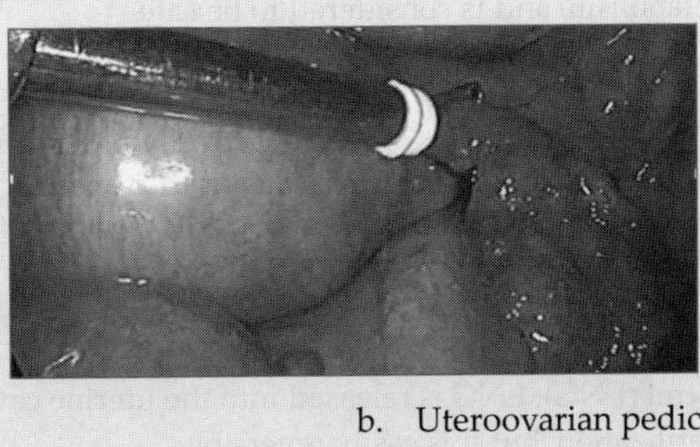

a. Tubal ligation
b. Uteroovarian pedicle ligation
c. Ectopic surgery
d. Hysterectomy

Ans. is 'a' Tubal ligation

LOW-DOSE PROGESTOGEN-ONLY PILL (POP)

Also k/a "minipill", is administered daily.

Contains norethisterone 350 mcg or norgestrel 75 mcg or LNG 30 mcg.

Precaution

- The tablet is taken daily without a break.
- The pill should be started within 5–7 days of the menstruation.
- Should be taken at the same time with the margin of 3 h on either side of the fixed time each day.
- If this regime is not taken any day, the woman continues with POP but observes extra precaution for 48 h.
- POP is started 21 days postpartum and soon after abortion. The woman needs to take precaution in the first 48 h in the first cycle.

Adverse Effects

- Strict daily compliance is a drawback.
- Irregular bleeding (20%)
- Amenorrhoea
- Depression
- Headache, migraine
- Weight gain
- Ectopic pregnancy
- Functional ovarian cysts besides a higher failure rate.

Contraindications

- Previous ectopic pregnancy
- Ovarian cyst
- Breast and genital cancers
- Abnormal vaginal bleeding
- Active liver disease
- Active arterial disease
- DVT
- Porphyria
- Liver tumor
- *Drugs*: Valproate, spironolactone and meprobamate.
- Because of osteopenia, it is contraindicated in adolescents and young women.

Advantages

Advantages of POP are that they can be recommended to:

- Lactating women
- Women over 35 years
- Those with focal migraine
- Those intolerant to oestrogen or oestrogen contraindicated
- Diabetic
- Hypertensive woman
- Sickle cell anaemia.
- As regards to return of fertility, it is faster than in COC users because ovulation is not suppressed in all cases (suppressed in 40%).

The use of newer generation of synthetic progestogen, namely Desogestrel, has been encouraging. It has no androgenic effect, no adverse effect on carbohydrate and lipid metabolism, and is considered to be safe.

Mode of Action of Mini-pills

- Cerazette suppresses ovulation in 97–100%, whereas other progesterone only pills suppress ovulation in only 40%.
  - It forms a thick plug of mucus in the cervical canal and acts as a barrier to sperms.
  - It increases tubal peristalsis and fertilized egg reaches the uterine cavity too early for implantation.

MIRENA

Mirena contains a total of 52 mg levonorgestrel (LNG). LNG is released into the uterine cavity at a rate of approximately 20 pg/day.

- The LNG IUD is about as effective as sterilization, but it is easily reversible.
- These devices act mainly by local progestogenic effects and act for up to 5 years.
- The ovarian function not disturbed by LNG 20.

The time periods for replacement for various IUDs are:

Device	Duration
Copper T 200	3 years
Copper T 380A	10 years
Multiload Cu 250	3 years
Multiload 375	5 years
LNG-IUD Mirena	5 years
Progestasert	1 year
Nova T	5 years

Complications of IUD

- **Increased bleeding** is the greatest disadvantage of IUDs and accounts for their removal in 2–10 per 100 users in the 1 year.
- **Misplaced IUD**: If the device is detected inside the peritoneal cavity, it should be removed as early as possible. Copper devices produce irrigative reactions, inflammations, and a lot of adhesions.
- **Infections**: Doxycycline 200 mg or, better still, azithromycin 500 mg, administered orally 1 h before insertion, reduces chance of infection.
- **Pregnancy:** As soon as pregnancy is confirmed, the IUD should be removed, if it can be done easily, to reduce the risk of pelvic infection and miscarriage—the most frequent complication of pregnancy with an IUD in place.
- **Ectopic pregnancy**

Failure Rates

Method	Failure rate
Male condom	4–14%
Female condom	18–20%
Copper LUD	0.5–1.5%
LNG LUD/Mirena	0.1–1%
OC pills	0.1–1%
DMPA	0.1–0.4%

POSTCOITAL (EMERGENCY) PILLS

Emergency contraception is used to prevent pregnancy after the act of an unprotected intercourse. It is an interceptive.

MOA

- Its main action is to make the endometrium unsuitable for implantation.
- It may also prevent or delay ovulation, and prevent fertilization of the egg by the sperms. It has, however, no role in the interruption of early pregnancy once conceived.
  - They are not abortifacients or contraceptives. They cannot interrupt an early pregnancy (they cannot cause an abortion).

Regimens

- Levonorgestrel 0.5 mg + ethinyl oestradiol 0.1 mg → within 72 hours of unprotected intercourse and repeated after 12 hours → Yuzpe method.
- Levonorgestrel alone 0.75 mg taken twice with 12 hour gap within 72 hours of unprotected intercourse → method of choice for emergency contraception.
- Mifepristone 600 mg single dose within 72 hours of unprotected intercourse.
- Other methods: progesterone only pill (mini pills), IUD insertion, high-dose estrogens.

POST COITAL CONTRACEPTION

Emergency Contraception Pills (ECPs) and Combined Oral Contraceptive Pills (COCs)

WHO recommends any of the following drugs for emergency contraception:

- ECPs with UPA, taken as a single dose of 30 mg;
- ECPs with LNG taken as a single dose of 1.5 mg, or alternatively, LNG taken in 2 doses of 0.75 mg each, 12 hours apart.
- COCs, taken as a split dose, one dose of 100 μg of ethinylestradiol plus 0.50 mg of LNG, followed by a second dose of 100 μg of ethinylestradiol plus 0.50 mg of LNG 12 hours later. (Yuzpe method)

Copper-bearing Intrauterine Devices

WHO recommends that a copper-bearing IUD, when used as an emergency contraceptive method, be inserted within 5 days of unprotected intercourse. This method is particularly appropriate for women who would like to start using a highly effective, long-acting, and reversible contraceptive method.

Mifepristone is a highly effective post-coital **contraceptive** up to 120 h unprotected intercourse and should be offered to women who present late for **emergency contraception** and find the IUCD an unacceptable method.

Danazol is a synthetic androgen and cannot be used as an emergency contraceptive.

Suppresses pituitary output of follicle-stimulating hormone (FSH) and luteinizing hormone (LH), resulting in regression and atrophy of normal and ectopic endometrial tissue **(treatment of endometriosis)**; decreases rate of growth of abnormal breast tissue; reduces attacks associated with hereditary angioedema by increasing levels of C4 component of complement **(treatment of hereditary angioedema).**

89. All of the following can be used for postcoital contraception *except*: *(NEET 2020)*

a. Danazol
b. RU 486
c. Cu200
d. High dose estrogens

Ans. is 'a' Danazol

ORAL CONTRACEPTIVE PILLS (OCP)

OCPs protect against:

- Endometrial cancer
- Uterine sarcomas
- Ovarian carcinoma
- Decrease the risk of colon cancer
- Regular OC pill users are protected from PIDs to the extent of 50%. By hindering the ascent of STD bacteria (including chlamydia) from the vagina upward by thickening cervical mucus and lessening uterine motility, as well as by obviating illegal abortions and delivery of children.
    - Studies have indicated that there is marginal increase in relative risk for dysplasia of cervix and invasive Ca and breast cancer after prolonged use of OC pills.

Side Effects of OCPs

1. **Breakthrough bleeding**: This is slightly more common with the lower-dose pills.

   Hypomenorrhea happens sometimes with low-dose pills. The women should be reassured that it is not harmful but rather good for health.
2. **Stroke and myocardial infarction**: Women who do not smoke, have their blood pressure checked, and do not have hypertension or diabetes are at no increased risk of myocardial infarction if they use low-dose COCs, irrespective of their age and duration of OC use.
3. **Breast and cervical cancer:** There is a small increase in risk of current users of the pill (relative risk 1.24), and the risk reduces gradually over the 10 years after discontinuing use.
4. **Liver tumor:** OCs increase the incidence of a rare benign liver tumor, namely, primary hepatocellular adenoma.

Contraceptive Rings

Nuvaring: It is a soft vaginal ring that releases 15 μg EE and 120 μg ENG, etonogestrel, the active metabolite of desogestrel, per day as a controlled delivery system.

A vaginal progesterone-only ring called "Progering" has been developed and has been undergoing clinical trials

LNG ring: It contains 5 mg LNG, 20 μg/day, is released; left inside vagina for 3 months continuously.

Method of Contraception in Heart Disease Patient

- The best method of contraception for a woman with heart disease is vasectomy of male partner if the family is complete or double barrier as a temporary method.
- OC pills and tubal ligation are absolutely contraindicated and heart disease is a relative contraindication for IUCD insertion

Important Points

- Hormonal contraceptive of choice in lactating mother → progesterone only pill (mini pill)
- Other methods for lactating mother → IUCDs, barrier methods and lactation amenorrhea method.
- Contraceptive method of choice for newly married couple → Combined oral contraceptive pills.
- Contraceptive method of choice in patients with diabetes or heart disease → Barrier methods (if family not complete) or terminal method/sterilization (if family complete).
- Persona is a natural family planning method which is based on measurement of LH and estrgen-3glucuronide (E3 G) in early morning.

Ulipristal

- **Ulipristal** (Ella) is a progesterone agonist/antagonist marketed for emergency contraception. It is available by prescription only. Its mechanism of action varies based on time of administration. When taken before ovulation, ulipristal delays or inhibits ovulation.
- Administration in the early luteal phase may decrease endometrial thickness and affect implantation of a fertilized egg.
- Ulipristal is labelled for use as an emergency contraceptive following unprotected sexual intercourse or contraceptive failure.
- One tablet (30-mg tablet) taken as soon as possible, within 120 hours (5 days) of unprotected sexual intercourse or contraceptive failure.
- This is a selective progesterone receptor modulator (SPRM)
- It has partial agonistic as well as antagonistic effects on the progesterone receptor.
- It also binds to the glucocorticoid receptor, but is only a weak anti-glucocorticoid relative to mifepristone, and has no relevant affinity to the estrogen, androgen and mineralocorticoid receptors.
- **Mechanism of action:** Blocking or delaying ovulation and delaying the maturation of the endometrium.
- **Uses:**
  - **For emergency contraception,** *30 mg tablet* is used within 120 hours (5 days) after an unprotected intercourse or contraceptive failure.
  - It has been shown to prevent about 60% of expected pregnancies, and prevents more pregnancies than emergency contraception with levonorgestrel.
  - **For uterine fibroids:** Ulipristal acetate is used for preoperative treatment of moderate to severe symptoms of uterine fibroids in adult women of reproductive age in a daily dose of 5 mg tablet for 13 weeks, effectively controlled excessive bleeding due to uterine fibroids and reduced the size of the fibroids.
  - **Side effects:**
    - Pain abdominal
    - Irregular menstruation
    - Nausea and headache after long-term administration (12 weeks)
  - **Contraindication:**
    - Pregnancy
    - Liver disease (Metabolized by CYP)

90. What is the dose of ulipristal acetate: *(NEET 2019)*

a. 300 mg
b. 30 mg
c. 300 μg
d. 30 μg

Ans. is 'b' 30 mg

91. Which of the following is an absolute CONTRAINDICATION to OCP use: *(NEET 2019)*

a. Chronic renal disease
b. DVT
c. Diabetes mellitus
d. History of amenorrhea

Ans. is 'b' DVT

92. Regarding progestine only pill incorrect is: *(NEET 2018)*

a Ovulation is stopped completely
b. Ovulation can occur some time
c. Make cervical mucosa thick
d. Interfere with implantation

Ans. is 'a' Ovulation is stopped completely

93. Failure rate or copper IUCD is:

a. 3–4%
b. 0.01–0.03%
c. 0.5–1.5%
d. 4–5%

Ans. is 'c' 0.5–1.5%

94. Emergency contraception prevents pregnancy by all of the following mechanisms *except*:

a. Delaying/inhibiting ovulation
b. Inhibiting fertilization
c. Preventing implantation of the fertilize egg
d. Interrupting an early pregnancy

Ans. is 'd' Interrupting an early pregnancy

95. Contraception of choice for woman with heart disease:

a. OC pills
b. IUCD
c. Barrier
d. Tubal ligation

Ans. is 'c' Barrier

ECTOPIC PREGNANCY

ECTOPIC PREGNANCY

In ectopic pregnancy the fertilized ovum is implanted and develops outside the normal endometrial cavity, the gestation grows and draws its blood supply from the site of abnormal implantation.

- M/c site of ectopic pregnancy is fallopian tube (97%).
- M/c site of ectopic pregnancy in fallopian tube → Ampulla of the fallopian tube.
- Ampulla > isthmus > infundibulum > interstitial

Management of Ectopic Pregnancy

- Positive urine pregnancy test indicates that the amenorrhea is due to pregnancy.
- Pain and shock in early pregnancy are mostly always due to ruptured ectopic.
- When the patient is in shock, the next immediate line of treatment is to resuscitate the patient and can treat shock with blood and IV fluids, and start preparations for surgery simultaneously.
- This should be followed by immediate exploratory laparotomy which is the definitive treatment.
- When the patient is in shock, the next immediate treatment should always be measures to correct the shock (blood for cross match and IV fluids: crystalloids and colloids).
- By the time you prepare the patient for exploration (alert the OT and shift the patient to OT), and start IV Fluid and also blood if ready.
- Medical management and laparoscopy are contraindicated in shock.
- *Expectant management*: Only observation is done hoping spontaneous resolution.

Criteria for Expectant Management of Ectopic Pregnancy

- Patient should be stable (no evidence of rupture/bleeding)
- Initial HCG levels < 1000 IU/l and subsequent levels are falling
- Gestational sac < 4 cm
- Absence of cardiac activity.

Risk of Ectopic Pregnancy

The most common cause is an antecedent ectopic pregnancy.

- *PID*: Infection caused by *Chlamydia trachomatis* and *Neisseria gonorrhoeal* increases the risk of ectopic pregnancy; history of salpingitis increases the risk of ectopic pregnancy 4–10 fold.
- Genital TB also increases the risk of ectopic pregnancy
- Contraception failure
- Tubal surgery
- History of previous ectopic pregnancy
- ART
- Pelvic adhesions
- Increasing age
- Smoking
  - Implantation within the tubal segment that penetrates the uterine wall results in an interstitial pregnancy.
  - These account for about 3% of all tubal gestations. Rupture may not occur until up to 16 weeks
  - Ampullary pregnancy generally ruptures at 8 weeks and isthmic at 6 weeks.

96. MC site of ectopic pregnancy:

a. Fallopian tube isthmus
b. Fallopian tube ampulla
c. Cervix
d. Ovary

Ans. is 'b' Fallopian tube ampulla

97. hCG levels at which expectant management of ectopic pregnancy can be done:

a. 10,000 IU/L
b. 1000 IU/L
c. 2500 IU/L
d. 5000 IU/L

Ans. is 'b' 1000 IU/L

98. A 21-year-old female presents to emergency ward with 2 months of amenorrhea with pain in abdomen and shock. BP 90/60 mm Hg and Hb 6 gm% urine pregnancy test is found positive next immediate line of treatment is:

a. Laparotomy
b. IV fluids and cross match
c. Medical management
d. Laparoscopy

Ans. is 'b' IV fluids and cross match

ENDOMETRIOSIS AND DYSMENORRHEA

ENDOMETRIOSIS

Endometriosis is defined as the presence of normal functional endometrial mucosa (glands and stroma) abnormally implanted in locations other than the uterine cavity.

It was first described by Von Rokitansky.

About one-third of women with endometriosis remain asymptomatic.

Clinical Features

The classical triad of symptoms are:

- Dysmenorrhea (may be exaggerated or occurring before menses due to PGF2 and thromboxane)
- Dyspareunia (mostly seen in endometriosis of rectovaginal septum or Pouch of Douglas and with fixed retroverted uterus)
- Infertility (Around 40–60% patients have infertility due to multiple factors like tubal adhesions, ovarian dysfunction, dyspareunia).

Other Features

- Menorrhagia and premenstrual spotting (50–60%)
- Pelvic pain or backache due to adhesions, scarring or impingement of nerves
- Lower abdominal or back pain
- Dyschezia *(pain on defecation)*: Often with cycles of diarrhoea and constipation, rectal bleeding in cases of involvement of colon and rectum.
- Pain on micturition and/or urinary frequency, cyclical haematuria if bladder is involved.

MC Sites in Order of Frequency

Ovaries (ovarian endometriosis = endometrioma = chocolate cyst of the ovaries) > POD > Uterosacral ligaments

Investigation

- Laparoscopy is the investigation of choice
- Laparoscopy findings in endometriosis are:
  - Chocolate cysts
  - Powder burn spots
  - Matchstick burnt spots
  - Blueberry lesion
  - Red/purple raspberry lesion
  - White lesion
  - Red/flame lesion
  - Sub ovarian adhesions

Theories for Development of Endometriosis

- *Samson's theory of retrograde menstruation*: The most accepted theory
- *Ivanoff and Meyer*: Celomic metaplasia
  - Hematogenous spread
  - Lymphatic spread (Halban's theory)
  - Direct implantation

99. Triad of symptoms of endometriosis are all *except*:

a. Infertility b. Dysmenorrhea
c. Dyspareunia d. Cyclical haematuria

Ans. is 'd' Cyclical haematuria

100. Endometriosis is:

a. Endometrium within the myometrium b. Functional endometrium outside the uterus
c. Myometrium within the endometrium d. Rare squamous variety of CA endometrium

Ans. is 'b' Functional endometrium outside the uterus

101. Investigation of choice for endometriosis:

a. USG b. CA 125
c. MRI d. Laparoscopy

Ans. is 'd' Laparoscopy

TROPHOBLASTIC DISEASES INCLUDING CHORIOCARCINOMA

GESTATIONAL TROPHOBLASTIC NEOPLASM

Refers to group of malignant neoplasm consisting of abnormal proliferation of trophoblastic tissue.

Aetiology: among all cases:

- 50% arises after molar pregnancy
- 25% arises after ectopic pregnancy or miscarriage
- 25% arises after term or preterm pregnancy

Risk Factors

- Age of female ≥ 40 years
- b-hCG levels > 105 mIU/mL
- Uterine size larger than gestational age
- B/L Theca luteal cyst > 6 cm
- Slow decline in b-hCG levels

Feature	Partial mole	Complete mole
Karyotype	69,XXX or 69,XXY	46XX is MC, followed by 46XX
Clinical presentation		
Diagnosis	Missed abortion	Molar gestation
Uterine size	Small for dates	Large for dates
Theca-lutein cysts	Rare	25–30%of cases
Initial hCG levels	<100,000 MIU/mL	>100,000 MIU/ml
Medical complications	Rare	Uncommon
Rate of subsequent GTN	1–5% of cases	15–20% of cases
Pathology		
Embryo-fetus	Often present	Absent
Amnion, fetal erythrocytes	Often present	Absent
Villous edema	Focal	Widespread
Trophoblastic proliferation	Focal, slight to moderate	Slight to severe
Trophoblastic atypia	Mild	Marked
p57 immunostaining	Positive	Negative

Classification: Based on histology:

Invasive Mole (Chorioadenoma Destruens)

- Arises from myometrial invasion of *H. mole* via direct extension through tissue or lymphatic channel.
- About 15% metastasize to the lung or vagina.

Choriocarcinoma

- Most malignant tumor of uterus.
- Characterized by abnormal trophoblastic hyperplasia and anaplasia, absence of chorionic villi, hemorrhage and necrosis
- With direct invasion into the myometrium and vascular invasion, resulting in spread to distant sites, lung (80%) > vagina (39%) > pelvis (20%) > liver (10%) and brain (10%) and less frequently kidney, GIT and spleen.

Placental Site Trophoblastic Tumour

- Extremely rare.
- Arises from the placental implantation site.
- Consists predominantly of mononuclear intermediate trophoblasts without chorionic villi infiltrating in sheets and cords between myometrial fibers.
- It tends to remain localized in the uterus for long periods before metastasizing.
- It has propensity for lymphatic metastasis and is resistant to chemotherapy
- Despite very aggressive chemotherapy, the majority of cases of Placental site trophoblastic tumor (PSTT) with metastases have a bad prognosis, whereas prognosis is excellent in non-metastatic cases where all lesions can surgically resect.

Epithelioid Trophoblastic Tumor

- Unusual type of trophoblastic tumor.
- Composed of chorionic type intermediate trophoblastic cells closely resemble to membranous chorion, has similar features of carcinoma.
- Presents as a discrete expansive nodule in the endomyometrium in contrast to PSTT.
- Diagnosis is typically made at advanced stages, with 50% of patients presenting with metastatic disease.

Clinical Features

- Elevated hCG: Only in cases of invasive mole or choriocarcinoma. At very high levels, hCG stimulation may cause hyperthyroidism, ovarian luteal cysts, hyperemesis, or pre-eclampsia.
- Abnormal uterine bleeding or amenorrhea.
- Abdominal/pelvic pain.
- Symptom caused by metastasis.

Investigation

Lab test: hCG, thyroid function test, liver and kidney function test

Pelvic Ultrasound

Invasive mole	A central uterine mass with very high diastolic blood flow and areas of cystic vascular spaces showing low-impedance flow that reveals invasion into the myometrium.
Choriocarcinoma	Appears as a mass enlarging the uterus, with a heterogenous appearance that correlates with areas of necrosis and hemorrhage. It is markedly hypervascular on colour Doppler and it may extend into the parametrium.
PSTT	It appears as a small heterogeneosly hyperechoic intrauterine mass with cystic spaces within the myometrium.
ETT	It appears as an irregular anechoic lacuna within the myometrium with low-resistance blood flow and the tumor border growing in an expansive fashion, invading the cervix or the myometrium deeply.

To Detect Metastasis

- **Chest radiograph:** It may produce the following four patterns:
  - An alveolar snow storm pattern (snowstorm appearance on USG–means H mole; snowstorm appearance on chest X-ray means choriocarcinoma)
  - Discrete rounded densities or canon ball appearance
  - Pleural effusion
  - An embolic pattern caused by pulmonary arterial occlusion.
- **Pelvic ultrasound:** To detect uterine extension
- **Abdominopelvic CT scan:** To rule out abdominal metastases.
- **MRI of the brain:** To detect lesions in the brain, if brain imaging is negative lumbar puncture may be indicated to measure the cerebrospinal fluid/plasma hCG ratio (normal value is <60:1)

Management of Low-risk GTN-Single agent regimen: Methotrexate (MTX), actinomycin D

Management of High-risk GTN: EMA/CO or MAC regimens

102. Gestational Trophoblastic neoplasm does not include: *(NEET 2019)*

a. Choriocarcinoma
b. Placental site trophoblastic tumor
c. Invasive mole
d. Partial mole

Ans. is 'd' Partial mole

103. Chromosome number of partial hydatidiform mole is: *(NEET 2019)*

a. 46 XX
b. 45 XO
c. 46 XXY
d. 69 XXX

Ans. is 'd' 69 XXX

104. Complete vesicular mole is associated theca-leutin cysts in what percentage of cases:

a. <5
b. 5–15
c. 20–40
d. 60–70

Ans. is 'c' 20–40

105. Patient with 3 months amenorrhoea, c/o hyperemesis and vaginal bleeding since one month. O/E = uterus 16 weeks with absent fetal heart sound. The diagnosis is:

a. Vesicular mole
b. Ectopic pregnancy
c. IUFD
d. Abruptio placentae

Ans. is 'a' Vesicular mole

DISORDERS OF MENSTRUATION

CRYPTOMENORRHEA

It is a condition in which there is periodic shedding of endometrium (menstruation) but the blood fails to come out of the genital tract due to outflow tract obstruction.

Causes

a. Congenital
Imperforate hymen: It is due to failure of disintegration of the central cells of Müllerian eminence that project into urogenital sinus
   - Transverse vaginal septum
   - Atresia of vagina, cervix.

b. *Acquired*:
Cervical stenosis (Following surgeries like conization, amputation or cancer).

c. *Pathology*:
The blood fails to come out of hymen → distends the vagina –4 hematocolpos → then uterus distends (hematometra) '→ hematosalpinx.

Clinical Features

- *In congenital variety*: The girl is around 14 to 16 years of age, presents with primary amenorrhea
- In acquired cases there would be secondary amenorrhea
- Periodic lower abdominal pain
- Urinary complaints like frequency, dysuria or retention of urine (hematocolpos leads to elongation of urethra) examination
- Abdominal examination reveals globular mass (distended uterus or full bladder) in supra-pubic region
- *Vulval examination*: Tense bulging hymen with bluish coloration
- Rectal examination reveals bulged vagina and uterine mass.

106. Cryptomenorrhea occurs in:

a. Fibroids
b. PCOS
c. Imperforate hymen
d. All of the above

Ans. is 'c' Imperforate hymen

IMPERFORATE HYMEN

Imperforate hymen — An imperforate hymen is one of the most common obstructive lesions of the female genital tract.

Diagnosis of an imperforate hymen may be made in neonates if a bulging introitus is noted at birth. The bulging is due to a mucocolpos from vaginal secretions due to stimulation by maternal estradiol. If the diagnosis is not made in the newborn period and the hymen remains imperforate, the mucus will be reabsorbed and the child usually remains asymptomatic until menarche.

At the usual age of menarche, the adolescent girl may present with amenorrhea (sometimes referred to as crypto-menarche), cyclic abdominal or pelvic pain, and hematocolpos, which may give the hymenal membrane a bluish discoloration. Marked distension of the vagina may also result in back pain, pain with defecation, or difficulties with urination.

On examination, there is typically a bulging obstruction of the vagina. It is important that the clinician does not assume that all bulging obstructive anomalies of the vagina are an imperforate hymen. The differential diagnosis includes: imperforate hymen (thin, fairly transparent membrane), agenesis of the lower vagina, or a low transverse vaginal septum.

The diagnosis can be confirmed with the use of a translabial or transperitoneal ultrasound to determine the distance from the obstruction to the level of the normal location of an introitus. If there is a thin structure (several millimeters) obstructing the introitus, then it is most likely the membrane of an imperforate hymen. But if obstructing structure is thicker, the diagnosis is not an imperforate hymen.

Transverse vaginal septa are often fenestrated and thus may not be associated with amenorrhea. Longitudinal vaginal septa are typically associated with uterine anomalies, such as septate uterus and uterus didelphys. The most common symptom associated with vaginal septa is difficulty with tampons or sexual intercourse. Imaging can help to delineate other reproductive tract anomalies occurring with a septum. Treatment is excision of the septum.

Total vaginal agenesis (Mayer-Rokitansky-Küster-Hauser syndrome) is usually accompanied by cervical and uterine agenesis and urologic anomalies. Ultrasound examination should be performed to assess the kidneys and confirm the presence of ovaries and the absence or presence of a uterus or uterine structures. Nonsurgical management is the preferred first line therapy for creation of a functional vagina (vaginal dilators); surgical treatment is also possible.

107. A 16-year-old girl presented with primary amenorrhea and cyclical abdomen pain. Perrectal examination revealed swelling in the upper vagina. What is the diagnosis? *(NEET 2020)*

a. MRKH syndrome
b. Vaginal atresia
c. Transverse vaginal septum
d. Imperforate hymen

Ans. is 'd' Imperforate hymen

PREDICTOR OF MENOPAUSE

- No single test for menopause is highly sensitive and specific.
- The best predictors that a woman will enter menopause within 4 years include
  - Age at least 50 years
  - Amenorrhea for 3 to 11 months
  - Menstrual cycle irregularity within 12 months.
- An increase in serum follicle-stimulating hormone (FSH) and decreases in estradiol are the endocrine changes that occur during the transition to menopause.
- As per the American Association of Clinical Endocrinologists, the diagnosis of menopause is confirmed by F levels >40 IU/L.
- In both males and females, primary hypogonadism results in an elevation of basal follicle-stimulating hormone (FSH) and luteinizing hormone (LH) levels.
- FSH and LH are generally elevated in:
  - Primary gonadal failure
  - Complete testicular feminization syndrome
  - Precocious puberty (either idiopathic or secondary to a central nervous system lesion)
  - Menopause (postmenopausal FSH levels are generally >40 IU/L)
  - Primary ovarian hypofunction in females.

108. Menopause is diagnosed by:

a. Estradiol < 20 pg/mL
b. Progesterone <40 ng/dL
c. FSH> 40 IU/L
d. LH> 20 IU/L

Ans. is 'c' FSH> 40 IU/L

MENORRHAGIA IN PERIMENOPAUSAL AGE GROUP

- It is necessary to rule out endometrial hyperplasia and cancer in this age group.
- Histopathological examination of endometrium is required, and therefore D and C should be done first.
- Alternatively, endometrial biopsy or hysteroscopy and biopsy can also be done, but always histopathological diagnosis is required in this age group.
- Depending on the endometrial pathology, hormonal treatment or surgery is advised.
- Never directly proceed with hysterectomy because the type of hysterectomy to be performed (simple/radical/TAH + BSO) will depend on the diagnosis.
- Progesterone (oral, injectables, and Mirena) may be used after excluding endometrial carcinomas

109. A 46-year-old P3L3 complains of menorrhagia since 3 months. Next line of management is:

a. D and C
b. Progesterone × 6 months
c. OC pills × 6 months
d. Hysterectomy

Ans. is 'a' D and C

Treatment **should not be initiated** until the etiology of AUB has been evaluated (or evaluation is underway) and premalignant or malignant disease excluded, as appropriate. Empiric treatment without evaluation may miss a primary etiology that may be corrected or mask symptoms of neoplastic disease. Invasive procedures may also be limited by insurance coverage or medical guidelines; for example, the National Health Service (NHS) in the United Kingdom advises against routine performance of dilation and curettage and hysterectomy for heavy menstrual bleeding.

AUB symptoms may persist until menopause. The goal of initial therapy is to control the bleeding, treat anemia (if present), and restore quality of life. Once this has been accomplished, some women are satisfied with continuing chronic medical therapy, while others desire a treatment that requires less maintenance or is definitive. The approach to treatment is generally stepwise:

- The primary etiology should be treated, if possible. This includes endocrine or infectious disorders that are treated medically (eg, polycystic ovarian syndrome or chronic endometritis) as well as structural lesions that are resectable via hysteroscopy (endometrial polyp, submucosal fibroid).
- The initial approach in women with chronic AUB is usually pharmacologic treatment. The choice of medication depends upon the factors listed above. For some women who do not wish to conceive in the next year, the LNg52/5 is used as first-line therapy.
- Secondary approaches are used for women who fail or cannot tolerate medical therapy or who prefer treatment options that do not require frequent dosing. Primary deciding factors are whether the patient is planning future childbearing and the level of invasiveness and risk associated with the procedure.

Women often choose surgical therapy after long-term medical therapy. A systematic review of eight randomized trials of women with heavy menstrual bleeding found that 58 percent of women randomly assigned to medical treatment underwent surgery by two years.

110. A 32-year-old woman is presented with complaint of heavy menstrual bleeding for 6 months which is not controlled by non-hormonal treatment. TVS and per rectal examination were normal. What is the next appropriate step in management? *(NEET 2020)*

a. Endometrial sampling
b. Endometrial ablation
c. Hormonal treatment
d. Hysterectomy

Ans. is 'c' Hormonal treatment

ENDOMETRIAL POLYP

A well circumscribed echogenic endometrial thickening with a central feeding vessel in a stalk is highly suggestive of an endometrial polyp. However, the central feeding vessel is not pathognomonic as it can occasionally be seen with atypical fibroids or endometrial carcinoma.

Uterine leiomyoma can be differential diagnosis especially if pedunculated and submucosal, although most leiomyomas tend to be hypoechoic on ultrasound.

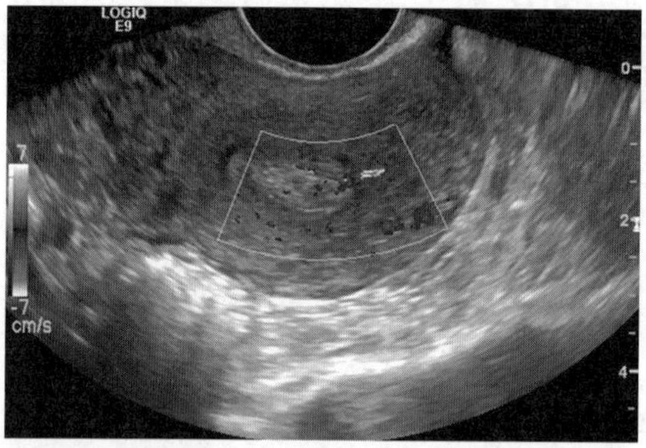

111. A middle aged woman presented with irregular intermenstrual bleeding. USG was done as shown below which revealed feeding vessel sign. What is the diagnosis? *(NEET 2020)*

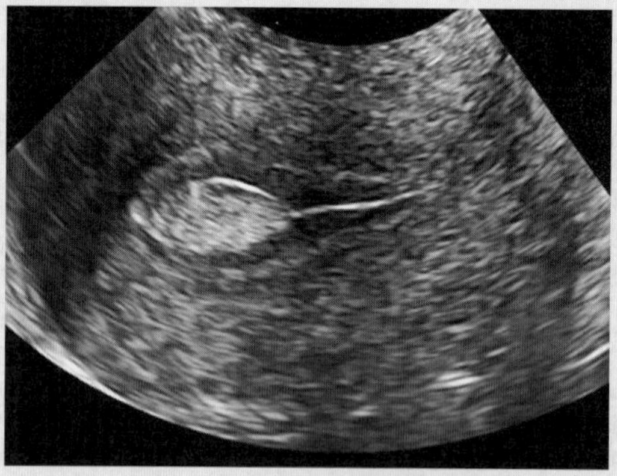

a. Endometrial polyp
b. Submucosal fibroid
c. CA endometrium
d. Endometrial hyperplasia

Ans. is 'a' Endometrial polyp

POLYPECTOMY

For routine outpatient hysteroscopy, the choice of distension medium between carbon dioxide and normal saline should be left to the discretion of the operator as neither is superior in reducing pain, although uterine distension with normal saline appears to reduce the incidence of vasovagal episodes. Uterine distension with normal saline allows improved image quality and allows outpatient diagnostic hysteroscopy to be completed more quickly compared with carbon dioxide. Operative outpatient hysteroscopy, using bipolar electrosurgery, requires the use of normal saline to act as both the distension and conducting medium.

112. Fluid used for hysteroscopic polypectomy using bipolar cautery is: *(NEET 2020)*

a. Glycine
b. NS
c. Dextrose
d. CO_2

Ans. is 'b' NS

GYNECOLOGICAL ONCOLOGY

CERVICAL CANCER

- Human papilloma virus (HPV) has been shown to be the **causative agent** of most **cervical cancers.**

HPV type	Causes
6, 11	Anogenital warts
31,33,35,51,52	CIN 1, 2, 3
16, 18,45,56	CIN 2,3 Invasive CA

- HP V-16 is the most common HPV seen in invasive CA and CIN2/3 and is found in 50% cases.
- HPV-16 is not very specific and is also the most common HPV type in women with normal cytology.
- HPV-18 is more specific than HPV-16 for invasive tumors.

Cervical Cancer Staging

Stage I:
The carcinoma is strictly confined to the cervix uteri (extension to the corpus should be disregarded) • **IA** Invasive carcinoma that can be diagnosed only by microscopy, with maximum depth of invasion <5 mm – **IA1** Measured stromal invasion <3 mm in depth – **IA2** Measured stromal invasion ≥3 mm and <5 mm in depth • **IB** Invasive carcinoma with measured deepest invasion ≥5 mm (greater than stage IA), lesion limited to the cervix uteri – **IB1** Invasive carcinoma ≥5 mm depth of stromal invasion and <2 cm in greatest dimension – **IB2** Invasive carcinoma ≥2 cm and <4 cm in greatest dimension – **IB3** Invasive carcinoma ≥4 cm in greatest dimension
Stage II:
The carcinoma invades beyond the uterus, but has not extended onto the lower third of the vagina or to the pelvic wall • **IIA** Involvement limited to the upper two-thirds of the vagina without parametrial involvement – **IIA1** Invasive carcinoma <4 cm in greatest dimension – **IIA2** Invasive carcinoma ≥4 cm in greatest dimension • **IIB** With parametrial involvement but not up to the pelvic wall
Stage III:
The carcinoma involves the lower third of the vagina and/or extends to the pelvic wall and/or causes hydro nephrosis or non-functioning kidney and/or involves pelvic and/or paraaortic lymph node • **IIIA** Carcinoma involves the lower third of the vagina, with no extension to the pelvic wall • **IIIB** Extension to the pelvic wall and/or hydro nephrosis or non-functioning kidney (unless known to be due to another cause) • **IIIC** Involvement of pelvic and/or paraaortic lymph nodes, irrespective of tumor size and extent (with r and p notations)c – **IIIC1** Pelvic lymph node metastasis only – **IIIC2** Para aortic lymph node metastasis
Stage IV:
The carcinoma has extended beyond the true pelvis or has involved (biopsy proven) the mucosa of the bladder or rectum. A bullous edema, as such, does not permit a case to be allotted to stage IV • IVA Spread of the growth to adjacent organs • IVB Spread to distant organs

Cervical Cancer Treatment

General Treatment for Primary Invasive Cervical Carcinoma

Cancer stage	Treatment
IA1b	Simple hysterectomy preferred if childbearing completed or Cervical conization
IA1b (with LVSI)	Modified radical hysterectomy and pelvic lymphadenectomy or Radical trachelectomy and pelvic lymphadenectomy for selected patients desiring fertility

Contd...

Contd...

Cancer stage	Treatment
IA2b,c	Radical hysterectomy and pelvic lymphadenectomy or Radical trachelectomy and pelvic lymphadenectomy for selected patients desiring fertility
IB1c Some IB2 IIA1	Radical hysterectomy and pelvic lymphadenectomy or radical trachelectomy and pelvic lymphadenectomy for selected patients desiring fertility or Chemoradiation
Bulky IB2 IIA2	Chemoradiation
IIB to IVA	Chemoradiation or rarely, pelvic exenteration
IVB	Palliative chemotherapy and/or palliative radiotherapy OR supportive care

Radiotherapy

Point A and Point B are in relation to radiotherapy for Ca Cervix

	Point A	Point B
Location	2 cm above and 2 cm lateral to external os	2 cm above and 5 cm lateral to external os
Structure present	Paracervical/parametrial lymph node	Obturator lymph node
Dose of radiation	7000–8000 cGY	6000 cY

Vaccines for Prevention of Cervical Cancer

	Gardasil	Cervirax
Type	Quadrivalent	Bivalent
Effective against HPV strains	6, 11, 16, 18	16, 18
Schedule	0, 2, 6 months	0, 1, 6 months
Route	Intramuscular	Itramuscular
Protects against	Carcinoma cervix and genital warts	Carcinoma cervix

113. Stage 1b cervical cancer is diagnosed in a young woman. Assuming that the cancer is confirmed to the cervix and that intraoperative biopsies are negative. Which of the following structure would not be removed during the radical hysterectomy:

a. Uterosacral and uterovesical ligaments
b. Pelvic nodes
c. The entire parametrium on both sides of the cervix
d. Both ovaries

Ans. is 'd' Both ovaries

114. In ca cervix treatment point A receives:

a. 3000 cGy
b. 5000 cGy
c. 7000 cGy
d. 10,000 cGy

Ans. is 'c' 7000 cGy

115. Therapeutic conisation is indicated in:

a. Microinvasive carcinoma cervix stage 1a1
b. CIN III
c. Unsatisfactory colposcopy with cervical dysplasia
d. Cervical metaplasia

Ans. is 'a' Microinvasive carcinoma cervix stage 1a1

116. Cervical cancer with involvement of upper vagina and parametrium is stage:

a. 1b
b. 2a
c. 2b
d. 3a

Ans. is 'c' 2b

117. GARDASIL vaccine is for:

a. HPV 16, 18
b. HSV
c. HPV 6, 11, 16, 18
d. Hepatitis B

Ans. is 'c' HPV 6, 11, 16, 18

Ovarian Tumors

WHO classification of ovarian tumors (major groups):

- *Common epithelial tumors*: Serous tumors
  - Mucinous tumors
  - Endometrioid tumors

- Clear cell (mesonephroid tumors)
- Brenner tumors
- Mixed epithelial tumors
- Undifferentiated carcinoma
- Unclassified epithelial tumors

❖ *Sex cord (gonadal stromal) tumors*:
- Granulosa stromal cell tumors, theca cell tumors
- Androblastomas: Sertoli-Leydig cell tumors
- Gynandroblastomas
- Unclassified

❖ Lipid (lipoid) cell tumors

❖ *Germ cell tumors*:
- Dysgerminoma
- Endodermal sinus tumor
- Embryonal carcinoma
- Polyembryoma
- Choriocarcinoma
- Teratoma
- Mixed forms

❖ *Gonadoblastoma*:
- Pure
- Mixed with dysgerminoma or other germ cell tumors

❖ Soft tissue tumors not specific to ovary

❖ Unclassified tumors

❖ Secondary (metastatic) tumors

❖ Tumor-like conditions.

118. Which is an epithelial cancer:

a. Endometrioid
b. Dysgerminoma
c. Granulose cell tumor
d. Leydig cell tumor

Ans. is 'a' Endometrioid

Endometrial Cancer

Risk Factors for Endometrial CA (Estrogen-dependent Tumor)

❖ Nulliparity
❖ Early menarche, late menopause
❖ Obesity
❖ Diabetes mellitus and hypertension
❖ Unopposed estrogen therapy/Anovulation
❖ Tamoxifen therapy
❖ Atypical endometrial hyperplasia
❖ Obesity, hypertension, and diabetes mellitus associated with CA endometrium = corpus CA syndrome OC pills, POP, DMPA, Mirena, Multiparty are all protective for CA endometrium

FIGO Grading of Endometrial Carcinoma

Histopathologic degree of differentiation:

❖ *G1*: < 5% nonsquamous or nonmorular growth pattern
❖ *G2*: 6–50% nonsquamous or nonmorular growth pattern
❖ *G3*: >50% nonsquamous or nonmorular growth pattern

Management of Ca Endometrium

a. Stage 1:
Surgery (total abdominal hysterectomy with bilateral salpingo-oophorectomy with lymph node sampling), followed by radiotherapy
Only patients with stage lA, grades 1 and 2 do not require postoperative radiotherapy.

b. Stage 2:
Modified radical hysterectomy, bilateral salpingo-oophorectomy with lymph node dissection, followed by radiotherapy.

c. Stages 3 and 4:
Debulking surgery followed by radiotherapy.

119. Choice of adjuvant treatment for endometrial carcinoma stage IA, grade I is:

a. Radiotherapy
b. Chemotherapy
c. Chemotherapy plus radiotherapy
d. No treatment

Ans. is 'd' No treatment

120. Grade 1 ca endometrium, there is presence of__________ % non-squamous growth:

a. <5
b. 6–25
c. 25–50
d. >50

Ans. is 'a' < 5

121. All are risk factors for ca endometrium *except*:

a. Tamoxifen
b. Multiparty
c. Obesity and hypertension
d. Late menopause

Ans. is 'b' Multiparty

Vaginal Cancer

Vaginal cancer is an uncommon cancer of the female reproductive system.

There are four types of vaginal cancer.

1. *Squamous cell carcinoma*: Squamous cell carcinoma can develop in the cells lining the vagina, most often in the area closest to the cervix. Squamous cell carcinoma makes up 85% to 90% of vaginal cancers. It develops slowly through a precancerous condition (changes in cells that may, but do not always, become cancer) called vaginal intraepithelial neoplasia or VAIN.
2. *Adenocarcinoma*: Adenocarcinoma begins in the vaginal gland tissue. It makes up about 5% to 10% of vaginal cancers.
3. *Clear cell adenocarcinoma*: This cancer occurs in women whose mothers took the drug diethylstilbestrol (DES) during pregnancy between the late 1940s and 1971. It is estimated that 1 woman out of 1,000 women exposed to DES will develop vaginal cancer.
4. *Melanoma*: Melanoma can begin on the skin of the vagina or other internal organs. Melanoma is usually found on skin exposed to the sun and often appears as a dark-colored tumor on the lower or outer parts of the vagina.

Modes of Spread of ca Vulva

a. *Direct*: Urethra, vagina, rectum, pelvic bones
b. *Lymphatic*: MC route of spread
   Lymphatics of labia to superficial, then deep inguinal nodes and then pelvic nodes
c. Hematogenous route rare and may occur in advanced cases

122. Most common variety of vaginal cancer is:

a. Adenocarcinoma
b. Squamous carcinoma
c. Melanoma
d. Clear cell

Ans. is 'b' Squamous carcinoma

123. Ca vulva spreads to all *except*:

a. Urethra
b. Deep inguinal nodes
c. Superficial inguinal nodes
d. Paraaortic nodes

Ans. is 'd' Paraaortic nodes

Tumor Markers

Cancer	Tumor marker
Endodermal sinus tumor/yolk sac tumor	AFP
Epithelial ovarian tumors (especially serous)	CA-125
Sertoli cell, leydig cell, hilus cell tumors	Testosterone
Dysgerminoma	LDH, alkaline phosphatase
Choriocarcinoma	HCG

124. Tumor marker for choriocarcinoma is:

a. CA 125
b. HCG
c. AFP
d. LDH

Ans. is 'b' HCG

125. Tumor marker for germ cell malignancy are all *except*:

a. LDH
b. Alkaline phosphatase
c. AFP
d. CA-125

Ans. is 'd' CA-125

POSTPARTUM HEMORRHAGE (PPH), UTERINE INVERSION AND SHOCK

POSTPARTUM HEMORRHAGE (PPH)

Definition: Postpartum Hemorrhage (PPH) is blood loss of more than 500 mL from the genital tract following vaginal delivery and more than 1000 mL following cesarean.

Types of PPH

Primary PPH

- Hemorrhage occurring within 24 hours following child birth.
- Most common cause: Atonic PPH

Secondary PPH

- Hemorrhage occurring after 24 hours and up to 6 weeks postpartum
- Most common cause: Retained placenta

Causes of PPH

1. **Atonic uterus:** most common cause
2. **Traumatic PPH**
3. **Coagulopathy (rare causes):** DIC and Hypofibrrinogenemia
4. **Retained product of conception**

Predisposing Factors of PPH

Atonic PPH	Traumatic PPH	Blood coagulopathy
Grand multipara	Instrumental delivery	Abruption
Malnutrition/Anemia	Vaginal birth after cesarean	Sepsis
Previous H/o atonic PPH	Face to pubis delivery	Intrauterine death
Antepartum hemorrhage	Precipitate labor	HELLP syndrome
Overdistended uterus due to multiple pregnancy	Macrosomia	Severe preeclampsia
Hydramnios		
Macrosomia		
Preeclampsia/hypertension		
Precipitate labour and prolonged labor (>12 hours)		
Uterine malformations or fibroid uterus		

Medical Management of PPH

Drug	Dose	Route	Adverse effects	Contraindications
Oxytocin	30–40 units in 500 mL of crystalloid; Start at 125 mL/hour;	IV- first line; IM- second line (10 units)	Nausea	Should not be given as IV bolus, but as continuous infusion otherwise no complication
15 methyl PGF2a or carbo prost (Best drug to control PPH)	0.25 mg; Every 15–20 mins. (maximum 8 doses, equal to 2 gm)	First line IM	• Nausea • Vomiting • Diarrhea • Chills	• Bronchial asthma; • Active cardiac, renal or hepatic disease
Methergine (for both prophylaxis and treatment of PPH)	0.5 mg; Every 2–4 hours	IM/IV-first line PO-second line	• Nausea • Vomiting Hypertension	• Hypertension • Preeclampsia
Misoprostol (PGE1)	200–1000 mcg (FIGO = 800 mcg oral); Single dose	PR- first line PO- second line	• Nausea • Vomiting • Fever • Tachycardia	Scarred uterus like previous cesarean scar

Surgical Management of PPH

Family completed: Hysterectomy

Family not completed:

- B lynch sutures
- Radiographic embolization of pelvic vessel

- ❖ Uterine artery and ovarian artery ligation
- ❖ Internal iliac artery ligation

↓

Hysterectomy done (if all fail)

126. PGF2 alpha maximum dose in PPH is: *(NEET 2019)*

a. 2000 μg b. 200 μg
c. 2 mg d. 20 mg

Ans. is 'c' 2 mg

SHEEHAN SYNDROME

Sheehan syndrome—Sheehan syndrome (ie, postpartum hypopituitarism) is a rare but potentially life-threatening complication. The pituitary gland is enlarged in pregnancy and prone to infarction from hypovolemic shock. Damage to the pituitary can be mild or severe, and can affect the secretion of one, several, or all of its hormones. A common presentation is a combination of failure to lactate postdelivery and amenorrhea or oligomenorrhea, but any of the manifestations of hypopituitarism (eg, hypotension, hyponatremia, hypothyroidism) can occur any time from the immediate postpartum period to years after delivery. If the patient remains hypotensive after control of hemorrhage and volume replacement, she should be evaluated and treated for adrenal insufficiency immediately; evaluation of other hormonal deficiencies can be deferred until four to six weeks postpartum.

127. A female sustained massive PPH during delivery and presented with failure of lactation and amenorrhea 1 year later. What is the likely diagnosis? *(NEET 2020)*

a. Pituitary adenoma b. Premature ovarian failure
c. Sheehan syndrome d. Simmonds syndrome

Ans. is 'c' Sheehan syndrome

Pituitary apoplexy—Sudden hemorrhage into the pituitary gland is called pituitary apoplexy. Hemorrhage often occurs into a pituitary adenoma. In one report, the prevalence of pituitary apoplexy among patients with nonfunctioning pituitary macroadenomas was 8 percent [68]. In its most dramatic presentation, apoplexy causes the sudden onset of excruciating headache, diplopia due to pressure on the oculomotor nerves, and hypopituitarism. All pituitary hormonal deficiencies can occur, but the sudden onset of ACTH and therefore cortisol deficiency is the most serious because it can cause life-threatening hypotension.

128. All of the following are seen in pituitary apoplexy *except*: *(NEET 2020)*

a. Shock b. Hypertension
c. unconsciousness d. Severe headache

Ans. is 'b' Hypertension

GYNECOLOGICAL DIAGNOSIS AND OPERATIVE SURGERY

PROLAPSE

Prolapse is defined as the displacement of an organ from its normal anatomical position.

Genital prolapse occurs due to weakness of the supports.

Symptoms

There may not be any symptoms even with severe degree of prolapse or the following symptoms may be present:

Generally postmenopausal or premenopausal multiparous women with complaints of:

- ❖ Something coming out through per vaginal fullness within the vagina which increases with straining.
- ❖ Backache or lower pelvic dragging pain during walking, working

The above 2 symptoms are usually relieved on lying down:

- ❖ Vaginal symptoms
- ❖ Bowel symptoms (In presence of rectocele)
- ❖ Sexual symptoms

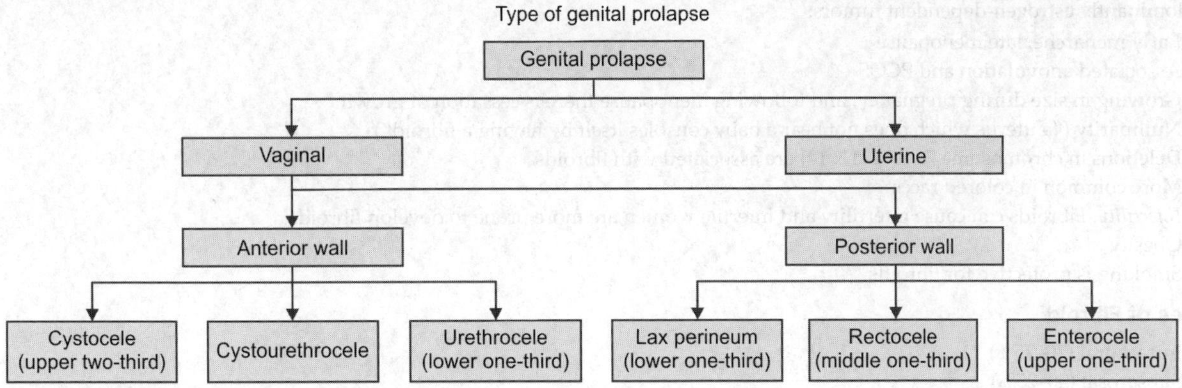

- Cystocele is the MC type of vaginal prolapsed

Enterocele Prevention

The goal of the Moschcowitz procedure is to fix and suture the strong connective tissue that normally supports the uterus to the top of the vagina, thus pre+enting it from "falling out." At the same time, the pouch between the rectum and the vagina is reduced with a purse-string type suture.
Enterocele formation can be prevented by Moschowitz's or Halban's surgeries, in both the POD is obliterated

Surgery

Vaginal hysterectomy with pelvic floor repair is done for vaginouterine prolapse in peri/post-menopausal women.
- First clamp includes uterosacral and Mackenrodt's ligament
- Second clamp includes uterine artery
- Third clamp includes cornual structures.

129. Upper two-third anterior vaginal wall prolapse is: *(NEET 2018)*

a. Cystocele b. Urethrocele
c. Rectocele d. Enterocele

Ans. is 'a' Cystocele

130. 55-year-old lady complaints of mass in the vagina, which is reducible and increases on defecation. The diagnosis is: *(NEET 2018)*

a. Rectal prolapse b. Uterine prolapse
c. Cervical fibroid d. Vaginal cancer

Ans. is 'b' Uterine prolapse

131. Moschowitz's surgery is done for: *(NEET 2018)*

a. Cervical cancer b. Fundal fibroids
c. Uterine prolapse d. Enterocele prevention

Ans. is 'd' Enterocele prevention

132. In vaginal hysterectomy, the first clamp includes: *(NEET 2018)*

a. Uterine artery b. Fallopian tube and round ligament
c. Uterosacral ligament d. None of the above

Ans. is 'c' Uterosacral ligament

FIBROMYOMAS

Fibromyomas (leiomyomas, fibroids or simply myomas) are generally benign uterine neoplasms, commonly encountered in gynecological practice (5–20% of women in the reproductive age group). They are slow growing tumors and take 3–5 years to be clinically palpable, unlike ovarian tumors. The presence of myoma causes hyperplasia of the myometrial wall.
- The cavity of the uterus is often distorted and enlarged. The endometrium tends to be thicker due to endometrial hyperplasia. The ovaries at times are enlarged, cystic and hyperemic with evidence of salpingo—oophoritis in about 15% cases.
- Cervical, submucous and broad ligament fibroids are usually single. Interstitial and subserous fibroids may be single or multiple, varying in size from a seedling fibroid to a huge neoplasm.

Etiology

Each myoma is derived from smooth muscle cell rests, either from vessel walls or uterine musculature. Although estrogen, progesterone growth hormone and possibly human placental lactogen have been implicated in the growth of myomas. The fibroids are often associated with adenomyosis, pelvic endometriosis and pelvic inflammatory disease.

Predominantly estrogen-dependent tumors:

- Early menarche, late menopause
- Associated anovulation and PCOS
- Growing in size during pregnancy, and following menopause there is cessation of growth
- Nulliparity ("a uterus which does not bear a baby consoles itself by having a fibroid")
- Deletions in chromosome 7 and t (12, 14) are associated with fibroids
- More common in colored races
- *Infertility*: Fibroids can cause infertility and infertile women are more prone to develop fibroids.
- Obesity
- Smoking is protective for fibroids.

Types of Fibroid

- Intramural (70–75%)
- Subserosal (20–25%)
- Submucosal (5%)

Management of Fibroids

- GnRH analogs (MC used)
- Danazol
- Progesterone (DMPA/Mirena/POP/low-dose OC pills)
- Mifepristone (RU-486) (fibroids are also partly progesterone dependent)
- Gestrinone
- Anastrozole (aromatase inhibitor)
- Asoprisnil (selective progesterone receptor modulator—SPRM)
- Ulipristal acetate—selective progesterone receptor modulators (SPRM).
- Submucous fibroids are located within muscle just below endometrium and distort endometrial cavity.
- Even small one may lead to menorrhagia and infertility.
- Surgery is indicated:
  - Who does not wish to conceive/family completed
  - Age >40 years
  - Uncontrolled menorrhagia/woman wants definitive treatment

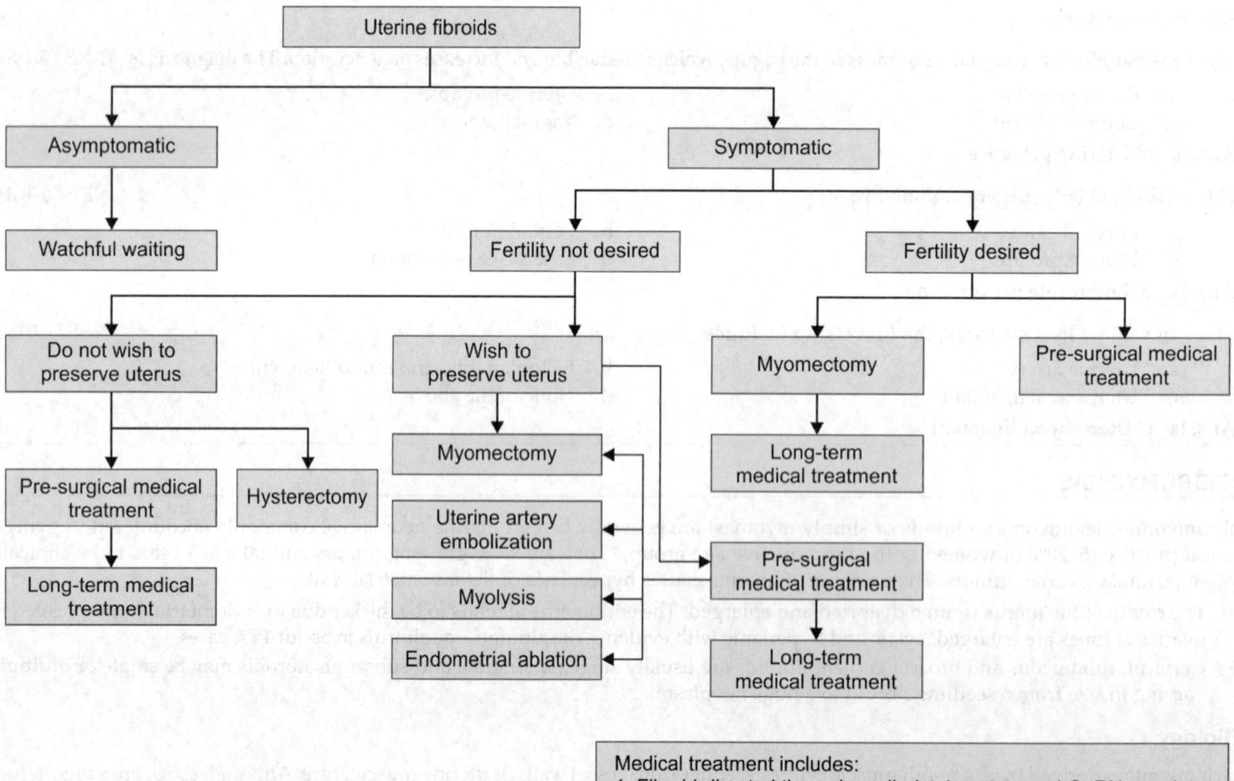

133. 60-year woman comes with third degree uterine prolapse. What will be the management: *(NEET 2019)*

a. Vaginal hysterectomy with pelvic floor repair
b. Pelvic floor repair
c. Sacrospinous fixation
d. Pessary

Ans. is 'a' Vaginal hysterectomy with pelvic floor repair

134. 45 years female with 3 months menorrhagia. USG showing 2 cm submucosal fibroid. Treatment options: *(NEET 2019)*

a. Ocp for 3 months
b. Progesterone for 3 months
c. Endometrial sampling
d. Hysterectomy

Ans. is 'd' Hysterectomy

135. Section of uterus showing what:

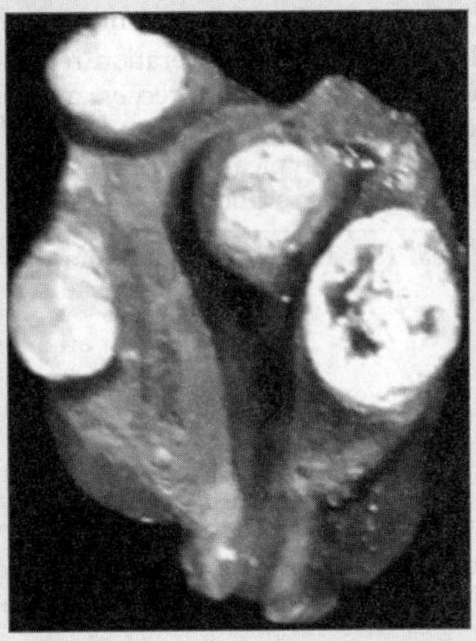

a. Leiomyoma
b. Endometrial polyp
c. Endometriosis
d. Leiomyosarcoma

Ans. is 'a' Leiomyoma

136. Most common type of the fibroid is:

a. Intramural
b. Subserosal
c. Submucosal
d. Cervical

Ans. is 'a' Intramural

137. Medical management of fibroids is with all except:

a. Progesterone
b. Mifepristone
c. Ulipristal acetate
d. Misoprostol

Ans. is 'd' Misoprostol

Perineal Tears

Perineal Tears are Classified into Four Categories

- *First-degree tear*: Laceration is limited to the fourchette and superficial perineal skin or vaginal mucosa.
- *Second-degree tear*: Laceration extends beyond fourchette, perineal skin and vaginal mucosa to perianal muscles and fascia, but not the anal sphincter.
- *Third-degree tear*: Couchette, perineal skin, vaginal mucosa, muscles, and anal sphincter are torn; third-degree tears may be further subdivided into three subcategories:
  - *3a*: partial tear of the external anal sphincter involving less than 50% thickness
  - *3b*: greater than 50% tear of the external anal sphincter
  - *3c*: internal sphincter is torn
- *Fourth-degree tear*: Fourchette, perineal skin, vaginal mucosa, muscles, anal sphincter, and rectal mucosa

138. If the anal sphincter is injured it is which degree of perineal tear:

a. First
b. Second
c. Third
d. Fourth

Ans. is 'c' Third

Traditionally, secondary repair of episiotomy breakdown was deferred for a minimum of two to three months. The purpose for delay was to allow sufficient time for revascularization of the wound edges and formation of scar tissue, which was thought to be of value during reanastomosis of the torn sphincter. However, few data support this approach and it commits the woman to an extended period of physical, social, and sexual disability because of continuous incontinence. Available evidence, although extremely limited and inconclusive, supports re-repair of both superficial and deep episiotomy dehiscence within the first two weeks following childbirth, which may result in a reduction in perineal pain during the healing process up to six months postdelivery and a reduction in dyspareunia.

Early repair of episiotomy breakdown has replaced the traditional approach and has overall success rates of 87 to 100 percent. Disadvantages of an early procedure include:

- ❖ It prolongs hospitalization early in the postpartum period, which could interfere with breastfeeding and maternal-infant bonding.
- ❖ It removes the possibility of spontaneous closure, which could occur in some cases.
- ❖ Some early attempts at repair may fail, resulting in a need for subsequent surgical procedures.

Women with delayed presentation of third- or fourth-degree laceration repairs are typically treated with antibiotics, undergo operative tissue debridement until healthy tissue is present, and then receive a secondary repair performed at around 3 months We believe this approach minimizes the risk of fistula formation and increases the likelihood of a successful repair, although supporting data are limited, particularly around choice of antibiotics. We typically use a first-generation cephalosporin unless there is evidence that more broad coverage is required (eg, fecal contamination of laceration).

139. A female presented with complete perineal tear 2 weeks after home delivery. What is the best management for her? *(NEET 2020)*

a. Immediate repair
b. Repair after 2 weeks
c. Repair after 6 weeks
d. Repair after 3 months

Ans. is 'd' Repair after 3 months

ADENOMYOSIS

Adenomyosis is a condition that involves the encroachment, or movement, of the endometrial tissue that lines the uterus into the muscles of the uterus. This makes the uterine walls grow thicker. It may lead to menorrhagia, dysmenorrhea and pain during intercourse.

Treatment Options

- ❖ Anti-inflammatory medications/NSAID:
  - These medications can help to reduce blood flow during period while also relieving severe cramps.
- ❖ Hormonal treatments
  - These include oral contraceptives pills, progestin-only contraceptives (oral, injection, or an intrauterine device), and GnRH-analogues such as leuprolide.
- ❖ Endometrial ablation
  - This involves techniques to remove or destroy the endometrium. However, this procedure may not work for everyone, since adenomyosis often invades the muscle more deeply.
- ❖ Uterine artery embolization
  - This is a procedure that prevents certain arteries from supplying blood to the affected area. With the blood supply cut-off, the adenomyosis shrinks.
- ❖ MRI-guided focused ultrasound surgery (MRgFUS)
  - MRgFUS uses precisely focused high-intensity waves to create heat and destroy the targeted tissue. The heat is monitored using MRI images in real time. Studies have shown this procedure to be successful in providing relief of symptoms. However, more studies are needed.
- ❖ Hysterectomy
  - The only way to completely cure this condition is to have a hysterectomy. This is often the treatment of choice for women with significant symptoms.
  - A hysterectomy is an operation to remove the uterus.
  - A woman may have a hysterectomy for different reasons, including: Uterine fibroids that cause pain, bleeding, or other problems.
  - More hysterectomies are done because of fibroids than any other problem of the uterus:
    - Uterine prolapse
    - Cancer of the uterus, cervix, or ovaries/fallopian tube
    - Endometriosis
    - DUB/menorrhagia
    - Chronic pelvic pain/chronic PID
    - Adenomyosis.

Obstetrics and Gynecology

140. 30-year-old woman with complaint of dysmenorrhoea, dyspareunia with chronic pelvic pain undergoes hysterectomy. From the cut section of hyster- ectomy specimen below identify the condition. *(NEET 2019)*

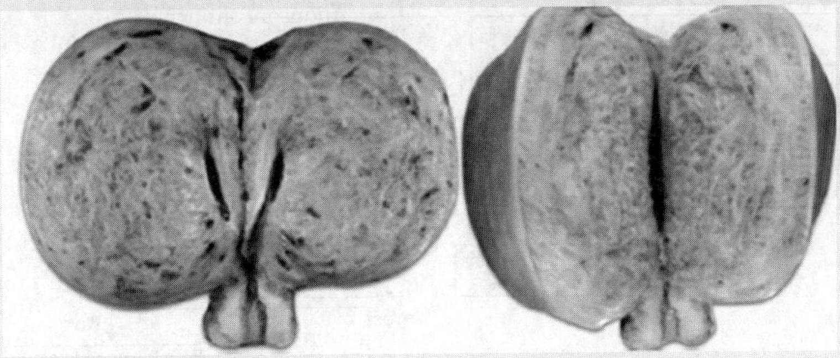

a. Adenomyosis
b. Fibroids
c. Leiomyoma
d. Endometriosis

Ans. is 'a' Adenomyosis

141. MC cause for hysterectomy is:

a. Prolapse
b. Fibroids
c. ca endometrium
d. Acute PID

Ans. is 'b' Fibroids

MULTIFETAL PREGNANCY

Sign for Chorionicity on USG

Dichorionic	Monochorionic
The "twin peak" sign or lambda sign (placenta intervenes between the membranes) indicate 2 fused placentas	T sign/inverted T sign (right angle relation between the placenta and foetal membrane)
Intervening membrane is >2 mm thick	Intervening membrane is <2 mm

142. Twin-peak sign is seen in:

a. All monozygotic twins
b. Monochorionic twins
c. Dichorionic twins
d. Siamese twins

Ans. is 'c' Dichorionic twins

MANAGEMENT OF TWIN PREGNANCIES

Criteria for the Diagnosis of Preeclampsia

Systolic blood pressure ≥ 140 mmHg or diastolic blood pressure ≥ 90 mmHg on at least 2 occasions at least 4 hours apart after 20 weeks of gestation in a previously normotensive patient AND the new onset of 1 or more of the following*:

- Proteinuria ≥ 0.3 g in a 24-hour urine specimen or protein/creatinine ratio ≥0.3 (mg/mg) (30 mg/mmol) in a random urine specimen or dipstick ≥2 + if a quantitative measurement is unavailable.
- Platelet count <100,000/microL
- Serum creatinine >1.1 mg/dL (97.2 micromol/L) or doubling of the creatinine concentration in the absence of other renal disease
- Liver transaminases at least twice the upper limit of the normal concentrations for the local laboratory
- Pulmonary edema
- Cerebral or visual symptoms (e.g new-onset and presistent headaches not accounted for by alternative diagnoses and not responding to usual doses of analgesies; blurred vision, flashing lights or sparks, scotomata)

For women at term (≥37+0 weeks) with preeclampsia without features of severe disease, we suggest delivery rather than expectant management. Delivery reduces the risk of maternal complications and is associated with a low risk of neonatal morbidity at this gestational age.

Preeclampsia is not an indication for cesarean delivery. Most patients with preeclampsia with or without severe features can be delivered vaginally. Cesarean should be reserved for usual obstetric indications

The algorithm for determining route of delivery in twin pregnancy:

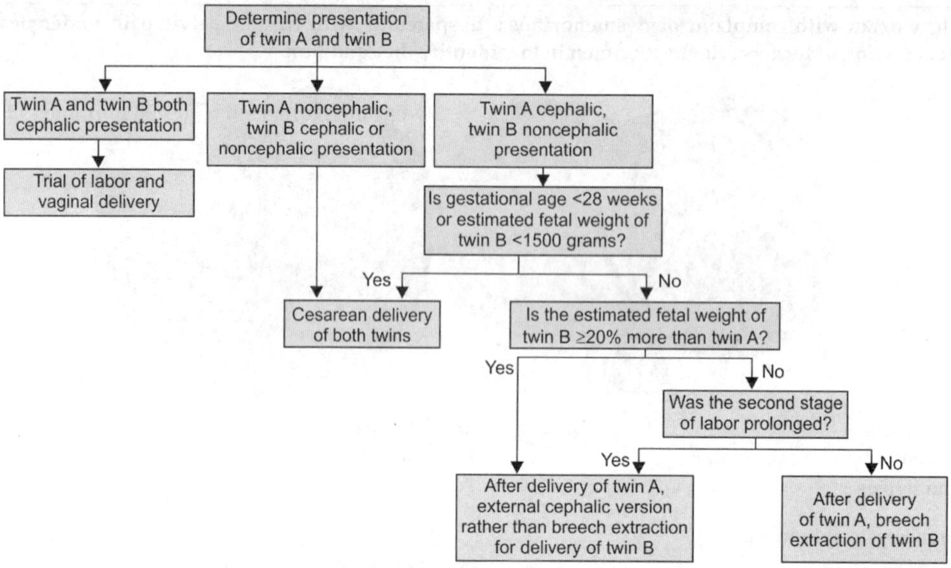

143. An antenatal woman with 38 weeks of pregnancy is presented with a twin pregnancy with first fetus in breech position. Her BP is 140/110 and urine dipstick for protein is 1+. What is the best management? *(NEET 2020)*

a. Immediate CS
b. Wait and watch until 40 weeks
c. Give antihypertensives and $MgSO_4$
d. Induction of labour with PGE2.

Ans. is 'a' Immediate CS

MEDICAL DISORDERS IN PREGNANCY

NATIONAL GUIDELINES FOR PREVENTION OF PARENT-TO-CHILD TRANSMISSION OF HIV

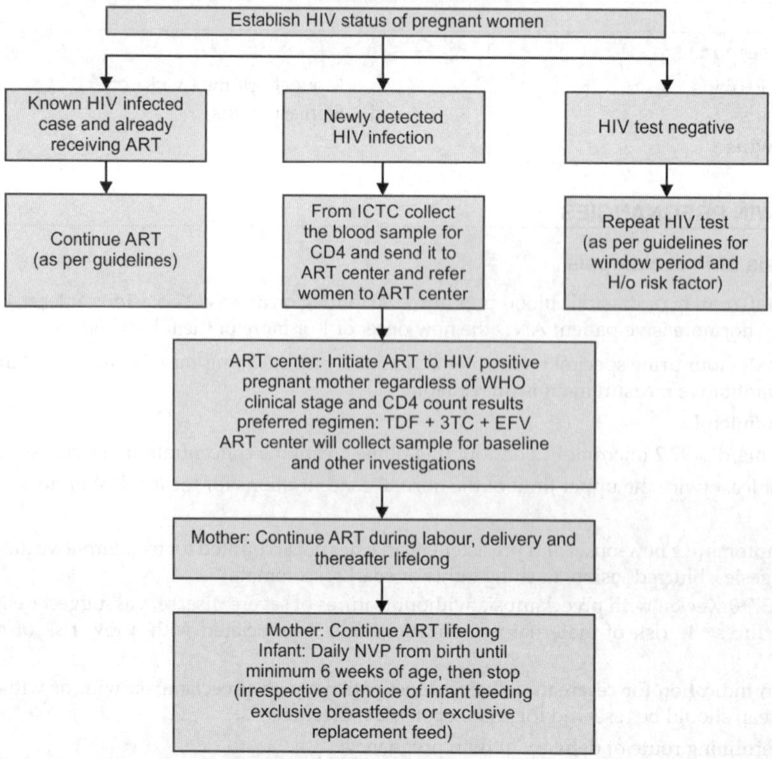

144. A female is found to be positive for HIV in pregnancy. How will you manage this case: *(NEET 2018)*

a. Start ART in second trimester and give till pregnancy
b. Start ART in immediately and give till pregnancy
c. Start ART in second trimester and continue lifelong
d. Start ART immediately and continue lifelong

Ans. is 'd' Start ART immediately and continue lifelong

High-risk Factors in Pregnancy

Reproductive history	Medical disorders in pregnancy	Previous surgery
• Two or more previous miscarriage or **previous induced abortion** • Previous stillbirth, neonatal death or birth of babies with congenital abnormality • Previous preterm labor or birth of a IUGR or macrosomic baby • Grand multiparity • Previous cesarean section or hysterotomy • Third stage abnormalities (PPH) • Previous infant with Rh isoimmunization or ABO incompatibility	*Diseases*: • Pulmonary disease—TB • Renal disease—Pyelonephritis • Thyroid disorders • Psychiatric illness • Cardiac disease • Epilepsy • Viral hepatitis • Preeclampsia • Eclampsia • Anemia • Infections in pregnancy	• Myomectomy • Repair of complete perineal tear • Repair of vesicovaginal fistula • Repair of stress incontinence • *Family history*: – Socioeconomic status—Patients belonging to low socioeconomic status have a higher incidence of anemia, preterm labor, growth retarded babies – Family history of diabetes, hypertension or multiple pregnancy and congenital malformation

145. Which of the following is not a high-risk pregnancy: *(NEET 2018)*

a. Previous history of manual removal or placenta
b. Anemia
c. Infertility history
d. Obesity

Ans. is 'a' Previous history of manual removal or placenta

ACUTE FATTY LIVER OF PREGNANCY

Acute fatty liver of pregnancy is usually seen in obese woman.

- It is more commonly seen in woman carrying a male fetus.
- The neonate is at risk of fatty infiltration of liver.
- It more commonly occurs in 3rd trimester.
- It may be associated with uric acid.

Etiology: It is associated with disorders of fatty acid transport and oxidation-deficiencyof LCHAD enzyme, i.e. long chair hydroxyl acyl coenzyme A dehydrogenase.

Risk Factors

- First pregnancy
- Male fetuses
- Preeclampsia
- Maternal obesity
- Multiple pregnancy.

Pathology: Liver is yellow, soft and greasy

- Swollen hepatocytes with central nuclei and cytoplasm filled with micro vesicular fat
- Acute yellow atrophy
- Minimal hepatocellular.

Clinical Features

- Patients present in the third trimester (generally at 37 weeks) with nonspecific symptoms like nausea, vomiting, anorexia, vague abdominal discomfort and malaise.
- In many women, persistent vomiting is the main symptom.
- AFP should also be suspected in any woman who presents with new onset nausea and malaise in third trimester.
- followed by jaundice (progressive in nature)
- In 50% cases—features of preeclampsia viz—hypertension, proteinuria and edema are present.
- In almost all severe cases, there is profound endothelial cell activation with capillary leakage causing hemoconcentration, hepatorenal syndrome, ascites, and sometimes pulmonary edema.
- Fetal death is more common in cases with severe hemoconcentration. Stillbirth possibly follows diminished uteroplacental perfusion, but is also related to more severe disease and acidosis.
- There is maternal leukocytosis and thrombocytopenia.
- The syndrome typically continues to worsen after diagnosis. Hypoglycemia is common, and obvious hepatic encephalopathy, severe coagulopathy, and some degree of renal failure develop in approximately half of women.

Investigation

Liver Function Tests

- Rise in serum bilirubin but less than 10 mg/dL
- Increase in SGOT and SGPT (< 1000 IU/L)
- Increase in alkaline phosphatase (moderately)
- Prothrombin time may be increased
- Clotting time prolonged
- In severe cases, there may be disseminated coagulation failure.

Renal Function Test

- ↑ S. creatinine (present in all patients)
- ↑ S. uric acid
- ↑ S. ammonia levels

Others

- Level of glucose (hypoglycemia)
- Platelet count
- Fibrinogen levels (<100 mg)

Management

- Rapid delivery is essential
- Mode of delivery—Induction of labor followed by vaginal delivery
- Since the patient has coagulopathy, hence cesarean section is avoided, but still in practice cesarean is very common.

Complication

- Maternal mortality 10–75%
- Hepatic dysfunction resolves automatically in the postpartum period.
- There are two associated complications which can develop during this period:
  - Transient diabetes insipidus
  - Acute pancreatitis

Fetal Prognosis

- Fetal prognosis is poor.
- If the fetuses survive, they may later on develop a Reye like syndrome of hepatic encephalopathy and severe hypoglycemia due to the defect in beta fatty acid oxidation.

146. Which of the following statement is correct about acute fatty liver of pregnancy: *(NEET 2019)*

a. Occurs in 1 in 1000 pregnancy
b. Mostly seen in last trimester
c. Common if female fetus is present
d. May be associated with decreased uric acid

Ans. is 'b' Mostly seen in last trimester

147. Acute fatty liver commonly seen is pregnancy at: *(NEET 2018)*

a. 3rd trimester
b. 1st trimester
c. Immediate postpartum
d. Intrapartum

Ans. is 'a' 3rd trimester

Hyperthyroidism in Pregnancy

- Graves' disease is the most common cause of hyperthyroidism in pregnancy.
- Hashimoto's thyroiditis is the most common cause of hypothyroidism in pregnancy.
- Complications associated with both hypo and hyperthyroidism in pregnancy:
  - Recurrent first trimester abortions
  - IUGR
  - Increased risk of preeclampsia
  - Abruption
  - Stillbirths, hydrops fetalis
  - Preterm labor
  - Hypothyroidism is also associated with cretinism.

Management

- ❖ Propylthiouracil is the DOC for hyperthyroidism in pregnancy.
- ❖ Methimazole and carbimazole used in early pregnancy have been associated with esophageal and choanal atresia, aplasia cutis, and fetal agranulocytosis. These drugs can be used in 2nd and 3rd trimester.
- ❖ Graves' disease is the most common cause of hyperthyroidism in pregnancy.
- ❖ Hashimoto's thyroiditis is the most common cause of hypothyroidism in pregnancy.

148. In a pregnant lady with hyperthyroidism, the safest drug to be used is:

a. Propylthiouracil b. Methimazole
c. Carbimazole d. Lugol's iodine

Ans. is 'a' Propylthiouracil

Clarke's Classification for Risk of Maternal Mortality in Cardiac Disorders

Cardiac disorder	Mortality (%)
Group 1: Minimal risk	
• Atrial septal defect • Ventricular septal defect • Patent ductus arteriosus • Pulmonic or tricuspid disease • Fallot tetralogy, corrected • Bioprosthetic value • Mitral stenosis, NYHA classes I and II	0–1
Group 2: Moderate risk	
• Mitral stenosis, NYHA classes III and IV • Aortic stenosi • Aortic coarctation without valvular involvement • Fallot tetralogy, uncorrected • Previous myocardial infarction • Marfan syndrome, normal aorta • Mitral stenosis with atrial fibrillation • Artificial value	5–15
Group 3: Major risk	
• Pulmonary hypertension (primary and secondary) • Aortic coarctation with valvular involvement • Marfan syndrome with aortic involvement • Eisenmenger's syndrome	25–50

WPW syndrome is a variety of tachyarrhythmia and can have a favorable outcome in pregnancy with digoxin, adenosine or calcium channel blockers.

149. Pregnancy is contraindicated in all of the following *except*:

a. Primary pulmonary hypertension b. Eisenmenger's syndrome
c. Marfan's with aortic root dilation d. WPW syndrome

Ans. is 'd' WPW syndrome

Hydrops Fetalis

Immune	
Rh incompatibility	
Nonimmune	
• Anemia	a-thalassemia, G-6PD deficiency
• Cardiac dysarrhythmias	Supraventricular tachycardia, AF, congenital heart block
• Structural cardiac defects	Tricuspid insufficient endocardial cushion defect, cardiomyopathy, hypoplastic left heart, premature closure of foramen ovale
• Vascular	Chorangioma of placenta, Twin-to-twin transfusion, umbilical artery aneurysm, thrombosis of renal or umbilical vein or WC
• Lymphatic	Lymphangiectasia, cystic hygroma, Noonan syndrome
• CNS	Encephalocele, intracranial hemorrhage
• Thoracic	Mediastinal teratoma, diaphragmatic hernia
• Teratomas	Choriocarcinoma, sacrococcygeal teratoma
• Tumor and storage diseases	Neuroblastoma, hepatoblastoma, Gaucher disease, Niemann-Pick disease, mucopolysaccharidosis
• Chromosomal	Trisomy 13, 15, 16, 18, 21
• Bone diseases	Osteogenesis imperfecta, skeletal dysplasia
• Congenital infections	CMV, rubella, toxoplasmosis, syphilis, parvovirus, leptospirosis, chagas disease
• Others	Congenital nephrosis, myotonic dystrophy, infant of diabetic mother, maternal therapy with indomethacin, hepatic fibroses

150. Cause of non-immune hydrops include all *except*:

a. Congenital heart block
b. Alpha thalassemia
c. Parvovirus infection
d. Congenital varicella infection

Ans. is 'd' Congenital varicella infection

RH-ISOIMMUNIZATION

Management of Alloimmunization in Subsequent Pregnancies

Pregnancies after the first alloimmunized pregnancy are characterized by increasingly severe fetalhemolytic disease due to the entry of fetal red cells into the maternal circulation at each delivery, which causes an anamnestic maternal antibody response. A woman whose prior pregnancy was complicated by the need for intrauterine fetal transfusion, fetal hydrops, preterm delivery because of severe fetalanemia, or neonatal exchange transfusion can expect development of severe fetalanemia in subsequent pregnancies with an RhD-positive fetus. The severe anemia occurs earlier in gestation than in the prior pregnancy.

Fetal *RHD* type should be determined early in gestation using cell-free DNA (cfDNA) and we should begin middle cerebral artery (MCA) peak systolic velocity (PSV) monitoring of *RHD*-positive fetuses at 16 to 18 weeks of gestation.

Measure MCA-PSV at one- to two-week intervals. The frequency is increased if indicated by multiples of the median (MoMs) approaching 1.5. An MCA-PSV ≤ 1.5 MoMs for gestational age is consistent with absence of moderate to severe anemia. If MCA-PSV remains at this level, we schedule delivery at 37 to 38 weeks of gestation.

- For pregnancies with MCA-PSV >1.5 MoMs for gestational age, obtain fetal blood by cordocentesis for hemoglobin determination and perform an intrauterine fetal transfusion if fetalhemoglobin is two standard deviations below the mean value for gestational age. Intrauterine transfusion is generally limited to pregnancies <35 weeks of gestation because after 35 weeks, intrauterine transfusion is considered riskier than delivery followed by postnatal transfusion therapy. At ≥ 35 weeks of gestation we would deliver a fetus with MCA-PSV >1.5 MoMs for gestational age.

151. In modern obstetric practice, the investigation done in a Rh-ve female with sensitization is? *(NEET 2020)*

a. MCA Doppler
b. Fetal blood sampling
c. Biophysical profile
d. Amniotic fluid spectrometry

Ans. is 'a' MCA Doppler

HYPERTENSIVE DISORDERS IN PREGNANCY

HYPERTENSIVE DISORDER DURING PREGNANCY

Definition: Systolic BP ≥ 140 mm of Hg or diastolic BP ≥ 90 mm of Hg on two occasions at-least 6 hours but no more than 7 days apart.

Pregnancy induced hypertension: normotensive woman conceived and become hypertensive

- **Preeclampsia:** Rise in B/P seen after 20 weeks of pregnancy + Proteinuria (>300 mg in 24 hours urine collection or >30 mg/dL in a random urine sample or > + 1 on.) + B/P comes back to normal within 12 weeks of delivery
- **Eclampsia:** Preeclampsia + seizure
- **Gestational Hypertension:** Preeclampsia not associated with proteinuria
- **Chronic hypertension in pregnancy:** hypertensive female has conceived rise in B/P seen before 20 weeks + No proteinuria + B/P does not come back to normal within 12 weeks of delivery.

HELLP syndrome: is a variant of preeclampsia defined by following criteria:

- Hemolysis identified by Burr cells and schistocytes on an abnormal peripheral smear,
- an elevated serum bilirubin (> 1.2 mg/dL) or LDH level (> 600 IU/L), or a low serum haptoglobin.
- Thrombocytopenia with platelets < 100,000/micro liter is the most consistent finding in HELLP syndrome.
- Elevated liver function tests (i.e transaminases) greater than two times the upper limit of normal (≥ 72 IU/L)

Management

- Pregnancy induced hypertension (Preeclampsia/Gestational hypertension) are raised BP conditions due to placental pathology (incomplete trophoblastic invasion) so their definitive treatment would be termination of pregnancy always.
- Antihypertensive of choice for chronic hypertension in pregnancy—Labetalol.
- Antihypertensive of choice for pregnancy-induced hypertension (Preeclampsia/Gestational hypertension) is Labetalol
- Antihypertensive of choice for hypertensive crisis is—Labetalol

Antihypertensives in Pregnancy

Safe	Contraindicated
Labetalol	ACE inhibitors
Calcium channel blockers	Diuretics
Hydralazine	Reserpine
Alpha methyldopa	Loratidine
Sodium nitroprusside	

Management of PIH/eclampsia

Mild PIH	Severe PIH	Eclampsia
Bed rest + diet control	Seizure prophylaxis – $MgSO_4$	Airway management
Termination of pregnancy done at 37 completed weeks of pregnancy	Antihypertensive BP should be b/w 140/90 to 155/105 mmHg	Drug to control seizures—$MgSO_4$
	Glucocorticoids—for lung maturation	Antihypertensive to control BP
	Definitive management—termination of pregnancy at 34 completed weeks	Definitive management—termination of pregnancy immediately
		Delivery should occur within 24 hours of 1st seizure

Prevention and Treatment of Convulsions with $MgSO_4$

- $MgSO_4$ is the drug of choice for prevention and management of convulsions in eclampsia
- **Regimens for $MgSO_4$**: IM loading dose Pritchard Regimen—5 gm (50% solution) in each buttock deep IM maintenance dose—5 gm (50%) deep IM on alternate buttock every 4 hours.
- IV loading dose 4–6 slow over 3–5 minutes at rate not more than 1 g/min. Maintenance dose – 1–2 gm/hr IV infusion
- Therapeutic range—4 to 7 mEq/L
- There is a narrow range at which therapeutic effect and toxic effects of magnesium occurs, therefore monitoring for magnesium toxicity is very essential.

Monitoring for Magnesium Toxicity

- Urine output should be at least 30 mL/hr
- Deep tendon reflexes (Patellar reflex) should be present
- Respiration rate should be more than 14/min.
- Pulse oximetry should be ≥96%.

Investigations in a Case of Preeclampsia

- Urine for proteins/albumin. 24 hours urine protein
- *CBC*: There is hemoconcentration so Hb values are false elevated. Low platelets indicate HELLP syndrome
- *Sr uric acid*: It is a biochemical marker of preeclampsia. Raised levels (>4.5 mg/dL) indicate renal involvement also correlate with severity of preeclampsia, volume contraction and fetal jeopardy.
- *LFT*: SGOT, SGPT, bilirubin
- *RFT*: Sr creatinine

Coagulation profile may be required in severe cases:
- BT
- CT
- PT, APTT
- Fibrinogen levels
- FDP

Management of Preeclampsia

- Antiseizure prophylaxis with magnesium sulphate is started.
- Careful assessment of maternal and fetal status followed by delivery is done.
- Administration of corticosteroids improves perinatal (↑ pulmonary maturity, ↓ IVH and ↓ necrotizing enterocolitis) and maternal (↑thrombocyte count, ↑ urinary output) outcome.
- Cesarean section is the common mode of delivery.
- Epidural anaesthesia can be used safely if the platelet count is >1,00,000/mm^3).

- Platelet transfusion should be given if the count is <50,000/mm³.
- Patient should be managed in an ICU until there is improvement in platelet count, urine output, BP and liver enzymes.
- Recurrence risk of HELLP syndrome is 3–19%.

Cesarean Section

The operation should be done by an experienced surgeon with the help of an expert anesthetist. Epidural anesthesia is preferred, unless there is coagulopathy. Indications:

1. When an urgent termination is indicated and the cervix is unfavorable (unripe and closed).
2. Severe preeclampsia with a tendency of prolonged induction delivery interval.
3. Associated complicating factors, such as elderly primigravidae, contracted pelvis, malpresentation, etc.

Management During Labor

- Blood pressure tends to rise during labor and convulsions may occur due to stress hormones (intraparturn eclampsia).
- The patient should be in bed.
- Antihypertensive drugs are given if the blood pressure becomes high.
- Blood pressure and urinary output are to be noted frequently so as to detect imminent eclampsia. Prophylactic $MgSO_4$ is started when systolic BP >160 diastolic >110, MAP >125 mm Hg. Careful monitoring of the fetal well-being is mandatory.
- Labor duration is curtailed by low rupture of the membranes in the first stage; and forceps or ventouse in second stage.
- Intravenous ergometrine following the delivery of the anterior shoulder is withheld as it may cause further rise of blood pressure.
- However, there is no contraindication of synto IM or slow IV and to keep the patient under dose observation for several hours.

Complications of Preeclampsia

Maternal	Fetal
Eclampsia	IUFD
Abruption	IUGR
Preterm labor	Oligohydramnios
HELLP Syndrome DIC	
Blindness	

152. Features of non-severe/mild preeclampsia are all *except*:

a. Diastolic BP < 100 mm Hg
b. Systolic BP < 160 mm Hg
c. Mild IUGR
d. No premonitory symptoms

Ans. is 'c' Mild IUGR

153. What is monitored in a patient of preeclampsia:

a. Uric acid
b. Platelet count
c. LFT
d. All of the above

Ans. is 'd' All of the above

154. Complications of preeclampsia are all *except*:

a. Post-datism
b. DIC
c. Blindness
d. None of the above

Ans. is 'a' Post-datism

PRETERM LABOR, PROM AND POST-DATED PREGNANCY

CERVICAL INCOMPETENCE

Characterised by:

- Painless cervical dilatation in the second or early third trimester
- Ballooning of the amniotic sac into the vagina
- Rupture of membranes and expulsion of a usually live fetus.
  - The usual timing is 16 to 24 weeks.
  - M/C cause of 2nd trimester recurrent abortion

Etiology

Congenital	Acquired
Developmental weakness of cervix	due to previous cervical trauma
Associated with uterine anomalies like septate uterus	Forcible dilatation during MTP and D and C
Following in utero exposure to diethyl stilbestrol	Conisation of cervix
	Cauterisation of cervix
	Amputation of cervix or Fothergill's operation

Diagnosis

History: The typical history of painless rupture of membranes followed by the quick delivery of a live fetus in mid-trimester is very suggestive.

Nonpregnant state	In pregnancy
The internal os allows the passage of a No. 8 Hegar's cervical dilator or Foley's catheter filled with 1 ml water without resistance	Transvaginal ultrasound is the ideal method to follow up and detect early incompetence
Premenstrual hysterocervicography will show the typical funnelling of the internal os	The normal cervical length at 14 weeks is 35 – 40 mm. A cervical length less than 25 mm, funnelling of the os, and os diameter > 1 cm on USG indicates cervical incompetence

Management

The treatment is surgical by a cervical circlage, which can be done prophylactically or in emergency (Rescue cerclage)

Time of Operation

Prophylactic cervical cerclage at 12-14 weeks (usually delayed so that miscarriage due to other causes can be eliminated)

OR

at least 2 weeks earlier than the lowest period of earlier loss (but never earlier than 10 weeks).

Procedures

Vaginal cerclage	Abdominal cerclage
• McDonald's operation • Shirodkar's operation	• Women with incompetent cervix due to severe trauma to cervix such as deep laceration, extensive conization or repeated LEP for treatment of Ca in situ. • H/O repetitive 2nd trimester loss and failed vaginal circlages. • In women with 2nd trimester losses and anatomic impossibility to place a vaginal circlage

Removal of circlage stitch: The stitch should be removed at 37 weeks or earlier if labor pain starts or features of abortion appears.

GLUCOCORTICOID THERAPY

Maternal administration of glucocorticoids is advocated where the pregnancy is less than 34 weeks. This helps in fetal lung maturation so that the incidence of RDS, IVH and NEC are minimized. This is beneficial when the delivery is delayed beyond 48 hours of the first dose.

- Benefit persists as long as 18 days.
- Either betamethasone (Betnesol) 12 mg IM 24 hours a part for two doses
  or
- Dexamethasone 6 mg IM every 12 hours for 4 doses is given.
- Betamethasone is the steroid of choice.
- Steroids (dexamethasone or betamethasone) are given to enhance fetal lung maturity and they also decrease the incidence of intraventricular hemorrhage
- Betamethasone is preferred over dexamethasone, as it also prevents periventricular leukomalacia

Risks of Antenatal Corticosteroid Use

- Premature rupture of the membranes especially with evidence of infection as the infection may flare-up
- Insulin-dependent diabetes mellitus, where patients need insulin dose readjustment
- Transient reduction of fetal breathing and body movements.

Contraindications

Chorioamnionitis and active infection in mother.

155. A 30-year-old is 14 weeks pregnant. She has two painless deliveries at 16 weeks earlier. Next line of management is: *(NEET 2018)*

a. Cervical encerclage
b. Evaluation for diabetes mellitus and thyroid disorders
c. Cervical length assessment
d. Tocolytics

Ans. is 'a' Cervical encerclage

156. Drug that is used for fetal lung maturity is: *(NEET 2018)*

a. Dexamethasone
b. Folic acid
c. Beclomethasone
d. None of the above

Ans. is 'a' Dexamethasone

OBSTRUCTED LABOR AND INTRAUTERINE DEATH

DIABETES IN PREGNANCY

Can be of two types:

1. **Gestational diabetes:**
   - Due to insulin resistance and effect of HPL hormone
   - These females will thus have high sugar levels at or after approx. 24 weeks of pregnancy.
2. **Overt diabetes:** patient of DM type-1 or DM type-2
   - Switch to insulin from oral hypoglycemic drugs
   - In diabetes patient free radical gets generate which leads to congenital malformation, in overt diabetes patient it starts generating from early weeks so congenital anomaly in fetus will be present in contrast to gestational diabetes where blood sugar level increases at 24 weeks (after organogenesis) so no congenital anomaly seen.

Diagnostic Criteria for Diabetes during Pregnancy

According to American diabetes association the criteria for diagnosis of overt diabetes during pregnancy is:

- Random plasma glucose >200 mg/dL + classic symptoms of diabetes
- Fasting blood glucose >125 mg/dL
- HbA1C > 6.5% d. Two or more abnormal values on 100 gm oral glucose tolerance test during pregnancy.

Screening for Diabetes during Pregnancy

Glucose Challenges Test (O Sullivan blood sugar screening test)

- Performed by orally administering 50 g of glucose irrespective of previous meal and measuring venous plasma glucose 1 hour later.
- Interpretation of result
  Plasma glucose Interpretation
  < 140 mg/dL—normal
  ≥ 140 mg/dL—GTT required
  ≥ 200 mg/dL—diabetes confirmed

Glucose tolerance test (to diagnose diabetes)

- Patients with abnormal screening test are followed by a 3 hours glucose tolerance test (GTT)
- The test is performed with 100 gm of glucose or 75 gm of glucose

Time	100 gm glucose	75 gm glucose
Fasting	95 mg/dL	92 mg/dL
1 hour	180 mg/dL	180 mg/dL
2 hours	155 mg/dL	153 mg/dL
3 hours	140 mg/dL	

Management

Diet Management

- Intake of caloric requirement is 25-35 kcal/kg body weight/day according to body mass index.
- Means should divide into 3 major and 3 minor meals.
- **Exercise:** 30 mins physical activity per day
- **Insulin:** DOC for diabetes in pregnancy.

Time of delivery

- ❖ Low risk patients—wait for spontaneous labor till maximum 40 weeks
- ❖ High risk patients—38 weeks—induce labor as IUD occurs mostly in last 2 weeks of pregnancy.
- ❖ Elective cesarian section should perform
- ❖ Macrosomia with weight > 4.5 kg (for predicting macrosomia, shoulder width > 14 cm, EFW > 4.5 kg on ultrasound)
- ❖ Demonstrable fetal compromise (severe IUGR)
- ❖ If fasting is 92–125 mg/dL it is diagnosed as GDM and if it is = 126 mg/dL it is designated as overt diabetes.

DIC

- ❖ Thromboplastin from the dead fetus can enter the maternal system and cause DIC.
- ❖ This only happens when the dead fetus is retained inside for 3–4 weeks.

Signs	Interval (after death)
Robert sign (gas in great vessels)	12 hours
Spalding sign (overlapping of skull bones)	1 week
Blair-Hartley/ball sign (hyperflexion/hyperextension of spine with overcrowding of ribs	3–4 weeks

Still Birth

Stillbirth is the birth of a new-born after 28th completed week (weighing 1000 gm or more) when the baby does not breathe or show any sign of life after delivery. It includes both fresh and macerated (antepartum) deaths.

Macrosomia

- ❖ Macrosomia is the term used to describe a large fetus.
- ❖ Macrosomia is associated with gestational diabetes (GDM) and maternal obesity
- ❖ The recommended definition is fetal (neonatal) weight exceeding two standard deviations or above 90th centile for the appropriate normal population.
- ❖ According to ACOG: birth weight of > 4500gm is called as macrosomia.
- ❖ In Indian context birth weight of > 4000 gm is called as macrosomia.

157. After IUFD, when does the mother develop DIC:

a. 48 hours
b. 1–2 weeks
c. 3–4 weeks
d. 6 weeks

Ans. is 'c' 3–4 weeks

158. Earliest sign after IUFD is:

a. Overlapping of skull bones
b. Hyperflexion of spine
c. Gas in great vessel
d. Overcrowding of ribs

Ans. is 'c' Gas in great vessel

159. In 34 weeks gestation the weight of baby was 3kg. The child shows following features may indicate associated condition macrosomic baby, weighing 5.3 kg, of a diabetic mother, looked plethoric (due to polycythemia), with plumpy face, buried eyes and excessive buccal fat. *(NEET 2019)*

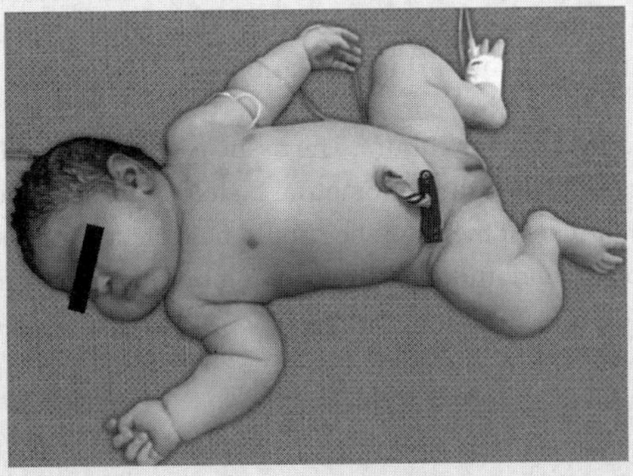

a. Anemia
b. Diabetes
c. APH
d. None

Ans. is 'b' Diabetes

Obstetrics and Gynecology

160. Overt gestational diabetes is defined as blood glucose more than_: *(NEET 2019)*

a. >200 mg/dL
b. >126 mg/dL
c. >100 mg/dL
d. >180 mg/dL

Ans. is 'b' >126 mg/dL

MALPRESENTATIONS AND HIGH-RISK PREGNANCIES

CEPHALOHEMATOMA

Cephalohematoma	Caput succedaneum
Hemorrhage of blood between the skull and the periosteum of a new-born baby	An edema of the scalp at the neonate's presenting part of the head
Same	Appears over the vertex of the new-born's head
Secondary to rupture of blood vessels crossing the periosteum due to prolonged second stage of labor or instrumental delivery, particularly ventouse.	As a result of pressure against the mother's cervix during labor
Because the swelling is subperiosteal its boundaries are limited by the individual bones	edema in caput succedaneum crosses the suture lines
Cephalohematoma usually appears on the second or third day after birth and disappears within weeks or months	It always presents at birth

161. True about cephalohematoma is:

a. Crosses the suture lines
b. Always presents at birth
c. Ventouse delivery is a risk factor
d. All of the above

Ans. is 'c' Ventouse delivery is a risk factor.

OPERATIVE OBSTETRICS, PHARMACOTHERAPEUTICS

DILATATION AND CURETTAGE

Obstetric indications of cervical dilatation are:

Prior to evacuation in missed abortion, incomplete abortion, evacuation of hydatidiform mole. It is also necessary in medical termination of pregnancy.

Curettage: is mainly diagnostic.
This is required in:

- Abnormal uterine bleeding (AUB) to study the hormonal pattern causing abnormal bleeding.
  Secondary amenorrhea to detect tubercular endometritis.
- Postmenopausal bleeding to rule out endometrial cancer.
- Endometrial cancer to study the endocervical tissue and the extent of spread. This helps in staging and deciding on treatment.
- Infertility: Until recently, DandC was performed premenstrual to detect if ovulation has occurred. Secretory endometrium indicates that ovulation has occurred. Proliferative endometrium in the premenstrual phase indicates non-ovulation.
  Now, ultrasound has replaced DandC for monitoring ovulation. It is however required if tubercular endometriosis is suspected.
  - The endometrial tissue is preserved in saline for culture. The tissue is also subjected to polymerase chain reaction.
  - Corpus luteal phase defect is diagnosed when the endometrial histology lags behind the menstrual date by 2 days.
- A menopausal woman on hormonal replacement therapy; she should be watched for endometrial hyperplasia and cancer.
- A woman on tamoxifen for breast cancer should undergo curettage 6-monthly to diagnose endometrial hyperplasia and cancer.

Therapeutic DandC is Indicated

To remove endometrial polyp (polypectomy).

Contraindications to DandC are:

Suspected pregnancy

Lower genital tract infection

Sequelae of DandC:
Infection of upper genital tract.
Asherman syndrome

DIFFERENCES BETWEEN FORCEPS AND VACUUM

Forceps	Vacuum
Traction force = +18 kg for primi, +13 kg for multi	Negative pressure = 0.8 kg/cm² (600 mm Hg)
Cervix should be fully dilate	Minimum 7 cm dilation
Less fetal but more maternal complications	More fetal but less maternal complications
Preferred in fetal distress	Less preferred (as vacuum takes time to build up)
Rotation forceps not applied nowadays	Vacuum causes rotation and extraction
Can be applied presentation and after coming head of breech	Cannot be applied on face presentation and after coming head of breech
Can be applied on preterm fetus	Contraindicated on preterm fetus (increase risk of intraventricular hemorrhage)
Can be applied in cases of fetal coagulopathy and if recent scalp blood sampling has been done	Contraindicated in cases of fetal coagulopathy and if recent scalp blood sampling has been done
Can be applied in cases of (IUFD)	Should not be applied as chignon formation will not occur in (IUFD)

- Penicillamine interferes with synthesis of collagen and elastin and can cause: Elastosis perforans serpiginosa and localized cutis laxa

162. Dilatation and curettage (D and C) is contraindicated in: *(NEET 2018)*

a. Pelvic inflammatory disease (PID)
b. Endometriosis
c. Ectopic pregnancy
d. None

Ans. is 'a' Pelvic inflammatory disease (PID)

163. Pressure created in vacuum is:

a. 12 kg
b. 0.2 kg/cm^2
c. 0.8 kg/cm^2
d. 18 kg

Ans. is 'c' 0.8 kg/cm^2

DIAGNOSIS IN OBSTETRICS

RUPTURE OF UTERUS

Disruption in the continuity of all uterine layers: endometrium, myometrium and serosa anytime beyond 28 weeks of pregnancy is called rupture of uterus.

Incidence

1 in 2000 to 1 in 200 deliveries. Rupture uterus from obstructed labor is becoming less because of improved obstetric care, but prevalence of scar rupture is increased because of increase in LSCS rates.

Etiology

1. Rupture of previous LSCS scar during VBAC is one of the commonest cause of rupture uterus today: LSCS scar generally ruptures in labor (mainly in second stage or towards end of first stage) and unlikely to rupture during pregnancy.
2. Spontaneous (intact or unscarred uterus)
3. Iatrogenic: mainly due to injudicious use of oxytocin or prostaglandins (for induction or augmentation of labor) and very rarely due to internal podalic version and destructive operations as they are not performed in modern day obstetrics.

164. In modern day obstetrics, most common cause of rupture uterus is:

a. Prolonged labor
b. Previous LSCS scar rupture
c. Forceps delivery
d. Internal podalic version

Ans. is 'b' Previous LSCS scar rupture

DOWN SYNDROME

TRIPLE MARKER TEST

- Triple Marker Test is a screening test
- done between 16 and 18 weeks of gestation
- mainly to identify a mother who is at a high risk of having a fetus with trisomy 21
- It involves estimation of 3 hormones: hCG, AFP, and unconjugated estriol (UE3)

Quadruple test: (hCG, APP, UE3, INHIBIN A) is also done in 2nd trimester

Double marker test: (hCG + PAPP A) is done in first trimester

Interpretation			
Trisomy	hCG	AFP	UE3
Down syndrome	↑	↓	↓
Edward syndrome	↓	↓	↓

USG Features of Down Syndrome (Soft Markers)

USF features of down syndrome (soft tissue markers)	
• Echogenic bowel	• Cystic hygroma
• Echogenic intracardiac foci	• ASPI VSD
• Duodena' atresia	• Ventriculomegaly
• Absent nasal bone	• Annular pancreas
• Single umbilical artery	• Increased nuchal fold thickness, increased NT
• Renal pyelectasis	• Congenital diaphragmatic hernia
• Exomphalos	• Sandal gap
• Choroid plexus cyst	• Fifth finger middle phalanx hypoplasia
• Short femur/humerus	

165. Triple marker test includes:

a. hCG, AFP, and unconjugated estriol
b. hCG, AFP, and unconjugated estradiol
c. hCG, PAPP-A, unconjugated estriol
d. Inhibin A, hCG and PAPP-A

Ans. is 'a' hCG, AFP, and unconjugated estriol

166. Which of the following is not a soft tissue marker of Down syndrome on USG:

a. Increase NT
b. Absent nasal bone
c. Exomphalos
d. Polydactyly

Ans. is 'd' Polydactyly

ELECTRONIC FHR MONITORING

FETAL HEART RATE DECELERATION

Features of Early Fetal Heart Rate Deceleration

Characteristics include gradual decrease in the heart rate with both onset and recovery coincident with the onset and recovery of the contraction. Early decelerations are due to head compression (stimulation of vagus nerve)

Features of Late Fetal Heart Rate Deceleration

Characteristics include gradual decrease in the heart rate with the nadir and recovery occurring after the end of the contraction. The nadir of the deceleration occurs 30 seconds or more after the onset-of-the deceleration. Late decelerations are due to uteroplacental insufficiency (fetal distress/hypoxia)

Features of Variable Fetal Heart Rate Decelerations

Characteristics include abrupt decrease in the heart rate with onset commonly varying with successive contractions. The decelerations measure 15 beats/mm for 15 seconds or longer with an onset-to nadir phase of less than 30 seconds. Total duration is less than 2 minutes. Variable decelerations are due to cord compression (oligohydramnios in labor)

167. Variable deceleration is seen in:

a. Head compression
b. Uteroplacental insufficiency
c. Cord compression
d. None of the above

Ans. is 'c' Cord compression

BIOPHYSICAL PROFILE

- It has 5 components.
- Biophysical profile components (Manning's score)
  - Nonstress test
  - Fetal breathing
  - Fetal movement
  - Fetal tone
  - Amniotic fluid volume

Component	Score 2	Score 0
Non stress test	Reactive NST = In a period of 20 minutes, there should be at least 2 accelerations of >15 bpm lasting for at least 15 seconds	0–1 acceleration in 20-40 minutes
Foetal breathing	>1 episode of rhythmic breathing lasting >30 second within 30 minutes	<30 second of breathing in 30 min
Amniotic fluid volume	Single vertical pocket >2 cm	Largest single vertical pocket <2 cm
Foetal tone	>1 episode of extension of fetal extremity with return to flexion, or opening or closing of hand within 30 minutes	No movements or no extension/ flexion
Fetal movement	>3 discrete body or limb movements within 30 minutes	<3 discrete movements

- Individual CNS centers that may regulate the biophysical activities appear to vary in their sensitivity to hypoxia. Accordingly, a "gradual hypoxia" model has been proposed in which the activities that first appear embryologically are the last to disappear with progressively worsening hypoxia.
- According to the gradual hypoxia model, FHR-R should be the first component of the BPP to become abnormal (i.e. to be lost) in hypoxic states. The gradual hypoxia concept would help explain the increased incidence of abnormal outcome as more biophysical activities decrease in occurrence and eventually disappear. Ultimately, the persistent and true lack of fetal tone should be associated with the highest perinatal death rate.

168. Modified Biophysical profile is:

a. NST + FETAL TONE
b. FETAL TONE+ AFI
c. NST + AFI
d. NST + FETAL TONE + AFI

Ans. is 'c' NST + AFI

169. If fetus is having hypoxia, which of the BPP parameter will be affected last:

a. Fetal tone
b. Fetal breathing movement
c. Fetal movements
d. NST

Ans. is 'a' Fetal tone

PARTOGRAPH

Explanation: The given partograph shows no cervical dilatation for first 2 hrs followed by 1 cm in next 2 hrs.

This is suggestive of prolonged active phase of first stage of labour (dilatation < 1 cm/hr). At 4 hrs, oxytocin was started and the contractions increased in intensity along with descent of fetal head. So the most likely pathology was inadequate uterine contractions.

Why not rupture uterus?—Would result in lost of fetal station and the head descent curve would be upsloping.

Why not maternal exhaustion?—In this case, the contractions would be normal in the beginning and lateral there would be a decrease in intensity.

Why not CPD ?—If there is CPD, there won't be descent of fetal head at any intensity of contractions.

170. Identify the condition based on the partograph shown? *(NEET 2020)*

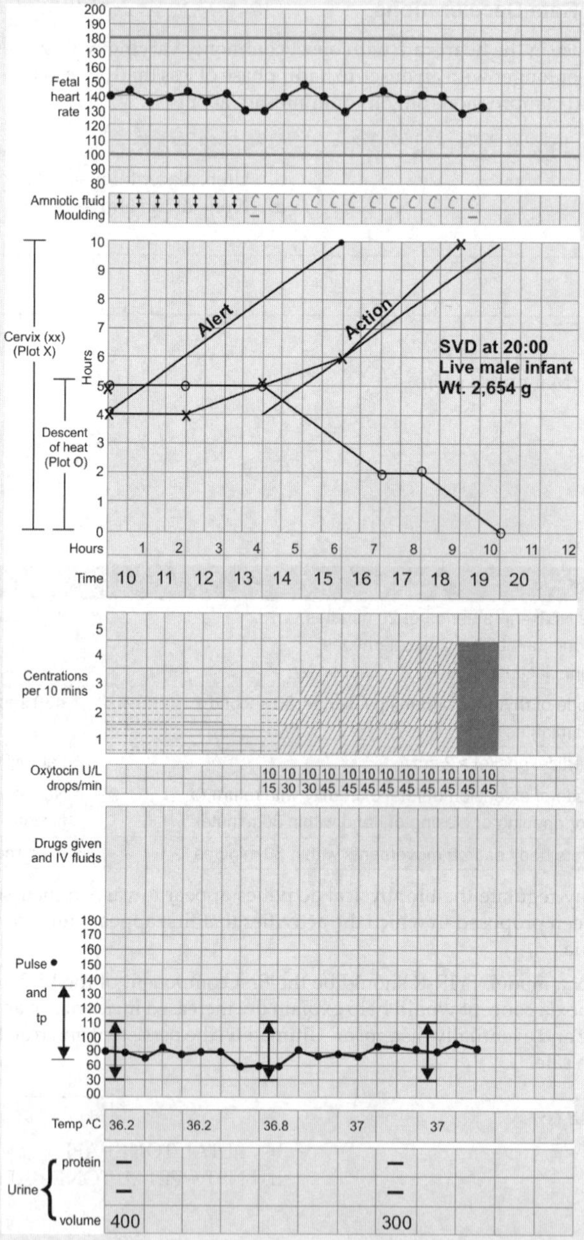

a. Rupture uterus
b. Maternal exhaustion
c. Inadequate uterine contractions
d. Cephalopelvic disproportion

Ans. is 'c' Inadequate uterine contractions

CHAPTER 15 Dermatology

LAYERS OF EPIDERMIS

- Basal layer/stratum germinativum – mitotically active keratinocytes.
- Stratum spinosum—spines have abundant desmosomes, Ca^{2+} dependent cell surface modification that promote adhesion of epidermal cells resistance to mechanical stress. Langerhans cells are found in stratum spinosum and function as epidermal macrophages (Antigen presenting cells). Thickening of stratum spinosum is called Acanthosis. Presence of intercellular edema in stratum spinosum is called spongiosis.
- *Granular layer:* Cells have basophilic keratinohyaline granules composed of profilaggrin keratin filament, loricrin.
- Stratum corneum—layer made of keratin
  - *Corneocyte*: Largest cell of epidermis.
  - Filaggrin responsible for keratin filament aggregation.
- Fifth layer-Stratum lucidum, between S. corneum and S. granulosum is found in palms and soles.

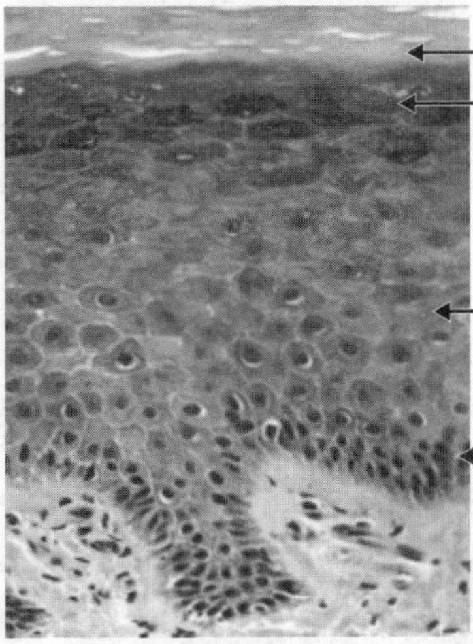

1. Langerhans cell are seen in which layer of skin:

a. Stratum basale
b. Stratum corneum
c. Stratum granulosum
d. Stratum spinosum

Ans. is 'd' Stratum spinosum

2. Increase in the thickness of the prickle cell layer of the epidermis is called:

a. Spongiosis
b. Acanthosis
c. Hypergranulosis
d. Hyperkeratosis

Ans. is 'b' Acanthosis

LEPROSY

Spectrum of manifestations in leprosy is summarized in the following table:

Feature	TT	BT	BB	BL	LL
Skin lesions					
Number	Single/few	Few	Several	Numerous	Innumerable
Size	Variable	May be large	Variable	Small	Small
Sensations	Anesthetic	Hypoesthetic	Hypoesthetic	Hypoesthetic	Normoesthetic
Symmetry	Asymmetrical	Asymmetrical	Bilateral, Asymmetrica	Nearly Symmetrical	Symmetrical
Morphology	Well-defined macule/plaque	Well-defined plaques with satellite lesions	Plaques with sloping edge (inverted saucer appearance	Macule, nodules, Ill defined plaques	Macule, nodules, Ill defined plaques
Nerves	Single trunk	Asymmetrical involvement of few nerves with thickening	Several nerves involved asymmetrically with thickening	Glove and stocking anesthesia	Symmetrical nerve thickening

Contd...

Contd...

Feature	TT	BT	BB	BL	LL
Reactions	Stable	Type I	Type I	Type I/II	Type II
Lepromin Test	+	+/–	–	–	–
Histology					
Granuloma	Well-defined epithelioid cell granulomas	Epithelioid cell granuloma	–	Ill-defined macrophage granulomas with many lymphocytes	Ill-defined foamy macrophage granulomas
Grenz Zone	–	+	++Q	++Q	++Q
AFB	–	–	+/–	+	++Q

NERVE BIOPSY

- A thickened sensory nerve is selected for biopsy. The suitable nerves include supraorbital branch of the fifth cranial nerve, supra-clavicular nerve, great auricular nerve of the forearm or thigh, sural nerve at the back of the leg or superficial peroneal nerve on the dorsum of the foot. The nerves usually chosen for biopsy are a branch of sural nerve at the level just above the ankle, or a branch of radial cutaneous nerve at the wrist region.

3. Identify the nerve thickened here in a leprosy patient:

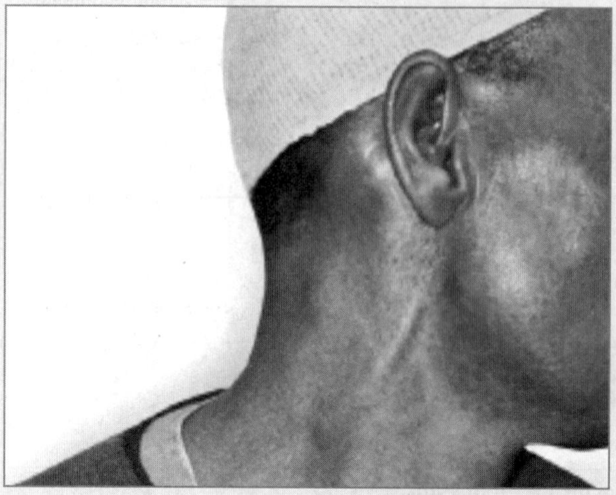

a. Greater auricular nerve
b. Facial nerve
c. Trigeminal nerve
d. Occipital nerve

Ans. is 'a' Greater auricular nerve

LUPUS VULGARIS

- Lupus vulgaris is a chronic form of skin TB seen in patients with moderate immunity to TB bacilli
- It is seen more common in females

Pathogenesis

- It occurs due to hematogenous, lymphatic, or contiguous spread from elsewhere in the body, or from exogenous inoculation.

Clinical Features

- It presents as single or few lesions which are well-demarcated, annular plaques which extend centrifugally. Periphery show erythematous deep seated nodules which on diascopy may stand out as apple jelly nodules. They are most commonly seen in buttocks, upper extremities and face. Center is depigmented with paper-thin scar with nodules.
- Papules may recur on the scarred areas, which enlarge and coalesce. This leads to the formation of large, firm, elevated plaques. At the periphery are small reddish-yellow or brown nodules.

Diagnosis

- Histologic examination and a positive culture for M. tuberculosis/bovis confirm the diagnosis
- Most prominent histopathologic feature: Typical granulomas

Complication

Secondary scarring and squamous cell carcinomas may develop rarely.

4. A 32-year-old lady from Chhattisgarh tribal area came with an erythematous indurated plaque with scarring on right side of face and extension to ear lobe. Most likely diagnosis:

a. Lepromatous leprosy
b. Molluscum leprosy
c. Lupus vulgaris
d. Pityriasis rubra pilaris

Ans. is 'c' Lupus vulgaris

Tuberculosis verrucosa cutis—Tuberculosis verrucosa cutis (TBVC, also known as prosectors wart, anatomic tuberculosis, verruca necrogenica, and warty tuberculosis) is a form of cutaneous TB that occurs after direct inoculation of the mycobacteria into the skin of a previously sensitized host with moderate to high immunity against the bacillus. Inoculation typically occurs from an exogenous source; rarely, inoculation may occur from the patient's own sputum.

In adults, TBVC most frequently develops on the acral extremities; the fingers and dorsum of the hands are commonly affected. The ankles or buttocks are frequent sites for lesion occurrence in children. TBVC on the lower lip, an unusual site, has been reported.

The skin lesions are usually solitary and manifest as painless, violaceous or brown-red, indurated warty plaques that range from 1 to 5 cm in diameter. TBVC grows via peripheral extension; central clearing and atrophy may or may not be present. Although ulceration is uncommon, fissures that exude purulent drainage or keratinous material may occur.

The treatment of cutaneous TB is the same as that for systemic TB. The administration of a course of multidrug therapy is the treatment of choice.

5. What is the best treatment for this condition? *(NEET 2020)*

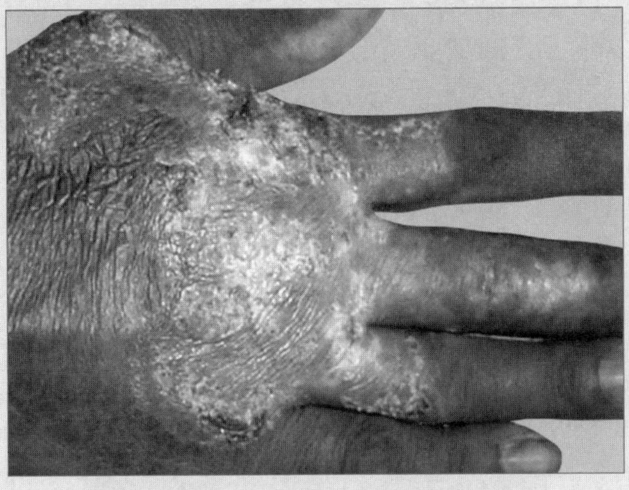

a. Oral steroids
b. Anti leprosy treatment
c. Antitubercular therapy
d. Oral terbinafine

Ans. is 'c' Antitubercular therapy

IMPETIGO

- Superficial skin infection
- Neutrophils collect beneath stratum corneum
- Macules → papules → rupture → erosions
- Dried sebum → "Honey-colored" crust
- Highly Contagious
- **Impetigo Contagiosa**
  - Most common form
  - Face and extremities
  - Caused by *Staph. aureus* and Beta-hemolytic streptococcus (mostly *S. pyogenes*)
  - Honey-crusted lesions
- **Bullous Impetigo**
  - Seen in children
  - Trunk is commonly involved
  - Caused by *Staph. aureus*

Treatment of Impetigo

Impetigo contagiosa
• Localized—Topical antibiotics like fusidic acid or mupirocin. • Extensive—Systemic antibiotics (erythromycin group to cover Staphylococcus and Streptococcus). If response is poor, oxacillin—clavulanic acid or cephalexin can be tried.
Bullous impetigo
• Localized—Topical fusidic acid or mupirocin • Extensive—Systemic antistaphylococcal antibiotics (flucloxacillin, amoxicillin clavulanic acid, methicillin or erythromycin)

6. **Treatment for impetigo includes all *except*:**
   a. Topical mupirocin
   b. Systemic erythromycin
   c. Topical gentamicin
   d. Systemic cephalosporins

Ans. is 'c' Topical gentamicin

SCABIES

Etiology: Sarcoptes scabiei spreads by prolonged and intimate contact

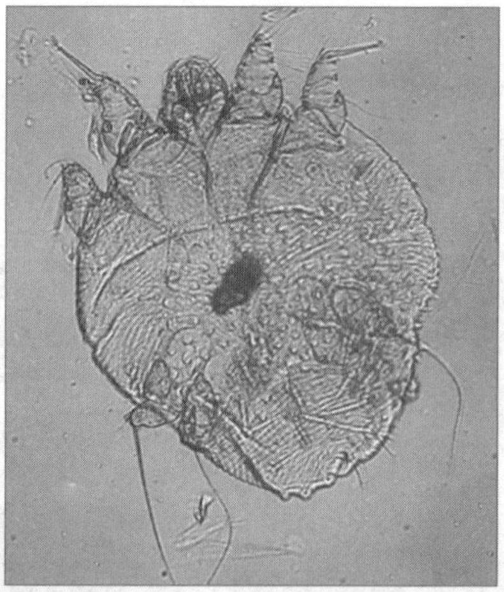

Morphology: Burrow (serpentine (S-shaped), thread like gray-brown line which represent the intraepidermal tunnel created by the moving female mite in stratum corneum) is characteristic lesion. Papulovesicles and nodules are also seen

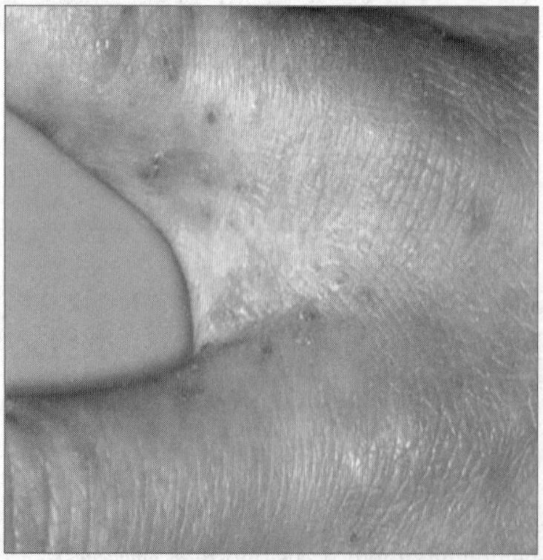

Site: Webs, wrists, ulnar aspect of forearms, breasts, scrotum and penis. Face, soles and palms spared in adults but characteristically involved in infants.

Complications: Secondary pyoderma and eczematisation.

Treatment: Permethrin (DOC) 5% / gamma benzene hexachloride 1%.: single application of the first two medications. Ivermectin is the only drug available for scabies.

7. Patient presents with pruritis of interdigits of left hand as shown in the image. Identify the condition: *(NEET 2019)*

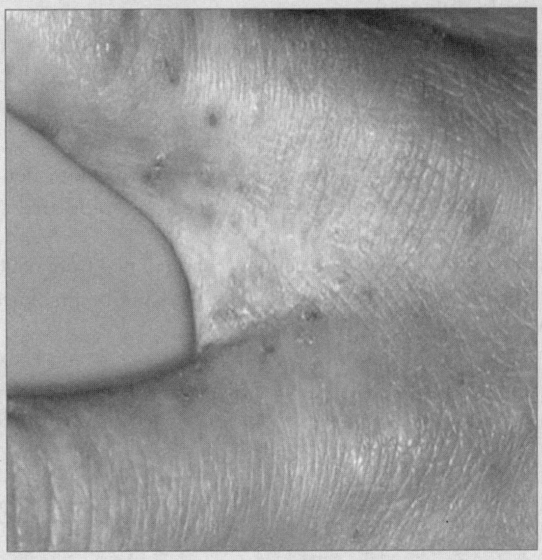

a. Scabies
b. Dermatitis herpatiformis
c. Xerotic dermatitis
d. Erythema multiforme

Ans. is 'a' Scabies

8. Which of the following is not true for scabies?

a. Wrist is common site in children
b. Burrows are intradermal lesions
c. Papules and pustules are due to hypersensitivity to mite
d. Itching is generalized

Ans. is 'b' Burrows are intradermal lesions

VESICULO-BULLOUS DISORDERS

Immunologically mediated bullous disorders

Disease	*Pemphigus vulgaris*	*Bullous pemphigoid*	*Linear IgA disease*	*Dermatitis herpetiformis*
Auto antigen	Desmoglein1,3	BP230, BP180	BPAg2	Epidermal and tissue transglutaminase
Clinical features	Flaccid blister denuded skin, oral lesions	Large tense blisters on flexor surfaces and trunk	Pruritic small papules on extensor surfaces occasionally larger acneiform blister in adults	Extremely pruritic small vesicles on elbows, knees Buttocks and posterior neck
Direct immunofluorescence Microscopy	Cells surface deposits of IgG and C3 on keratinocytes in fishnet pattern	Linear band of IgG and /or C3 in epidermal basement membrane	Linear band of IgA, in epidermal basement membrane	Granular deposits of IgA in dermal papillae
Histology	Epidermal acantholytic blister in stratum spinosum(suprabasal layer)	Subepidermal blister with an eosinophil rich infiltrate in perivascular and vesicular sites	Subepidermal blister with neutrophils in dermal papillae	Subepidermal blister with neutrophils in dermal papillae
Associations	HLA-DR4 and DRW6	HLA-DQ	HLA B8 (+) TNF2 allele	Subclinical gluten sensitive enteropathy 100%) HLA-B8 (60%)/DRW (95%) and HLA–DQW2 haplotype (95–100%)

9. Which of the following disease is closely related to enteropathy?

a. Linear IgA disease
b. Pemphigus foliaceous
c. Dermatitis herpetiformis
d. Erythema multiforme

Ans. is 'c' Dermatitis herpetiformis

PAPULOSQUAMOUS DISORDERS

Clinical Features of Psoriasis (Psoriasis Vulgaris)

- Psoriasis occurs at all ages, most patients are young or middle aged adults.
- The typical lesion is round plaque which is well-defined and has Profuse, silvery white, powdery scales (Candle drop scales) -> Loosely adherent and easily drops.
- Plaque is often surrounded by a hypopigmented halo – Ring of Woronoff
- Psoriatic lesions may develop at the site of trauma—Koebner's or isomorphic phenomenon.
- When a psoriatic lesion is scratched with the point of a dissecting forceps, a candle-grease like scale can be repeatedly produced even from the non-scaling lesions - Candle-grease sign
- Commonly involves nails – Causes nail pitting and oncholysis (separation of nail from nailbed)
- Lesions are bilaterally symmetrical. Psoriasis favors extensors areas, pressure points (knee, elbow), scalp, lumbosacral area and back. Face involvement is uncommon.

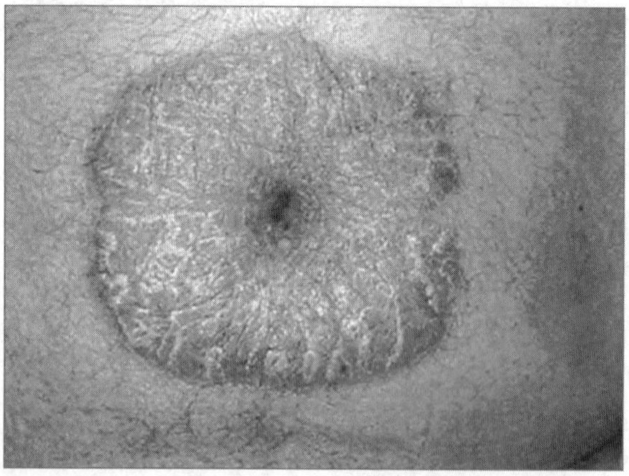

Psoriatic plaque with Woronoff ring (hypopigmented halo)

Treatment of psoriasis vulgaris

	Treatment of choice	*Alternatives in resistant cases*
Localized (<10% BSA)	Topical coal tar + salicylic acid Topical dithranol (short constant)	Topical steroids + salicylic acid
Moderate extensive (10-30% BSA)	Narrow band UVB therapy PUVA/PUVA sol	Methotrexate
Extensive (>30% BSA)	Topical low-mid potency steroids	
Palmoplantar psoriasis	Topical high potency steroid combined with salicylic acid even under occlusion	Methotrexate (small dose) in debilitating cases

10. Which of the following nail findings is seen in the condition shown below?

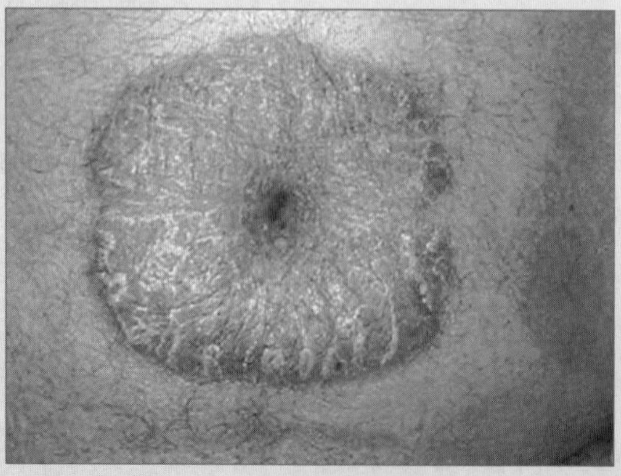

a. Pterygium
b. Pigmentation
c. Pitting
d. Ridges

Ans. is 'c' Pitting

LICHEN PLANUS

Etiology

- Etiology is unknown
- Cutaneous eruptions resembling LP (lichenoid eruptions) may be caused by:
  1. Drugs, e.g. gold, antimalarials (Chloroquine), thiazide diuretics, penicillamine, phenothiazines and rarely NSAIDs
  2. Contact sensitizer
  3. Hepatitis C infection
  4. Chronic graft versus host reaction

Characteristic Histopathology in Lichen Planus

- Basal epidermal cell degeneration causing saw tooth appearance and eosinophilic bodies (civatte body)
- Max Joseph spaces due to basal cell degeneration.
- Subepidermal band of lymphocytes and histiocytes
- Thickening of granular layer of epidermis

Clinical Features

Cutaneous Lesions

- 5Ps- Pink (purple or violaceous), plain topped (flat), polygonal, pruritic papule, which often has a whitish lacework pattern on its surface (Wickham's striae)
- Lesions have a predilection for wrist, shins, lower back and genitalia
- Face is generally not involved.
- Isomorphic or Koebner's phenomenon- new lesions appear in sites of trauma.

Mucosal Lesions

- Buccal mucosa is commonly involved
- Oral lesions show a white lacework pattern.

Nail Changes

- Pterygium- Wing shaped projection of proximal nail fold onto nail bed, splitting and destroying nailplate.
- Longitudinal ridges on nailplates with increased brittleness is seen in early cases. This is called onychorrhexia.
- Thinning, tenting and distal splitting of nail plates
- Complete destruction of nail plate may result.
- Annular lesions are seen in genital mucosa.
- Scalp involvement may cause cicatricial alopecia.

Course and Complications:

- It is usually self limiting, resolving in 6 months to 2 years duration.
- Lesions heal, leaving behind hyperpigmented patches.
- Nail and hair loss is irreversible.
- Very rarely chronic ulcerative lesions may develop into squamous cell carcinoma.

Treatment

- Topical steroids are given for symptomatic relief.

11. Civatte bodies are a feature of:

a. Lichen simplex chronicus b. Lichen planus
c. Lichen sclerosus d. All of the above

Ans. is 'b' Lichen planus

ATOPIC DERMATITIS (AD)

- It is a type of endogenous eczema triggered by exogenous agents.
- Lesion are extremely pruritic, recurrent, symmetric.
- Family history of atopy is present and the condition usually starts in childhood
- Clinical features vary depending upon the age:
  1. *Infantile phase*: Intensely itchy papules and vesicles, starting on the face, but can involve any part of the body except the diaper area.
  2. *Childhood phase*: leathery, itchy plaques mainly on the elbow and knee flexors. Often a reversed extensor pattern in seen.
  3. *Adult phase*: Itchy, lichenified plaques, involving the cubital and popliteal fossae.

- Differential diagnosis include contact dermatitis, psoriasis, and seborrheic dermatitis.
- Criteria for diagnosing atopic dermatitis includes one mandatory and five major criteria
- Mandatory criteria includes evidence of pruritic skin, including the report by a parent of a child rubbing or scratching.
- In addition to itchy skin, three or more of the following are needed to make the diagnosis:
  - History of skin creases being involved. These include: antecubital fossae, popliteal fossae, neck, areas around eyes, fronts of ankles.
  - History of asthma or hay fever (or history of atopic disease in a first-degree relative for children <4 years of age).
  - The presence of generally dry skin within the past year.
  - Symptoms beginning in a child before the age of two years. This criterion is not used to make the diagnosis in a child who is under four years old.
  - Visible dermatitis involving flexural surfaces. For children under four years of age, this criterion is met by dermatitis affecting the cheeks or forehead and outer aspects of the extremities.

12. In this child with asthmatic mother, identify this condition:

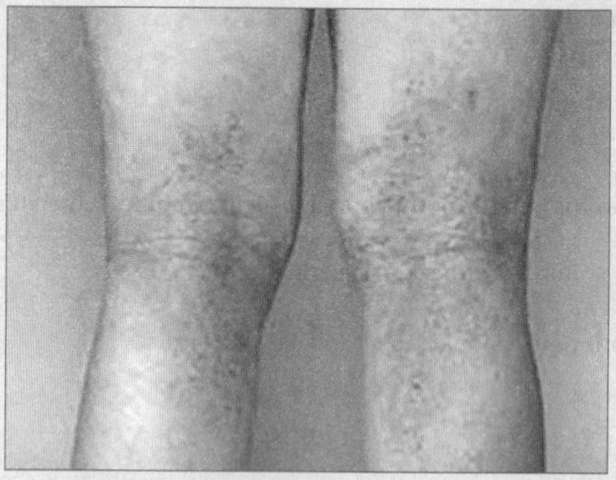

a. Atopic dermatitis
b. SLE
c. Erythema
d. TEN

Ans. is 'a' Atopic dermatitis

VITILIGO

Clinical Features

- Depigmented macules that may be chalky or milky white color
- The depigmentation may be partial and occasionally, three shades (white, light brown and dark brown) are seen in the same lesion representing the different stages of evolution- called trichome vitiligo.
- Macules have a scalloped margin and form geographical lesions on fusion.
- Leukotrichia: In the older lesions, the hair may lose their pigment
- Koebner's (isomorphic) phenomenon: Trauma results in new lesions of depigmentation

Sites of Lesions

- Occurs in any part of the body
- Areas subjected to repeated friction and trauma are frequently affected, e.g., the dorsal aspect of hands and feet, knees and elbows.

Vitiligo is associated with autoimmune diseases: Alopecia areata, Pernicious anemia, Diabetes mellitus, Addison disease, Hyperthyroidism (Grave's disease), Hypothyroidism (Hashimoto thyroiditis)

Patterns of vitiligo	Characteristic features
1. Vitiligo vulgaris	• Most common type • Widespread involvement with positive family history
2. Segmental vitiligo	• Depigmentation is dermatomal, most frequently along the distribution of trigeminal nerve • Occurs in children • Not associated with autoimmune diseases • Stable course, i.e. lesions increase initially (6-12 months) and then remain static. • Leukotrichia on the depigmented areas as well as away from vitiliginous areas frequently seen. Margins are feathery. • Response to treatment is not satisfactory
3. Acrofacial vitiligo	• Involves acral areas (palms, soles and periungual areas) and facial areas (around eyes and lips) • Resistant to therapy due to absence of hair in affected parts
4. Lip-tip vitiligo	• Lips, tips of penis, vulva and nipples are involved
5. Vitiligo universalis	• Widespread vitiligo, usually associated with multiple endocrinopathies.

Treatment

- Photochemotherapy involving use of psoralens in combination with UVA exposure (PUVA) forms the mainstay of therapy in vitiligo.
- Topical corticosteroids are the 1st line of treatment for children. It is indicated for single lesion, especially of recent origin.

13. Vitiligo is commonly associated with:

a. Celiac sprue b. PCOD
c. Diabetes d. Alpha-1 antitrypsin deficiency

Ans. is 'c' Diabetes

DERMATOMYOSITIS

- It is the commonest type of inflammatory myopathy.
- More common in females.
- Associated with HLA types B8, B14 and DR3. Juvenile DM is associated with HLA DR3. Production anti-Jo-I antibodies is strongly associated with HLA DR3.

Cutaneous Signs of Dermatomyositis

- *Gottron's papules*: Lilac or violaceous papules on knuckles and dorsa of hands
- *Gottron's sign*: Violaceous erythema with edema over shoulders, arms and forearms
- *Heliotrope sign*: Violaceous erythema with edema over eyelids, periorbital region
- *Poikiloderma*: Atrophy of skin, hypopigmentation, dilated blood vessels over trunk
- *Mechanic hand*: Symmetrical hyperkeratosis on ulnar aspect of thumb and radial aspect of fingers
- *Shawl sign*: Violaceous erythema extending from dorsolateral aspect of hands, forearms and arms to shoulders and neck.
- *'V' sign*: Violaceous erythema in a V-shaped distribution over anterior neck and chest.
- *Holster sign*: B/I symmetrical, patchy macular violaceous erythema displaying a reticuloid or levidoid array over the lateral aspect of upper thigh and hips.
- *Calcinosis cutis*: Calcium deposits in skin (in juvenile variant)
- *Miscellaneous signs*: Photosensitivity, vasculitis, panniculitis, Nail-fold telangiectasia

14. Which of the following is not a feature of dermatomyositis?

a. 'V' sign b. Holster sign
c. Pokiloderma d. Groove sign

Ans. is 'd' Groove sign

ALOPECIA AREATA

Non cicatricial, non inflammatory alopecia which can affect any hair-bearing area
Also known as spot baldness or 'Davey Kirts syndrome'
It is often associated with other autoimmune diseases e.g., myxoedema, pernicious anemia etc.

Genetic Factors

- Family history is present in 10–20% of cases.
- Inheritance is polygenic, with a strong association with HLA DR4, DQ3

Pathology

- It is an autoimmune disease, mediated by CD8+ T-cells affecting hair follicles (forming peribulbar infiltrates called "swarm of bees") and nails.
- Higher incidence is seen in autoimmune polyglandular syndrome type 1 (APS-l, autoimmune polyendocrinopathy-candidiasis –ectodermal dystrophy syndrome) and Down's syndrome.

Clinical Features

- It can start at any age; males and females are equally affected.
- Characteristically presents with a discoid patch of alopecia, which shows no scaling, inflammation or atrophy.
- Short easily extractable broken hairs known as exclamation mark hairs are seen at margins of bald patch.
- Most frequently seen on scalp, mustache and beard area.

Alopecia totalis	Total or almost total loss of scalp hair
Alopecia universalis	Loss of all body hair
Ophiasis	Alopecia along scalp margin
Sisaipho pattern	Hair loss spares the sides and back of head

- It preferentially spares white hairs.
- This results in a dramatic change in hair colour if alopecia progress rapidly. It is called "going white overnight phenomenon"
- Nail Involvement: most common finding is fine pitting, and roughening of nail plate, known as trachyonychia.

Treatment

If there are only a few lesions which are less than 6 months old, no treatment is needed. A few lesions lasting more than 6 months are treated with topical steroids or topical PUVA. Extensive lesions require systemic steroids.

15. Identify the condition: *(NEET 2019)*

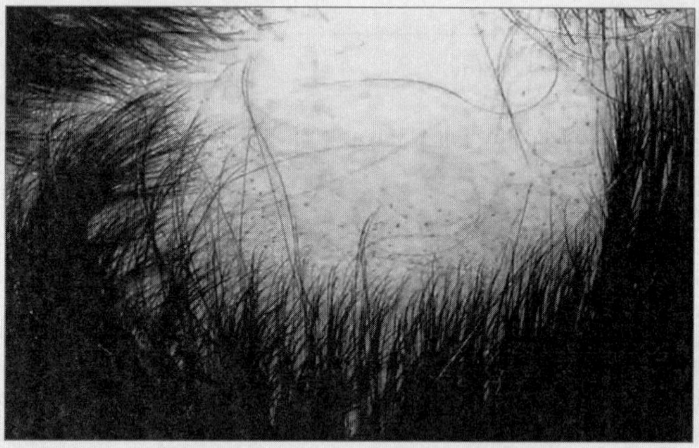

a. Sebaceous cyst
b. Alopecia areata
c. Trichotillomania
d. Tinea capitis

Ans. is 'b' Alopecia areata

ACANTHOSIS NIGRICANS

- Acanthosis nigricans is associated with obesity and insulin resistance in majority of the patients.
- Acanthosis is diffuse epidermal hyperplasia (thickening of the skin).
- Implies increased thickness of the Malpighian layer (stratum basale and stratum spinosum).
- Occurs primarily in flexural areas as velvety hyperpigmentation.
- Commonly seen in axilla.
- May be a reflection of endocrinopathy such as acromegaly, cushing's syndrome, polycystic ovarian syndrome and GIT malignancy.

16. Which of the following is true regarding the condition depicted in the image?

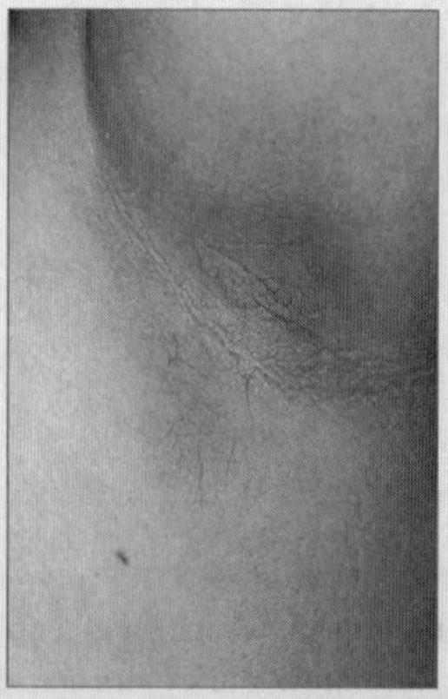

a. May be an indication of skin malignancy
b. Hypopigmentation
c. May be associated with insulin-resistant diabetes mellitus
d. Commonly occurs in lean and thin

Ans. is 'c' May be associated with insulin-resistant diabetes mellitus

Previously Asked Facts

- Langer's lines, also called cleavage lines, is a term used to define the direction within the human skin along which the skin has the least flexibility. Incisions made parallel to Langer's lines generally heal better and produce less scarring.
- Volcano sign: Morphologic feature of Old World cutaneous leishmaniasis. The lesion starts as a small nontender papule, which enlarges in size and ulcerates in the center. The border of the crusted ulcer often has an erythematous rim and is called as "Volcano sign"
- Actinomycete is an anaerobe causing multiple abscesses with discharging sinuses, demonstrating sulphur granules in pus.
- Tinea cruris (Jock itch) is dermatophytic infection of groin and adjacent skin most commonly caused by Trichophyton rubrum and Epidermophyton floccosum.
- Treatment of choice for cutaneous candidiasis is Topical (nystatin, clotrimazole, ketoconazole, amphotericin)
- A Warthin- Finkeldey cell is a type of giant multinucleate cell found in hyperplastic lymph nodes early in the course of measles.
- Munro's microabscesses are seen in psoriasis.
- Multiple erythematous annular lesions with peripheral scales arranged predominantly on trunk are characteristic of pityriasis rubra pilaris. Treatment of choice is topical steroids and salicylic acid.
- Koebner's phenomenon (isomorphic phenomenon)—New lesions of the original disease develop at sites of trauma (scratches, surgical incision and injury). Common examples – Lichen planus, psoriasis, vitilligo, lichen nitidus, pityriasis rubra pilaris.

KOEBNER'S PHENOMENON

Koebner phenomenon — Repeated mechanical trauma (friction) and other types of physical trauma such as scratching, chronic pressure, or cuts along with allergic or irritant contact reactions may trigger similar skin lesions on areas such as the neck, elbows, and ankles. This is known as the Koebner phenomenon, also called «isomorphic response,» which describes the development of skin disease in sites of skin trauma.

17. Identify the given condition: *(NEET 2020)*

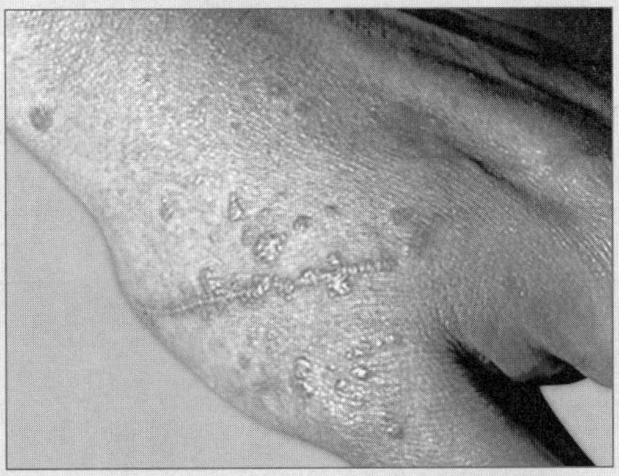

a. Isomorphic phenomenon
b. Nikolsky's sign
c. Auspitz sign
d. Woronoff sign

Ans. is 'a' Isomorphic phenomenon

- Pseudo-Koebner's (Pseudo-isomorphic) phenomenon—This is due to autoinoculations and is seen in infections (warts, molluscum contagiosum) and eczematous lesions.
- Most common metal responsible for contact dermatitis is Nickel.
- Darier's sign—Gentle rubbing or stroking of affected skin results in itching, erythema and wheal formation within 2–5 min. It is caused by the release of histamine from the mast cells. Seen in urticaria pigmentosa.
- Telogen effluvium—Diffuse decrease in hair density secondary to rapid conversion of anagen to telogen hair. Precipitated by stressful events, illness, fever, pregnancy, crash diet, medications; hair can be shed 2–6 months after precipitant.

Treatment options for acne

Drug/Acne	Mild		Moderate		Severe
	Comedonal	Papular/Pustular	Papular/Pustular	Nodular	Nodular/Conglobate
1st choice	Topical retinoid	Topical retinoid + Topical antimicrobial (clindamycin)	Topical retinoid + Oral antibiotic ± Benzoyl peroxide	Topical retinoid + Oral antibiotic ± Benzoyl peroxide	Oral isotretinoin
Alternatives for females	Topical retinoid	Topical retinoid + Topical antimicrobial (clindamycin)	Oral antiandrogen + topical retinoid ± topical antimicrobial (clindamycin)	Oral antiandrogen + topical retinoid ± oral antibiotic	High dose oral antiandrogen + topical retinoid ± topical antimicrobial (clindamycin)

Dermatology

VIRAL WARTS

External anogenital warts are typically found on the vulva, penis, groin, perineum, anal skin, perianal skin, and/or suprapubic skin. The CA can be single or multiple, flat, dome-shaped, cauliflower-shaped, filiform, fungating, pedunculated, cerebriform, plaque-like, smooth (especially on the penile shaft), verrucous, or lobulated. The color varies; warts may be white, skin-colored, erythematous (pink or red), violaceous, brown, or hyperpigmented. Anogenital warts are usually soft to palpation and can range from 1 mm to more than several centimeters in diameter. The warts are typically asymptomatic but can occasionally be pruritic.

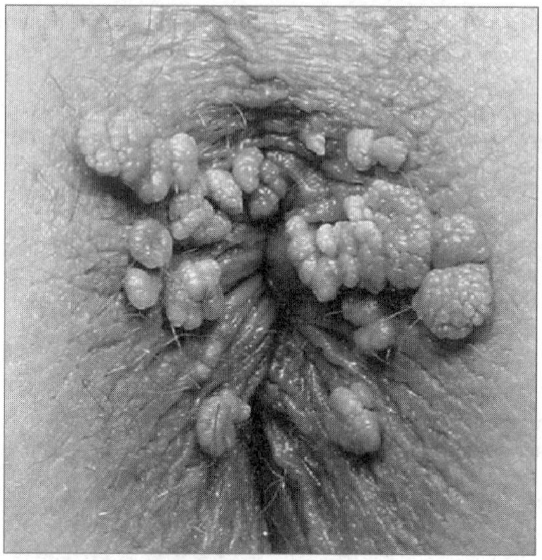

Condyloma Accuminatum

External anogenital warts can be accompanied by involvement of the cervix or urethra. CA may also develop in the anal canal, typically manifesting as small flat-topped to globoid-shaped papules, usually distal to the dentate line.

Sexually transmitted diseases such as molluscumcontagiosum, which typically manifests as umbilicated small papules, and condylomalatum of syphilis, which typically manifests as single or multiple moist, gray-white papules or plaques, may enter the differential diagnosis.

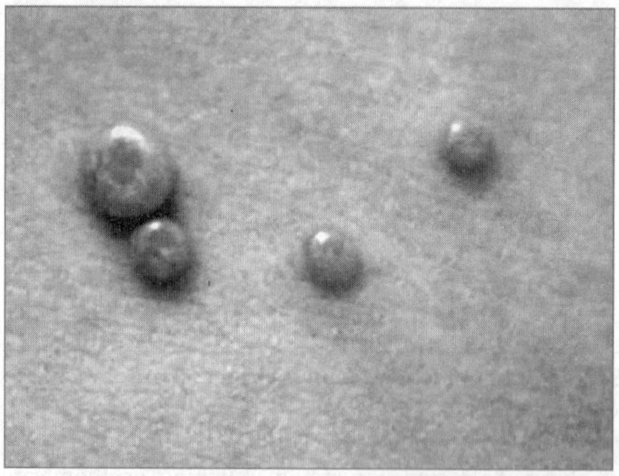

Molluscum Contagiosum

18. A female presented with soft, sessile and warty lesions on vulva, which were spreading to other parts. What is the diagnosis? *(NEET 2020)*

a. Condyloma acuminata
b. Chancroid
c. Molluscum contagiosum
d. Herpes genitalis

Ans. is 'a' Condyloma acuminata

DLE

DLE classically presents with erythematous-to-violaceous, scaly plaques with prominent follicular plugging that often results in scarring and atrophy (see the images below). **DLE may occur in the absence of systemic disease, or it may occur in association with systemic lupus erythematosus (SLE).**

Dermatology

19. Identify the given condition: *(NEET 2020)*

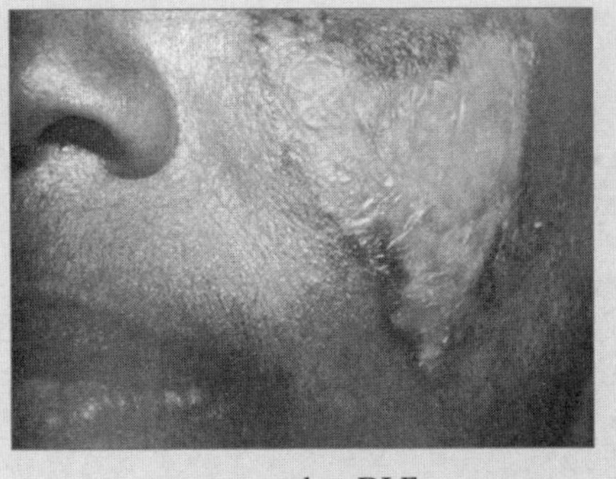

a. SLE
b. DLE
c. Lichen planus
d. Lupus vulgaris

Ans. is 'b' DLE

ICTHYOSIS

Lamellar ichthyosis and congenital ichthyosiform erythroderma — Although initially considered separate entities, lamellar ichthyosis (LI) and congenital ichthyosiform erythroderma (CIE) show clinical and genetic overlap. Most cases are caused by mutations in one of several genes.

LI and CIE typically present at birth with a collodion membrane a tight translucent membrane covering the newborn's body that sheds in the first few weeks of life with emollient application. In LI, the collodion membrane is replaced by thick hyperkeratosis with dark, plate-like adherent scales. Ectropion is prominent and palmoplantar keratoderma (thickening of the palms and soles) of varying severity is usually present. The hyperkeratosis may impair the sweat gland function, resulting in hypohidrosis. In CIE, scaling tends to be milder than in LI, with variable erythroderma and ectropion

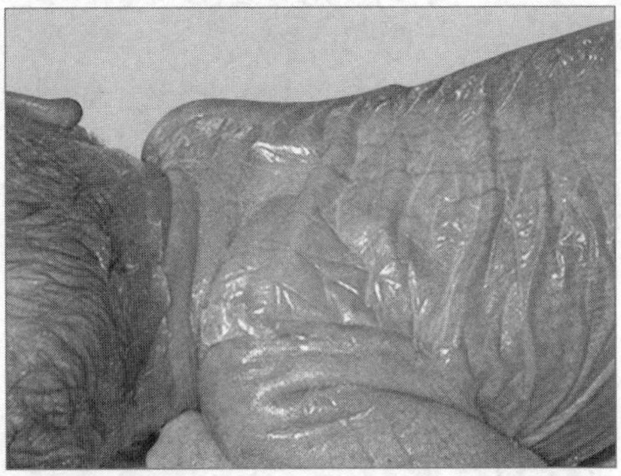

This infant appears encased in a taut, shiny stratum corneum, with underlying generalized erythroderma.

20. A child is presented to OPD with lesions shown below. At birth, the child was found to be wrapped in a membrane. What is the diagnosis? *(NEET 2020)*

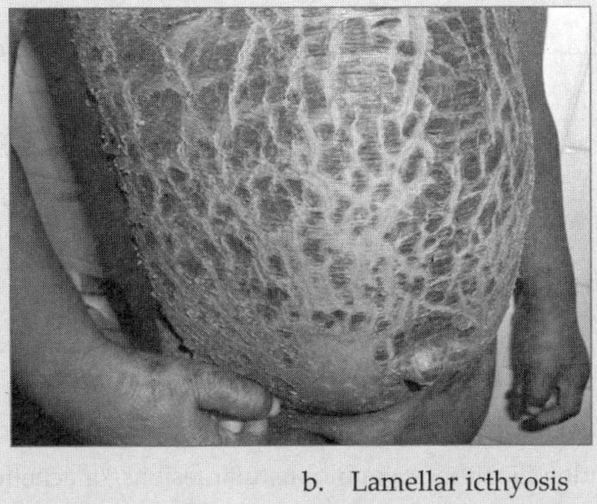

a. Epidermal hyperkeratosis
b. Lamellar icthyosis
c. Icthyosis vulgaris
d. X linked icthyosis

Ans. is 'b' Lamellar icthyosis

TINEA

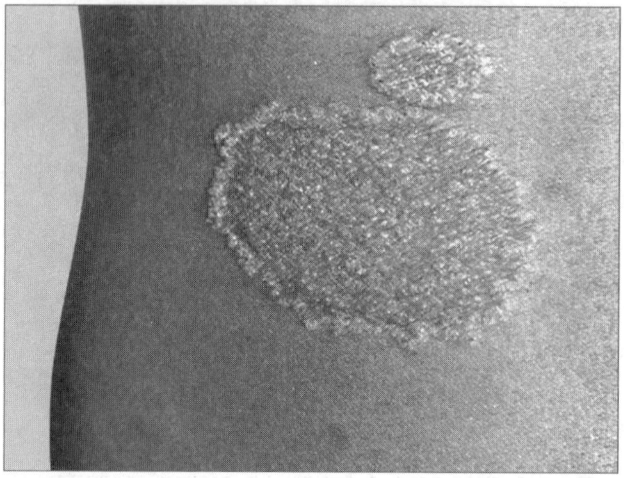

Tinea corporis often begins as a pruritic, circular or oval, erythematous, scaling patch or plaque that spreads centrifugally. Central clearing follows, while an active, advancing, raised border remains. The result is an annular (ring-shaped) plaque from which the disease derives its common name (ringworm).

21. Identify this intensely itchy lesion on trunk? *(NEET 2020)*

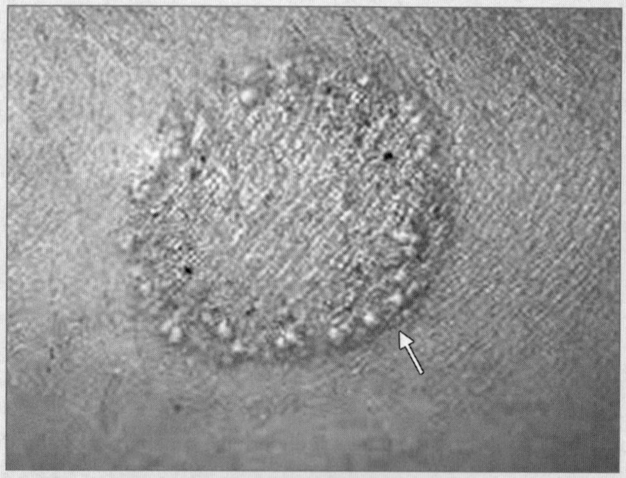

a. Tinea
b. DLE
c. Lichen planus
d. Psoriasis

Ans. is 'a' Tinea

BEHCET DISEASE

Diagnostic criteria for Behcet disease

Recurrent oral ulceration: Minor aphthous, major aphthous, or herpetiform

ulceration recurring at least 3 times in one 12 mo period

Plus 2 of the following:

- Recurrent genital ulcers: Aphthous ulceration or scarring
- Eye lesions Anterior uveitis, posterior uveitis, cells in vitreous on slit-lamp examination, or retinal vasculitis
- Skin lesions: Erythema nodosum, pseudofolliculitis or papulopustular lesions, or acneiform nodules in postadolescent patient not on corticosteroid treatment
- Pathergy Skin reaction to a needle prick observed by physician at 2448 hr

Sweet syndrome also known as acute febrile neutrophilic dermatosis is a skin disease characterized by sudden onset fever, elevated WBC count, tender, red well-demarcated papules with dense infiltrates by neutrophils on histologic examination. Genital ulcers are rare.

Reiter's Syndrome (now known as Reactive Arthritis) develops in response to an infection and characterized by a triad of arthritis, conjunctivitis, and nonspecific urethritis. Not associated with aphthous ulcers.

Pyoderma gangrenosum is a rare, inflammatory skin disease where painful pustules or nodules become ulcers that progressively grow. It is not infectious. At least half of all pyoderma gangrenosum patients suffer from immune-mediated diseases like, ulcerative colitis, rheumatoid arthritis, and multiple myeloma (MM). Hallmark of pyoderma gangrenosum is pathergy (appearance of new lesions at sites of trauma, including surgical wounds).

22. A patient presented with multiple superficial oral ulcers that are recurrent. On examination, genital ulcers are also present. What is the diagnosis? *(NEET 2020)*

a. Behcet disease
b. Sweet syndrome
c. Reiters disease
d. Pyoderma gangrenosum

Ans. is 'a' Behcet disease

CHAPTER 16

Anesthesia

CAPNOGRAPHY

Rebreathing

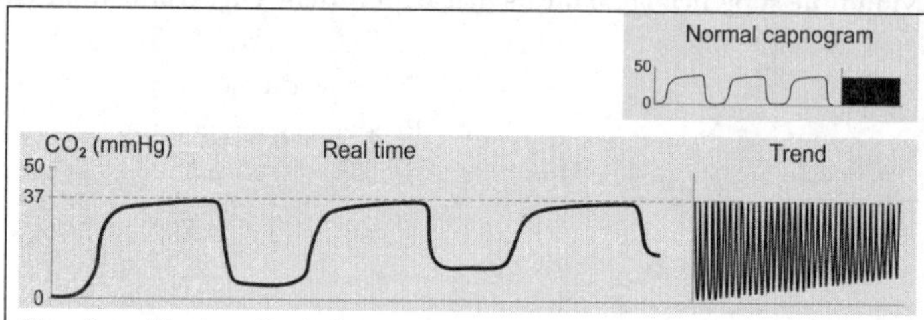

Elevation of the baseline indicates rebreathing (may also show a corresponding increase in $ETCO_2$)

Possible causes:
- Faulty expiratory valve
- Inadequate inspiratory flow
- Malfunction of a CO_2 absorber system
- Partial rebreathing circuits
- Insufficient expiratory time

Muscle Relaxants (Curare Cleft)

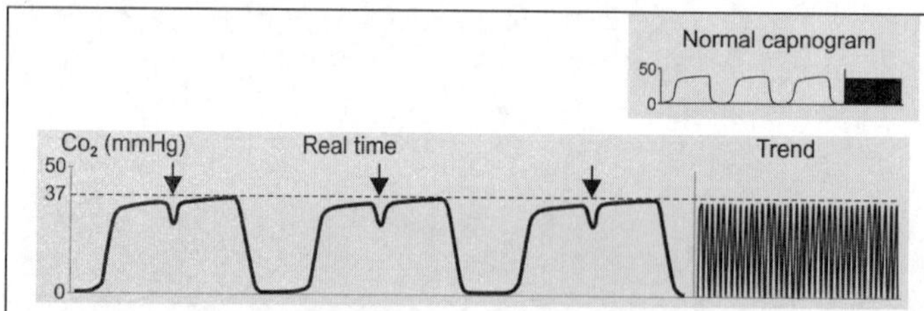

Cleft are seen in the plateau portion of the capnogram. They appear when the action of the muscle relaxant begins to subside and spontaneous ventilation returns

Characteristics:
- Depth of the cleft is inversely proportional to the degree of drug activity
- Position is fairly constant on the same patient but not necessarily present with every breath

Obstruction in Breathing Circuit or Airway

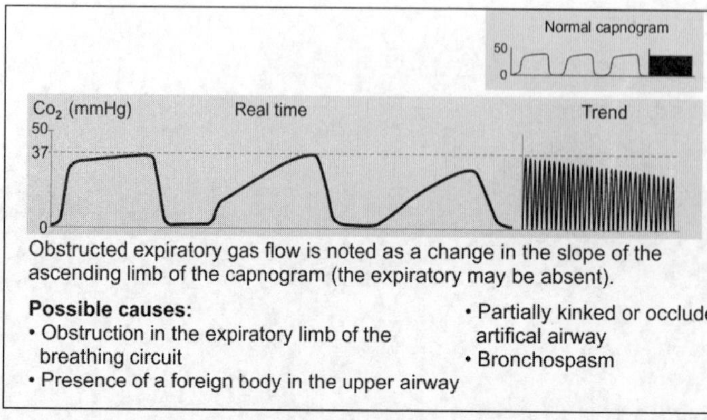

Obstructed expiratory gas flow is noted as a change in the slope of the ascending limb of the capnogram (the expiratory may be absent).

Possible causes:
- Obstruction in the expiratory limb of the breathing circuit
- Presence of a foreign body in the upper airway
- Partially kinked or occluded artifical airway
- Bronchospasm

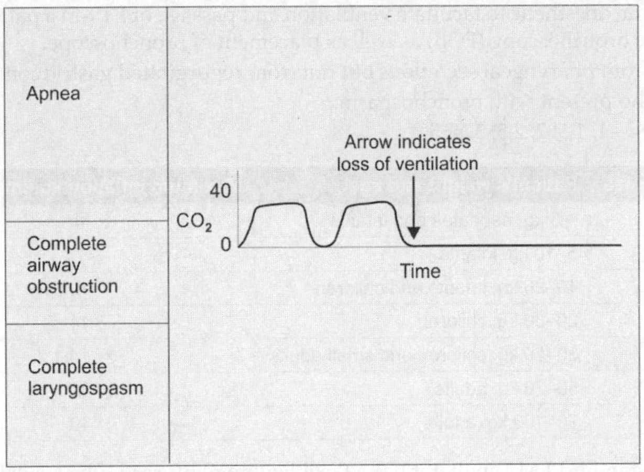

1. What does the following capnograph indicate? *(NEET 2020)*

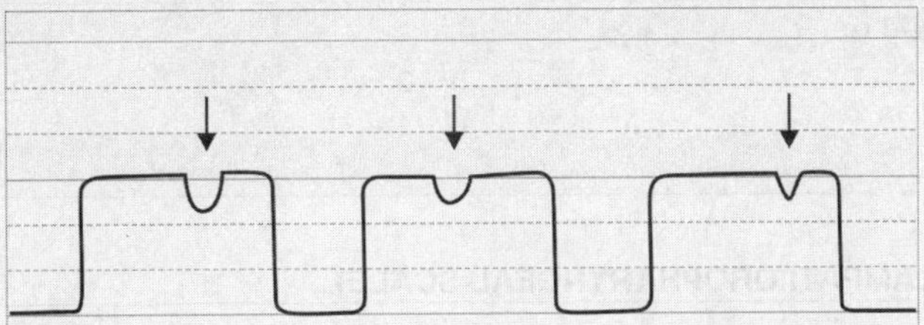

a. CO_2 rebreathing
b. Return of spontaneous breathing
c. Bronchospasm
d. Apnea spells

Ans. is 'b' Return of spontaneous breathing

PIN INDEX SYSTEM

This is the safety mechanism so that one cylinder cannot be fitted at the other's position.

Color identification of medical gas cylinders

Name of gas	*Body*	*Shoulder*	*Pin index*
Air	Grey	White and black quarter	1, 5
Carbon dioxide (Conc. >7.5%)	Grey	Grey	1, 6
Oxygen	Black	White	2, 5
Carbon dioxide (Conc. <7.5%)	Grey	Grey	2, 6
Nitrous oxide	Blue	Blue	3, 5
Entonox (50% O_2 + 50% N_2O)	Blue	Blue and White	Single pin

2. Pin index system is a safety feature adopted in anesthesia machines to prevent:

a. Incorrect attachment of anesthesia machines
b. Incorrect attachment of anesthesia face masks
c. Incorrect inhalation agent delivery
d. Incorrect gas cylinder attachment

Ans. is 'd' Incorrect gas cylinder attachment

3. Blue cylinder with blue and white collar is for:

a. Oxygen
b. Air
c. Nitrogen
d. Entonox

Ans. is 'd' Entonox

LARYNGEAL MASK AIRWAY (LMA)

- It is a device used to secure the airway to facilitate gas exchange.
- Also known as Brain mask (named after its inventor-Archie Brain).
- It has 3 parts: an inflatable mask, mask inflation line and airway tube
- It is mostly used to maintain patent airway in patients who are breathing spontaneously.

- *Uses*: During administration of an anesthetic to facilitate ventilation and passage of ETT in a patient with difficult airway and to aid in ventilation during fiber optic bronchoscopy (FOB) as well as placement of bronchoscope.
- LMA offers partial protection from pharyngeal secretions but not from regurgitated gastric contents.
- It cannot be used in patients who present with bronchospasm.
- It is available in 7 different sizes—1, 1.5, 2, 2.5, 3, 4, 5.

Mask size	Patient's weight and age	Maximum inflation volume (in mL)
1	< 5 kg, neonates and infants	4
1.5	5–10 kg, infants	7
2	10–20 kg, infants and children	10
2.5	20–30 kg, children	14
3	30–50 kg, children and small adults	14
4	50–70 kg, adults	30
5	70–100 kg, adults	40

- The flexible LMA differs from standard LMA in that it has a flexible wire reinforced tube available in sizes 2, 2.5, 3, 4, and 5.
- A tracheal tube can be passed through it to intubate trachea

4. Size of LMA for a 15 kg child is:

a. 1
b. 2
c. 3
d. 4

Ans. is 'b' 2

MALLAMPATI SCORE (MALLAMPATI OROPHARYNGEAL SCALE)

- Mallampati grading is used to evaluate the visibility of tonsil and tonsillar fossa which in turn assess the adequate mouth opening depending upon the grade.
- Mallampati scoring is used for assessing difficulty during intubation.
- Mallampati score is divided into four grades

Class 1	Class 2	Class 3	Class 4
Soft palate, uvula, faucial pillars and posterior pharyngeal wall are visible	Lower part of faucial pillar and uvula are masked by the base of tongue Upper part of faucial pillars and soft palate are visible.	Only soft palate is visible	None of the structure is visible. Only hard palate is visible

5. Modified Mallampati grading is used in assessment of:

a. Difficult intubation
b. Airway obstruction
c. Death due to aspiration
d. Mobility of cervical spine

Ans. is 'a' Difficult intubation

Preoperative Modifications of Pre-existing Drugs

Drugs which can be stopped	Drugs which can be continued till the day of surgery
• Conventional dose aspirin and clopidogrel (antiplatelets)—1 week before surgery • Oral anticoagulants—4 days before and switch to heparin, which is stopped 12 hours prior to surgery • Oral hypoglycemic (metformin)—48 hours before surgery and switch to insulin • AT-II antagonists (losartan)—1 day prior • Lithium—48–72 hours before surgery • MAO inhibitors —3 weeks before surgery	• Antianginal (except aspirin) • Antiepileptics • Antihypertensives (except AT –II antagonists) • Levodopa • Digitalis • TCAs • Low dose aspirin

Note: Antiplatelet drugs like clopidogrel and conventional dose of aspirin should be stopped 7 days prior to surgery. But low dose aspirin can be continued till the day of surgery.

6. American anesthetic association says that clopidogrel should be withheld how many days before surgery?

a. 1 day
b. 1 week
c. 3 weeks
d. 4 weeks

Ans. is 'b' 1 week

Anesthesia

MUSCLE RELAXANTS

- Longest acting neuromuscular blocker→ Pancuronium (duration of action 120–180 minutes).
- Shortest and fastest acting neuromuscular blocker→ Succinylcholine (duration of act 5–8 minutes)
- Shortest acting competitive (nondepolarizing) neuromuscular blocker→ Mivacurium (duration of action 12–18 minutes).
- Fastest acting nondepolarizing blocker→ Rocuronium (can be used for endotracheal intubation as an alternative to SCh).
- Histamine release is caused by→ d-Tc (maximum tendency), succinylcholine, mivacurium, doxacuri atracurium. Tubocurarine can cause bronchoconstriction.
- Virtually no histamine release→ Pancuronium.
- Vagal block is caused by→ Pancuronium (maximal), rocuronium, gallamine.
- Vagal stimulation is caused by→ Succinylcholine (can cause bradycardia).
- Ganglion block is caused by→ d-Tc (maximum)
- Ganglion stimulation is caused by→ Succinylcholine
- Most commonly used muscle relaxant for routine surgery→ Vecuronium.
- Most potent skeletal muscle relaxant→ Doxacurium.
- Least potent skeletal muscle relaxant→ Succinylcholine
- Least potent nondepolarising muscle relaxant→ Rocuronium.
- MR of choice for intubation→ SCh (1st choice), Rapacuronium (2nd choice), Rocuronium (3rd choice).
- Mivacurium is the only nondepolarizing blocker that is metabolized by plasma cholinesterase.
- Rocuronium produces pain on injection

7. Which of the following is a weak skeletal muscle relaxant?

a. Atracurium
b. Rocuronium
c. Suxamethonium
d. Rapacuronium

Ans. is 'c' Suxamethonium

DANTROLENE

- Centrally acting muscle relaxant which acts by interfering with excitation-contraction coupling in the muscle fibers.
- *Mechanism of Action*: Blocks RyR1 Ca-release channels in the sarcoplasmic reticulum of skeletal muscle
- *Effects*: Reduces actin-myosin interaction and weakens skeletal muscle contraction
- *Clinical applications*
  - *Intravenous*: Malignant hyperthermia. Drugs causing malignant hyperthermia—Succinylcholine, Desflurane, Tricyclic antidepressants, Halothane, Cyclopropane, Phenothiazines, Isoflurane, Ether, Lignocaine, Enflurane, Methoxyflurane, Sevoflurane and MAO inhibitors
  - *Oral*: Spasm due to cerebral palsy, spinal cord injury, multiple sclerosis
- *Adverse-effects*
  - Muscular weakness is the dose limiting side effect.
  - Sedation, malaise, light headedness; Troublesome diarrhea is another problem.
  - Long term use causes dose dependent serious liver toxicity in 0.1—0.5% patients.

8. Malignant hyperthermia is associated with all of the following *except*:

a. Succinylcholine
b. Dantrolene
c. Halothane
d. Methoxyflurane

Ans. is 'b' Dantrolene

INTRAVENOUS ANESTHETICS

Ketamine

- Produces dissociative anaesthesia and cataleptic state
- Acts on NMDA receptor, dose is 2 mg/kg IV
- Onset of action—30 to 60 s, T1/2–2–3 hours
- Patient regains consciousness early because of redistribution

Advantages and Uses of Ketamine

- Induction agent of choice for:
  - Asthmatics, shock
  - Constrictive pericarditis, cardiac tamponade (Ketamine causes tachycardia and increases cardiac output in these conditions)
  - Right to left shunt like tetralogy of Fallot (Ketamine by causing hypertension increases the afterload there by decreasing the right to left shunt fraction)
- Can be used as sole agent for minor procedures
- Since pharyngeal and laryngeal reflexes are preserved when ketamine is used, it is the preferred agent for patients with full stomach

Contraindications

- Since it increases ICT and IOP, it is avoided in head injury, intracranial space occupying lesion, eye injury.
- Since it increases myocardial oxygen demand and BP, it is avoided in ischemic heart disease, vascular aneurysm and hypertension.
- It is avoided in psychiatric patients due to its hallucinogenic properties.

9. Ketamine is contraindicated in:

a. Status asthmaticus
b. Obstetric hemorrhage
c. Glaucoma
d. Shock

Ans. is 'c' Glaucoma

ETOMIDATE

- Short-acting intravenous anesthetic agent; induction agent
- Fast onset of action – 30-60 seconds
- Modulates $GABA_A$ receptor – blocks neuroexcitation
- Used for short procedures
- Used in emergency settings (Propofol is now the drug of choice)
- Used for conscious sedation and Rapid Sequence Intubation
- Major advantage of etomidate – Relatively hemodynamically neutral; useful in hypotensive patients
- In patients with traumatic brain injury, it decreases intracranial pressure and maintan a normal arterial pressure
- Adverse effect – Blocks cortisol synthesis

10. Which of the following is not cardiodepressive? *(NEET 2019)*

a. Propofol
b. Thiopentone
c. Ketamine
d. Etomidate

Ans. is 'd' Etomidate

INHALATIONAL ANESTHETICS

Minimum Alveolar Concentration (MAC)

- MAC, the minimum alveolar concentration is defined as the minimum alveolar concentration of anaesthetic at 1 atmosphere (atm), which produces immobility in 50% of subjects exposed to a noxious stimulus, usually a skin incision.
- MAC is a measure of potency of anesthetic agent. Higher the MAC, lower the potency.
- MAC of various agents are given below:

Agent	MAC
Nitrous oxide	104
Desflurane	6.6
Sevoflurane	1.8
Enflurane	1.63
Isoflurane	1.17
Halothane	0.75

Variation of MAC with age is depicted in the following graph

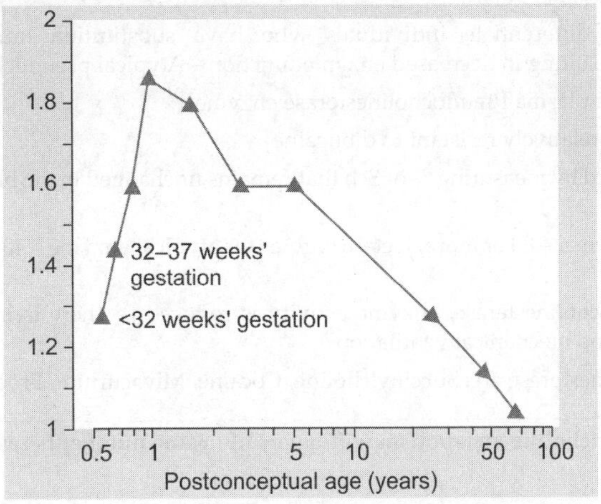

As shown, MAC increases up to an age of one year and then gradual decline to values lesser then those in neonates. The lower MAC in neonates compared with infants may be related to immaturity of the central nervous system and attenuation of the pain response due to high levels of plasma peptides (beta-endorphin and beta-lipoprotein). The higher MAC in infants compared with older children and adults may be due to an increase in the brain water content.

11. MAC of an anesthetic agent is the measure of its:

a. Potency
b. Speed of induction and recovery
c. Lipid solubility
d. Toxicity

Ans. is 'a' Potency

NITROUS OXIDE (DINITROGEN MONOXIDE/N_2O)

N_2O is a colorless, odorless gas which is heavier than air

- It was discovered by Joseph Priestley in 1774.
- It is non-flammable, but it supports combustion when a flammable material is present.
- It is the least potent agent currently in use, with a MAC of 105%
- *Adverse effect*: Bone marrow depression
- Used for labour analgesia, painful dressing and changing thoracotomy drains

Anesthetic Properties

- N_2O is highly insoluble in blood resulting in rapid equilibration between blood levels and alveolar anesthetic concentrations causing rapid induction and rapid emergence.
- N_2O is almost completely eliminated by the lungs (minimal diffusion through the skin), mostly unchanged.

Uses

- Weak anesthetic agent, poor muscle relaxant activity with good analgesic effect.
- Frequently used in conc. of 50% to provide analgesia and mild sedation in outpatient dentistry.
- Reduces the dose of inhalational anesthetics required.
- N_2O exchanges with N_2 in any air-containing cavity in the body. Because of differential blood: Gas partition coefficients, nitrous oxide enters the cavity faster than nitrogen escapes, increasing the volume and/or pressure in the cavity.
- It is therefore contraindicated in pneumothorax, obstructed middle ear, air embolus, obstructed loop of bowel, intraocular air bubble, pulmonary bulla and intracranial air.

Second gas effect	Diffusion hypoxia (Fink effect)
N_2O is rapidly taken up from alveoli, increasing the concentration of co-administered halogenated anesthetics; it speeds up the induction	During recovery, N_2O can diffuse from blood into the alveoli, reducing the concentration of O_2. To avoid hypoxia, 100% O_2 rather than air should be administered when N_2O is discontinued.

12. Anesthetic agent which can lead to bone marrow depression is:

a. Halothane
b. N_2O
c. Ether
d. Isoflurane

Ans. is 'b' N_2O

DIBUCAINE NUMBER

- Dibucaine number is used to differentiate individuals who have substitution mutations of the bytyrylcholinesterase (pseudocholinesterase) enzyme resulting in decreased enzyme function – Atypical pseudocholinesterase
- When given IV, Dibucaine inhibits plasma Pseudocholinesterase enzyme.
- Atypical Pseudo-cholinesterase is relatively resistant to dibucaine
- Extent of activity can be determined by measuring % of Sch that remains unchanged in the blood after a standard dose of Dibucaine – given as Dibucaine Number
- Values of Dibucaine number – Normal – 80 or more; Heterozygotes for atypical enzyme – 40–60; Homozygotes for atypical enzyme – 20 or less
- In patients with Atypical pseudocholinesterase, enzyme activity is reduced → there is increase in duration of neuromuscular blockade → may necessitate post-op mechanical ventilation
- Drugs hydrolized by pseudocholinesterase are: Succinylcholine, Cocaine, Mivacurium, Procaine, Bambuterol, Remifentanil

13. A patient with normal succinylcholine metabolism will have Dibucaine number between:

a. 20–30
b. 40–45
c. 50–60
d. 70–80

Ans. is 'd' 70–80

SPINAL ANESTHESIA

- In spinal anesthesia LA is injected into subarachnoid space (space between pia matter and arachnoid matter).
- Structure pierced during SA (from outside in) – Skin → subcutaneous tissue→ Supraspinous and intraspinous ligament→ Ligamentum flavum→ Dura mater → Arachnoid mater.
- Site of spinal anesthesia is L2–3 or L3–4 intervertebral space in adult (In adult spinal cord ends at lower border of L1 vertebra). In children it is L4–5 intervertebral space (spinal cord ends at lower border L3 vertebra in children).
- Total spinal anesthesia results when the level of block is above the cervical region, thus involving the entire spinal cord and occasionally the brainstem during either spinal or accidental intrathecal injection during epidural anesthesia. It is manifested as bradycardia, hypotension, dyspnea, difficulty in swallowing and loss of consciousness.
- Onset of analgesia is approximately 15–30 minutes in an epidural, while it is approximately 5 minutes in spinal anesthesia.

14. Which of the following is true about spinal anesthesia?

a. Onset of analgesia takes about 15 minutes
b. Anesthesia is injected in subarachnoid space
c. Most common complication is PDPH
d. May lead to intra-operative tachycardia

Ans. is 'b' Anesthesia is injected in subarachnoid space

BISPECTRAL INDEX

- The bispectral index is a statistically based, empirically derived complex parameter. It is a weighted sum of several electroencephalographic subparameters; like EEG signals, eye blinks, etc.
- BIS is the most common method used to know the depth of anesthesia.
- The BIS monitor provides a single dimensionless number, which ranges from 0 (equivalent to EEG silence) to 100. A BIS value between 40 and 60 indicates an appropriate level for general anesthesia.

BIS value	Interpretation
80–100	Awake
60–80	Moderate sedation
40–60	General anesthesia (no awareness)
<40	Deep anesthesia

15. Which of the following is the most common method used to know the depth of anesthesia? *(NEET 2019)*

a. BIS
b. Esophageal contractility
c. Depressed responses
d. BP

Ans. is 'a' BIS

Previously Asked Facts

- Term anesthesia was coined by Wendell Holmes.
- Circuit of choice for spontaneous ventilation in adult →Mapleson A (Magill circuit)
- Circuit of choice for controlled ventilation in adult →Mapleson D (Bain circuit)
- Circuit of choice for children → Type F, i.e. Jackson-Rees (first choice) and type E, i.e. Ayre's T piece (second choice)
- Co-axial system → Mapleson C (Water's to and fro)
- Succinylcholine can cause dangerous hyperkalemia
- *Pain on injection*: Intra-arterial – Thiopental; On intravenous injection – Propofol, Methohexital, Thiopental (without thrombophlebitis), Etomidate (with thrombophlebitis)
- Desflurane and isoflurane when used for induction cause respiratory irritation due to their pungent smell leading to breath holding and coughing. Halothane and sevoflurane do not cause such effects.
- Anesthetic agent of choice in bronchial asthma patients – Ketamine (Bronchodilator)
- Inhalational agent of choice in asthmatics – Halothane
- Anesthetic agent contraindicated in acute intermittent porphyria – Thiopentone, Etomidate
- Safest anesthetic agent in porphyria patient – Propofol

Anesthesia in liver disease	
Intravenous induction	Thiopentone or propofol
Inhalational agents	Isoflurane (volatile agent of choice for maintenance)
Muscle relaxants	Cisatracurium/atracurium (muscle relaxants of choice)

- Anesthetic of choice for induction for day care procedures is Propofol.
- Etomidate has the highest incidence of nausea and vomiting amongst inducing agents.
- Intra-arterial Thiopentone injection leads to Ischemia.
- All inhalational agent cause mild hepatotoxicity by decreasing hepatic blood flow. Direct hepatotoxicity (Hepatitis and Hepatic necrosis) is caused by Halothane, Chloroform, Carbon tetrachloride and methoxyflurane. Isoflurane is the agent of choice in liver disease as it has least effect on hepatic blood flow.
- Articaine, prilocaine and benzocaine can cause Methemoglobinemia.
- Succinyl choline increases in all pressures→ intraocular, intracranial, BP, and intra-abdominal.
- Bupivacaine is the most cardiotoxic local anesthetic agent.
- Benzocaine and cocaine are used only in topical anesthesia.
- Local anesthetics act by inhibiting Na^+ channels from inside.
- Central neuraxial block pertains to local anesthetics placed around the nerves of the central nervous system. Examples are spinal anesthesia, epidural anesthesia and caudal anesthesia.
- Adductor pollicis muscle supplied by ulnar nerve is most commonly utilized muscle for neuromuscular monitoring.

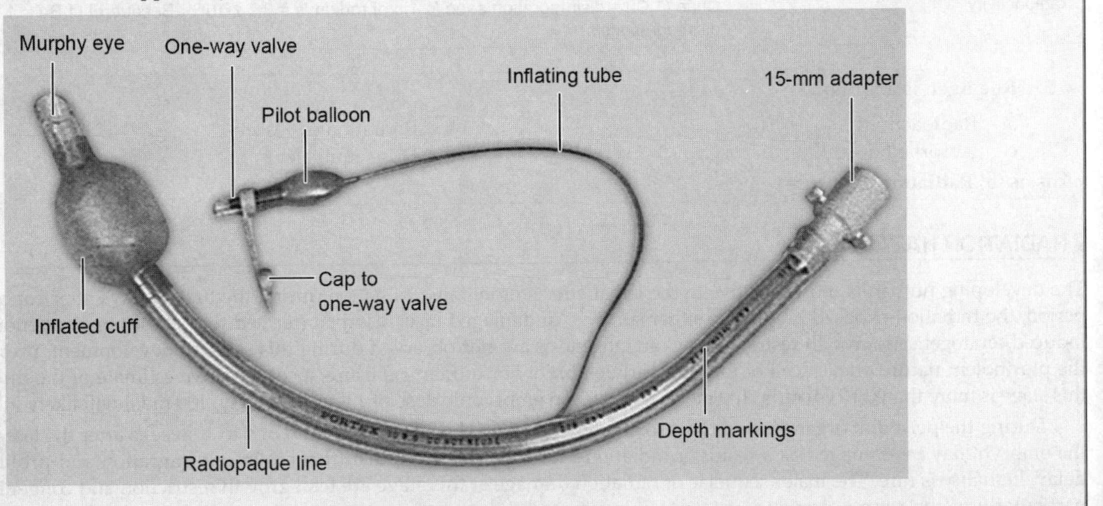

Parts of endotracheal tube

CHAPTER 17 Radiology

USG MICKEY MOUSE SIGN

The Mickey Mouse sign representing the normal anatomy of the common femoral artery, common femoral vein and great saphenous vein at the saphenofemoral junction on ultrasound.

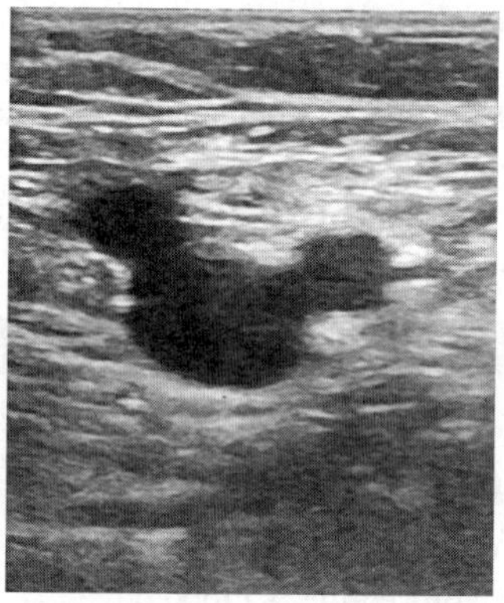

1. The relationship of femoral artery, femoral vein and saphenous vein at saphenofemoral junction is known as: ***(NEET 2020)***

a. Mickey mouse sign
b. Stemmers sign
c. Tillaux sign
d. String sign

Ans. is 'a' Mickey mouse sign

RADIATION

Radiation units	Conventional unit	SI unit
Total radiation exposure	Roentgen	Coulomb/Kg
Absorbed radiation	Rad	Gray (1 Gy = 100 Rad)
Biological effectiveness or equivalence	Rem	Sievert (1 Sv = 100 Rem)
Radioactivity	Curie (1 Cu = disintegration seen in 1 g of radium/s = 3.7 x 10^{10} disintegrations/s)	Becquerel (1 Bq = 1 disintegration/s)

2. Roentgen is a unit of:

a. Radioactivity
b. Radiation exposure
c. Absorbed dose
d. Dose equivalent

Ans. is 'b' Radiation exposure

RADIATION HAZARDS

The developing human is most sensitive to the lethal effects of ionizing radiation during the first 14 days after conception. During this period, the radiation-exposed pregnancy either survives undamaged or is resorbed (termed the "all or none" phenomenon). Radiation-induced teratogenesis, growth restriction, or carcinogenesis are **not** observed during this stage of development, presumably because of the pluripotent nature of each cell of the very early embryo. For human exposure, a conservative estimate of the threshold for death at this stage is more than 0.10 Gy rads (100 mGy, 10 rads). An embryonic dose of 1 Gy (1000 mGy, 100 rads) will likely kill 50% of embryos.

During the period of organogenesis (approximately 2 to 8 weeks after conception or 4 to 10 weeks after the last menstrual period), the embryo may be damaged as a result of radiation-induced cell death, disturbances in cell migration and proliferation, or mitotic delay. Lethality is rare. The major sequelae of radiation damage at this stage are fetal growth restriction and congenital malformations, particularly of the central nervous system (e.g., microcephaly, gross eye abnormalities), which may be associated with intellectual disability. Microcephaly is the most frequently cited manifestation of radiation injury in utero. In the absence of any of these findings, the presence of other types of malformations in humans should not be attributed to radiation exposure. Carcinogenesis and an increase in the frequency of naturally occurring genetic mutations are other potential effects.

Fetal Dose

Effects of dose less than 0.05 Gy: Diagnostic imaging studies typically expose the fetus to less than 0.05 Gy (50 mGy, 5 rads), and there is **no** evidence of an increased risk of fetal anomalies, intellectual disability, growth restriction, or pregnancy loss from ionizing radiation at this dose level. The margin of safety is augmented by the fact that most human exposures from diagnostic imaging will be fractionated over a period of time; this type of exposure is less harmful than a single large acute exposure.

3. A pregnant lady underwent single accidental exposure to X-ray at 7 weeks of gestation. What advice will you give to her? *(NEET 2020)*

a. Continue pregnancy
b. Termination of pregnancy
c. Preinvasive investigation
d. Karyotyping

Ans. is 'a' Continue pregnancy

THERMOLUMINESCENT DOSIMETER BADGE

Thermoluminescent dosimeter (TLD) is a passive radiation detection device that is used for personal dose monitoring or to measure patient dose.

A **TLD** measures ionizing radiation exposure by measuring the amount of visible light emitted from a crystal in the detector when the crystal is heated. The amount of light emitted is dependent upon the radiation exposure.

4. Personal monitoring of radiation dose is done as: *(NEET 2020)*

a. Lead shields
b. TLD badge
c. LINAC
d. Gamma camera

Ans. is 'b' TLD badge

MODALITIES USING NON-IONIZING RADIATION

- USG
- Doppler
- MRI
- MRCP
- Thermography—Infrared rays

MODALITIES USING IONIZING RADIATION

- Gamma rays
  - Radioisotope studies/Scintigraphy (Tc scan)
  - PET
  - SPECT (Single Photon Emmission)
  - Bone Scan (Tc 99m MDP), DMSA
- X-rays
  - Radiographs
  - Fluoroscopy—Video of X-rays
  - Angiography
  - Mammography
  - CT scan
  - Barium studies
  - IVP, MCU, RGU
  - ERCP
  - DEXA Scan
  - HSG

5. Non-ionizing radiation among the following is:

a. MRI
b. CT scan
c. X-ray
d. Position emission scintigraphy

Ans. is 'a' MRI

GENERAL RADIOLOGY

BARIUM STUDIES FOR GIT

Use Barium Sulphate suspension

Barium Swallow: Pharynx + esophagus

- IOC for swallowing disorder–Fluoroscopic barium swallow

Radiology

Barium meal: Stomach + Duodenum

Barium meal follow through (BMFT): Small intestine

- *Jejunum*: Valvulae conniventes (mucosal circular folds, feathery appearance, closely placed complete rings)
- *Ileum*: Featureless, central position

Barium enema: Colon

- Peripheral position, Haustrae (Incomplete rings, more distance between folds)

Modifications in Barium Contrast

- *Tracheoesophageal fistula/Aspiration*: Non-ionic iodinated contrast (Iohexol, Iomeprol)/Dilute barium is used (to prevent pulmonary edema)
- *Leak/Perforation*: Ionic (Sodium diatrizoate)/Non-ionic iodinated contrast is used (to prevent peritonitis)

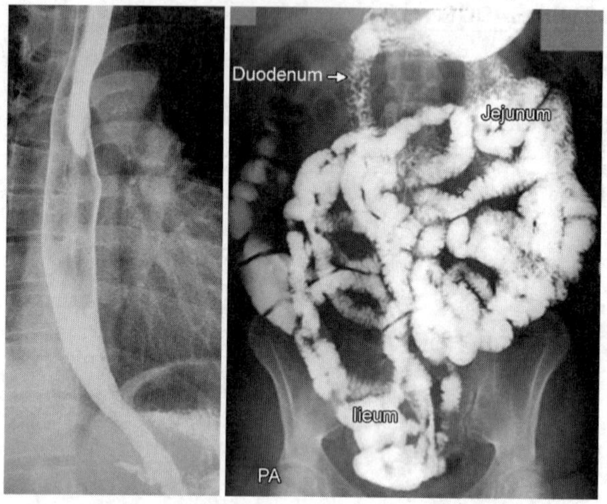

Barium swallow, Barium meal follow through

6. Identify the radiological procedure shown below: *(NEET 2019)*

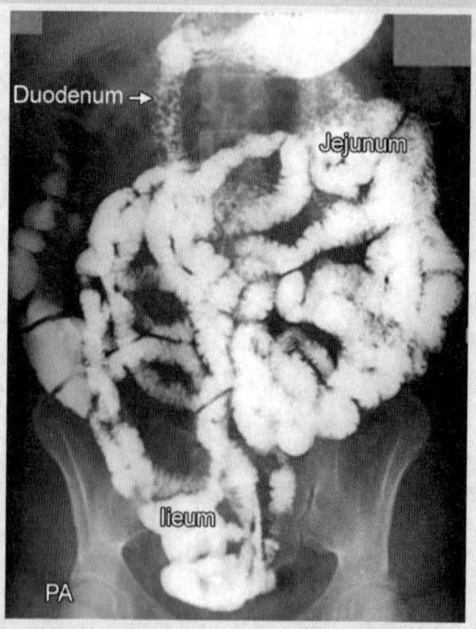

a. Barium meal follow through
b. Barium enema
c. Enteroclysis
d. Proctography

Ans. is 'a' Barium meal follow through

7. What would be the contrast of choice in esophageal perforation?

a. Gadolinium
b. Iohexol
c. Barium
d. Water

Ans. is 'b' Iohexol

8. Barium meal follow through is helpful in diagnosing:

a. Colonic stricture
b. Ileal stricture
c. Rectal stricture
d. Esophageal stricture

Ans. is 'b' Ileal stricture

MRI SEQUENCES

T1WI	T2WI
Time taken for 63% of longitudinal magnetization to be recovery (T1 Recovery Time)	Time taken for 63% of transverse magnetization to be decayed; i.e. 37% to be left (T2 Decay Time)
Depends on Spin-Lattice interaction	Depends on Spin-Spin interaction
Short TE Short TR	Long TE Long TR
Good for anatomy	Good for pathology
CSF—Hypointense Gray matter—Gray White matter—White	CSF/Fluid–Hyperintense Gray matter–White White matter-Gray
Most pathologies are hypointense	Most pathologies are hyperintense

Tissue	T1-weighted	T2-weighted
CSF	Dark	Bright
Muscle	Gray	Dark gray
Spinal cord	Gray	Light gray
Fat (subcutaneous tissue)	Bright	Light
Disk (if intact and hydrated)	Gray	Bright
Air (pharynx)	Very dark	Very dark
Inflammation (edema, infarction, demyelination)	Dark	Bright

9. T2 image in MRI is:

a. Good to detect pathology
b. Good to detect anatomy
c. Good for both
d. Good for none

Ans. is 'a' Good to detect pathology

10. CSF in T1 weight MRI gives following appearance:

a. Hypointense
b. Hyperintense
c. Isointense
d. None

Ans. is 'a' Hypointense

COMPUTED TOMOGRAPHY IMAGE

- **Principle:** Linear attenuation of X-rays
- **Beer Lambert's Law:** $I = I_o e^{-mx}$
  - I – Initial X-ray intensity
  - I_o – Final X-ray intensity
  - m – Linear attenuation co-efficient of material
  - X – Length of X-ray path
- **CT Number-Hounsfield Units (HU)**
  - Obtained by measured attenuation co-efficients
  - Based on arbitrary values: Water – 0 HU; Air –1000 HU
- **HU values**
  - –1000 – Air
  - –100 – Fat
  - 0 – Water/CSF
  - 60–70 – Acute bleed
  - 130–Contrast
  - 200–250–Calcification
  - 400–1000–Cortical bone

11. Hounsfield number for water is:

a. 0
b. +100
c. –100
d. –80

Ans. is 'a' 0

SYSTEMIC RADIOLOGY

CARDIOTHORACIC RADIOLOGY

Shapes of Heart in Congenital Heart Disease

Shape	Disease	Pathology
Snowman heart/Figure of 8	Supracardiac TAPVC	Dilated vein on left, Brachiocephalic vein in middle and SVC on right → Head of Snowman Enlarged RA → Body of Snowman
Egg on string/egg on side	D-TGA (Transposition of great arteries)	Narrowed vascular pedicle with atrial enlargement
Boot-shaped heart/Cor en sabot	TOF (Tetralogy of Fallot)	Upturned apex d/t right ventricular hypertrophy and concave pulmonary artery
Box-shaped heart	Ebstein's Anomaly	Huge right atrium – Wall-to-wall cardiomegaly

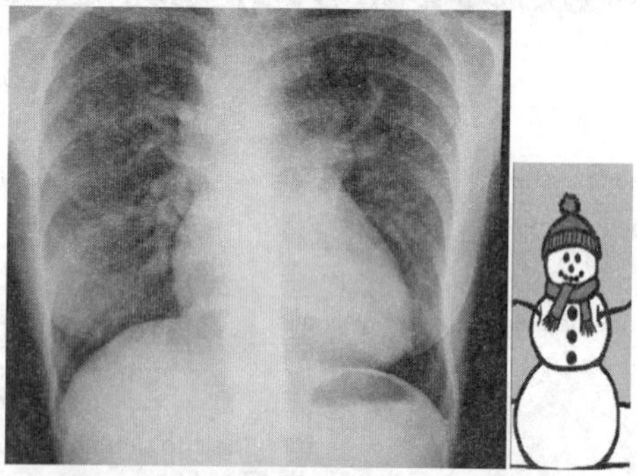

Snowman heart in supracardiac TAPVC

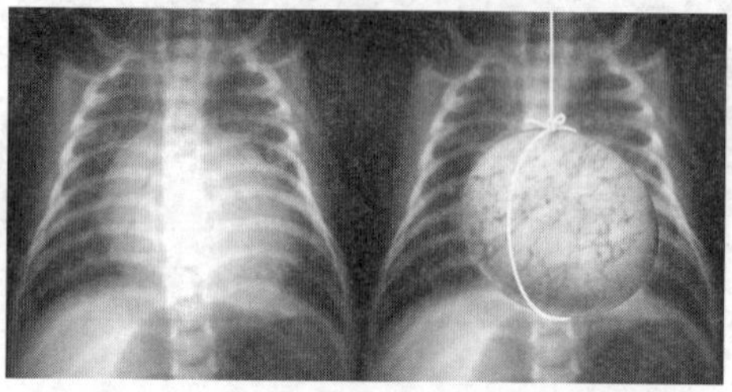

Egg on String appearance in D-TGA

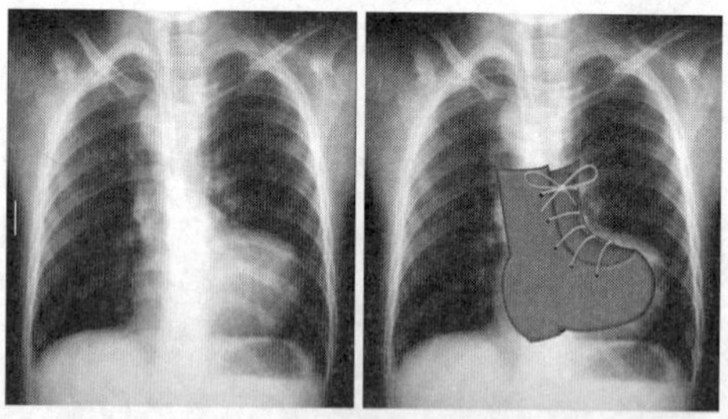

Boot-shaped heart in TOF

12. Boot-shaped heart in TOF is due to: *(NEET 2019)*

a. Left atrial enlargement
b. Right atrial enlargement
c. Right ventricular hypertrophy
d. Biventricular hypertrophy

Ans. is 'c' Right ventricular hypertrophy

TOTAL ANOMALY PULMONARY VENOUS RETURN (TAPVC)

A number of entities can present as **cyanotic congenital heart disease**. These can be divided into those with increased (pulmonary plethora) or decreased pulmonary vascularity:

- ❖ **Increased pulmonary vascularity (pulmonary plethora)**
  - **Total anomalous pulmonary venous return (TAPVR) (types I and II)**
  - Transposition of the great arteries (TGA)
  - Truncus arteriosus (types I, II and III)
  - Single ventricle without pulmonary stenosis
- ❖ **Decreased pulmonary vascularity (pulmonary oligemia)**
  - Tetralogy of Fallot
  - *Hypoplastic right heart syndrome*: Pulmonary vascularity dependent on systemic collaterals
    - Tricuspid atresia
    - Hypoplastic right ventricle
    - Pulmonary atresia or severe stenosis
  - Ebstein anomaly with atrial septal defect
  - Many other combined and infrequent anomalies such as
    - Double outlet right ventricle (DORV) with pulmonary stenosis
    - Single ventricle with pulmonary stenosis
    - Pentalogy of Cantrell

The most important cyanotic congenital heart defects can be remembered with the five Ts mnemonic.

13. All of the following produce pulmonary oligemia *except*: *(NEET 2020)*

a. TAPVC b. TOF
c. ASD d. Tricuspid atresia

Ans. is 'a' TAPVC

Coarctation of Aorta (CoA)

This is the figure of 3 sign seen in coarctation of Aorta

The **figure 3 sign** is formed by prestenotic dilatation of the aortic arch and left subclavian artery, indentation at the coarctation site (also known as the "tuck"), and post-stenotic dilatation of the descending aorta.

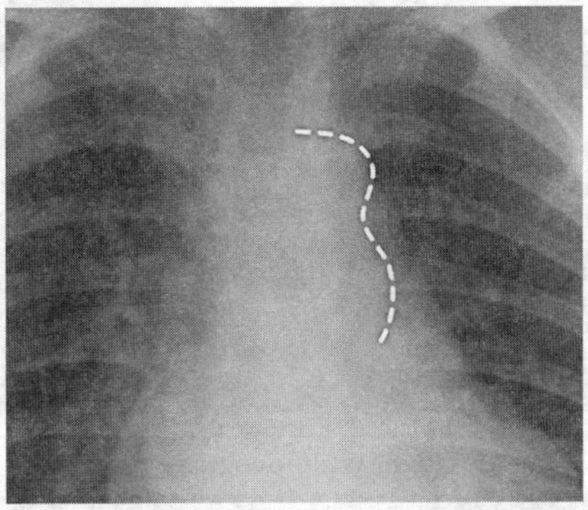

"Figure of 3 sign" of coarctation

14. The following abnormality of aortic knuckle is seen in: *(NEET 2020)*

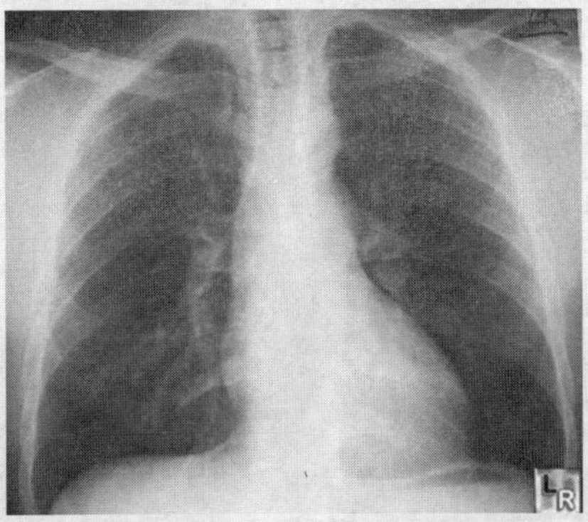

a. TGA b. PDA
c. CoA d. PAH

Ans. is 'c' CoA

Miliary Nodules (Millet Seed Opacities)

- TB, histoplasmosis
- Metastases
- Sarcoidosis
- Healed varicella pneumonia
- Pulmonary hemosiderosis

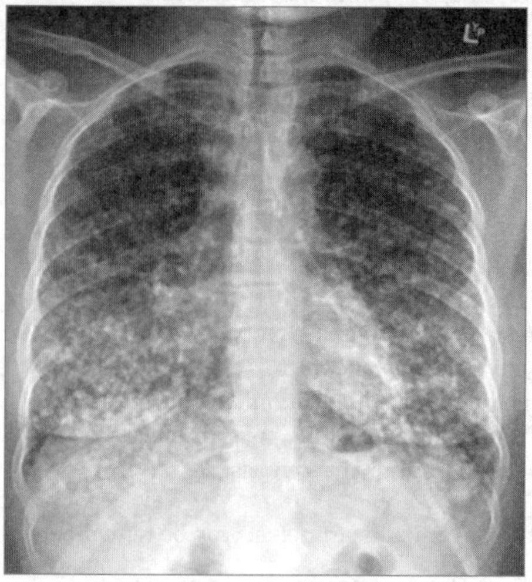

TREE-IN-BUD Appearance (Multiple Areas of Centrilobular Nodules with a Linear Branching Pattern)

- Endobronchial spread of TB
- Active infections

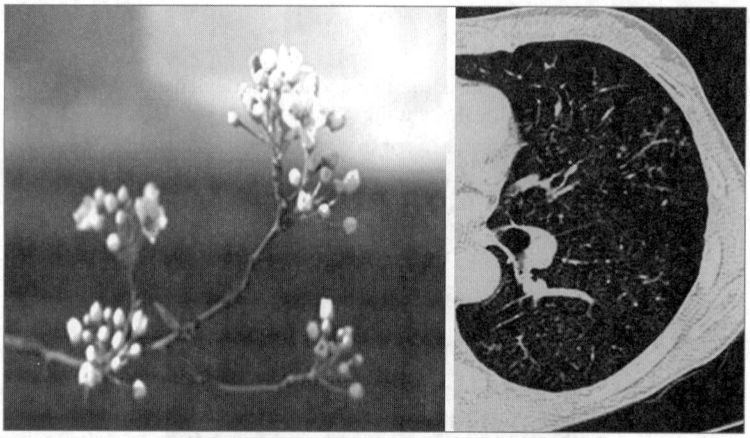

15. Identify the infection from the chest X-ray of patient with low grade fever:

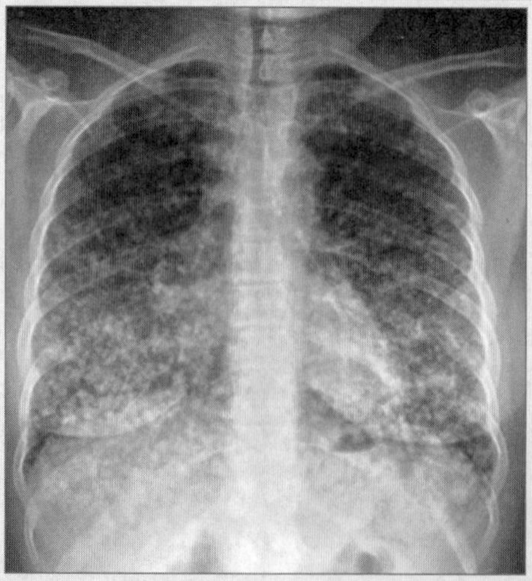

a. ILD
b. Bronchopneumonia
c. Miliary TB
d. Consolidation

Ans. is 'c' Miliary TB

CONGESTIVE HEART FAILURE (CHF) X-RAY

The chest radiograph remains the most practical and useful method of radiologically assessing and quantifying pulmonary edema, which is commonly caused due to left ventricular failure.

Features useful for broadly assessing pulmonary edema on a plain chest radiograph include:

- Central pulmonary venous congestion
  - Upper lobe pulmonary venous diversion/pulmonary venous engorgement/Stag's antler sign (Cephalization of blood flow)
- *Increased cardiothoracic ratio/cardiac Silhouette size*: Useful for assessing for an underlying cardiogenic cause or association
- Features of pulmonary interstitial edema:
  - Peribronchial cuffing and perihilar haze
  - Septal lines/Kerley lines
  - Thickening of interlobar fissures
- Features of pulmonary alveolar edema:
  - Air space opacification classically in a batwing distribution
  - May have air bronchograms
- Pleural effusions and fluid in interlobar fissures (including, vanishing, pulmonary pseudotumor)

16. All of the following are seen in an X-ray of LV failure *except*: *(NEET 2020)*

a. Cephalization of blood flow
b. Kerley B lines
c. Cardiomegaly
d. Oligemic lung fields

Ans. is 'd' Oligemic lung fields

Pulmonary Embolism

Work-up

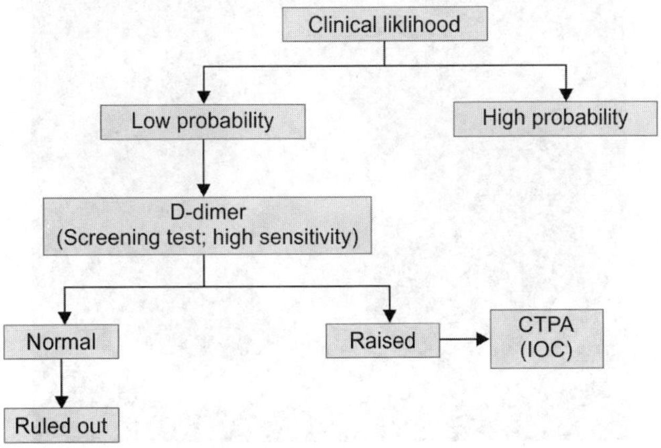

CTPA: CT pulmonary angiography; IOC: Investigation of choice

PE in Pregnancy

- D-dimer not used for screening. USG is used to r/o DVT.
- V/Q SCAN is preferred over CTPA – d/t less fetal dose in V/Q scan

Findings

- Chest X-ray – Normal in 30%
  - *Hampton's Hump*: Peripheral wedge-shaped opacity due to infarct
  - *Westermark sign*: Focal oligemia
  - *Fleischner's sign*: Prominent central pulmonary artery
- CTPA – Imaging done when contrast in pulmonary artery
- V/Q Scan – Ventilation-perfusion scan; nuclear scan

- *Ventilation*: Technegas, xenon, krypton
- *Perfusion*: Tc 99m-MAA (Macro-aggregates of albumin), Tc 99m labeled RBCs
- *V-Q mismatch*: Normal ventilation, ↓ perfusion

❖ Saddle thrombus – At bifurcation of pulmonary artery

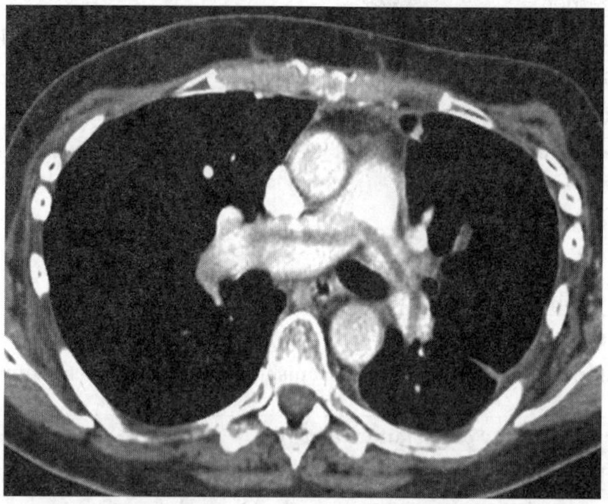

17. A 45-year-old female presented with chest pain and breathless in the ER and below is the representative CT section. What is the most likely cause of her symptoms?

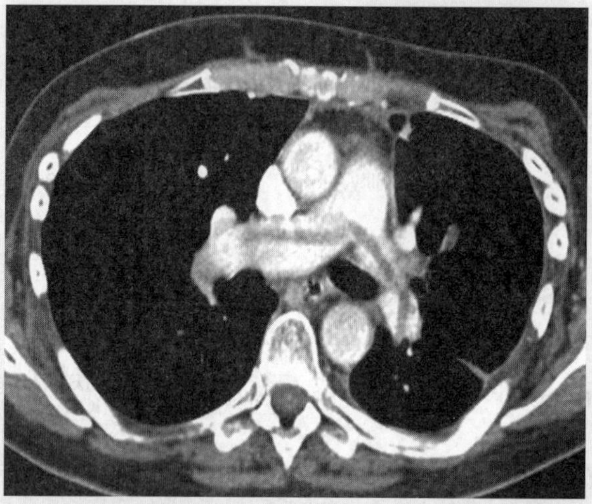

a. Aortic dissection b. Pulmonary embolism
c. Aortic aneurysm d. Budd- Chiari syndrome

Ans. is 'b' Pulmonary embolism

Pulmonary Edema

Grading of PVH/Pulm edema	PCWP (mm Hg)		Findings
	Acute	*Chronic*	
0 – Normal chest radiograph	8–12		
1 – Cephalization of blood flow	12–19	15–25	>3 mm vessels in 1st ICS
2 – Interstitial edema	20–25	25–30	Kerley lines, peribronchial cuffing, pleural effusion
3 – Alveolar edema	>25	>30	'Batwing' consolidation/GGOs

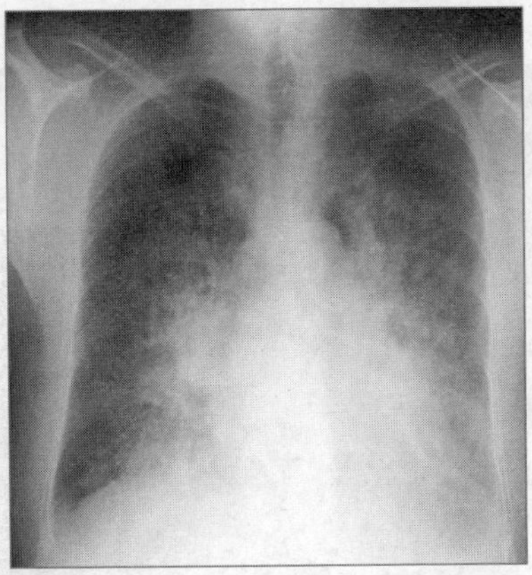

Batwing opacities in pulmonary edema

18. Radiographic sign characteristic of pulmonary edema is:

a. Westermark's sign
b. Hampton's hump
c. Palla sign
d. Bat wing sign

Ans. is 'd' Bat wing sign

ABDOMINAL RADIOLOGY

Anatomy

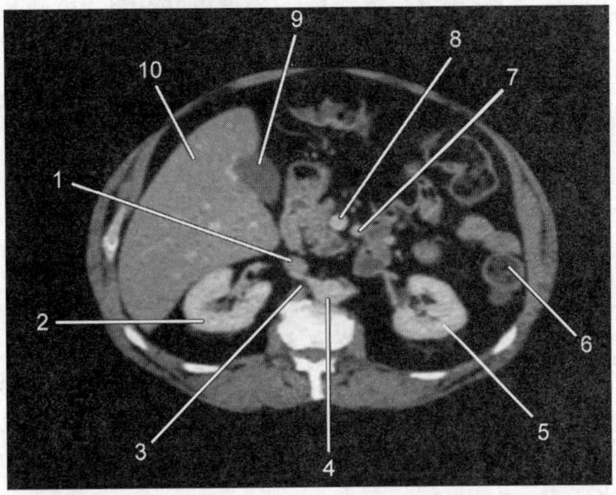

CECT Abdomen axial section; (1) Inferior vena cava; (2) Right kidney; (3) Origin of the right renal artery; (4) Aorta; (5) Left kidney; (6) Left colon; (7) Superior mesenteric artery; (8) Superior mesenteric vein; (9) Gallbladder; (10) Liver.

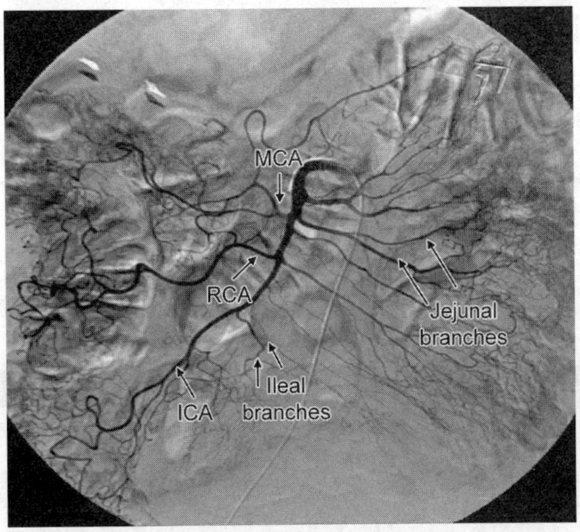

Superior mesenteric artery angiography branches

19. CT scan of abdomen showing the structure marked is:

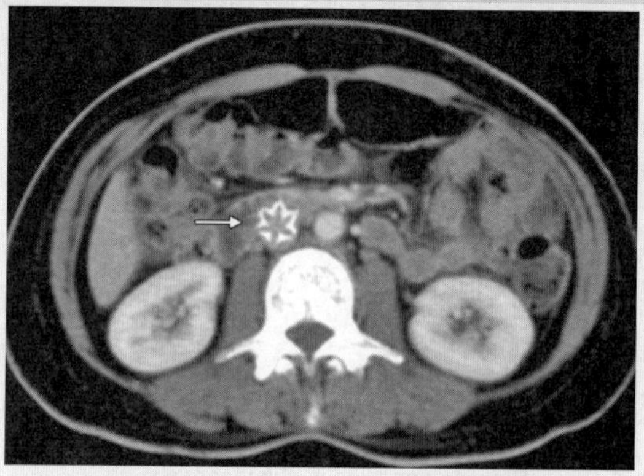

a. SVC
b. IVC
c. Aorta
d. Thoracic duct

Ans. is 'b' IVC

20. Which artery has been shown in the following CT angiographic image?

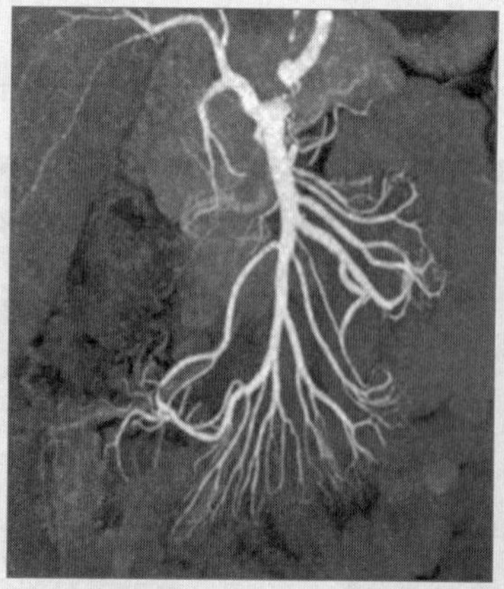

a. Superior mesenteric artery
b. Inferior mesenteric artery
c. Inferior rectal artery
d. Coeliac artery

Ans. is 'a' Superior mesenteric artery

Chronic Pancreatitis Imaging

- IOC – CT (for Ca^{2+}) + MRCP (Secretin stimulated – for duct)
- IOC – MRCP > CT
- Gold standered/Best/Most sensitive investigation – Endoscopic USG
- Calcification, fibrosis, strictures present
- ERCP – 'Chain of lakes/String of pearls/String of beads'

21. Chain of lakes appearance is seen in:

a. Acute pancreatitis
b. Chronic pancreatitis
c. Carcinoma pancreas
d. Ductal adenoma

Ans. is 'b' Chronic pancreatitis

Important Radiological Appearances in Abdominal Imaging

Radiological appearance	Seen in
Spider leg appearance on IVP	Adult Polycystic Kidney Disease
Cobra head appearance on IVP	Ureterocele
Drooping Lily sign on IVP	Duplicated collecting system

Contd...

Contd...

Radiological appearance	Seen in
Flower vase appearance on IVP	Horse shoe kidney
Apple core lesion on Barium enema	Ca colon
Claw appearance on Barium enema	Intussusception
Saw tooth appearance	Colonic diverticula
Cork screw appearance on Barium swallow	Diffuse esophageal spasm
Bird's beak appearance on Barium swallow	Achalasia cardia
Rat-tail appearance on Barium swallow	Carcinoma esophagus
String sign of Kantor	Crohn's disease
Thumb printing sign	Ischemic colitis

22. Cork screw appearance on radiography is seen in:

a. Achalasia cardia
b. Carcinoma esophagus
c. Hiatus hernia
d. Diffuse esophageal spasm

Ans. is 'd' Diffuse esophageal spasm

Hysterosalpingography

- Best time – 6th to 10th day of menstrual cycle (not to be done during menstruation; risk of damage to undiagnosed pregnancy after 10th day)
- A radiopaque dye is injected through the cannula into the uterine cavity under direct vision with fluoroscopic screen; 15 mL of the medium is usually adequate to visualize the uterine cavity and the tubes.
- If the tubes are patent, the medium is usually adequate to exit through the abdominal ostia and smear the adjacent bowel.

23. Name the investigation shown in the given image:

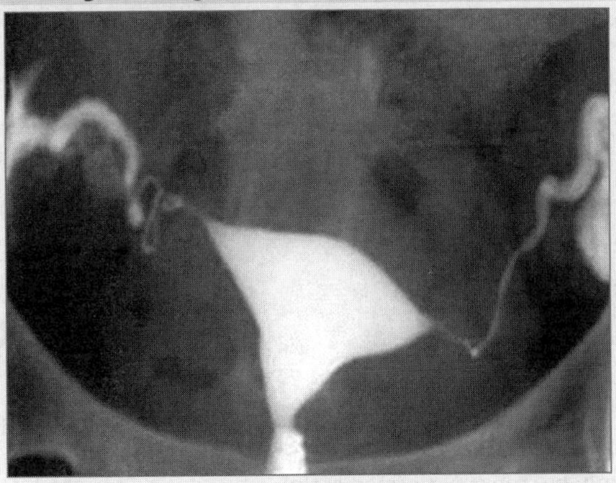

a. MR HSG
b. CT HSG
c. Conventional HSG
d. USG HSG

Ans. is 'c' Conventional HSG

NEURORADIOLOGY

NCCT Head in Infarct—Investigation of Choice

- **Acute infarct**
  - Wedge-shaped hypodensity involving both GM and WM
  - *Hyperdense artery sign*: Most common in MCA
  - *Sylvian dot sign*: Hyperdense MCA in cross-section
  - Loss of GM-WM differentiation
    - Loss of insular ribbon sign
    - Disappearing basal ganglia sign
- **Subacute Infarct:** ↓HU, ↑mass effect
- **Chronic Infarct**: ↓HU, volume loss

Lacunar Infarcts

- ❖ Chronic HTN
- ❖ Basal ganglia, thalamus, internal capsule

Embolic infarcts: Gray atter-White matter interface

Watershed infarcts: 'Vascular border zones'; hypoperfusion

- ❖ Deep WM parallel to lateral ventricles

24. Identify the condition in the below image.

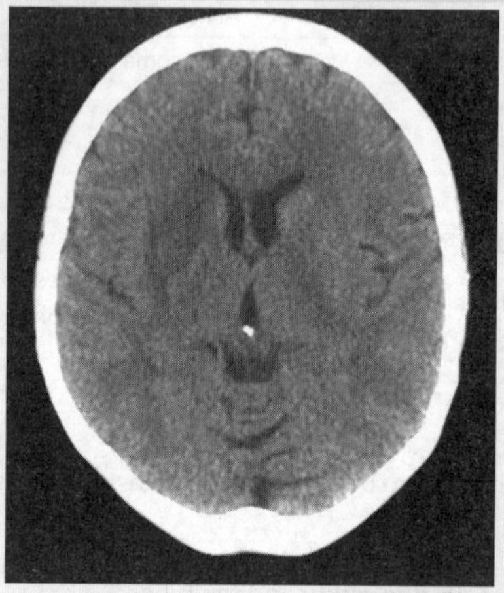

a. Lacunar infarct
b. Multiple Sclerosis
c. Brain tumor
d. Intracerebral hemorrhage

Ans. is 'a' Lacunar infarct

Explanation: NCCT shows hypodensity involving right basal ganglia; s/o lacunar infarct.

SUBARACHNOID HEMORRHAGE NCCT

Intracranial hemorrhage (**ICH**) is a collective term encompassing many different conditions characterized by the extravascular accumulation of blood within different intracranial spaces. A simple categorization is based on location:

- ❖ **Intra-axial hemorrhage**
  - Intracerebral hemorrhage
- ❖ **Extra-axial hemorrhage**
  - Extradural hemorrhage (EDH)
  - Subdural hemorrhage (SDH)
  - Subarachnoid hemorrhage (SAH)
  - Intraventricular hemorrhage (IVH)

CT scan is almost always the first imaging modality used to assess patients with suspected intracranial hemorrhage. Fortunately acute blood is markedly hyperdense compared to brain parenchyma, and as such usually poses little difficulty in diagnosis (provided the amount of blood is large enough, and the scan is performed early).

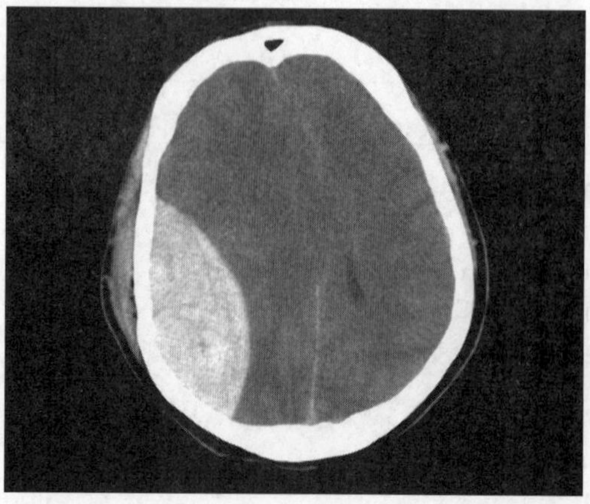

Extradural hemorrhage

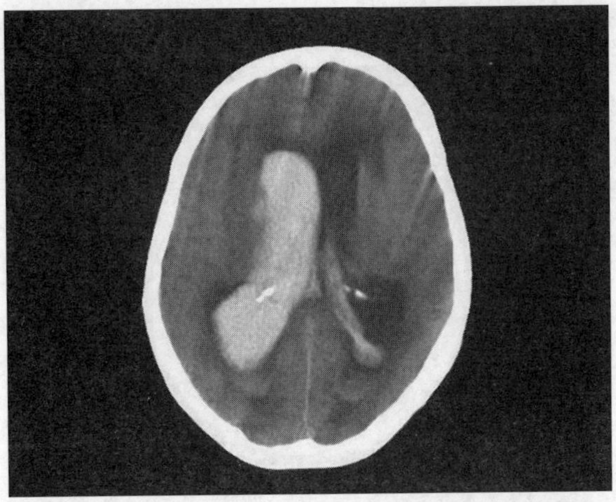

Intraventricular hemorrhage

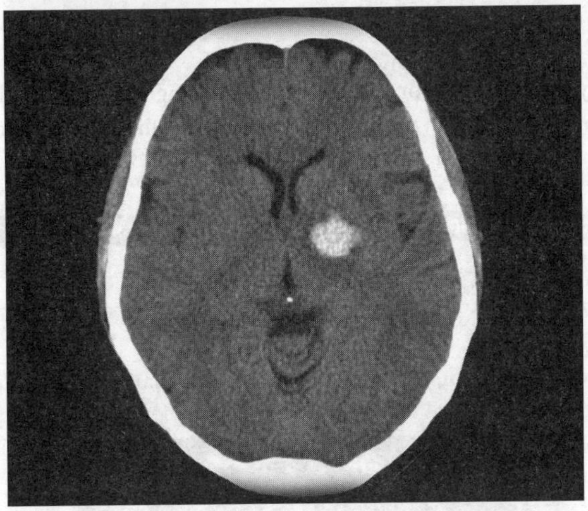

Intracranial hemorrhage

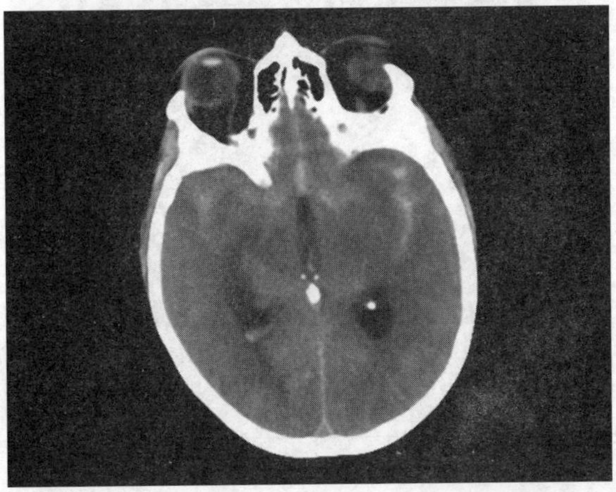

Subarachnoid hemorrhage

The diagnosis of SAH is suspected when a hyperdense material is seen filling the subarachnoid space. Most commonly this is apparent around the circle of Willis, on account of the majority of berry aneurysms occurring in this region (~65%), or in the Sylvian fissure (~30%).

Subarachnoid hemorrhages are grouped into four categories according to the amount of blood on unenhanced CT by the modified Fisher scale.

25. An elderly patient presented with severe headache and neck rigidity. CT is shown below. What is the diagnosis? *(NEET 2020)*

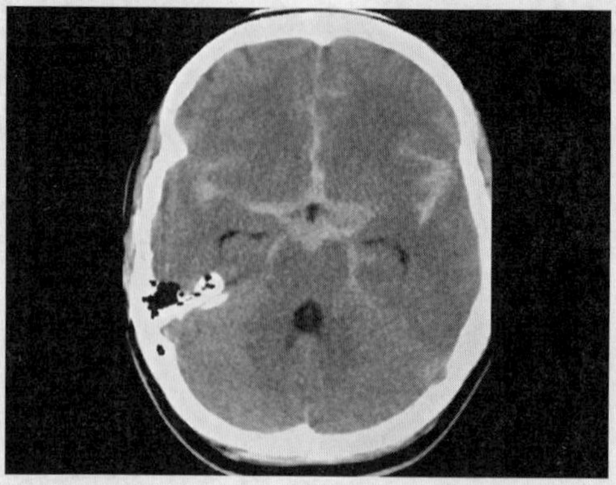

a. EDH
b. SDH
c. SAH
d. Meningitis

Ans. is 'c' SAH

Craniopharyngioma

- Rare, usually suprasellar, partially calcified, solid, or mixed solid-cystic benign tumors that arise from remnants of Rathke's pouch.
- Bimodal distribution, occurring predominantly in children but also between the ages of 55 and 65 years.
- They present with headaches, visual impairment, and impaired growth in children and hypopituitarism in adults.
- Two types

Adamantinomatous (90% cases)	Papillary (10% cases)
Children <10 years	Adults
Cystic (Machine-Oil fluid)	Solid
Invasive	Non-invasive

26. 8-year-old child with bitemporal hemianopia. His IQ is normal. His visual acuity is diminished. The radiological image of this patient is shown below. What is the most likely diagnosis?

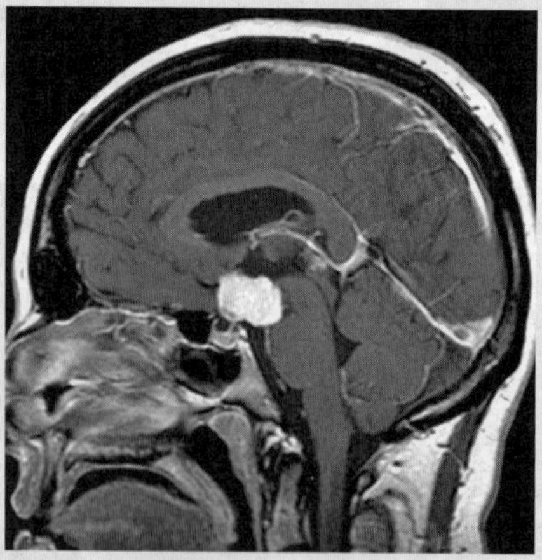

a. Craniopharyngioma
b. Optic glioma
c. Pineal tumor
d. Torus tubaris

Ans. is 'a' Craniopharyngioma

CRANIOPHARYNGIOMA CT

Craniopharyngiomas are relatively benign (WHO grade I) neoplasms that typically arise in the sellar/suprasellar region. They account for ~1–5% of primary brain tumors, and can occur anywhere along the infundibulum (from the floor of the third ventricle to the pituitary gland).

Although craniopharyngiomas are found in patients of all ages, there is a bimodal distribution. The first peak occurs between the ages of 5–15 years and a second smaller peak occurs in adults aged over 40 years old.

Clinical presentation is variable on account of the variable location and size of the tumor. Presenting complaints include:

❖ Headaches and raised intracranial pressure
❖ Visual symptoms
  • 20% of children
  • 80% of adults
❖ Hormonal imbalances
  • Short stature and delayed puberty in children
  • Decreased libido
  • Amenorrhea
  • Diabetes insipidus
❖ Behavioral change due to frontal or temporal extension

27. A child presented with defective vision and headache and CT showed suprasellar mass with calcification. What is the diagnosis? *(NEET 2020)*

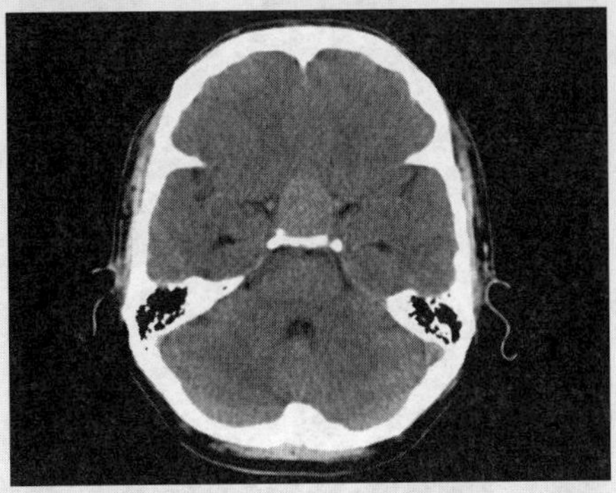

a. Meningioma
b. Craniopharyngioma
c. Astrocytoma
d. Oligodendroglioma

Ans. is 'b' Craniopharyngioma

Vein of Galen Malformation (VOGM)

❖ AV malformation with deep arteries opening into vein of Galen
❖ Child presents with
  • Hydrocephalus
  • Midline swelling in region of great cerebral vein/vein of Galen
  • High output congestive heart failure
❖ Radiographic features:
  • *Antenatal ultrasound*: The dilated median prosencephalic vein (MPV) appears as an anechoic structure in the midline posteriorly and demonstrates prominent flow on doppler examination
  • Dilated feeding and draining vessels appear as flow voids on T2-weighted MRI

28. Identify the condition shown is the CT scan image below:

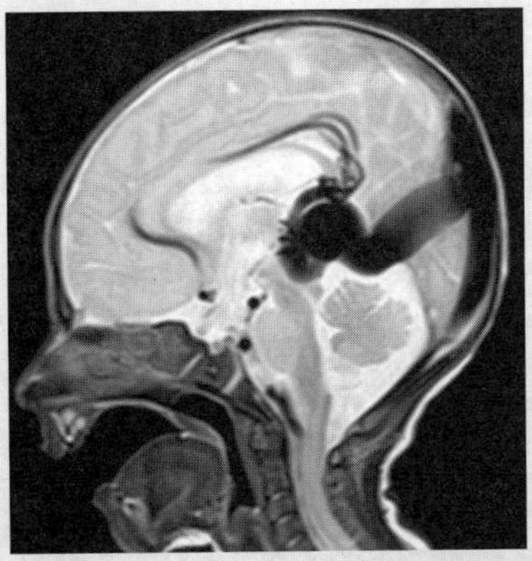

a. Dandy Walker syndrome
b. Vein of Galen malformation
c. Arnold Chiari malformation
d. Cerebellar vermis malformation

Ans. is 'b' Vein of Galen malformation

Orbital Blowout Fracture

- Fracture of one of the walls of orbit but orbital rim (the most anterior bony margin of orbit) remains intact
- Results from blunt trauma to central orbit
- May present with diplopia, enophthalmos, orbital emphysema
- Inferior wall blowout fractures are the most common
- Prolapse of orbital fat and inferior rectus muscle can be seen—Teardrop sign

29. A patient presented with history of diplopia and restricted eye movements. A clinical image and CT image is shown below. What will be the diagnosis? *(NEET 2019)*

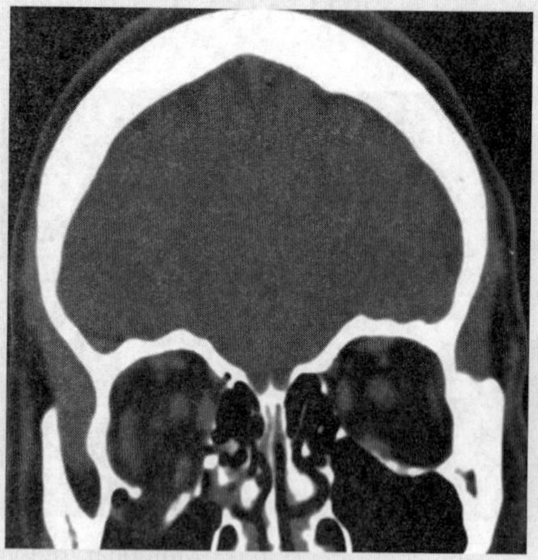

a. Le-Fort fracture
b. Fracture maxilla
c. Fracture zygomatic
d. Blowout fracture

Ans. is 'd' Blowout fracture

RADIOTHERAPY

DOSE-DEPTH CURVE

- **Electron beam**: Deposit most of radiation dose in superficial tissue—Used in CUTANEOUS T-cell LYMPHOMA (Mycosis Fungoides); Eyelids and Lips tumors; Intraoperative RT
- **Proton beam**: Deposit most of dose deep in tissue peaking suddenly–**Bragg's Peak**—used in deep seated Brain Tumor; skull base Chordoma
- **X-rays/Gamma rays**: High entry dose and low exit dose
- MC method of intraoperative radiotherapy—Electron beam
- MC method of radiotherapy—X-rays

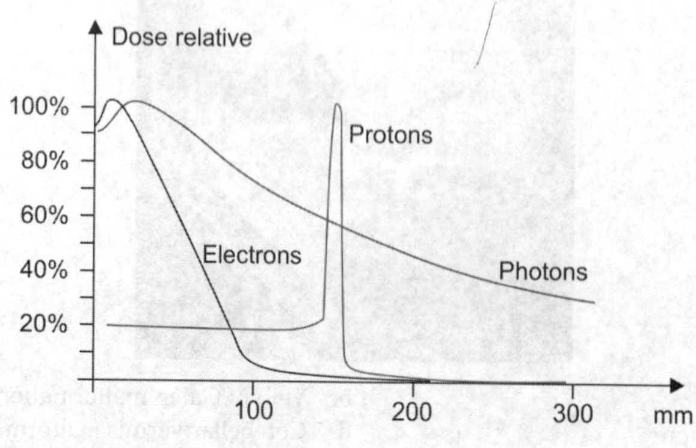

30. Bragg's peak effect is seen in:

a. X-rays
b. Neutron
c. Protons
d. Electron

Ans. is 'c' Protons

31. Most commonly used radiation in radiotherapy is:

a. X-rays
b. Beta rays
c. Alpha
d. Electron

Ans. is 'a' X-rays

TYPES OF RADIOTHERAPY

- **Teletherapy**: Source of radiation is distant from the patient. Can be given by
  - X-ray beams (Linear acceleration)
  - *Gamma rays*: Cobalt—60 beam or Cesium—137
  - *Particulate beams*: Electron beam, Proton beam
- **Brachytherapy**: Radiation source in close contact with tumor

Interstitial—Source inserted into tumor tissue—prostate Ca	
Removable implant	***Permanent implant***
Iridium-192	**Gold-198**
Cesium-137	**I-125**
Radium-226	**Radon-222**
Co-60	**Palladium-103**
Intracavitary—Source inserted into body cavity Ca cervix, uterus, esophageal, lung Ca	
Removable implant (Long half life)	***Permanent implant (Short half life)***
Co-60	Colloidal Gold
Cesium-137	I-131
Radium-226	

- **Systemic radiotherapy:** Radioisotopes are given systemically (IV)

32. Permanent implant for brachytherapy are all *except*:

a. Cesium-131
b. Gold-198
c. Radon-222
d. Iridium-192

Ans. is 'd' Iridium-192

Explanation: Cesium-137 is used as removable implant; Cesium-131 is used as permanent implant in interstitial radiotherapy.

REMOTE AFTERLOADERS

This term is used in reference to Brachytherapy

Remote afterloading brachytherapy systems automatically administer a radioisotope directly to cancerous tissue, thereby minimizing the radiation dose to surrounding tissue and eliminating the radiation exposure to hospital staff. The amount of the radiation dose varies with the brachytherapy method chosen for treatment delivery: low-dose-rate (LDR) brachytherapy uses an implanted source that delivers a dose of 40 to 60 centigrays (cGy) per hour over several days; high-dose-rate (HDR) brachytherapy uses a traveling (stepping) source that delivers a dose greater than 100 cGy per minute for 5 to 30 minutes; pulsed-dose-rate (PDR) brachytherapy uses a cable-driven source delivering a dose of up to about 300 cGy per hour for 10 to 30 minutes, repeated over several days.

33. "Remote afterloaders" is employed with reference to: *(NEET 2020)*

a. EBRT
b. Brachytherapy
c. Proton beam therapy
d. Nuclear scintigraphy

Ans. is 'b' Brachytherapy

RADIOTHERAPY PRINCIPLES

Radiotherapy (RT) is a treatment modality that delivers energy to kill malignant cells in the area specifically targeted by the clinician.

Radiotherapy primarily damages the DNA of cancer cells by ionizing the atoms that make up the DNA chain. Ionizations result in broken atomic and molecular bonds; the generation of double-strand breaks in DNA is considered the dominant factor that causes cellular lethality.

Both malignant and normal cells in the treatment field are subject to the ionizing effects of **radiation**. Normal cells generally are better able to repair damage caused by **radiation** at the cellular level, using molecular machinery that detects DNA breaks and mutations and repairs them. In contrast, many malignant cells lack these molecular mechanisms and, therefore, are preferentially damaged by **radiation**. However, normal tissues have limits on the dose of **radiation** that they can safely withstand; these limits determine the maximum dose that can be safely administered during a course of treatment.

Acute RT-related cystitis can be a common complication with conventionally dosed pelvic RT, although the incidence is highly variable. It can be associated with irritative voiding symptoms (dysuria, frequency, urgency, and nocturia) and bladder spasms. It is due to RT-induced bladder inflammation and edema, which can compromise urothelial integrity. When they occur during RT, the symptoms typically resolve in one to two weeks after completing therapy.

- ❖ Late GU toxicities generally arise as a result of RT-induced epithelial and **microvascular changes,** which can lead to changes in bladder physiology. These can result in a similar spectrum of lower urinary tract symptoms to that seen in the acute phase, such as urgency and frequency, which is often attributed to bladder overactivity or contraction. With significant contraction, bladder dysfunction can result in urge incontinence. However, at expected doses of external beam radiation therapy (EBRT) employed for gynecologic cancers (40 to 50 Gy), the likelihood of serious lasting side effects is low.
- ❖ The **small bowel is very sensitive to the early effects of RT**, and when it is contained within the RT field, radiation injury can present acutely as nausea and vomiting. However, the treatment of acute radiation injury is largely symptomatic.
- ❖ The symptoms of late GI toxicity include chronic diarrhea, malabsorption, recurrent bouts of ileus or obstruction, and the development of mucosal telangiectasias or ulcerations. Advances in radiation techniques, including use of intensity-modulated RT and image-guided brachytherapy, show promise in reducing the incidence and severity of late GI toxicity.
- ❖ **Vaginal toxicity is common for women undergoing treatment** for cervical and uterine cancer, in which cases, either pelvic RT or vaginal brachytherapy (VBT) is often administered. This can lead to sexual dysfunction and interfere with quality of life.
- ❖ Radiation to the ovaries may lead to infertility or premature menopause. The dose necessary to eliminate 50% of remaining oocytes has been determined to be between 2 and 4 Gy. Due to these risks, for women who are premenopausal and aged <40 years old, laparoscopic ovarian transposition is often employed before a course of pelvic radiation.
- ❖ Acute skin reactions range from erythema and soreness to moist desquamation, and on rare occasion, ulceration. High-energy photons (10 to 18 Mv) and multi-field arrangements are typically used with pelvic radiotherapy. Both of these factors have a skin-sparing effect on the distribution of radiation dose

34. A female with stage 2B cervical cancer underwent radiotherapy. Which of the following is true regarding it? *(NEET 2020)*

a. Small vessels are resistant to radiation
b. Dose of radiation at a point is inversely proportional to the square of its distance from the source
c. Spares actively dividing cells
d. Rectal and vaginal mucosa are resistant to radiation

Ans. is 'b' Dose of radiation at a point is inversely proportional to the square of its distance from the source

IODINE RADIO-ISOTOPES

	Half-life	Uses	Emmission
I^{131}	8 days	• Radio-ablation of thyroid (Ca, graves) • Systemic radiotherapy of Ca thyroid	Beta (destroy cancer and thyroid cells) + Gamma emitter. Most carcinogenic isotope of thyroid
I^{125}	60 days	• Brachytherapy of prostate • Radioimmunoassay for hormones	
I^{124}	4 days	• PET	Positron emitter
I^{123}	13 hours	Thyroid scintigraphy (Functional scans of thyroid– RAIU in western countries)	

Radioactive iodine is administered orally as well as parentally i.e. IV, SC and IM. Although most commonly it is administered orally in the form of a solution or rarely as capsule.

35. Mode of administration of radioactive iodine is:

a. Intravenous
b. Subcutaneous
c. Oral
d. All of the above

Ans. is 'd' All of the above

NUCLEAR MEDICINE

CARDIAC SCINTIGRAPHY

Myocardial Perfusion Scintigraphy

- ❖ Isotope goes to perfused myocardium
- ❖ Thallium-201, Tc^{99m}-Tetrofosmin, Tc^{99m}-Sestamibi (MIBI scan)
- ❖ Stress (Treadmill, Dobutamine) Thallium study increases sensitivity for decreased perfusion areas
- ❖ Ischemic areas Cold

Myocardial Infarct Scintigraphy

- **Infarct:** Binding agent
- **Tc^{99m}:** Pyrophosphate
- **Infarct:** Hot
  - Gold Std. Investigation for Myocardial Function—MRI
  - Nuclear Imaging technique for Myocardial Function—MUGA scan/Radionuclide ventriculography (with Tc-99m labeled RBCs)
  - Delayed enhanced MRI—New Gold Std. for Myocardial Viability (Earlier – PET)

Gallium-67 Scan

- Taken up by lymphocytes
- Used in:
  - Occult abscess
  - Lambda and panda sign in sarcoidosis
  - Acute myocarditis

36. Acute myocarditis scintigraphy is done with:

a. Thallium
b. Technetium
c. Gallium
d. None

Ans. is 'c' Gallium

HALF-LIFE OF SOME IMPORTANT RADIOISOTOPES

- Phosphorus (P-32)–14.3 days
- Strontium (Sr)–28 days
- Yttrium (Y-90)–2.54 days
- Radium (Ra-226)–1622 years
- Iodine (I-131)–8 days
- Iridium (Ir-192)–74.5 days
- Cobalt (Co-60)–5.2 years
- Cesium (Cs-137)–30 years
- Technetium (Tc-99)–6 hours
- Tritium–12.3 years

37. Half life of tritium is:

a. 10.2 years
b. 12.3 years
c. 15.5 years
d. 20.7 years

Ans. is 'b' 12.3 years

STEREOTACTIC RADIOSURGERY

- Large dose of radiation is deposited in single fraction with high precision
- Gamma knife – Uses Co-60
  - Helmet around patient which determines xyz coordinates of the lesion – Leksell frame
- Stereotactic radio surgery (SRS) uses – Solitary brain mets; trigeminal neuralgia; AVM; pituitary adenoma; CP angle meningioma/schwannoma
- Advantage of stereotactic radiosurgery are:
  - Achieve tumor ablation without surgery
  - Damage to nearby structure is minimized as radiation is delivered to focused area
  - Tumor ablation can be achieved in difficult location, e.g. brain
- Cyber knife – Uses Linac (Linear accelerator; X-rays)
  - No leksell frame; robotic manipulator is used; continued image guidance

Stereotactic body radiotherapy (SBRT)	Stereotactic radiosurgery (SRS)
Cyberknife	Gamma-knife
Linac (X-rays)	Cobalt (γ-rays)
Whole body	Brain only
Frameless	Frame around head

38. Gamma knife utilizes:

a. Strontium 89
b. I-131
c. Cobalt -60
d. P-32

Ans. is 'c' Cobalt-60

39. All are true about stereotactic radiosurgery *except*:

a. X-rays are used
b. A form of radiotherapy
c. Used in AV malformation
d. Damage to nearby structures is significant

Ans. is 'd' Damage to nearby structures is significant

Previously Asked Facts

- Thickness of lead apron is 0.5 mm
- Maximum permissible whole body radiation exposure per year is 1 mSv.
- Ionising/Damaging power – Alpha > Beta > Gamma
- Penetration power – Neutrons > Gamma > Beta > Alpha
- Safe light in radiographic dark room should be Red
- Hair-on-end/Crew-cut appearance of skull – Diploic space widening; seen in all hemolytic anemias; Best in Thalassemia
- Soap-bubble appearances
  - Around knee – GCT
  - Mandible – Ameloblastoma
  - Abdominal X-ray – Meconium Ileus
  - MRI Brain – Cryptococcal meningitis
  - Antenatal scan – Multi-cystic dysplastic kidney
- Photosensitive material used in X-ray film is silver bromide
- Stenver's view is used for internal auditory canal
- Snow-storm appearance on chest X-ray – Silicosis
- Normal cardiac borders on Chest X-ray PA view (superior to inferior)
  - Right – SVC, right atrium, IVC
  - Left – Aortic knuckle, left pulmonary artery. Left auricle (Not atrium), left ventricle
- The keyhole sign is an ultrasonographic sign seen in boys with posterior urethral valves. It refers to the appearance of the dilated proximal urethra.
- Central dot sign refers to tiny dots which is actually portal vein within dilated hepatic bile ducts on CT; seen in Caroli's disease.
- 'Snow storm appearance' or 'bunch of grapes appearance' on USG is characteristic of molar pregnancy
- Most commonly used investigation to diagnose urinary tract obstruction—USG
- Most commonly used initial investigation of urinary tract malignancies (kidney, bladder)—USG
- Investigation of choice for hydronephrosis—USG
- Investigation of choice for pyonephrosis—USG
- Investigation of choice for vesicourethral reflex—voiding cystourethrogram
- Investigation of choice for posterior urethral valve—voiding cystourethrogram
- Best method to visualize posterior urethra—voiding cystourethrogram
- Investigation of choice for renal and ureteric stones—NCCT KUB
- Investigation of choice for diagnosis and staging of RCC—Contrast - enhanced CT
- CT Head giving tram track appearance is diagnostic of Sturge-Weber syndrome
- On antenatal USG, lemon sign – Anterior indentation of frontal bones; Banana sign – Wrapping of cerebellum around brainstem due to herniation – Both signs are seen with Chiari malformations and Spina bifida.
- Bone-within-bone appearance is seen in Osteopetrosis
- Onion peel periosteal reaction is seen in Ewing's sarcoma
- Father of modern radiology - Gosta Forssell
- Inventor of CT scan – Godfrey Hounsfield

CHAPTER 18 Psychiatry

NORMAL PRESSURE HYDROCEPHALUS

Normal pressure hydrocephalus (NPH) refers to a condition of pathologically enlarged ventricular size with normal opening pressures on lumbar puncture. NPH is a form of communicating hydrocephalus and is distinguished from obstructive or noncommunicating hydrocephalus, in which there is a structural blockage of the cerebrospinal fluid (CSF) circulation within the ventricular system (e.g., stenosis of aqueduct of Sylvius).

NPH is associated with a classic triad of dementia, gait disturbance, and urinary incontinence. Because this clinical syndrome is potentially reversible by the placement of a ventriculoperitoneal (VP) shunt.

Parkinson disease dementia: Cognitive impairment and dementia related to Parkinson disease typically present as a later-stage finding, at a time when typical motor features (e.g., tremor, bradykinesia, rigidity) are prominent. Patients with a triad of dementia, gait dysfunction, and urinary incontinence due to Parkinson disease dementia rather than NPH are therefore usually distinguishable by these additional Parkinsonian signs.

1. An elderly female was brought by her family with complaints that she has started forgetting the things and started wetting the bed. On examination she had a broad based Gait. What is the diagnosis? *(NEET 2020)*

a. Alzheimers
b. Frontotemporal dementia
c. Normal pressure hydrocephalus
d. Parkinsonism

Ans. is 'c' Normal pressure hydrocephalus

MENTAL HEALTH CARE ACT

2. What is the maximum duration of voluntary stay in a hospital as per Mental Health Care Act? *(NEET 2020)*

a. 48 hrs
b. 14 days
c. 30 days
d. 60 days

Ans. is 'c' 30 days

Explanation: Guidelines of Mental Health Care Act 2017: page 35/51

https://drive.google.com/file/d/1_GenaH46pUPfcY1TxP7JnuCh4aWLXdB2/view?usp=sharing

1. The person is in eligible to receive care and treatment as an independent patient because the person is unable to make mental healthcare and treatment decisions independently and needs very high support from his nominated representative in making decisions.
2. The admission of a person with mental illness to a mental health establishment under this section shall be limited to a period of thirty days.
3. At the end of the period mentioned under subsection (2), or earlier, if the person no longer meets the criteria for admission as stated in sub-section (1), the patient shall no longer remain in the establishment under this section.
4. On the expiry of the period of thirty days referred to in subsection (2), the person may continue to remain admitted in the mental health establishment in accordance with the provisions of section 90.

SCHIZOPHRENIA

Poor prognostic factors
1. Insidious onset 2. Onset < 20 years of age (early onset) 3. Absence of stress or 4. Poor premorbid adjustment 5. Disorganized, simple, undifferentiated subtypes 6. Chronic course (>2 years) 7. Absence of depression 8. Predominance of negative symptoms 9. Family history of schizophrenia 10. Past history of schizophrenia 11. Asthenic (thin) physique 12. Male sex 13. Single, divorced 14. Poor social support 15. Flat or blunted affect 16. Absence of proper treatment or poor response to the treatment 17. Institutionalization (long-term hospitalization) 18. Evidence of ventricular enlargement on cranial CT scan

3. Poor prognosis of schizophrenia is seen in:

a. Female sex
b. Presence of depression
c. Acute onset
d. Predominance of negative symptoms

Ans. is 'd' Predominance of negative symptoms

HALLUCINATIONS

- Perceptions in the absence of external stimuli (e.g., seeing a light that is not actually present).
- Contrast with misperceptions (e.g., illusions) of real external stimuli.
- Types include:
  - *Auditory*: More commonly due to psychiatric illness (e.g., schizophrenia) than medical illness.
  - *Visual*: More commonly due to medical illness (e.g., drug intoxication) than psychiatric illness.
  - *Tactile*: Common in alcohol withdrawal and stimulant use (e.g., "cocaine crawlies," a type of delusional parasitosis).
  - *Olfactory*: Often occur as an aura of temporal lobe epilepsy (e.g., burning rubber) and in brain tumors.
  - *Gustatory*: Rare, but seen in epilepsy.
  - *Hypnagogic*: Occurs while going to sleep. Sometimes seen in narcolepsy.
  - *Hypnopompic*: Occurs while waking from sleep ("get pumped up in the morning"). Sometimes seen in narcolepsy.

4. Hallucination is:

a. Altered perception of real object
b. Perception without external stimulus
c. False, firm [unshakable] belief
d. Transient state of altered sensorium

Ans. is 'b' Perception without external stimulus

TACTILE HALLUCINATION

Cocaine Bugs

Also known as **Magnan's sign** and **Magnan-Saury's sign**. All three terms refer to a tactile hallucination consisting of a crawling foreign body beneath or upon the skin that is associated with the chronic use of cocaine.

Body Stuffer

Heroin poisoning occurs most commonly when an individual unintentionally overdoses on the drug. Poisoning may also occur in a "body packer," "body pusher," or "body stuffer." Body packers, also called "mules," are people who swallow and pack their GI tracts with bags of heroin in order to smuggle the illegal drug from one country to another. Body pushers conceal the drugs in their rectum and/or vagina. In both of these groups, the drugs are carefully packaged for safe passage, but poisoning occurs if the packages rupture. Body packing or pushing should be suspected in persons who are found unconscious at airports, during international flights, or soon after a trip to endemic countries.

Body stuffers, on the other hand, are people who ingest all the drugs in their possession in order to conceal the evidence from the police. Because these packages are typically not designed for safe GI transport, they easily rupture and frequently cause poisoning.

5. A patient of cocaine addiction complains of itching and sensation of insects crawling under his skin. What is the diagnosis? *(NEET 2020)*

a. Magnan syndrome
b. Body stuffer syndrome
c. Malory Weiss syndrome
d. Tourette syndrome

Ans. is 'a' Magnan syndrome

DEPRESSION

	Adjustment disorder	Major depressive disorder	Dysthymia (persistent depressive disorder)	Cyclothymia
Stressor	Definite stressor present ++	Stressor +/–	+/–	+/–
Duration	Not more than 6 months	2 weeks	At least 2 years (in children 1 year)	At least 2 years (in children 1 year)
Criterion	Symptoms triggered within 3 months of stressor Marked distress out of proportion to severity of the stressor	At least one out of depressed mood (or irritable mood) or loss of interest must be present Plus at least 4 out of following must be present • Significant weight loss (5% in a month)	Depressed mood must be present with 2/6 criteria • Poor appetite or overeating • Insomnia or hypersomnia • Low energy or fatigue • Low self-esteem	Multiple periods of hypomanic and depressive symptoms never meeting criteria of a hypomania and depression disorders. These symptoms are present for 50% of the time Symptoms free period should not be >2 months at a stretch

Contd...

Contd...

	Adjustment disorder	Major depressive disorder	Dysthymia (persistent depressive disorder)	Cyclothymia
	Criteria for Depression should not be met	• Insomnia or hypersomnia • Feelings of restlessness or being slowed down • Fatigue • Feelings of worthlessness or excessive or inappropriate guilt • Decreased concentration • Suicidal thoughts	• Poor concentration or difficulty making decisions • Feelings of hopelessness • Symptoms free period should not be >2 months at a stretch	

Diagnose as follows:

- *With pure dysthymic syndrome*: Full criteria for a major depressive episode have never been met in at least the preceding 2 years.
- *Dysthymia with persistent major depressive episode*: Full criteria for a major depressive episode have been met throughout the preceding 2-year period.

Treatment Modalities for Depression

1 *Drugs*: The treatment of major depression usually requires starting pharmacotherapy with antidepressants:
   - Tricyclic antidepressants (TCAs): Imipramine, Amitriptyline, Trimipramine, Clomipramine, Desipramine, Nortriptyline, Amoxapine, Reboxetine;
   - SSRI (selective serotonin reuptake inhibitors): Fluoxetine, Paroxetine, Sertaline, Citalopram, Escitalopram. These drugs devoid of side effects seen with TCAs and are safe in elderly;
   - Atypical antidepressants: Trazodone, Mianserine, Mitrazapine, Venlafaxine, Duloxetine, Tianeptine, Amineptine, Bupropion.
2. *Electroconvulsive therapy (ECT)*: Indications of ECT in depression are: Suicidal risk, Depression with psychotic feature, Resistant depression, Severe agitated or stuporous depression with lack of self-care.
3. *Psychotherapy*: Supportive psychotherapy, cognitive behavioral psychotherapy

Choice of Anti-depressants

- There is no ideal antidepressant. First choice is determined by side effect profile least objectionable to patient's physical status, severity of disorder including self-harm, patient preference and nature of any associated illness.
- Since SSRIs are comparatively free of side effects and are not costly, they are generally recommended as first choice antidepressants. Where there is a previous history of response to a specific drug or class, the best first choice is that antidepressant.

6. Treatment of choice for acute depression is:

a. SSRIs b. Alprazolam
c. ECT d. Psychotherapy

Ans. is 'a' SSRIs

7. Duration of the disease for the diagnosis of dysthymia is:

a. 2 years b. 4 years
c. 6 years d. 8 years

Ans. is 'a' 2 years

DSM-5 diagnostic criteria for a major depressive episode
A. Five (or more) of the following symptoms have been present during the same two-week period and represent a change from previous functioning; at least one of the symptoms is either (1) depressed mood or (2) loss of interest or pleasure. *Note*: Do not include symptoms that are clearly attributable to another medical condition.
1. Depressed mood most of the day, nearly every day, as indicated by either subjective report (e.g, feels sad, empty, hopeless) or observations made by others (e.g., appears tearful). (*Note*: In children and adolescents, can be irritable mood.)
2. Markedly diminished interest or pleasure in all, or almost all, activities most of the day, nearly every day (as indicated by either subjective account or observation)
3. Significant weight loss when not dieting or weight gain (e.g., a change of more than 5% of body weight in a month), or decrease or increase in appetite nearly every day. (*Note*: In children, consider failure to make expected weight gain.)
4. Insomnia or hypersomnia nearly every day
5. Psychomotor agitation or retardation nearly every day (observable by others, not merely subjective feelings of restlessness or being slowed down)
6. Fatigue or loss of energy nearly every day
7. Feelings of worthlessness or excessive or inappropriate guilt (which may be delusional) nearly every day (not merely self-reproach or guilt about being sick)

Contd...

Contd...

DSM-5 diagnostic criteria for a major depressive episode
8. Diminished ability to think or concentrate, or indecisiveness, nearly every day (either by their subjective account or as observed by others)
9. Recurrent thoughts of death (not just fear of dying), recurrent suicidal ideation without a specific plan, or a suicide attempt or a specific plan for committing suicide
B. The symptoms cause clinically significant distress or impairment in social, occupational, or other important areas of functioning.
C. The episode is not attributable to the direct physiological effects of a substance or to another medical condition. *Note*: Criteria A through C represent a major depressive episode. *Note*: Responses to a significant loss (e.g., bereavement, financial ruin, losses from a natural disaster, a serious medical illness or disability) may include the feelings of intense sadness, rumination about the loss, insomnia, poor appetite, and weight loss noted in Criterion A, which may resemble a depressive episode. Although such symptoms may be understandable or considered appropriate to the loss, the presence of a major depressive episode in addition to the normal response to a significant loss should also be carefully considered. This decision inevitably requires the exercise of clinical judgement based on the individual's history and the cultural norms for the expression of distress in the context of loss.
D. The occurence of the major depressive episode is not better explained by schizoaffective disorder, schizophrenia, schizophreniform disorder, delusoinal disorder, or other specified and unspecified schizophrenia spectrum and other psychotic disorders.
E. There has never been a manic or hypomanic episode. *Note*: This exclusion does not apply if all of the manic-like or hypomanic-like epsidoes are substance-induced or are attributable to the physiological effects of another medical condition.

Unipolar major depression with psychotic features, schizophrenia, and schizoaffective disorder can all present with delusions and hallucinations. However, in unipolar psychotic depression, delusions and hallucinations occur only during an episode of major depression. By contrast, in schizophrenia and schizoaffective disorder, psychotic symptoms can and do occur in the absence of major depression.

8. A patient presents with persistence sadness of mood, loss of desire to do anything and feeling of low energy for 6 months. He gets awake early in the morning and does not feel like eating anything. Recently since 2 weeks, he also started ex-periencing voices telling him to end his life. What is the diagnosis? *(NEET 2020)*

a. Schizophrenia
b. Depression with psychosis
c. Delusional disorder
d. Dysthymia

Ans. is 'b' Depression with psychosis

OBSESSIVE COMPULSIVE DISORDER (OCD)

- OCD involves recurrent, intrusive, and distressing thoughts, images or impulses (Obsession) and repetitive mental or behavioral acts (Compulsion) performed to reduce stress arising from the obsession.
- Defense mechanisms for OCD are isolation, undoing and reaction formation
- Obsessions are recognized as one's own idea but is Ego-alien (foreign to one's personality). Attempts to suppress them results in distress.

Types of OCD

1. Washers (most common)
2. Checkers
3. Pure obsession
4. Obsession slowness

Most common obsessions:

1. Contamination
2. Pathological doubt
3. Somatic
4. Need for symmetry
5. Aggressive
6. Sexual

Most common compulsions:

1. Checking
2. Washing
3. Counting
4. Need to ask for confess
5. Symmetry and precision
6. Hoarding

Management of OCD

1. *Behaviour Therapy (BT)*:
   - It is the treatment of choice for OCD
   - Exposure and response prevention is the preferred and principal approach. It is most effective in compulsions.
   - Other methods are flooding, thought stopping, systemic desensitization, implosion therapy, modeling, and aversive conditioning.
2. *Pharmacotherapy*: Drug of choice: SSRI
3. *Psychotherapy*: Supportive psychotherapy is given.
4. *ECT*: For extreme cases that are resistant and chronically debilitating, ECT and psychosurgery are considerations.
5. *Psychosurgery*:
   - Procedures: Stereotactic limbic leucotomy (cingulotomy), stereotactic subcaudate tractotomy (capsulotomy)

Prognosis of OCD

- A poor prognosis is indicated by yielding to (rather than resisting) compulsions, childhood onset, bizarre compulsions, need for hospitalization, coexisting major depressive disorder, delusional beliefs, presence of overvalued ideas (i.e. some acceptance of obsessions and compulsions), presence of a personality disorder (especially schizotypal personality disorder) and presence of comorbid hoarding disorder.
- A good prognosis is indicated by good social and occupational adjustment, presence of a precipitating event and episodic nature of the symptoms.
- The obsessional content does not seem to be related to the prognosis.

9. Which of the following is the poor prognostic factor for OCD? *(NEET 2019)*

a. Magical thinking
b. Dirt contamination
c. Pathological doubt
d. Hoarding

Ans. is 'd' Hoarding

10. Recurrent thought of doing something are known as:

a. Obsession
b. Compulsion
c. Preoccupation
d. Confabulations

Ans. is 'a' Obsession

POST-TRAUMATIC STRESS DISORDER (PTSD)

- According to ICD-10, this disorder arises as a delayed protracted response to an exceptionally stressful or catastrophic life event or situation, which is likely to cause pervasive distress in any person (e.g. disasters, war, rape or torture, serious accident)
- PTSD is characterized by recurrent and intrusive recollections of the stressful event, either in flashbacks (images, thoughts, or perceptions) or in dreams. There is an associated sense of re-experiencing of the stressful event. There is marked avoidance of the events or situations that arouse recollections of the stressful event, along with marked symptoms of anxiety. There is also partial amnesia for some aspects of the event.
- *Treatment*: Supportive psychotherapy, Cognitive behavior therapy

11. A group of 4 teenagers while going for a trip met a car accident. Out of four, 3 people died on the spot. Surviving girl was admitted in an ICU for 3 months. After being discharged she often gets up in night and feels terrified. She says that she sees same events in her dreams. She is now afraid of the cars. The diagnosis is:

a. Anxiety disorder
b. Phobia
c. Conversion disorder
d. Post-traumatic stress disorder

Ans. is 'd' Post-traumatic stress disorder

GENERALIZED ANXIETY DISORDER

- This is characterized by excessive anxiety and worry which are persistent and generalized and not restricted to any specific situation or object.
- Duration of symptoms should be at least 6 months.
- Associated with at least three symptoms from following (Along with anxiety):
  - Restlessness or feeling keyed up
  - Difficulty concentrating
  - Muscle tension
  - Irritability
  - Easily fatigued
  - Sleep disturbance
- Benzodiazepines are the drug of choice.

12. Meena, a 42-year-old divorced lady, lives with her mother. She has no significant past medical history, but she frequently makes appointment with her GP problems experienced by her. She complains of feeling 'stressed' all the time and constantly worries about 'anything and everything'. This is also affecting her performance at her work. She describes herself as always having been a 'worrier' but her anxiety has become much worse in the past 12 months since her mother became unwell, and she no longer feels that she feels tension in her shoulders, stomach and legs, her heart races and sometimes she finds it difficult to breathe. Her sleep is poor with difficulty getting off to sleep due to worrying and frequent wakening. She feels tired and irritable. She does not drink any alcohol. Most likely diagnosis is:

a. Panic disorder
b. Generalized anxiety disorder
c. Depression
d. Conversion disorder

Ans. is 'b' Generalized anxiety disorder

PANIC DISORDER

Panic disorder: DSM-5 diagnostic criteria for panic disorder are described below.

- Recurrent unexpected panic attacks
- At least one of the attacks has been followed by a month or more of one or both of the following:
  - Persistent concern or worry about additional panic attacks or their consequences (e.g., losing control, having a heart attack, "going crazy").
  - A significant maladaptive change in behavior related to the attacks (e.g., behaviors designed to avoid having panic attacks, such as avoidance of exercise or unfamiliar situations).
- The disturbance is not attributable to the physiological effects of a substance (e.g., medication or illicit drug) or another medical condition (e.g., hyperthyroidism, cardiopulmonary disorders).
- The disturbance is not better explained by another mental disorder. As examples, the panic attacks do not occur only in response to:
  - Feared social situations, as in social anxiety disorder
  - Circumscribed phobic objects or situations, as in specific phobia
  - Obsessions, as in obsessive-compulsive disorder
  - Reminders of traumatic events, as in posttraumatic stress disorder
  - Separation from attachment figures, as in separation anxiety disorder

13. A young female presents with tachycardia, palpitations and an impending sense of death. Her physical examination is absolutely normal. She keeps worrying about trivial things all the time. What is the diagnosis? *(NEET 2020)*

a. Panic disorder
b. Conversion disorder
c. Somatoform disorder
d. Malingering

Ans. is 'a' Panic disorder

ALCOHOL WITHDRAWAL SYMPTOMS

- *Common symptoms*: Hangover (MC) on the next morning, fine tremor, nausea, vomiting, weakness, anxiety and restlessness.
- Three severe withdrawal syndrome are delirium tremens, Alcoholic hallucinosis, and alcoholic seizure (fits).

1. Delirium tremens
   - Delirium tremens is the most severe alcohol withdrawal syndrome. It occurs usually within 2–4 days of alcohol abstinence. It is characterized by:
     - Clouding of consciousness with disorientation in time and place.
     - Poor attention span and distractibility
     - Visual (and also auditory) hallucination, and illusion. Tactile hallucination of insect crawling under the skin (formication) may also occur.
     - Marked autonomic disturbances with tachycardia, sweating, hypertension, mydriasis, coarse tremors.
   - Benzodiazepines are the drugs of choice for delirium tremens. Chlordiazepoxide is the agent of choice with diazepam as an alternative.
2. Alcoholic seizures (rum fits)
   - Generalized tonic clonic seizures occur, usually 12–48 hours after a heavy bout of drinking. Benzodiazepines are the drugs of choice for alcoholic seizures.
3. Alcoholic hallucinosis
   - Alcoholic hallucinosis is characterized by the presence of hallucinations in the presence of clear consciousness. Develops within 12–24 hours after drinking stops.
   - Order of hallucinations in alcohol withdrawal is auditory > visual > tactile.

14. A 40-year-old male with history of alcohol abuse for 20 years is brought to the hospital emergency with complains of fearfulness, talking to self, aggressive behavior, tremulousness and saying that there insects crawling under his skin. Physical examination shows tachycardia, palpitations, sweating, and high grade fever. He is unable to recognize few of his family members. There is history of drinking alcohol two days prior to the onset of the present complaints. He is most likely suffering from:

a. Delirium tremens
b. Alcoholic hallucinosis
c. Schizophrenia
d. Seizure disorder

Ans. is 'a' Delirium tremens

Psychiatry

DELIRIUM

- It is characterized by reduced ability to focus, sustain, or shift attention
- Clouding of consciousness, impairment of immediate recall and recent memory, with relatively intact remote memory, disorientation in time, place or person are characteristic features.
- Symptoms are rapid in onset and often fluctuant
- Speech is disorganized (rambling, irrelevant, illogical speech)
- Psychomotor disturbances: Rapid shifts from hypoactivity to hyperactivity; increased reaction time; enhanced startle reaction
- Insomnia, nocturnal worsening of symptoms, disturbing dreams and nightmares which may continue as hallucinations and illusions after awakening are other features.

	Delirium	Dementia
Course	Acute	Insidious
Consciousness	Clouded	Usually normal
Orientation	Disturbed	Normal
Memory	Immediate retention disturbed	Immediate retention normal
Comprehension	Impaired	Impaired only in late stage
Sleep wake cycle	Disturbed	Normal
Perception	Visual illusions and hallucinations common	Hallucinations may occur

15. Difference between dementia and delirium is:

a. Attention is impaired in delirium
b. Consciousness is impaired in dementia
c. Orientation is normal in dementia
d. All of the above

Ans. is 'a' Attention is impaired in delirium

PERSONALITY DISORDERS

Personality disorders are organized into three "clusters" in both the DSM-IV-TR and DSM-5. The disorders in each cluster share key features or have overlap in terms of the characteristics of individuals who are diagnosed within that cluster.

'Cluster A'

The "Cluster A" personality disorders are characterized by odd or eccentric behavior. Individuals with the personality disorders in this cluster tend to experience major disruptions in relationships because their behavior may be perceived as peculiar, suspicious or detached. The "Cluster A" personality disorders include:

- *Schizotypal personality disorder*: Exhibit marked eccentricities of thought, perception, and behavior
- *Paranoid personality disorder*: It is characterized by generalized mistrust and suspiciousness about the motives and actions of others and a tendency to interpret them as malevolent
- *Schizoid personality disorder*: Lack of interpersonal relationship and the lack of desire to obtain such relationships

'Cluster B'

The "Cluster B" personality disorders are characterized by dramatic or erratic behavior. Individuals with the personality disorders in this cluster lend to either experience very intense emotions or engage in extremely impulsive, theatrical, promiscuous or law-breaking behaviors. The "Cluster B" personality disorders include:

- *Borderline personality disorder*: Pervasive pattern of unstable and intense interpersonal relationship, self-perception and mood. The patient makes recurrent suicidal threats and gestures.
- *Histrionic personality disorder*: Excessive emotionality and attention-seeking behaviour
- *Antisocial personality disorder*: Disregard for and violation of the rights of the other and the rules of the society
- *Narcissistic personality disorder*: Ideas of grandiosity and require admiration from others

'Cluster C'

The "Cluster C" personality disorders are characterized by anxiety. Individuals with the personality disorders in this cluster tend to experience pervasive anxiety and/or fearfulness. 'The "Cluster C" personality disorders include:

- Dependent personality disorder
- Obsessive-compulsive personality disorder
- Avoidant personality disorder

16. A 40-year-old married male thinks that he is multitalented and is always overconfident. He never listens to his family or friends. In fact whenever anyone gives him any advice, he thinks that they have some motive against him. He is always suspicious of his wife. All these are features of:

a. Borderline personality disorder
b. Schizoid personality disorder
c. Paranoid personality disorder
d. Histrionic personality disorder

Ans. is 'c' Paranoid personality disorder

17. A 24-year-old girl named Heena is often flamboyantly dressed and goes out on dates frequently. Although she changed boyfriend almost monthly, but she used to plan her marriage and future with each of them with equal enthusiasm and optimism. She would often make stories to seek attention. She would feel uncomfortable at big parties leave them midway. Heena made promises to other people that were impossible to keep but seemed to be aimed at winning their approval; when she broke the promise, she usually made up a story designed to elicit sympathy and compassion. Diagnosis is:

a. Borderline personality disorder
b. Histrionic personality disorder
c. Dependent personality disorder
d. Antisocial personality disorder

Ans. is 'b' Histrionic personality disorder

18. Borderline personality is characterized by:

a. Unstable and intense interpersonal relationship
b. Violation of the rules
c. Grandiose
d. Attention seeking behavior

Ans. is 'a' Unstable and intense interpersonal relationship

POLYSOMNOGRAPHY

- Polysomnography is a continuous, comprehensive recording of physiological parameters during sleep.
- It is recorded at night for 6–8 hrs.
- Parameters monitored are EEG, EOG, submental EMG, nasal-oral air fowl respiratory effort, hemoglobin saturation, heart rhythm and leg movements during sleep.
- Muscle tension and movements subside with deeper sleep and can also be used to diagnose periodic limb movement disorder and restless leg syndrome.

Indications

- Diagnosis of sleep-related breathing disorders
- Positive airway pressure titration and assessment of treatment efficacy
- Evaluation of sleep-related behaviors that are violent or may potentially harm the patient or bed partner

19. Sleep disturbances are diagnosed by:

a. Polysomnography
b. Oximetry
c. Echocardiography
d. Orthography

Ans. is 'a' Polysomnography

SOMNAMBULISM

- Somnambulism is a disorder of sleep arousal.
- It generally occurs in deep nonrapid eye movement (NREM) (stages 3 and 4) sleep and, thus, most often takes place in the first third of the night when these sleep stages are most common.
- The event may last from several minutes to an hour.
- There is complete amnesia about the event after waking up from sleep.
- Somnambulism can consist of very complex motor activity of which walking is just one element.
- Somnambulism may be precipitated by a variety of conditions such as insufficient sleep resulting from an irregular sleep schedule, staying up late, giving up a daily nap or waking early in the morning.

20. Not true about somnambulism among the following is: *(NEET 2019)*

a. Sleep walking
b. It occurs during NREM sleep
c. Disorder of sleep arousal
d. Only low level motor skill/function is present

Ans. is 'd' Only low level motor skill/function is present

AUTISTIC DISORDER

- It is characterized by qualitative impairment in reciprocal social interaction, delayed and aberrant communication skills and a restricted repertoire of activities and interests, with normal development.
- By definition, the onset is before the age of 3 years.
- More common in boys

Clinical Features

Autism (marked impairment in reciprocal social and interpersonal interaction)

- Absent social smile, lack of eye-to-eye-contact, lack of awareness of others existence or feelings; treats people as furniture, lack of attachment to parents and absence of separation anxiety, no or abnormal social play; prefers solitary games. Marked impairment in making friends, lack of imitative behaviour, absence of fear in presence of danger,

Marked impairment in language and non-verbal communication:

- Lack of verbal or facial response to sounds or voices; might be thought as deaf initially. Absent or delayed speech, abnormal speech patterns and content. Presence of echolalia, perseveration, poor articulation and pronominal reversal is common. Remote memory is usually good. Abstract thinking is impaired.

Abnormal behavioral characteristics:

- Mannerisms, Stereotyped behaviour such as head-banging, bodyspinning, lining-up objects, rocking, clapping, twirling, etc. Ritualistic and compulsive behaviour. Resistance to even the slightest change in the environment. Attachment may develop to inanimate objects. Hyperkinesis is commonly associated.

Mental retardation: > 50% of these children have moderate to profound mental retardation.

21. Autistic spectrum disorder:

a. Defective communication
b. Absent separation anxiety
c. Impaired concentration
d. More common in girls

Ans. is 'a' Defective communication

ATTENTION DEFICIT HYPERACTIVITY DISORDER (ADHD)

- Most common psychiatric problem in school-age population. It usually arises in the first 5 years of life and is three times more common in boys than in girls.
- Frequent symptoms of hyperactivity/impulsivity to a degree that is maladaptive and inconsistent with development level
- Present in more than one setting (school/home)
- Persist for at least six months
- Present before age of 12 years
- Impairs social/school functioning

Six (or more) of the following symptoms of inattention	*Six (or more) of the following symptoms of hyperactivity/impulsivity*
1. Often make careless mistakes	1. Often fidgets or squirms
2. Often has difficulty sustaining attention	2. Often leaves seat
3. Often does not listen	3. Often moves excessively (may feel restless)
4. Often fails to follow through on instruction or of finish tasks	4. Often has difficulty playing or engaging in leisure activities quietly
5. Often has difficulty organizing tasks and activities	5. Is often "on the go"
6. Often avoids tasks requiring sustained attention	6. Often talks excessively impulsivity
7. Often loses things	7. Often blurts out answers
8. Often is easily distracted by external stimuli	8. Often has difficulty awaiting turn
9. Often is forgetful in daily activities	9. Often interrupts or intrudes on others

22. A 10-year-old boy is so restless all the time. In the school, rest of the class is unable to concentrate because of him. He is hardly ever in his seat be it at home or school. He has difficulty in playing quietly. He does not listen to his mother at all. The most likely diagnosis is?

a. Attention-deficit hyperactivity disorder
b. Conduct disorder
c. Depressive disorder
d. Schizophrenia

Ans. is 'a' Attention-deficit hyperactivity disorder

Polygraph

- A polygraph, popularly referred to as a lie detector test, is a device or procedure that measures and records several physiological indicators such as blood pressure, pulse, respiration, and skin conductivity while a person is asked and answers a series of questions.

- The belief underpinning the use of the polygraph is that deceptive answers will produce physiological responses that can be differentiated from those associated with non-deceptive answers.
- There are, however, no specific physiological reactions associated with lying, making it difficult to identify factors that separate liars from truth tellers

23. Test based on the principle of physiological responses associated with a suspect's reaction to a question, is: *(NEET 2019)*

a. Narco analysis
b. Brain mapping
c. Truth serum testing
d. Polygraph

Ans. is 'd' Polygraph

FACTITIOUS DISORDER (MUNCHAUSEN SYNDROME)

- It is also known as hospital addiction, hospital hoboes, or Professional patient.
- Patients who repeatedly simulate or fake diseases (intentional for the sole purpose of obtaining medical attention). There is no other recognizable motive (in contrast malingering).
- Characterized by a restless journey from doctor to doctor and hospital to hospital, an ever-changing list of complaints and symptoms. Patient tries to maintain sick role to obtain medical attention. There may be evidence of earlier treatment usually surgical procedure, example multiple surgical scars (grid iron abdomen).
- The patients distort their clinical histories, laboratory tests reports and even facts about other aspects of their life, i.e. pseudologia fantastica.
- Patient has eagerness to undergo various tests, investigations and procedures.

24. A 25-year-old male c/o recurrent abdominal pain but biochemical assays and ultrasound abdomen is normal. He also complains of constant headache. He suddenly complains of loss of vision of bilateral eyes. Ophthalmologist finds nothing on examination. Symptoms are most probably due to:

a. Bilateral optic neuritis
b. Posterior inferior cerebellar artery infarct
c. Malingering
d. Factitious disorder

Ans. is 'd' Factitious disorder

Previously Asked Facts

- *Delusional Disorder*: One or more delusion lasting > 1 month, but without a mood disorder or other psychotic symptoms. Daily functioning, including socialization, may be impacted by the pathological, fixed belief but is otherwise unaffected. Can be shared by individuals in close relationships.
- Anhedonia is inability to experience pleasure
- Dramatic self-mutilation occurring in schizophrenia has also been called Von-Gogh syndrome
- Decreased levels of serotonin and norepinephrine are seen in Depression. Increase in epinephrine levels are seen in mania.
- Beck's cognitive triad represents three types of negative thoughts present in depression. The triad involves negative thoughts about: The self (i.e. the self is worthless) ; The world/environment (i.e. the world is unfair, helpless), and The future (i.e. the future is hopeless)
- Drug of choice for panic disorders—SSRIs; Drug of choice for acute panic attack—Benzodiazepines.
- Kleptomania is irresistible desire to steal things.
- Irresistible urge to drink alcohol is called Dipsomania.
- Agoraphobia refers to fear of crowds.
- Methadone is used as maintenance therapy for opioid addiction.
- Schizophrenia is associated with 3 types of personality disorders, i.e. schizoid, borderline and paranoid.
- Othello syndrome (morbid jealously) is delusion of Infidelity
- Drug of choice for Tourette Syndrome is Haloperidol
- Stanford Binet scale is a cognitive ability and intelligence test that is used to diagnose developmental or intellectual deficiencies in young children.
- Expression and consequent release of previously repressed emotion is called as Abreaction
- Most common side effect of unmodified Electro Convulsive Therapy (ECT) is fracture at T4–T8.
- Hypochondriasis is preoccupation with fear for a serious illness
- Freud coined the term "The Ego and The Id" and divided the mental apparatus (Personality) into three dynamic structures – The Id based on Pleasure principle, The Ego based on Reality principle, The Superego based on Idealism principle.

CHAPTER 19 Pediatrics

FETAL CIRCULATION

1. All are true about fetal circulation *except*: *(NEET 2020)*

a. Right umbilical vein disappears after birth
b. Functional closure of foramen ovale occurs soon after birth
c. Umbilical artery regresses to form medial umbilical ligament
d. Anatomical closure of ductus arteriosus occurs by 1 month.

Ans. is 'a' Right umbilical vein disappears after birth

Fate of the Umbilical Veins

In the normal fetus, the right umbilical vein begins to obliterate around the fourth week of gestation and disappears by the seventh week of gestation.

The neonate's left umbilical vein is completely obliterated and is replaced by a fibrous cord called the round ligament of the liver within a week

Fate of the Foramen Ovale

At birth, the right to left shunt provided by the foramen ovale ceases to function when changes in atrial pressure bring the overlapping portions of the septum primum (valve of the foramen ovale) and the septum secundum into apposition. The primary cause of septal apposition (closure of the foramen ovale) appears to be the result of an abrupt decrease in right atrial pressure which is associated with the sudden termination of placental circulation at birth, Le., clamping or tying the umbilical cord. Apposition may also be enhanced by the increase in left atrial pressure which is associated with the onset of pulmonary function, Le., increased perfusion and venous return.

Fate of the Ductus Arteriosus Postnatal Circulation

The ductus arteriosus begins to close almost immediately after birth and may be closed functionally within a few hours; complete obliteration of the lumen and fibrosis may require three or four weeks. It persists throughout life as the ligamentum arteriosum.

Fate of the Umbilical Arteries

The umbilical artery regresses after birth. A portion obliterates to become the medial umbilical ligament (be careful not to confuse this with the median umbilical ligament, a different structure that represents the remnant of the embryonic urachus). A portion remains open as a branch of the anterior division of the internal iliac artery.

Adult remnants of fetal circulatory structures

Fetal structure	***Adult remnant***
Foramen ovale	*Fossa ovalis* of the heart
Ductus arteriosus	*Ligamentum arteriosum*
Left umbilical vein	
Extra-hepatic portion Intra-hepatic portion (ductus venosus)	*Ligamentum tereshepatis* *Ligamentum venosum*
Left and right umbilical arteries	
Proximal portions Distal portions	Umbilical branches of internal iliac arteries Medial umbilical ligaments

KAWASAKI DISEASE

2. A child of 7 years presented with fever for 5 days along with conjunctivitis, rash over the palms and soles, red tongue and unilateral cervical lymphadenopathy. What is the diagnosis? *(NEET 2020)*

a. Kawasaki disease
b. Scarlet fever
c. Bacterial conjunctivitis
d. HSP

Ans. is 'a' Kawasaki disease

The classic clinical criteria for Kawasaki disease

- **Fever persisting at least 5 days**
- **Presence of at least 4 principal features:**
  - Changes in extremities
    - Acute: Erythema of palms, soles, edema of hands, feet
    - Subacute: periungal peeling in weeks 2 and 3 of illness
  - Polymorphous exanthem
  - Bilateral bulbar conjunctival injection without exudates
  - Changes in lips and oral cavity: erythema, lip cracking, strawberry tongue
  - Cervical lymphadenopathy (>1.5cm), usually unilateral
- **Exclusion of other diseases with similar findings**

The clinical scenario clearly fits the diagnostic criteria for Kawasaki disease. Scarlet fever (caused by streptococcus) is a close differential and needs to be ruled out before establishing the diagnosis.

Kawasaki disease	Scarlet fever
Fever responds poorly to antipyretics	Respond s well to antipyretics
Painful adenopathy	Painful adenopathy
Non-specific polymorphous rash	Rash blanches, may be in the form of fine papillae (sandpaper rash) or Pastia lines (marked in skin folds)
May lead to aneurysm formation	Not associated with aneurysm formation

Bacterial conjunctivitis is exudative and usually not associated with generalized rash, red tongue and cervical lymphadenopathy.

HSP (Henoch Schonlein Purpura) is the most common childhood vasculitis, involves small sized blood vessels (compared with Kawasaki disease which is a medium vessel vasculitis) and manifests with palpable purpuric rash generally over the lower limbs and buttocks region. Other features include pain abdomen with gross/microscopic hematuria.

3. First stool after birth is green due to: *(NEET 2020)*

a. Bilirubin
b. Biliverdin
c. Meconium
d. Gut flora

Ans. is 'c' Meconium

Explanation: Meconium is the earliest stool of a neonate. Unlike later feces, meconium is composed of materials ingested during the time the infant spends in the uterus: intestinal epithelial cells, lanugo, mucus, amniotic fluid, bile and water.

The gut of a newborn is sterile, therefore no gut flora contributes to the first stool.

GROWTH AND DEVELOPMENT

FONTANELLES

	Time of fusion
Anterior fontanelle	$1^{1/2}$–2 years
Posterior fontanelle	2–6 months
Anterolateral (Sphenoidal) fontanelle	2–3 months
Posterolateral (Mastoid) fontanelle	12 months

4. Last fontanelle to fuse in a child is: *(NEET 2018)*

a. Anterior
b. Posterior
c. Medial
d. Lateral

Ans. is 'a' Anterior

DEVELOPMENTAL MILESTONES

Gross Motor

Age	Milestone
3 mo	Neck holding
5 mo	Rolls over
6 mo	Sits in tripod position
8 mo	Sits without support

Contd...

Pediatrics

Contd...

Age	Milestone
10 mo	Stands with support
12 mo	Stands without support
15 mo	Walks alone
18 mo	Runs
2 yr	Walks up and downstairs, 2 feet per step
3 yr	Rides tricycle, alternate feet going upstairs
4 yr	Hops on one foot, alternate feet going downstairs

Fine Motor

Age	Milestone
4 mo	Bidextrous approach
6 mo	Unidextrous approach
9 mo	Immature pincer grasp
12 mo	Mature pincer grasp
15 mo	Imitates scribbling, tower of 2 blocks, drinks from cup
18 mo	Scribbles, tower of 3 blocks, feeds with spoon
2 yr	Tower of 6 blocks, vertical and circular strokes, undresses, turn pages of book one at a time
3 yr	Tower of 9 blocks, copies circle, dresses
4 yr	Copies cross, bridge with blocks
5 yr	Copies triangle, gate with blocks

Social and Adaptive

Age	Milestone
2 mo	Social smile
3 mo	Recognizes mother
6 mo	Stranger anxiety, inhibits to no
9 mo	Waves bye bye, repeats activity when appreciated
12 mo	Comes when called, plays simple ball game
15 mo	Jargon, points to objects of interest
18 mo	Copies parents in task
2 yr	Asks for food, drink, toilet
3 yr	Shares toys, knows full name and gender
4 yr	Plays cooperatively in group, goes to toilet alone
5 yr	Helps in household tasks

Language

Age	Milestone
1 mo	Alerts to sound
3 mo	Coos
4 mo	Laughs loud
6 mo	Monosyllables
9 mo	Bisyllables
12 mo	1–2 words with meaning
18 mo	8–10 words vocabulary
2 yr	2–3 word sentences, uses pronouns
3 yr	Asks questions
4 yr	Sings song, tell stories
5 yr	Asks meaning of words

5. What is the age of the child who draws a circle and builds tower of 7 cubes?

a. 1 year
b. 2 years
c. 2 ½ years
d. 3 years

Ans. is 'd' 3 years

6. Bidextrous grip is seen at what age? *(NEET 2019)*

a. 4 months
b. 5 months
c. 6 months
d. 7 months

Ans. is 'a' 4 months

7. Vocabulary of a 1 year old child is:

a. Limited to a bisyllable sound like baba, mama
b. 2 words with meaning
c. 10 words with meaning
d. Simple sentence

Ans. is 'b' 2 words with meaning

8. Which of the following can be done by an 18 months old baby?

a. Making tower of 9 cubes
b. Can use 10 words with meaning
c. Ride tricycle
d. Turn pages of book one at a time

Ans. is 'b' Can use 10 words with meaning

SHORT STATURE

Constitutional Delay in Growth

- The most common cause of short stature in mid childhood period but the ultimate height is normal.
- Their birth weight and height are normal. Strong family history of parents having short stature in childhood with delay in onset of puberty is usually present.
- The average growth velocity is normal and ultimate growth potential is adequate.
- The bone age is less than chronological age
- Upper segment and lower segment ratio is normal.

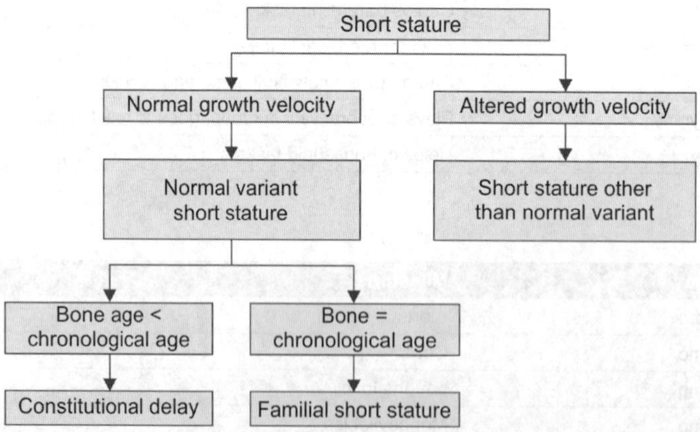

9. If chronological age > skeletal age with normal growth velocity, then the final height that is expected to be achieved is:

a. Normal
b. Less because of small bones
c. More than expected
d. Less because of epiphyseal closure due to accelerated growth velocity

Ans. is 'a' Normal

NEONATOLOGY

RESPIRATORY DISTRESS SYNDROME

10. A premature baby develops respiratory distress syndrome. Which cells are defective in this baby? *(NEET 2020)*

a. Type 1 alveolar pneumocytes
b. Type 2 alveolar pneumocytes
c. Capillary endothelial cells
d. Bronchial mucosal cells

Ans. is 'b' Type 2 alveolar pneumocytes

Surfactant is synthesized within the alveolar type II pneumocytes starting with phospholipid synthesis in the endoplasmic reticulum, then is processed through the Golgi apparatus to the lamellar bodies. Phospholipids combine with the surfactant proteins SP-B and SP-C to form the surfactant lipoprotein complex within the lamellar bodies. Lamellar bodies localize to the apical surface of the type II cell and are released into the alveoli by exocytosis.

The protein content of surfactant from preterm lung is low relative to the amount of surfactant lipid. In general, type II cells with lamellar bodies appear in the human lung after 20 weeks with very little surfactant protein mRNA expression until later in gestation. The expression of the four surfactant proteins varies with gestational age: SP-A increases after 32 weeks gestation, SP-B increases after 34 weeks gestation, SP-C mRNA is highly expressed at the tip of branching airways during early lung development, and expression of SP-D mRNA is low until late gestation.

In the preterm infant, both a decrease in the quantity and quality of surfactant contributes to decreased surfactant activity, resulting in RDS.

11. A premature infant delivered at 32 weeks presents with respiratory distress after birth. Which of the following is deficient in him? *(NEET 2020)*

a. Dipalmitoylphosphatidylcholine
b. Dipalmitoyl ethanolamine
c. Sphingomyelin
d. Cardiolipin

Ans. is 'a' Dipalmitoylphosphatidylcholine

Pulmonary surfactant is a complex mixture that is mostly composed of lipids (90 percent), primarily phospholipids, and approximately 10 percent proteins.

- **Lipid:** Approximately 70 percent of the lipid in surfactant is phosphatidylcholine species. Of this, approximately 60 percent is disaturatedpalmitoylphosphatidyl choline, the main component of surfactant that lowers alveolar surface tension.
- **Protein:** Four surfactant-specific proteins have been identified, and their functions have been partly elucidated. They include the hydrophobic surfactant proteins SP-B and SP-C, and the hydrophilic proteins SP-A and SP-D

PRIMITIVE CNS REFLEXES

Reflex	Description	Age of appearance	Age of disappearance
Moro	Light drop of head → sudden extension followed by flexion of arms and legs	28–32 weeks gestation	3–6 months
Grasp	Placing finger in palm results in flexing of infant's fingers	28 weeks gestation	2–3 months
Rooting	Tactile stimulus at side of mouth → mouth pursues the stimulus	32 weeks gestation	Less prominent after 1 month
Asymmetrical tonic neck	With infant supine, turning of the head results in ipsilateral extension of arm and leg with flexion of opposite extremities in a 'fencing' posture	35 weeks gestation	6 months
Parachute	Infant is suspended face down by the chest. When infant is moved toward a table, the arms extend as if to protect self	8 months postnatal	Remains throughout life

12. True about tonic neck reflex is:

a. Extension of arm on ipsilateral side, flexion on contralateral side
b. Extension of arm on contralateral side, flexion on ipsilateral side
c. Extension of arm on both sides
d. Flexion of arms on both sides

Ans. is 'a' Extension of arm on ipsilateral side, flexion on contralateral side

13. Asymmetric tonic neck reflex disappears at what age?

a. 2 months
b. 3 months
c. 6 months
d. 8 months

Ans. is 'c' 6 months

NEONATAL JAUNDICE

Criteria for Physiological Jaundice

- Clinical jaundice appears after 24 hours of age.
- Total bilirubin rises by less than 5 mg/dL per day (no sudden rise).

- ❖ Peak bilirubin occurs at 3–5 days of age, with a total bilirubin of no more than 15 mg/dL
- ❖ Clinical jaundice is resolved by 1 week in term infants and 2 weeks in preterm infants

Management of Neonate Presenting with Jaundice

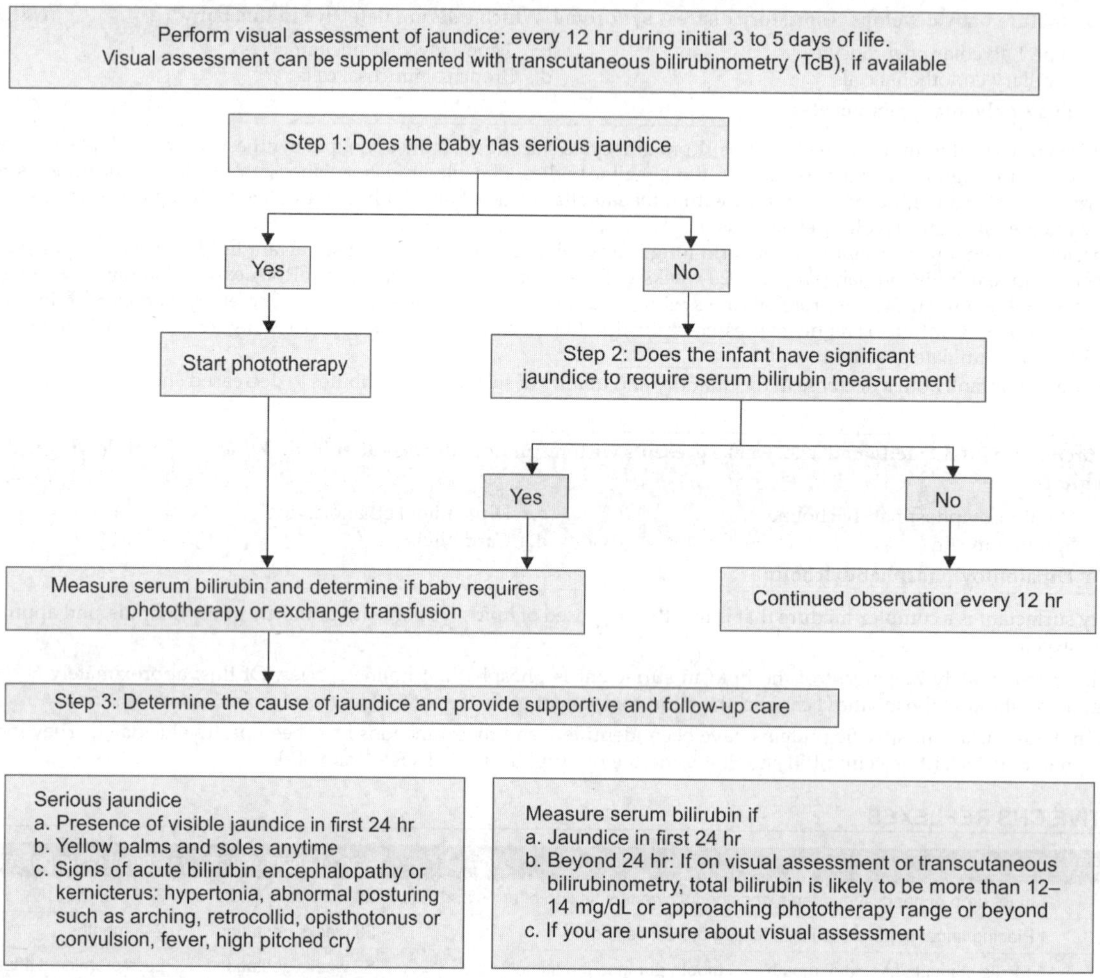

14. At what age is physiological jaundice seen?

a. At birth
b. One week of life
c. One month of age
d. One year of age

Ans. is 'b' One week of life

Pediatrics

15. A term newborn 2700 gm weight, presented with jaundice on 5th day of life with S.bilirubin levels 14 mg%. What is the appropriate management? *(NEET 2020)*

a. Phototherapy
b. Exchange transfusion
c. Routine newborn care
d. Stop breast feeding for 2 days

Ans. is 'c' Routine newborn care

- ❖ Neonatal hyperbilirubinemia cut offs for phototherapy and exchange transfusion vary with gestational age and day of life.
- ❖ NICE (National Institute of health and Clinical Excellence) guidelines, 2016, have given these cut off values in graphical and tabular forms for gestational ages 23 weeks to ≥38 weeks.
- ❖ These values are given in micromoles/litre. To obtain values in mg/dL (unit used in the Indian scenario and asked in the question) the value in micromoles/litre is divided by 17.1.
- ❖ E.g. In a neonate born at 37 weeks gestation, on day 4 of life, the cut off for phototherapy is 270 micromole/L which is equal to 15.8mg/dL (270/17.1) (See graph below)

Treatment threshold graph for babies with neonatal jaundice

Baby's name ______ Date of birth ______

Hospital number ______ Time of birth ______ Direct Antiglobulin Test ______ **37 weeks gestation**

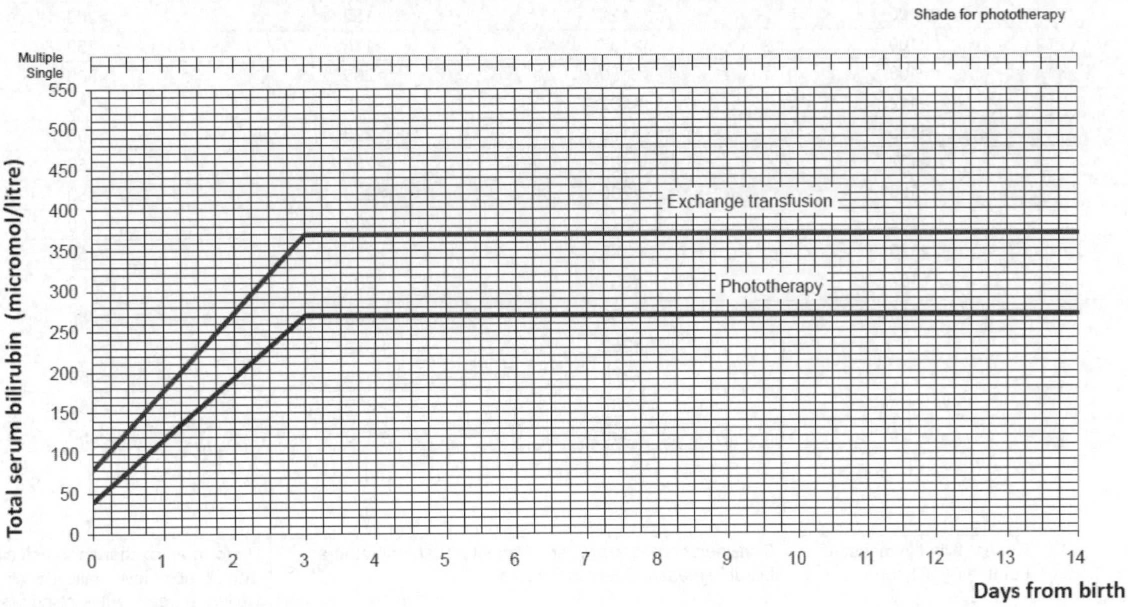

Key Points for Answering Such Questions

- For a newborn mentioned as term use cut offs for ≥38 weeks. (graph given below)
- Cut off values for both phototherapy and exchange transfusion plateau after day 3 (72hrs) of life at all gestations. (except for term newborns in whom the phototherapy cut off plateaus at day 4 of life).
- The cut off for phototherapy in term newborns is 20.4mg% after day 4 of life
- The cut off for exchange transfusion in term newborns is 26.3mg% after day 3 of life

Treatment threshold graph for babies with neonatal jaundice

Baby's name ______ Date of birth ______

Hospital number ______ Time of birth ______ Direct Antiglobulin Test ______ **>=38 weeks gestation**

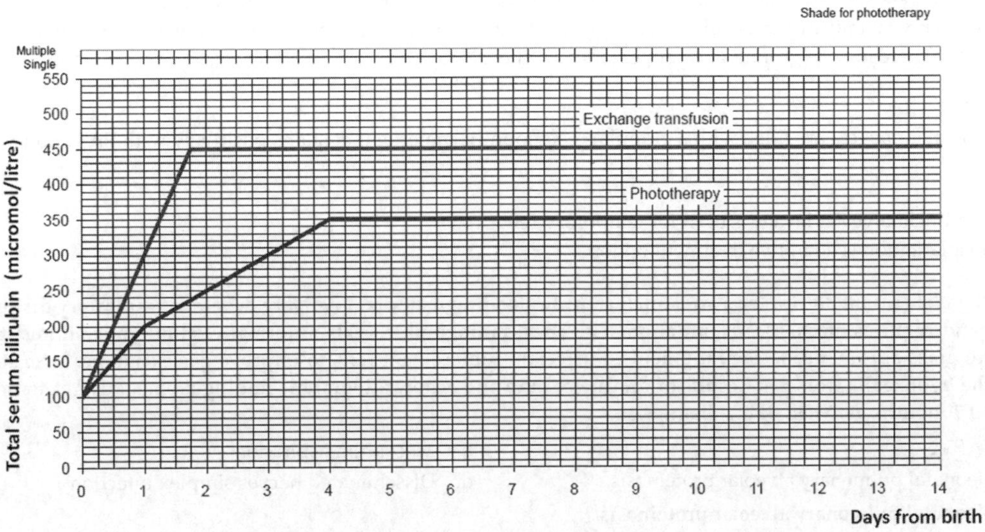

Therefore in the above question a serum bilirubin level of 14mg% in a term baby is below cut off for both phototherapy and exchange transfusion. It is suggestive of physiological jaundice and does not mandate cessation of breast feeding.

Consensus-based bilirubin thresholds for the management of babies of 38 weeks or more gestational age with hyperbilirubinaemia				
Age (hours)	***Bilirubin measurement (micromol/litre)***			
0			>100	>100
6	>100	>112	>125	>150
12	>100	>125	>150	>200
18	>100	>137	>175	>250
24	>100	>150	>200	>300
30	>112	>162	>212	>350
36	>125	>175	>225	>400
42	>137	>187	>237	>450
48	>150	>200	>250	>450
54	>162	>212	>262	>450
60	>175	>225	>275	>450
66	>187	>237	>287	>450
72	>200	>250	>300	>450
78		>262	>312	>450
84		>275	>325	>450
90		>287	>337	>450
96+		>300	>350	>450
	↓	↓	↓	↓
Action	Repeat bilirubin measurement in 6–12 hours	Consider phototherapy and repeat bilirubin measurement in 6 hours	Start phototherapy	Perform an exchange transfusion unless the bilirubin level falls below threshold while the treatment is being prepared

PULMONARY ALVEOLAR PROTEINOSIS

It is characterized by intra-alveolar accumulation of pulmonary surfactant.

Pathogenesis

There is impairment of the rapid spread and absorption of the phospholipid due to the absence of protein B. The alveoli thus fail to expand, resulting in respiratory distress.

Clinical Manifestation

- There are two different types of presentations:
  - Fatal form: Presents immediately after birth (congenital PAP)
  - Gradually progressive form: Presenting in older infants & children.
- Newborn may present with respiratory distress, and the presentation mimics pneumonia, generalized bacterial infection, respiratory distress syndrome and total anomalous pulmonary venous return with obstruction. Usually newborn is full term and may have positive family history. Child usually present with respiratory distress immediately after birth which does not respond to surfactant. There may be ground glass appearance on chest X-ray.

Investigations

Lung biopsy: Distal air spaces are filled with a granular, eosinophilic material that stains positively with PAS and is diastase resistant.

Treatment

- Repeated bronchoalveolar lavage is used for temporary relief.
- Lung transplantation is definitive treatment option.

16. A 3.3 kg male infant born at term after an uncomplicated pregnancy and delivery develops respiratory distress shortly after birth and requires mechanical ventilation. The chest radiograph reveals a normal cardiothymic silhouette but a diffuse ground glass appearance to the lung fields. Surfactant replacement fails to improve gas exchange. Over the first week of life, the hypoxemia worsens. Results of routine culture and echocardiographic finding are negative. A term female sibling died at 1 month age. Most likely diagnosis:

a. TAPVC
b. Meconium aspiration
c. Neonatal pulmonary alveolar proteinosis
d. Disseminated herpes simplex infection

Ans. is 'c' Neonatal pulmonary alveolar proteinosis

NEONATAL RESUSCITATION

Neonatal Resuscitation Algorithm: 2015 Update

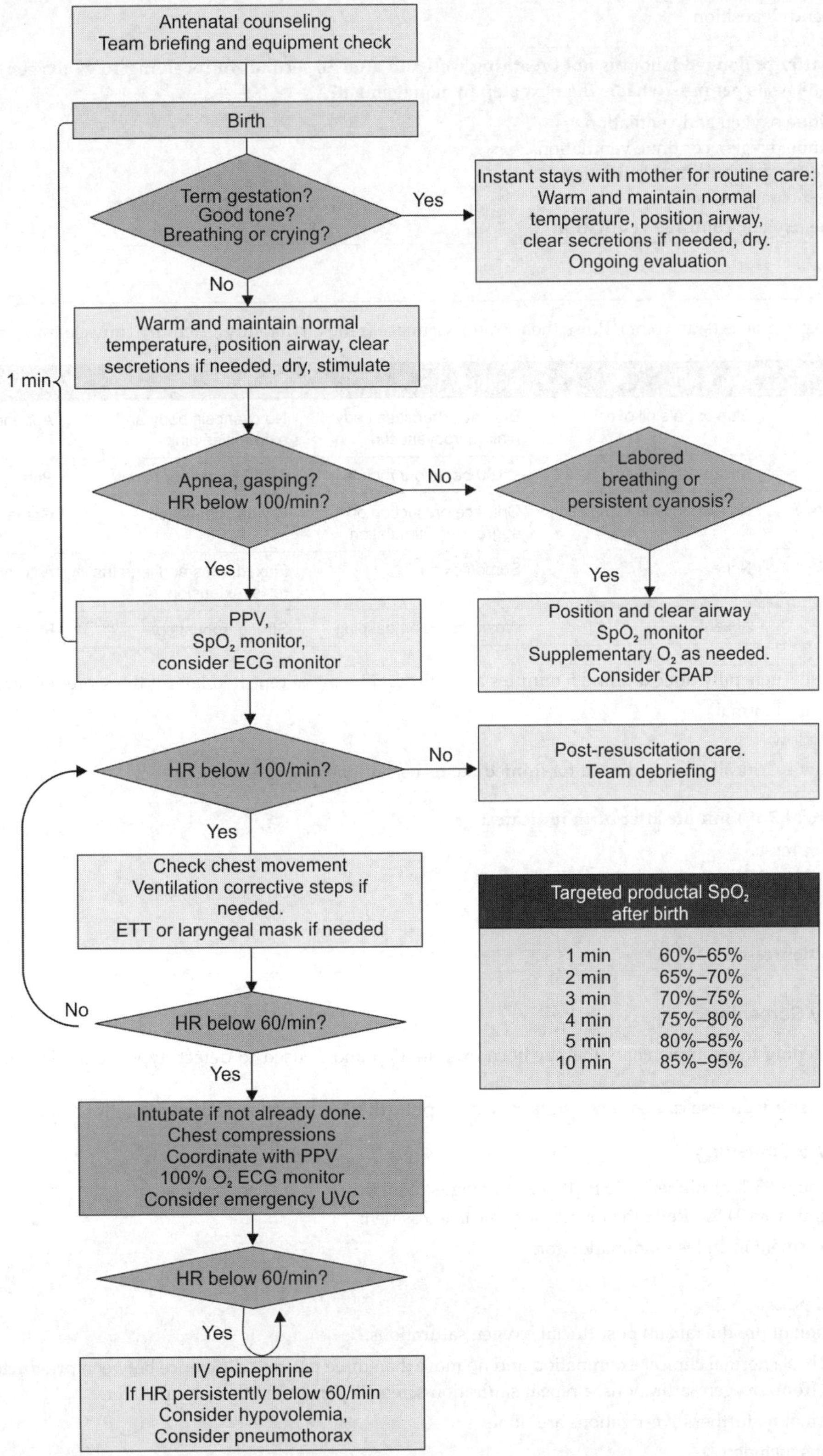

Targeted productal SpO_2 after birth	
1 min	60%–65%
2 min	65%–70%
3 min	70%–75%
4 min	75%–80%
5 min	80%–85%
10 min	85%–95%

The "Initial Steps" of resuscitation include the following:
1. *Warmth*: By placing the baby under a radiant warmer.
2. *Positioning*: Placed on her back or side with the neck slightly extended with the help of a shoulder roll.
3. *Clearing the airway*: Always suction Mouth before Nose to prevent aspiration. ('M' before 'N')
4. Dry, Stimulate and Reposition

17. A newborn after prolonged labour is not breathing well and after 30 seconds of receiving 100% oxygen by bag and mask, heart rate is 88 beats per min, what is the next step in management?

a. Discontinue oxygen and ventilation
b. Discontinue oxygen, continue ventilation
c. Continue oxygen, continue ventilation
d. Start chest compressions

Ans. is 'c' Continue oxygen, continue ventilation

APGAR SCORE

APGAR stands for Appearance (skin color), Pulse (heart rate), Grimace (reflex irritability), Activity (muscle tone), and Respiration.

	Score of 0	Score of 1	Score of 2	Component of backronym
Skin color	Blue or pale all over	Blue at extremities body pink (acrocyanosis)	No cyanosis body and extremities pink	Appearance
Pulse rate	Absent	< 100 beats per minute	> 100 Beats per minute	Pulse
Reflex irritability grimace	No response to stimulation	Grimace on suction or aggressive stimulation	Cry on stimulation	Grimace
Activity	None	Some flexion	Flexed arms and legs that resist extension	Activity
Respiratory effort	Absent	Weak, irregular, gasping	Strong, robust cry	Respiration

Interpretation: The test is generally done at 1 and 5 minutes after birth and may be repeated later if the score remains low.
- Score 7 and above – Normal
- Score 4-6 – Fairly low
- Score 3 and below – Critically low and need for immediate resuscitation

18. APGAR score of 3 at 1 minute after birth indicates: *(NEET 2019)*

a. Mildly depressed
b. Further resuscitation not needed
c. Severely depressed
d. Normal

Ans. is 'c' Severely depressed

Newborn Oximetry Screening

- The oxygen screening test complements the newborn examination and is used to detect hypoxaemia in infants who otherwise appear well.
- Screening may identify diverse causes and results may prompt further examination and investigation.

Results of Oximetry Screening

1. Oxygen saturation is 95 % or higher – No further screening is required
2. Oxygen saturation is 90–94 % - Refer the infant for clinical assessment
   - Clinical assessment includes examination for:
     - Murmurs
     - Femoral pulses
     - Evaluation of pre-ductal and post-ductal oxygen saturations.
   - If the infant has a normal clinical examination and no more than three per cent difference between **pre-ductal (right hand)** and **post-ductal (foot)** oxygen saturations, a repeat saturation screen is performed three hours later.
   - If any abnormality, further investigations are done.
   - Investigations include:

- Four limb blood pressure
- Echocardiogram (echo); a normal electrocardiogram (ECG) may not exclude a cardiac lesion
- Chest X-ray.

❖ If the repeat screen has saturations of 90–94 per cent, admit the infant to the SCN for further assessment as this is usually indicative of an underlying pathology.

3. Oxygen saturation is less than 90% – Urgent referral to pediatric team and cardiology referral

Newborn Oximetry Screening

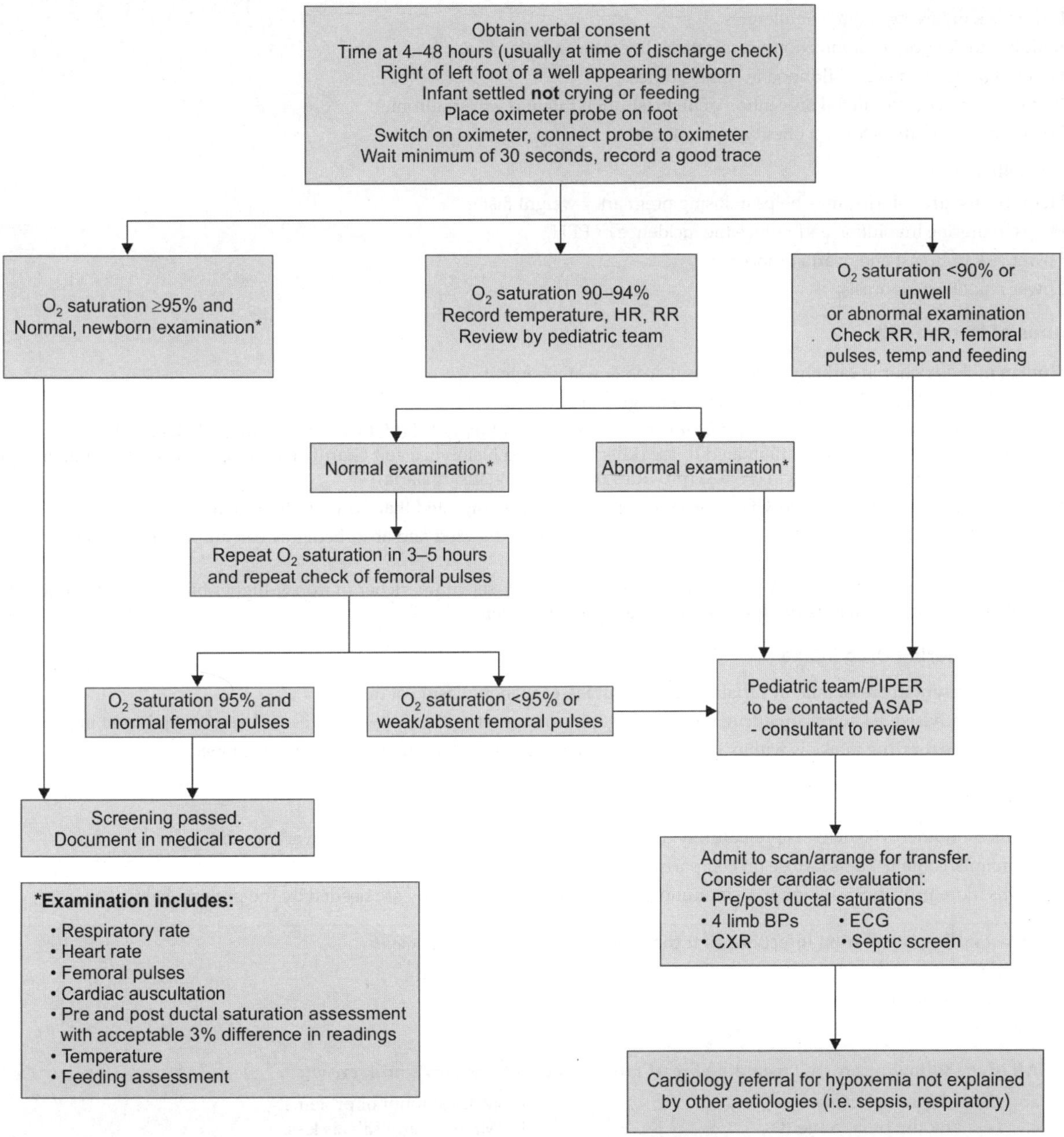

19. Where to look for pre-ductal O_2 saturation in PDA in a 3 minute born infant? *(NEET 2019)*

a. Left upper limb
b. Left lower limb
c. Right upper limb
d. Right lower limb

Ans. is 'c' Right upper limb

NUTRITION

BREASTFEEDING

Benefits of Breastfeeding

For the baby

- Breast milk provides the ideal nutrition for infants.
- Breast milk contains antibodies and other factors that boosts immunity.
- Lower risk of having asthma or allergies.
- Reduced incidence of ear infections, respiratory illnesses, and diarrhea.
- Higher IQ scores in later childhood in some studies.
- It may also have a role in the prevention of SIDS (sudden infant death syndrome).
- Lower the risk of diabetes and obesity in adulthood.

For the mother:

- Helps burn extra calories, thus helps in losing pregnancy weight faster.
- Helps in uterine involution and reduce the incidence of PPH.
- Lower risk of breast and ovarian cancer.
- Lower risk of osteoporosis.

Features of Human Milk

- Human milk is richer in carbohydrate (lactose), iron & water content
- Cow's milk is richer in fat, protein, calcium & energy content
- Breast milk contains several anti-infective factors—Antibodies secretory IgA, IgM, Lysozyme, Antistaphylococcal factor, Lactoferrin (inhibits growth of *E. Coli*), Bile stimulated lipase (kills entamoeba histolytica and Giardia lamblia), Bifidus factor (inhibits growth of *E. Coli*), Para amino-benzoic acid (PABA) (provides protection against malaria).
- *Human milk proteins*: More cystine & taurine; less methionine; better digested than cow's milk proteins
- *Human milk fats*: Higher levels of PUFAs, esp., linoleic acid; better digested and absorbed; low calcium content but better absorbed than cow's milk
- Human milk is richer in Vitamin A & C; richer in copper, cobalt & selenium; richer in iron & higher bioavailability; high calcium/phosphorus ratio; human milk has lesser sodium; less protein content

Breastfeeding during Drug Intake

The drugs are present in breast milk in variable amount but lesser than in plasma of mother.
Breastfeeding is advised 3-4 hours after drug intake so that plasma concentration is lesser and so is drug less in breast milk of mother
The optimum time for drug intake is within 30–60 minutes after nursing and 3–4 hours before the next feed.

Preterm Milk

- The milk of mother who delivers prematurely differs from the milk of a mother who delivers at term.
- Preterm milk contains: Less lactose (in comparison to term milk).
- Contains more protein S, sodium, iron, immunoglobulins and calories as they are needed by the preterm baby.

20. Breast milk protects from infections as it contains all of the following *except*:

a. IgE
b. Lactoferrin
c. Bifidus factor
d. PABA

Ans. is 'a' IgE

21. All of the following are true regarding breast milk as compared to cow's milk *except*:

a. Contains more lactose
b. More amount of proteins
c. Less amount of fat content
d. Minerals and salts is less

Ans. is 'b' More amount of proteins

22. Which of the following is true regarding premature milk as compared to mature milk?

a. Less lactose
b. Less iron
c. Less immunoglobulins
d. Less sodium

Ans. is 'a' Less lactose

PROTEIN ENERGY MALNUTRITION (PEM)

- Marasmus and kwashiorkor are due to deficiency of proteins and calories.
- **Kwashiorkor**
  - Represents the uncompensated phase of PEM.
  - Characterized by classical 'triad' of edema (Due to hypoalbuminemia), markedly retarded growth and psychomotor (mental) changes.
- **Marasmus**
  - Prolonged deficiency of calories and proteins. Thus there is excessive catabolism of adipose tissue and muscle protein.
  - Characterized by gross wasting of muscle and subcutaneous tissues resulting in emaciation and marked stunting. There is no edema.
  - Body weight is less than 60% of expected.
  - Fat in adipose tissues is severely depleted. However the buccal pad of fat is preserved till the malnutrition becomes extreme because a higher proportion of saturated fatty acids is stored there and the saturated fat is the last to be depleted.
  - Skin is dry, scaly and inelastic with wrinkles. The hair is hypopigmented. Abdomen is distended due to wasting and hypotonia of abdominal wall muscles.
  - The child is alert but irritable and may show voracious appetite.
  - Marasmus represents the compensated phase of PEM.

23. Features of marasmus are all *except*:

a. Absence of anasarca
b. Increased appetite
c. Excessive catabolism of adipose tissue and muscle protein
d. Uncompensated phase of PEM

Ans. is 'd' Uncompensated phase of PEM

24. Which of the following rules out protein energy malnutrition? *(NEET 2020)*

a. BMI > 17
b. Normal lean body mass
c. Normal skinfold thickness
d. Normal ECF volume

Ans. is 'b' Normal lean body mass

WHO Criteria for Malnutrition

	Moderate malnutrition	Severe malnutrition
Symmetrical edema	No	Yes
Weight for height	-2SD to -3SD	<-3SD (severe wasting)
Height for age	-2SD to -3SD	<-3SD (severe stunting)

BMI is not used as a marker of labelling malnutrition as presence of edema may falsely lead to higher estimated BMI. Skin fold thickness and ECF fluid volume are unreliable in the presence of generalized edema in children with severe malnutriton.

KWASHIORKOR

25. A 2-year-old baby of 6.7 kg weight belongs to a daily worker who feeds him only milk and rice. His Hb is 6 gm%, s.albumin is 2 gm% with distended abdomen but no proteinuria. What is the diagnosis? *(NEET 2020)*

a. Marasmus
b. Kwashiorkor
c. Iron def. anemia
d. Indian childhood cirrhosis

Ans. is 'b' Kwashiorkor

Kwashiorkor is a form of severe protein malnutrition characterized by edema. It is caused by sufficient calorie intake, but with insufficient protein consumption, which distinguishes it from marasmus. In the above question the 2 years old has a weight of 6.7 Kg against a target weight of approximately 10 Kg (assuming birth weight to be 2.5 Kg and rough estimate of weight at 2 years to be 4 times the birth weight). Therefore the child is undernourished. His calorie and protein intake is low as indicated by his socio-economic status (born to a daily worker) and history of intake of only milk and rice based diet. Low Hb and Albumin (in the absence of proteinuria) are markers of chronic malnutrition. Although the child also has anaemia and might have iron deficiency, the entire clinical picture fits better with kwashiorkor. Therefore Kwashiorkor is the most likely diagnosis

INDICATORS OF MALNUTRITION

Indicator	Parameter	Interpretation
Stunting	Low height for age	Chronic malnutrition
Wasting	Low weight for height	Acute malnutrition
Under weight	Low weight for age	Both acute & chronic malnutrition

Severe Acute Malnutrition

- Severe acute malnutrition (SAM) among children 6–59 months of age is defined by World Health Organization (WHO) and UNICEF as any of the following:
  1. Weight-for-height below –3 standard deviation (SD or Z scores) of the median WHO growth reference
  2. Visible severe wasting
  3. Presence of bipedal edema
  4. Mid-upper arm circumference below 11.5 cm
- This classification is used to identify children at high risk of death.
- Children having SAM require urgent attention & management in the hospital.

26. Severe acute malnutrition as per WHO criteria:

a. Weight for age less than median – 2 SD
b. Weight for height less than median + 2 SD
c. Weight for age less than median + 3 SD
d. Weight for height less than median – 3 SD

Ans. is 'd' Weight for height less than median – 3 SD

DEHYDRATION

ASSESSMENT OF DEHYDRATION IN A PATIENT WITH DIARRHOEA

Parameters	No dehydration	Some dehydration	Severe dehydration
Appearance	Well, alert	Restless, irritable	Lethargic, or unconscious, floppy
Eyes	Normal	Sunken	Very sunken
Thirst	Drinks normally, not thirsty	Thirsty, drinks eagerly	Drinks poorly or not able to drink
Skin pinch	Goes back quickly (< 1 second)	Goes back slowly (1 second)	Goes back very slowly (2 seconds)

Treatment Plan A: Treatment of 'No Dehydration'

Oral redehydration therapy to prevent dehydration (Plan A)		
Age	*Amount of ORS or other culturally appropriate ORT fluids to give after each loose stool*	*Amount of ORS to provide for use at home*
< 24 months	50–100 mL	500 mL/day
2–10 years	100–200 mL	1000 mL/day
> 10 years	Ad lib	2000 mL/day

Treatment Plan B: Treatment of 'Some Dehydration'

- The daily fluid requirements in children are calculated as follows:
  - Up to 10 kg = 100 mL/kg
  - 10–20 kg = 50 mL/kg
  - > 20 kg = 20 mL/kg
  - As an example, the daily fluid requirement in a child weighing 15 kg will be 1250 mL (first 10 kg, 10 × 100 = 1000 mL; another 5 kg, 5 × 250 mL, total 1000 + 250 = 1250 mL).
    - Deficit replacement or rehydration therapy is calculated as 75 mL/kg of ORS, to be given over 4 hr.
    - If after 4 hr, the child still has some dehydration then another treatment with ORS (as in rehydration therapy) is to be given. This therapy is effective in 95% cases.

Treatment Plan C: Children with 'Severe Dehydration'

- Intravenous fluids should be started immediately using Ringer lactate with 5% dextrose. Normal saline or plain Ringer solution may be used as an alternative. A total of 100 mL/kg of fluid is given, over 6 hr in children <12 months and over 3 hr in children >12 months as shown below. ORS solution should be started simultaneously if the child can take orally.

Age	30 mL/kg	70 mL/kg
< 12 months	1 hour	5 hours
> 12 months	30 minutes	2 ½ minutes

27. A 15 month child weighing 6 kg is suffering from acute gastroenteritis along with signs of sunken eyes and skin pitch goes back in 2 seconds. What will be your management?

a. RL infusion 120 mL in the first hour followed by 360 mL in the next 5 hours
b. RL infusion 180 mL in the first hour followed by 420 mL in the next 5 hours
c. RL infusion 180 mL in the first hour followed by 480 mL in the next 2 hours
d. RL infusion 240 mL in the first hour followed by 360 mL in the next 5 hours

Ans. is 'b' RL infusion 180 mL in the first hour followed by 420 mL in the next 5 hours

The child shows signs of severe dehydration and has to treated with Plan C.

28. What is the grade of dehydration if a child demonstrates excessive thirst and decreased urine output?

a. No dehydration
b. Mild dehydration
c. Moderate dehydration
d. Severe dehydration

Ans. is 'b' Mild dehydration

GENETICS

WILLIAM SYNDROME

29. A child presents with coarse facial features, hypercalcemia and an audible murmur suggestive of supravalvular AS. Chromosomal analaysis reveal deletion of chr 7q11.23. What is the diagnosis? *(NEET 2020)*

a. Williams syndrome
b. Hunters syndrome
c. Liddle syndrome
d. Barters syndrome

Ans. is 'a' Williams Syndrome

Williams syndrome (WS) is a genetic disorder that affects many parts of the body. It is caused by a genetic abnormality, specifically a deletion of about 27 genes from the long arm of one of the two chromosome 7s. Facial features frequently include a broad forehead, short nose and full cheeks, an appearance that has been described as "elfin".

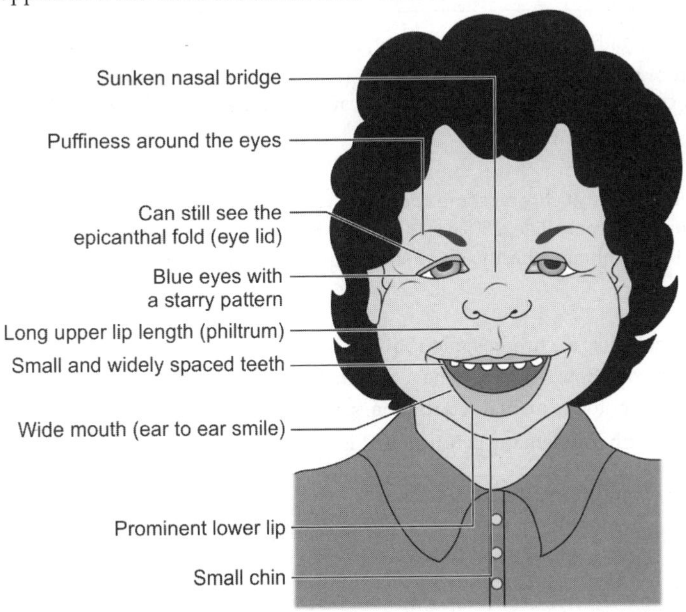

Mild to moderate intellectual disability, problems with visual spatial tasks such as drawing is typical, verbal skills are generally relatively unaffected.

Often have an outgoing personality, interact readily with strangers, and appear happy. Problems with teeth, heart problems, especially supravalvular aortic stenosis, and periods of high blood calcium are common.

Mucopolysaccharidosis type II (MPS II), also known as Hunter syndrome, occurs almost exclusively in males (X-Linked recessive). Between ages 2 and 4, they also develop coarse facies with full lips, large rounded cheeks, a broad nose, and an enlarged tongue. The vocal cords enlarge, which results in a deep, hoarse voice. Other features include macrocephaly, hydrocephalus, hepatosplenomegaly, umbilical hernia, inguinal hernia, hearing loss, recurrent ear infections, carpal tunnel syndrome, valvular heart disease, spinal stenosis, short stature, contractures, dysostosis multiplex and sleep apnoea.

Bartter syndrome and Liddle syndrome are renal tubular disorders with genetic basis. These generally present with fluid, electrolyte abnormalities and no dysmorphism.

DOWN SYNDROME

- In 95% of cases of Down Syndrome, there is trisomy of chromosome 21. Extra chromosome is of maternal in origin. 1% have mosaic with 46 chromosomes. 4% have Robertsonian translocation - t(22:21), t(14:21), t(15:21).

Clinical Features of Down Syndrome

- Most striking feature in the neonate is hypotonia
- Mental retardation, short stature
- *Cranio-facial*: Brachycephaly, epicanthic fold, protruding tongue, small ears, upward sloping palpebral fissures (Mongoloid slant), Brushfield spots in iris.
- *Limbs*: Fifth finger clinodactyly, single palmar crease (Simian crease), wide gap between first and second toes (sandal gap).
- *Congenital heart disease*: Common AV canal, ostium primum/endocardial cushion defect type ASD (most common), VSD, PDA, Fallot's tetralogy.
- *GIT*: Anal atresia, Duodenal atresia, Hirschsprung disease, annular pancreas.
- Increased incidence of leukemia (1%). Leukemias common are ALL (most common), AML (M7-AML) transient myeloproliferative disorders, and juvenile CML.
- *Others*: Early onset of Alzheimer's disease, decreased immunity with recurrent infections, obesity, DM, hypothyroidism (most common endocrine abnormality).

30. Which of the following is not a feature of Down syndrome?

a. Hypotonia
b. Infections
c. Female infertility
d. Early onset Alzheimer's disease

Ans. is 'c' Female infertility

GENOMIC IMPRINTING

- In this scenario, one of the allele (either maternal or paternal) is silenced and only the counterpart remains active.
- When the allele inherited from mother is silenced/inactivated (paternal allele is active), it is called maternal genomic imprinting. When paternal allele is silenced (maternal allele is active) it is called paternal genomic imprinting.

Important examples of genomic imprinting are:

- **Prader-Willi syndrome**
  - Loss of function of paternal allele at chromosome 15q11-q13.
  - 75% cases from deletion of paternal allele; 25% cases from maternal uniparental disomy
  - They are characterized by hypotonia, obesity, short stature, mental retardation, hypogonadism, hyperphagia, and short hand and feet.
- **Angelman syndrome**
  - Loss of function of maternal allele at chromosome 15q11-q13
  - Majority of cases caused by deletion; 3-5% cases have paternal uniparental disomy.
  - They are characterized by hypotonia, mental retardation, seizures, ataxia, and inappropriate laughter (Happy puppets).
- Other examples include – Beckwith-Wiedemann syndrome, Russell-Silver syndrome.

31. Which chromosome is involved in Angelman syndrome?

a. chr 13
b. chr 15
c. chr 18
d. chr 21

Ans. is 'b' chr 15

FRAGILE X SYNDROME

- Fragile X syndrome is associated with a fragile site on chromosome X (Xq29.3)
- X-linked dominant disorder
- Abnormal FMR1 gene on long arm of X chromosome
- Increase in triple nucleotide CGG sequence – Normal <55 repeats; full mutation >200 repeats → leads to DNA methylation and silencing of FMR1 gene
- More severe among males

- 2nd most common genetic cause of intellectual disability (MC is Down syndrome)
- About 20% of women who are carriers for the fragile X pre-mutation are affected by fragile X-related primary ovarian insufficiency.
- Individuals with FXS may present anywhere on a continuum from learning disabilities in the context of a normal intelligence Quotient (IQ) to severe intellectual disability with an average IQ of 40 in males who have complete silencing of FMR1 gene
- Fragile sites are regions of chromosomes that show a tendency to separate or break under particular growth conditions.
- Presents with mental retardation, macro-orchidism (large testicles) and characteristic facial features (long face, large prominent ears, prominent jaw).

32. True about Fragile X syndrome:

a. Triple nucleotide CAG sequence mutation
b. 10% female carriers mentally retarded
c. Males have IQ 20-40
d. Gain of function mutation

Ans. is 'c' Males have IQ 20-40

CYSTIC FIBROSIS

Autosomal Recessive Disease

Mutated Gene –CFTR (Cystic Fibrosis Transmembrane Regulator)

- ATP ion transporter
- *Epithelial cells*: Hydrates mucosal surfaces (lungs, GI tract); pumps Cl^- out of cells
- Sweat glands: Removes NaCl from sweat; makes sweat hypotonic
- *Most common mutation*: delta F508

Pathophysiology

- Ducts of mucus-secreting glands (GI, lungs) are obstructed due to increase in viscosity of secretions leading to glandular dilatation and destruction
- Serous glands like sweat glands are not obstructed in CF; there are abnormal concentrations of inorganic ions used for diagnosis

Presentation

- Usually diagnosed < 2 years of age
- *Lung disease*: Recurrent infections, bronchitis, bronchiectasis
- Meconium ileus
- *Pancreatic insufficiency*: Chronic pancreatitis, Diabetes, Steatorrhea, deficiencies of fat-soluble vitamins (A, D, E, K)
- Biliary disease
- Infertility

Diagnosis

- Sweat Chloride Test
  - Pilocarpine iontophoresis
  - Electrode placed over pilocarpine gauze on skin
  - Small electrical current drives pilocarpine into skin
  - Sweating occurs
  - Chloride content analysed – High chloride level suggests CF
- DNA testing – done if sweat test positive
- Nasal transepithelial potential difference
  - More negative nasal voltage in CF patients
  - Useful in rare CF patients with negative sweat test

Treatment

- Promote airway clearance (Inhaled saline, N-acetylcysteine, Inhaled DNase)
- Antibiotics for exacerbations
- Pancreatic enzyme replacement

33. Which of the following exocrine glandular ducts are not obstructed in cystic fibrosis? *(NEET 2019)*

a. Pancreas
b. Lung
c. Sweat glands
d. All of the above

Ans. is 'c' Sweat glands

IMMUNIZATION

NATIONAL IMMUNIZATION SCHEDULE

National Immunization Schedule (NIS) for infants, children and pregnant women				
Vaccine	***When to give***	***Dose***	***Route***	***Site***
For pregnant women				
TT-1	Early in pregnancy	0.5 mL	Intramuscular	Upper arm
TT-2	4 weeks after TT-1*	0.5 mL	Intramuscular	Upper arm
TT-Booster	If received 2 TT doses in a pregnancy within the last 3 years*	0.5 mL	Intramuscular	Upper arm
For infants				
BCG	At birth or as early as possible till one year of age	0.1 mL (0.05 mL until 1 month age)	intradermal	Left upper arm
Hepatitis B—Birth dose	At birth or as early as possible within 24 hours	0.5 mL	intramuscular	Antero-lateral side of mid-thigh
OPV-0	At birth or as early as possible within the first 15 days	2 drops	Oral	Oral
OPV 1, 2 and 3	At 6 weeks, 10 weeks and 14 weeks (OPV can be given till 5 years of age)	2 drops	Oral	Oral
Pentavalent 1, 2 and 3	At 6 weeks, 10 weeks and 14 weeks (can be given till one year of age)	0.5 mL	Intramuscular	Antero-lateral side of mid-thigh
Rotavirus#	At 6 weeks, 10 weeks and 14 weeks (can be given till one year of age)	5 drops	Oral	Oral
IPV	Two fractional dose at 6 and 14 weeks of age	0.1 mL	Intradermal two fractional dose	Intradermal right upper arm
Measles/MR 1st dose$	9 completed months–12 months. (can be given till 5 years of age)	0.5 mL	Sub-cutaneous	Right upper arm
JE-1**	9 completed months–12 months	0.5 mL	Sub-cutaneous	Left upper arm
Vitamin A (1st dose)	At 9 completed months with measles—Rubella	1 mL (1 lakh IU)	Oral	Oral
For children				
DPT Booster-1	16-24 months	0.5 mL	Intramuscular	Antero-lateral side of mid thigh
Measles/MR 2nd dose $	16-24 months	0.5 mL	Subcutaneous	Right upper arm
OPV Booster	16-24 months	2 drops	Oral	Oral
JE-2	16-24 months	0.5 mL	Subcutaneous	Left-upper arm
Vitamin A*** (2nd to 9th dose)	16-18 months. Then one dose every 6 months up to the age of 5 years	2 mL (2 lakh IU)	Oral	Oral
DPT Booster-2	5-6 years	0.5 mL	Intramuscular	Upper arm
TT	10 years and 16 years	0.5 mL	Intramuscular	Upper arm

*Give TT-2 or booster doses before 16 weeks of pregnancy. However, give these even if more than 36 weeks have passed. Give TT to a woman in labour, if she has not previously received TT.

**JE Vaccine is introduced in select endemic districts after the campaign.

***The 2nd to 9th doses of vitamin A can be administered to children 1-5 years old during biannual rounds, in collaboration with ICDS.

#Phased introduction, at present in Andhra Pradesh, Haryana, Himachal Pradesh and Orissa from 2016 and expanded in Madhya Pradesh, Assam, Rajasthan, and Tripura in February 2017 and planned in Tamil Nadu and Uttar Pradesh in 2017.

$Phased introduction, at present in five states namely Karnataka, Tamil Nadu, Goa, Lakshadweep and Puducherry (As of Feb' 2017).

Catch-up Immunization

	At evaluation	After 1 mo	After 2 mo	After 6 mo
Age <7 yrs	BCG, OPV, DTP, Hep B	OPV, DTP, Hep B	MMR, Typhoid	DTP, Hep B
Age > 7 yrs	Tdap, Hep B	dT, Hep B	MMR, Typhoid	Hep B

Simultaneous administration and interval for immunization	
Combination	***Recommendation***
≥ 2 killed antigens	Give simultaneously or at any interval (exception—cholera and yellow fever, 3–4 weeks gap)
Killed and live antigens	Can be given simultaneously or at any interval
≥ 2 live antigens	4 weeks minimum interval if not given together, ***except OPV and* BCG, MMR**
IG and corresponding antigen	For MMR–3 months interval For HepB, tetanus, Rabies—can be given simultaneously

34. Time gap between 2 live vaccines is:

a. 2 weeks
b. 4 weeks
c. 8 weeks
d. 6 weeks

Ans. is 'b' 4 weeks

SYSTEMIC DISORDERS

MEASLES

35. A child presented with the following findings in oral cavity and skin rash as show below. What is the likely complication? *(NEET 2020)*

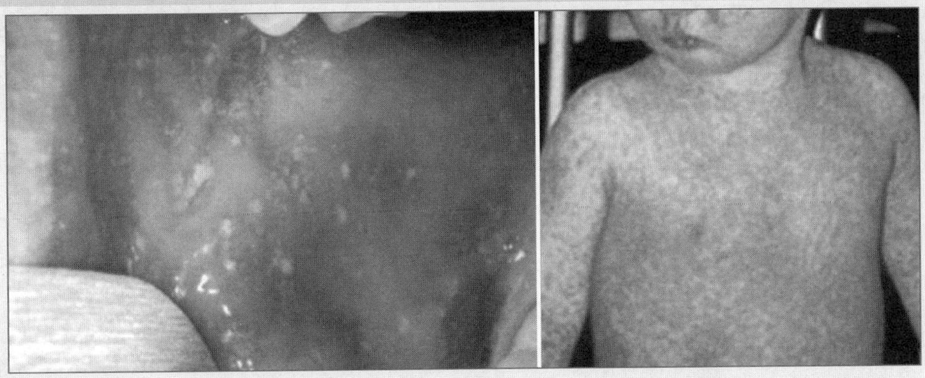

a. Acute myocarditis
b. Acute epididymoorchitis
c. Acute hepatitis
d. Acute nephritis

Ans. is 'a' Acute myocarditis

Complications in Patients with Measles

- Acute otitis media (Most common)
- Pneumonia (Most common cause of death in Measles)
- Croup, tracheitis, and bronchiolitis
- Diarrhea and vomiting
- Febrile seizures
- Encephalitis
- Hemorrhagic measles or "black measles."
- Myocarditis (rare complication of measles)
- Subacute sclerosing panencephalitis (SSPE) is a chronic complication.

PNEUMONIA

36. A 2 years old baby weighing 11 kg had fever, cough, fast breathing and chest indrawing. His RR was 38/min. under what category of IMNCI is he classified for pneumonia and what is the management? *(NEET 2020)*

a. No pneumonia; send him home with advice on follow up
b. Pneumonia; give oral amoxicillin
c. Severe pneumonia; immediate referral to higher centre
d. Very severe pneumonia; give first dose of antibiotic and refer to higher centre

Ans. is 'b' Pneumonia; give oral amoxicillin

Pediatrics

Diagnosis and Assessment of Severity of Pneumonia: 2 Months to 5 Years

Clinical category	Essential features
Severe Pneumonia	Central cyanosis, not able to breast feed or drink, convulsions, lethargy, unconsciousness, severe respiratory distress (head nodding)
Pneumonia	Fast breathing < 2 months ≥ 60 2–12 months ≥ 50 12–59 months ≥ 40 With or without chest indrawing, with oxygen saturation > 92%
No Pneumonia	No fast breathing and no indicatiors of severe pneumonia

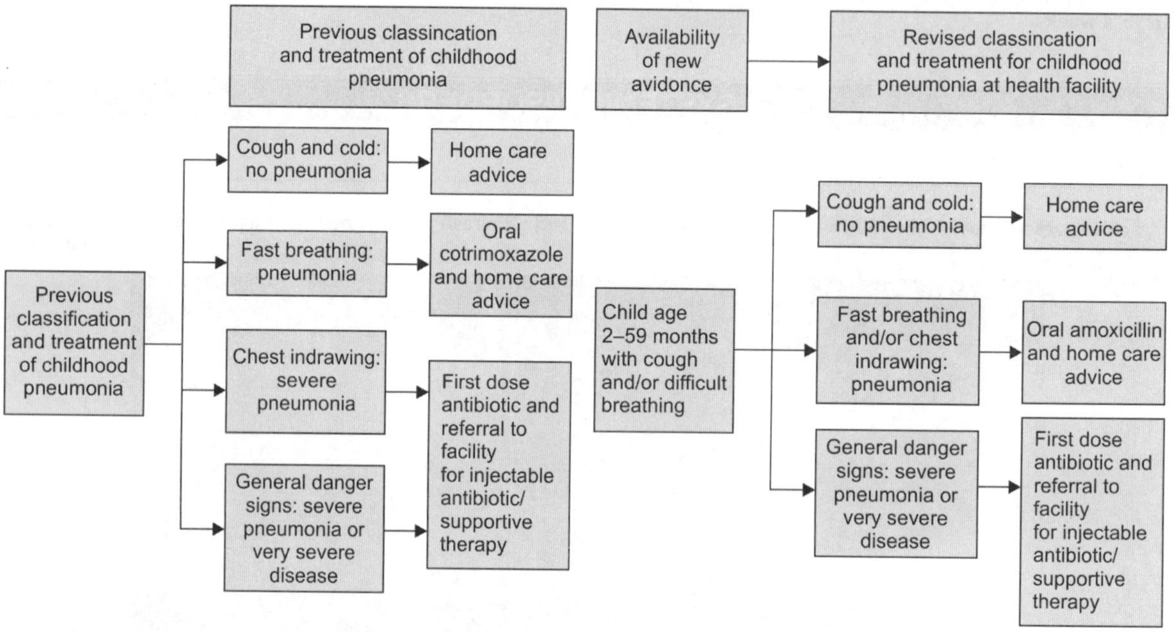

HEMODYNAMICS OF ASD

- Blood flows from left atrium to right atrium because left atrium has slightly higher pressure than right atrium—Left to right shunt.
- Blood passes at as narrow pressure difference—No shunt murmur.
- Volume overload to right atrium—Right atrial dilatation and hypertrophy.
- During diastole large amount of blood passes from right atrium to right ventricle through tricuspid valve—Delayed diastolic murmur and accentuation of first heart sound.
- Volume overload to right ventricle—Right ventricular hypertrophy that produces parasternal heave.
- Large blood volume passes through pulmonary valve—Pulmonary ejection systolic murmur.
- Prolonged blood passage along pulmonary valve causes delayed closure of pulmonary valve P2 is delayed and accentuated, wide split and fixed S2.
- Increased blood flow through pulmonary circulation—Pulmonary plethora
- The left atrium is not enlarged because it decompresses itself by shunting blood to right atrium. The left atrium may enlarge once Eisenmenger's syndrome develops and a reversal of shunt is seen across the defect.

HEMODYNAMICS OF PDA

- In PDA, blood flows from aorta to pulmonary artery because aortic pressure is higher than pulmonary artery pressure—Left to right shunt.
- Pressure gradient between aorta and pulmonary artery is maintained throughout the cardiac cycle (during systole and diastole)—Continuous murmur
- Larger blood volume passes through pulmonary circulation—pulmonary plethora
- Increased flow after passing through lung reaches the left atrium and causes volume overload—Left atrial dilatation and hypertrophy.
- Increased blood volume passes from left atrium to left ventricle through mitral valve — Accentuation of S1 and delayed diastolic murmur.

- ❖ Left ventricle receives larger amount of blood that results in volume overload—Left ventricle enlargement.
- ❖ Extra volume passes through aortic area cause delayed closure of aortic valve which may close even after pulmonary valve (normal pulmonary valves close after aortic valves). Paradoxical splitting of S2, i.e., A2 occurs after P2 (Normally A2 occurs before P2).
- ❖ Large left ventricular volume ejected into the aorta results in dilatation of the ascending aorta—Aortic ejection click.
- ❖ Large volume of blood passes through normal aortic valve—Aortic ejection systolic murmur (but it is masked by continuous murmur).
- ❖ Factors stimulating closure of ductus arteriosus – Increase in O_2 tension at birth and Decrease in concentration of prostaglandins at birth.

37. Which of the following is not seen in ASD?

a. Left atrial enlargement
b. Right atrial enlargement
c. Pulmonary hypertension
d. Widely split S2

Ans. is 'a' Left atrial enlargement

38. Which of the following is not seen in patent ductus arteriosus?

a. Left atrial hypertrophy
b. Left ventricular enlargement
c. Continuous murmur
d. Attenuated S1

Ans. is 'd' Attenuated S1

CONGENITAL RUBELLA SYNDROME

The classic triad for congenital rubella syndrome is:

- ❖ Sensorineural deafness (58% of patients)
- ❖ Eye abnormalities—especially retinopathy, cataract, glaucoma, and microphthalmia (43% of patients)
- ❖ Congenital heart disease—especially pulmonary artery stenosis and patent ductus arteriosus (50% of patients)

Other manifestations of CRS may include:

- ❖ Spleen, liver, or bone marrow problems (some of which may disappear shortly after birth)
- ❖ Intellectual disability
- ❖ Small head size (microcephaly)
- ❖ Eye defects
- ❖ Low birth weight
- ❖ Thrombocytopenic purpura
- ❖ Extramedullary hematopoiesis (presents as a characteristic blueberry muffin rash)
- ❖ Hepatomegaly
- ❖ Micrognathia
- ❖ Skin lesions.

39. Most characteristic cardiovascular defect seen in rubella:

a. Pulmonary artery stenosis
b. Coarctation of aorta
c. Ankylosing spondylitis
d. Rheumatic fever

Ans. is 'a' Pulmonary artery stenosis

CONGENITAL HYPERTROPHIC PYLORIC STENOSIS (CHPS)

- ❖ Hypertrophic pyloric stenosis is the most common surgical disorder of the gastrointestinal tract in infants.
- ❖ The pylorus is thickened and elongated with narrowing of its lumen due to hypertrophy of the circular muscle fibers of pylorus.

Clinical Presentation

- ❖ Non-bilious projectile vomiting
- ❖ More common in boys than girls.
- ❖ Most patients present with vomiting starting beyond 3 weeks of age.
- ❖ Recurrent and persistent vomiting causes dehydration, malnutrition and hypochloremic alkalosis.
- ❖ As the stomach muscles contract to overcome the obstruction, a vigorous peristaltic wave can be seen to move from left hypochondrium to umbilicus, particularly on examination after feeding.
- ❖ A firm olive-shaped mass is palpable in the mid epigastrium in 75–80% infants, especially after feeds.

Evaluation

- ❖ Ultrasound abdomen is the investigation of choice and shows muscle thickness of > 4 mm and pylorus length of > 16 mm. The ultrasound is 100% sensitive and nearly 90% specific in diagnosis of hypertrophic pyloric stenosis.
- ❖ However, in case of doubt, an upper GI barium study can show a consistent elongation of the pyloric channel or an upper GI endoscopy is performed.

Management

- The treatment includes rapid correction of dehydration and electrolyte abnormalities.
- The treatment of choice is surgical; a pyloromyotomy (Ramstedt operation) is performed.

40. The abdominal mass swelling of pyloric stenosis can be best felt by:

a. Above umbilicus
b. When baby is being fed milk
c. From right to left upper quadrant
d. When baby is sleeping

Ans. is 'b' When baby is being fed milk

BEHAVIOURAL DISORDERS IN CHILDREN

Breath Holding Spells

- Paroxysmal event occurring in 0.1–5% of healthy children from the age of 6 months to 6 years
- Breath-holding occurs during expiration and is reflexive (not volitional) in nature.
- *Cyanotic spells*: More common and is provoked in response to frustration and anger precipitated by upsetting or scolding infant/child
- *Pallid spells*: Initiated by painful experience, e.g falling and striking the head
- The only treatment is support and reassurance to parents

Rett's Syndrome

- Age of onset is around 5 months.
- Development may proceed normally until 1 yr of age, when regression of language and motor milestones become apparent–characteristic feature
- Acquired microcephaly (Declaration of head growth due to significantly reduced brain weight)
- Most children develop peculiar sighing respirations with intermittent periods of apnea that may be associated with cyanotic breath-holding spells.
- Autistic behaviour is a typical finding in all patients.
- Generalized tonic-clonic convulsions occur in the majority.
- Feeding disorder and poor weight gain are common.
- Cardiac arrhythmias may result in sudden, unexpected death.

41. All of the following are features of Rett's syndrome *except*:

a. Microcephaly
b. Regression of milestones
c. Cardiac arrhythmias
d. Focal convulsions

Ans. is 'd' Focal convulsions

Previously Asked Facts

- Delayed eruption is failure of teeth to appear by 13 months.
- Degenerative diseases of the brain generally cause regression of both motor and cognitive function (global regression).
- The best reference for growth monitoring in children is NCHS (National Centre for Health Statistics) standards.
- Meconium plug syndrome when meconium plug causes obstruction of colon. It is seen in Hirschsprung disease, maternal DM, maternal preeclampsia, prematurity, sepsis, hypothyroidism.
- Meconium ileus when meconium plug obstruct ileum. It is seen in cystic fibrosis.
- Weight of an infant doubles by 5 months and quadruples by 2 years of age.
- Hypovolemia is the most common cause of shock in children
- Sodium content in Ringer lactate is 130 mEq of sodium is 1000 mL of fluid.
- Earliest symptom of Tay-Sachs disease is hyperacusis.
- *Body proportions*: In infants, the upper segment is greater than the lower segment and the height is greater than the arm span.

Infantile body proportion	Reverse infantile body proportion
Achondroplasia	Eunuchoidism
Cretinism	Marfan syndrome
	Homocystinuria
	Klinefelter's syndrome
	Frohlich's syndrome

- Tyrosinase is the enzyme deficient in albinism.
- Maternal syphilis can be transmitted throughout pregnancy, more commonly during later pregnancy. Pathognomonic features include skeletal lesions, snuffles, pneumonia alba, notched central incisors (Hutchinson's teeth), keratitis, saber shins and frontal bossing. Though the typical Hutchinson's triad includes interstitial keratitis, eighth nerve involvement, Hutchinson's teeth.
- A child with recurrent urinary tract infection is most likely to have vesico-ureteric reflux.
- VSD is the commonest congenital heart disease.
- Most important prognostic marker of tetralogy of Fallot is Pulmonary stenosis.
- HbA (Adult Hb) = $\alpha_2\beta_2$; HbF (Fetal Hb) = a_2g_2
- *Physiologic Anemia of Infancy*: Hemoglobin drops to low point at age 6 to 8 weeks due to Erythropoietin nadir. Term infants: Hemoglobin drops to 9–11 g/dL; Preterm infants: Hemoglobin drops to 7–9 g/dL
- Most common cause of cranial irradiation in children is ALL
- Sacrococcygeal teratoma is the most common tumor in fetus. Most common presentation is with an abnormal, obvious protruding mass from the sacral area.
- Rotavirus is the single most common cause of diarrhea amongst children in both developed and developing world.
- ETEC is the single most common cause of bacterial diarrhea amongst children in the developing world.
- *Tachypnea is defined as*: Respiratory rate > 60/min less than 2 months of age; > 50/min 2-12 months of age; > 40/min > 12 months of age
- Transient tachypnea of the newborn is a benign self-limiting to delayed clearance of lung fluid. TTN follows uneventful normal vaginal delivery or a cesarean delivery. Chest X-ray shows hyperaerated lung fields.
- Most common cause of renal scarring in children is Vesico-ureteric reflux.
- In a newborn, chest compressions are given using the two thumbs or two fingers (middle and index fingers) to apply pressure on lower third of sternum.
- *Bag and Mask Ventilation is contraindicated in*: Congenital diaphragmatic hernia, Tracheo-esophageal fistula and Meconium aspiration syndrome.

DR. APURV MEHRA
Aspiring to Serve Humanity

Dr. Apurv Mehra

Orthopedic Surgeon | International Faculty of Ortho | Renowned Author | Motivational Speake

Helpline Nos:

Vidya Jeevan Orthopedics Centre

Most Trusted Centre For Ethical Practice

For Appointments 8800222008 | 8800222014 | Landline No: 011-41512008

Mail Reports / X-rays / MRI to vjortho14@gmail.com

Dr. Apurv Mehra's Orthopedics (ODD)

For UG / PG Aspirants (Medical & FMGE)

ODD Helpline: Call | Whatsapp 8800605979 | 9999664864

Mail: drapurv@gmail.com

Cerebellum Academy

An Institute For The Students By The Teachers

For NEET PG | FMGE Exam Preparation

Helpline Nos: 8800222009 | 8800605979

Dr. Apurv Mehra's Conceptual Orthopedics App

Exclusively for Ortho Residents And practitioners

CO helpline: Call| Whatsapp 9999664864 | 8447540715

Mail: drapurv@conceptualorthopedics.com

Conceptual Surgery App

Exclusively For Surgery Residents

CO helpline: Call| Whatsapp 9999664864 | 8447540715

Mail: drapurv@theconceptualsurgery.com

Releasing Soon - Conceptual Anesthesia App

Exclusively For Anesthesia Residents & Practitioners

CA Helpline Nos: 9999664864 | 7217774639

For Any Academic / Unacademic Doubt

Helpline: No Call | Whatsapp 8800605979 | 9999664864

Mail to: drapurv@gmail.com

Dr. Apurv Mehra Linktree